Contents in Brief

P9-DXZ-551

*The following content can be found online at www.davisplus.com:
- Psychopharmacology
- Relaxation Therapy
- Complementary Therapies
- Forensic Nursing
- Controlled Drug Categories and Pregnancy Categories
- Sample Client Teaching Guides

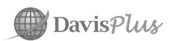

Get the most out of your textbook and resources online at **DavisPlus** to prepare for class, clinical, and professional success.

Gain access to your complete text online with the Davis Digital Version. Quickly search for the content you need and add notes, highlights, and bookmarks. Redeem your *Plus* Code to access your **DavisPlus** Premium resources.

STEP 1.
Preview what you'll learn

Objectives

Read the **Objectives** now to see exactly what you'll be learning in each chapter. Then, after you read the chapter, revisit the section and assess your progress. Can you correctly define and explain all of the key points?

Chapter Outline, Key Terms, & Core Concepts

Take a look at the **Chapter Outline** and **Key Terms** sections at the beginning of every chapter to see what you will be learning and what **Core Concepts** to focus on.

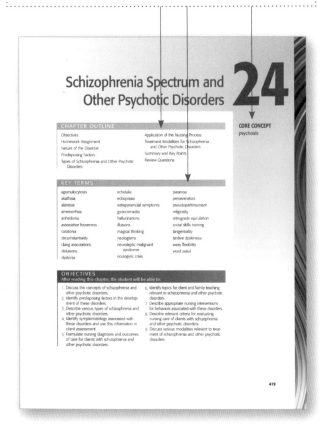

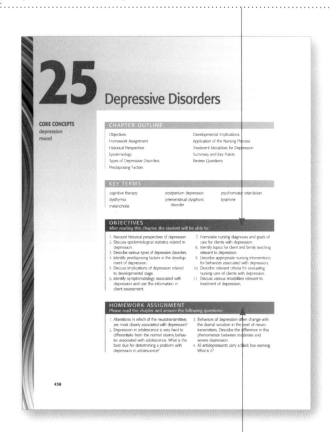

Homework Assignment

Take a few moments to review the **Homework Assignment** before you begin the chapter. When you've finished reading the chapter, complete the assignment to reinforce what you've learned.

Quality and Safety Education for Nurses (QSEN) Activities

Stay up to date—attain the knowledge, skills, and attitudes you need to fulfill the initiative's most current quality and safety competencies.

BOX 24-4 QSEN TEACHING STRATEGY

Assignment: Using Evidence to Address Clinical Problems
Intervention With a Combative Client

Competency Domain: Evidence-Based Practice

Learning Objectives: Student will:
- Differentiate clinical opinion from research and evidence summaries.
- Explain the role of evidence in determining the best clinical practice for intervening with combative cl
- Identify gaps between what is observed in the treatment setting to what has been identified as best p
- Discriminate between valid and invalid reasons for modifying evidence-based clinical practice based o
  expertise or other reasons.
- Participate effectively in appropriate data collection and other research activities.
- Acknowledge own limitations in knowledge and clinical expertise before determining when to deviat
  evidence-based best practices.

NEW! Communication Exercises Boxes

Practice your communication skills with **clinical scenarios** to prepare for the real world of nursing practice.

💬 Communication Exercises

1. Hal, a patient on the psychiatric unit, has a diagnosis of schizophrenia. He lives in a halfway house, where last evening he began yelling that "aliens were on the way to take over our bodies! The message is coming through loud and clear!" The residence supervisor became frightened and called 911. Hal tells the nurse, "I'm special! I get messages from a higher being! We are in for big trouble!"

   How would the nurse respond appropriately to this statement by Hal?

2. The nurse notices that Hal is sitting off to himself in a corner of the dayroom. He appears to be talking to himself and tilts his head to the side as if listening to something.

   How would the nurse intervene with Hal in this situation?

3. Hal says to the nurse, "We must choose to take a ride. All alone we slip and slide. Now it's time to

Table 24-4 | CARE PLAN FOR THE CLIENT WITH SCHIZOPHRENIA

NURSING DIAGNOSIS: DISTURBED SENSORY PERCEPTION: AUDITORY/VISUAL

RELATED TO: Panic anxiety, extreme loneliness, and withdrawal into the self

EVIDENCED BY: Inappropriate responses, disordered thought sequencing, rapid mood swings, poor concentration, disorientation

OUTCOME CRITERIA	NURSING INTERVENTIONS	RATIONALE
Short-Term Goal • Client will discuss content of hallucinations with nurse or therapist within 1 week. **Long-Term Goal** • Client will be able to define and test reality, reducing or eliminating the occurrence of hallucinations. This goal may not be realistic for the individual with severe and persistent illness who has experienced auditory hallucinati for many years. A more realistic goal may be: • Client will verbalize understanding that the voices are a result of his or her illness and demonstrate ways to	1. Observe client for signs of hallucinations (listening pose, laughing or talking to self, stopping in midsentence). Ask, "Are you hearing the voices again?" 2. Avoid touching the client without warning him or her that you are about to do so. ...titude of acceptance will ...ge the client to share the ...of the hallucination with ... "What do you hear the ...saying to you?" ... Do not reinforce the hallucination. Use "the voices" instead of words like "they" that imply validation. Let client know	1. Early intervention may prevent aggressive response to command hallucinations. 2. Client may perceive touch as threatening and may respond in an aggressive manner. 3. This is important to prevent possible injury to the client or others from command hallucinations. 4. It is important for the nurse to be honest, and the client must accept the perception as unreal before hallucinations can be eliminated.

Therapeutic Communication Icon

Find helpful interventions and guidance on how to speak to your patients—just look for this icon in the Care Plan sections.

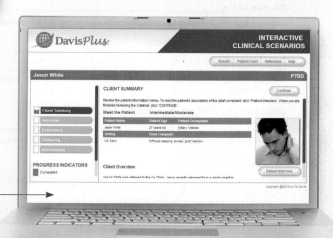

Interactive Clinical Scenarios Online at 🌐 DavisPlus *

Work through the nursing process with client summaries, multiple-choice questions with rationales, drag-and-drop activities, and more!

Summary and Key Points

- Of all mental illness, schizophrenia undoubtedly results in the greatest amount of personal, emotional, and social costs. It presents an enormous threat to life and happiness, yet it remains an enigma to the medical community.
- For many years there was little agreement as to a definition of the concept of schizophrenia. The *DSM-5* (APA, 2013) identifies specific criteria for diagnosis of the disorder.
- The initial symptoms of schizophrenia most often occur in early adulthood. Development of the disorder can be viewed in four phases: (1) the premorbid phase, (2) the prodromal phase, (3) the active phase (schizophrenia), and (4) the resid-

STEP 3.
Build your confidence

Summary and Key Points

Too busy to take notes? Refer to the **Summary** and **Key Points** section at the end of every chapter for a recap of the most important concepts.

NCLEX-Style Test Bank
Online at 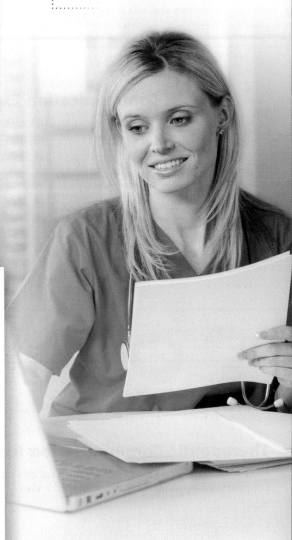 DavisPlus*

Practice makes perfect! Quiz yourself and assess your progress with a wealth of questions, including alternate-item-format questions.

SAMPLE CLIENT TEACHING GUIDES

BENZODIAZEPINES

Patient Medication Instruction Sheet

Patient Name_____ Drug Prescribed_____

Directions for Use_____

Examples and Uses of this Medicine:
Benzodiazepines are used to treat moderate to severe anxiety: alprazolam [Xanax], chlordiazepoxide [Librium], clonazepam [Klonopin], clorazepate [Tranxene], diazepam [Valium], lorazepam [Ativan], and oxazepam. Some are used to treat insomnia (sleeplessness): flurazepam [Dalmane], temazepam [Restoril], estazolam, quazepam [Doral], and triazolam [Halcion]. Some are used for muscle spasms and to treat seizure disorders.

Before Using this Medicine, Be Sure to tell your Doctor if you:

- Are allergic to any medicine
- Have glaucoma
- Are pregnant, plan to be, or are breastfeeding
- Are taking any other medications

Side Effects of this Medicine:

REPORT THE FOLLOWING SIDE EFFECTS TO YOUR DOCTOR IMMEDIATELY:

- Mental confusion or depression
- Hallucinations (seeing, hearing, or feeling things not there)
- Skin rash or itching
- Sore throat and fever
- Unusual excitement, nervousness, irritability, or trouble sleeping

SIDE EFFECTS THAT MAY OCCUR BUT NOT REQUIRE A DOCTOR'S ATTENTION UNLESS THEY PERSIST LONGER THAN A FEW DAYS:

Client Teaching Guide
Online at DavisPlus

Review the crucial information your patients need to know, including possible side effects and what to do before, during, and after taking medication.

*A *Plus* Code in the front of each new book unlocks Davis*Plus* Premium Content. (Access can also be purchased at Davis*Plus*.FADavis.com.)

Lists of Movies

Take a visual approach—watch the movies listed in every chapter to better understand the conditions and behaviors you may not encounter in clinical.

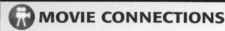

🎬 MOVIE CONNECTIONS

I Never Promised You a Rose Garden (schizophrenia) • *A Beautiful Mind* (schizophrenia) • *The Fisher King* (schizophrenia) • *Bennie & Joon* (schizophrenia) • *Out of Darkness* (schizophrenia) • *Conspiracy Theory* (delusional disorder) • *The Fan* (delusional disorder)

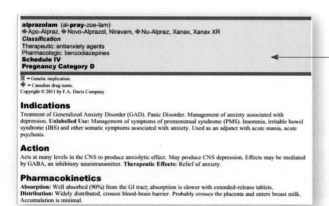

alprazolam (al-**pray**-zoe-lam)
Apo-Alpraz, Novo-Alprazol, Niravam, Nu-Alpraz, Xanax, Xanax XR
Classification
Therapeutic: antianxiety agents
Pharmacologic: benzodiazepines
Schedule IV
Pregnancy Category D

= Genetic implication.
= Canadian drug name.
Copyright © 2011 by F.A. Davis Company

Indications
Treatment of Generalized Anxiety Disorder (GAD). Panic Disorder. Management of anxiety associated with depression. **Unlabelled Use:** Management of symptoms of premenstrual syndrome (PMS). Insomnia, irritable bowel syndrome (IBS) and other somatic symptoms associated with anxiety. Used as an adjunct with acute mania, acute psychosis.

Action
Acts at many levels in the CNS to produce anxiolytic effect. May produce CNS depression. Effects may be mediated by GABA, an inhibitory neurotransmitter. **Therapeutic Effects:** Relief of anxiety.

Pharmacokinetics
Absorption: Well absorbed (90%) from the GI tract; absorption is slower with extended-release tablets.
Distribution: Widely distributed, crosses blood-brain barrier. Probably crosses the placenta and enters breast milk. Accumulation is minimal.

Psychotropic Drug Monographs
Online at 🌐 DavisPlus

Attach these handy, printable monographs to your care plans or take them into clinical rotations. Patient safety information, classifications, indications, actions, and nursing implications are easy to find on each psychotropic drug monograph from the trusted Davis's Drug Guide for Nurses® database.

More resources for **SUCCESS!**

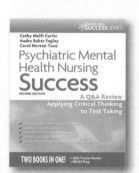

Curtis, Fegley, & Tuzo
Psychiatric Mental Health Nursing Success
A Q&A Review Applying Critical Thinking to Test Taking

Course Review & NCLEX Prep!
Multiple-choice and alternate-item-format questions assure your mastery of psychiatric mental health nursing knowledge while honing your critical-thinking and test-taking skills. Perfect for classroom exams and the NCLEX, too.

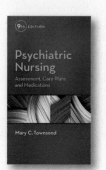

Townsend
Psychiatric Nursing
Assessment, Care Plans and Medications

Practical diagnoses + patient safety.
The first half provides the diagnostic information you need to create a care plan; the second half covers the safe prescription and administration of psychotropic medications.

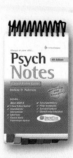

Pedersen
Psych Notes
Clinical Pocket Guide

Includes DSM-5 Content!
Quickly find crucial, yet succinct information on all aspects of psychiatric mental health nursing—from basic behavioral theories to psychiatric and crisis interventions.

Visit **www.FADavis.com** for details.

Psychiatric Mental Health Nursing:

Concepts of Care in Evidence-Based Practice

EIGHTH EDITION

Mary C. Townsend, DSN, PMHCNS-BC
Clinical Specialist/Nurse Consultant
Adult Psychiatric Mental Health Nursing

Former Assistant Professor and
Coordinator, Mental Health Nursing
Kramer School of Nursing
Oklahoma City University
Oklahoma City, Oklahoma

F.A. Davis Company • Philadelphia

F. A. Davis Company
1915 Arch Street
Philadelphia, PA 19103
www.fadavis.com

Printed in the United States of America

Last digit indicates print number: 10 9 8 7 6 5 4 3 2 1

Publisher, Nursing: Robert G. Martone
Director of Content Development: Darlene D. Pedersen
Content Project Manager: Jacalyn C. Clay
Electronic Project Editor: Katherine E. Crowley
Cover Design: Carolyn O'Brien

As new scientific information becomes available through basic and clinical research, recommended treatments and drug therapies undergo changes. The author(s) and publisher have done everything possible to make this book accurate, up to date, and in accord with accepted standards at the time of publication. The author(s), editors, and publisher are not responsible for errors or omissions or for consequences from application of the book, and make no warranty, expressed or implied, in regard to the contents of the book. Any practice described in this book should be applied by the reader in accordance with professional standards of care used in regard to the unique circumstances that may apply in each situation. The reader is advised always to check product information (package inserts) for changes and new information regarding dose and contraindications before administering any drug. Caution is especially urged when using new or infrequently ordered drugs.

Library of Congress Control Number: 2014944300
ISBN: 978-0-8036-4092-4

THIS BOOK IS DEDICATED TO:

FRANCIE

God made sisters for sharing laughter

and wiping tears

Contributors

Lois Angelo, MSN, APRN, BC
ED Care Manager
Newton Wellesley Hospital
Newton, Massachusetts

Cathy Melfi Curtis, MSN, RN-BC
Nursing Educator Consultant
Charleston, South Carolina

Tona Leiker, PhD, APRN-CNS, CNE
Clinical Nurse Specialist
Wesley Medical Center
Wichita, Kansas

Karyn I. Morgan, RN, MSN, CNS
Senior Instructor, Mental Health Nursing
The University of Akron
Akron, Ohio
and
CNS, Intensive Outpatient Psychiatry
Summa Health System
Akron, Ohio

Carol Norton Tuzo, MSN, RN-BC
Nursing Educator Consultant
Charleston, South Carolina

Reviewers

Theresa Aldelman
Bradley University
Peoria, Illinois

Fredrick Astle
University of South Carolina
Columbia, South Carolina

Carol Backstedt
Baton Rouge Community College
Baton Rouge, Louisiana

Elizabeth Bailey
Clinton Community College
Pittsburgh, New York

Sheryl Banak
Baptist Health Schools - Little Rock
Little Rock, Arkansas

Joy A. Barham
Northwestern State University
Shreveport, Louisiana

Barbara Barry
Cape Fear Community College
Wilmington, North Carolina

Carole Bomba
Harper College
Palatine, Illinois

Judy Bourrand
Samford University
Birmingham, Alabama

Susan Bowles
Barton Community College
Great Bend, Kansas

Wayne Boyer
College of the Desert
Palm Desert, California

Joyce Briggs
Ivy Tech Community College
Columbus, Indiana

Toni Bromley
Rogue Community College
Grants Pass, Oregon

Terrall Bryan
North Carolina A & T State University
Greensboro, North Carolina

Ruth Burkhart
New Mexico State University/Dona Ana Community College
Las Cruces, New Mexico

Annette Cannon
Platt College
Aurora, Colorado

Deena Collins
Huron School of Nursing
Cleveland, Ohio

Martha Colvin
Georgia College & State University
Milledgeville, Georgia

Mary Jean Croft
St. Joseph School of Nursing
Providence, Rhode Island

Connie Cupples
Union University
Germantown, Tennessee

Karen Curlis
State University of New York Adirondack
Queensbury, New York

Nancy Cyr
North Georgie College and State University
Dahlonega, Georgia

Carol Danner
Baptist Health Schools Little Rock - School of Nursing
Little Rock, Arkansas

Carolyn DeCicco
Our Lady of Lourdes School of Nursing
Camden, New Jersey

Leona Dempsey, PhD, APNP (ret.), PMHCS-BC
University of Wisconsin Oshkosh
Oshkosh, Wisconsin

Debra J. DeVoe
Our Lady of Lourdes School of Nursing
Camden, New Jersey

Victoria T. Durkee, PhD, APRN
University of Louisiana at Monroe
Monroe, Louisiana

J. Carol Elliott

St. Anselm College
Fairfield, California

Sandra Farmer

Capital University
Columbus, Ohio

Patricia Freed

Saint Louis University
St. Louis, Missouri

Diane Gardner

University of West Florida
Pensacola, Florida

Maureen Gaynor

Saint Anselm College
Manchester, New Hampshire

Denise Glenore

West Coast University
Riverside, California

Sheilia R. Goodwin

Winston Salem State University
Salem, North Carolina

Janine Graf-Kirk

Trinitas School of Nursing
Elizabeth, New Jersey

Susan B. Grubbs

Francis Marion University
Florence, South Carolina

Elizabeth Gulledge

Jacksonville State University
Jacksonville, Alabama

Kim Gurcan

Columbus Practical School of Nursing
Columbus, Ohio

Patricia Jean Hedrick Young

Washington Hospital School of Nursing
Washington, Pennsylvania

Melinda Hermanns

University of Texas at Tyler
Tyler, Texas

Alison Hewig

Victoria College
Victoria, Texas

Cheryl Hilgenberg

Millikin University
Decatur, Illinois

Lori Hill

Gadsden State Community College
Gadsden, Alabama

Ruby Houldson

Illinois Eastern Community College
Olney, Illinois

Eleanor J. Jefferson

Community College of Denver
Platt College
Metropolitan St. College
Denver, Colorado

Dana Johnson

Mesa State College/Grand Junction Regional Center
Grand Junction, Colorado

Janet Johnson

Fort Berthold Community College
New Town, North Dakota

Nancy Kostin

Madonna University
Livonia, Michigan

Linda Lamberson

University of Southern Maine
Portland, Maine

Irene Lang

Bristol Community College
Fall River, Massachusetts

Rhonda Lansdell

Northeast MS Community College
Baldwyn, Mississippi

Jacqueline Leonard

Franciscan University of Steubenville
Steubenville, Ohio

Judith Lynch-Sauer

University of Michigan
Ann Arbor, Michigan

Glenna Mahoney

University of Saint Mary
Leavenworth, Kansas

Jacqueline Mangnall

Jamestown College
Jamestown, North Dakota

Lori A. Manilla

Hagerstown Community College
Hagerstown, Maryland

Patricia Martin

West Kentucky Community and Technical College
Paducah, Kentucky

Christine Massey

Barton College
Wilson, North Carolina

Joanne Matthews
University of Kentucky
Lexington, Kentucky

Joanne McClave
Wayne Community College
Goldsboro, North Carolina

Mary McClay
Walla Walla University
Portland, Oregon

Susan McCormick
Brazosport College
Lake Jackson, Texas

Shawn McGill
Clovis Community College
Clovis, New Mexico

Margaret McIlwain
Gordon College
Barnesville, Georgia

Nancy Miller
Minneapolis Community and Technical College
Minneapolis, Minnesota

Vanessa Miller
California State University Fullerton
Fullerton, California

Mary Mitsui
Emporia State University
Emporia, Kansas

Cheryl Moreland, MS, RN
Western Nevada College
Carson City, Nevada

Daniel Nanguang
El Paso Community College
El Paso, Texas

Susan Newfield
West Virginia University
Morgantown, West Virginia

Dorothy Oakley
Jamestown Community College
Olean, New York

Christie Obritsch
University of Mary
Bismarck, North Dakota

Sharon Opsahl
Western Technical College
La Crosse, Wisconsin

Vicki Paris
Jackson State Community College
Jackson, Tennessee

Lillian Parker
Clayton State University
Morrow, Georgia

JoAnne M. Pearce, MS, RN
Idaho State University
Pocatello, Idaho

Karen Peterson
DeSales University
Center Valley, Pennsylvania

Carol Pool
South Texas College
McAllen, Texas

William S. Pope
Barton College
Wilson, North Carolina

Karen Pounds
Northeastern University
Boston, Massachusetts

Konnie Prince
Victoria College
Victoria, Texas

Susan Reeves
Tennessee Technological University
Cookeville, Tennessee

Debra Riendeau
Saint Joseph's College of Maine
Lewiston, Maine

Sharon Romer
South Texas College
McAllen, Texas

Lisa Romero
Solano Community College
Fairfield, California

Donna S. Sachse
Union University
Germantown, Tennessee

Betty Salas
Otero Junior College
La Junta, Colorado

Sheryl Samuelson, PhD, RN
Millikin University
Decatur, Illinois

John D. Schaeffer
San Joaquin Delta College
Stockton, California

Mindy Schaffner
Pacific Lutheran University
Tacoma, Washington

Becky Scott
Mercy College of Northwest Ohio
Toledo, Ohio

Janie Shaw
Clayton State University
Morrow, Georgia

Lori Shaw
Nebraska Methodist College
Omaha, Nebraska

Joyce Shea
Fairfield University
Fairfield, Connecticut

Judith Shindul-Rothschild
Boston College
Chestnut Hill, Massachusetts

Audrey Silveri
UMass Worcester Graduate School of Nursing
Worcester, Massachusetts

Brenda Smith, MSN, RN
North Georgia College and State University
Dahlonega, Georgia

Janet Somlyay
University of Wyoming
Laramie, Wyoming

Charlotte Strahm, DNSc, RN, CNS-PMH
Purdue North Central
Westville, Indiana

Jo Sullivan
Centralia College
Centralia, Washington

Kathleen Sullivan
Boise State University
Boise, Idaho

Judy Traynor
Jefferson Community College
Watertown, New York

Claudia Turner
Temple College
Temple, Texas

Suzanne C. Urban
Mansfield University
Mansfield, Pennsylvania

Dorothy Varchol
Cincinnati State
Cincinnati, Ohio

Connie M. Wallace
Nebraska Methodist College
Omaha, Nebraska

Sandra Wardell
Orange County Community College
Middletown, New York

Susan Warmuskerken
West Shore Community College
Scottville, Michigan

Roberta Weseman
East Central College
Union, Missouri

Margaret A. Wheatley
Case Western Reserve University, FPB School of
Nursing
Cleveland, Ohio

Jeana Wilcox
Graceland University
Independence, Missouri

Jackie E. Williams
Georgia Perimeter College
Clarkston, Georgia

Rita L. Williams, MSN, RN, CCM
Langston University School of Nursing & Health
Professions
Langston, Oklahoma

Rodney A. White
Lewis and Clark Community College
Godfrey, Illinois

Vita Wolinsky
Dominican College
Orangeburg, New York

Marguerite Wordell
Kentucky State University
Frankfort, Kentucky

Jan Zlotnick
City College of San Francisco
San Francisco, California

Acknowledgments

Robert G. Martone, Publisher, Nursing, F. A. Davis Company, for your sense of humor and continuous optimistic outlook about the outcome of this project.

Jacalyn Clay, Content Project Manager, Nursing, F.A. Davis Company, for all your help and support in preparing the manuscript for publication.

Sharon Lee, Production Manager, F. A. Davis Company, and Matt Rosenquist, Graphic World Inc, for your support and competence in the final editing and production of the manuscript.

The nursing educators, students, and clinicians, who provide critical information about the usability of the textbook, and offer suggestions for improvements. Many changes have been made based on your input.

To those individuals who critiqued the manuscript for this edition and shared your ideas, opinions, and suggestions for enhancement. I sincerely appreciate your contributions to the final product.

My daughters, Kerry and Tina, for all the joy you have provided me and all the hope that you instill in me. I'm so thankful that I have you.

My grandchildren, Meghan, Matthew, and Catherine, for showing me what life is truly all about. I am blessed by your very presence.

My furry friends, Angel, Max, Riley, and Charlie, for the pure pleasure you bring into my life every day that you live.

My husband, Jim, who gives meaning to my life in so many ways. You are the one whose encouragement keeps me motivated, whose support gives me strength, and whose gentleness gives me comfort.

Contents

UNIT 5
Psychiatric/Mental Health Nursing of Special Populations   703

***The following content can be found online at
www.davisplus.com:**

• Psychopharmacology

• Relaxation Therapy

• Complementary Therapies

• Forensic Nursing

• Controlled Drug Categories and Pregnancy Categories

• Sample Client Teaching Guides

To the Instructor

Currently in progress, implementation of the recommendations set forth by the New Freedom Commission on Mental Health has given enhanced priority to mental health care in the United States. Moreover, at the 65th meeting of the World Health Assembly (WHA) in May 2012, India, Switzerland, and the United States cosponsored a resolution requesting that the World Health Organization, in collaboration with member countries, develop a global mental health action plan. This resolution was passed at the 66th WHA in May 2013. By their support of this resolution, member countries have expressed their commitment for "promotion of mental health, prevention of mental disorders, and early identification, care, support, treatment, and recovery of persons with mental disorders." With the passage of this resolution, mental health services may now be available for millions who have been without this type of care.

Many nurse leaders see this period of mental health-care reform as an opportunity for nurses to expand their roles and assume key positions in education, prevention, assessment, and referral. Nurses are, and will continue to be, in key positions to assist individuals to attain, maintain, or regain optimal emotional wellness.

As it has been with each new edition of *Psychiatric Mental Health Nursing: Concepts of Care in Evidence-Based Nursing*, the goal of this eighth edition is to bring to practicing nurses and nursing students the most up-to-date information related to neurobiology, psychopharmacology, and evidence-based nursing interventions. Notable in this edition are changes associated with the recently-published fifth edition of the American Psychiatric Association's *Diagnostic and Statistical Manual of Mental Disorders (DSM-5)*.

Content and Features New to the Eighth Edition

All content has been updated to reflect the current state of the discipline of nursing.

All psychiatric diagnostic content is reflective of the newly published American Psychiatric Association's *Diagnostic and Statistical Manual of Mental Disorders, 5th Edition* (2013).

All nursing diagnoses are current with the NANDA-I *2012-2014 Nursing Diagnoses Definitions and Classifications*.

Six "Communication Exercises" boxes—one each following the chapters on Neurocognitive Disorders,

Substance Use and Addictive Disorders, Schizophrenia, Depressive Disorders, Personality Disorders, and Survivors of Abuse or Neglect. These exercises portray clinical scenarios that allow the student to practice communication skills with clients. Examples of answers appear in an appendix at the back of the book.

New content on factitious disorder, Munchausen syndrome, and hoarding disorder.

New chapter on "Trauma- and Stressor-Related Disorders" (to correlate with *DSM-5*).

New chapter on "Military Families."

New chapter on "The Recovery Model" in the Therapeutic Approaches unit of the textbook. Additional content on the Recovery Model in chapters on Schizophrenia and Bipolar Disorder.

Updated and new psychotropic drugs approved since the publication of the seventh edition. These are included in the specific diagnostic chapters to which they apply and in the psychopharmacology chapter found on davisplus.com.

Features That Have Been Retained in the Eighth Edition

The concept of **holistic nursing** is retained in the eighth edition. An attempt has been made to ensure that the physical aspects of psychiatric/mental health nursing are not overlooked. In all relevant situations, the mind/body connection is addressed.

Nursing process is retained in the eighth edition as the tool for delivery of care to the individual with a psychiatric disorder or to assist in the primary prevention or exacerbation of mental illness symptoms. The six steps of the nursing process, as described in the American Nurses Association *Standards of Clinical Nursing Practice*, are used to provide guidelines for the nurse. These standards of care are included for the *DSM-5* diagnoses, as well as those on the aging individual, the bereaved individual, survivors of abuse and neglect, and military families, and as examples in several of the therapeutic approaches. The six steps include:

Assessment: Background assessment data, including a description of symptomatology, provides an extensive knowledge base from which the nurse may draw when performing an assessment. Several assessment tools are also included.

Diagnosis: Analysis of the data is included, from which nursing diagnoses common to specific psychiatric disorders are derived.

Outcome Identification: Outcomes are derived from the nursing diagnoses and stated as measurable goals.

Planning: A plan of care is presented with selected nursing diagnoses for the *DSM-5* diagnoses, as well as for the elderly client, the bereaved individual, victims of abuse and neglect, military veterans and their families, the elderly homebound client, and the primary caregiver of the client with a chronic mental illness. The planning standard also includes tables that list topics for educating clients and families about mental illness. Concept map care plans are included for all major psychiatric diagnoses.

Implementation: The interventions that have been identified in the plan of care are included along with rationales for each. Case studies at the end of each *DSM-5* chapter assist the student in the practical application of theoretical material. Also included as a part of this particular standard is Unit 3 of the textbook, "Therapeutic Approaches in Psychiatric Nursing Care." This section of the textbook addresses psychiatric nursing intervention in depth, and frequently speaks to the differentiation in scope of practice between the basic level psychiatric nurse and the advanced practice level psychiatric nurse.

Evaluation: The evaluation standard includes a set of questions that the nurse may use to assess whether the nursing actions have been successful in achieving the objectives of care.

Other features of this eighth edition:

- **Internet references** for each *DSM-5* diagnosis, with website listings for information related to the disorder.
- **Tables that list topics for client/family education** (in the clinical chapters).
- **Boxes that include current research studies** with implications for evidence-based nursing practice (in the clinical chapters).
- **Assigning nursing diagnoses to client behaviors** (diagnostic chapters and Appendix F).
- **Taxonomy and diagnostic criteria from the *DSM-5* (2013).** Used throughout the text.
- **All references have been updated throughout the text.** Classical references are distinguished from general references.
- **Boxes with definitions of core concepts** appear throughout the text.
- **Comprehensive glossary.**
- **Answers to end-of-chapter review questions** (Appendix A).
- **Answers to communication exercises** (Appendix B).
- **Sample client teaching guides** (online at www.davisplus.com).
- **Website.** An F.A. Davis/Townsend website that contains additional nursing care plans that do not appear in the text, links to psychotropic medications,

concept map care plans, and neurobiological content and illustrations, as well as student resources including practice test questions, learning activities, concept map care plans, and client teaching guides.

Additional Educational Resources

Faculty may also find the following teaching aids that accompany this textbook helpful:

Instructor Resources at www.davisplus.com:

- **Multiple choice questions** (including new format questions reflecting the latest NCLEX blueprint).
- **Lecture outlines** for all chapters
- **Learning activities** for all chapters (including answer key)
- **Answers to the Critical Thinking Exercises** from the textbook
- **PowerPoint Presentation** to accompany all chapters in the textbook
- **Answers to the Homework Assignment Questions** from the textbook
- **Case studies for use with student teaching**

Additional chapters on Psychopharmacology, Relaxation Therapy, Complementary Therapies, and Forensic Nursing are online at www.davisplus.com.

It is hoped that the revisions and additions to this eighth edition continue to satisfy a need within psychiatric/mental health nursing practice. The mission of this textbook has been, and continues to be, to provide both students and clinicians with up-to-date information about psychiatric/mental health nursing. The user-friendly format and easy-to-understand language, for which we have received many positive comments, have been retained in this edition. I hope that this eighth edition continues to promote and advance the commitment to psychiatric/mental health nursing.

Mary C. Townsend

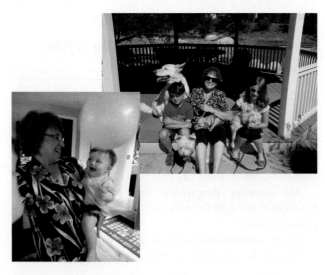

Basic Concepts in Psychiatric/Mental Health Nursing

1 The Concept of Stress Adaptation

CORE CONCEPTS

adaptation
maladaptation
stressor

KEY TERMS

"fight or flight" syndrome
general adaptation syndrome

precipitating event
predisposing factors

OBJECTIVES
After reading this chapter, the student will be able to:

1. Define *adaptation* and *maladaptation*.
2. Identify physiological responses to stress.
3. Explain the relationship between stress and "diseases of adaptation."
4. Describe the concept of stress as an environmental event.
5. Explain the concept of stress as a transaction between the individual and the environment.
6. Discuss adaptive coping strategies in the management of stress.

HOMEWORK ASSIGNMENT
Please read the chapter and answer the following questions:

1. How are the body's physiological defenses affected when under sustained stress? Why?
2. In the view of stress as an environmental event, what aspects are missing when considering an individual's response to a stressful situation?
3. In their study, what event did Miller and Rahe find produced the highest level of stress reaction in their subjects?
4. What is the initial step in stress management?

Psychologists and others have struggled for many years to establish an effective definition of the term *stress*. This term is used loosely today and still lacks a definitive explanation. Stress may be viewed as an individual's reaction to any change that requires an adjustment or response, which can be physical, mental, or emotional. Responses directed at stabilizing internal biological processes and preserving self-esteem can be viewed as healthy adaptations to stress.

Roy (1976) defined an adaptive response as behavior that maintains the integrity of the individual. Adaptation is viewed as positive and is correlated with a healthy response. When behavior disrupts the integrity of the individual, it is perceived as maladaptive.

Maladaptive responses by the individual are considered to be negative or unhealthy.

Various 20th-century researchers contributed to several different concepts of stress. Three of these concepts include stress as a biological response, stress as an environmental event, and stress as a transaction between the individual and the environment. This chapter includes an explanation of each of these concepts.

CORE CONCEPT

Stressor

A biological, psychological, social, or chemical factor that causes physical or emotional tension and may be a factor in the etiology of certain illnesses.

Stress as a Biological Response

In 1956, Hans Selye published the results of his research concerning the physiological response of a biological system to a change imposed on it. Since his initial publication, he has revised his definition of stress, calling it "the state manifested by a specific syndrome which consists of all the nonspecifically-induced changes within a biologic system" (Selye, 1976). This syndrome of symptoms has come to be known as the "**fight or flight**" **syndrome**. Schematics of these biological responses, both initially and with sustained stress, are presented in Figures 1-1 and 1-2. Selye called this general reaction of the body to stress the **general adaptation syndrome**. He described three distinct stages of the reaction:

1. **Alarm Reaction Stage.** During this stage, the physiological responses of the "fight or flight" syndrome are initiated.
2. **Stage of Resistance.** The individual uses the physiological responses of the first stage as a defense in the attempt to adapt to the stressor. If adaptation occurs, the third stage is prevented or delayed. Physiological symptoms may disappear.

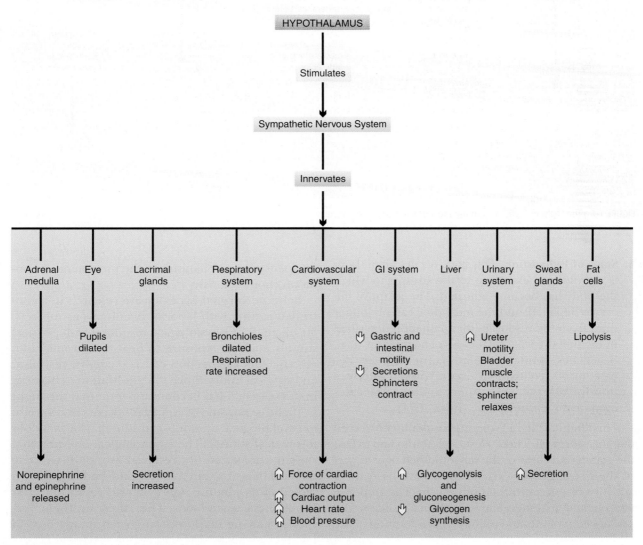

FIGURE 1–1 The "fight or flight" syndrome: the initial stress response.

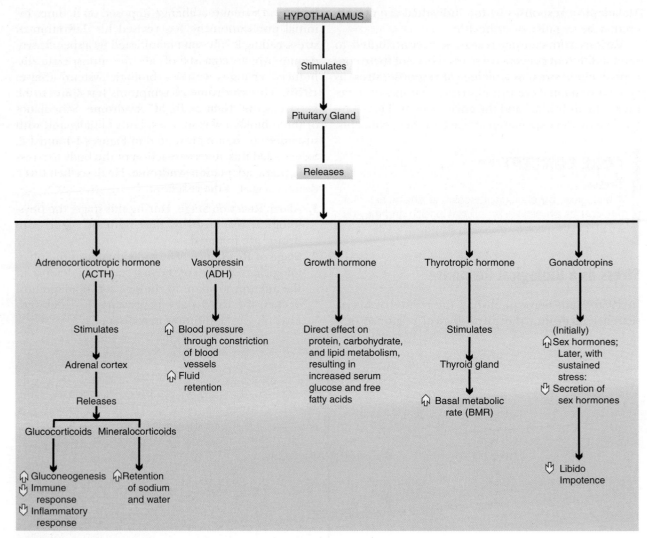

FIGURE 1–2   The "fight or flight" syndrome: the sustained stress response.

3. **Stage of Exhaustion.** This stage occurs when there is a prolonged exposure to the stressor to which the body has become adjusted. The adaptive energy is depleted, and the individual can no longer draw from the resources for adaptation described in the first two stages. Diseases of adaptation (e.g., headaches, mental disorders, coronary artery disease, ulcers, colitis) may occur. Without intervention for reversal, exhaustion, and in some cases even death, ensues (Selye, 1956, 1974).

This "fight or flight" response undoubtedly served our ancestors well. Those *Homo sapiens* who had to face the giant grizzly bear or the saber-toothed tiger as part of their struggle for survival must have used these adaptive resources to their advantage. The response was elicited in emergency situations, used in the preservation of life, and followed by restoration of the compensatory mechanisms to the pre-emergent condition (homeostasis).

Selye performed his extensive research in a controlled setting with laboratory animals as subjects. He elicited the physiological responses with physical stimuli, such as exposure to heat or extreme cold, electric shock, injection of toxic agents, restraint, and surgical injury. Since the publication of his original research, it has become apparent that the "fight or flight" syndrome of symptoms occurs in response to psychological or emotional stimuli, just as it does to physical stimuli. The psychological or emotional stressors are often not resolved as rapidly as some physical stressors, and therefore the body may be depleted of its adaptive energy more readily than it is from physical stressors. The "fight or flight" response may be inappropriate, even dangerous, to the lifestyle of today, in which stress has been described as a psychosocial state that is pervasive, chronic, and relentless. It is this chronic response that maintains the body in the aroused condition for extended periods of time that promotes susceptibility to diseases of adaptation.

CORE CONCEPT

Adaptation

Adaptation is said to occur when an individual's physical or behavioral response to any change in his or her internal or external environment results in preservation of individual integrity or timely return to equilibrium.

Stress as an Environmental Event

A second concept defines stress as the "thing" or "event" that triggers the adaptive physiological and psychological responses in an individual. The event creates change in the life pattern of the individual, requires significant adjustment in lifestyle, and taxes available personal resources. The change can be either positive, such as outstanding personal achievement, or negative, such as being fired from a job. The emphasis here is on *change* from the existing steady state of the individual's life pattern.

Miller and Rahe (1997) have updated the original Social Readjustment Rating Scale devised by Holmes and Rahe in 1967. Just as in the earlier version, numerical values are assigned to various events, or changes, that are common in people's lives. The updated version reflects an increased number of stressors not identified in the original version. In the new study, Miller and Rahe found that women react to life stress events at higher levels than men, and unmarried people gave higher scores than married people for most of the events. Younger subjects rated more events at a higher stress level than older subjects. A high score on the Recent Life Changes Questionnaire (RLCQ) places the individual at greater susceptibility to physical or psychological illness. The questionnaire may be completed considering life stressors within a 6-month or 1-year period. Six-month totals equal to or greater than 300 life change units (LCUs) or 1-year totals equal to or greater than 500 LCUs are considered indicative of a high level of recent life stress, thereby increasing the risk of illness for the individual. The RLCQ is presented in Table 1-1.

It is unknown whether stress overload merely predisposes a person to illness or actually precipitates it, but there does appear to be a causal link (Pelletier, 1992). Life changes questionnaires have been criticized because they do not consider the individual's perception of the event. Individuals differ

TABLE 1–1 The Recent Life Changes Questionnaire

LIFE CHANGE EVENT	LCU	LIFE CHANGE EVENT	LCU
HEALTH		**HOME AND FAMILY**	
An injury or illness which:		Major change in living conditions	42
Kept you in bed a week or more, or sent you to the hospital	74	Change in residence:	
		Move within the same town or city	25
Was less serious than above	44	Move to a different town, city, or state	47
Major dental work	26	Change in family get-togethers	25
Major change in eating habits	27	Major change in health or behavior of family member	55
Major change in sleeping habits	26		
Major change in your usual type/ amount of recreation	28	Marriage	50
		Pregnancy	67
WORK		Miscarriage or abortion	65
Change to a new type of work	51	Gain of a new family member:	
Change in your work hours or conditions	35	Birth of a child	66
		Adoption of a child	65
Change in your responsibilities at work:		A relative moving in with you	59
More responsibilities	29	Spouse beginning or ending work	46
Fewer responsibilities	21		
Promotion	31		

Continued

TABLE 1–1   The Recent Life Changes Questionnaire—cont'd

LIFE CHANGE EVENT	LCU	LIFE CHANGE EVENT	LCU
Demotion	42	Child leaving home:	
Transfer	32	To attend college	41
		Due to marriage	41
Troubles at work:		For other reasons	45
With your boss	29	Change in arguments with spouse	50
With coworkers	35		
With persons under your supervision	35	In-law problems	38
Other work troubles	28	Change in the marital status of your parents:	
Major business adjustment	60	Divorce	59
		Remarriage	50
Retirement	52	Separation from spouse:	
Loss of job:		Due to work	53
Laid off from work	68	Due to marital problems	76
Fired from work	79	Divorce	96
Correspondence course to help you in your work	18	Birth of grandchild	43
		Death of spouse	119
PERSONAL AND SOCIAL		Death of other family member:	
Change in personal habits	26	Child	123
Beginning or ending school or college	38	Brother or sister	102
Change of school or college	35	Parent	100
Change in political beliefs	24	**FINANCIAL**	
Change in religious beliefs	29	Major change in finances:	
Change in social activities	27	Increased income	38
Vacation	24	Decreased income	60
		Investment and/or credit difficulties	56
New, close, personal relationship	37	Loss or damage of personal property	43
Engagement to marry	45	Moderate purchase	20
Girlfriend or boyfriend problems	39	Major purchase	37
Sexual difficulties	44	Foreclosure on a mortgage or loan	58
"Falling out" of a close personal relationship	47		
An accident	48		
Minor violation of the law	20		
Being held in jail	75		
Death of a close friend	70		
Major decision regarding your immediate future	51		
Major personal achievement	36		

SOURCE: Miller and Rahe (1997), with permission.

in their reactions to life events, and these variations are related to the degree to which the change is perceived as stressful. These types of instruments also fail to consider the individual's coping strategies and available support systems at the time when the life change occurs. Positive coping mechanisms and strong social or familial support can reduce the intensity of the stressful life change and promote a more adaptive response.

Stress as a Transaction Between the Individual and the Environment

This concept of stress emphasizes the *relationship* between the individual and the environment. Personal characteristics and the nature of the environmental event are considered. This illustration parallels the modern concept of the etiology of disease. No longer is causation viewed solely as an external entity; whether or not illness occurs depends also on the receiving organism's susceptibility. Similarly, to predict psychological stress as a reaction, the properties of the person in relation to the environment must be considered.

Precipitating Event

Lazarus and Folkman (1984) define *stress* as a relationship between the person and the environment that is appraised by the person as taxing or exceeding his or her resources and endangering his or her well-being. A **precipitating event** is a stimulus arising from the internal or external environment and is perceived by the individual in a specific manner. Determination that a particular person-environment relationship is stressful depends on the individual's cognitive appraisal of the situation. *Cognitive appraisal* is an individual's evaluation of the personal significance of the event or occurrence. The event "precipitates" a response on the part of the individual, and the response is influenced by the individual's perception of the event. The *cognitive response* consists of a primary appraisal and a secondary appraisal.

Individual's Perception of the Event
Primary Appraisal

Lazarus and Folkman (1984) identify three types of primary appraisal: irrelevant, benign-positive, and stressful. An event is judged *irrelevant* when the outcome holds no significance for the individual. A *benign-positive* outcome is one that is perceived as producing pleasure for the individual. *Stress* appraisals include harm/loss, threat, and challenge. *Harm/loss* appraisals refer to damage or loss already experienced by the individual. Appraisals of a *threatening* nature are perceived as anticipated harms or losses.

When an event is appraised as *challenging*, the individual focuses on potential for gain or growth, rather than on risks associated with the event. Challenge produces stress even though the emotions associated with it (eagerness and excitement) are viewed as positive, and coping mechanisms must be called upon to face the new encounter. Challenge and threat may occur together when an individual experiences these positive emotions along with fear or anxiety over possible risks associated with the challenging event.

When stress is produced in response to harm/loss, threat, or challenge, a secondary appraisal is made by the individual.

Secondary Appraisal

This secondary appraisal is an assessment of skills, resources, and knowledge that the person possesses to deal with the situation. The individual evaluates by considering the following:

- Which coping strategies are available to me?
- Will the option I choose be effective in this situation?
- Do I have the ability to use that strategy in an effective manner?

The interaction between the primary appraisal of the event that has occurred and the secondary appraisal of available coping strategies determines the quality of the individual's adaptation response to stress.

Predisposing Factors

A variety of elements influence how an individual perceives and responds to a stressful event. These **predisposing factors** strongly influence whether the response is adaptive or maladaptive. Types of predisposing factors include genetic influences, past experiences, and existing conditions.

Genetic influences are those circumstances of an individual's life that are acquired through heredity. Examples include family history of physical and psychological conditions (strengths and weaknesses) and temperament (behavioral characteristics present at birth that evolve with development).

Past experiences are occurrences that result in learned patterns that can influence an individual's adaptation response. They include previous exposure to the stressor or other stressors, learned coping responses, and degree of adaptation to previous stressors.

Existing conditions incorporate vulnerabilities that influence the adequacy of the individual's physical, psychological, and social resources for dealing with adaptive demands. Examples include current health status, motivation, developmental maturity, severity and duration of the stressor, financial and educational resources, age, existing coping strategies, and a support system of caring others.

This transactional model of stress/adaptation will serve as a framework for the process of nursing in this text. A graphic display of the model is presented in Figure 1-3.

CORE CONCEPT
Maladaptation
Maladaptation occurs when an individual's physical or behavioral response to any change in his or her internal or external environment results in disruption of individual integrity or in persistent disequilibrium.

Stress Management*

The growth of stress management into a multimillion-dollar-a-year business attests to its importance in our society. Stress management involves the use of coping strategies in response to stressful situations. Coping strategies are adaptive when they protect the individual from harm (or additional harm) or strengthen the individual's ability to meet challenging situations. Adaptive responses help restore homeostasis to the body and impede the development of diseases of adaptation.

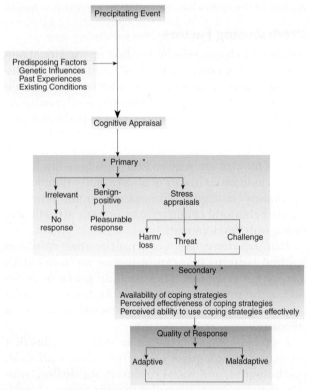

FIGURE 1-3 Transactional model of stress/adaptation.

---

*Techniques of stress management are discussed at greater length in Unit 3 of this text.

Coping strategies are considered maladaptive when the conflict being experienced goes unresolved or intensifies. Energy resources become depleted as the body struggles to compensate for the chronic physiological and psychological arousal being experienced.

The effect is a significant vulnerability to physical or psychological illness.

Adaptive Coping Strategies
Awareness

The initial step in managing stress is awareness—to become aware of the factors that create stress and the feelings associated with a stressful response. Stress can be controlled only when one recognizes that it is being experienced. As one becomes aware of stressors, he or she can omit, avoid, or accept them.

Relaxation

Individuals experience relaxation in different ways. Some individuals relax by engaging in large motor activities, such as sports, jogging, and physical exercise. Still others use techniques such as breathing exercises and progressive relaxation to relieve stress. (A discussion of relaxation therapy may be found online at www.DavisPlus.com.

Meditation

Practiced 20 minutes once or twice daily, meditation has been shown to produce a lasting reduction in blood pressure and other stress-related symptoms (Davis, Eshelman, & McKay, 2008). Meditation involves assuming a comfortable position, closing the eyes, casting off all other thoughts, and concentrating on a single word, sound, or phrase that has positive meaning to the individual. The technique is described in detail online at www.DavisPlus.com.

Interpersonal Communication With Caring Other

As previously mentioned, the strength of one's available support systems is an existing condition that significantly influences the adaptability of coping with stress. Sometimes just "talking the problem out" with an individual who is empathetic is sufficient to interrupt escalation of the stress response. Writing about one's feelings in a journal or diary can also be therapeutic.

Problem Solving

An extremely adaptive coping strategy is to view the situation objectively (or to seek assistance from another individual to accomplish this if the anxiety level is too high to concentrate). After an objective assessment of the situation, the problem-solving/decision-making model can be instituted as follows:

■ Assess the facts of the situation.
■ Formulate goals for resolution of the stressful situation.

- Study the alternatives for dealing with the situation.
- Determine the risks and benefits of each alternative.
- Select an alternative.
- Implement the alternative selected.
- Evaluate the outcome of the alternative implemented.
- If the first choice is ineffective, select and implement a second option.

Pets

Studies show that those who care for pets, especially dogs and cats, are better able to cope with the stressors of life (Allen, Blascovich, & Mendes, 2002; Barker, Knisely, McCain, & Best, 2005). The physical act of stroking or petting a dog or cat can be therapeutic. It gives the animal an intuitive sense of being cared for and at the same time gives the individual the calming feeling of warmth, affection, and interdependence with a reliable, trusting being. One study showed that among people who had had heart attacks, pet owners had one-fifth the death rate of those who did not have pets (Friedmann & Thomas, 1995). Another study revealed evidence that individuals experienced a statistically significant drop in blood pressure in response to petting a dog or cat (Whitaker, 2000).

Music

It is true that music can "soothe the savage beast." Creating and listening to music stimulate motivation, enjoyment, and relaxation. Music can reduce depression and bring about measurable changes in mood and general activity.

Summary and Key Points

- Stress has become a chronic and pervasive condition in the United States today.
- Adaptive behavior is viewed as behavior that maintains the integrity of the individual, with a timely return to equilibrium. It is viewed as positive and is correlated with a healthy response.
- When behavior disrupts the integrity of the individual or results in persistent disequilibrium, it is perceived as maladaptive. Maladaptive responses by the individual are considered to be negative or unhealthy.
- A stressor is defined as a biological, psychological, social, or chemical factor that causes physical or emotional tension and may be a factor in the etiology of certain illnesses.
- Hans Selye identified the biological changes associated with a stressful situation as the "fight or flight" syndrome.

- Selye called the general reaction of the body to stress the "general adaptation syndrome," which occurs in three stages: the alarm reaction stage, the stage of resistance, and the stage of exhaustion.
- When individuals remain in the aroused response to stress for an extended period of time, they become susceptible to diseases of adaptation, some examples of which include headaches, mental disorders, coronary artery disease, ulcers, and colitis.
- Stress may also be viewed as an environmental event. This results when a change from the existing steady state of the individual's life pattern occurs.
- When an individual experiences a high level of life change events, he or she becomes susceptible to physical or psychological illness.
- Limitations of the environmental concept of stress include failure to consider the individual's perception of the event, coping strategies, and available support systems at the time when the life change occurs.
- Stress is more appropriately expressed as a transaction between the individual and the environment that is appraised by the individual as taxing or exceeding his or her resources and endangering his or her well-being.
- The individual makes a cognitive appraisal of the precipitating event to determine the personal significance of the event or occurrence.
- Primary cognitive appraisals may be irrelevant, benign-positive, or stressful.
- Secondary cognitive appraisals include assessment and evaluation by the individual of skills, resources, and knowledge to deal with the stressful situation.
- Predisposing factors influence how an individual perceives and responds to a stressful event. They include genetic influences, past experiences, and existing conditions.
- Stress management involves the use of adaptive coping strategies in response to stressful situations in an effort to impede the development of diseases of adaptation.
- Examples of adaptive coping strategies include developing awareness, relaxation, meditation, interpersonal communication with caring other, problem solving, pets, and music.

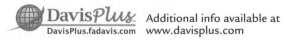

DavisPlus™ Additional info available at
DavisPlus.fadavis.com www.davisplus.com

Review Questions
Self-Examination/Learning Exercise

*Select the answer that is **most** appropriate for questions 1 through 5. In question 6, identify the category in which each example belongs.*

1. Sondra, who lives in Maine, hears on the evening news that 25 people were killed in a tornado in south Texas. Sondra experiences no anxiety upon hearing of this stressful situation. This is most likely because Sondra:
   a. Is selfish and does not care what happens to other people.
   b. Appraises the event as irrelevant to her own situation.
   c. Assesses that she has the skills to cope with the stressful situation.
   d. Uses suppression as her primary defense mechanism.

2. Cindy regularly develops nausea and vomiting when she is faced with a stressful situation. Which of the following is most likely a predisposing factor to this maladaptive response by Cindy?
   a. Cindy inherited her mother's "nervous" stomach.
   b. Cindy is fixed in a lower level of development.
   c. Cindy has never been motivated to achieve success.
   d. When Cindy was a child, her mother pampered her and kept her home from school when she was ill.

3. When an individual's stress response is sustained over a long period, the endocrine system involvement results in which of the following?
   a. Decreased resistance to disease.
   b. Increased libido
   c. Decreased blood pressure.
   d. Increased inflammatory response.

4. Management of stress is extremely important in today's society because:
   a. Evolution has diminished human capability for "fight or flight."
   b. The stressors of today tend to be ongoing, resulting in a sustained response.
   c. We have stress disorders that did not exist in the days of our ancestors.
   d. One never knows when one will have to face a grizzly bear or saber-toothed tiger in today's society.

5. Nancy has just received a promotion on her job. She is very happy and excited about moving up in her company, but she has been experiencing anxiety since receiving the news. Her primary appraisal is that she most likely views the situation as which of the following?
   a. Benign-positive
   b. Irrelevant
   c. Challenging
   d. Threatening

6. Precipitating stressors, past experiences, existing conditions, and genetic influences are components of the Transactional Model of Stress Adaptation, and influence an individual's response to stress. Identify each of these conditions in the following examples.
   a. Precipitating stressor
   b. Past experience
   c. Existing conditions
   d. Genetic influences

   _____ Mr. T is fixed in a lower level of development.

   _____ Mr. T's father had diabetes mellitus.

   _____ Mr. T has been fired from his last five jobs.

   _____ Mr. T's baby was stillborn last month.

References

Allen, K., Blascovich, J., & Mendes, W.B. (2002). Cardiovascular reactivity and the presence of pets, friends, and spouses: The truth about cats and dogs. *Psychosomatic Medicine, 64,* 727–739.

Barker, S.B., Knisely, J.S., McCain, N.L., & Best, A.M. (2005). Measuring stress and immune response in healthcare professionals following interaction with a therapy dog: A pilot study. *Psychological Reports, 96,* 713–729.

Davis, M.D., Eshelman, E.R., & McKay, M. (2008). *The relaxation and stress reduction workbook* (6th ed.). Oakland, CA: New Harbinger Publications.

Friedmann, E., & Thomas, S.A. (1995). Pet ownership, social support, and one-year survival after acute myocardial infarction in the cardiac arrhythmia suppression trial. *American Journal of Cardiology, 76*(17), 1213.

Miller, M.A., & Rahe, R.H. (1997). Life changes scaling for the 1990s. *Journal of Psychosomatic Research, 43*(3), 279–292.

Pelletier, K.R. (1992). *Mind as healer, mind as slayer: A holistic approach to preventing stress disorders.* New York, NY: Dell.

Whitaker, J. (2000). Pet owners are a healthy breed. *Health & Healing, 10*(10), 1–8.

Classical References

Holmes, T., & Rahe, R. (1967). The social readjustment rating scale. *Journal of Psychosomatic Research, 11,* 213–218.

Lazarus, R.S., & Folkman, S. (1984). *Stress, appraisal and coping.* New York, NY: Springer Publishing.

Roy, C. (1976). *Introduction to nursing: An adaptation model.* Englewood Cliffs, NJ: Prentice-Hall.

Selye, H. (1956). *The stress of life.* New York, NY: McGraw-Hill.

Selye, H. (1974). *Stress without distress.* New York, NY: Signet Books.

Selye, H. (1976). *The stress of life* (rev. ed.). New York, NY: McGraw Hill.

2 Mental Health/Mental Illness: Historical and Theoretical Concepts

CHAPTER OUTLINE

KEY TERMS

anticipatory grieving
bereavement overload
defense mechanisms
  compensation
  denial
  displacement
  identification
  intellectualization

introjection
isolation
projection
rationalization
reaction formation
regression
repression
sublimation

suppression
undoing
humors
mental health
mental illness
neurosis
psychosis
"ship of fools"

OBJECTIVES
After reading this chapter, the student will be able to:

1. Discuss the history of psychiatric care.
2. Define *mental health* and *mental illness*.
3. Discuss cultural elements that influence attitudes toward mental health and mental illness.
4. Describe psychological adaptation responses to stress.
5. Identify correlation of adaptive/maladaptive behaviors to the mental health/mental illness continuum.

HOMEWORK ASSIGNMENT
Please read the chapter and answer the following questions:

1. Explain the concepts of *incomprehensibility* and *cultural relativity*.
2. Describe some symptoms of panic anxiety.
3. Jane was involved in an automobile accident in which both her parents were killed. When you ask her about it, she says she has no memory of the accident. What ego defense mechanism is she using?
4. In what stage of the grieving process is the individual with delayed or inhibited grief fixed?

The consideration of mental health and mental illness has its basis in the cultural beliefs of the society in which the behavior takes place. Some cultures are quite liberal in the range of behaviors that are considered acceptable, whereas others have very little tolerance for behaviors that deviate from the cultural norms.

A study of the history of psychiatric care reveals some shocking truths about past treatment of individuals with mental illness. Many were kept in control by means that today could be considered less than humane.

This chapter deals with the evolution of psychiatric care from ancient times to the present. **Mental health** and **mental illness** are defined, and the psychological adaptation to stress is explained in terms of the two major responses: anxiety and grief. Behavioral responses and their placement along the mental health/mental illness continuum are discussed.

Historical Overview of Psychiatric Care

Primitive beliefs regarding mental disturbances took several views. Some thought that an individual with mental illness had been dispossessed of his or her soul and that the only way wellness could be achieved was if the soul returned. Others believed that evil spirits or supernatural or magical powers had entered the body. The "cure" for these individuals involved a ritualistic exorcism to purge the body of these unwanted forces. This often consisted of brutal beatings, starvation, or other torturous means. Still others considered that the individual with mental illness may have broken a taboo or sinned against another individual or God, for which ritualistic purification was required or various types of retribution were demanded. The correlation of mental illness to demonology or witchcraft led to some individuals with mental illness being burned at the stake.

The position of these ancient beliefs evolved with increasing knowledge about mental illness and changes in cultural, religious, and sociopolitical attitudes. The work of Hippocrates, about 400 B.C., began the movement away from belief in the supernatural. Hippocrates associated insanity and mental illness with an irregularity in the interaction of the four body fluids—blood, black bile, yellow bile, and phlegm. He called these body fluids **humors**, and associated each with a particular disposition. Disequilibrium among these four humors was thought to cause mental illness, and it was often treated by inducing vomiting and diarrhea with potent cathartic drugs.

During the Middle Ages (A.D. 500 to 1500), the association of mental illness with witchcraft and the supernatural continued to prevail in Europe. During this period, many people with severe mental illness were sent out to sea on sailing boats with little guidance to search for their lost rationality. The expression **"ship of fools"** was derived from this operation.

During the same period in the Middle Eastern Islamic countries, however, a change in attitude began to occur, from the perception of mental illness as the result of witchcraft or the supernatural to the idea that these individuals were actually ill.

This notion gave rise to the establishment of special units for clients with mental illness within general hospitals, as well as residential institutions specifically designed for this purpose. They can likely be considered the first asylums for individuals with mental illness.

Colonial Americans tended to reflect the attitudes of the European communities from which they had emigrated. Particularly in the New England area, individuals were punished for behavior attributed to witchcraft. In the 16th and 17th centuries, institutions for people with mental illness did not exist in the United States, and care of these individuals became a family responsibility. Those without family or other resources became the responsibility of the communities in which they lived and were incarcerated in places where they could do no harm to themselves or others.

The first hospital in America to admit clients with mental illness was established in Philadelphia in the middle of the 18th century. Benjamin Rush, often called the father of American psychiatry, was a physician at the hospital. He initiated the provision of humanistic treatment and care for clients with mental illness. Although he included kindness, exercise, and socialization, he also employed harsher methods such as bloodletting, purging, various types of physical restraints, and extremes of temperatures, reflecting the medical therapies of that era.

The 19th century brought the establishment of a system of state asylums, largely the result of the work of Dorothea Dix, a former New England schoolteacher, who lobbied tirelessly on behalf of the mentally ill population. She was unfaltering in her belief that mental illness was curable and that state hospitals should provide humanistic therapeutic care. This system of hospital care for individuals with mental illness grew, but the mentally ill population grew faster. The institutions became overcrowded and understaffed, and conditions deteriorated. Therapeutic care reverted to custodial care. These state hospitals provided the largest resource for individuals with mental illness until the initiation of the community health movement of the 1960s (see Chapter 36).

The emergence of psychiatric nursing began in 1873 with the graduation of Linda Richards from the nursing program at the New England Hospital for Women and Children in Boston. She has come to be known as the first American psychiatric nurse. During her career, Richards was instrumental in the establishment of a number of psychiatric hospitals and the first school of psychiatric nursing at the McLean Asylum in Waverly, Massachusetts, in

1882. The focus in this school, and those that followed, was "training" in how to provide custodial care for clients in psychiatric asylums—training that did not include the study of psychological concepts. Significant change did not occur until 1955, when incorporation of psychiatric nursing into their curricula became a requirement for all undergraduate schools of nursing.

Nursing curricula emphasized the importance of the nurse-patient relationship and therapeutic communication techniques. Nursing intervention in the somatic therapies (e.g., insulin and electroconvulsive therapy) provided impetus for the incorporation of these concepts into nursing's body of knowledge.

With the apparently increasing need for psychiatric care in the aftermath of World War II, the government passed the National Mental Health Act of 1946. This legislation provided funds for the education of psychiatrists, psychologists, social workers, and psychiatric nurses. Graduate-level education in psychiatric nursing was established during this period. Also significant at this time was the introduction of antipsychotic medications, which made it possible for psychotic clients to more readily participate in their treatment, including nursing therapies.

Knowledge of the history of psychiatric/mental health care contributes to the understanding of the concepts presented in this chapter and those in Chapter 3, which describe the theories of personality development according to various 19th-century and 20th-century leaders in the psychiatric/mental health movement. Modern American psychiatric care has its roots in ancient times. A great deal of opportunity exists for continued advancement of this specialty within the practice of nursing.

Mental Health

A number of theorists have attempted to define the concept of mental health. Many of these concepts deal with various aspects of individual functioning. Maslow (1970) emphasized an individual's motivation in the continuous quest for self-actualization. He identified a "hierarchy of needs," the lower ones requiring fulfillment before those at higher levels can be achieved, with self-actualization being fulfillment of one's highest potential. An individual's position within the hierarchy may reverse from a higher level to a lower level based on life circumstances. For example, an individual facing major surgery who has been working on tasks to achieve self-actualization may become preoccupied, if only temporarily, with the need for physiological safety. A representation of this needs hierarchy is presented in Figure 2-1.

Maslow described self-actualization as being "psychologically healthy, fully human, highly evolved, and fully mature." He believed that "healthy," or "self-actualized," individuals possessed the following characteristics:

■ An appropriate perception of reality
■ The ability to accept oneself, others, and human nature
■ The ability to manifest spontaneity
■ The capacity for focusing concentration on problem solving
■ A need for detachment and desire for privacy
■ Independence, autonomy, and a resistance to enculturation
■ An intensity of emotional reaction
■ A frequency of "peak" experiences that validates the worthwhileness, richness, and beauty of life
■ An identification with humankind
■ The ability to achieve satisfactory interpersonal relationships
■ A democratic character structure and strong sense of ethics
■ Creativeness
■ A degree of nonconformance

Jahoda (1958) identified a list of six indicators that she suggested are a reflection of mental health:

1. **A Positive Attitude Toward Self.** This includes an objective view of self, including knowledge and acceptance of strengths and limitations. The individual feels a strong sense of personal identity and a security within the environment.

2. **Growth, Development, and the Ability to Achieve Self-actualization.** This indicator correlates with whether the individual successfully achieves the tasks associated with each level of development (see Erikson, Chapter 3). With successful achievement in each level, the individual gains motivation for advancement to his or her highest potential.

3. **Integration.** The focus here is on maintaining an equilibrium or balance among various life processes. Integration includes the ability to adaptively respond to the environment and the development of a philosophy of life, both of which help the individual maintain anxiety at a manageable level in response to stressful situations.

4. **Autonomy.** This refers to the individual's ability to perform in an independent, self-directed manner. The individual makes choices and accepts responsibility for the outcomes.

5. **Perception of Reality.** Accurate reality perception is a positive indicator of mental health. This includes perception of the environment without

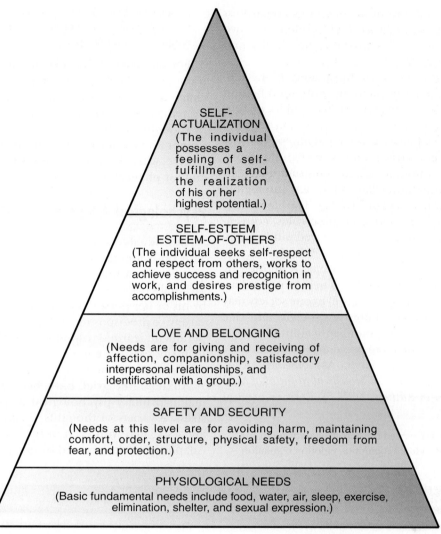

FIGURE 2-1 Maslow's hierarchy of needs.

distortion, as well as the capacity for empathy and social sensitivity—a respect and concern for the wants and needs of others.

6. **Environmental Mastery.** This indicator suggests that the individual has achieved a satisfactory role within the group, society, or environment. It suggests that he or she is able to love and accept the love of others. When faced with life situations, the individual is able to strategize, make decisions, change, adjust, and adapt. Life offers satisfaction to the individual who has achieved environmental mastery.

Black and Andreasen (2011) define mental health as:

> a state of being that is relative rather than absolute. The successful performance of mental functions shown by productive activities, fulfilling relationships with other people, and the ability to adapt to change and to cope with adversity. (p. 608)

Robinson (1983) has offered the following definition of mental health:

> a dynamic state in which thought, feeling, and behavior that is age-appropriate and congruent with the local and cultural norms is demonstrated. (p. 74)

For purposes of this text, and in keeping with the framework of stress/adaptation, a modification of Robinson's definition of mental health is considered. Thus, *mental health* is viewed as "the successful adaptation to stressors from the internal or external environment, evidenced by thoughts, feelings, and behaviors that are age-appropriate and congruent with local and cultural norms."

Mental Illness

A universal concept of mental illness is difficult, because of the cultural factors that influence such a definition. However, certain elements are associated with individuals' perceptions of mental illness, regardless of cultural origin. Horwitz (2002) identifies two of these elements as (1) incomprehensibility and (2) cultural relativity.

Incomprehensibility relates to the inability of the general population to understand the motivation behind the behavior. When observers are unable to find meaning or comprehensibility in behavior, they are likely to label that behavior as mental illness. Horwitz states, "Observers attribute labels of mental illness when the rules, conventions, and understandings they use to interpret behavior fail to find any intelligible motivation behind an action" (p. 17). The element of *cultural relativity* considers that these rules, conventions, and understandings are conceived within an individual's own particular culture. Behavior that is considered "normal" and "abnormal" is defined by one's cultural or societal norms. Therefore, a behavior that is recognized as mentally ill in one society may be viewed as "normal" in another society, and vice versa. Horwitz identified a number of cultural aspects of mental illness, which are presented in Box 2-1.

The American Psychiatric Association (APA), 2013), in its *Diagnostic and Statistical Manual of Mental Disorders, Fifth Edition (DSM-5)*, defines mental disorder as:

> a syndrome characterized by clinically significant disturbance in an individual's cognitions, emotion regulation, or behavior that reflects a dysfunction in the psychological, biological, or developmental processes underlying mental functioning. (p. 20)

For purposes of this text, and in keeping with the framework of stress/adaptation, *mental illness* will be characterized as "maladaptive responses to stressors from the internal or external environment, evidenced by thoughts, feelings, and behaviors that are incongruent with the local and cultural norms, and that interfere with the individual's social, occupational, and/or physical functioning."

Psychological Adaptation to Stress

All individuals exhibit some characteristics associated with both mental health and mental illness at any given point in time. Chapter 1 described how an individual's response to stressful situations is influenced by his or her personal perception of the event and a variety of predisposing factors, such as heredity, temperament, learned response patterns, developmental maturity, existing coping strategies, and support systems of caring others.

Anxiety and grief have been described as two major, primary psychological response patterns to stress. A variety of thoughts, feelings, and behaviors are associated with each of these response patterns. Adaptation is determined by the degree to which the

---

BOX 2-1 Cultural Aspects of Mental Illness

1. Usually members of the lay community, rather than a psychiatric professional, initially recognize that an individual's behavior deviates from the societal norms.
2. People who are related to an individual or who are of the same cultural or social group are less likely to label an individual's behavior as mentally ill than someone who is relationally or culturally distant. Relatives (or people of the same cultural or social group) try to "normalize" the behavior; that is, they try to find an explanation for the behavior.
3. Psychiatrists see a person with mental illness most often when the family members can no longer deny the illness and often when the behavior is at its worst. The local or cultural norms define pathological behavior.
4. Individuals in the lowest social class usually display the highest amount of mental illness symptoms. However, they tend to tolerate a wider range of behaviors that deviate from societal norms and are less likely to consider these behaviors as indicative of mental illness. Mental illness labels are most often applied by psychiatric professionals.
5. The higher the social class, the greater the recognition of mental illness behaviors. Members of the higher social classes are likely to be self-labeled or labeled by family

members or friends. Psychiatric assistance is sought near the first signs of emotional disturbance.
6. The more highly educated the person, the greater the recognition of mental illness behaviors. However, even more relevant than the *amount* of education is the *type* of education. Individuals in the more humanistic types of professions (lawyers, social workers, artists, teachers, nurses) are more likely to seek psychiatric assistance than professionals such as business executives, computer specialists, accountants, and engineers.
7. In terms of religion, Jewish people are more likely to seek psychiatric assistance than are Catholics or Protestants.
8. Women are more likely than men to recognize the symptoms of mental illness and seek assistance.
9. The greater the cultural distance from the *mainstream* of society (i.e., the fewer the ties with *conventional* society), the greater the likelihood of negative response by society to mental illness. For example, immigrants have a greater distance from the mainstream than the native born, ethnic minorities greater than the dominant culture, and "bohemians" greater than the bourgeoisie. They are more likely to be subjected to coercive treatment, and involuntary psychiatric commitments are more common.

Adapted from Horwitz, A.V. (2002). *The social control of mental illness.* Clinton Corners, NY: Percheron Press.

thoughts, feelings, and behaviors interfere with an individual's functioning.

> ## CORE CONCEPT
> **Anxiety**
> A diffuse apprehension that is vague in nature and is associated with feelings of uncertainty and helplessness.

Anxiety

Feelings of anxiety are so common in our society that they are almost considered universal. Anxiety arises from the chaos and confusion that exists in the world today. Fears of the unknown and conditions of ambiguity offer a perfect breeding ground for anxiety to take root and grow. Low levels of anxiety are adaptive and can provide the motivation required for survival. Anxiety becomes problematic when the individual is unable to prevent the anxiety from escalating to a level that interferes with the ability to meet basic needs.

Peplau (1963) described four levels of anxiety: mild, moderate, severe, and panic. It is important for nurses to be able to recognize the symptoms associated with each level to plan for appropriate intervention with anxious individuals.

- **Mild Anxiety.** This level of anxiety is seldom a problem for the individual. It is associated with the tension experienced in response to the events of day-to-day living. Mild anxiety prepares people for action. It sharpens the senses, increases motivation for productivity, increases the perceptual field, and results in a heightened awareness of the environment. Learning is enhanced and the individual is able to function at his or her optimal level.
- **Moderate Anxiety.** As the level of anxiety increases, the extent of the perceptual field diminishes. The moderately anxious individual is less alert to events occurring in the environment. The individual's attention span and ability to concentrate decrease, although he or she may still attend to needs with direction. Assistance with problem solving may be required. Increased muscular tension and restlessness are evident.
- **Severe Anxiety.** The perceptual field of the severely anxious individual is so greatly diminished that concentration centers on one particular detail only or on many extraneous details. Attention span is extremely limited, and the individual has much difficulty completing even the simplest task. Physical symptoms (e.g., headaches, palpitations, insomnia) and emotional symptoms (e.g., confusion, dread, horror) may be evident. Discomfort is experienced to the degree that virtually all overt behavior is aimed at relieving the anxiety.
- **Panic Anxiety.** In this most intense state of anxiety, the individual is unable to focus on even one detail in the environment. Misperceptions are common, and a loss of contact with reality may occur. The individual may experience hallucinations or delusions. Behavior may be characterized by wild and desperate actions or extreme withdrawal. Human functioning and communication with others is ineffective. Panic anxiety is associated with a feeling of terror, and individuals may be convinced that they have a life-threatening illness or fear that they are "going crazy," are losing control, or are emotionally weak. Prolonged panic anxiety can lead to physical and emotional exhaustion and can be a life-threatening situation.

A synopsis of the characteristics associated with each of the four levels of anxiety is presented in Table 2-1.

Behavioral Adaptation Responses to Anxiety

A variety of behavioral adaptation responses occur at each level of anxiety. Figure 2-2 depicts these behavioral responses on a continuum of anxiety ranging from mild to panic.

Mild Anxiety

At the mild level, individuals employ any of a number of coping behaviors that satisfy their needs for comfort. Menninger (1963) described the following types of coping mechanisms that individuals use to relieve anxiety in stressful situations:

- Sleeping
- Yawning
- Eating
- Drinking
- Physical exercise
- Daydreaming
- Smoking
- Laughing
- Crying
- Cursing
- Pacing
- Nail biting
- Foot swinging
- Finger tapping
- Fidgeting
- Talking to someone with whom one feels comfortable

Undoubtedly there are many more responses too numerous to mention here, considering that each individual develops his or her own unique ways to relieve anxiety at the mild level. Some of these behaviors are more adaptive than others.

Mild-to-Moderate Anxiety

Sigmund Freud (1961) identified the ego as the reality component of the personality that governs problem solving and rational thinking. As the level of anxiety increases, the strength of the ego is tested, and energy is mobilized to confront the threat. Anna Freud (1953) identified a number of **defense mechanisms** employed by the ego in the face of threat to biological or psychological integrity. Some of these ego defense mechanisms are more adaptive than others, but all are used either consciously or unconsciously as a protective device for

TABLE 2–1 Levels of Anxiety

LEVEL	PERCEPTUAL FIELD	ABILITY TO LEARN	PHYSICAL CHARACTERISTICS	EMOTIONAL/BEHAVIORAL CHARACTERISTICS
Mild	Heightened perception (e.g., noises may seem louder; details within the environment are clearer) Increased awareness Increased alertness	Learning is enhanced	Restlessness Irritability	May remain superficial with others Rarely experienced as distressful Motivation is increased
Moderate	Reduction in perceptual field Reduced alertness to environmental events (e.g., someone talking may not be heard; part of the room may not be noticed)	Learning still occurs, but not at optimal ability Decreased attention span Decreased ability to concentrate	Increased restlessness Increased heart and respiration rate Increased perspiration Gastric discomfort Increased muscular tension Increase in speech rate, volume, and pitch	A feeling of discontent May lead to a degree of impairment in interpersonal relationships as individual begins to focus on self and the need to relieve personal discomfort
Severe	Greatly diminished; only extraneous details are perceived, or fixation on a single detail may occur May not take notice of an event even when attention is directed by another	Extremely limited attention span Unable to concentrate or problem-solve Effective learning cannot occur	Headaches Dizziness Nausea Trembling Insomnia Palpitations Tachycardia Hyperventilation Urinary frequency Diarrhea	Feelings of dread, loathing, horror Total focus on self and intense desire to relieve the anxiety
Panic	Unable to focus on even one detail within the environment Misperceptions of the environment common (e.g., a perceived detail may be elaborated and out of proportion)	Learning cannot occur Unable to concentrate Unable to comprehend even simple directions	Dilated pupils Labored breathing Severe trembling Sleeplessness Palpitations Diaphoresis and pallor Muscular incoordination Immobility or purposeless hyperactivity Incoherence or inability to verbalize	Sense of impending doom Terror Bizarre behavior, including shouting, screaming, running about wildly, clinging to anyone or anything from which a sense of safety and security is derived Hallucinations; delusions Extreme withdrawal into self

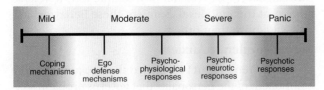

FIGURE 2-2 Adaptation responses on a continuum of anxiety.

the ego in an effort to relieve mild-to-moderate anxiety. They become maladaptive when they are used by an individual to such a degree that there is interference with the ability to deal with reality, with effective interpersonal relations, or with occupational performance.

Maladaptive use of defense mechanisms promotes disintegration of the ego. The major ego defense mechanisms identified by Anna Freud are discussed here and summarized in Table 2-2.

1. **Compensation** is the covering up of a real or perceived weakness by emphasizing a trait one considers more desirable.

EXAMPLES:

(a) A handicapped boy who is unable to participate in sports compensates by becoming a great scholar. (b) A young man who is the shortest among members of his peer group views this as a deficiency and compensates by being overly aggressive and daring.

TABLE 2–2 Ego Defense Mechanisms

DEFENSE MECHANISM	EXAMPLE	DEFENSE MECHANISM	EXAMPLE
COMPENSATION Covering up a real or perceived weakness by emphasizing a trait one considers more desirable.	A physically handicapped boy is unable to participate in football, so he compensates by becoming a great scholar.	**RATIONALIZATION** Attempting to make excuses or formulate logical reasons to justify unacceptable feelings or behaviors.	John tells the rehab nurse, "I drink because it's the only way I can deal with my bad marriage and my worse job."
DENIAL Refusing to acknowledge the existence of a real situation or the feelings associated with it.	A woman drinks alcohol every day and cannot stop, failing to acknowledge that she has a problem.	**REACTION FORMATION** Preventing unacceptable or undesirable thoughts or behaviors from being expressed by exaggerating opposite thoughts or types of behaviors.	Jane hates nursing. She attended nursing school to please her parents. During career day, she speaks to prospective students about the excellence of nursing as a career.
DISPLACEMENT The transfer of feelings from one target to another that is considered less threatening or that is neutral.	A client is angry with his physician, does not express it, but becomes verbally abusive with the nurse.	**REGRESSION** Retreating in response to stress to an earlier level of development and the comfort measures associated with that level of functioning.	When 2-year-old Jay is hospitalized for tonsillitis he will drink only from a bottle, even though his mom states he has been drinking from a cup for 6 months.
IDENTIFICATION An attempt to increase self-worth by acquiring certain attributes and characteristics of an individual one admires.	A teenager who required lengthy rehabilitation after an accident decides to become a physical therapist as a result of his experiences.	**REPRESSION** Involuntarily blocking unpleasant feelings and experiences from one's awareness.	An accident victim can remember nothing about his accident.
INTELLECTUALIZATION An attempt to avoid expressing actual emotions associated with a stressful situation by using the intellectual processes of logic, reasoning, and analysis.	S's husband is being transferred with his job to a city far away from her parents. She hides anxiety by explaining to her parents the advantages associated with the move.	**SUBLIMATION** Rechanneling of drives or impulses that are personally or socially unacceptable into activities that are constructive.	A mother whose son was killed by a drunk driver channels her anger and energy into being the president of the local chapter of Mothers Against Drunk Driving.
INTROJECTION Integrating the beliefs and values of another individual into one's own ego structure.	Children integrate their parents' value system into the process of conscience formation. A child says to a friend, "Don't cheat. It's wrong."	**SUPPRESSION** The voluntary blocking of unpleasant feelings and experiences from one's awareness.	Scarlett O'Hara says, "I don't want to think about that now. I'll think about that tomorrow."
ISOLATION Separating a thought or memory from the feeling, tone, or emotion associated with it.	A young woman describes being attacked and raped, without showing any emotion.	**UNDOING** Symbolically negating or canceling out an experience that one finds intolerable.	Joe is nervous about his new job and yells at his wife. On his way home he stops and buys her some flowers.
PROJECTION Attributing feelings or impulses unacceptable to one's self to another person.	Sue feels a strong sexual attraction to her track coach and tells her friend, "He's coming on to me!"		

2. **Denial** is the refusal to acknowledge the existence of a real situation or the feelings associated with it.

EXAMPLES:

(a) A woman has been told by her family doctor that she has a lump in her breast. An appointment is made for her with a surgeon; however, she does not keep the appointment and goes about her activities of daily living with no evidence of concern. (b) Individuals continue to smoke cigarettes even though they have been told of the health risks involved.

3. **Displacement** is the transferring of feelings from one target to another that is considered less threatening or neutral.

EXAMPLES:

(a) A man who is passed over for promotion on his job says nothing to his boss but later belittles his son for not making the basketball team. (b) A boy who is teased and hit by the class bully on the playground comes home after school and kicks his dog.

4. **Identification** is an attempt to increase self-worth by acquiring certain attributes and characteristics of an individual one admires.

EXAMPLES

(a) A teenage girl emulates the mannerisms and style of dress of a popular female rock star. (b) The young son of a famous civil rights worker adopts his father's attitudes and behaviors with the intent of pursuing similar aspirations.

5. **Intellectualization** is an attempt to avoid expressing actual emotions associated with a stressful situation by using the intellectual processes of logic, reasoning, and analysis.

EXAMPLES:

(a) A man whose brother is in a cardiac intensive care unit following a severe myocardial infarction (MI) spends his allotted visiting time in discussion with the nurse, analyzing test results and making a reasonable determination about the pathophysiology that may have occurred to induce the MI. (b) A young psychology professor receives a letter from his fiancée breaking off their engagement. He shows no emotion when discussing this with his best friend. Instead he analyzes his fiancée's behavior and tries to reason why the relationship failed.

6. **Introjection** is the internalization of the beliefs and values of another individual such that they symbolically become a part of the self to the extent that the feeling of separateness or distinctness is lost.

EXAMPLES:

(a) A small child develops her conscience by internalizing what the parents believe is right and wrong. The parents

literally become a part of the child. The child says to a friend while playing, "Don't hit people. It's not nice!" (b) A psychiatric client claims to be the Son of God, drapes himself in sheet and blanket, "performs miracles" on other clients, and refuses to respond unless addressed as Jesus Christ.

7. **Isolation** is the separation of a thought or a memory from the feeling, tone, or emotions associated with it (sometimes called emotional isolation).

EXAMPLES:

(a) A young woman describes being attacked and raped by a street gang. She displays an apathetic expression and no emotional tone. (b) A physician is able to isolate her feelings about the eventual death of a terminally ill cancer client by focusing her attention instead on the chemotherapy that will be given.

8. **Projection** is the attribution of feelings or impulses unacceptable to one's self to another person. The individual "passes the blame" for these undesirable feelings or impulses to another, thereby providing relief from the anxiety associated with them.

EXAMPLES:

(a) A young soldier who has an extreme fear of participating in military combat tells his sergeant that the others in his unit are "a bunch of cowards." (b) A businessperson who values punctuality is late for a meeting and states, "Sorry I'm late. My assistant forgot to remind me of the time. It's so hard to find good help these days."

9. **Rationalization** is the attempt to make excuses or formulate logical reasons to justify unacceptable feelings or behaviors.

EXAMPLES:

(a) A self-employed person deliberately neglects to report part of her income to the Internal Revenue Service, and justifies it to herself by saying, "It's okay. Everybody does it." (b) A young man is unable to afford the sports car he wants so desperately. He tells the salesperson, "I'd buy this car but I'll be getting married soon. This is really not the car for a family man."

10. **Reaction formation** is the prevention of unacceptable or undesirable thoughts or behaviors from being expressed by exaggerating opposite thoughts or types of behaviors.

EXAMPLES:

(a) The young soldier who has an extreme fear of participating in military combat volunteers for dangerous frontline duty. (b) A secretary is sexually attracted to her boss and feels an intense dislike toward his wife. She treats her boss with detachment and aloofness while performing her secretarial duties and is overly courteous, polite, and flattering to his wife when she comes to the office.

11. **Regression** is the retreating to an earlier level of development and the comfort measures associated with that level of functioning.

EXAMPLES:

(a) When his mother brings his new baby sister home from the hospital, 4-year-old Tommy, who had been toilet trained for more than a year, begins to wet his pants, cry to be held, and suck his thumb. (b) A person who is depressed may withdraw to his or her room, curl up in a fetal position on the bed, and sleep for long periods of time.

12. **Repression** is the involuntary blocking of unpleasant feelings and experiences from one's awareness.

EXAMPLES:

(a) A woman cannot remember being sexually assaulted when she was 15 years old. (b) A teenage boy cannot remember driving the car that was involved in an accident in which his best friend was killed.

13. **Sublimation** is the rechanneling of drives or impulses that are personally or socially unacceptable (e.g., aggressiveness, anger, sexual drives) into activities that are more tolerable and constructive.

EXAMPLES:

(a) A teenage boy with strong competitive and aggressive drives becomes the star football player on his high school team. (b) A young unmarried woman with a strong desire for marriage and a family achieves satisfaction and success in establishing and operating a day-care center for preschool children.

14. **Suppression** is the voluntary blocking of unpleasant feelings and experiences from one's awareness.

EXAMPLES:

(a) Scarlett O'Hara says, "I'll think about that tomorrow." (b) A young woman who is depressed about a pending divorce proceeding tells the nurse, "I just don't want to talk about the divorce. There's nothing I can do about it anyway."

15. **Undoing** is the act of symbolically negating or canceling out a previous action or experience that one finds intolerable.

EXAMPLES:

(a) A man spills some salt on the table, then sprinkles some over his left shoulder to "prevent bad luck." (b) A man who is anxious about giving a presentation at work yells at his wife during breakfast. He stops on his way home from work that evening to buy her a dozen red roses.

Moderate-to-Severe Anxiety

Anxiety at the moderate-to-severe level that remains unresolved over an extended period of time can contribute to a number of physiological disorders. The *DSM-5* (APA, 2013) describes these disorders under the category of "Psychological Factors Affecting Other Medical Conditions." The psychological factors may exacerbate symptoms of, delay recovery from, or interfere with treatment of the medical condition. The condition may be initiated or exacerbated by an environmental situation that the individual perceives as stressful. Measurable pathophysiology can be demonstrated. It is thought that psychological and behavioral factors may affect the course of almost every major category of disease, including, but not limited to, cardiovascular, gastrointestinal, neoplastic, neurological, and pulmonary conditions.

Severe Anxiety

Extended periods of repressed severe anxiety can result in psychoneurotic patterns of behaving. **Neurosis** is no longer considered a separate category of mental disorder. However, the term sometimes is still used in the literature to further describe the symptomatology of certain disorders and to differentiate from behaviors that occur at the more serious level of *psychosis*. Neuroses are psychiatric disturbances, characterized by excessive anxiety that is expressed directly or altered through defense mechanisms. It appears as a symptom, such as an obsession, a compulsion, a phobia, or a sexual dysfunction (Sadock & Sadock, 2007). The following are common characteristics of people with neuroses:

■ They are aware that they are experiencing distress.
■ They are aware that their behaviors are maladaptive.
■ They are unaware of any possible psychological causes of the distress.
■ They feel helpless to change their situation.
■ They experience no loss of contact with reality.

The following disorders are examples of psychoneurotic responses to anxiety as they appear in the *DSM-5:*

1. **Anxiety Disorders.** Disorders in which the characteristic features are symptoms of anxiety and avoidance behavior (e.g., phobias, panic disorder, generalized anxiety disorder, and separation anxiety disorder).
2. **Somatic Symptom Disorders.** Disorders in which the characteristic features are physical symptoms for which there is no demonstrable organic pathology. Psychological factors are judged to play a significant role in the onset, severity, exacerbation, or maintenance of the symptoms (e.g., somatic symptom disorder, illness anxiety disorder, conversion disorder, and factitious disorder).

3. **Dissociative Disorders.** Disorders in which the characteristic feature is a disruption in the usually integrated functions of consciousness, memory, identity, or perception of the environment (e.g., dissociative amnesia, dissociative identity disorder, and depersonalization-derealization disorder).

Panic Anxiety

At this extreme level of anxiety, an individual is not capable of processing what is happening in the environment, and may lose contact with reality. **Psychosis** is defined as "a severe mental disorder characterized by gross impairment in reality testing, typically manifested by delusions, hallucinations, disorganized speech, or disorganized or catatonic behavior" (Black & Andreasen, 2011, p. 618). The following are common characteristics of people with psychoses:

■ They exhibit minimal distress (emotional tone is flat, bland, or inappropriate).
■ They are unaware that their behavior is maladaptive.
■ They are unaware of any psychological problems.
■ They are exhibiting a flight from reality into a less stressful world or into one in which they are attempting to adapt.

Examples of psychotic responses to anxiety include the schizophrenic, schizoaffective, and delusional disorders.

> ### CORE CONCEPT
> **Grief**
> Grief is a subjective state of emotional, physical, and social responses to the loss of a valued entity.

Grief

Most individuals experience intense emotional anguish in response to a significant personal loss. A loss is anything that is perceived as such by the individual. Losses may be real, in which case they can be substantiated by others (e.g., death of a loved one, loss of personal possessions), or they may be perceived by the individual alone, unable to be shared or identified by others (e.g., loss of the feeling of femininity following mastectomy). Any situation that creates change for an individual can be identified as a loss. Failure (either real or perceived) also can be viewed as a loss.

The loss, or anticipated loss, of anything of value to an individual can trigger the grief response. This period of characteristic emotions and behaviors is called *mourning*. The "normal" mourning process is adaptive and is characterized by feelings of sadness, guilt, anger, helplessness, hopelessness, and despair. Indeed, an absence of mourning after a loss may be considered maladaptive.

Stages of Grief

Kübler-Ross (1969), in extensive research with terminally ill patients, identified five stages of feelings and behaviors that individuals experience in response to a real, perceived, or anticipated loss:

Stage 1—Denial. This is a stage of shock and disbelief. The response may be one of "No, it can't be true!" The reality of the loss is not acknowledged. Denial is a protective mechanism that allows the individual to cope in an immediate time frame while organizing more effective defense strategies.

Stage 2—Anger. "Why me?" and "It's not fair!" are comments often expressed during the anger stage. Envy and resentment toward individuals not affected by the loss are common. Anger may be directed at the self or displaced on loved ones, caregivers, and even God. There may be a preoccupation with an idealized image of the lost entity.

Stage 3—Bargaining. During this stage, which is usually not visible or evident to others, a "bargain" is made with God in an attempt to reverse or postpone the loss: "If God will help me through this, I promise I will go to church every Sunday and volunteer my time to help others." Sometimes the promise is associated with feelings of guilt for not having performed satisfactorily, appropriately, or sufficiently.

Stage 4—Depression. During this stage, the full impact of the loss is experienced. The sense of loss is intense, and feelings of sadness and depression prevail. This is a time of quiet desperation and disengagement from all association with the lost entity. It differs from *pathological* depression, which occurs when an individual becomes fixed in an earlier stage of the grief process. Rather, stage 4 of the grief response represents advancement toward resolution.

Stage 5—Acceptance. The final stage brings a feeling of peace regarding the loss that has occurred. It is a time of quiet expectation and resignation. The focus is on the reality of the loss and its meaning for the individuals affected by it.

All individuals do not experience each of these stages in response to a loss, nor do they necessarily experience them in this order. Some individuals' grieving behaviors may fluctuate, and even overlap, between stages.

Anticipatory Grief

When a loss is anticipated, individuals often begin the work of grieving before the actual loss occurs. Most people re-experience the grieving behaviors once the loss occurs, but having this time to prepare for the loss can facilitate the process of mourning, actually decreasing the length and intensity of the response. Problems arise, particularly in anticipating the death of a loved one, when family members experience **anticipatory grieving** and the mourning process is completed prematurely. They disengage emotionally from the dying person, who may then experience feelings of rejection by loved ones at a time when this psychological support is so necessary.

Resolution

The grief response can last from weeks to years. It cannot be hurried, and individuals must be allowed to progress at their own pace. In the loss of a loved one, grief work usually lasts for at least a year, during which the grieving person experiences each significant "anniversary" date for the first time without the loved one present.

Length of the grief process may be prolonged by a number of factors. If the relationship with the lost entity had been marked by ambivalence or if there had been an enduring "love-hate" association, reaction to the loss may be burdened with guilt. Guilt lengthens the grief reaction by promoting feelings of anger toward the self for having committed a wrongdoing or behaved in an unacceptable manner toward that which is now lost, and perhaps the grieving person may even feel that his or her behavior has contributed to the loss.

Anticipatory grieving is thought to shorten the grief response in some individuals who are able to work through some of the feelings before the loss occurs. If the loss is sudden and unexpected, mourning may take longer than it would if individuals were able to grieve in anticipation of the loss.

Length of the grieving process is also affected by the number of recent losses experienced by an individual and whether he or she is able to complete one grieving process before another loss occurs. This is particularly true for elderly individuals who may be experiencing numerous losses, such as spouse, friends, other relatives, independent functioning, home, personal possessions, and pets, in a relatively short time. Grief accumulates, and this represents a type of **bereavement overload**, which for some individuals presents an impossible task of grief work.

Resolution of the process of mourning is thought to have occurred when an individual can look back on the relationship with the lost entity and accept both the pleasures and the disappointments (both the positive and the negative aspects) of the association (Bowlby & Parkes, 1970). Disorganization and emotional pain have been experienced and tolerated. Preoccupation with the lost entity has been replaced with energy and the desire to pursue new situations and relationships.

Maladaptive Grief Responses

Maladaptive responses to loss occur when an individual is not able to satisfactorily progress through the stages of grieving to achieve resolution. These responses usually occur when an individual becomes fixed in the denial or anger stage of the grief process. Several types of grief responses have been identified as pathological. They include responses that are prolonged, delayed or inhibited, or distorted. The *prolonged* response is characterized by an intense preoccupation with memories of the lost entity for *many years after the loss has occurred*. Behaviors associated with the stages of denial or anger are manifested, and disorganization of functioning and intense emotional pain related to the lost entity are evidenced.

In the *delayed or inhibited* response, the individual becomes fixed in the denial stage of the grieving process. The emotional pain associated with the loss is not experienced, but anxiety disorders (e.g., phobias, somatic symptom disorders) or sleeping and eating disorders (e.g., insomnia, anorexia) may be evident. The individual may remain in denial for many years until the grief response is triggered by a reminder of the loss or even by another, unrelated loss.

The individual who experiences a *distorted* response is fixed in the anger stage of grieving. In the distorted response, all the normal behaviors associated with grieving, such as helplessness, hopelessness, sadness, anger, and guilt, are exaggerated out of proportion to the situation. The individual turns the anger inward on the self, is consumed with overwhelming despair, and is unable to function in normal activities of daily living. Pathological depression is a distorted grief response.

Mental Health/Mental Illness Continuum

Anxiety and grief have been described as two major, primary responses to stress. In Figure 2-3, both of these responses are presented on a continuum according to degree of symptom severity. Disorders as they appear in the *DSM-5* are identified at their appropriate placement along the continuum.

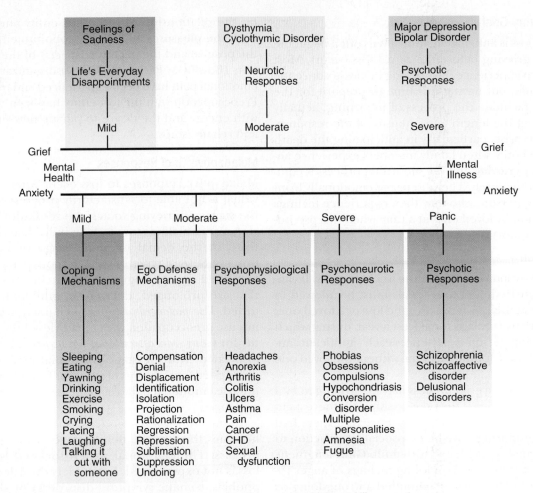

FIGURE 2-3 Conceptualization of anxiety and grief responses along the mental health/mental illness continuum.

Summary and Key Points

■ Psychiatric care has its roots in ancient times, when etiology was based in superstition and ideas related to the supernatural.

■ Treatments were often inhumane and included brutal beatings, starvation, or other torturous means.

■ Hippocrates associated insanity and mental illness with an irregularity in the interaction of the four body fluids (humors)—blood, black bile, yellow bile, and phlegm.

■ Conditions for care of the mentally ill have improved, largely because of the influence of leaders such as Benjamin Rush, Dorothea Dix, and Linda Richards, whose endeavors provided a model for more humanistic treatment.

■ Maslow identified a "hierarchy of needs" that individuals seek to fulfill on their quest to self-actualization (one's highest potential).

■ For purposes of this text, the definition of *mental health* is viewed as "the successful adaptation to stressors from the internal or external environment, evidenced by thoughts, feelings, and behaviors that are age-appropriate and congruent with local and cultural norms."

■ In determining mental illness, individuals are influenced by *incomprehensibility* of the behavior; that is, whether or not they are able to understand the motivation behind the behavior.

■ Another consideration is *cultural relativity*. The "normality" of behavior is determined by cultural and societal norms.

■ For purposes of this text, the definition of *mental illness* is viewed as "maladaptive responses to stressors from the internal or external environment, evidenced by thoughts, feelings, and behaviors that are incongruent with the local and cultural norms, and that interfere with the individual's social, occupational, and/or physical functioning."

■ Anxiety and grief have been described as two major, primary psychological response patterns to stress.

■ Peplau defined anxiety by levels of symptom severity: mild, moderate, severe, and panic.

■ Behaviors associated with levels of anxiety include coping mechanisms, ego defense mechanisms, psychophysiological responses, psychoneurotic responses, and psychotic responses.

■ Grief is described as a response to loss of a valued entity. Loss is anything that is perceived as such by the individual.

■ Kübler-Ross, in extensive research with terminally ill patients, identified five stages of feelings and behaviors that individuals experience in response to a real, perceived, or anticipated loss: denial, anger, bargaining, depression, and acceptance.

■ Anticipatory grief is grief work that is begun, and sometimes completed, before the loss occurs.

■ Resolution is thought to occur when an individual is able to remember and accept both the positive and negative aspects associated with the lost entity.

■ Grieving is thought to be maladaptive when the mourning process is prolonged, delayed or inhibited, or becomes distorted and exaggerated out of proportion to the situation. Pathological depression is considered to be a distorted reaction.

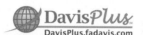 Additional info available at
DavisPlus.fadavis.com   www.davisplus.com

Review Questions
Self-Examination/Learning Exercise

*Select the answer that is **most** appropriate for each of the following questions.*

1. Three years ago, Anna's dog, Lucky, whom she had had for 16 years, was hit by a car and killed. Anna's daughter reports that since that time, Anna has lost weight, rarely leaves her home, and just sits and talks about Lucky. Anna's behavior would be considered maladaptive because:
   a. It has been more than three years since Lucky died.
   b. Her grief is too intense just over the loss of a dog.
   c. Her grief is interfering with her functioning.
   d. People in this culture would not comprehend such behavior over loss of a pet.

2. Based on the information in Question 1, Anna's grieving behavior would most likely be considered to be:
   a. Delayed
   b. Inhibited
   c. Prolonged
   d. Distorted

3. Anna is diagnosed with major depressive disorder. She is most likely fixed in which stage of the grief process?
   a. Denial
   b. Anger
   c. Depression
   d. Acceptance

4. Anna, who is 72 years old, is of the age when she may have experienced many losses coming close together. What is this called?
   a. Bereavement overload
   b. Normal mourning
   c. Isolation
   d. Cultural relativity

5. Anna, age 72, has been grieving the death of her dog, Lucky, for 3 years. She is not able to take care of her activities of daily living, and wants only to make daily visits to Lucky's grave. Her daughter has likely put off seeking help for Anna because:
   a. Women are less likely to seek help for emotional problems than men.
   b. Relatives often try to "normalize" the behavior, rather than label it mental illness.
   c. She knows that all older people are expected to be a little depressed.
   d. She is afraid that the neighbors "will think her mother is crazy."

Continued

Review Questions—cont'd
Self-Examination/Learning Exercise

6. Anna's dog, Lucky, got away from her while they were taking a walk. He ran into the street and was hit by a car. Anna cannot remember any of these circumstances of his death. This is an example of what defense mechanism?
   a. Rationalization
   b. Suppression
   c. Denial
   d. Repression

7. Lucky sometimes refused to obey Anna, and indeed did not come back to her when she called to him on the day he was killed. But Anna continues to insist, "He was the very best dog. He always minded me. He always did everything I told him to do." This represents the defense mechanism of:
   a. Sublimation
   b. Compensation
   c. Reaction Formation
   d. Undoing

8. Anna has been a widow for 20 years. Her maladaptive grief response to the loss of her dog may be attributed to which of the following? (Select all that apply.)
   a. Unresolved grief over loss of her husband.
   b. Loss of several relatives and friends over the last few years.
   c. Repressed feelings of guilt over the way in which Lucky died.
   d. Inability to prepare in advance for the loss.

9. For what reason would Anna's illness be considered a neurosis rather than a psychosis?
   a. She is unaware that her behavior is maladaptive.
   b. She exhibits inappropriate affect (emotional tone).
   c. She experiences no loss of contact with reality.
   d. She tells the nurse, "There is nothing wrong with me!"

10. Which of the following statements by Anna might suggest that she is achieving resolution of her grief over Lucky's death?
   a. "I don't cry anymore when I think about Lucky."
   b. "It's true. Lucky didn't always mind me. Sometimes he ignored my commands."
   c. "I remember how it happened now. I should have held tighter to his leash!"
   d. "I won't ever have another dog. It's just too painful to lose them."

References

American Psychiatric Association. (2013). *Diagnostic and statistical manual of mental disorders* (5th ed.). Washington, DC: American Psychiatric Publishing.

Black, D.W., & Andreasen, N.C. (2011). *Introductory textbook of psychiatry* (5th ed.). Washington, DC: American Psychiatric Publishing.

Horwitz, A.V. (2002). *The social control of mental illness.* Clinton Corners, NY: Percheron Press.

Robinson, L. (1983). *Psychiatric nursing as a human experience* (3rd ed.). Philadelphia, PA: WB Saunders.

Sadock, B.J., & Sadock, V.A. (2007). *Synopsis of psychiatry: Behavioral sciences/clinical psychiatry* (10th ed.). Baltimore, MD: Lippincott Williams & Wilkins.

Classical References

Bowlby, J., & Parkes, C.M. (1970). Separation and loss. In E.J. Anthony & C. Koupernik (Eds.), *International yearbook for child psychiatry and allied disciplines: The child and his family* (Vol. 1). New York, NY: John Wiley & Sons.

Freud, A. (1953). *The ego and mechanisms of defense.* New York, NY: International Universities Press.

Freud, S. (1961). The ego and the id. In *Standard edition of the complete psychological works of Freud* (Vol. XIX). London, UK: Hogarth Press.

Jahoda, M. (1958). *Current concepts of positive mental health.* New York, NY: Basic Books.

Kübler-Ross, E. (1969). *On death and dying.* New York, NY: Macmillan.

Maslow, A. (1970). *Motivation and personality* (2nd ed.). New York, NY: Harper & Row.

Menninger, K. (1963). *The vital balance.* New York, NY: Viking Press.

Peplau, H. (1963). A working definition of anxiety. In S. Burd & M. Marshall (Eds.), *Some clinical approaches to psychiatric nursing.* New York, NY: Macmillan.

Foundations for Psychiatric/Mental Health Nursing

3 Theoretical Models of Personality Development

KEY TERMS

cognitive development
cognitive maturity
counselor
ego

id
libido
psychodynamic nursing
superego

surrogate
symbiosis
technical expert
temperament

OBJECTIVES
After reading this chapter, the student will be able to:

1. Define *personality*.
2. Identify the relevance of knowledge associated with personality development to nursing in the psychiatric/mental health setting.
3. Discuss the major components of the following developmental theories:
   a. Psychoanalytic theory—Freud
   b. Interpersonal theory—Sullivan

   c. Theory of psychosocial development—Erikson
   d. Theory of object relations development—Mahler
   e. Cognitive development theory—Piaget
   f. Theory of moral development—Kohlberg
   g. A nursing model of interpersonal development—Peplau

HOMEWORK ASSIGNMENT
Please read the chapter and answer the following questions:

1. Which part of the personality as described by Freud is developed as the child internalizes the values and morals set forth by primary caregivers?
2. According to Erikson, what happens when the adolescent does not master the tasks of *identity vs. role confusion*?
3. According to Mahler's theory, the individual with borderline personality disorder harbors fears of abandonment and underlying rage based on fixation in what stage of development?
4. When Joey sees an old woman struggling with a heavy bag of groceries, he runs to help her carry them to her car. This describes behavior at which stage of moral development?

Black and Andreasen (2011) define *personality* as "the characteristic way in which a person thinks, feels, and behaves; the ingrained pattern of behavior that each person evolves, both consciously and unconsciously, as his or her style of life or way of being" (p. 612).

Nurses must have a basic knowledge of human personality development to understand maladaptive behavioral responses commonly seen in psychiatric clients. Developmental theories identify behaviors associated with various *stages* through which individuals pass, thereby specifying what is appropriate or inappropriate at each developmental level.

Specialists in child development believe that infancy and early childhood are the major life periods for the origination and occurrence of developmental change. Specialists in life-cycle development believe that people continue to develop and change throughout life, thereby suggesting the possibility for renewal and growth in adults.

Developmental stages are identified by age. Behaviors can then be evaluated by whether or not they are recognized as age-appropriate. Ideally, an individual successfully fulfills all the tasks associated with one stage before moving on to the next stage (at the appropriate age). Realistically, however, this seldom happens. One reason is related to **temperament**, or the inborn personality characteristics that influence an individual's manner of reacting to the environment, and ultimately his or her developmental progression (Chess & Thomas, 1986). The environment may also influence one's developmental pattern. Individuals who are reared in a dysfunctional family system often have retarded ego development. According to specialists in life-cycle development, behaviors from an unsuccessfully completed stage can be modified and corrected in a later stage.

Stages overlap, and an individual may be working on tasks associated with several stages at one time. When an individual becomes fixed in a lower level of development, with age-inappropriate behaviors focused on fulfillment of those tasks, psychopathology may become evident. Only when personality traits become inflexible, and personality functioning becomes individually and interpersonally impaired, do they constitute *personality disorders*.

CORE CONCEPT

Personality

The combination of character, behavioral, temperamental, emotional, and mental traits that are unique to each specific individual.

Psychoanalytic Theory

Sigmund Freud (1961), who has been called the father of psychiatry, is credited as the first to identify development by stages. He considered the first 5 years of a child's life to be the most important, because he believed that an individual's basic character had been formed by the age of 5.

Freud's personality theory can be conceptualized according to structure and dynamics of the personality, topography of the mind, and stages of personality development.

Structure of the Personality

Freud organized the structure of the personality into three major components: the **id**, **ego**, and **superego**. They are distinguished by their unique functions and different characteristics.

Id

The *id* is the locus of instinctual drives—the "pleasure principle." Present at birth, it endows the infant with instinctual drives that seek to satisfy needs and achieve immediate gratification. Id-driven behaviors are impulsive and may be irrational.

Ego

The *ego*, also called the *rational self* or the "reality principle," begins to develop between the ages of 4 and 6 months. The ego experiences the reality of the external world, adapts to it, and responds to it. As the ego develops and gains strength, it seeks to bring the influences of the external world to bear upon the id, to substitute the reality principle for the pleasure principle (Marmer, 2003). A primary function of the ego is one of mediator; that is, to maintain harmony among the external world, the id, and the superego.

Superego

If the id is identified as the pleasure principle, and the ego the reality principle, the *superego* might be referred to as the "perfection principle." The superego, which develops between ages 3 and 6 years, internalizes the values and morals set forth by primary caregivers. Derived out of a system of rewards and punishments, the superego is composed of two major components: the *ego-ideal* and the *conscience*. When a child is consistently rewarded for "good" behavior, the self-esteem is enhanced, and the behavior becomes part of the ego-ideal; that is, it is internalized as part of his or her value system. The conscience is formed when the child is punished consistently for "bad" behavior. The child learns what is considered morally right or wrong from feedback received from parental figures and from society or culture. When moral and ethical principles or even internalized ideals and values are disregarded, the conscience generates a feeling of guilt within the individual. The superego is important in the socialization of the individual because it assists the ego in the control of id impulses. When the superego becomes rigid and punitive, problems with low self-confidence and low self-esteem arise. Examples of behaviors associated with these components of the personality are presented in Box 3-1.

Topography of the Mind

Freud classified all mental contents and operations into three categories: the conscious, the preconscious, and the unconscious.

■ The *conscious* includes all memories that remain within an individual's awareness. It is the smallest of the three categories. Events and experiences that are easily remembered or retrieved are considered to be within one's conscious awareness. Examples include telephone numbers, birthdays of self and significant others, the dates of special holidays, and what one had for lunch today. The conscious mind is thought to be under the control of the ego, the rational and logical structure of the personality.

■ The *preconscious* includes all memories that may have been forgotten or are not in present awareness but with attention can be readily recalled into consciousness. Examples include telephone numbers or addresses once known but little used and

feelings associated with significant life events that may have occurred at sometime in the past. The preconscious enhances awareness by helping to *suppress* unpleasant or nonessential memories from consciousness. It is thought to be partially under the control of the superego, which helps to suppress unacceptable thoughts and behaviors.

■ The *unconscious* includes all memories that one is unable to bring to conscious awareness. It is the largest of the three topographical levels. Unconscious material consists of unpleasant or nonessential memories that have been *repressed* and can be retrieved only through therapy, hypnosis, and with certain substances that alter awareness and have the capacity to restructure repressed memories. Unconscious material may also emerge in dreams and in seemingly incomprehensible behavior.

Dynamics of the Personality

Freud believed that *psychic energy* is the force or impetus required for mental functioning. Originating in the id, it instinctually fulfills basic physiological needs. Freud called this psychic energy (or the drive to fulfill basic physiological needs such as hunger, thirst, and sex) the **libido**. As the child matures, psychic energy is diverted from the id to form the ego and then from the ego to form the superego. Psychic energy is distributed within these three components, with the ego retaining the largest share to maintain a balance between the impulsive behaviors of the id and the idealistic behaviors of the superego. If an excessive amount of psychic energy is stored in one of these personality components, behavior will reflect that part of the personality. For instance, impulsive behavior prevails when excessive psychic energy is stored in the id. Over-investment in the ego reflects self-absorbed, or narcissistic, behaviors; an excess within the superego results in rigid, self-deprecating behaviors.

Freud used the terms *cathexis* and *anticathexis* to describe the forces within the id, ego, and superego that are used to invest psychic energy in external sources to satisfy needs. Cathexis is the process by which the id invests energy into an object in an attempt to achieve gratification. An example is the individual who instinctively turns to alcohol to relieve stress. Anticathexis is the use of psychic energy by the ego and the superego to control id impulses. In the example cited, the ego would attempt to control the use of alcohol with rational thinking, such as, "I already have ulcers from drinking too much. I will call my AA counselor for support. I will not drink." The superego would exert control with thinking such as "I shouldn't drink. If I drink, my family will be hurt and angry. I should think of how it affects them. I'm such a weak person." Freud believed that

---

BOX 3-1 Structure of the Personality

BEHAVIORAL EXAMPLES

Id	Ego	Superego
"I found this wallet; I will keep the money."	"I already have money. This money doesn't belong to me. Maybe the person who owns this wallet doesn't have any money."	"It is never right to take something that doesn't belong to you."
"Mom and Dad are gone. Let's party!!!!!"	"Mom and Dad said no friends over while they are away. Too risky."	"Never disobey your parents."
"I'll have sex with whomever I please, whenever I please."	"Promiscuity can be very dangerous."	"Sex outside of marriage is always wrong."

an imbalance between cathexis and anticathexis resulted in internal conflicts, producing tension and anxiety within the individual. Freud's daughter Anna devised a comprehensive list of defense mechanisms believed to be used by the ego as a protective device against anxiety in mediating between the excessive demands of the id and the excessive restrictions of the superego (see Chapter 2).

Freud's Stages of Personality Development

Freud described formation of the personality through five stages of *psychosexual* development. He placed much emphasis on the first 5 years of life and believed that characteristics developed during these early years bore heavily on one's adaptation patterns and personality traits in adulthood. Fixation in an early stage of development will almost certainly result in psychopathology. An outline of these five stages is presented in Table 3-1.

Oral Stage: Birth to 18 Months

During the oral stage, behavior is directed by the id, and the goal is immediate gratification of needs. The focus of energy is the mouth, with behaviors that include sucking, chewing, and biting. The infant feels a sense of attachment and is unable to differentiate the self from the person who is providing the mothering. This includes feelings such as anxiety. Because of this lack of differentiation, a pervasive feeling of anxiety on the part of the mother may be passed on to her infant, leaving the child vulnerable to similar feelings of insecurity. With the beginning of development of the ego at age 4 to 6 months, the infant starts to view the self as separate from the mothering figure. A sense of security and the ability to trust others is derived from the gratification of fulfilling basic needs during this stage.

Anal Stage: 18 Months to 3 Years

The major task in the anal stage is gaining independence and control, with particular focus on the excretory function. Freud believed that the manner in which the parents and other primary caregivers approach the task of toilet training may have far-reaching effects on the child in terms of values and personality characteristics. When toilet training is strict and rigid, the child may choose to retain the feces, becoming constipated. Adult retentive personality traits influenced by this type of training include stubbornness, stinginess, and miserliness. An alternate reaction to strict toilet training is for the child to expel feces in an unacceptable manner or at inappropriate times. Far-reaching effects of this behavior pattern include malevolence, cruelty to others, destructiveness, disorganization, and untidiness.

Toilet training that is more permissive and accepting attaches the feeling of importance and desirability to feces production. The child becomes extroverted, productive, and altruistic.

Phallic Stage: 3 to 6 Years

In the phallic stage, the focus of energy shifts to the genital area. Discovery of differences between genders results in a heightened interest in the sexuality of self and others. This interest may be manifested in sexual self-exploratory or group-exploratory play. Freud proposed that the development of the *Oedipus complex* (males) or *Electra complex* (females) occurred during this stage of development. He described this as the child's unconscious desire to eliminate the parent of the same gender and to possess the parent of the opposite gender for him- or herself. Guilt feelings result with the emergence of the superego during these years. Resolution of this internal conflict occurs when the child develops a strong identification with the parent of the same gender and internalizes that parent's attitudes, beliefs, and value system.

Latency Stage: 6 to 12 Years

During the elementary school years, the focus changes from egocentrism to more interest in group activities, learning, and socialization with peers. Sexuality is not absent during this period but remains obscure and

TABLE 3–1 **Freud's Stages of Psychosexual Development**		
AGE	STAGE	MAJOR DEVELOPMENTAL TASKS
Birth–18 months	Oral	Relief from anxiety through oral gratification of needs
18 months–3 years	Anal	Learning independence and control, with focus on the excretory function
3–6 years	Phallic	Identification with parent of same gender; development of sexual identity; focus on genital organs
6–12 years	Latency	Sexuality repressed; focus on relationships with same-gender peers
13–20 years	Genital	Libido reawakened as genital organs mature; focus on relationships with members of the opposite gender

imperceptible to others. The preference is for same-gender relationships, even rejecting members of the opposite gender.

Genital Stage: 13 to 20 Years

In the genital stage, the maturing of the genital organs results in a reawakening of the libidinal drive. The focus is on relationships with members of the opposite gender and preparations for selecting a mate. The development of sexual maturity evolves from self-gratification to behaviors deemed acceptable by societal norms. Interpersonal relationships are based on genuine pleasure derived from the interaction rather than from the more self-serving implications of childhood associations.

Relevance of Psychoanalytic Theory to Nursing Practice

Knowledge of the structure of the personality can assist nurses who work in the mental health setting. The ability to recognize behaviors associated with the id, the ego, and the superego assists in the assessment of developmental level. Understanding the use of ego defense mechanisms is important in making determinations about maladaptive behaviors, in planning care for clients to assist in creating change (if desired), or in helping clients accept themselves as unique individuals.

CLINICAL PEARL Assessing Patient Behaviors

Id Behaviors
Those behaviors that follow the principle of "if it feels good, do it." Social and cultural acceptability are not considered. It reflects a need for immediate gratification. Individuals with a strong id show little if any remorse for their unacceptable behavior.

Ego Behaviors
Behaviors that reflect the rational part of the personality. An effort is made to delay gratification and to satisfy societal expectations. The ego uses defense mechanisms to cope and regain control over id impulses.

Superego Behaviors
Behaviors that are somewhat uncompromising and rigid. Based on morality and society's values. Behaviors of the superego strive for perfection. Violation of the superego's standards generates guilt and anxiety in an individual who has a strong superego.

Interpersonal Theory

Harry Stack Sullivan (1953) believed that individual behavior and personality development are the direct result of interpersonal relationships. Before the development of his own theoretical framework, Sullivan embraced the concepts of Freud. Later, he changed the focus of his work from the *intrapersonal* view of Freud to one with a more *interpersonal* flavor

in which human behavior could be observed in social interactions with others. His ideas, which were not universally accepted at the time, have been integrated into the practice of psychiatry through publication only since his death in 1949. Sullivan's major concepts include the following:

■ *Anxiety* is a feeling of emotional discomfort, toward the relief or prevention of which all behavior is aimed. Sullivan believed that anxiety is the "chief disruptive force in interpersonal relations and the main factor in the development of serious difficulties in living" (p. XV). It arises out of one's inability to satisfy needs or to achieve interpersonal security.

■ *Satisfaction of needs* is the fulfillment of all requirements associated with an individual's physiochemical environment. Sullivan identified examples of these requirements as oxygen, food, water, warmth, tenderness, rest, activity, sexual expression—virtually anything that, when absent, produces discomfort in the individual.

■ *Interpersonal security* is the feeling associated with relief from anxiety. When all needs have been met, one experiences a sense of total well-being, which Sullivan termed *interpersonal security*. He believed individuals have an innate need for interpersonal security.

■ *Self-system* is a collection of experiences, or security measures, adopted by the individual to protect against anxiety. Sullivan identified three components of the self-system, which are based on interpersonal experiences early in life:

  ■ The "*good me*" is the part of the personality that develops in response to positive feedback from the primary caregiver. Feelings of pleasure, contentment, and gratification are experienced. The child learns which behaviors elicit this positive response as it becomes incorporated into the self-system.

  ■ The "*bad me*" is the part of the personality that develops in response to negative feedback from the primary caregiver. Anxiety is experienced, eliciting feelings of discomfort, displeasure, and distress. The child learns to avoid these negative feelings by altering certain behaviors.

  ■ The "*not me*" is the part of the personality that develops in response to situations that produce intense anxiety in the child. Feelings of horror, awe, dread, and loathing are experienced in response to these situations, leading the child to deny these feelings in an effort to relieve anxiety. These feelings, having then been denied, become "not me," but someone else. This withdrawal from emotions has serious implications for mental disorders in adult life.

Sullivan's Stages of Personality Development

Sullivan described six stages of personality development. An outline of the stages of personality development according to Sullivan's interpersonal theory is presented in Table 3-2.

Infancy: Birth to 18 Months

During the beginning stage, the major developmental task for the child is the gratification of needs. This is accomplished through activity associated with the mouth, such as crying, nursing, and thumb sucking.

Childhood: 18 Months to 6 Years

At ages 18 months to 6 years, the child learns that interference with fulfillment of personal wishes and desires may result in delayed gratification. He or she learns to accept this and feel comfortable with it, recognizing that delayed gratification often results in parental approval, a more lasting type of reward. Tools of this stage include the mouth, the anus, language, experimentation, manipulation, and identification.

Juvenile: 6 to 9 Years

The major task of the juvenile stage is formation of satisfactory relationships within peer groups. This is accomplished through the use of competition, cooperation, and compromise.

Preadolescence: 9 to 12 Years

The tasks at the preadolescence stage focus on developing relationships with persons of the same gender. One's ability to collaborate with and show love and affection for another person begins at this stage.

Early Adolescence: 12 to 14 Years

During early adolescence, the child is struggling with developing a sense of identity that is separate and independent from the parents. The major task is formation of satisfactory relationships with members of the opposite gender. Sullivan saw the emergence of lust in response to biological changes as a major force occurring during this period.

Late Adolescence: 14 to 21 Years

The late adolescent period is characterized by tasks associated with the attempt to achieve interdependence within the society and the formation of a lasting, intimate relationship with a selected member of the opposite gender. The genital organs are the major developmental focus of this stage.

Relevance of Interpersonal Theory to Nursing Practice

The interpersonal theory has significant relevance to nursing practice. Relationship development, which is a major concept of this theory, is a major psychiatric nursing intervention. Nurses develop therapeutic relationships with clients in an effort to help them generalize this ability to interact successfully with others.

Knowledge about the behaviors associated with all levels of anxiety and methods for alleviating anxiety helps nurses to assist clients achieve interpersonal security and a sense of well-being. Nurses use the concepts of Sullivan's theory to help clients achieve a higher degree of independent and interpersonal functioning.

Theory of Psychosocial Development

Erik Erikson (1963) studied the influence of social processes on the development of the personality. He described eight stages of the life cycle during which individuals struggle with developmental "crises." Specific tasks associated with each stage must be completed for resolution of the crisis and for emotional growth to

TABLE 3–2 **Stages of Development in Sullivan's Interpersonal Theory**		
AGE	STAGE	MAJOR DEVELOPMENTAL TASKS
Birth–18 months	Infancy	Relief from anxiety through oral gratification of needs
18 months–6 years	Childhood	Learning to experience a delay in personal gratification without undue anxiety
6–9 years	Juvenile	Learning to form satisfactory peer relationships
9–12 years	Preadolescence	Learning to form satisfactory relationships with persons of same gender; initiating feelings of affection for another person
12–14 years	Early adolescence	Learning to form satisfactory relationships with persons of the opposite gender; developing a sense of identity
14–21 years	Late adolescence	Establishing self-identity; experiencing satisfying relationships; working to develop a lasting, intimate opposite-gender relationship

occur. An outline of Erikson's stages of psychosocial development is presented in Table 3-3.

Erikson's Stages of Personality Development

Trust versus Mistrust: Birth to 18 Months

Major Developmental Task

From birth to 18 months, the major task is to develop a basic trust in the mothering figure and learn to generalize it to others.

■ Achievement of the task results in self-confidence, optimism, faith in the gratification of needs and desires, and hope for the future. The infant learns to trust when basic needs are met consistently.

■ Nonachievement results in emotional dissatisfaction with the self and others, suspiciousness, and difficulty with interpersonal relationships. The task remains unresolved when primary caregivers fail to respond to the infant's distress signal promptly and consistently.

Autonomy versus Shame and Doubt: 18 Months to 3 Years

Major Developmental Task

The major task during the ages of 18 months to 3 years is to gain some self-control and independence within the environment.

■ Achievement of the task results in a sense of self-control and the ability to delay gratification, and a feeling of self-confidence in one's ability to perform. Autonomy is achieved when parents encourage and provide opportunities for independent activities.

■ Nonachievement results in a lack of self-confidence, a lack of pride in the ability to perform, a sense of being controlled by others, and a rage against the self. The task remains unresolved when primary caregivers restrict independent behaviors, both physically and verbally, or set the child up for failure with unrealistic expectations.

Initiative versus Guilt: 3 to 6 Years

Major Developmental Task

During the ages of 3 to 6 years the goal is to develop a sense of purpose and the ability to initiate and direct one's own activities.

■ Achievement of the task results in the ability to exercise restraint and self-control of inappropriate social behaviors. Assertiveness and dependability increase, and the child enjoys learning and personal achievement. The conscience develops, thereby controlling the impulsive behaviors of the id. Initiative is achieved when creativity is encouraged and performance is recognized and positively reinforced.

■ Nonachievement results in feelings of inadequacy and a sense of defeat. Guilt is experienced to an excessive degree, even to the point of accepting liability in situations for which one is not responsible. The

TABLE 3-3	**Stages of Development in Erikson's Psychosocial Theory**	
AGE	STAGE	MAJOR DEVELOPMENTAL TASKS
Infancy (Birth–18 months)	Trust vs. mistrust	To develop a basic trust in the mothering figure and learn to generalize it to others
Early childhood (18 months–3 years)	Autonomy vs. shame and doubt	To gain some self-control and independence within the environment
Late childhood (3–6 years)	Initiative vs. guilt	To develop a sense of purpose and the ability to initiate and direct own activities
School age (6–12 years)	Industry vs. inferiority	To achieve a sense of self-confidence by learning, competing, performing successfully, and receiving recognition from significant others, peers, and acquaintances
Adolescence (12–20 years)	Identity vs. role confusion	To integrate the tasks mastered in the previous stages into a secure sense of self
Young adulthood (20–30 years)	Intimacy vs. isolation	To form an intense, lasting relationship or a commitment to another person, cause, institution, or creative effort
Adulthood (30–65 years)	Generativity vs. stagnation	To achieve the life goals established for oneself, while also considering the welfare of future generations
Old age (65 years–death)	Ego integrity vs. despair	To review one's life and derive meaning from both positive and negative events, while achieving a positive sense of self-worth

child may view him- or herself as evil and deserving of punishment. The task remains unresolved when creativity is stifled and parents continually expect a higher level of achievement than the child produces.

Industry versus Inferiority: 6 to 12 Years

Major Developmental Task

The major task for 6- to 12-year-olds is to achieve a sense of self-confidence by learning, competing, performing successfully, and receiving recognition from significant others, peers, and acquaintances.

■ Achievement of the task results in a sense of satisfaction and pleasure in the interaction and involvement with others. The individual masters reliable work habits and develops attitudes of trustworthiness. He or she is conscientious, feels pride in achievement, and enjoys play but desires a balance between fantasy and "real world" activities. Industry is achieved when encouragement is given to activities and responsibilities in the school and community, as well as those within the home, and recognition is given for accomplishments.

■ Nonachievement results in difficulty in interpersonal relationships because of feelings of personal inadequacy. The individual can neither cooperate and compromise with others in group activities nor problem solve or complete tasks successfully. He or she may become either passive and meek or overly aggressive to cover up for feelings of inadequacy. If this occurs, the individual may manipulate or violate the rights of others to satisfy his or her own needs or desires; he or she may become a workaholic with unrealistic expectations for personal achievement. This task remains unresolved when parents set unrealistic expectations for the child, when discipline is harsh and tends to impair self-esteem, and when accomplishments are consistently met with negative feedback.

Identity versus Role Confusion: 12 to 20 Years

Major Developmental Task

At 12 to 20 years, the goal is to integrate the tasks mastered in the previous stages into a secure sense of self.

■ Achievement of the task results in a sense of confidence, emotional stability, and a view of the self as a unique individual. Commitments are made to a value system, to the choice of a career, and to relationships with members of both genders. Identity is achieved when adolescents are allowed to experience independence by making decisions that influence their lives. Parents should be available to offer support when needed but should gradually relinquish control to the maturing individual in an effort to encourage the development of an independent sense of self.

■ Nonachievement results in a sense of self-consciousness, doubt, and confusion about one's role in life. Personal values or goals for one's life are absent. Long-term commitments to relationships with others are nonexistent. A lack of self-confidence is often expressed by delinquent and rebellious behavior. Entering adulthood, with its accompanying responsibilities, may be an underlying fear. This task can remain unresolved for many reasons. Examples include the following:
  ■ When independence is discouraged by the parents and the adolescent is nurtured in the dependent position
  ■ When discipline within the home has been overly harsh, inconsistent, or absent
  ■ When there has been parental rejection or frequent shifting of parental figures

Intimacy versus Isolation: 20 to 30 Years

Major Developmental Task

The objective for 20- to 30-year-olds is to form an intense, lasting relationship or a commitment to another person, a cause, an institution, or a creative effort (Murray, Zentner, & Yakimo, 2009).

■ Achievement of the task results in the capacity for mutual love and respect between two people and the ability of an individual to pledge a total commitment to another. The intimacy goes far beyond the sexual contact between two people. It describes a commitment in which personal sacrifices are made for another, whether it be another person or, if one chooses, a career or other type of cause or endeavor to which an individual elects to devote his or her life. Intimacy is achieved when an individual has developed the capacity for giving of oneself to another. This is learned when one has been the recipient of this type of giving within the family unit.

■ Nonachievement results in withdrawal, social isolation, and aloneness. The individual is unable to form lasting, intimate relationships, often seeking intimacy through numerous superficial sexual contacts. No career is established; he or she may have a history of occupational changes (or may fear change and thus remain in an undesirable job situation). The task remains unresolved when love in the home has been deprived or distorted through the younger years (Murray et al., 2009). One fails to achieve the ability to give of the self without having been the recipient early on from primary caregivers.

Generativity versus Stagnation or Self-Absorption: 30 to 65 Years

Major Developmental Task

The major task at this stage is to achieve the life goals established for oneself while also considering the welfare of future generations.

■ Achievement of the task results in a sense of gratification from personal and professional achievements and from meaningful contributions to others. The individual is active in the service of and to society. Generativity is achieved when the individual expresses satisfaction with this stage in life and demonstrates responsibility for leaving the world a better place in which to live.

■ Nonachievement results in lack of concern for the welfare of others and total preoccupation with the self. He or she becomes withdrawn, isolated, and highly self-indulgent, with no capacity for giving of the self to others. The task remains unresolved when earlier developmental tasks are not fulfilled and the individual does not achieve the degree of maturity required to derive gratification out of a personal concern for the welfare of others.

Ego Integrity versus Despair: 65 Years to Death

Major Developmental Task

Between the age of 65 years and death, the goal is to review one's life and derive meaning from both positive and negative events, while achieving a positive sense of self.

■ Achievement of the task results in a sense of self-worth and self-acceptance as one reviews life goals, accepting that some were achieved and some were not. The individual derives a sense of dignity from his or her life experiences and does not fear death, rather viewing it as another stage of development. Ego integrity is achieved when individuals have successfully completed the developmental tasks of the other stages and have little desire to make major changes in how their lives have progressed.

■ Nonachievement results in a sense of self-contempt and disgust with how life has progressed. The individual would like to start over and have a second chance at life. He or she feels worthless and helpless to change. Anger, depression, and loneliness are evident. The focus may be on past failures or perceived failures. Impending death is feared or denied, or ideas of suicide may prevail. The task remains unresolved when earlier tasks are not fulfilled: self-confidence, a concern for others, and a strong sense of self-identity were never achieved.

Relevance of Psychosocial Development Theory to Nursing Practice

Erikson's theory is particularly relevant to nursing practice in that it incorporates sociocultural concepts into the development of personality. Erikson provides a systematic, stepwise approach and outlines specific tasks that should be completed during each stage. This information can be used quite readily in psychiatric/mental health nursing. Many individuals with mental health problems are still struggling to achieve tasks from a number of developmental stages. Nurses can plan care to assist these individuals to fulfill these tasks and move on to a higher developmental level.

> **CLINICAL PEARL**　During assessment, nurses can determine if a client is experiencing difficulties associated with specific life tasks as described by Erikson. Knowledge about a client's developmental level, along with other assessment data, can help to identify accurate nursing interventions.

Theory of Object Relations

Margaret Mahler (Mahler, Pine, & Bergman, 1975) formulated a theory that describes the separation-individuation process of the infant from the maternal figure (primary caregiver). She describes this process as progressing through three major phases, and she further delineates phase III, the separation-individuation phase, into four subphases. Mahler's developmental theory is outlined in Table 3-4.

Phase I: The Autistic Phase (Birth to 1 Month)

In the autistic phase, also called *normal autism*, the infant exists in a half-sleeping, half-waking state and does not perceive the existence of other people or an external environment. The fulfillment of basic needs for survival and comfort is the focus and is merely accepted as it occurs.

Phase II: The Symbiotic Phase (1 to 5 Months)

Symbiosis is a type of "psychic fusion" of mother and child. The child views the self as an extension of the mother, but with a developing awareness that it is she who fulfills the child's every need. Mahler suggested that absence of, or rejection by, the maternal figure at this phase can lead to symbiotic psychosis.

Phase III: Separation-Individuation (5 to 36 Months)

This third phase represents what Mahler calls the "psychological birth" of the child. *Separation* is defined as the physical and psychological attainment of a

TABLE 3–4	**Stages of Development in Mahler's Theory of Object Relations**	
AGE	PHASE/SUBPHASE	MAJOR DEVELOPMENTAL TASKS
Birth–1 month	I. Normal autism	Fulfillment of basic needs for survival and comfort
1–5 months	II. Symbiosis	Development of awareness of external source of need fulfillment
	III. Separation-Individuation	
5–10 months	a. Differentiation	Commencement of a primary recognition of separateness from the mothering figure
10–16 months	b. Practicing	Increased independence through locomotor functioning; increased sense of separateness of self
16–24 months	c. Rapprochement	Acute awareness of separateness of self; learning to seek "emotional refueling" from mothering figure to maintain feeling of security
24–36 months	d. Consolidation	Sense of separateness established; on the way to object constancy (i.e., able to internalize a sustained image of loved object/person when it is out of sight); resolution of separation anxiety

sense of personal distinction from the mothering figure. *Individuation* occurs with a strengthening of the ego and an acceptance of a sense of "self," with independent ego boundaries. Four subphases through which the child evolves in his or her progression from a symbiotic extension of the mothering figure to a distinct and separate being are described.

Subphase 1: Differentiation (5 to 10 Months)

The differentiation phase begins with the child's initial physical movements away from the mothering figure. A primary recognition of separateness commences.

Subphase 2: Practicing (10 to 16 Months)

With advanced locomotor functioning, the child experiences feelings of exhilaration from increased independence. He or she is now able to move away from, and return to, the mothering figure. A sense of omnipotence is manifested.

Subphase 3: Rapprochement (16 to 24 Months)

This third subphase, rapprochement, is extremely critical to the child's healthy ego development. During this time, the child becomes increasingly aware of his or her separateness from the mothering figure, while the sense of fearlessness and omnipotence diminishes. The child, now recognizing the mother as a separate individual, wishes to reestablish closeness with her but shuns the total re-engulfment of the symbiotic stage. The need is for the mothering figure to be available to provide "emotional refueling" on demand.

Critical to this subphase is the mothering figure's response to the child. If the mothering figure is available to fulfill emotional needs as they arise, the child develops a sense of security in the knowledge that he or she is loved and will not be abandoned. However, if emotional needs are inconsistently met or if the mother rewards clinging, dependent behaviors and withholds nurturing when the child demonstrates independence, feelings of rage and a fear of abandonment develop and often persist into adulthood.

Subphase 4: Consolidation (24 to 36 Months)

With achievement of the consolidation subphase, a definite individuality and sense of separateness of self are established. Objects are represented as whole, with the child having the ability to integrate both "good" and "bad." A degree of object constancy is established as the child is able to internalize a sustained image of the mothering figure as enduring and loving, while maintaining the perception of her as a separate person in the outside world.

Relevance of Object Relations Theory to Nursing Practice

Understanding of the concepts of Mahler's theory of object relations helps the nurse assess the client's level of individuation from primary caregivers. The emotional problems of many individuals can be traced to lack of fulfillment of the tasks of separation/individuation. Examples include problems related to dependency and excessive anxiety. The individual with borderline personality disorders is thought to be fixed in the rapprochement phase of development, harboring fears of abandonment and underlying rage. This knowledge is important in the provision of nursing care to these individuals.

Cognitive Development Theory

Jean Piaget (Piaget & Inhelder, 1969) has been called the father of child psychology. His work concerning **cognitive development** in children is based on the premise that human intelligence is an extension of biological adaptation, or one's ability to adapt psychologically to the environment. He believed that human intelligence progresses through a series of stages that are related to age, demonstrating at each successive stage a higher level of logical organization than at the previous stages.

From his extensive studies of cognitive development in children, Piaget discovered four major stages, each of which he believed to be a necessary prerequisite for the one that follows. An outline is presented in Table 3-5.

Stage 1: Sensorimotor (Birth to 2 Years)

At the beginning of his or her life, the child is concerned only with satisfying basic needs and comforts. The self is not differentiated from the external environment. As the sense of differentiation occurs, with increasing mobility and awareness, the mental system is expanded. The child develops a greater understanding regarding objects within the external environment and their effects upon him or her. Knowledge is gained regarding the ability to manipulate objects and experiences within the environment. The sense of *object permanence*—the notion that an object will continue to exist when it is no longer present to the senses—is initiated.

Stage 2: Preoperational (2 to 6 years)

Piaget believed that preoperational thought is characterized by egocentrism. Personal experiences are thought to be universal, and the child is unable to accept the differing viewpoints of others. Language development progresses, as does the ability to attribute special meaning to symbolic gestures (e.g., bringing a storybook to mother is a symbolic invitation to have a story read). Reality is often given to inanimate objects. Object permanence culminates in the ability to conjure up mental representations of objects or people.

Stage 3: Concrete Operations (6 to 12 Years)

The ability to apply logic to thinking begins in this stage; however, "concreteness" still predominates. An understanding of the concepts of reversibility and spatiality is developed. For example, the child recognizes that changing the shape of objects does not necessarily change the amount, weight, volume, or the ability of the object to return to its original form. Another achievement of this stage is the ability to classify objects by any of their several characteristics. For example, he or she can classify all poodles as dogs but recognizes that all dogs are not poodles.

The concept of a lawful self is developed at this stage as the child becomes more socialized and rule conscious. Egocentrism decreases, the ability to cooperate in interactions with other children increases, and understanding and acceptance of established rules grow.

Stage 4: Formal Operations (12 to 15+ Years)

At this stage, the individual is able to think and reason in abstract terms. He or she can make and test hypotheses using logical and orderly problem solving. Current situations and reflections of the future are idealized, and a degree of egocentrism returns during this stage. There may be some difficulty reconciling idealistic hopes with more rational prospects. Formal operations, however, enable individuals to distinguish

TABLE 3–5 **Piaget's Stages of Cognitive Development**		
AGE	STAGE	MAJOR DEVELOPMENTAL TASKS
Birth–2 years	Sensorimotor	With increased mobility and awareness, development of a sense of self as separate from the external environment; the concept of object permanence emerges as the ability to form mental images evolves
2–6 years	Preoperational	Learning to express self with language; development of understanding of symbolic gestures; achievement of object permanence
6–12 years	Concrete operations	Learning to apply logic to thinking; development of understanding of reversibility and spatiality; learning to differentiate and classify; increased socialization and application of rules
12–15+ years	Formal operations	Learning to think and reason in abstract terms; making and testing hypotheses; capability of logical thinking and reasoning expand and are refined; cognitive maturity achieved

between the ideal and the real. Piaget's theory suggests that most individuals achieve **cognitive maturity**, the capability to perform all mental operations needed for adulthood, in middle to late adolescence.

Relevance of Cognitive Development Theory to Nursing Practice

Nurses who work in psychiatry are likely to be involved in helping clients, particularly depressed clients, with techniques of cognitive therapy. In cognitive therapy, the individual is taught to control thought distortions that are considered to be a factor in the development and maintenance of mood disorders. In the cognitive model, depression is characterized by a triad of negative distortions related to expectations of the environment, self, and future. In this model, depression is viewed as a distortion in cognitive development, the self is unrealistically devalued, and the future is perceived as hopeless. Therapy focuses on changing "automatic thoughts" that occur spontaneously and contribute to the distorted affect. Nurses who assist with this type of therapy must have knowledge of how cognition develops in order to help clients identify the distorted thought patterns and make the changes required for improvement in affective functioning (see Chapter 19).

Theory of Moral Development

Lawrence Kohlberg's (1976) stages of moral development are not closely tied to specific age groups. Research was conducted with males ranging in age from 10 to 28 years. Kohlberg believed that each stage is necessary and basic to the next stage and that all individuals must progress through each stage sequentially. He defined three major levels of moral development, each of which is further subdivided into two stages. An outline of Kohlberg's developmental stages is presented in Table 3-6. Most people do not progress through all six stages.

Level I: Preconventional Level (Prominent from Ages 4 to 10 Years)

Stage 1: Punishment and Obedience Orientation

At the punishment and obedience orientation stage, the individual is responsive to cultural guidelines of good or bad and right or wrong, but primarily in terms of the known related consequences. Fear of punishment is likely to be the incentive for conformity (e.g., "I'll do it, because if I don't I can't watch TV for a week").

Stage 2: Instrumental Relativist Orientation

Behaviors at the instrumental relativist orientation stage are guided by egocentrism and concern for self. There is an intense desire to satisfy one's own needs, but occasionally the needs of others are considered. For the most part, decisions are based on personal benefits derived (e.g., "I'll do it if I get something in return," or occasionally, ". . . because you asked me to").

TABLE 3–6 **Kohlberg's Stages of Moral Development**		
LEVEL/AGE*	STAGE	DEVELOPMENTAL FOCUS
I. Preconventional (common from age 4–10 years)	1. Punishment and obedience orientation	Behavior motivated by fear of punishment
	2. Instrumental relativist orientation	Behavior motivated by egocentrism and concern for self
II. Conventional (common from age 10–13 years, and into adulthood)	3. Interpersonal concordance orientation	Behavior motivated by expectations of others; strong desire for approval and acceptance
	4. Law and order orientation	Behavior motivated by respect for authority
III. Postconventional (can occur from adolescence on)	5. Social contract legalistic orientation	Behavior motivated by respect for universal laws and moral principles; guided by internal set of values
	6. Universal ethical principle orientation	Behavior motivated by internalized principles of honor, justice, and respect for human dignity; guided by the conscience

*Ages in Kohlberg's theory are not well defined. The stage of development is determined by the motivation behind the individual's behavior.

Level II: Conventional Level (Prominent From Ages 10 to 13 Years and Into Adulthood)*

Stage 3: Interpersonal Concordance Orientation

Behavior at the interpersonal concordance orientation stage is guided by the expectations of others. Approval and acceptance within one's societal group provide the incentive to conform (e.g., "I'll do it because you asked me to," ". . . because it will help you," or ". . . because it will please you").

Stage 4: Law and Order Orientation

In the law and order orientation stage, there is a personal respect for authority. Rules and laws are required and override personal principles and group mores. The belief is that all individuals and groups are subject to the same code of order, and no one shall be exempt (e.g., "I'll do it because it is the law").

Level III: Postconventional Level (Can Occur From Adolescence Onward)

Stage 5: Social Contract Legalistic Orientation

Individuals who reach stage 5 have developed a system of values and principles that determine for them what is right or wrong; behaviors are acceptably guided by this value system, provided they do not violate the human rights of others. They believe that all individuals are entitled to certain inherent human rights, and they live according to universal laws and principles. However, they hold the idea that the laws are subject to scrutiny and change as needs within society evolve and change (e.g., "I'll do it because it is the moral and legal thing to do, even though it is not my personal choice").

Stage 6: Universal Ethical Principle Orientation

Behavior at stage 6 is directed by internalized principles of honor, justice, and respect for human dignity. Laws are abstract and unwritten, such as the "Golden Rule," "equality of human rights," and "justice for all." They are not the concrete rules established by society. The conscience is the guide, and when one fails to meet the self-expected behaviors, the personal consequence is intense guilt. The allegiance to these ethical principles is so strong that the individual will stand by them even knowing that negative consequences will result (e.g., "I'll do it because I believe it is the right thing to do, even though it is illegal and I will be imprisoned for doing it").

---

*Eighty percent of adults are fixed in level II, with a majority of women in stage 3 and a majority of men in stage 4.

Relevance of Moral Development Theory to Nursing Practice

Moral development has relevance to psychiatric nursing in that it affects critical thinking about how individuals ought to behave and treat others. Moral behavior reflects the way a person interprets basic respect for other persons, such as the respect for human life, freedom, justice, or confidentiality. Psychiatric nurses must be able to assess the level of moral development of their clients in order to be able to help them in their effort to advance in their progression toward a higher level of developmental maturity.

A Nursing Model–Hildegard E. Peplau

Peplau (1991) applied interpersonal theory to nursing practice and, most specifically, to nurse-client relationship development. She provided a framework for "psychodynamic nursing," the interpersonal involvement of the nurse with a client in a given nursing situation. Peplau stated, "Nursing is helpful when both the patient and the nurse grow as a result of the learning that occurs in the nursing situation" (p. ix).

Peplau correlated the stages of personality development in childhood to stages through which clients advance during the progression of an illness. She also viewed these interpersonal experiences as learning situations for nurses to facilitate forward movement in the development of personality. She believed that when there is fulfillment of psychological tasks associated with the nurse-client relationship, the personalities of both can be strengthened. Key concepts include the following:

■ *Nursing* is a human relationship between an individual who is sick, or in need of health services, and a nurse especially educated to recognize and to respond to the need for help.

■ **Psychodynamic nursing** is being able to understand one's own behavior, to help others identify felt difficulties, and to apply principles of human relations to the problems that arise at all levels of experience.

■ *Roles* are sets of values and behaviors that are specific to functional positions within social structures. Peplau identifies the following *nursing roles*:

  ■ A *stranger.* A nurse is at first a stranger to the client. The client is also a stranger to the nurse. Peplau (1991) stated:

Respect and positive interest accorded a stranger is at first nonpersonal and includes the same ordinary courtesies that are accorded to a new guest who has been brought into any situation. This principle implies: (1) accepting the patient as he is; (2) treating the patient as an emotionally able stranger and relating to him on this basis until evidence shows him to be otherwise. (p. 44)

■ A *resource person* is one who provides specific, needed information that helps the client understand his or her problem and the new situation.

■ A **counselor** is one who listens as the client reviews feelings related to difficulties he or she is experiencing in any aspect of life. "Interpersonal techniques" have been identified to facilitate the nurse's interaction in the process of helping the client solve problems and make decisions concerning these difficulties.

■ A *teacher* is one who identifies learning needs and provides information to the client or family that may aid in improvement of the life situation.

■ A *leader* is one who directs the nurse-client interaction and ensures that appropriate actions are undertaken to facilitate achievement of the designated goals.

■ A **technical expert** is one who understands various professional devices and possesses the clinical skills necessary to perform the interventions that are in the best interest of the client.

■ A **surrogate** is one who serves as a substitute figure for another.

Phases of the nurse-client relationship are stages of overlapping roles or functions in relation to health problems, during which the nurse and client learn to work cooperatively to resolve difficulties. Peplau identified four phases:

■ *Orientation* is the phase during which the client, nurse, and family work together to recognize, clarify, and define the existing problem.

■ *Identification* is the phase after which the client's initial impression has been clarified and when he or she begins to respond selectively to those who seem to offer the help that is needed. Clients may respond in one of three ways: (1) on the basis of participation or interdependent relations with the nurse, (2) on the basis of independence or isolation from the nurse, or (3) on the basis of helplessness or dependence on the nurse (Peplau, 1991).

■ *Exploitation* is the phase during which the client proceeds to take full advantage of the services offered to him or her. Having learned which services are available, feeling comfortable within the setting, and serving as an active participant in his or her own health care, the client exploits the services available and explores all possibilities of the changing situation.

■ *Resolution* occurs when the client is freed from identification with helping persons and gathers strength to assume independence. Resolution is the direct result of successful completion of the other three phases.

Peplau's Stages of Personality Development

Psychological tasks are developmental lessons that must be learned on the way to achieving maturity of the personality. Peplau (1991) identified four psychological tasks that she associated with the stages of infancy and childhood described by Freud and Sullivan. She stated:

> When psychological tasks are successfully learned at each era of development, biological capacities are used productively and relations with people lead to productive living. When they are not successfully learned they carry over into adulthood and attempts at learning continue in devious ways, more or less impeded by conventional adaptations that provide a superstructure over the baseline of actual learning. (p. 166)

In the context of nursing, Peplau (1991) related these four psychological tasks to the demands made on nurses in their relations with clients. She maintained that:

> Nursing can function as a maturing force in society. Since illness is an event that is experienced along with feelings that derive from older experiences but are reenacted in the relationship of nurse to patient, the nurse-patient relationship is seen as an opportunity for nurses to help patients to complete the unfinished psychological tasks of childhood in some degree. (p. 159)

Peplau's psychological tasks of personality development include the four stages outlined in the following paragraphs. An outline of the stages of personality development according to Peplau's theory is presented in Table 3-7.

Learning to Count on Others

Nurses and clients first come together as strangers. Both bring to the relationship certain "raw materials," such as inherited biological components, personality characteristics (*temperament*), individual intellectual capacity, and specific cultural or environmental influences. Peplau relates these to the same "raw materials" with which an infant comes into this world. The newborn is capable of experiencing *comfort* and *discomfort*. He or she soon learns to communicate feelings in a way that results in the fulfillment of comfort needs by the mothering figure who provides love and care unconditionally. However, fulfillment of these dependency needs is inhibited when goals of the mothering figure become the focus, and love and care are contingent on meeting the needs of the caregiver rather than the infant.

TABLE 3–7 Stages of Development in Peplau's Interpersonal Theory

AGE	STAGE	MAJOR DEVELOPMENTAL TASKS
Infancy	Learning to count on others	Learning to communicate in various ways with the primary caregiver in order to have comfort needs fulfilled
Toddlerhood	Learning to delay satisfaction	Learning the satisfaction of pleasing others by delaying self-gratification in small ways
Early childhood	Identifying oneself	Learning appropriate roles and behaviors by acquiring the ability to perceive the expectations of others
Late childhood	Developing skills in participation	Learning the skills of compromise, competition, and cooperation with others; establishment of a more realistic view of the world and a feeling of one's place in it

Clients with unmet dependency needs regress during illness and demonstrate behaviors that relate to this stage of development. Other clients regress to this level because of physical disabilities associated with their illness. Peplau believed that when nurses provide unconditional care, they help these clients progress toward more mature levels of functioning. This may involve the role of "surrogate mother," in which the nurse fulfills needs for the client with the intent of helping him or her grow, mature, and become more independent.

Learning to Delay Satisfaction

Peplau related this stage to that of toddlerhood, or the first step in the development of interdependent social relations. Psychosexually, it is compared to the anal stage of development, when a child learns that, because of cultural mores, he or she cannot empty the bowels for relief of discomfort at will, but must delay to use the toilet, which is considered more culturally acceptable. When toilet training occurs too early or is very rigid, or when appropriate behavior is set forth as a condition for love and caring, tasks associated with this stage remain unfulfilled. The child feels powerless and fails to learn the satisfaction of pleasing others by delaying self-gratification in small ways. He or she may also exhibit rebellious behavior by failing to comply with demands of the mothering figure in an effort to counter the feelings of powerlessness. The child may accomplish this by withholding the fecal product or failing to deposit it in the culturally acceptable manner.

Peplau cited Fromm (1949) in describing the following potential behaviors of individuals who have failed to complete the tasks of the second stage of development:

■ Exploitation and manipulation of others to satisfy their own desires because they are unable to do so independently

■ Suspiciousness and envy of others; directing hostility toward others in an effort to enhance their own self-image

■ Hoarding and withholding possessions from others; miserliness

■ Inordinate neatness and punctuality

■ Inability to relate to others through sharing of feelings, ideas, or experiences

■ Ability to vary the personality characteristics to those required to satisfy personal desires at any given time

When nurses observe these types of behaviors in clients, it is important to encourage full expression and to convey unconditional acceptance. When the client learns to feel safe and unconditionally accepted, he or she is more likely to let go of the oppositional behavior and advance in the developmental progression. Peplau (1991) stated:

> Nurses who aid patients to feel safe and secure, so that wants can be expressed and satisfaction eventually achieved, also help them to strengthen personal power that is needed for productive social activities. (p. 207)

Identifying Oneself

"A concept of self develops as a product of interaction with adults" (Peplau, 1991, p. 211). A child learns to structure self-concept by observing how others interact with him or her. Roles and behaviors are established out of the child's perception of the expectations of others. When children perceive that adults expect them to maintain more-or-less permanent roles as infants, they perceive themselves as helpless and dependent. When the perceived expectation is that the child must behave in a manner beyond his or her maturational level, the child is deprived of the fulfillment of emotional and growth needs at the lower levels of development. Children who are given freedom to respond to situations and experiences unconditionally (i.e., with behaviors that are appropriate to their feelings) learn to improve on and reconstruct behavioral responses at their own individual pace. Peplau (1991) stated, "The ways in which adults appraise the child and the way he functions in relation to his experiences and perceptions are taken in or introjected and become the child's view of himself" (p. 213).

In nursing, it is important for the nurse to recognize cues that communicate how the client feels about him- or herself and about the presenting medical problem. In the initial interaction, it is difficult for the nurse to perceive the "wholeness" of the client, because the focus is on the condition that has caused him or her to seek help. Likewise, it is difficult for the client to perceive the nurse as a "mother (or father)" or "somebody's wife (or husband)" or as having a life aside from being there to offer assistance with the immediate presenting problem. As the relationship develops, nurses must be able to recognize client behaviors that indicate unfulfilled needs and provide experiences that promote growth. For example, the client who very proudly announces that she has completed activities of daily living independently and wants the nurse to come and inspect her room may still be craving the positive reinforcement associated with lower levels of development.

Nurses must also be aware of the predisposing factors that they bring to the relationship. Attitudes and beliefs about certain issues can have a deleterious effect on the client and interfere not only with the therapeutic relationship but also with the client's ability for growth and development. For example, a nurse who has strong beliefs against abortion may treat a client who has just undergone an abortion with disapproval and disrespect. The nurse may respond in this manner without even realizing he or she is doing so. Attitudes and values are introjected during early development and can be integrated so completely as to become a part of the self-system. Nurses must have knowledge and appreciation of their own concept of self in order to develop the flexibility required to accept all clients as they are, unconditionally. Effective resolution of problems that arise in the interdependent relationship can be the means for both client and nurse to reinforce positive personality traits and modify those more negative views of self.

Developing Skills in Participation

Peplau cited Sullivan's (1953) description of the "juvenile" stage of personality development (ages 6 through 9). During this stage, the child develops the capacity to "compromise, compete, and cooperate" with others. These skills are considered basic to one's ability to participate collaboratively with others. If a child tries to use the skills of an earlier level of

development (e.g., crying, whining, demanding), he or she may be rejected by peers of this juvenile stage. As this stage progresses, children begin to view themselves through the eyes of their peers. Sullivan (1953) called this "consensual validation." Preadolescents take on a more realistic view of the world and a feeling of their place in it. The capacity to love others (besides the mother figure) develops at this time and is expressed in relation to one's self-acceptance.

Failure to develop appropriate skills at any point along the developmental progression results in an individual's difficulty with participation in confronting the recurring problems of life. It is not the responsibility of the nurse to teach solutions to problems, but rather to help clients improve their problem-solving skills so that they may achieve their own resolution. This is accomplished through development of the skills of competition, compromise, cooperation, consensual validation, and love of self and others. Nurses can assist clients to develop or refine these skills by helping them to identify the problem, define a goal, and take the responsibility for performing the actions necessary to reach that goal. Peplau (1991) stated:

> Participation is required by a democratic society. When it has not been learned in earlier experiences, nurses have an opportunity to facilitate learning in the present and thus to aid in the promotion of a democratic society. (p. 259)

Relevance of Peplau's Model to Nursing Practice

Peplau's model provides nurses with a framework to interact with clients, many of whom are fixed in—or because of illness have regressed to—an earlier level of development. She suggested roles that nurses may assume to assist clients to progress, thereby achieving or resuming their appropriate developmental level. Appropriate developmental progression arms the individual with the ability to confront the recurring problems of life. Nurses serve to facilitate learning of that which has not been learned in earlier experiences.

Summary and Key Points

- Growth and development are unique with each individual and continue throughout the life span.
- Personality is defined as the combination of character, behavioral, temperamental, emotional, and mental traits that are unique to each specific individual.
- Sigmund Freud, who has been called the father of psychiatry, believed the basic character has been formed by the age of 5.
- Freud's personality theory can be conceptualized according to structure and dynamics of the personality,

topography of the mind, and stages of personality development.

■ Freud's structure of the personality includes the id, ego, and superego.

■ Freud classified all mental contents and operations into three categories: the conscious, the preconscious, and the unconscious.

■ Harry Stack Sullivan, author of the *Interpersonal Theory of Psychiatry*, believed that individual behavior and personality development are the direct result of interpersonal relationships. Major concepts include *anxiety, satisfaction of needs, interpersonal security,* and *self-system.*

■ Erik Erikson studied the influence of social processes on the development of the personality.

■ Erikson described eight stages of the life cycle from birth to death. He believed that individuals struggled with developmental "crises," and that each must be resolved for emotional growth to occur.

■ Margaret Mahler formulated a theory that describes the separation-individuation process of the infant from the maternal figure (primary caregiver). Stages of development describe the progression of the child from birth to object constancy at age 36 months.

■ Jean Piaget has been called the father of child psychology. He believed that human intelligence progresses through a series of stages that are related to age, demonstrating at each successive stage a higher level of logical organization than at the previous stages.

■ Lawrence Kohlberg outlined stages of moral development. His stages are not closely tied to specific age groups or the maturational process. He believed that moral stages emerge out of our own thinking and the stimulation of our mental processes.

■ Hildegard Peplau provided a framework for "psychodynamic nursing," the interpersonal involvement of the nurse with a client in a given nursing situation.

■ Peplau identified the nursing roles of stranger, resource person, counselor, teacher, leader, technical expert, and surrogate.

■ Peplau described four psychological tasks that she associated with the stages of infancy and childhood as identified by Freud and Sullivan.

■ Peplau believed that nursing is helpful when both the patient and the nurse grow as a result of the learning that occurs in the nursing situation.

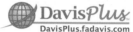 **DavisPlus** Additional info available at
DavisPlus.fadavis.com   www.davisplus.com

Review Questions
Self-Examination/Learning Exercise

*Select the answer that is **most** appropriate for each of the following questions:*

1. Mr. J. is a new client on the psychiatric unit. He is 35 years old. Theoretically, in which level of psychosocial development (according to Erikson) would you place Mr. J.?
   a. Intimacy vs. isolation
   b. Generativity vs. self-absorption
   c. Trust vs. mistrust
   d. Autonomy vs. shame and doubt

2. Mr. J. has been diagnosed with schizophrenia. He refuses to eat, and told the nurse he knew he was "being poisoned." According to Erikson's theory, in what developmental stage would you place Mr. J.?
   a. Intimacy vs. isolation
   b. Generativity vs. self-absorption
   c. Trust vs. mistrust
   d. Autonomy vs. shame and doubt

3. Janet, a psychiatric client diagnosed with borderline personality disorder, has just been hospitalized for threatening suicide. According to Mahler's theory, Janet did not receive the critical "emotional refueling" required during the rapprochement phase of development. What are the consequences of this deficiency?
   a. She has not yet learned to delay gratification.
   b. She does not feel guilt about wrongdoings to others.
   c. She is unable to trust others.
   d. She has internalized rage and fears of abandonment.

Review Questions—cont'd
Self-Examination/Learning Exercise

4. John is on the Alcohol Treatment Unit. He walks into the dayroom where other clients are watching a program on TV. He picks up the remote and changes the channel and says, "That's a stupid program! I want to watch something else!" In what stage of development is John fixed according to Sullivan's interpersonal theory?
   a. Juvenile. He is learning to form satisfactory peer relationships.
   b. Childhood. He has not learned to delay gratification.
   c. Early adolescence. He is struggling to form an identity.
   d. Late adolescence. He is working to develop a lasting relationship.

5. Adam has antisocial personality disorder. He says to the nurse, "I'm not crazy. I'm just fun-loving. I believe in looking out for myself. Who cares what anyone thinks? If it feels good, do it!" Which of the following describes the psychoanalytical structure of Adam's personality?
   a. Weak id, strong ego, weak superego
   b. Strong id, weak ego, weak superego
   c. Weak id, weak ego, punitive superego
   d. Strong id, weak ego, punitive superego

6. Larry, who has antisocial personality disorder, feels no guilt about violating the rights of others. He does as he pleases without thought to possible consequences. In which of Peplau's stages of development would you place Larry?
   a. Learning to count on others
   b. Learning to delay gratification
   c. Identifying oneself
   d. Developing skills in participation

7. Danny has been diagnosed with schizophrenia. On the unit he appears very anxious, paces back and forth, and darts his head from side to side in a continuous scanning of the area. He has refused to eat, making some barely audible comment related to "being poisoned." In planning care for Danny, which of the following would be the primary focus for nursing?
   a. To decrease anxiety and develop trust
   b. To set limits on his behavior
   c. To ensure that he gets to group therapy
   d. To attend to his hygiene needs

8. The nurse has just admitted Nancy to the psychiatric unit. The psychiatrist has diagnosed Nancy with major depressive disorder. The nurse says to Nancy, "Please tell me what it was like when you were growing up." Which nursing role described by Peplau is the nurse fulfilling in this instance?
   a. Surrogate
   b. Resource person
   c. Counselor
   d. Technical Expert

9. The nurse has just admitted Nancy to the psychiatric unit. The psychiatrist has diagnosed Nancy with major depressive disorder. The nurse says to Nancy, "What questions do you have about being here on the unit?" Which nursing role described by Peplau is the nurse fulfilling in this instance?
   a. Resource person
   b. Counselor
   c. Surrogate
   d. Technical Expert

Continued

Review Questions—cont'd
Self-Examination/Learning Exercise

10. The nurse has just admitted Nancy to the psychiatric unit. The psychiatrist has diagnosed Nancy with major depressive disorder. The nurse says to Nancy, "Some changes will have to be made in your behavior. I care about what happens to you." Which nursing role described by Peplau is the nurse fulfilling in this instance?
    a. Counselor
    b. Surrogate
    c. Technical Expert
    d. Resource Person

References

Black, D.W., & Andreasen, N.C. (2011). *Introductory textbook of psychiatry* (5th ed.). Washington, DC: American Psychiatric Publishing.

Marmer, S.S. (2003). Theories of the mind and psychopathology. In R.E. Hales & S.C. Yudofsky (Eds.), *Textbook of clinical psychiatry* (4th ed.) pp. 107–154. Washington, DC: American Psychiatric Publishing.

Murray, R.B., Zentner, J.P., & Yakimo, R. (2009). *Health promotion strategies through the life span* (8th ed.). Upper Saddle River, NJ: Prentice Hall.

Peplau, H.E. (1991). *Interpersonal relations in nursing.* New York, NY: Springer.

Classical References

Chess, S., & Thomas, A. (1986). *Temperament in clinical practice.* New York, NY: Guilford Press.

Erikson, E. (1963). *Childhood and society* (2nd ed.). New York, NY: WW Norton.

Freud, S. (1961). The ego and the id. *Standard edition of the complete psychological works of Freud* (Vol. XIX). London, UK: Hogarth Press.

Fromm, E. (1949). *Man for himself.* New York, NY: Farrar & Rinehart.

Kohlberg, L. (1976). Moral stages and moralization: The cognitive-development approach. In T. Lickona (Ed.), *Moral development and behavior: Theory, research, and social issues* (pp. 170–205). New York, NY: Holt, Rinehart and Winston.

Mahler, M., Pine, F., & Bergman, A. (1975). *The psychological birth of the human infant.* New York, NY: Basic Books.

Piaget, J., & Inhelder, B. (1969). *The psychology of the child.* New York, NY: Basic Books.

Sullivan, H.S. (1953). *The interpersonal theory of psychiatry.* New York, NY: WW Norton.

Concepts of Psychobiology 4

CORE CONCEPTS

genetics
neuroendocrinology
psychobiology
psychoimmunology
psychotropic medication

KEY TERMS

axon
cell body
circadian rhythms
dendrites
genotype
limbic system

neurons
neurotransmitter
phenotype
receptor sites
synapse

OBJECTIVES
After reading this chapter, the student will be able to:

1. Identify gross anatomical structures of the brain and describe their functions.
2. Discuss the physiology of neurotransmission in the central nervous system.
3. Describe the role of neurotransmitters in human behavior.
4. Discuss the association of endocrine functioning to the development of psychiatric disorders.
5. Describe the role of genetics in the development of psychiatric disorders.
6. Discuss the correlation of alteration in brain functioning to various psychiatric disorders.
7. Identify various diagnostic procedures used to detect alteration in biological functioning that may be contributing to psychiatric disorders.
8. Discuss the influence of psychological factors on the immune system.
9. Discuss historical perspectives related to psychopharmacology.
10. Describe the physiological mechanism by which various psychotropic medications exert their effects.
11. Discuss the implications of psychobiological concepts to the practice of psychiatric/mental health nursing.

HOMEWORK ASSIGNMENT
Please read the chapter and answer the following questions:

1. A dramatic reduction in which neurotransmitter is most closely associated with Alzheimer's disease?
2. Anorexia nervosa has been associated with a primary dysfunction of which structure of the brain?
3. Many psychotropics work by blocking the reuptake of neurotransmitters. Describe the process of *reuptake*.
4. What psychiatric disorder may be linked to chronic hypothyroidism?

In recent years, a greater emphasis has been placed on the study of the organic basis for psychiatric illness. This "neuroscientific revolution" has placed an emphasis on the biological basis of behavior, and several mental illnesses are now being considered as physical disorders that are the result of malfunctions and/or malformations of the brain.

This is not to imply that psychosocial and sociocultural influences are totally discounted. Such a notion would negate the transactional model of stress/adaptation on which the framework of this textbook is conceptualized.

The systems of biology, psychology, and sociology are not mutually exclusive—they are interacting systems. This is clearly indicated by the fact that individuals experience biological changes in response to various environmental events. Indeed, each of these disciplines may be, at various times, most appropriate for explaining behavioral phenomena.

This chapter focuses on the role of neurophysiological, neurochemical, genetic, and endocrine influences on psychiatric illness. A discussion of psychopharmacology is included, and various diagnostic procedures used to detect alteration in biological function that may contribute to psychiatric illness are identified. The implications for psychiatric/mental health nursing are discussed.

CORE CONCEPT

Psychobiology

The study of the biological foundations of cognitive, emotional, and behavioral processes.

The Nervous System: An Anatomical Review

The Brain

The brain has three major divisions, subdivided into six major parts:

1. Forebrain
   a. Cerebrum
   b. Diencephalon
2. Midbrain
   a. Mesencephalon
3. Hindbrain
   a. Pons
   b. Medulla
   c. Cerebellum

Each of these structures is discussed individually. A summary is presented in Table 4-1.

Cerebrum

The cerebrum consists of a right and left hemisphere and constitutes the largest part of the human brain.

TABLE 4–1 Structure and Function of the Brain

STRUCTURE	PRIMARY FUNCTION
I. THE FOREBRAIN A. Cerebrum	Composed of two hemispheres separated by a deep groove that houses a band of 200 million neurons called the corpus callosum. The outer shell is called the cortex. It is extensively folded and consists of billions of neurons. The left hemisphere appears to deal with logic and solving problems. The right hemisphere may be called the "creative" brain and is associated with affect, behavior, and spatial-perceptual functions. Each hemisphere is divided into four lobes.
1. Frontal lobes	Voluntary body movement, including movements that permit speaking, thinking and judgment formation, and expression of feelings.
2. Parietal lobes	Perception and interpretation of most sensory information (including touch, pain, taste, and body position).
3. Temporal lobes	Hearing, short-term memory, and sense of smell; expression of emotions through connection with limbic system.
4. Occipital lobes	Visual reception and interpretation.
B. Diencephalon 1. Thalamus	Connects cerebrum with lower brain structures. Integrates all sensory input (except smell) on way to cortex; some involvement with emotions and mood.
2. Hypothalamus	Regulates anterior and posterior lobes of pituitary gland; exerts control over actions of the autonomic nervous system; regulates appetite and temperature.
3. Limbic system	Consists of medially placed cortical and subcortical structures and the fiber tracts connecting them with one another and with the hypothalamus. It is sometimes called the "emotional brain"—associated with feelings of fear and anxiety; anger and aggression; love, joy, and hope; and with sexuality and social behavior.

TABLE 4–1	**Structure and Function of the Brain—cont'd**
STRUCTURE	PRIMARY FUNCTION
II. THE MIDBRAIN A. Mesencephalon	Responsible for visual, auditory, and balance ("righting") reflexes.
III. THE HINDBRAIN A. Pons	Regulation of respiration and skeletal muscle tone; ascending and descending tracts connect brain stem with cerebellum and cortex.
B. Medulla	Pathway for all ascending and descending fiber tracts; contains vital centers that regulate heart rate, blood pressure, and respiration; reflex centers for swallowing, sneezing, coughing, and vomiting.
C. Cerebellum	Regulates muscle tone and coordination and maintains posture and equilibrium.

The right and left hemispheres are connected by a deep groove, which houses a band of 200 million **neurons** (nerve cells) called the *corpus callosum*. Because each hemisphere controls different functions, information is processed through the corpus callosum so that each hemisphere is aware of the activity of the other.

The surface of the cerebrum consists of gray matter and is called the cerebral cortex. The gray matter is so called because the neuron cell bodies of which it is composed look gray to the eye. These gray matter cell bodies are thought to be the actual thinking structures of the brain. Another pair of masses of gray matter called *basal ganglia* is found deep within the cerebral hemispheres. They are responsible for certain subconscious aspects of voluntary movement, such as swinging the arms when walking, gesturing while speaking, and regulating muscle tone (Scanlon & Sanders, 2011).

The cerebral cortex is identified by numerous folds, called *gyri*, and deep grooves between the folds, called *sulci*. This extensive folding extends the surface area of the cerebral cortex, and thus permits the presence of millions more neurons than would be possible without it (as is the case in the brains of some animals, such as dogs and cats). Each hemisphere of the cerebral cortex is divided into the frontal lobe, parietal lobe, temporal lobe, and occipital lobe. These lobes, which are named for the overlying bones in the cranium, are identified in Figure 4-1.

The Frontal Lobes

Voluntary body movement is controlled by the impulses through the frontal lobes. The right frontal lobe controls motor activity on the left side of the body and the left frontal lobe controls motor activity on the

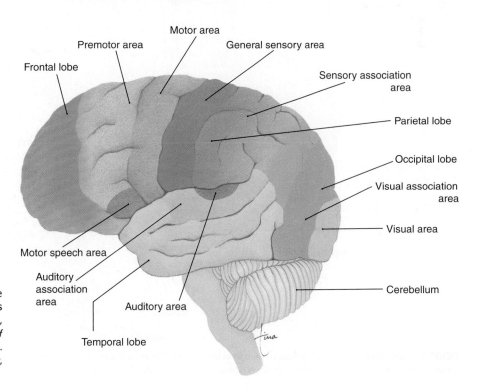

FIGURE 4-1 Left cerebral hemisphere showing some of the functional areas that have been mapped. (From Scanlon, V.C., & Sanders, T. [2011]. *Essentials of anatomy and physiology* [6th ed.]. Philadelphia, PA: F.A. Davis Company, with permission.)

right side of the body. Movements that permit speaking are also controlled by the frontal lobe, usually only on the left side (Scanlon & Sanders, 2011). The frontal lobe may also play a role in the emotional experience, as evidenced by changes in mood and character after damage to this area. The alterations include fear, aggressiveness, depression, rage, euphoria, irritability, and apathy and are likely related to a frontal lobe connection to the **limbic system**. The frontal lobe may also be involved (indirectly through association fibers linked to primary sensory areas) in thinking and perceptual interpretation of information.

The Parietal Lobes

Somatosensory input occurs in the parietal lobe area of the brain. These include touch, pain and pressure, taste, temperature, perception of joint and body position, and visceral sensations. The parietal lobes also contain association fibers linked to the primary sensory areas through which interpretation of sensory-perceptual information is made. Language interpretation is associated with the left hemisphere of the parietal lobe.

The Temporal Lobes

The upper anterior temporal lobe is concerned with auditory functions, while the lower part is dedicated to short-term memory. The sense of smell has a connection to the temporal lobes, as the impulses carried by the olfactory nerves end in this area of the brain. The temporal lobes also play a role in the expression of emotions through an interconnection with the limbic system. The left temporal lobe, along with the left parietal lobe, is involved in language interpretation.

The Occipital Lobes

The occipital lobes are the primary area of visual reception and interpretation. Visual perception, which gives individuals the ability to judge spatial relationships such as distance and to see in three dimensions, is also processed in this area. Language interpretation is influenced by the occipital lobes through an association with the visual experience.

Diencephalon

The second part of the forebrain is the diencephalon, which connects the cerebrum with lower structures of the brain. The major components of the diencephalon include the thalamus, the hypothalamus, and the limbic system. These structures are identified in Figures 4-2 and 4-3.

Thalamus

The thalamus integrates all sensory input (except smell) on its way to the cortex. This helps the cerebral cortex interpret the whole picture very rapidly, rather

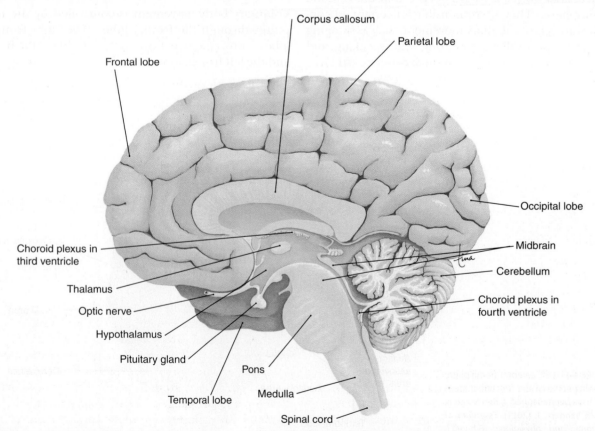

FIGURE 4-2   Midsagittal section of the brain as seen from the left side. This medial plane shows internal anatomy as well as the lobes of the cerebrum. (From Scanlon, V.C., & Sanders, T. [2011]. *Essentials of anatomy and physiology* [6th ed.]. Philadelphia, PA: F.A. Davis Company, with permission.)

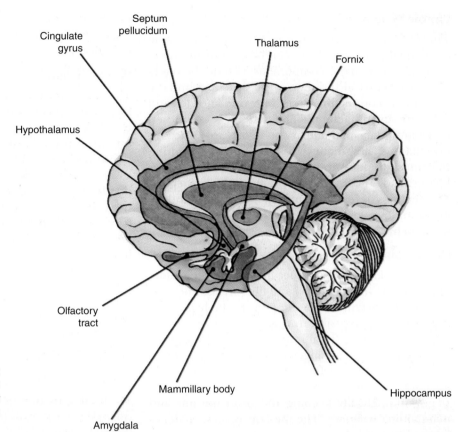

FIGURE 4–3 Structures of the limbic system. (Adapted from Scanlon, V.C., & Sanders, T. [2011]. *Essentials of anatomy and physiology* [6th ed.]. Philadelphia, PA: F.A. Davis Company, with permission.)

than experiencing each sensation individually. The thalamus is also involved in temporarily blocking minor sensations, so that an individual can concentrate on one important event when necessary. For example, an individual who is studying for an examination may be unaware of the clock ticking in the room, or even of another person walking into the room, because the thalamus has temporarily blocked these incoming sensations from the cortex.

Hypothalamus

The hypothalamus is located just below the thalamus and just above the pituitary gland and has a number of diverse functions.

1. **Regulation of the Pituitary Gland.** The pituitary gland consists of two lobes: the posterior lobe and the anterior lobe.
   a. *The posterior lobe* of the pituitary gland is actually extended tissue from the hypothalamus. The posterior lobe stores antidiuretic hormone (which helps to maintain blood pressure through regulation of water retention) and oxytocin (the hormone responsible for stimulation of the uterus during labor and the release of milk from the mammary glands). Both of these hormones are produced in the hypothalamus. When the hypothalamus detects the body's need for these

hormones, it sends nerve impulses to the posterior pituitary for their release.
   b. *The anterior lobe* of the pituitary gland consists of glandular tissue that produces a number of hormones used by the body. These hormones are regulated by "releasing factors" from the hypothalamus. When the hormones are required by the body, the releasing factors stimulate the release of the hormone from the anterior pituitary and the hormone in turn stimulates its target organ to carry out its specific functions.

2. **Direct Neural Control over the Actions of the Autonomic Nervous System.** The hypothalamus regulates the appropriate visceral responses during various emotional states. The actions of the autonomic nervous system are described later in this chapter.

3. **Regulation of Appetite.** Appetite is regulated through response to blood nutrient levels.

4. **Regulation of Temperature.** The hypothalamus senses internal temperature changes in the blood that flows through the brain. It receives information through sensory input from the skin about external temperature changes. The hypothalamus then uses this information to promote certain types of responses (e.g., sweating or shivering) that help to maintain body temperature within the normal range.

Limbic System

The part of the brain known as the limbic system consists of portions of the cerebrum and the diencephalon. The major components include the medially placed cortical and subcortical structures and the fiber tracts connecting them with one another and with the hypothalamus. The system is composed of the amygdala, mammillary body, olfactory tract, hypothalamus, cingulate gyrus, septum pellucidum, thalamus, hippocampus, and fornix. This system has been called "the emotional brain" and is associated with feelings of fear and anxiety; anger, rage, and aggression; love, joy, and hope; and with sexuality and social behavior.

Mesencephalon

Structures of major importance in the mesencephalon, or midbrain, include nuclei and fiber tracts. The mesencephalon extends from the pons to the hypothalamus and is responsible for integration of various reflexes, including visual reflexes (e.g., automatically turning away from a dangerous object when it comes into view), auditory reflexes (e.g., automatically turning toward a sound that is heard), and righting reflexes (e.g., automatically keeping the head upright and maintaining balance). The mesencephalon is identified in Figure 4-2.

Pons

The pons is a bulbous structure that lies between the midbrain and the medulla (Fig. 4-2). It is composed of large bundles of fibers and forms a major connection between the cerebellum and the brainstem. It also contains the central connections of cranial nerves V through VIII and centers for respiration and skeletal muscle tone.

Medulla

The medulla is the connecting structure between the spinal cord and the pons and all of the ascending and descending fiber tracts pass through it. The vital centers are contained in the medulla, and it is responsible for regulation of heart rate, blood pressure, and respiration. Also in the medulla are reflex centers for swallowing, sneezing, coughing, and vomiting. It also contains nuclei for cranial nerves IX through XII. The medulla, pons, and midbrain form the structure known as the brainstem. These structures are identified in Figure 4-2.

Cerebellum

The cerebellum is separated from the brainstem by the fourth ventricle but has connections to the brainstem through bundles of fiber tracts. It is situated just below the occipital lobes of the cerebrum (Figs. 4-1 and 4-2). The functions of the cerebellum are concerned with involuntary movement, such as muscular tone and coordination and the maintenance of posture and equilibrium.

Nerve Tissue

The tissue of the central nervous system (CNS) consists of nerve cells called neurons that generate and transmit electrochemical impulses. The structure of a neuron is composed of a cell body, an axon, and dendrites. The **cell body** contains the nucleus and is essential for the continued life of the neuron. The **dendrites** are processes that transmit impulses toward the cell body, and the **axon** transmits impulses away from the cell body. The axons and dendrites are covered by layers of cells called *neuroglia* that form a coating, or "sheath," of myelin. *Myelin* is a phospholipid that provides insulation against short-circuiting of the neurons during their electrical activity and increases the velocity of the impulse. The white matter of the brain and spinal cord is so called because of the whitish appearance of the myelin sheath over the axons and dendrites. The gray matter is composed of cell bodies that contain no myelin.

The three classes of neurons include afferent (sensory), efferent (motor), and interneurons. The *afferent neurons* carry impulses from receptors in the internal and external periphery to the CNS, where they are then interpreted into various sensations. The *efferent neurons* carry impulses from the CNS to *effectors* in the periphery, such as muscles (that respond by contracting) and glands (that respond by secreting). A schematic of afferent and efferent neurons is presented in Figure 4-4.

Interneurons exist entirely within the CNS, and 99 percent of all nerve cells belong to this group. They may carry only sensory or motor impulses, or they may serve as integrators in the pathways between afferent and efferent neurons. They account in large part for thinking, feelings, learning, language, and memory. The directional pathways of afferent, efferent, and interneurons are presented in Figure 4-5.

Synapses

Information is transmitted through the body from one neuron to another. Some messages may be processed through only a few neurons, while others may require thousands of neuronal connections. The neurons that transmit the impulses do not actually touch each other. The junction between two neurons is called a **synapse**. The small space between the axon terminals of one neuron and the cell body or dendrites of another is called the *synaptic cleft*. Neurons conducting impulses toward the synapse are called *presynaptic neurons* and those conducting impulses away are called *postsynaptic neurons*.

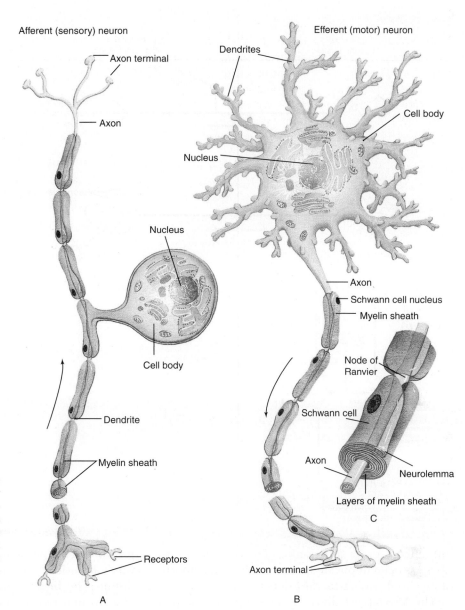

FIGURE 4-4 Neuron structure. **(A)** A typical sensory neuron. **(B)** A typical motor neuron. The arrows indicate the direction of impulse transmission. **(C)** Details of the myelin sheath and neurolemma formed by Schwann cells. (From Scanlon, V.C., & Sanders, T. [2011]. *Essentials of anatomy and physiology* [6th ed.]. Philadelphia, PA: F.A. Davis Company, with permission.)

A chemical, called a **neurotransmitter**, is stored in the axon terminals of the presynaptic neuron. An electrical impulse through the neuron causes the release of this neurotransmitter into the synaptic cleft. The neurotransmitter then diffuses across the synaptic cleft and combines with **receptor sites** that are situated on the cell membrane of the postsynaptic neuron. The result of the combination of neurotransmitter-receptor site is the determination of whether or not another electrical impulse is generated. If one is generated, the result is called an *excitatory response* and the electrical impulse moves on to the next synapse, where the same process recurs. If another electrical impulse is not generated by the neurotransmitter-receptor site combination, the result is called an *inhibitory response*, and synaptic transmission is terminated.

The cell body or dendrite of the postsynaptic neuron also contains a chemical *inactivator* that is specific to the neurotransmitter that has been released by the presynaptic neuron. When the synaptic transmission has been completed, the chemical inactivator quickly inactivates the neurotransmitter to prevent unwanted, continuous impulses, until a new impulse from the presynaptic neuron releases more neurotransmitter. A schematic representation of a synapse is presented in Figure 4-6.

Autonomic Nervous System

The autonomic nervous system (ANS) is actually considered part of the peripheral nervous system. Its regulation is integrated by the hypothalamus, however, and therefore the emotions exert a great deal of

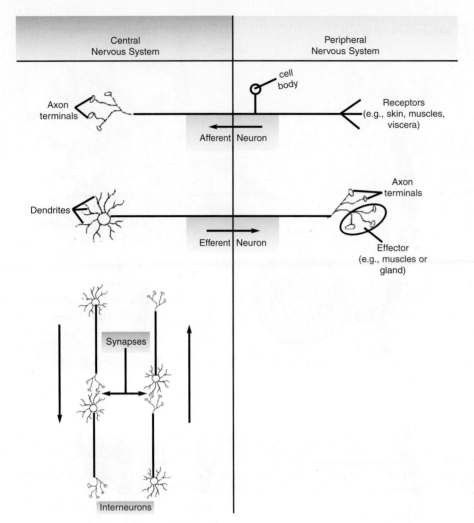

FIGURE 4–5 Directional pathways of neurons.

influence over its functioning. For this reason, the ANS has been implicated in the etiology of a number of psychophysiological disorders.

The ANS has two divisions: the sympathetic and the parasympathetic. The sympathetic division is dominant in stressful situations and prepares the body for the "fight or flight" response that was discussed in Chapter 1. The neuronal cell bodies of the sympathetic division originate in the thoracolumbar region of the spinal cord. Their axons extend to the chains of sympathetic ganglia where they synapse with other neurons that subsequently innervate the visceral effectors. This results in an increase in heart rate and respirations and a decrease in digestive secretions and peristalsis. Blood is shunted to the vital organs and to skeletal muscles to ensure adequate oxygenation.

The neuronal cell bodies of the parasympathetic division originate in the brainstem and the sacral segments of the spinal cord, and extend to the parasympathetic ganglia where the synapse takes place either very close to or actually in the visceral organ being innervated. In this way, a very localized response is possible. The parasympathetic division dominates when an individual is in a relaxed, nonstressful condition. The heart and respirations are maintained at a normal rate and secretions and peristalsis increase for normal digestion. Elimination functions are promoted. A schematic representation of the autonomic nervous system is presented in Figure 4-7.

Neurotransmitters

Neurotransmitters were described during the explanation of synaptic activity. They are being discussed separately and in detail because of the essential function they play in the role of human emotion and behavior and because they are the target for mechanism of action of many of the psychotropic medications.

Neurotransmitters are chemicals that convey information across synaptic clefts to neighboring target cells. They are stored in small vesicles in the axon terminals of neurons. When the action potential, or electrical impulse, reaches this point, the neurotransmitters are released from the vesicles. They

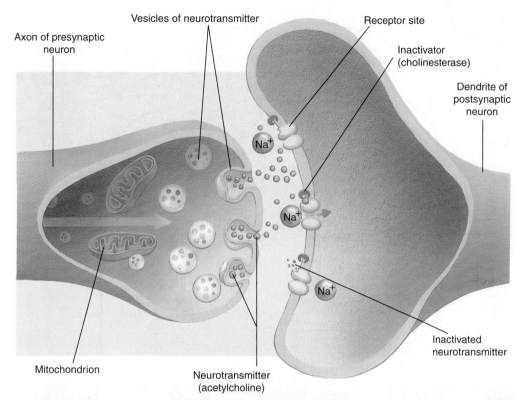

Vesicles of neurotransmitter

Axon of presynaptic
neuron

Receptor site

Inactivator
(cholinesterase)

Dendrite of
postsynaptic
neuron

Na⁺

Na⁺

Na⁺

Inactivated
neurotransmitter

Mitochondrion

Neurotransmitter
(acetylcholine)

FIGURE 4-6 Impulse transmission at a synapse. The arrow indicates the direction of electrical impulses. (From Scanlon, V.C., & Sanders, T. [2011]. *Essentials of anatomy and physiology* [6th ed.]. Philadelphia, PA: F.A. Davis Company, with permission.)

cross the synaptic cleft and bind with receptor sites on the cell body or dendrites of the adjacent neuron to allow the impulse to continue its course or to prevent the impulse from continuing. After the neurotransmitter has performed its function in the synapse, it either returns to the vesicles to be stored and used again, or it is inactivated and dissolved by enzymes. The process of being stored for reuse is called *reuptake*, a function that holds significance for understanding the mechanism of action of certain psychotropic medications.

Many neurotransmitters exist in the central and peripheral nervous systems, but only a limited number have implications for psychiatry. Major categories include cholinergics, monoamines, amino acids, and neuropeptides. Each of these is discussed separately and summarized in Table 4-2.

Cholinergics

Acetylcholine

Acetylcholine was the first chemical to be identified and proven as a neurotransmitter. It is a major effector chemical in the ANS, producing activity at all sympathetic and parasympathetic presynaptic nerve terminals and all parasympathetic postsynaptic nerve terminals. It is highly significant in the neurotransmission that occurs at the junctions of nerve and

muscles. Acetylcholinesterase is the enzyme that destroys acetylcholine or inhibits its activity.

In the CNS, acetylcholine neurons innervate the cerebral cortex, hippocampus, and limbic structures. The pathways are especially dense through the area of the basal ganglia in the brain.

Functions of acetylcholine are manifold and include sleep, arousal, pain perception, the modulation and coordination of movement, and memory acquisition and retention (Gilman & Newman, 2003). Cholinergic mechanisms may have some role in certain disorders of motor behavior and memory, such as Parkinson's disease, Huntington's disease, and Alzheimer's disease.

Monoamines

Norepinephrine

Norepinephrine is the neurotransmitter that produces activity at the sympathetic postsynaptic nerve terminals in the ANS resulting in the "fight or flight" responses in the effector organs. In the CNS, norepinephrine pathways originate in the pons and medulla and innervate the thalamus, dorsal hypothalamus, limbic system, hippocampus, cerebellum, and cerebral cortex. When norepinephrine is not returned for storage in the vesicles of the axon terminals, it is metabolized and inactivated by the enzymes monoamine

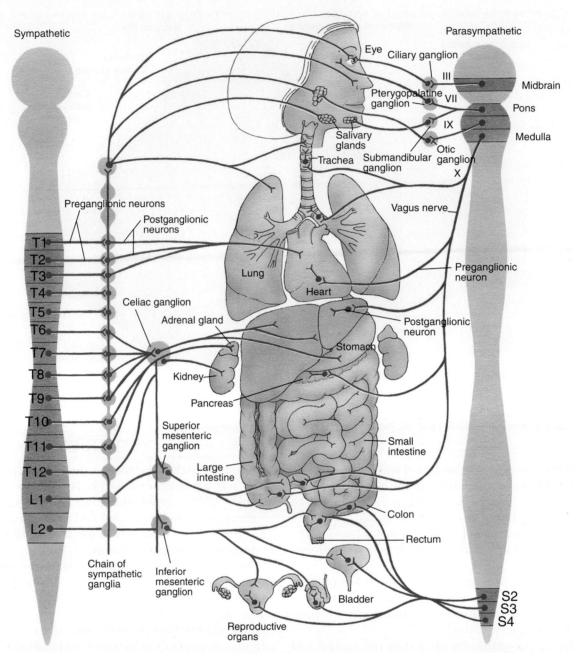

FIGURE 4–7   The autonomic nervous system. The sympathetic division is shown on the left, and the parasympathetic division is shown on the right (both divisions are bilateral). (From Scanlon, V.C., & Sanders, T. [2011]. *Essentials of anatomy and physiology* [6th ed.]. Philadelphia, PA: F.A. Davis Company, with permission.)

oxidase (MAO) and catechol-*O*-methyl-transferase (COMT).

The functions of norepinephrine include the regulation of mood, cognition, perception, locomotion, cardiovascular functioning, and sleep and arousal (Gilman & Newman, 2003). The activity of norepinephrine also has been implicated in certain mood disorders such as depression and mania, in anxiety states, and in schizophrenia (Sadock & Sadock, 2007).

Dopamine

Dopamine pathways arise from the midbrain and hypothalamus and terminate in the frontal cortex, limbic system, basal ganglia, and thalamus. Dopamine neurons in the hypothalamus innervate the posterior pituitary and those from the posterior hypothalamus project to the spinal cord. As with norepinephrine, the inactivating enzymes for dopamine are MAO and COMT.

Dopamine functions include regulation of movements and coordination, emotions, voluntary decision-making ability, and because of its influence on the pituitary gland, it inhibits the release of prolactin (Sadock & Sadock, 2007). Increased levels of dopamine are associated with mania (Dubovsky, Davies, & Dubovsky, 2003) and schizophrenia (Black & Andreasen, 2011).

TABLE 4–2 Neurotransmitters in the Central Nervous System

NEUROTRANSMITTER	LOCATION/FUNCTION	POSSIBLE IMPLICATIONS FOR MENTAL ILLNESS
I. CHOLINERGICS A. Acetylcholine	*ANS:* Sympathetic and parasympathetic presynaptic nerve terminals; parasympathetic postsynaptic nerve terminals *CNS:* Cerebral cortex, hippocampus, limbic structures, basal ganglia *Functions:* Sleep, arousal, pain perception, movement, memory	*Increased levels:* Depression *Decreased levels:* Alzheimer's disease, Huntington's disease, Parkinson's disease
II. MONOAMINES A. Norepinephrine	*ANS:* Sympathetic postsynaptic nerve terminals *CNS:* Thalamus, hypothalamus, limbic system, hippocampus, cerebellum, cerebral cortex *Functions:* Mood, cognition, perception, locomotion, cardiovascular functioning, sleep and arousal	*Decreased levels:* Depression *Increased levels:* Mania, anxiety states, schizophrenia
B. Dopamine	Frontal cortex, limbic system, basal ganglia, thalamus, posterior pituitary, and spinal cord *Functions:* Movement and coordination, emotions, voluntary judgment, release of prolactin	*Decreased levels:* Parkinson's disease and depression *Increased levels:* Mania and schizophrenia
C. Serotonin	Hypothalamus, thalamus, limbic system, cerebral cortex, cerebellum, spinal cord *Functions:* Sleep and arousal, libido, appetite, mood, aggression, pain, perception, coordination, judgment	*Decreased levels:* Depression *Increased levels:* Anxiety states
D. Histamine	Hypothalamus *Functions:* Wakefulness; pain sensation and inflammatory response	*Decreased levels:* Depression
III. AMINO ACIDS A. Gamma-amino-butyric acid (GABA)	Hypothalamus, hippocampus, cortex, cerebellum, basal ganglia, spinal cord, retina *Function:* Slowdown of body activity	*Decreased levels:* Huntington's disease, anxiety disorders, schizophrenia, and various forms of epilepsy
B. Glycine	Spinal cord and brainstem *Function:* Recurrent inhibition of motor neurons	*Toxic levels:* "glycine encephalopathy" decreased levels are correlated with spastic motor movements
C. Glutamate and Aspartate	Pyramidal cells of the cortex, cerebellum, and the primary sensory afferent systems; hippocampus, thalamus, hypothalamus, spinal cord *Functions:* Relay of sensory information and in the regulation of various motor and spinal reflexes	*Decreased levels:* Schizophrenia *Increased levels:* Huntington's disease, temporal lobe epilepsy, spinal cerebellar degeneration, anxiety disorders, depressive disorders
IV. NEUROPEPTIDES A. Endorphins and Enkephalins	Hypothalamus, thalamus, limbic structures, midbrain, and brainstem; enkephalins are also found in the gastrointestinal tract *Functions:* Modulation of pain and reduced peristalsis (enkephalins)	Modulation of dopamine activity by opioid peptides may indicate some link to the symptoms of schizophrenia
B. Substance P	Hypothalamus, limbic structures, midbrain, brainstem, thalamus, basal ganglia, and spinal cord; also found in gastrointestinal tract and salivary glands *Function:* Regulation of pain	*Decreased levels:* Huntington's disease and Alzheimer's disease *Increased levels:* Depression

Continued

TABLE 4–2 **Neurotransmitters in the Central Nervous System—cont'd**		
NEUROTRANSMITTER	LOCATION/FUNCTION	POSSIBLE IMPLICATIONS FOR MENTAL ILLNESS
C. Somatostatin	Cerebral cortex, hippocampus, thalamus, basal ganglia, brainstem, and spinal cord *Functions:* Depending on part of the brain being affected, stimulates release of dopamine, serotonin, norepinephrine, and acetylcholine, and inhibits release of norepinephrine, histamine, and glutamate. Also acts as a neuromodulator for serotonin in the hypothalamus.	*Decreased levels:* Alzheimer's disease *Increased levels:* Huntington's disease

Serotonin

Serotonin pathways originate from cell bodies located in the pons and medulla and project to areas including the hypothalamus, thalamus, limbic system, cerebral cortex, cerebellum, and spinal cord. Serotonin that is not returned to be stored in the axon terminal vesicles is catabolized by the enzyme MAO.

Serotonin may play a role in sleep and arousal, libido, appetite, mood, aggression, and pain perception. The serotoninergic system has been implicated in the etiology of certain psychopathological conditions including anxiety states, mood disorders, and schizophrenia (Sadock & Sadock, 2007).

Histamine

The role of histamine in mediating allergic and inflammatory reactions has been well documented. Its role in the CNS as a neurotransmitter has only recently been confirmed, and the availability of information is limited. The highest concentrations of histamine are found within various regions of the hypothalamus. Histaminic neurons in the posterior hypothalamus are associated with sustaining wakefulness (Gilman & Newman, 2003). The enzyme that catabolizes histamine is MAO. Although the exact processes mediated by histamine within the central nervous system are uncertain, some data suggest that histamine may play a role in depressive illness.

Amino Acids

Inhibitory Amino Acids

Gamma-Aminobutyric Acid Gamma-aminobutyric acid (GABA) has a widespread distribution in the CNS, with high concentrations in the hypothalamus, hippocampus, cortex, cerebellum, and basal ganglia of the brain, in the gray matter of the dorsal horn of the spinal cord, and in the retina. Most GABA is associated with short inhibitory interneurons, although some long-axon pathways within the brain also have been identified. GABA is catabolized by the enzyme GABA transaminase.

Inhibitory neurotransmitters, such as GABA, prevent postsynaptic excitation, interrupting the progression of the electrical impulse at the synaptic junction. This function is significant when slowdown of body activity is advantageous. Enhancement of the GABA system is the mechanism of action by which the benzodiazepines produce their calming effect.

Alterations in the GABA system have been implicated in the etiology of anxiety disorders, movement disorders (e.g., Huntington's disease), and various forms of epilepsy.

Glycine The highest concentrations of glycine in the CNS are found in the spinal cord and brainstem. Little is known about the possible enzymatic metabolism of glycine.

Glycine appears to be the neurotransmitter of recurrent inhibition of motor neurons within the spinal cord, and is possibly involved in the regulation of spinal and brainstem reflexes. It has been implicated in the pathogenesis of certain types of spastic disorders and in "glycine encephalopathy," which is known to occur with toxic accumulation of the neurotransmitter in the brain and cerebrospinal fluid (Hamosh, Scharer, & Van Hove, 2009).

Excitatory Amino Acids

Glutamate and Aspartate Glutamate and aspartate appear to be primary excitatory neurotransmitters in the pyramidal cells of the cortex, the cerebellum, and the primary sensory afferent systems. They are also found in the hippocampus, thalamus, hypothalamus, and spinal cord. Glutamate and aspartate are inactivated by uptake into the tissues and through assimilation in various metabolic pathways.

Glutamate and aspartate function in the relay of sensory information and in the regulation of various motor and spinal reflexes. Alteration in these systems has been implicated in the etiology of certain neurodegenerative disorders, such as Huntington's disease, temporal lobe epilepsy, and spinal cerebellar degeneration. Recent studies have implicated increased levels of glutamate in anxiety and depressive disorders and decreased levels in schizophrenia (Bunney, Bunney, & Carlsson, 2012; Ouellet-Plamondon & George, 2012).

Neuropeptides

Numerous neuropeptides have been identified and studied. They are classified by the area of the body in which they are located or by their pharmacological or functional properties. Although their role as neurotransmitters has not been clearly established, it is known that they often coexist with the classic neurotransmitters within a neuron; however, the functional significance of this coexistence still requires further study. Hormonal neuropeptides are discussed in the section of this chapter on neuroendocrinology.

Opioid Peptides

Opioid peptides, which include the endorphins and enkephalins, have been widely studied. Opioid peptides are found in various concentrations in the hypothalamus, thalamus, limbic structures, midbrain, and brainstem. Enkephalins are also found in the gastrointestinal (GI) tract. Opioid peptides are thought to have a role in pain modulation, with their natural morphine-like properties. They are released in response to painful stimuli, and may be responsible for producing the analgesic effect following acupuncture. Opioid peptides alter the release of dopamine and affect the spontaneous activity of the dopaminergic neurons. These findings may have some implication for opioid peptide–dopamine interaction in the etiology of schizophrenia.

Substance P

Substance P was the first neuropeptide to be discovered. It is present in high concentrations in the hypothalamus, limbic structures, midbrain, and brainstem, and is also found in the thalamus, basal ganglia, and spinal cord. Substance P has been found to be highly concentrated in sensory fibers, and for this reason is thought to play a role in sensory transmission, and particularly in the regulation of pain. Substance P abnormalities have been associated with Huntington's disease, Alzheimer's disease, and mood disorders (Sadock & Sadock, 2007).

Somatostatin

Somatostatin (also called growth hormone–inhibiting hormone) is found in the cerebral cortex, hippocampus, thalamus, basal ganglia, brainstem, and spinal cord, and has multiple effects on the CNS. In its function as a neurotransmitter, somatostatin exerts both stimulatory and inhibitory effects. Depending on the part of the brain being affected, it has been shown to stimulate dopamine, serotonin, norepinephrine, and acetylcholine, and inhibit norepinephrine, histamine, and glutamate. It also acts as a neuromodulator for serotonin in the hypothalamus, thereby regulating its

release (i.e., determining whether it is stimulated or inhibited). It is possible that somatostatin may serve this function for other neurotransmitters as well. High concentrations of somatostatin have been reported in brain specimens of clients with Huntington's disease, and low concentrations in those with Alzheimer's disease.

CORE CONCEPT

Neuroendocrinology

Study of the interaction between the nervous system and the endocrine system, and the effects of various hormones on cognitive, emotional, and behavioral functioning.

Neuroendocrinology

Human endocrine functioning has a strong foundation in the CNS, under the direction of the hypothalamus, which has direct control over the pituitary gland. The pituitary gland has two major lobes—the anterior lobe (also called the *adenohypophysis*) and the posterior lobe (also called the *neurohypophysis*). The pituitary gland is only about the size of a pea, but despite its size and because of the powerful control it exerts over endocrine functioning in humans, it is sometimes called the "master gland." (Figure 4-8 shows the hormones of the pituitary gland and their target organs.) Many of the hormones subject to hypothalamus-pituitary regulation may have implications for behavioral functioning. Discussion of these hormones is summarized in Table 4-3.

Pituitary Gland

The Posterior Pituitary (Neurohypophysis)

The hypothalamus has direct control over the posterior pituitary through efferent neural pathways. Two hormones are found in the posterior pituitary: vasopressin (antidiuretic hormone) and oxytocin. They are actually produced by the hypothalamus and stored in the posterior pituitary. Their release is mediated by neural impulses from the hypothalamus (Fig. 4-9).

Antidiuretic Hormone

The main function of antidiuretic hormone (ADH) is to conserve body water and maintain normal blood pressure. The release of ADH is stimulated by pain, emotional stress, dehydration, increased plasma concentration, and decreases in blood volume. An alteration in the secretion of this hormone may be a factor in the polydipsia observed in about 10 to 15 percent of hospitalized psychiatric patients. Other factors correlated with this behavior include adverse effects of

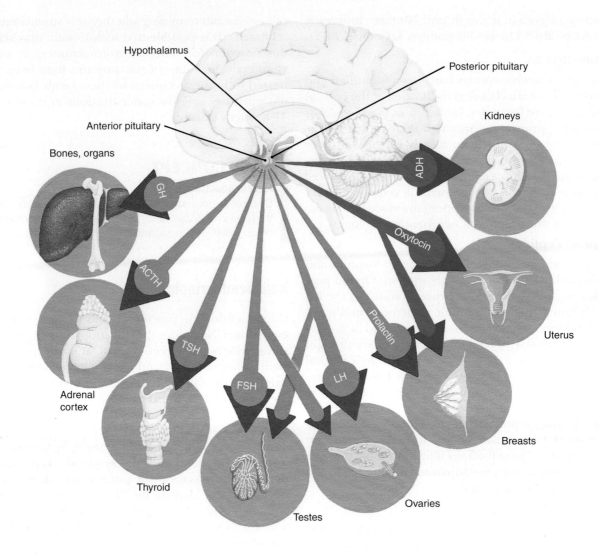

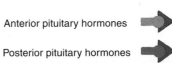

FIGURE 4–8 Hormones of the pituitary gland and their target organs. (From Scanlon, V.C., & Sanders, T. [2011]. *Essentials of anatomy and physiology* [6th ed.]. Philadelphia, PA: F.A. Davis Company, with permission.)

TABLE 4–3 **Hormones of the Neuroendocrine System**				
HORMONE	LOCATION AND STIMULATION OF RELEASE	TARGET ORGAN	FUNCTION	POSSIBLE BEHAVIORAL CORRELATION TO ALTERED SECRETION
Antidiuretic hormone (ADH)	Posterior pituitary; release stimulated by dehydration, pain, stress	Kidney (causes increased reabsorption)	Conservation of body water and maintenance of blood pressure	Polydipsia; altered pain response; modified sleep pattern
Oxytocin	Posterior pituitary; release stimulated by end of pregnancy; stress; during sexual arousal	Uterus; breasts	Contraction of the uterus for labor; release of breast milk	May play role in stress response by stimulation of ACTH

TABLE 4–3 Hormones of the Neuroendocrine System—cont'd

HORMONE	LOCATION AND STIMULATION OF RELEASE	TARGET ORGAN	FUNCTION	POSSIBLE BEHAVIORAL CORRELATION TO ALTERED SECRETION
Growth hormone (GH)	Anterior pituitary; release stimulated by growth hormone–releasing hormone from hypothalamus	Bones and tissues	Growth in children; protein synthesis in adults	Anorexia nervosa
Thyroid-stimulating hormone (TSH)	Anterior pituitary; release stimulated by thyrotropin-releasing hormone from hypothalamus	Thyroid gland	Stimulation of secretion of needed thyroid hormones for metabolism of food and regulation of temperature	*Increased levels:* insomnia, anxiety, emotional liability *Decreased levels:* fatigue, depression
Adrenocorticotropic hormone (ACTH)	Anterior pituitary; release stimulated by corticotropin-releasing hormone from hypothalamus	Adrenal cortex	Stimulation of secretion of cortisol, which plays a role in response to stress	*Increased levels:* mood disorders, psychosis *Decreased levels:* depression, apathy, fatigue
Prolactin	Anterior pituitary; release stimulated by prolactin-releasing hormone from hypothalamus	Breasts	Stimulation of milk production	*Increased levels:* depression, anxiety, decreased libido, irritability
Gonadotropic hormones	Anterior pituitary; release stimulated by gonadotropin-releasing hormone from hypothalamus	Ovaries and testes	Stimulation of secretion of estrogen, progesterone, and testosterone; role in ovulation and sperm production	*Decreased levels:* depression and anorexia nervosa *Increased testosterone:* increased sexual behavior and aggressiveness
Melanocyte-stimulating hormone (MSH)	Anterior pituitary; release stimulated by onset of darkness	Pineal gland	Stimulation of secretion of melatonin	*Increased levels:* depression

psychotropic medications and features of the behavioral disorder itself. ADH also may play a role in learning and memory, in alteration of the pain response, and in the modification of sleep patterns.

Oxytocin

Oxytocin stimulates contraction of the uterus at the end of pregnancy and stimulates release of milk from the mammary glands (Scanlon & Sanders, 2011). It is also released in response to stress and during sexual arousal. Its role in behavioral functioning is unclear, although it is possible that oxytocin may act in certain situations to stimulate the release of adrenocorticotropic hormone (ACTH), thereby playing a key role in the overall hormonal response to stress.

The Anterior Pituitary (Adenohypophysis)

The hypothalamus produces *releasing hormones* that pass through capillaries and veins of the hypophyseal portal system to capillaries in the anterior pituitary, where they stimulate secretion of specialized hormones. This pathway is presented in Figure 4-9. The hormones of the anterior pituitary gland regulate multiple body functions and include growth hormone, thyroid-stimulating hormone, ACTH, prolactin, gonadotropin-stimulating hormone, and melanocyte-stimulating hormone. Most of these hormones are regulated by a *negative feedback mechanism*. Once the hormone has exerted its effects, the information is "fed back" to the anterior pituitary, which inhibits the release, and ultimately decreases the effects, of the stimulating hormones.

Growth Hormone

The release of growth hormone (GH), also called somatotropin, is stimulated by growth hormone–releasing hormone (GHRH) from the hypothalamus. Its release is inhibited by growth hormone–inhibiting hormone (GHIH), or somatostatin, also from the hypothalamus. It is responsible for growth in children,

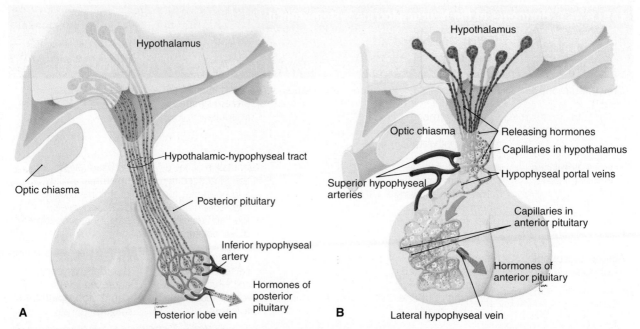

FIGURE 4–9 Structural relationships of hypothalamus and pituitary gland. **(A)** Posterior pituitary stores hormones produced in the hypothalamus. **(B)** Releasing hormones of the hypothalamus circulate directly to the anterior pituitary and influence its secretions. Notice the two networks of capillaries. (From Scanlon, V.C., & Sanders, T. [2011]. *Essentials of anatomy and physiology* [6th ed.]. Philadelphia, PA: F.A. Davis Company, with permission.)

as well as continued protein synthesis throughout life. During periods of fasting, it stimulates the release of fat from the adipose tissue to be used for increased energy. The release of GHIH is stimulated in response to periods of hyperglycemia. GHRH is stimulated in response to hypoglycemia and to stressful situations. During prolonged stress, GH has a direct effect on protein, carbohydrate, and lipid metabolism, resulting in increased serum glucose and free fatty acids to be used for increased energy. There has been some indication of a possible correlation between abnormal secretion of growth hormone and anorexia nervosa.

Thyroid-Stimulating Hormone

Thyrotropin-releasing hormone (TRH) from the hypothalamus stimulates the release of thyroid-stimulating hormone (TSH), or thyrotropin, from the anterior pituitary. TSH stimulates the thyroid gland to secrete triiodothyronine (T_3) and thyroxine (T_4). Thyroid hormones are integral to the metabolism of food and the regulation of temperature.

A correlation between thyroid dysfunction and altered behavioral functioning has been studied. Early reports in the medical literature associated hyperthyroidism with irritability, insomnia, anxiety, restlessness, weight loss, and emotional liability, and in some instances with progressing to delirium or psychosis. Symptoms of fatigue, decreased libido, memory impairment, depression, and suicidal ideations have been associated with chronic hypothyroidism. Studies have correlated various forms of thyroid dysfunction with mood disorders, anxiety, eating disorders, schizophrenia, and neurocognitive disorder.

Adrenocorticotropic Hormone

Corticotropin-releasing hormone (CRH) from the hypothalamus stimulates the release of ACTH from the anterior pituitary. ACTH stimulates the adrenal cortex to secrete cortisol. The role of cortisol in human behaviors is not well understood, although it seems to be secreted under stressful situations. Disorders of the adrenal cortex can result in hyposecretion or hypersecretion of cortisol.

Addison's disease is the result of hyposecretion of the hormones of the adrenal cortex. Behavioral symptoms of hyposecretion include mood changes with apathy, social withdrawal, impaired sleep, decreased concentration, and fatigue. Hypersecretion of cortisol results in Cushing's disease and is associated with behaviors that include depression, mania, psychosis, and suicidal ideation. Cognitive impairments also have been commonly observed.

Prolactin

Serum prolactin levels are regulated by prolactin-releasing hormone (PRH) and prolactin-inhibiting hormone (PIH) from the hypothalamus. Prolactin stimulates milk production by the mammary glands in the presence of high levels of estrogen and progesterone during pregnancy. Behavioral symptoms associated with hypersecretion of prolactin include depression, decreased libido, stress intolerance, anxiety, and increased irritability.

Gonadotropic Hormones

The gonadotropic hormones are so called because they produce an effect on the gonads—the ovaries and the testes. The gonadotropins include follicle-stimulating hormone (FSH) and luteinizing hormone (LH), and their release from the anterior pituitary is stimulated by gonadotropin-releasing hormone (GnRH) from the hypothalamus. In women, FSH initiates maturation of ovarian follicles into the ova and stimulates their secretion of estrogen. LH is responsible for ovulation and the secretion of progesterone from the corpus luteum. In men, FSH initiates sperm production in the testes, and LH increases secretion of testosterone by the interstitial cells of the testes (Scanlon & Sanders, 2011). The gonadotropins are regulated by a negative feedback of gonadal hormones at the hypothalamic or pituitary level.

Limited evidence exists to correlate gonadotropins to behavioral functioning, although some observations have been made to warrant hypothetical consideration. Studies have indicated decreased levels of testosterone, LH, and FSH in depressed men. Increased sexual behavior and aggressiveness have been linked to elevated testosterone levels in both men and women. Decreased plasma levels of LH and FSH commonly occur in patients with anorexia nervosa. Supplemental estrogen therapy has resulted in improved mentation and mood in some depressed women.

Melanocyte-Stimulating Hormone

Melanocyte-stimulating hormone (MSH) from the hypothalamus stimulates the pineal gland to secrete melatonin. The release of melatonin appears to depend on the onset of darkness and is suppressed by light. Studies of this hormone have indicated that environmental light can affect neuronal activity and influence *circadian rhythms*. Correlation between abnormal secretion of melatonin and symptoms of depression has led to the implication of melatonin in the etiology of seasonal affective disorder (SAD), in which individuals become depressed only during the fall and winter months when the amount of daylight decreases.

Circadian Rhythms

Human biological rhythms are largely determined by genetic coding, with input from the external environment influencing the cyclic effects. **Circadian rhythms** in humans follow a near-24-hour cycle and may influence a variety of regulatory functions, including the sleep-wakefulness cycle, body temperature regulation, patterns of activity such as eating and drinking, and hormone secretion. The 24-hour rhythms in humans

are affected to a large degree by the cycles of lightness and darkness. This occurs because of a "pacemaker" in the brain that sends messages to other systems in the body and maintains the 24-hour rhythm. This endogenous pacemaker appears to be the suprachiasmatic nuclei of the hypothalamus. These nuclei receive projections of light through the retina, and in turn stimulate electrical impulses to various other systems in the body, mediating the release of neurotransmitters or hormones that regulate bodily functioning.

Most of the biological rhythms of the body operate over a period of about 24 hours, but cycles of longer lengths have been studied. For example, women of menstruating age show monthly cycles of progesterone levels in the saliva, of skin temperature over the breasts, and of prolactin levels in the plasma of the blood (Hughes, 1989).

Some rhythms may even last as long as a year. These circannual rhythms are particularly relevant to certain medications, such as cyclosporine, that appears to be more effective at some times than others during the period of about a year (Hughes, 1989). One clinical study showed that administration of chemotherapy during the appropriate circadian phase can significantly increase the efficacy and decrease the toxic effects of certain cytotoxic agents (Lis et al., 2003).

The Role of Circadian Rhythms in Psychopathology

Circadian rhythms may play a role in psychopathology. Because many hormones have been implicated in behavioral functioning, it is reasonable to believe that peak secretion times could be influential in predicting certain behaviors. The association of depression with increased secretion of melatonin during darkness hours has already been discussed. External manipulation of the light-dark cycle and removal of external time cues often have beneficial effects on mood disorders.

Symptoms that occur in the premenstrual cycle have also been linked to disruptions in biological rhythms. A number of the symptoms associated with premenstrual dysphoric disorder (PMDD) strongly resemble those attributed to depression, and hormonal changes have been implicated in the etiology. Some of these changes include progesterone-estrogen imbalance, increase in prolactin and mineralocorticoids, high level of prostaglandins, decrease in endogenous opiates, changes in metabolism of biogenic amines (serotonin, dopamine, norepinephrine, acetylcholine), and variations in secretion of glucocorticoids or melatonin.

Sleep disturbances are common in both depression and PMDD. Because the sleep-wakefulness cycle is probably the most fundamental of biological rhythms, it will be discussed in greater detail. A representation of bodily functions affected by 24-hour biological rhythms is presented in Figure 4-10.

Sleep

The sleep-wakefulness cycle is genetically determined rather than learned and is established some time after birth. Even when environmental cues such as the ability to detect light and darkness are removed, the human sleep-wakefulness cycle generally develops about a 25-hour periodicity, which is close to the 24-hour normal circadian rhythm.

Sleep can be measured by the types of brain waves that occur during various stages of sleep activity. Dreaming episodes are characterized by rapid eye movement and are called REM sleep. The sleep-wakefulness cycle is represented by six distinct stages.

1. **Stage 0: Alpha Rhythm.** This stage of the sleep-wakefulness cycle is characterized by a relaxed,

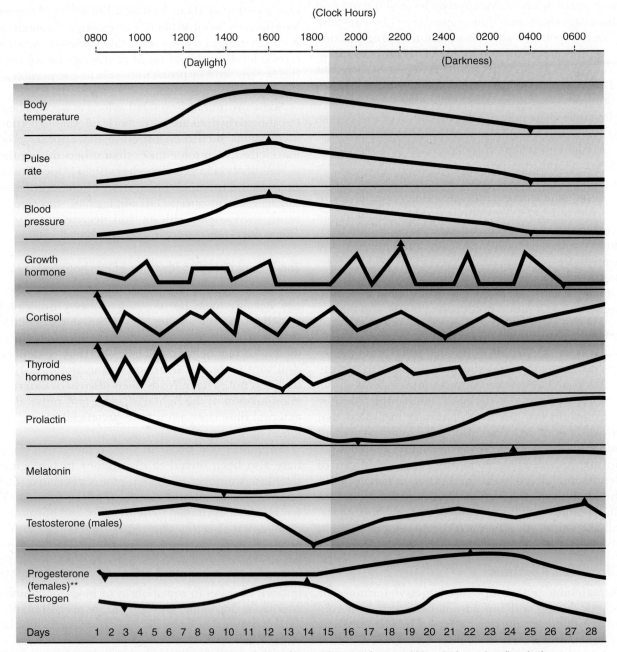

* ▼ indicates low point and ▲ indicates peak time of these biological factors within a 24-hour circadian rhythm.
** The female hormones are presented on a monthly rhythm because of their influence on the reproductive cycle.
  Daily rhythms of female gonadotropins are difficult to assay and are probably less significant than monthly.

FIGURE 4–10 Circadian biological rhythms.

waking state with eyes closed. The alpha brain wave rhythm has a frequency of 8 to 12 cycles per second.

2. **Stage 1: Beta Rhythm.** Stage 1 characterizes the "transition" into sleep, or a period of dozing. Thoughts wander, and there is a drifting in and out of sleep. Beta brain wave rhythm has a frequency of 18 to 25 cycles per second.

3. **Stage 2: Theta Rhythm.** This stage characterizes the manner in which about half of sleep time is spent. Eye movement and muscular activity are minimal. Theta brain wave rhythm has a frequency of 4 to 7 cycles per second.

4. **Stage 3: Delta Rhythm.** This is a period of deep and restful sleep. Muscles are relaxed, heart rate and blood pressure fall, and breathing slows. No eye movement occurs. Delta brain wave rhythm has a frequency of 1.5 to 3 cycles per second.

5. **Stage 4: Delta Rhythm.** This is the stage of deepest sleep. Individuals who suffer from insomnia or other sleep disorders often do not experience this stage of sleep. Eye movement and muscular activity are minimal. Delta waves predominate.

6. **REM Sleep: Beta Rhythm.** The dream cycle occurs during REM sleep. Eyes dart about beneath closed eyelids, moving more rapidly than when awake. The brain wave pattern is similar to that of stage 1 sleep. Heart and respiration rates increase and blood pressure may increase or decrease. Muscles are hypotonic during REM sleep.

Stages 2 through REM repeat themselves throughout the cycle of sleep. One is more likely to experience longer periods of stages 3 and 4 sleep early in the cycle and longer periods of REM sleep later in the sleep cycle. Most people experience REM sleep about four to five times during the night. The amount of REM sleep and deep sleep decreases with age, while the time spent in drowsy wakefulness and dozing increases.

Neurochemical Influences

A number of neurochemicals have been shown to influence the sleep-wakefulness cycle. Several studies have revealed information about the sleep-inducing characteristics of serotonin. L-tryptophan, the amino acid precursor to serotonin, has been used for many years as an effective sedative-hypnotic to induce sleep in individuals with sleep-onset disorder. Serotonin and norepinephrine both appear to be most active during non-REM sleep, whereas the neurotransmitter acetylcholine is activated during REM sleep (Skudaev, 2010). The exact role of GABA in sleep facilitation is unclear, although the sedative effects of drugs that enhance GABA transmission, such as the benzodiazepines, suggest that this neurotransmitter plays an important role in regulation of sleep and arousal. Some studies have suggested that acetylcholine induces and prolongs REM sleep, whereas histamine appears to have an inhibitory effect. Neuroendocrine mechanisms seem to be more closely tied to circadian rhythms than to the sleep-wakefulness cycle. One exception is growth hormone secretion, which exhibits increases during the early sleep period and may be associated with slow-wave sleep (Van Cauter et al., 1992).

CORE CONCEPT

Genetics

Study of the biological transmission of certain characteristics (physical and/or behavioral) from parent to offspring.

Genetics

Human behavioral genetics seeks to understand both the genetic and environmental contributions to individual variations in human behavior (McInerney, 2008). This type of study is complicated by the fact that behaviors, like all complex traits, involve *multiple genes*.

The term **genotype** refers to the total set of genes present in an individual at the time of conception, and coded in the DNA. The physical manifestations of a particular genotype are designated by characteristics that specify a specific **phenotype**. Examples of phenotypes include eye color, height, blood type, language, hair type, and method of communication. As evident by the examples presented, phenotypes are not *only* genetic, but may also be acquired (i.e., influenced by the environment) or a combination of both. It is likely that many psychiatric disorders are the result of a combination of genetics and environmental influences.

Investigators who study the etiological implications for psychiatric illness may explore several risk factors. Studies to determine if an illness is *familial* compare the percentages of family members with the illness to those in the general population or within a control group of unrelated individuals. These studies estimate the prevalence of psychopathology among relatives, and make predictions about the predisposition to an illness based on familial risk factors. Schizophrenia, bipolar disorder, major depressive disorder, anorexia nervosa, panic disorder, somatic symptom disorder, antisocial personality disorder, and alcoholism are examples of psychiatric illness in which familial tendencies have been indicated.

Studies that are purely genetic in nature search for a specific gene that is responsible for an individual having a particular illness. A number of disorders exist in which the mutation of a specific gene or change in the number or structure of a chromosome has been associated with the etiology. Examples include Huntington's disease, cystic fibrosis, phenylketonuria, Duchenne's muscular dystrophy, and Down syndrome.

The search for genetic links to certain psychiatric disorders continues. Risk factors for early-onset Alzheimer's disease have been linked to mutations on chromosomes 21, 14, and 1 (National Institute on Aging, 2012). Other studies have linked a gene in the region of chromosome 19 that produces apolipoprotein E (ApoE) with late-onset Alzheimer's disease. Additional research is required before definitive confirmation can be made.

In addition to familial and purely genetic investigations, other types of studies have been conducted to estimate the existence and degree of genetic and environmental contributions to the etiology of certain psychiatric disorders. Twin studies and adoption studies have been successfully employed for this purpose.

Twin studies examine the frequency of a disorder in monozygotic (genetically identical) and dizygotic (fraternal; not genetically identical) twins. Twins are called *concordant* when both members suffer from the same disorder in question. Concordance in monozygotic twins is considered stronger evidence of genetic involvement than it is in dizygotic twins. Disorders in which twin studies have suggested a possible genetic link include alcoholism, schizophrenia, major depressive disorder, bipolar

disorder, anorexia nervosa, panic disorder, and obsessive-compulsive disorder (Baker, 2004; Gill, 2004; O'Donovan, 2012).

Adoption studies allow comparisons to be made of the influences of genetics versus environment on the development of a psychiatric disorder. Knowles (2003) describes the following four types of adoption studies that have been conducted:

1. The study of adopted children whose biological parent(s) had a psychiatric disorder but whose adoptive parent(s) did not.
2. The study of adopted children whose adoptive parent(s) had a psychiatric disorder but whose biological parent(s) did not.
3. The study of adoptive and biological relatives of adopted children who developed a psychiatric disorder.
4. The study of monozygotic twins reared apart by different adoptive parents.

Disorders in which adoption studies have suggested a possible genetic link include alcoholism, schizophrenia, major depression, bipolar disorder, attention-deficit/hyperactivity disorder, and antisocial personality disorder (Knowles, 2003).

A summary of various psychiatric disorders and the possible biological influences discussed in this chapter is presented in Table 4-4. Various diagnostic procedures used to detect alteration in biological functioning that may contribute to psychiatric disorders are presented in Table 4-5.

TABLE 4–4 Biological Implications of Psychiatric Disorders

ANATOMICAL BRAIN STRUCTURES INVOLVED	NEUROTRANSMITTER HYPOTHESIS	POSSIBLE ENDOCRINE CORRELATION	IMPLICATIONS OF CIRCADIAN RHYTHMS	POSSIBLE GENETIC LINK
SCHIZOPHRENIA				
Frontal cortex, temporal lobes, limbic system	Dopamine hyperactivity; decreased glutamate	Decreased prolactin levels	May correlate antipsychotic medication administration to times of lowest level	Twin, familial, and adoption studies suggest genetic link
DEPRESSIVE DISORDERS				
Frontal lobes, limbic system, temporal lobes	Decreased levels of norepinephrine, dopamine, and serotonin; increased glutamate	Increased cortisol levels; thyroid hormone hyposecretion; increased melatonin	DST* used to predict effectiveness of antidepressants; melatonin linked to depression during periods of darkness	Twin, familial, and adoption studies suggest a genetic link
BIPOLAR DISORDER				
Frontal lobes, limbic system, temporal lobes	Increased levels of norepinephrine and dopamine in acute mania	Some indication of elevated thyroid hormones in acute mania		Twin, familial, and adoption studies suggest a genetic link

TABLE 4–4 Biological Implications of Psychiatric Disorders—cont'd

ANATOMICAL BRAIN STRUCTURES INVOLVED	NEUROTRANSMITTER HYPOTHESIS	POSSIBLE ENDOCRINE CORRELATION	IMPLICATIONS OF CIRCADIAN RHYTHMS	POSSIBLE GENETIC LINK
PANIC DISORDER Limbic system, midbrain	Increased levels of norepinephrine; decreased GABA activity	Elevated levels of thyroid hormones	May have some application for times of medication administration	Twin and familial studies suggest a genetic link
ANOREXIA NERVOSA Limbic system, particularly the hypothalamus	Decreased levels of norepinephrine, serotonin, and dopamine	Decreased levels of gonadotropins and growth hormone; increased cortisol levels	DST* often shows same results as in depression	Twin and familial studies suggest a genetic link
OBSESSIVE-COMPULSIVE DISORDER Limbic system, basal ganglia (specifically caudate nucleus)	Decreased levels of serotonin	Increased cortisol levels	DST* often shows same results as in depression	Twin studies suggest a possible genetic link
ALZHEIMER'S DISEASE Temporal, parietal, and occipital regions of cerebral cortex; hippocampus	Decreased levels of acetylcholine, norepinephrine, serotonin, and somatostatin	Decreased corticotropin-releasing hormone	Decreased levels of acetylcholine and serotonin may inhibit hypothalamic-pituitary axis and interfere with hormonal releasing factors	Familial studies suggest a genetic predisposition; late-onset disorder linked to marker on chromosome 19; early-onset to chromosomes 21, 14, and 1

*DST = dexamethasone suppression test. Dexamethasone is a synthetic glucocorticoid that suppresses cortisol secretion via the feedback mechanism. In this test, 1 mg of dexamethasone is administered at 11:30 p.m. and blood samples are drawn at 8 a.m., 4 p.m., and 11 p.m. on the following day. A plasma value greater than 5 mcg/dL suggests that the individual is not suppressing cortisol in response to the dose of dexamethasone. This is a positive result for depression and may have implications for other disorders as well.

TABLE 4–5 Diagnostic Procedures Used to Detect Altered Brain Functioning

EXAM	TECHNIQUE USED	PURPOSE OF THE EXAM AND POSSIBLE FINDINGS
Electroencephalography (EEG)	Electrodes are placed on the scalp in a standardized position. Amplitude and frequency of beta, alpha, theta, and delta brain waves are graphically recorded on paper by ink markers for multiple areas of the brain surface.	Measures brain electrical activity; identifies dysrhythmias, asymmetries, or suppression of brain rhythms; used in the diagnosis of epilepsy, neoplasm, stroke, metabolic, or degenerative disease.
Computerized EEG mapping	EEG tracings are summarized by computer-assisted systems in which various regions of the brain are identified and functioning is interpreted by color coding or gray shading.	Measures brain electrical activity; used largely in research to represent statistical relationships between individuals and groups or between two populations of subjects (e.g., patients with schizophrenia vs. control subjects).
Computed tomographic (CT) scan	CT scan may be used with or without contrast medium. X-rays are taken of various transverse planes of the brain while a computerized analysis produces a precise reconstructed image of each segment.	Measures accuracy of brain structure to detect possible lesions, abscesses, areas of infarction, or aneurysm. CT has also identified various anatomical differences in patients with schizophrenia, neurocognitive disorders, and bipolar disorder.

Continued

TABLE 4–5	Diagnostic Procedures Used to Detect Altered Brain Functioning–cont'd	
EXAM	TECHNIQUE USED	PURPOSE OF THE EXAM AND POSSIBLE FINDINGS
Magnetic resonance imaging (MRI)	Within a strong magnetic field, the nuclei of hydrogen atoms absorb and reemit electromagnetic energy that is computerized and transformed into image information. No radiation or contrast medium is used.	Measures anatomical and biochemical status of various segments of the brain; detects brain edema, ischemia, infection, neoplasm, trauma, and other changes such as demyelination. Morphological differences have been noted in brains of patients with schizophrenia as compared with control subjects.
Positron emission tomography (PET)	The patient receives an intravenous (IV) injection of a radioactive substance (type depends on brain activity to be visualized). The head is surrounded by detectors that relay data to a computer that interprets the signals and produces the image.	Measures specific brain functioning, such as glucose metabolism, oxygen utilization, blood flow, and, of particular interest in psychiatry, neurotransmitter-receptor interaction.
Single photon emission computed tomography (SPECT)	The technique is similar to PET, but longer-acting radioactive substance must be used to allow time for a gamma-camera to rotate about the head and gather the data, which are then computer assembled into a brain image.	Measures various aspects of brain functioning, as with PET; has also been used to image activity of cerebrospinal fluid circulation.

CORE CONCEPT

Psychoimmunology

The branch of medicine that studies the effects of psychological and social factors on the functioning of the immune system.

Psychoimmunology

Normal Immune Response

Cells responsible for *nonspecific* immune reactions include neutrophils, monocytes, and macrophages. They work to destroy the invasive organism and initiate and facilitate damaged tissue. If these cells are not effective in accomplishing a satisfactory healing response, *specific* immune mechanisms take over.

Specific immune mechanisms are divided into two major types: the cellular response and the humoral response. The controlling elements of the cellular response are the T lymphocytes (T cells); those of the humoral response are called B lymphocytes (B cells). When the body is invaded by a specific antigen, the T cells, and particularly the CD4 T lymphocytes (also called *helper T cells*), become sensitized to and specific for the foreign antigen. These antigen-specific CD4 T cells divide many times, producing antigen-specific CD4 T cells with other functions. One of these, the *killer T cell*, destroys viruses that reproduce inside other cells by puncturing the cell membrane of the host cell and allowing the contents of the cell, including viruses, to spill out into the bloodstream, where they can be engulfed by macrophages. Another cell produced through division of the CD4 T cells is the *suppressor T cell*, which serves to stop the immune response once the foreign antigen has been destroyed (Scanlon & Sanders, 2011).

The humoral response is activated when antigen-specific CD4 T cells communicate with the B cells in the spleen and lymph nodes. The B cells in turn produce the antibodies specific to the foreign antigen. Antibodies attach themselves to foreign antigens so that they are unable to invade body cells. These invader cells are then destroyed without being able to multiply.

Implications of the Immune System in Psychiatric Illness

In studies of the biological response to stress, it has been hypothesized that individuals become more susceptible to physical illness following exposure to a stressful stimulus or life event (see Chapter 1). This response is thought to be due to the effect of increased glucocorticoid release from the adrenal cortex following stimulation from the hypothalamic-pituitary-adrenal axis during stressful situations. The result is a suppression in lymphocyte proliferation and function.

Studies have shown that nerve endings exist in tissues of the immune system. The CNS has connections in both bone marrow and the thymus, where immune system cells are produced, and in the spleen and lymph nodes, where those cells are stored.

Growth hormone, which may be released in response to certain stressors, may enhance immune functioning, whereas testosterone is thought to inhibit immune functioning. Increased production of epinephrine and norepinephrine occurs in response to stress, and may decrease immunity. Serotonin has demonstrated both enhancing and inhibitory effects on immunity (Irwin, 2000).

Studies have correlated a decrease in lymphocyte functioning with periods of grief, bereavement, and depression, associating the degree of altered immunity with severity of the depression. A number of research studies have been conducted attempting to correlate the onset of schizophrenia to abnormalities of the immune system. These studies have considered autoimmune responses, viral infections, and immunogenetics (Sadock & Sadock, 2007). The role of these factors in the onset and course of schizophrenia remains unclear. Immunological abnormalities have also been investigated in a number of other psychiatric illnesses, including alcoholism, autism spectrum disorder, and neurocognitive disorder.

Evidence exists to support a correlation between psychosocial stress and the onset of illness. Research is still required to determine the specific processes involved in stress-induced modulation of the immune system.

Psychopharmacology

The middle of the 20th century identifies a pivotal period in the treatment of individuals with mental illness. It was during this time that the phenothiazine class of antipsychotics was introduced into the United States. Before that time they had been used in France as preoperative medications. As Dr. Henri Laborit of the Hospital Boucicaut in Paris stated,

> It was our aim to decrease the anxiety of the patients to prepare them in advance for their postoperative recovery. With these new drugs, the phenothiazines, we were seeing a profound psychic and physical relaxation . . . a real indifference to the environment and to the upcoming operation. It seemed to me these drugs must have an application in psychiatry. (Sage, 1984)

Indeed they have had a significant application in psychiatry. Not only have they helped many individuals to function effectively, but they have also provided researchers and clinicians with information to study the origins and etiologies of mental illness. Knowledge gained from learning how these drugs work has promoted advancement in understanding how

behavioral disorders develop. Dr. Arnold Scheibel, director of the UCLA Brain Research Institute, stated,

> [When these drugs came out] there was a sense of disbelief that we could actually do something substantive for the patients . . . see them for the first time as sick individuals and not as something bizarre that we could literally not talk to. (Sage, 1984)

CORE CONCEPT

Psychotropic Medication
Medication that affects psychic function, behavior, or experience.

Historical Perspectives

Historically, reaction to and treatment of individuals with mental illness ranged from benign involvement to interventions some would consider inhumane. Individuals with mental illness were feared because of common beliefs associating them with demons or the supernatural. They were looked upon as loathsome and often were mistreated.

Beginning in the late 18th century, a type of "moral reform" in the treatment of persons with mental illness began to occur. Community and state hospitals concerned with the needs of persons with mental illness were established. Considered a breakthrough in the humanization of care, these institutions, however well intentioned, fostered the concept of custodial care. Clients were ensured the provision of food and shelter but received little or no hope of change for the future. As they became increasingly dependent on the institution to fill their needs, the likelihood of their return to the family or community diminished.

The early part of the 20th century saw the advent of the somatic therapies in psychiatry. Individuals with mental illness were treated with insulin shock therapy, wet sheet packs, ice baths, electroconvulsive therapy, and psychosurgery. Before 1950, sedatives and amphetamines were the only significant psychotropic medications available. Even these had limited use because of their toxicity and addicting effects. Since the 1950s, the development of psychopharmacology has expanded to include widespread use of antipsychotic, antidepressant, and antianxiety medications. Research into how these drugs work has provided an understanding of the etiology of many psychiatric disorders.

Psychotropic medications are not intended to "cure" the mental illness. Most mental health practitioners who prescribe these medications for their clients use them as an adjunct to individual or group psychotherapy. Although their contribution to psychiatric care cannot be minimized, it must be emphasized that psychotropic medications relieve physical and behavioral symptoms. They do not resolve emotional problems.

Role of the Nurse

Ethical and Legal Implications

Nurses must understand the ethical and legal implications associated with the administration of psychotropic medications. Laws differ from state to state, but most adhere to the client's right to refuse treatment. Exceptions exist in emergency situations when it has been determined that clients are likely to harm themselves or others.

Assessment

A thorough baseline assessment must be conducted before a client is placed on a regimen of psychopharmacological therapy. A history and physical examination (see Chapter 9), an ethnocultural assessment (see Chapter 6), and a comprehensive medication assessment (see Box 4-1) are all essential components of this database.

Medication Administration and Evaluation

For the client in an inpatient setting, as well as for many others in partial hospitalization programs, day treatment centers, home health care, and other settings, the nurse is the key health-care professional in direct contact with the individual receiving the chemotherapy. Medication administration is followed by a careful evaluation, including continuous monitoring for side effects and adverse reactions. The nurse also evaluates the therapeutic effectiveness of the medication. It is essential for the nurse to have a thorough knowledge of psychotropic medications to be able to anticipate potential problems and outcomes associated with their administration.

Client Education

The information associated with psychotropic medications is copious and complex. An important role of the nurse is to translate that complex information into terms that can be easily understood by the client. Clients must understand why the medication has been prescribed, when it should be taken, and what they may expect in terms of side effects and possible adverse reactions. They must know whom to contact when they have a question and when it is important to report to their physician. Medication education encourages client cooperation and

---

BOX 4-1 Medication Assessment Tool

Date _____ Client's Name _____ Age _____

Marital Status _____ Children _____ Occupation _____

Presenting Symptoms (subjective & objective) _____
_____

Diagnosis (DSM-5) _____

Current Vital Signs: Blood Pressure: Sitting _____/_____ ; Standing _____/_____; Pulse_____ ;

Respirations _____ Height _____ Weight _____

CURRENT/PAST USE OF PRESCRIPTION DRUGS (Indicate with "c" or "p" beside name of drug whether current or past use):

Name	Dosage	How Long Used	Why Prescribed	By Whom	Side Effects/Results
_____	_____	_____	_____	_____	_____
_____	_____	_____	_____	_____	_____
_____	_____	_____	_____	_____	_____

CURRENT/PAST USE OF OVER-THE-COUNTER DRUGS (Indicate with "c" or "p" beside name of drug whether current or past use):

Name	Dosage	How Long Used	Why Prescribed	By Whom	Side Effects/Results
_____	_____	_____	_____	_____	_____
_____	_____	_____	_____	_____	_____
_____	_____	_____	_____	_____	_____

CURRENT/PAST USE OF STREET DRUGS, ALCOHOL, NICOTINE, AND/OR CAFFEINE (Indicate with "c" or "p" beside name of drug):

Name	Amount Used	How Often Used	When Last Used	Effects Produced
_____	_____	_____	_____	_____
_____	_____	_____	_____	_____
_____	_____	_____	_____	_____

BOX 4-1 Medication Assessment Tool—cont'd

Any allergies to food or drugs?_____

Any special diet considerations?_____

Do you have (or have you ever had) any of the following? If yes, provide explanation on the back of this sheet.

	Yes No		Yes No		Yes No
Difficulty swallowing	__ __	Chest pain	__ __	Sexual dysfunction	__ __
Delayed wound healing	__ __	Blood clots/pain in legs	__ __	Lumps in your breasts	__ __
Constipation problems	__ __	Fainting spells	__ __	Blurred or double vision	__ __
Urination problems	__ __	Swollen ankles/legs/hands	__ __	Ringing in the ears	__ __
Recent change in		Asthma	__ __	Insomnia	__ __
elimination patterns	__ __	Varicose veins	__ __	Skin Rashes	__ __
Weakness or tremors	__ __	Numbness/tingling		Diabetes	__ __
Seizures	__ __	(location?)	__ __	Hepatitis (or other liver	
Headaches	__ __	Ulcers	__ __	disease)	__ __
Dizziness	__ __	Nausea/vomiting	__ __	Kidney disease	__ __
High blood pressure	__ __	Problems with diarrhea	__ __	Glaucoma	__ __
Palpitations	__ __	Shortness of breath	__ __		

Are you pregnant or breast feeding?_____ Date of last menses_____ Type of contraception used_____

Describe any restrictions/limitations that might interfere with your use of medication for your current problem. _____
_____

Prescription orders: Patient teaching related to medications prescribed:

Lab work or referrals prescribed:

Nurse's signature _____   **Client's signature** _____

---

promotes accurate and effective management of the treatment regimen.

How Do Psychotropics Work?

Most of the medications have their effects at the neuronal synapse, producing changes in neurotransmitter release and the receptors to which they bind (see Figure 4-11). Researchers hypothesize that most antidepressants work by blocking the reuptake of neurotransmitters, specifically, serotonin and norepinephrine. *Reuptake* is the process of neurotransmitter inactivation by which the neurotransmitter is reabsorbed into the presynaptic neuron from which it had been released. Blocking the reuptake process allows more of the neurotransmitter to be available for neuronal transmission. This mechanism of action may also result in undesirable side effects (see Table 4-6). Some antidepressants also block receptor sites that are unrelated to their mechanisms of action. These include alpha-adrenergic, histaminergic, and muscarinic cholinergic receptors. Blocking these receptors is also associated with the development of certain side effects.

Antipsychotic medications block dopamine receptors, and some affect muscarinic cholinergic, histaminergic, and alpha-adrenergic receptors. The "atypical" (or novel) antipsychotics block a specific serotonin receptor. Benzodiazepines facilitate the transmission of the inhibitory neurotransmitter gamma-aminobutyric acid (GABA). The psychostimulants work by increasing norepinephrine, serotonin, and dopamine release.

Although each psychotropic medication affects neurotransmission, the specific drugs within each class have varying neuronal effects. Their exact mechanisms of action are unknown. Many of the neuronal effects occur acutely; however, the therapeutic effects may take weeks for some medications such as antidepressants and antipsychotics. Acute alterations in neuronal function do not fully explain how these medications work. Long-term neuropharmacological reactions to increased norepinephrine and serotonin levels relate more to their mechanisms of action. Recent research suggests that the therapeutic effects are related to the nervous system's adaptation to increased levels of neurotransmitters. These adaptive changes result from a homeostatic mechanism, much like a thermostat, that regulates the cell and maintains equilibrium.

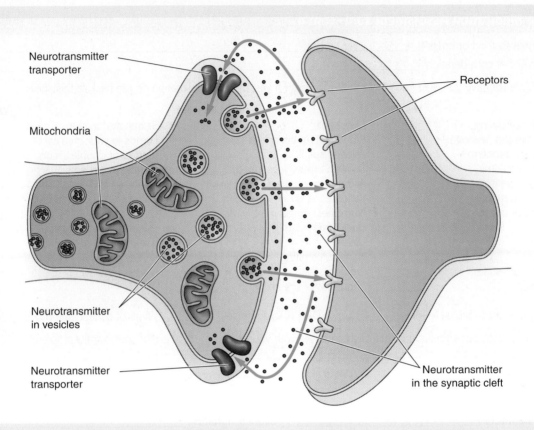

FIGURE 4–11 Area of synaptic transmission that is altered by drugs.

The transmission of electrical impulses from the axon terminal of one neuron to the dendrite of another is achieved by the controlled release of neurotransmitters into the synaptic cleft. Neurotransmitters include serotonin, norepinephrine, acetylcholine, dopamine, glutamate, gamma-aminobutyric acid (GABA), and histamine, among others. Prior to its release, the neurotransmitter is concentrated into specialized synaptic vesicles. Once fired, the neurotransmitter is released into the synaptic cleft where it encounters receptors on the postsynaptic membrane. Each neurotransmitter has receptors specific to it alone. Some neurotransmitters are considered to be excitatory, whereas others are inhibitory, a feature that determines whether another action potential will occur. In the synaptic cleft, the neurotransmitter rapidly diffuses, is catabolized by enzymatic action, or is taken up by the neurotransmitter transporters and returned to vesicles inside the axon terminal to await another action potential.

Psychotropic medications exert their effects in various ways in this area of synaptic transmission. Reuptake inhibitors block reuptake of the neurotransmitters by the transporter proteins, thus resulting in elevated levels of extracellular neurotransmitter. Drugs that inhibit catabolic enzymes promote excess buildup of the neurotransmitter at the synaptic site.

Some drugs cause receptor blockade, thereby resulting in a reduction in transmission and decreased neurotransmitter activity. These drugs are called antagonists. Drugs that increase neurotransmitter activity by direct stimulation of the specific receptors are called agonists.

TABLE 4–6 Effects of Psychotropic Medications on Neurotransmitters

EXAMPLE OF MEDICATION	ACTION ON NEUROTRANSMITTER AND/OR RECEPTOR	PHYSIOLOGICAL EFFECTS	SIDE EFFECTS
SSRIs	Inhibit reuptake of serotonin (5-HT)	Reduces depression Controls anxiety Controls obsessions	Nausea, agitation, headache, sexual dysfunction
Tricyclic antidepressants	Inhibit reuptake of 5-HT Inhibit reuptake of NE Block NE (α_1) receptor Block ACh receptor Block H_1 receptor	Reduces depression Relief of severe pain Prevent panic attacks	Sexual dysfunction (NE & 5-HT) Sedation, weight gain (H_1) Dry mouth, constipation, blurred vision, urinary retention (ACh) Postural hypotension and tachycardia (α_1)

TABLE 4–6	**Effects of Psychotropic Medications on Neurotransmitters–cont'd**		
EXAMPLE OF MEDICATION	ACTION ON NEUROTRANSMITTER AND/OR RECEPTOR	PHYSIOLOGICAL EFFECTS	SIDE EFFECTS
MAO inhibitors	Increase NE and 5-HT by inhibiting the enzyme that degrades them (MAO-A)	Reduces depression Controls anxiety	Sedation, dizziness Sexual dysfunction Hypertensive crisis (interaction with tyramine)
Trazodone and nefazodone	5-HT reuptake block 5-HT$_2$ receptor antagonism Adrenergic receptor blockade	Reduces depression Reduces anxiety	Nausea (5-HT) Sedation (5-HT$_2$) Orthostasis (α_1) Priapism (α_2)
SSNRIs: venlafaxine, desvenlafaxine, duloxetine, and levomilnacipran	Potent inhibitor of 5-HT and NE reuptake Weak inhibitor of D reuptake	Reduces depression Relieves pain of neuropathy (duloxetine) Relieves anxiety (venlafaxine)	Nausea (5-HT) ↑ sweating (NE) Insomnia (NE) Tremors (NE) Sexual dysfunction (5-HT)
Bupropion	Inhibits reuptake of NE and D	Reduces depression Aid in smoking cessation ↓ symptoms of ADHD	Insomnia, dry mouth, tremor, seizures
Antipsychotics: phenothiazines and haloperidol	Strong D$_2$ receptor blockade Weaker blockade of ACh, H$_1$, α_1-adrenergic, and 5-HT$_2$ receptors	Relief of psychosis Relief of anxiety (Some) provide relief from nausea and vomiting and intractable hiccoughs	Blurred vision, dry mouth, decreased sweating, constipation, urinary retention, tachycardia (ACh) EPS (D$_2$) ↑ plasma prolactin (D$_2$) Sedation; weight gain (H$_1$) Ejaculatory difficulty (5-HT$_2$) Postural hypotension (α; H$_1$)
Antipsychotics (Novel): aripiprazole, asenapine, clozapine, iloperidone, lurasidone, olanzepine, paliperidone, quetiapine, risperdone, ziprasidone	Receptor antagonism of 5-HT$_1$ and 5-HT$_2$ D$_1$–D$_5$ (varies with drug) H$_1$ α_1-adrenergic muscarinic (ACh)	Relief of psychosis (with minimal or no EPS) Relief of anxiety Relief of acute mania	Potential with some of the drugs for mild EPS (D$_2$) Sedation, weight gain (H$_1$) Orthostasis and dizziness (α-adrenergic) Blurred vision, dry mouth, decreased sweating, constipation, urinary retention, tachycardia (ACh)
Antianxiety: benzodiazepines	Binds to BZ receptor sites on the GABA$_A$ receptor complex; increases receptor affinity for GABA	Relief of anxiety Sedation	Dependence (with long-term use) Confusion; memory impairment; motor incoordination
Antianxiety: Buspirone	5-HT$_{1A}$ agonist D$_2$ agonist D$_2$ antagonist	Relief of anxiety	Nausea, headache, dizziness Restlessness

ACh, acetylcholine; ADHD, attention-deficit/hyperactivity disorder; BZ, benzodiazepine; D, dopamine; EPS, extrapyramidal symptoms; GABA, gamma-aminobutyric acid; H, histamine; 5-HT, 5-hydroxytryptamine (serotonin); MAO, monoamine oxidase; NE, norepinephrine; SNRI, serotonin-norepinephrine reuptake inhibitor; SSRI, selective serotonin reuptake inhibitor.

Implications for Nursing

The discipline of psychiatric/mental health nursing has always spoken of its role in holistic health care, but historical review reveals that emphasis has been placed on treatment approaches that focus on psychological and social factors. Psychiatric nurses must integrate knowledge of the biological sciences into their practices if they are to ensure safe and effective care to people with mental illness. In the Surgeon General's Report on Mental Health (U.S. Department of Health and Human Services, 1999), Dr. David Satcher wrote:

> The mental health field is far from a complete understanding of the biological, psychological, and sociocultural bases of development, but development

clearly involves interplay among these influences. Understanding the process of development requires knowledge, ranging from the most fundamental level—that of gene expression and interactions between molecules and cells—all the way up to the highest levels of cognition, memory, emotion, and language. The challenge requires integration of concepts from many different disciplines. A fuller understanding of development is not only important in its own right, but it is expected to pave the way for our ultimate understanding of mental health and mental illness and how different factors shape their expression at different stages of the life span. (pp. 61–62)

To ensure a smooth transition from a psychosocial focus to one of biopsychosocial emphasis, nurses must have a clear understanding of the following:

■ *Neuroanatomy and neurophysiology*: the structure and functioning of the various parts of the brain and their correlation to human behavior and psychopathology.
■ *Neuronal processes*: the various functions of the nerve cells, including the role of neurotransmitters, receptors, synaptic activity, and informational pathways.
■ *Neuroendocrinology*: the interaction of the endocrine and nervous systems, and the role that the endocrine glands and their respective hormones play in behavioral functioning.
■ *Circadian rhythms*: the regulation of biochemical functioning over periods of rhythmic cycles and its influence in predicting certain behaviors.
■ *Genetic influences*: the hereditary factors that predispose individuals to certain psychiatric disorders.
■ *Psychoimmunology*: the influence of stress on the immune system and its role in the susceptibility to illness.
■ *Psychopharmacology*: the increasing use of psychotropic drugs in the treatment of mental illness, demanding greater knowledge of psychopharmacological principles and nursing interventions necessary for safe and effective management.
■ *Diagnostic technology*: the importance of keeping informed about the latest in technological procedures for diagnosing alterations in brain structure and function.

Why are these concepts important to the practice of psychiatric/mental health nursing? The interrelationship between psychosocial adaptation and physical functioning has been established. Integrating biological and behavioral concepts into psychiatric nursing practice is essential for nurses to meet the complex needs of clients with mental illness. Psychobiological perspectives must be incorporated into nursing practice, education, and research to attain the evidence-based outcomes necessary for the delivery of competent care.

Summary and Key Points

■ It is important for nurses to understand the interaction between biological and behavioral factors in the development and management of mental illness.
■ Psychobiology is the study of the biological foundations of cognitive, emotional, and behavioral processes.
■ The limbic system has been called "the emotional brain." It is associated with feelings of fear and anxiety; anger, rage, and aggression; love, joy, and hope; and with sexuality and social behavior.
■ The three classes of neurons include afferent (sensory), efferent (motor), and interneurons. The junction between two neurons is called a synapse.
■ Neurotransmitters are chemicals that convey information across synaptic clefts to neighboring target cells. Many neurotransmitters have implications in the etiology of emotional disorders and in the pharmacological treatment of those disorders.
■ Major categories of neurotransmitters include cholinergics, monoamines, amino acids, and neuropeptides.
■ The endocrine system plays an important role in human behavior through the hypothalamic-pituitary axis.
■ Hormones and their circadian rhythm of regulation significantly influence a number of physiological and psychological life cycle phenomena, such as moods, sleep and arousal, stress response, appetite, libido, and fertility.
■ Research continues to validate the role of genetics in psychiatric illness.
■ Familial, twin, and adoption studies suggest that genetics may be implicated in the etiology of schizophrenia, bipolar disorder, depressive disorder, panic disorder, anorexia nervosa, alcoholism, and obsessive-compulsive disorder.
■ Psychoimmunology examines the impact of psychological factors on the immune system.
■ Evidence exists to support a link between psychosocial stressors and suppression of the immune response.
■ Technologies such as magnetic resonance imagery (MRI), computed tomographic (CT) scan, positron emission tomography (PET), and electroencephalography (EEG) are used as diagnostic tools for detecting alterations in psychobiological functioning.

■ Psychotropic medications have given many individuals a chance to function effectively.

■ Nurses must understand the ethical and legal implications associated with the administration of psychotropic medications, and knowledge of the physiological mechanisms by which psychotropic medications exert their effects.

■ Integrating knowledge of the expanding biological focus into psychiatric nursing is essential if nurses are to meet the changing needs of today's psychiatric clients.

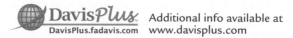

Additional info available at
www.davisplus.com

Review Questions
Self-Examination/Learning Exercise

*Select the answer that is **most** appropriate for each of the following questions:*

1. Which of the following parts of the brain is associated with multiple feelings and behaviors and is sometimes referred to as the "emotional brain?"
   a. Frontal lobe
   b. Thalamus
   c. Hypothalamus
   d. Limbic System

2. Which of the following parts of the brain is concerned with visual reception and interpretation?
   a. Frontal lobe
   b. Parietal lobe
   c. Temporal lobe
   d. Occipital lobe

3. Which of the following parts of the brain is associated with voluntary body movement, thinking and judgment, and expression of feeling?
   a. Frontal lobe
   b. Parietal lobe
   c. Temporal lobe
   d. Occipital lobe

4. Which of the following parts of the brain integrates all sensory input (except smell) on the way to the cortex?
   a. Temporal lobe
   b. Thalamus
   c. Limbic system
   d. Hypothalamus

5. Which of the following parts of the brain deals with sensory perception and interpretation?
   a. Hypothalamus
   b. Cerebellum
   c. Parietal lobe
   d. Hippocampus

6. Which of the following parts of the brain is concerned with hearing, short-term memory, and sense of smell?
   a. Temporal lobe
   b. Parietal lobe
   c. Cerebellum
   d. Hypothalamus

Continued

Review Questions—cont'd
Self-Examination/Learning Exercise

7. Which of the following parts of the brain has control over the pituitary gland and autonomic nervous system, as well as regulation of appetite and temperature?
   a. Temporal lobe
   b. Parietal lobe
   c. Cerebellum
   d. Hypothalamus

8. At a synapse, the determination of further impulse transmission is accomplished by means of which of the following?
   a. Potassium ions
   b. Interneurons
   c. Neurotransmitters
   d. The myelin sheath

9. A decrease in which of the following neurotransmitters has been implicated in depression?
   a. GABA, acetylcholine, and aspartate
   b. Norepinephrine, serotonin, and dopamine
   c. Somatostatin, substance P, and glycine
   d. Glutamate, histamine, and opioid peptides

10. Which of the following hormones has been implicated in the etiology of mood disorder with seasonal pattern?
    a. Increased levels of melatonin
    b. Decreased levels of oxytocin
    c. Decreased levels of prolactin
    d. Increased levels of thyrotropin

11. Psychotropic medications that block the reuptake of serotonin may result in which of the following side effects?
    a. Dry mouth
    b. Constipation
    c. Blurred vision
    d. Sexual dysfunction

12. Psychotropic medications that block the acetylcholine receptor may result in which of the following side effects?
    a. Dry mouth
    b. Sexual dysfunction
    c. Nausea
    d. Priapism

13. Psychotropic medications that are strong blockers of the D_2 receptor are more likely to result in which of the following side effects?
    a. Sedation
    b. Urinary retention
    c. Extrapyramidal symptoms
    d. Hypertensive crisis

References

Baker, C. (2004). *Behavioral genetics.* Washington, DC: American Association for the Advancement of Science.

Black, D.W., & Andreasen, N.C. (2011). *Introductory textbook of psychiatry* (5th ed.). Washington, DC: American Psychiatric Publishing.

Bunney, B.G., Bunney, W.E., & Carlsson, A. (2012). Schizophrenia and glutamate: An update. *Neuropsychopharmacology: The fifth generation of progress.* Retrieved from http://www.acnp.org/g4/gn401000116/ch114.html

Dubovsky, S.L., Davies, R., & Dubovsky, A.N. (2003). Mood disorders. In R.E. Hales & S.C. Yudofsky (Eds.), *Textbook of clinical psychiatry* (4th ed.) (pp. 439–542). Washington, DC: American Psychiatric Publishing.

Gill, M. (2004). Genetic approaches to the understanding of mental illness. *Genes and Mental Health.* Public symposium, October 9, 2004, Department of Psychiatry. Dublin, Ireland: Trinity College.

Gilman, S., & Newman, S.W. (2003). *Essentials of clinical neuroanatomy and neurophysiology* (10th ed.). Philadelphia, PA: F.A. Davis.

Hamosh, A., Scharer, G., & Van Hove, J. (2009). Glycine encephalopathy. *GeneReviews.* National Library of Medicine. Retrieved from http://www.ncbi.nlm.nih.gov/books/NBK1357

Hughes, M. (1989). *Body clock: The effects of time on human health.* New York, NY: Andromeda Oxford.

Irwin, M. (2000). Psychoneuroimmunology of depression. In F.E. Bloom & D.J. Kupfer (Eds.), *Psychopharmacology—The fourth generation of progress.* Nashville, TN: American College of Neuropsychopharmacology.

Knowles, J.A. (2003). Genetics. In R.E. Hales & S.C. Yudofsky (Eds.), *Textbook of psychiatry* (4th ed.) (pp. 3–65). Washington, DC: American Psychiatric Publishing.

Lis, C.G., Grutsch, J.F., Wood, P., You, M., Rich, I., & Hrushesky, W.J. (2003). Circadian timing in cancer treatment: The biological foundation for an integrative approach. *Integrative Cancer Therapies, 2*(2), 105–111.

McInerney, J. (2008). Behavioral genetics. *The Human Genome Project.* Retrieved from http://www.ornl.gov/sci/techresources/Human_Genome/elsi/behavior.shtml

National Institute on Aging. (2012). The Alzheimer's Disease Education and Referral Center. *Alzheimer's disease genetics.* Retrieved from http://www.nia.nih.gov/alzheimers/publication/alzheimers-disease-genetics-fact-sheet

O'Donovan, M. (2012). Genes and mental disorders. *Genetic Futures News.* Retrieved from http://www.geneticfutures.com/cracked/info/sheet3.asp

Ouellet-Plamondon, C., & George, T.P. (2012). Glutamate and psychiatry in 2012—up, up and away! *Psychiatric Times, 29*(12), 1–5.

Sadock, B.J., & Sadock, V.A. (2007). *Synopsis of psychiatry: Behavioral sciences/clinical psychiatry* (10th ed.). Philadelphia, PA: Lippincott Williams & Wilkins.

Sage, D.L. (Producer). (1984). *The Brain: Madness* [Television Broadcast]. Washington, DC: Public Broadcasting Company.

Scanlon, V.C., & Sanders, T. (2011). *Essentials of anatomy and physiology* (6th ed.). Philadelphia, PA: F.A. Davis.

Skudaev, S. (2010). The neurophysiology and neurochemistry of sleep. Retrieved from http://www.healthstairs.com/sleep3.php

U.S. Department of Health and Human Services. (1999). *Mental Health: A report of the Surgeon General—Executive Summary.* Rockville, MD: U.S. Department of Health and Human Services.

Van Cauter, E., Kerkhofs, M., Caufriez, A., Van Onderbergen, A., Thorner, M.O. & Copinschi, G. (1992). A quantitative estimation of growth hormone secretion in normal man: Reproducibility and relation to sleep and time of day. *Journal of Clinical Endocrinology and Metabolism, 74,* 1441–1450.

5

Ethical and Legal Issues in Psychiatric/Mental Health Nursing

KARYN I. MORGAN AND MARY C. TOWNSEND

CORE CONCEPTS

bioethics

ethics

moral behavior

right

values

values clarification

KEY TERMS

advocacy	defamation of character	natural law
assault	ethical dilemma	negligence
autonomy	ethical egoism	nonmaleficence
battery	false imprisonment	privileged communication
beneficence	informed consent	slander
Christian ethics	justice	statutory law
civil law	Kantianism	tort
common laws	libel	utilitarianism
criminal law	malpractice	veracity

OBJECTIVES

After reading this chapter, the student will be able to:

1. Differentiate among e*thics, morals, values,* and *rights*.
2. Discuss ethical theories including *utilitarianism, Kantianism, Christian ethics, natural law* theories, and *ethical egoism*.
3. Define *ethical dilemma*.
4. Discuss the ethical principles of *autonomy, beneficence, nonmaleficence, justice*, and *veracity*.
5. Use an ethical decision-making model to make an ethical decision.
6. Describe ethical issues relevant to psychiatric/mental health nursing.
7. Define *statutory law* and *common law*.
8. Differentiate between *civil law* and *criminal law*.
9. Discuss legal issues relevant to psychiatric/mental health nursing.
10. Differentiate between *malpractice* and *negligence*.
11. Identify behaviors relevant to the psychiatric/mental health setting for which specific malpractice action could be taken.

HOMEWORK ASSIGNMENT

Please read the chapter and answer the following questions:

1. Malpractice and negligence are examples of what kind of law?
2. What charges may be brought against a nurse for confining a client against his or her wishes (outside of an emergency situation)?
3. Which ethical theory espouses that what is right and good is what is best for the individual making the decision?
4. Name the three major elements of informed consent.

Nurses are constantly faced with the challenge of making difficult decisions regarding good and evil or life and death. Complex situations frequently arise in caring for individuals with mental illness, and nurses are held to the highest level of legal and ethical accountability in their professional practice. This chapter presents basic ethical and legal concepts and their relationship to psychiatric/mental health nursing. A discussion of ethical theory is presented as a foundation upon which ethical decisions may be made. The American Nurses' Association (ANA) (2001) has established a code of ethics for nurses to use as a framework within which to make ethical choices and decisions (Box 5-1).

Because legislation determines what is *right* or *good* within a society, legal issues pertaining to psychiatric/mental health nursing are also discussed in this chapter. Definitions are presented, along with rights of psychiatric clients of which nurses must be aware. Nursing competency and client care accountability are compromised when the nurse has inadequate knowledge about the laws that regulate the practice of nursing.

Knowledge of the legal and ethical concepts presented in this chapter will enhance the quality of care the nurse provides in his or her psychiatric/mental health nursing practice and will also protect the nurse within the parameters of legal accountability. Indeed, the very right to practice nursing carries with it the responsibility to maintain a specific level of competency and to practice in accordance with certain ethical and legal standards of care.

CORE CONCEPTS

Ethics is a branch of philosophy that deals with systematic approaches to distinguishing right from wrong behavior (Butts & Rich, 2008). **Bioethics** is the term applied to these principles when they refer to concepts within the scope of medicine, nursing, and allied health.

Moral behavior is defined as conduct that results from serious critical thinking about how individuals ought to treat others. Moral behavior reflects the way a person interprets basic respect for other persons, such as the respect for autonomy, freedom, justice, honesty, and confidentiality.

Values are personal beliefs about what is important and desirable (Butts & Rich, 2008). **Values clarification** is a process of self-exploration through which individuals identify and rank their own personal values. This process increases awareness about why individuals behave in certain ways. Values clarification is important in nursing to increase understanding about why certain choices and decisions are made over others and how values affect nursing outcomes.

A **right** is defined as "a valid, legally recognized claim or entitlement, encompassing both freedom from government interference or discriminatory treatment and an entitlement to a benefit or service" (Levy and Rubenstein, 1996). A right is *absolute* when there is no restriction whatsoever on the individual's entitlement. A *legal right* is one on which the society has agreed and formalized into law. Both the National League for Nursing (NLN) and the American Hospital Association (AHA) have established guidelines of patients' rights. Although these are not considered legal documents, nurses and hospitals are considered responsible for upholding these rights of patients.

BOX 5-1 American Nurses' Association Code of Ethics for Nurses

1. The nurse, in all professional relationships, practices with compassion and respect for the inherent dignity, worth and uniqueness of every individual, unrestricted by consideration of social or economic status, personal attributes, or the nature of health problems.
2. The nurse's primary commitment is to the patient whether an individual, family, group or community.
3. The nurse promotes, advocates for and strives to protect the health, safety, and rights of the patient.
4. The nurse is responsible and accountable for individual nursing practice and determines the appropriate delegation of tasks consistent with the nurse's obligation to provide optimum patient care.
5. The nurse owes the same duties to self as to others, including the responsibility to preserve integrity and safety, to maintain competence, and to continue personal and professional growth.
6. The nurse participates in establishing, maintaining, and improving healthcare environments and conditions of employment conducive to the provision of quality healthcare and consistent with the values of the profession through individual and collective action.
7. The nurse participates in the advancement of the profession through contributions to practice, education, administration, and knowledge development.
8. The nurse collaborates with other health professionals and the public in promoting community, national, and international efforts to meet health needs.
9. The profession of nursing, as represented by associations and their members, is responsible for articulating nursing values, for maintaining the integrity of the profession and its practice, and for shaping social policy.

Ethical Considerations

Theoretical Perspectives

An *ethical theory* is a moral principle or a set of moral principles that can be used in assessing what is morally right or morally wrong (Ellis & Hartley, 2012). These principles provide guidelines for ethical decision making.

Utilitarianism

The basis of **utilitarianism** is "the greatest-happiness principle." This principle holds that actions are right to the degree that they tend to promote happiness and wrong as they tend to produce the reverse of happiness. Thus, the good is happiness and the right is that which promotes the good. Conversely, the wrongness of an action is determined by its tendency to bring about unhappiness. An ethical decision based on the utilitarian view looks at the end results of the decision. Action is taken based on the end results that produced the most good (happiness) for the most people.

Kantianism

Named for philosopher Immanuel Kant, **Kantianism** is directly opposed to utilitarianism. Kant argued that it is not the consequences or end results that make an action right or wrong; rather it is the principle or motivation on which the action is based that is the morally decisive factor. Kantianism suggests that our actions are bound by a sense of duty. This theory is often called *deontology* (from the Greek word *deon*, which means "that which is binding; duty"). Kantian-directed ethical decisions are made out of respect for moral law. For example, "I make this choice because it is morally right and my duty to do so" (not because of consideration for a possible outcome).

Christian Ethics

This approach to ethical decision making is focused on the way of life and teachings of Jesus Christ. It advances the importance of virtues such as love, forgiveness, and honesty. One basic principle often associated with Christian ethics is known as the golden rule: "Do unto others as you would have them do unto you." The imperative demand of **Christian ethics** is that all decisions about right and wrong should be centered in love for God and in treating others with the same respect and dignity with which we would expect to be treated.

Natural Law Theory

Natural law theory is based on the writings of St. Thomas Aquinas. It advances the idea that decisions about right versus wrong are self-evident and determined by human nature. The theory espouses that, as rational human beings, we inherently know the difference between good and evil (believed to be knowledge that is given to man from God), and this knowledge directs our decision making.

Ethical Egoism

Ethical egoism espouses that what is right and good is what is best for the individual making the decision. An individual's actions are determined by what is to his or her own advantage. The action may not be best for anyone else involved, but consideration is only for the individual making the decision.

Ethical Dilemmas

An **ethical dilemma** is a situation that requires an individual to make a choice between two equally unfavorable alternatives (Catalano, 2012). Evidence exists to support both moral "rightness" and moral "wrongness" related to a certain action. The individual who must make the choice experiences conscious conflict regarding the decision.

Not all ethical issues are dilemmas. An ethical dilemma arises when there is no clear reason to choose one action over another. Ethical dilemmas generally create a great deal of emotion. Often the reasons supporting each side of the argument for action are logical and appropriate. The actions associated with both sides are desirable in some respects and undesirable in others. In most situations, taking no action is considered an action taken.

Ethical Principles

Ethical principles are fundamental guidelines that influence decision making. The ethical principles of autonomy, beneficence, nonmaleficence, veracity, and justice are helpful and used frequently by health-care workers to assist with ethical decision making.

Autonomy

The principle of **autonomy** arises from the Kantian duty of respect for persons as rational agents. This viewpoint emphasizes the status of persons as autonomous moral agents whose right to determine their destinies should always be respected. This presumes that individuals are always capable of making independent choices for themselves. Health-care workers know this is not always the case. Children, comatose individuals, and people with serious mental illness are examples of clients who are incapable of making informed choices. In these instances, a representative of the individual is usually asked to intervene and give consent. However, health-care workers must ensure that respect for an individual's autonomy is not disregarded in favor of what another person may view as best for the client.

Beneficence

Beneficence refers to one's duty to benefit or promote the good of others. Health-care workers who act in their clients' interests are beneficent, provided their actions really do serve the client's best interest. In fact, some duties do seem to take preference over other duties. For example, the duty to respect the autonomy of an individual may be overridden when that individual has been deemed harmful to self or others. Aiken (2004) stated, "The difficulty that sometimes arises in implementing the principle of beneficence lies in determining what exactly is good for another and who can best make that decision" (p. 109).

Peplau (1991) recognized client **advocacy** as an essential role for the psychiatric nurse. The term *advocacy* means acting in another's behalf—being a supporter or defender. Being a client advocate in psychiatric nursing means helping the client fulfill needs that, without assistance and because of the client's illness, may go unfulfilled. Individuals with mental illness are not always able to speak for themselves. Nurses serve in this manner to protect the client's rights and interests. Strategies include educating clients and their families about their legal rights, ensuring that clients have sufficient information to make informed decisions or to give informed consent, and assisting clients to consider alternatives and supporting them in the decisions they make. Additionally, nurses may act as advocates by speaking on behalf of individuals with mental illness to secure essential mental health services.

Nonmaleficence

Nonmaleficence is the requirement that health-care providers do no harm to their clients, either intentionally or unintentionally (Aiken, 2004). Some philosophers suggest that this principle is more important than beneficence; that is, they support the notion that it is more important to avoid doing harm than it is to do good. In any event, ethical dilemmas often arise when a conflict exists between an individual's rights and what is thought to best represent the welfare of the individual. An example of this conflict might occur when a psychiatric client refuses antipsychotic medication (consistent with his or her rights), and the nurse must then decide how to maintain client safety while psychotic symptoms continue.

Justice

The principle of **justice** has been referred to as the "justice as fairness" principle. It is sometimes referred to as *distributive justice*, and its basic premise lies with the right of individuals to be treated equally regardless of race, sex, marital status, medical diagnosis, social standing, economic level, or religious belief (Aiken, 2004). The concept of justice reflects a duty to treat all individuals equally and fairly. When applied to health care, this principle suggests that all resources within the society (including health-care services) ought to be distributed evenly without respect to socioeconomic status. Thus, according to this principle, the vast disparity in the quality of care dispensed to the various classes within our society would be considered unjust. A more equitable distribution of care for all individuals would be favored.

Veracity

The principle of **veracity** refers to one's duty to always be truthful. Aiken (2004) stated, "Veracity requires that the health-care provider tell the truth and not intentionally deceive or mislead clients" (p. 109). There are times when limitations must be placed on this principle, such as when the truth would knowingly produce harm or interfere with the recovery process. Being honest is not always easy, but rarely is lying justified. Clients have the right to know about their diagnosis, treatment, and prognosis.

A Model for Making Ethical Decisions

The following is a set of steps that may be used in making an ethical decision. These steps closely resemble the steps of the nursing process.

1. **Assessment:** Gather the subjective and objective data about a situation. Consider personal values as well as values of others involved in the ethical dilemma.
2. **Problem identification:** Identify the conflict between two or more alternative actions.
3. **Planning:**
   a. Explore the benefits and consequences of each alternative.
   b. Consider principles of ethical theories.
   c. Select an alternative.
4. **Implementation:** Act on the decision made and communicate the decision to others.
5. **Evaluation:** Evaluate outcomes.

A schematic of this model is presented in Figure 5-1. A case study using this decision-making model is presented in Box 5-2. If the outcome is acceptable, action continues in the manner selected. If the outcome is unacceptable, benefits and consequences of the remaining alternatives are reexamined, and steps 3 through 7 in Box 5-2 are repeated.

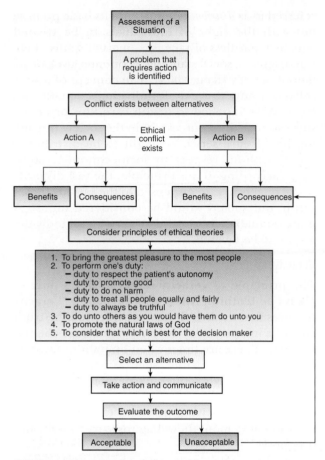

FIGURE 5–1 Ethical decision-making model.

Ethical Issues in Psychiatric/Mental Health Nursing

The Right to Refuse Medication

The AHA's (1992) Patient's Bill of Rights states: "The patient has the right to refuse treatment to the extent permitted by law, and to be informed of the medical consequences of his action." In psychiatry, refusal of treatment primarily concerns the administration of psychotropic medications. "To the extent permitted by law" may be defined within the U.S. Constitution and several of its amendments (e.g., the First Amendment, which addresses the rights of speech, thought, and expression; the Eighth Amendment, which grants the right to freedom from cruel and unusual punishment; and the Fifth and Fourteenth Amendments, which grant due process of law and equal protection for all). In psychiatry, "the medical consequences of his action" may include such steps as involuntary commitment, legal competency hearing, or client discharge from the hospital.

Although many courts are supporting a client's right to refuse medications in the psychiatric area, some limitations do exist. Weiss-Kaffie and Purtell (2001) stated:

> The treatment team must determine that three criteria be met to force medication without client consent. The client must exhibit behavior that is dangerous to self or others; the medication ordered by

---

BOX 5-2 Ethical Decision Making—A Case Study

STEP 1: ASSESSMENT
Tonja is a 17-year-old girl who is currently on the psychiatric unit with a diagnosis of conduct disorder. Tonja reports that she has been sexually active since she was 14. She had an abortion when she was 15 and a second one just 6 weeks ago. She states that her mother told her she has "had her last abortion," and that she has to start taking birth control pills. She asks her nurse, Kimberly, to give her some information about the pills and to tell her how to go about getting some. Kimberly believes Tonja desperately needs information about birth control pills, as well as other types of contraceptives, but the psychiatric unit is part of a Catholic hospital, and hospital policy prohibits distributing this type of information.

STEP 2: PROBLEM IDENTIFICATION
A conflict exists between the client's need for information, the nurse's desire to provide that information, and the institution's policy prohibiting the provision of that information.

STEP 3: ALTERNATIVES—BENEFITS AND CONSEQUENCES
1. Alternative 1: Give the client information and risk losing job.

2. Alternative 2: Do not give client information and compromise own values of holistic nursing.
3. Alternative 3: Refer client to another source outside the hospital and risk reprimand from supervisor.

STEP 4: CONSIDER PRINCIPLES OF ETHICAL THEORIES
1. Alternative 1: Giving the client information would certainly respect the client's autonomy and would benefit the client by decreasing her chances of becoming pregnant again. It would not be to the best advantage of Kimberly, in that she would likely lose her job. And according to the beliefs of the Catholic hospital, the natural laws of God would be violated.
2. Alternative 2: Withholding information restricts the client's autonomy. It has the potential for doing harm, in that without the use of contraceptives, the client may become pregnant again (and she implies that this is not what she wants). Kimberly's Christian ethic is violated in that this action is not what she would want "done unto her."
3. Alternative 3: A referral would respect the client's autonomy, would promote good, would do no harm (except perhaps to Kimberly's ego from the possible reprimand),

---

BOX 5-2 Ethical Decision Making—A Case Study—cont'd

and this decision would comply with Kimberly's Christian ethic.

STEP 5: SELECT AN ALTERNATIVE
Alternative 3 is selected based on the ethical theories of utilitarianism (does the most good for the greatest number), Christian ethics (Kimberly's belief of "Do unto others as you would have others do unto you"), and Kantianism (to perform one's duty), and the ethical principles of autonomy, beneficence, and nonmaleficence. The success of this decision depends on the client's follow-through with the referral and compliance with use of the contraceptives.

STEP 6: TAKE ACTION AND COMMUNICATE
Taking action involves providing information in writing for Tonja, perhaps making a phone call and setting up an appointment for her with Planned Parenthood. Communicating suggests sharing the information with Tonja's mother. Communication also includes documentation of the referral in the client's chart.

STEP 7: EVALUATE THE OUTCOME
An acceptable outcome might indicate that Tonja did indeed keep her appointment at Planned Parenthood and is complying with the prescribed contraceptive regimen. It might also include Kimberly's input into the change process in her institution to implement these types of referrals to other clients who request them.

An unacceptable outcome might be indicated by Tonja's lack of follow-through with the appointment at Planned Parenthood or lack of compliance in using the contraceptives, resulting in another pregnancy. Kimberly may also view a reprimand from her supervisor as an unacceptable outcome, particularly if she is told that she must select other alternatives should this situation arise in the future. This may motivate Kimberly to make another decision—that of seeking employment in an institution that supports a philosophy more consistent with her own.

---

the physician must have a reasonable chance of providing help to the client; and clients who refuse medication must be judged incompetent to evaluate the benefits of the treatment in question. (p. 361)

The Right to the Least-Restrictive Treatment Alternative

Health-care personnel must attempt to provide treatment in a manner that least restricts the freedom of clients. The "restrictiveness" of psychiatric therapy can be described in the context of a continuum, based on severity of illness. Clients may be treated on an outpatient basis, in day hospitals, or through voluntary or involuntary hospitalization. Symptoms may be treated with verbal rehabilitative techniques and move successively to behavioral techniques, chemical interventions, mechanical restraints, or electroconvulsive therapy. The problem appears to arise in selecting the least restrictive means among involuntary chemical intervention, seclusion, and mechanical restraints. Sadock and Sadock (2007) stated:

> Distinguishing among these interventions on the basis of restrictiveness proves to be a purely subjective exercise fraught with personal bias. Moreover, each of these three interventions is both more and less restrictive than each of the other two. Nevertheless, the effort should be made to think in terms of restrictiveness when deciding how to treat patients. (p. 1376)

Legal Considerations

The Patient Self-determination Act, as part of the Omnibus Budget Reconciliation Act of 1990,

went into effect on December 1, 1991. Cady (2010) states:

> The Patient Self-determination Act requires healthcare facilities to provide clear written information for every patient concerning his/her legal rights to make healthcare decisions, including the right to accept or refuse treatment. (p. 118)

Box 5-3 lists the rights of patients affirmed by this law.

Nurse Practice Acts

The legal parameters of professional and practical nursing are defined within each state by the state's nurse practice act. These documents are passed by the state legislature and in general are concerned with such provisions as the following:

■ The definition of important terms, including the definition of nursing and the various types of nurses recognized
■ A statement of the education and other training or requirements for licensure and reciprocity
■ Broad statements that describe the scope of practice for various levels of nursing (APN, RN, LPN)
■ Conditions under which a nurse's license may be suspended or revoked, and instructions for appeal
■ The general authority and powers of the state board of nursing

Most nurse practice acts are general in their terminology and do not provide specific guidelines for practice. Nurses must understand the scope of practice that is protected by their license, and should seek

---

BOX 5-3 Patient Self-determination Act–Patient Rights

1. The right to appropriate treatment and related services in a setting and under conditions that are the most supportive of such person's personal liberty and restrict such liberty only to the extent necessary consistent with such person's treatment needs, applicable requirements of law, and applicable judicial orders.
2. The right to an individualized, written treatment or service plan (such plan to be developed promptly after admission of such person), the right to treatment based on such plan, the right to periodic review and reassessment of treatment and related service needs, and the right to appropriate revision of such plan, including any revision necessary to provide a description of mental health services that may be needed after such person is discharged from such program or facility.
3. The right to ongoing participation, in a manner appropriate to a person's capabilities, in the planning of mental health services to be provided (including the right to participate in the development and periodic revision of the plan).
4. The right to be provided with a reasonable explanation, in terms and language appropriate to a person's condition and ability to understand the person's general mental and physical (if appropriate) condition, the objectives of treatment, the nature and significant possible adverse effects of recommended treatment, the reasons why a particular treatment is considered appropriate, and reasons why access to certain visitors may not be appropriate, and any appropriate and available alternative treatments, services, and types of providers of mental health services.

5. The right not to receive a mode or course of treatment in the absence of informed, voluntary, written consent to treatment except during an emergency situation or as permitted by law when the person is being treated as a result of a court order.
6. The right not to participate in experimentation in the absence of informed, voluntary, written consent (includes human subject protection).
7. The right to freedom from restraint or seclusion, other than as a mode or course of treatment or restraint or seclusion during an emergency situation with a written order by a responsible mental health professional.
8. The right to a humane treatment environment that affords reasonable protection from harm and appropriate privacy with regard to personal needs.
9. The right to access, on request, to such person's mental health-care records.
10. The right, in the case of a person admitted on a residential or inpatient care basis, to converse with others privately, to have convenient and reasonable access to the telephone and mail, and to see visitors during regularly scheduled hours. (For treatment purposes, specific individuals may be excluded.)
11. The right to be informed promptly and in writing at the time of admission of these rights.
12. The right to assert grievances with respect to infringement of these rights.
13. The right to exercise these rights without reprisal.
14. The right of referral to other providers upon discharge.

Adapted from the U.S. Code, Title 42, Section 10841, The Public Health and Welfare, 1991.

---

assistance from legal counsel if they are unsure about the proper interpretation of a nurse practice act.

Types of Law

There are two general categories or types of law that are of most concern to nurses: statutory law and common law. These laws are identified by their source or origin.

Statutory Law

A **statutory law** is a law that has been enacted by a legislative body, such as a county or city council, state legislature, or the U.S. Congress. An example of statutory law is the nurse practice acts.

Common Law

Common laws are derived from decisions made in previous cases. These laws apply to a body of principles that evolve from court decisions resolving various controversies. Because common law in the United States has been developed on a state basis, the law on specific subjects may differ from state to state. An example of a common law might be how different states

deal with a nurse's refusal to provide care for a specific client.

Classifications Within Statutory and Common Law

Broadly speaking, there are two kinds of unlawful acts: civil and criminal. Both statutory law and common law have civil and criminal components.

Civil Law

Civil law protects the private and property rights of individuals and businesses. Private individuals or groups may bring a legal action to court for breach of civil law. These legal actions are of two basic types: torts and contracts.

Torts

A **tort** is a violation of a civil law in which an individual has been wronged. In a tort action, one party asserts that wrongful conduct on the part of the other has caused harm, and seeks compensation for harm suffered. A tort may be *intentional* or *unintentional*. Examples of unintentional torts are malpractice and negligence actions. An example of an intentional tort is the touching of another person without that person's consent. Intentional touching (e.g., a medical treatment) without the client's consent can result in a charge of battery, an intentional tort.

Contracts

In a contract action, one party asserts that the other party, in failing to fulfill an obligation, has breached the contract, and either compensation or performance of the obligation is sought as remedy. An example is an action by a mental health professional whose clinical privileges have been reduced or terminated in violation of an implied contract between the professional and a hospital.

Criminal Law

Criminal law provides protection from conduct deemed injurious to the public welfare. It provides for punishment of those found to have engaged in such conduct, which commonly includes imprisonment, parole conditions, a loss of privilege (such as a license), a fine, or any combination of these (Ellis & Hartley, 2012). An example of a violation of criminal law is the theft by a hospital employee of supplies or drugs.

Legal Issues in Psychiatric/Mental Health Nursing

Confidentiality and Right to Privacy

The Fourth, Fifth, and Fourteenth Amendments to the U.S. Constitution protect an individual's privacy. Most states have statutes protecting the confidentiality of client records and communications. The only individuals who have a right to observe a client or have access to medical information are those involved in his or her medical care.

HIPPA

Until 1996, client confidentiality in medical records was not protected by federal law. In August 1996, President Clinton signed the Health Insurance Portability and Accountability Act (HIPAA) into law. Under this law, individuals have the rights to access their medical records, to have corrections made to their medical records, and to decide with whom their medical information may be shared. The actual document belongs to the facility or the therapist, but the information contained therein belongs to the client.

This federal privacy rule pertains to data that is called *protected health information* (PHI) and applies to most individuals and institutions involved in health care. Notice of privacy policies must be provided to clients upon entry into the health-care system. PHI is individually identifiable health information indicators that "relate to past, present, or future physical or mental health or condition of the individual, or the past, present, or future payment for the provision of health care to an individual; and (1) that identifies the individual; or (2) with respect to which there is a reasonable basis to believe the information can be used to identify the individual" (U.S. Department of Health and Human Services, 2003). These specific identifiers are listed in Box 5-4.

Pertinent medical information may be released without consent in a life-threatening situation. If information is released in an emergency, the following information must be recorded in the client's record: date of disclosure, person to whom information was disclosed, reason for disclosure, reason written consent could not be obtained, and the specific information disclosed.

Most states have statutes that pertain to the doctrine of **privileged communication**. Although the codes

---

BOX 5-4 Protected Health Information (PIH): Individually Identifiable Indicators

1. Names
2. Postal address information, (except state), including street address, city, county, precinct, and zip code
3. All elements of dates (except year) for dates directly related to an individual, including birth date, admission date, discharge date, date of death; and all ages over 89 and all elements of dates (including year) indicative of such age, except that such ages and elements may be aggregated into a single category of age 90 or older
4. Telephone numbers
5. Fax numbers
6. Electronic mail addresses
7. Social Security numbers
8. Medical record numbers
9. Health plan beneficiary numbers
10. Account numbers
11. Certificate/license numbers
12. Vehicle identifiers and serial numbers, including license plate numbers
13. Device identifiers and serial numbers
14. Web Universal Resource Locators (URLs)
15. Internet protocol (IP) address numbers
16. Biometric identifiers, including finger and voice prints
17. Full face photographic images and any comparable images
18. Any other unique identifying number, characteristic, or code

From U.S. Department of Health and Human Services (2003). Standards for privacy of individually identifiable health information. *Washington, DC: Author.*

differ markedly from state to state, most grant certain professionals privileges under which they may refuse to reveal information about, and communications with, clients. In most states, the doctrine of privileged communication applies to psychiatrists and attorneys; in some instances, psychologists, clergy, and nurses are also included.

In certain instances nurses may be called on to testify in cases in which the medical record is used as evidence. In most states, the right to privacy of these records is exempted in civil or criminal proceedings. Therefore, it is important that nurses document with these possibilities in mind. Strict record keeping using statements that are objective and nonjudgmental, having care plans that are specific in their prescriptive interventions, and keeping documentation that describes those interventions and their subsequent evaluation all serve the best interests of the client, the nurse, and the institution should questions regarding care arise. Documentation very often weighs heavily in malpractice case decisions.

The right to confidentiality is a basic one, and especially so in psychiatry. Although societal attitudes are improving, individuals have experienced discrimination in the past for no other reason than for having a history of emotional illness. Nurses working in psychiatry must guard the privacy of their clients with great diligence.

Exception: A Duty to Warn (Protection of a Third Party)

There are exceptions to the laws of privacy and confidentiality. One of these exceptions stems from the 1974 case of *Tarasoff v. Regents of the University of California*. The incident from which this case evolved came about in the late 1960s. A young man from Bengal, India (Mr. P.), who was a graduate student at the University of California (UC), Berkeley, fell in love with another university student (Ms. Tarasoff). Because she was not interested in an exclusive relationship with Mr. P., he became very resentful and angry. He began to stalk her and to record some of their conversations in an effort to determine why she didn't love him. He soon became very depressed and neglected his health, appearance, and studies.

Ms. Tarasoff spent the summer of 1969 in South America. During this time Mr. P. entered therapy with a psychologist at UC. He confided in the psychologist that he intended to kill his former girlfriend (identifying her by name) when she returned from vacation. The psychologist recommended civil commitment for Mr. P., claiming he was suffering from acute and severe paranoid schizophrenia. Mr. P. was picked up by the campus police but released a short time later because he appeared rational and promised to stay away

from Ms. Tarasoff. Neither Ms. Tarasoff nor her parents received any warning of the threat of Mr. P.'s intention to kill her.

When Ms. Tarasoff returned to campus in October 1969, Mr. P. resumed his stalking behavior and eventually stabbed her to death. Ms. Tarasoff's parents sued the psychologist, several psychiatrists, and the university for failure to warn. The case was referred to the California Supreme Court, which ruled that a mental health professional has a duty not only to a client, but also to individuals who are being threatened by that client. The Court stated:

> Once a therapist does in fact determine, or under applicable professional standards should have determined, that a patient poses a serious danger of violence to others, he bears a duty to exercise reasonable care to protect the foreseeable victim of that danger. While the discharge of this duty of due care will necessarily vary with the facts of each case, in each instance the adequacy of the therapist's conduct must be measured against the traditional negligence standard of reasonable care under the circumstances. (*Tarasoff v. Regents of University of California*, 1974a)

The defendants argued that warning the woman or her family would have breached professional ethics and violated the client's right to privacy. But the court ruled that "the confidential character of patient-psychotherapist communications must yield to the extent that disclosure is essential to avert danger to others. The protective privilege ends where the public peril begins" (*Tarasoff v. Regents of University of California*, 1974b).

In 1976, the California Supreme Court expanded the original case ruling (now referred to as *Tarasoff I*). The second ruling (known as *Tarasoff II*) broadened the ruling of "duty to warn" to include "duty to protect." They stated that, under certain circumstances, a therapist might be required to warn an individual, notify police, or take whatever steps are necessary to protect the intended victim from harm. This duty to protect can also "occur in instances when patients, because of their vulnerable state and their inability to distinguish potentially harmful situations, must be protected by healthcare providers" (Guido, 2010, p. 413).

The Tarasoff rulings created a great deal of controversy in the psychiatric community regarding breach of confidentiality and the subsequent negative impact on the client-therapist relationship. However, most states now recognize that therapists have ethical and legal obligations to prevent their clients from harming themselves or others. Many states have passed their own variations on the original "protect and warn" legislation, but in most cases, courts have outlined the following guidelines for therapists to follow in determining their obligation to take protective measures:

1. Assessment of a threat of violence by a client toward another individual
2. Identification of the intended victim
3. Ability to intervene in a feasible, meaningful way to protect the intended victim

When these guidelines apply to a specific situation, it is reasonable for the therapist to notify the victim, law enforcement authorities, and/or relatives of the intended victim. They may also consider initiating voluntary or involuntary commitment of the client in an effort to prevent potential violence.

Implications for Nursing Advanced practice psychiatric nurses who are licensed to practice independently would be held to the same duty as other therapists. Generalist psychiatric nurses who are not acting independently, but rather under the supervision of a psychiatrist, nevertheless have a responsibility to protect a third party who is being threatened by the client. If a client confides in the nurse the potential for harm to an intended victim, it is the duty of the nurse to report this information to the psychiatrist or to other team members. This is not a breach of confidentiality and the nurse may be considered negligent for failure to do so. All members of the treatment team must be made aware of the potential danger that the client poses to self or others. Detailed written documentation of the situation is also essential.

Informed Consent

According to law, all individuals have the right to decide whether to accept or reject treatment. A healthcare provider can be charged with assault and battery for providing life-sustaining treatment to a client when the client has not agreed to it. The rationale for the doctrine of **informed consent** is the preservation and protection of individual autonomy in determining what will and will not happen to the person's body (Guido, 2010).

Informed consent is a client's permission granted to a physician to perform a therapeutic procedure, before which information about the procedure has been presented to the client with adequate time given for consideration about the pros and cons. The client should receive information such as what treatment alternatives are available; why the physician believes this treatment is most appropriate; the possible outcomes, risks, and adverse effects; the possible outcome should the client select another treatment alternative; and the possible outcome should the client choose to have no treatment. An example of a treatment in the psychiatric area that requires informed consent is electroconvulsive therapy.

There are some conditions under which treatment may be performed without obtaining informed consent. A client's refusal to accept treatment may be challenged under the following circumstances: (Aiken, 2004; Guido, 2010; Levy & Rubenstein, 1996; Mackay, 2001):

1. When a client is mentally incompetent to make a decision and treatment is necessary to preserve life or avoid serious harm
2. When refusing treatment endangers the life or health of another
3. During an emergency, in which a client is in no condition to exercise judgment
4. When the client is a child (consent is obtained from parent or surrogate)
5. In the case of therapeutic privilege: Information about a treatment may be withheld if the physician can show that full disclosure would
   a. hinder or complicate necessary treatment
   b. cause severe psychological harm, or
   c. be so upsetting as to render a rational decision by the client impossible

Although most clients in psychiatric/mental health facilities are competent and capable of giving informed consent, those with severe psychiatric illness do not possess the cognitive ability to do so. If an individual has been legally determined to be mentally incompetent, consent is obtained from the legal guardian. Difficulty arises when no legal determination has been made, but the individual's current mental state prohibits informed decision making (e.g., the person who is psychotic, unconscious, or inebriated). In these instances, informed consent is usually obtained from the individual's nearest relative, or if none exist and time permits, the physician may ask the court to appoint a conservator or guardian. When time does not permit court intervention, permission may be sought from the hospital administrator.

A client or guardian always has the right to withdraw consent after it has been given. When this occurs, the physician should inform (or re-inform) the client about the consequences of refusing treatment. If treatment has already been initiated, the physician should terminate treatment in a way least likely to cause injury to the client and inform the client or guardian of the risks associated with interrupted treatment (Guido, 2010).

The nurse's role in obtaining informed consent is usually defined by agency policy. A nurse may sign the consent form as witness for the client's signature. However, legal liability for informed consent lies with the physician. The nurse acts as client advocate to ensure that the following three major elements of informed consent have been addressed:

1. **Knowledge:** The client has received adequate information on which to base his or her decision.
2. **Competency:** The individual's cognition is not impaired to an extent that would interfere with decision making or, if so, that the individual has a legal representative.
3. **Free will:** The individual has given consent voluntarily without pressure or coercion from others.

Restraints and Seclusion

An individual's privacy and personal security are protected by the Patient Self-determination Act of 1991. This legislation includes a set of patient rights, one of which is an individual's right to freedom from restraint or seclusion except in an emergency situation. The use of seclusion and restraint as a therapeutic intervention for psychiatric patients has been controversial and many efforts have been made through federal and state regulations and through standards set forth by accrediting bodies to minimize or eliminate its use. Because there have been injuries and deaths associated with restraint and seclusion, this treatment requires careful attention when it is used. Further, the laws, regulations, accreditation standards, and hospital policies are frequently being revised so it is important for anyone practicing in inpatient psychiatric settings to be well informed in each of these areas.

In psychiatry, the term *restraints* generally refers to a set of leather straps that are used to restrain the extremities of an individual whose behavior is out of control and who poses an immediate risk to the physical safety and psychological well-being of the individual and others. It is important to note, however, that the current generally accepted definition of restraint refers not only to leather restraints but rather to any manual method or medication used to restrict a person's freedom of movement (The Joint Commission, 2010). Restraints are never to be used as punishment or for the convenience of staff. Other measures to decrease agitation, such as "talking down" (verbal intervention) and chemical restraints (tranquilizing medication) are usually tried first. If these interventions are ineffective, mechanical restraints may be instituted (although some controversy exists as to whether chemical restraints are indeed less restrictive than mechanical restraints). *Seclusion* is another type of physical restraint in which the client is confined alone in a room from which he or she is unable to leave. The room is usually minimally furnished with items to promote the client's comfort and safety.

The Joint Commission, an association that accredits health-care organizations, has established specific standards regarding the use of seclusion and restraint. Some examples of current standards include the following (The Joint Commission, 2010):

1. Seclusion or restraint is discontinued at the earliest possible time regardless of when the order is scheduled to expire.
2. Unless state law is more restrictive, orders for restraint or seclusion must be renewed every 4 hours for adults ages 18 and older, every 2 hours for children and adolescents ages 9 to 17, and every hour for children younger than 9 years. Orders may be renewed according to these time limits for a maximum of 24 consecutive hours.
3. An in-person evaluation (by a physician, clinical psychologist, or other licensed independent practitioner responsible for the care of the patient) must be conducted within 1 hour of initiating restraint or seclusion. Appropriately trained registered nurses and physician assistants may also conduct this assessment but they must consult with the physician.
4. Patients who are simultaneously restrained and secluded must be continuously monitored by trained staff, either in person or through audio or video equipment positioned near the patient.
5. Staff who are involved in restraining and secluding patients are trained to monitor the physical and psychological well-being of the patient including (but not limited to) respiratory and circulatory status, skin integrity, and vital signs.

The laws, regulations, accreditation standards, and hospital policies pertaining to restraint and seclusion share a common priority of maintaining patient safety for a procedure that has the potential to incur injury or death. The importance of close and careful monitoring cannot be overstated.

False imprisonment is the deliberate and unauthorized confinement of a person within fixed limits by the use of verbal or physical means (Ellis & Hartley, 2012). Health-care workers may be charged with false imprisonment for restraining or secluding—against the wishes of the client—anyone having been admitted to the hospital voluntarily. Should a voluntarily admitted client decompensate to a point that restraint or seclusion for protection of self or others is necessary, court intervention to determine competency and involuntary commitment is required to preserve the client's rights to privacy and freedom.

Commitment Issues

Voluntary Admissions

Each year, more than one million persons are admitted to health-care facilities for psychiatric treatment; of these admissions, approximately two-thirds are considered voluntary. To be admitted voluntarily, an individual makes direct application to the institution for services and may stay as long as treatment is deemed necessary. He or she may sign out of the hospital at any time unless, following a mental status examination, the health-care professional determines that the client may be harmful to self or others and recommends that the admission status be changed from voluntary to involuntary. Although these types of admissions are considered voluntary, it is important to ensure that the individual comprehends the meaning of his or her actions, has not been coerced in any manner, and is willing to proceed with admission.

Involuntary Commitment

Because involuntary hospitalization results in substantial restrictions of the rights of an individual, the admission process is subject to the guarantee of the Fourteenth Amendment to the U.S. Constitution that provides citizens protection against loss of liberty and ensures due process rights (Weiss-Kaffie & Purtell, 2001). Involuntary commitments are made for various reasons. Most states commonly cite the following criteria:

■ In an emergency situation (for the client who is dangerous to self or others)
■ For observation and treatment of mentally ill persons
■ When an individual is unable to take care of basic personal needs (the "gravely disabled")

Under the Fourth Amendment, individuals are protected from unlawful searches and seizures without probable cause. Therefore, the individual seeking the involuntary commitment must show probable cause why the client should be hospitalized against his or her wishes; that is, the person must show that there is cause to believe that the person would be dangerous to self or others, is mentally ill and in need of treatment, or is gravely disabled.

Emergency Commitments

Emergency commitments are sought when an individual manifests behavior that is clearly and imminently dangerous to self or others. These admissions are usually instigated by relatives or friends of the individual, police officers, the court, or health-care professionals. Emergency commitments are time-limited, and a court hearing for the individual is scheduled, usually within 72 hours. At that time the court may decide that the client may be discharged; or, if deemed necessary, and voluntary admission is refused by the client, an additional period of involuntary commitment may be ordered. In most instances, another hearing is scheduled for a specified time (usually in 7 to 21 days).

The Mentally Ill Person in Need of Treatment

A second type of involuntary commitment is for the observation and treatment of mentally ill persons in need of treatment. Most states have established definitions of what constitutes "mentally ill" for purposes of state involuntary admission statutes. Some examples include individuals who, because of severe mental illness, are:

■ Unable to make informed decisions concerning treatment
■ Likely to cause harm to self or others
■ Unable to fulfill basic personal needs necessary for health and safety

In determining whether commitment is required, the court looks for substantial evidence of abnormal conduct—evidence that cannot be explained as the result of a physical cause. There must be "clear and convincing evidence" as well as "probable cause" to substantiate the need for involuntary commitment to ensure that an individual's rights under the Constitution are protected. The U.S. Supreme Court, in *O'Connor v. Donaldson*, held that the existence of mental illness alone does not justify involuntary hospitalization. State standards require a specific impact or consequence to flow from the mental illness that involves danger or an inability to care for one's own needs. These clients are entitled to court hearings with representation, at which time determination of commitment and length of stay are considered. Legislative statutes governing involuntary commitments vary from state to state.

Involuntary Outpatient Commitment

Involuntary outpatient commitment (IOC) is a court-ordered mechanism used to compel a person with mental illness to submit to treatment on an outpatient basis. A number of eligibility criteria for commitment to outpatient treatment have been cited (Appelbaum, 2001; Maloy, 1996; Torrey & Zdanowicz, 2001). Some of these include:

■ A history of repeated decompensation requiring involuntary hospitalization
■ Likelihood that without treatment the individual will deteriorate to the point of requiring inpatient commitment
■ Presence of severe and persistent mental illness (e.g., schizophrenia or bipolar disorder) and limited awareness of the illness or need for treatment
■ The presence of severe and persistent mental illness contributing to a risk of becoming homeless, incarcerated, or violent, or of committing suicide
■ The existence of individualized treatment plan likely to be effective and a service provider who has agreed to provide the treatment

Most states have already enacted IOC legislation or currently have resolutions that speak to this topic on their agendas. Most commonly, clients who are committed into the IOC programs are those with severe and persistent mental illness, such as schizophrenia. The rationale behind the legislation is to improve preventive care and reduce the number of readmissions and lengths of hospital stays of these clients. The need for this kind of legislation arose after it was recognized that patients with schizophrenia who did not meet criteria for involuntary hospital treatment were, in some cases, ultimately dangerous to themselves or others. In New York, public attention to this need arose after a man with schizophrenia who had stopped taking his medication pushed a young woman into the path of a subway train. He would not have met criteria for involuntary hospitalization until he was deemed dangerous to others, but advocates for this legislation argued that there should be provisions to prevent violence rather than waiting until it happens. The subsequent law governing IOC in New York became known as Kendra's Law in reference to the woman who was pushed to her death. Opponents of this legislation fear that it may violate the individual rights of psychiatric clients without significant improvement in outcomes.

Some research studies have attempted to evaluate whether IOC improves care, reduces lengths of stay in the hospital, and/or reduces episodes of violence. One study at Bellevue hospital in New York found no difference in treatment outcomes between court-ordered outpatient treatment and voluntary outpatient treatment (Steadman et al., 2001). Other studies have shown positive outcomes, including a decrease in hospital readmissions, with IOC (Ridgely, Borum, & Petrila, 2001; Swartz et al., 2001). Continuing research is required to determine if IOC will improve treatment compliance and enhance quality of life in the community for individuals with severe and persistent mental illness.

The Gravely Disabled Client

A number of states have statutes that specifically define the "gravely disabled" client. For those that do not use this label, the description of the individual who, because of mental illness, is unable to take care of basic personal needs is very similar.

Gravely disabled is generally defined as a condition in which an individual, as a result of mental illness, is in danger of serious physical harm resulting from inability to provide for basic needs such as food, clothing, shelter, medical care, and personal safety. Inability to care for oneself cannot be established by showing that an individual lacks the resources to provide the necessities of life. Rather, it is the inability to make use of available resources.

Should it be determined that an individual is gravely disabled, a guardian, conservator, or committee will be appointed by the court to ensure the management of the person and his or her estate. To legally restore competency then requires another court hearing to reverse the previous ruling. The individual whose competency is being determined has the right to be represented by an attorney.

Nursing Liability

Mental health practitioners—psychiatrists, psychologists, psychiatric nurses, and social workers—have a duty to provide appropriate care based on the standards of their professions and the standards set by law. The standards of care for psychiatric/mental health nursing are presented in Chapter 9.

Malpractice and Negligence

The terms **malpractice** and **negligence** are often used interchangeably. Negligence has been defined as:

> The failure to exercise the standard of care that a reasonably prudent person would have exercised in a similar situation; any conduct that falls below the legal standard established to protect others against unreasonable risk of harm, except for conduct that is intentionally, wantonly, or willfully disregardful of others' rights. (Garner, 2011)

Any person may be negligent. In contrast, malpractice is a specialized form of negligence applicable only to professionals.

Black's Law Dictionary defines malpractice as:

> An instance of negligence or incompetence on the part of a professional. To succeed in a malpractice claim, a plaintiff must also prove proximate cause and damages. (Garner, 2011)

In the absence of any state statutes, common law is the basis of liability for injuries to clients caused by acts of malpractice and negligence of individual practitioners. In other words, most decisions of negligence in the professional setting are based on legal precedent (decisions that have previously been made about similar cases) rather than any specific action taken by the legislature.

To summarize, when the breach of duty is characterized as malpractice, the action is weighed against the professional standard. When it is brought forth as negligence, action is contrasted with what a reasonably prudent professional would have done in the same or similar circumstances.

Austin (2011) cites the following basic elements of a nursing malpractice lawsuit:

1. A duty to the patient existed, based on the recognized standard of care.

2. A breach of duty occurred, meaning that the care rendered was not consistent with the recognized standard of care.
3. The client was injured.
4. The injury was directly caused by the breach of a standard of care.

For the client to prevail in a malpractice claim, each of these elements must be proved. Juries' decisions are generally based on the testimony of expert witnesses, because members of the jury are laypeople and cannot be expected to know what nursing interventions should have been carried out. Without the testimony of expert witnesses, a favorable verdict usually goes to the defendant nurse.

Types of Lawsuits That Occur in Psychiatric Nursing

Most malpractice suits against nurses are civil actions; that is, they are considered breach of conduct actions on the part of the professional, for which compensation is being sought. The nurse in the psychiatric setting should be aware of the types of behaviors that may result in charges of malpractice.

Basic to the psychiatric client's hospitalization is his or her right to confidentiality and privacy. A nurse may be charged with *breach of confidentiality* for revealing aspects about a client's case, or even for revealing that an individual has been hospitalized, if that person can show that making this information known resulted in harm.

When shared information is detrimental to the client's reputation, the person sharing the information may be liable for **defamation of character**. When the information is in writing, the action is called **libel**. Oral defamation is called **slander**. Defamation of character involves communication that is malicious and false (Ellis & Hartley, 2012). Occasionally, libel arises out of critical, judgmental statements written in the client's medical record. Nurses need to be very objective in their charting, backing up all statements with factual evidence.

Invasion of privacy is a charge that may result when a client is searched without probable cause. Many institutions conduct body searches on clients with mental illness as a routine intervention. In these cases, there should be a physician's order and written rationale showing probable cause for the intervention. Many institutions are reexamining their policies regarding this procedure.

Assault is an act that results in a person's genuine fear and apprehension that he or she will be touched without consent. **Battery** is the unconsented touching of another person. These charges can result when a treatment is administered to a client against his or her wishes and outside of an emergency situation. Harm or injury need not have occurred for these charges to be legitimate.

For confining a client against his or her wishes, and outside of an emergency situation, the nurse may be charged with false imprisonment. Examples of actions that may invoke these charges include locking an individual in a room; taking a client's clothes for purposes of detainment against his or her will; and retaining in mechanical restraints a competent voluntary client who demands to be released.

Avoiding Liability

Hall and Hall (2001) suggested the following proactive nursing actions in an effort to avoid nursing malpractice:

1. Responding to the patient
2. Educating the patient
3. Complying with the standard of care
4. Supervising care
5. Adhering to the nursing process
6. Documenting carefully
7. Following up by evaluating the care that was given

In addition, it is a positive practice to develop and maintain a good interpersonal relationship with the client and his or her family. Some clients appear to be more "suit prone" than others. Suit-prone clients are often very critical, complaining, uncooperative, and even hostile. A natural response by the staff to these clients is to become defensive or withdrawn. Either of these behaviors increases the likelihood of a lawsuit should an unfavorable event occur (Ellis & Hartley, 2012). No matter how high the degree of technical competence and skill of the nurse, his or her insensitivity to a client's complaints and failure to meet the client's emotional needs often influence whether or not a lawsuit is generated. A great deal depends on the psychosocial skills of the health-care professional.

> **CLINICAL PEARLS**
> • Always put the client's rights and welfare first.
> • Develop and maintain a good interpersonal relationship with each client and his or her family.

Summary and Key Points

- *Ethics* is a branch of philosophy that addresses methods for determining the rightness or wrongness of one's actions.
- *Bioethics* is the term applied to these principles when they refer to concepts within the scope of medicine, nursing, and allied health.
- *Moral behavior* is defined as conduct that results from serious critical thinking about how individuals ought to treat others.

- *Values* are personal beliefs about what is important or desirable.
- A *right* is defined as "a valid, legally recognized claim or entitlement, encompassing both freedom from government interference or discriminatory treatment and an entitlement to a benefit or service."
- The ethical theory of *utilitarianism* is based on the premise that what is right and good is that which produces the most happiness for the most people.
- The ethical theory of *Kantianism* suggests that actions are bound by a sense of duty, and that ethical decisions are made out of respect for moral law.
- The code of *Christian ethics* is that all decisions about right and wrong should be centered in love for God and in treating others with the same respect and dignity with which we would expect to be treated.
- The moral precept of the *natural law theory* is "do good and avoid evil." Good is viewed as that which is inscribed by God into the nature of things. Evil acts are never condoned, even if they are intended to advance the noblest of ends.
- *Ethical egoism* espouses that what is right and good is what is best for the individual making the decision.
- Ethical principles include autonomy, beneficence, nonmaleficence, veracity, and justice.
- An *ethical dilemma* is a situation that requires an individual to make a choice between two equally unfavorable alternatives.

- Ethical issues may arise in psychiatric/mental health nursing around the right to refuse medication and the right to the least-restrictive treatment alternative.
- *Statutory laws* are those that have been enacted by legislative bodies, and common laws are derived from decisions made in previous cases. Both types of laws have civil and criminal components.
- *Civil law* protects the private and property rights of individuals and businesses, and *criminal law* provides protection from conduct deemed injurious to the public welfare.
- Legal issues in psychiatric/mental health nursing center around confidentiality and the right to privacy, informed consent, restraints and seclusion, and commitment issues.
- Nurses are accountable for their own actions in relation to legal issues, and violation can result in malpractice lawsuits against the physician, the hospital, and the nurse.
- Developing and maintaining a good interpersonal relationship with the client and his or her family appears to be a positive factor when the question of malpractice is being considered.

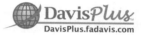 **DavisPlus** DavisPlus.fadavis.com   Additional info available at www.davisplus.com

Review Questions
Self-Examination/Learning Exercise

*Select the answer that is **most** appropriate for each of the following questions.*

1. Nurse Jones decides to go against family wishes and tell the client of his terminal status because that is what she would want if she were the client. Which of the following ethical theories is considered in this decision?
   a. Kantianism
   b. Christian ethics
   c. Natural law theories
   d. Ethical egoism

2. Nurse Jones decides to respect family wishes and not tell the client of his terminal status because that would bring the most happiness to the most people. Which of the following ethical theories is considered in this decision?
   a. Utilitarianism
   b. Kantianism
   c. Christian ethics
   d. Ethical egoism

Review Questions—cont'd
Self-Examination/Learning Exercise

3. Nurse Jones decides to tell the client of his terminal status because she believes it is her duty to do so. Which of the following ethical theories is considered in this decision?
   a. Natural law theories
   b. Ethical egoism
   c. Kantianism
   d. Utilitarianism

4. The nurse assists the physician with electroconvulsive therapy on his client who has refused to give consent. With which of the following legal actions might the nurse be charged because of this nursing action?
   a. Assault
   b. Battery
   c. False imprisonment
   d. Breach of confidentiality

5. A competent, voluntary client has stated he wants to leave the hospital. The nurse hides his clothes in an effort to keep him from leaving. With which of the following legal actions might the nurse be charged because of this nursing action?
   a. Assault
   b. Battery
   c. False imprisonment
   d. Breach of confidentiality

6. Joe is very restless and is pacing a lot. The nurse says to Joe, "If you don't sit down in the chair and be still, I'm going to put you in restraints!" With which of the following legal actions might the nurse be charged because of this nursing action?
   a. Defamation of character
   b. Battery
   c. Breach of confidentiality
   d. Assault

7. For which of the following reasons may an individual be considered *gravely disabled*? (Select all that apply.)
   a. A person, because of mental illness, cannot fulfill basic needs.
   b. A mentally ill person is in danger of physical harm based on inability to care for self.
   c. A mentally ill person lacks the resources to provide the necessities of life.
   d. A mentally ill person is unable to make use of available resources to meet daily living requirements.

8. Which of the following statements is (are) correct regarding the use of restraints? (Select all that apply.)
   a. Restraints may never be initiated without a physician's order.
   b. Orders for restraints must be reissued by a physician every 2 hours for children and adolescents.
   c. Clients in restraints must be observed and assessed every hour for issues regarding circulation, nutrition, respiration, hydration, and elimination.
   d. An in-person evaluation must be conducted within 1 hour of initiating restraints.

9. Guidelines relating to "duty to warn" state that a therapist should consider taking action to warn a third party when his or her client: (Select all that apply.)
   a. Threatens violence toward another individual
   b. Identifies a specific intended victim
   c. Is having command hallucinations
   d. Reveals paranoid delusions about another individual

Continued

Review Questions—cont'd
Self-Examination/Learning Exercise

10. Attempting to calm an angry client by using "talk therapy" is an example of which of the following clients' rights?
    a. The right to privacy
    b. The right to refuse medication
    c. The right to the least-restrictive treatment alternative
    d. The right to confidentiality

References

Aiken, T.D. (2004). *Legal, ethical, and political issues in nursing* (2nd ed.). Philadelphia, PA: F.A. Davis.

American Hospital Association (AHA). (1992). *A patient's bill of rights.* Chicago, IL: American Hospital Association.

American Nurses' Association (ANA). (2001). *Code of ethics for nurses with interpretive statements.* Washington, DC: ANA.

Appelbaum, P.S. (2001, March). Thinking carefully about outpatient commitment. *Psychiatric Services, 52* (3), 347–350.

Austin, S. (2011). Stay out of court with proper documentation. *Nursing2011, 41*(4), 25–29.

Butts, J., & Rich, K. (2008). *Nursing ethics: Across the curriculum and into practice* (2nd ed.). Sudbury, MA: Jones and Bartlett.

Cady, R.F. (2010). A review of basic patient rights in psychiatric care. *JONA's Healthcare Law, Ethics, and Regulation, 12*(4), 117–125.

Catalano, J.T. (2012). *Nursing now! Today's issues, tomorrow's trends* (6th ed.). Philadelphia, PA: F.A. Davis.

Ellis, J.R., & Hartley, C.L. (2012). *Nursing in today's world: Challenges, issues, and trends* (10th ed.). Philadelphia, PA: Lippincott Williams & Wilkins.

Garner, B.A. (Ed.). (2011). *Black's law dictionary: Fourth pocket edition.* St. Paul, MN: West Group.

Guido, G.W. (2010). *Legal and ethical issues in nursing* (5th ed.). Upper Saddle River, NJ: Pearson.

Hall, J.K., & Hall, D. (2001). Negligence specific to nursing. In M.E. O'Keefe (Ed.), *Nursing practice and the law: Avoiding malpractice and other legal risks* (pp. 132–149). Philadelphia: F.A. Davis.

Levy, R.M., & Rubenstein, L.S. (1996). *The rights of people with mental disabilities.* Carbondale, IL: Southern Illinois University Press.

Mackay, T.R. (2001). Informed consent. In M.E. O'Keefe (Ed.), *Nursing practice and the law: Avoiding malpractice and other legal risks* (pp. 199–213). Philadelphia, PA: F.A. Davis.

Maloy, K.A. (1996). Does involuntary outpatient commitment work? In B.D. Sales & S.A. Shah (Eds.), *Mental health and law: Research, policy and services* (pp. 41–74). Durham, NC: Carolina Academic Press.

Patient Self-determination Act—Patient Rights. (1991). U.S. Code, Title 42, Section 10841, The Public Health and Welfare.

Peplau, H.E. (1991). *Interpersonal relations in nursing: A conceptual frame of reference for psychodynamic nursing.* New York, NY: Springer.

Ridgely, M.S., Borum, R., & Petrila, J. (2001). *The effectiveness of involuntary outpatient treatment: Empirical evidence and the experience of eight states.* Santa Monica, CA: Rand Publications.

Sadock, B.J., & Sadock, V.A. (2007). *Synopsis of psychiatry: Behavioral sciences/clinical psychiatry* (10th ed.). Philadelphia, PA: Lippincott Williams & Wilkins.

Steadman, H., Gounis, K., Dennis, D., Hopper, K., Roche, B., Swartz, M., & Robbins, P. (2001). Assessing the New York City involuntary outpatient commitment pilot program. *Psychiatric Services, 52*(3), 330–336.

Swartz, M., Swanson, J., Hiday, V., Wagner, H.R., Burns, B., & Borum, R. (2001). A randomized controlled trial of outpatient commitment in North Carolina. *Psychiatric Services, 52*(3), 325–329.

Tarasoff v. Regents of University of California et al. (1974a), 551 P.d 345.

Tarasoff v. Regents of University of California et al. (1974b), 554 P.d 347.

The Joint Commission. (2010). *The comprehensive accreditation manual for hospitals: The official handbook* (January, 2010). Oakbrook Terrace, IL: Joint Commission Resources.

Torrey, E.F., & Zdanowicz, M. (2001). Outpatient commitment: What, why, and for whom. *Psychiatric Services, 52*(3), 337–341.

U.S. Department of Health and Human Services (USDHHS). (2003). *Standards for privacy of individually identifiable health information.* Washington, DC: Author.

Weiss-Kaffie, C.J. & Purtell, N.E. (2001). Psychiatric nursing. In M.E. O'Keefe (Ed.), *Nursing Practice and the law: Avoiding malpractice and other legal risks* (pp. 352–371). Philadelphia, PA: F.A. Davis.

Cultural and Spiritual Concepts Relevant to Psychiatric/Mental Health Nursing

6

KARYN I. MORGAN AND MARY C. TOWNSEND

CORE CONCEPTS

culture
ethnicity
religion
spirituality

KEY TERMS

culture-bound syndromes
curandera
curandero
density

distance
folk medicine
shaman
stereotyping

territoriality
yin and yang

OBJECTIVES
After reading this chapter, the student will be able to:

1. Define and differentiate between *culture* and *ethnicity*.
2. Identify cultural differences based on six characteristic phenomena.
3. Describe cultural variances, based on the six phenomena, for:
   a. Northern European Americans
   b. African Americans
   c. Native Americans
   d. Asian/Pacific Islander Americans
   e. Latino Americans
   f. Western European Americans
   g. Arab Americans
   h. Jewish Americans
4. Apply the nursing process in the care of individuals from various cultural groups.
5. Define and differentiate between *spirituality* and *religion*.
6. Identify clients' spiritual and religious needs.
7. Apply the six steps of the nursing process to individuals with spiritual and religious needs.

HOMEWORK ASSIGNMENT
Please read the chapter and answer the following questions:

1. Which cultural group may use a medicine man (or woman) called a *shaman*?
2. Restoring a balance between opposite forces is a fundamental concept of Asian health practices. What is this called?
3. Name five types of human spiritual needs.
4. What is the largest ethnic minority group in the United States?
5. What is the perception of mental illness in the Arab culture?

Cultural Concepts

What is culture? How does it differ from ethnicity? Why are these questions important? The answers lie in the changing face of America. Immigration is not new in the United States. Indeed, most U.S. citizens are either immigrants or descendants of immigrants and the number of foreign-born residents in this country continues to grow on a yearly basis. This pattern persists because of the many individuals who want to take advantage of the technological growth and upward mobility that exists in this country. A breakdown of cultural groups in the United States is presented in Figure 6-1.

CORE CONCEPTS

Culture describes a particular society's entire way of living, encompassing shared patterns of belief, feeling, and knowledge that guide people's conduct and are passed down from generation to generation. **Ethnicity** is a somewhat narrower term and relates to people who identify with each other because of a shared heritage (Griffith, Gonzalez, & Blue, 2003).

Knowledge related to culture and ethnicity is important because these influences affect human behavior, its interpretation, and the response to it. Therefore it is essential for nurses to understand the effects of these cultural influences if they are to work effectively with the diverse population. Caution must be taken, however, not to assume that all individuals who share a culture or ethnic group are identical or exhibit behaviors perceived as characteristic of the group. This constitutes **stereotyping** and must be avoided. Many variations and subcultures occur within a culture. These differences may be related to status, ethnic background, residence, religion, education, or other factors. Every individual must be appreciated for his or her uniqueness.

This chapter explores the ways in which various cultures differ. The nursing process is applied to the delivery of psychiatric/mental health nursing care for individuals from the following cultural groups: Northern European Americans, African Americans, Native Americans, Asian/Pacific Islander Americans, Latino Americans, Western European Americans, Arab Americans, and Jewish Americans.

How Do Cultures Differ?

It is difficult to generalize about any one specific group in a country that is known for its heterogeneity. Within our American "melting pot" any or all characteristics could apply to individuals within any or all of the cultural groups represented. As these differences continue to be integrated, one American culture will eventually emerge. This is already evident in certain regions of the country today, particularly in the urban coastal areas. However, some differences still do exist, and it is important for nurses to be aware of certain cultural influences that may affect individuals' behaviors and beliefs, particularly as they apply to health care.

Giger (2013) describes six cultural phenomena that vary with application and use yet are evidenced among all cultural groups: (1) communication, (2) space, (3) social organization, (4) time, (5) environmental control, and (6) biological variations.

Communication

All verbal and nonverbal behavior in connection with another individual is communication. Therapeutic communication has always been considered an essential part of the nursing process and represents a critical element in the curricula of most schools of nursing. Communication has its roots in culture. Cultural mores, norms, ideas, and customs provide the basis for our way of thinking. Cultural values are learned and differ from society to society. Communication is expressed through language (the spoken and written word), paralanguage (the voice quality, intonation, rhythm, and speed of the spoken word), and gestures (touch, facial expression, eye movements, body posture, and physical appearance). The nurse who is planning care must have an understanding of the client's needs and expectations as they are being communicated. As a third

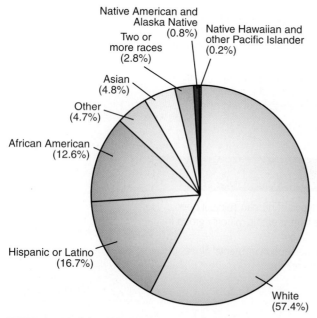

FIGURE 6–1 Breakdown of cultural groups in the United States. (Source: U.S. Census Bureau, 2012.)

Native American and Alaska Native (0.8%)
Two or more races (2.8%)
Native Hawaiian and other Pacific Islander (0.2%)
Asian (4.8%)
Other (4.7%)
African American (12.6%)
Hispanic or Latino (16.7%)
White (57.4%)

party, an interpreter often complicates matters, but one may be necessary when the client does not speak the same language as the nurse. Interpreting is a very complex process, however, that requires a keen sensitivity to cultural nuances, and not just the translating of words into another language. Tips for facilitating the communication process when using an interpreter are presented in Box 6-1.

Space

Spatial determinants relate to the place where the communication occurs and encompass the concepts of *territoriality*, *density*, and *distance*. **Territoriality** refers to the innate tendency to own space. The need for territoriality is met only if the individual has control of a space, can establish rules for that space, and is able to defend the space against invasion or misuse by others. **Density**, which refers to the number of people within a given environmental space, can influence interpersonal interaction. **Distance** is the means by which various cultures use space to communicate. Hall (1966) identified three primary dimensions of space in interpersonal interactions in the Western culture: the intimate zone (0 to 18 inches), the personal zone (18 inches to 3 feet), and the social zone (3 to 6 feet).

Social Organization

Cultural behavior is socially acquired through a process called *enculturation*, which involves acquiring knowledge and internalizing values (Giger, 2013). Children are acculturated by observing adults within their social organizations. Social organizations include families, religious groups, and ethnic groups.

Time

An awareness of the concept of time is a gradual learning process. Some cultures place great importance on values that are measured by clock time. Punctuality and efficiency are highly valued in the United States, whereas some cultures are actually scornful of clock time. For example, some rural people in Algeria label the clock as the "devil's mill" and therefore have no notion of scheduled appointment times or meal times (Giger, 2013). They are totally indifferent to the passage of clock time, and they despise haste in all human endeavors. Other cultural implications regarding time have to do with perception of time orientation. Whether individuals are present oriented or future oriented in their perception of time influences many aspects of their lives.

Environmental Control

The variable of environmental control has to do with the degree to which individuals perceive that they have control over their environment. Cultural beliefs and practices influence how an individual responds to his or her environment during periods of wellness and illness. To provide culturally appropriate care, the nurse should not only respect the individual's unique beliefs, but should also have an understanding of how these beliefs can be used to promote optimal health in the client's environment.

BOX 6-1 **Using an Interpreter**

When using an interpreter, keep the following points in mind:

- Address the client directly rather than speaking to the interpreter. Maintain eye contact with the client to ensure the client's involvement.
- Do not interrupt the client and the interpreter. At times their interaction may take longer because of the need to clarify, and descriptions may require more time because of dialect differences or the interpreter's awareness that the client needs more preparation before being asked a particular question.
- Ask the interpreter to give you verbatim translations so that you can assess what the client is thinking and understanding.
- Avoid using medical jargon that the interpreter or client may not understand.
- Avoid talking or commenting to the interpreter at length; the client may feel left out and distrustful.
- Be aware that asking intimate or emotionally laden questions may be difficult for both the client and the interpreter. Lead up to these questions slowly. Always ask permission to discuss these topics first, and prepare the interpreter for the content of the interview.
- When possible, allow the client and the interpreter to meet each other ahead of time to establish some rapport. If possible, try to use the same interpreter for succeeding interviews with the client.
- If possible, request an interpreter of the same gender as the client and of similar age. To make good use of the interpreter's time, decide beforehand which questions you will ask. Meet with the interpreter briefly before going to see the client so that you can let the interpreter know what you are planning to ask. During the session, face the client and direct your questions to the client, not the interpreter.

SOURCE: Gorman, L.M., & Sultan, D.F. (2008). Psychosocial nursing for general patient care (3rd ed.). *Philadelphia, PA: F.A. Davis, with permission.*

Biological Variations

Biological differences exist among people in various racial groups. These differences include body structure (both size and shape), skin color, physiological responses to medication, electrocardiographic patterns, susceptibility to disease, and nutritional preferences and deficiencies. Giger (2013) suggests that nurses who possess factual knowledge about biological variations among diverse groups are better able to provide culturally appropriate health care.

Application of the Nursing Process

Background Assessment Data

A cultural assessment tool for gathering information related to culture and ethnicity that is important in the planning of client care is provided in Box 6-2.

Northern European Americans

Northern European Americans have their origins in England, Ireland, Wales, Finland, Sweden, Norway, Germany, Poland, and the Baltic states of Estonia, Latvia, and Lithuania. English is their primary language. Their language may also include words and phrases that reflect the influence of the languages spoken in the countries of their heritage. The descendants of these immigrants now make up what is considered the dominant cultural group in the United States today. Specific dialects and rate of speech are common to various regions of the country. Northern European Americans value territory. Personal space preference is about 18 inches to 3 feet.

With the advent of technology and widespread mobility, less emphasis has been placed on the cohesiveness of the family. Data on marriage, divorce,

---

BOX 6-2 Cultural Assessment Tool

Client's name _____ Ethnic origin _____
Address _____ Birthdate _____
Name of significant other _____ Relationship _____
Primary language spoken _____ Second language spoken _____
How does client usually communicate with people who speak a different language? _____
Is an interpreter required? _____ Available? _____
Highest level of education achieved: _____ Occupation: _____
Presenting problem: _____
Has this problem ever occurred before? _____
  If so, in what manner was it handled previously? _____
What is the client's usual manner of coping with stress? _____
Who is (are) the client's main support system(s)? _____
Describe the family living arrangements: _____
Who is the major decision maker in the family? _____
Describe client's/family members' roles within the family. _____

Describe religious beliefs and practices: _____
  Are there any religious requirements or restrictions that place limitations on the client's care? _____
  If so, describe: _____
Who in the family takes responsibility for health concerns? _____
Describe any special health beliefs and practices: _____

From whom does family usually seek medical assistance in time of need? _____
Describe client's usual emotional/behavioral response to:
  Anxiety: _____
  Anger: _____
  Loss/change/failure: _____
  Pain: _____
  Fear: _____
Describe any topics that are particularly sensitive or that the client is unwilling to discuss (because of cultural taboos): _____

Describe any activities in which the client is unwilling to participate (because of cultural customs or taboos): _____

What are the client's personal feelings regarding touch? _____
What are the client's personal feelings regarding eye contact? _____
What is the client's personal orientation to time? (past, present, future) _____

BOX 6-2 **Cultural Assessment Tool—cont'd**

Describe any particular illnesses to which the client may be bioculturally susceptible (e.g., hypertension and sickle cell anemia in African Americans):

_____

Describe any nutritional deficiencies to which the client may be bioculturally susceptible (e.g., lactose intolerance in Native and Asian Americans) _____

Describe client's favorite foods: _____

Are there any foods the client requests or refuses because of cultural beliefs related to this illness (e.g., "hot" and "cold" foods for Latino Americans and Asian Americans)? If so, please describe: _____

_____

Describe client's perception of the problem and expectations of health care:_____

_____

_____

---

and remarriage in the United States show that about half of first marriages end in divorce (CDC, 2012). The value that was once placed on religion also seems to be diminishing in the American culture. With the exception of a few months following the terrorist attacks of September 11, 2001, when attendance increased, there was a steady decline reported in church attendance from 1992 to 2008 (Gallup, 2008). However, a more recent Gallup poll indicates that there has been a slight rise in church attendance—up from 42.8 percent in 2009 to 43.1 percent in 2010 (Gallup, 2012). Punctuality and efficiency are highly valued in the culture that promoted the work ethic, and most within this cultural group tend to be future oriented (Murray, Zentner, & Yakimo, 2009).

Northern European Americans, particularly those who achieve middle-class socioeconomic status, value preventive medicine and primary health care. This value follows along with the socioeconomic group's educational level, successful achievement, and financial capability to maintain a healthy lifestyle. Most recognize the importance of regular physical exercise.

A typical diet for many Northern European Americans is high in fats and cholesterol and low in fiber. Americans, in general, are learning about the health benefits of reducing fats and increasing nutrients in their diet. However, they still enjoy fast food, which conforms to their fast-paced lifestyles.

The United States, viewed as a "melting pot" of multiple worldwide ethnic groups, has its own unique culture that impacts the health and care of individuals. It is important that the nurse is self-aware of these conscious/unconscious attitudes and values within the U.S. culture when caring for clients, and also how these characteristics can impact mental health/illness. Characteristics common to the U.S. culture are presented in Box 6-3.

BOX 6-3 **Characteristics Common to the Culture of the United States**

1. **Individuality**—Independent, ambitious, self-reliant, control over one's life, desire for individual choices result in long-term debates concerning government control of health care, school choice, possession of personal firearms, etc.
2. **Perfectionism**—Strong emphasis on achievement in school, jobs, sports, and physical beauty.
3. **Direct Communication**—Display of emotions is proper, within limits. Constructive criticism is considered helpful for others. Vast public use of social media provides instant connections that can strengthen or hinder relationships.
4. **Time Adherence**—Punctuality is important, activities organized around specific schedules, hurried, active lifestyles causing difficulty with relaxation, stress tolerance, and physical fitness.
5. **Informality/Friendliness**—Common use of first name when addressing others. Many friendly expressions such as "let's get together soon" and "drop by anytime" are sincere at the time, but because of busy lifestyles are not meant literally.
6. **Consumerism**—Mass luxuries, growth of comfort pleasures, need for material goods, standardized "high end" designer products—homes, clothing, automobiles are desired in all income levels; long distance travel vacations, vast accumulation of goods leading to economic stress and excessive debt; overconsumption in food practices resulting in increased obesity and decreased overall health.
7. **Social Challenges**—Suburban tract housing, widespread drive-through dining, frequent relocations, solo car travel, decreased family and community connections, mall shopping vs. local shopping; increase in bullying behaviors in school/workplace and proliferation of violence and traumatic events within the family and community.

Contributed by Lois Angelo, Assistant Professor, Massachusetts College of Pharmacy and Health Sciences, Boston, Mass.

African Americans

The language dialect of some African Americans is different from what is considered standard English. The origin of the black dialect is not clearly understood but is thought to be a combination of various African languages and the languages of other cultural groups (e.g., Dutch, French, English, and Spanish) present in the United States at the time of its settlement. Personal space tends to be smaller than that of the dominant culture.

Patterns of discrimination date back to the days of slavery, and evidence of segregation still exists, usually in the form of predominantly black neighborhoods, churches, and schools, which are still visible in some U.S. cities. Some African Americans find it difficult to assimilate into the mainstream culture and choose to remain within their own social organization.

The most recent survey by the U.S. Census Bureau revealed that 47 percent of African American family households were headed by a woman (U.S. Census Bureau, 2012). Social support systems may be large and include sisters, brothers, aunts, uncles, cousins, boyfriends, girlfriends, neighbors, and friends. Many African Americans have a strong religious orientation, with the vast majority practicing some form of Protestantism (Pew Forum on Religion and Public Life, 2009).

African Americans who have assimilated into the dominant culture are likely to be well educated, professional, and future oriented. Some who have not become assimilated may believe that planning for the future is hopeless, a belief based on their previous experiences and encounters with racism and discrimination (Cherry & Giger, 2013). Among this group, some may be unemployed or have low-paying jobs, with little expectation for improvement. They are unlikely to value time or punctuality to the same degree as the dominant cultural group, which may result in their being labeled as irresponsible.

Some African Americans, particularly those from the rural South, may reach adulthood never having encountered a physician. They may receive their medical care from the local folk practitioner known as "granny" or "the old lady," or a "spiritualist." Incorporated into the system of **folk medicine** is the belief that health is a gift from God, whereas illness is a punishment from God or a retribution for sin and evil. Historically, African Americans have turned to folk medicine either because they could not afford the cost of mainstream medical treatment or because of the insensitive treatment by caregivers in the health-care delivery system.

Hypertension occurs more frequently, and sickle cell disease occurs predominantly, in African Americans. Hypertension carries a strong hereditary risk factor, whereas sickle cell disease is genetically derived. Alcoholism is a serious problem among members of the black community, leading to a high incidence of alcohol-related illness and death (Cherry & Giger, 2013).

The diet of most African Americans differs little from that of the mainstream culture. However, some African Americans follow their heritage and still enjoy what has come to be known as "soul" food, which includes items such as poke salad, collard greens, beans, corn, fried chicken, black-eyed peas, grits, okra, and cornbread. These foods are now considered typical Southern fare and are regularly consumed and enjoyed by most individuals who inhabit the southern region of the United States.

Native Americans

The federal government currently recognizes 566 American Indian tribes and Alaska Native groups. Approximately 200 tribal languages are still spoken, some by only a few individuals and others by many (Bureau of Indian Affairs [BIA], 2012). Fewer than half of these individuals still live on reservations, but many return regularly to participate in family and tribal life and sometimes to retire.

Touch is an aspect of communication that is not the same among Native Americans as in the dominant American culture. Some Native Americans view the traditional handshake as somewhat aggressive. Instead, if a hand is offered to another, it may be accepted with a light touch or just a passing of hands. Some Native Americans will not touch a dead person (Hanley, 2013).

Native Americans may appear silent and reserved. They may be uncomfortable expressing emotions because the culture encourages keeping private thoughts to oneself. Eye contact is avoided and considered rude (Purnell, 2009).

The concept of space is very concrete to Native Americans. Living space is often crowded with members of both nuclear and extended families. A large network of kin is very important to Native Americans. However, a need for extended space exists, as demonstrated by a distance of many miles between individual homes or camps.

The primary social organizations of Native Americans are the family and the tribe. From infancy, Native American children are taught the importance of these units. Traditions are passed down by the elderly, and children are taught to respect tradition and to honor wisdom.

Most Native Americans are very present-time oriented. The concept of time is very casual, and tasks are accomplished, not with the notion of a particular time in mind, but merely in a present-oriented time frame. Not only are Native Americans not ruled by the clock, some do not even own clocks.

Religion and health practices are intertwined in the Native American culture. The medicine man (or woman) is called the **shaman** and may use a variety of methods in his or her practice. Some use crystals to diagnose illness, some sing and perform healing ceremonies, and some use herbs and other plants or roots to create remedies with healing properties. The Native American healers and U.S. Indian Health Service have worked together with mutual respect for many years. Hanley (2013) relates that a Native American healer may confer with a physician regarding the care of a client in the hospital. Research studies have continued to show the importance of each of these health-care approaches in the overall wellness of Native American people.

The risks of illness and premature death from alcoholism, diabetes, tuberculosis, heart disease, accidents, homicide, suicide, pneumonia, and influenza are dramatically higher for Native Americans than for the U.S. population as a whole. The risks of illness and premature death from alcoholism alone are reported as 552 percent higher (Indian Health Service [IHS], 2013). Alcoholism is not only a significant problem among Native Americans but it may also be related to a number of other serious problems such as depression, automobile accidents, homicides, spouse and child abuse, and suicides.

Nutritional deficiencies are not uncommon among tribal Native Americans. Fruits and green vegetables are often scarce in many of the federally defined Indian geographical regions. Meat and corn products are identified as preferred foods. Fiber intake is relatively low, while fat intake is often of the saturated variety. A large number of Native Americans living on or near reservations recognized by the federal or state government receive commodity foods supplied by the U.S. Department of Agriculture's food distribution program (U.S. Department of Agriculture, 2012).

Asian/Pacific Islander Americans

Asian Americans comprise 4.8 percent of the U.S. population. The Asian American culture includes peoples (and their descendants) from Japan, China, Vietnam, the Philippines, Thailand, Cambodia, Korea, Laos, India, and the Pacific Islands. Although this discussion relates to these peoples as a single culture, it is important to keep in mind that a multiplicity of differences regarding attitudes, beliefs, values, religious practices, and language exist among these subcultures.

Many Asian Americans, particularly Japanese, are third- and even fourth-generation Americans. These individuals are likely to be acculturated to the U.S. culture. Kuo and Roysircar-Sodowsky (2000) describe three patterns common to Asian Americans in their attempt to adjust to the American culture:

1. **The traditionalists:** These individuals tend to be the older generation Asians who hold on to the traditional values and practices of their native culture. They have strong internalized Asian values. Primary allegiance is to the biological family.
2. **The marginal people:** These individuals reject the traditional values and totally embrace Western culture. Often they are members of the younger generations.
3. **Asian Americans:** These individuals incorporate traditional values and beliefs with Western values and beliefs. They become integrated into the American culture, while maintaining a connection with their ancestral culture.

The languages and dialects of Asian Americans are very diverse. In general, they do share a similar belief in harmonious interaction. To raise one's voice is likely to be interpreted as a sign of loss of control. The English language is very difficult to master, and even bilingual Asian Americans may encounter communication problems because of the differences in meaning assigned to nonverbal cues, such as facial gestures, verbal intonation and speed, and body movements. In Asian cultures, touching during communication has historically been considered unacceptable. However, with the advent of Western acculturation, younger generations of Asian Americans accept touching as more appropriate than did their ancestors. Eye contact is often avoided as it connotes rudeness and lack of respect in some Asian cultures. Acceptable personal and social spaces are larger than in the dominant American culture. Some Asian Americans have a great deal of difficulty expressing emotions. Because of their reserved public demeanor, Asian Americans may be perceived as shy, cold, or uninterested.

The family is the ultimate social organization in traditional Asian American culture, and loyalty to family is emphasized above all else. Children are expected to obey and honor their parents. Misbehavior is perceived as bringing dishonor to the entire family. Filial piety (one's social obligation or duty to one's parents) is held in high regard. Failure to fulfill these obligations can create a great deal of guilt and shame in an individual. A chronological hierarchy exists with the elderly maintaining positions of authority. Several generations, or even extended families, may share a single household.

Although education is highly valued among Asian Americans, many remain undereducated. Religious beliefs and practices are diverse and exhibit influences of Taoism, Buddhism, Confucianism, Islam, Hinduism, and Christianity.

Many Asian Americans value both a past and a present orientation. Emphasis is placed on the wishes of one's ancestors, while adjusting to demands of the present. Little value is given to prompt adherence to schedules or rigid standards of activities.

Restoring the balance of **yin and yang** is the fundamental concept of Asian health practices. Yin and yang represent opposite forces of energy, such as negative/positive, dark/light, cold/hot, hard/soft, and feminine/masculine. The belief is that illness occurs when there is a disruption in the balance of these energy forces. In medicine, the opposites are expressed as "hot" and "cold," and health is the result of a balance between hot and cold elements (Xu & Chang, 2013). Food, medicines, and herbs are classified according to their hot and cold properties and are used to restore balance between yin and yang (cold and hot), thereby restoring health.

Rice, vegetables, and fish are the main staple foods of Asian Americans. Milk is seldom consumed because a large majority of Asian Americans experience lactose intolerance. With Western acculturation, their diet is changing, and unfortunately, with more meat being consumed, the percentage of fat in the diet is increasing.

Many Asian Americans believe that psychiatric illness is merely behavior that is out of control. They view this as a great shame to the individual and the family. They often attempt to manage the ill person on their own until they can no longer handle the situation. It is not uncommon for Asian Americans to somaticize. Expressing mental distress through various physical ailments may be viewed as more acceptable than expressing true emotions.

The incidence of alcohol dependence is low among Asians. This may be a result of a possible genetic intolerance of the substance. Some Asians develop unpleasant symptoms, such as flushing, headaches, and palpitations, on drinking alcohol. Research indicates that this is due to an isoenzyme variant that quickly converts alcohol to acetaldehyde and the absence of an isoenzyme that is needed to oxidize acetaldehyde. This results in a rapid accumulation of acetaldehyde that produces the unpleasant symptoms (Wall et al., 1997).

Latino Americans

Latino Americans are the fastest growing group of people in the United States, comprising 16.7 percent of the population (U.S. Census Bureau, 2012). They represent the largest ethnic minority group.

Latino Americans trace their ancestry to countries such as Mexico, Spain, Puerto Rico, Cuba, and other countries of Central and South America. The common language is Spanish, spoken with a number of dialects by the various peoples. Touch is a common form of communication among Latinos; however, they are very modest and are likely to withdraw from any infringement on their modesty.

Traditional Latino Americans are very group oriented and often interact with large groups of relatives. Touching and embracing are common modes of communication. The family is the primary social organization and includes nuclear family members as well as numerous extended family members. The traditional nuclear family is male dominated, and the father possesses ultimate authority.

Latino Americans tend to be focused on the present time. The concept of being punctual and giving attention to activities that concern the future are perceived as less important than activities in the present time.

Roman Catholicism is the predominant religion among Latino Americans. Most Latinos identify with the Roman Catholic Church, even if they do not attend services. Religious beliefs and practices are likely to be strong influences in their lives. Especially in times of crisis, such as in cases of illness and hospitalization, Latino Americans rely on priests and the family to carry out important religious rituals, such as promise making, offering candles, visiting shrines, and offering prayers (Spector, 2013).

Folk beliefs regarding health are a combination of elements incorporating views of Roman Catholicism and Indian and Spanish beliefs. The folk healer is called a **curandero** (male) or **curandera** (female). Among traditional Latino Americans, the *curandero* is believed to have a gift from God for healing the sick and is often the first contact made when illness is encountered. Treatments used include massage, diet, rest, suggestions, practical advice, indigenous herbs, prayers, magic, and supernatural rituals (Owen, Gonzalez, & Espereat, 2013). Many Latino Americans still subscribe to the "hot and cold theory" of disease. This concept is similar to the Asian perception of yin and yang discussed earlier in this chapter. Diseases and the foods and medicines used to treat them are classified as "hot" or "cold," and the intention is to restore the body to a balanced state.

One national study revealed that the lifetime prevalence for selected psychiatric disorders is 36.8 percent for U.S.-born Latinos, which is higher than the prevalence for Latinos in the United States who are immigrants from other countries (Alegria et al., 2007). The authors theorized that this may be related to stress experienced as they attempt to assimilate to the economic and cultural ideals in the United States while still maintaining minority group status. They also noted that the Puerto Rican subgroup manifests a higher incidence of depression, substance abuse, and anxiety disorders (particularly post-traumatic stress disorder) when compared to Cuban, Mexican, or other Latino groups. These prevalence rates may even be conservative, because "certain symptoms of psychiatric disorders among immigrant populations (e.g., *ataque de nervios*) would not be represented in the diagnostic batteries used with the general population" (Kaplan, 2007, p. 2). As this cultural group, and particularly U.S.-born Latino Americans, continues to grow in number, mental health professionals will need to develop awareness of this increased risk for illness and sensitivity to the cultural values that may impact seeking treatment.

Western European Americans

Western European Americans have their origin in France, Italy, and Greece. Each of these cultures possesses its own language, in which a number of dialects are noticeable. Western Europeans are considered to be very warm and affectionate people. They tend to be physically expressive, using a lot of body language, including hugging and kissing.

Like Latino Americans, Western European Americans are very family oriented. They interact in large groups, and it is not uncommon for several generations to live together or in close proximity. A strong allegiance to the cultural heritage exists, and it is not uncommon, particularly among Italians, to find settlements of immigrants clustering together.

Roles within the family are clearly defined, with the man as the head of the household. Traditional Western European women view their role as mother and homemaker, and children are prized and cherished. The elderly are held in positions of respect and often are cared for in the home rather than placed in nursing homes.

Roman Catholicism is the predominant religion for French and Italian people, Greek Orthodox for the Greek community. A number of religious traditions are observed surrounding rites of passage. Masses and rituals are observed for births, first communions, marriages, anniversaries, and deaths.

Western Europeans tend to be present-time oriented, with a somewhat fatalistic view of the future. A priority is placed on the here and now, and whatever happens in the future is perceived as God's will.

Most Western European Americans follow health beliefs and practices of the dominant American culture, but some folk beliefs and superstitions still endure. Spector (2013) reports the following superstitions and practices of Italians as they relate to health and illness:

1. Congenital abnormalities can be attributed to the unsatisfied desire for food during pregnancy.
2. If a woman is not given food that she craves or smells, the fetus will move inside, and a miscarriage can result.
3. If a pregnant woman bends or turns or moves in a certain way, the fetus may not develop normally.
4. A woman must not reach during pregnancy because reaching can harm the fetus.
5. Sitting in a draft can cause a cold that can lead to pneumonia.

Food is very important in the Western European American culture. Italian, Greek, and French cuisine is world famous, and food is used in a social manner, as well as for nutritional purposes. Wine is consumed by all (even the children, who are given a mixture of water and wine) and is the beverage of choice with meals. However, among Greek Americans, drunkenness engenders social disgrace on the individual and the family (Purnell, 2009).

Arab Americans*

Arab Americans trace their ancestry and traditions to the nomadic desert tribes of the Arabian Peninsula. The Arab countries include Algeria, Bahrain, Comoros, Djibouti, Egypt, Iraq, Jordan, Kuwait, Lebanon, Libya, Mauritania, Morocco, Oman, Palestine, Qatar, Saudi Arabia, Somalia, Sudan, Syria, Tunisia, United Arab Emirates, and Yemen.

First-wave immigrants, primarily Christians, came to the United States between 1887 and 1913 seeking economic opportunity. First-wave immigrants and their descendants typically resided in urban centers of the Northeast. Second-wave immigrants entered the United States after World War II. Most are refugees from nations beset by war and political instability. This group includes a large number of professionals and individuals seeking educational degrees who have subsequently remained in the United States. Most are Muslims and favor professional occupations.

Arabic is the official language of the Arab world. Although English is a common second language, language and communication can pose formidable problems in health-care settings. Communication is highly contextual, where unspoken expectations are more important than the actual spoken words. While conversing, individuals stand close together, maintain steady eye contact, and touch (only between members of the same gender) the other's hand or shoulder.

Speech may be loud and expressive and characterized by repetition and gesturing, particularly when involved in serious discussions. Observers witnessing impassioned communication may incorrectly assume that members of this culture are argumentative, confrontational, or aggressive. Privacy is valued, and

---

*This section on Arab Americans is adapted from Kulwicki, A.D., & Ballout, S. (2013). People of Arab heritage. In L.D. Purnell (Ed.), *Transcultural health care: A culturally competent approach* (4th ed.). © F.A. Davis. Used with permission.

many resist disclosure of personal information to strangers, especially when it relates to familial disease conditions. Among friends and relatives, Arabs express feelings freely. Devout Muslim men may not shake hands with women. When an Arab man is introduced to an Arab woman, the man waits for the woman to extend her hand.

Punctuality is not taken seriously except in cases of business or professional meetings. Social events and appointments tend not to have a fixed beginning or end.

Gender roles are clearly defined. The man is the head of the household and women are subordinate to men. Men are breadwinners, protectors, and decision makers. Women are responsible for the care and education of children and for the maintenance of a successful marriage by tending to their husbands' needs.

The family is the primary social organization, and children are loved and indulged. The father is the disciplinarian and the mother is an ally and mediator. Loyalty to one's family takes precedence over personal needs. Sons are responsible for supporting elderly parents.

Women value modesty, especially devout Muslims, for whom modesty is expressed with their attire. Many Muslim women view the practice of *hijab*, covering the body except for one's face and hands, as offering them protection in situations in which the genders mix.

Sickle cell disease and the thalassemias are common in the eastern Mediterranean. Sedentary lifestyle and high fat intake among Arab Americans place them at higher risk for cardiovascular diseases. The rates of cholesterol testing, colorectal cancer screening, and uterine cancer screening are low; however, in recent years, the rate of mammography screening has increased.

Arab cooking shares many general characteristics. Spices and herbs include cinnamon, allspice, cloves, ginger, cumin, mint, parsley, bay leaves, garlic, and onions. Bread accompanies every meal and is viewed as a gift from God. Lamb and chicken are the most popular meats. Muslims are prohibited from eating pork and pork products. Food is eaten with the right hand because it is regarded as clean. Eating and drinking at the same time is viewed as unhealthy. Eating properly, consuming nutritious foods, and fasting are believed to cure disease. Gastrointestinal complaints are the most frequent reason for seeking health care. Lactose intolerance is common.

Most Arabs are Muslims. Islam is the religion of most Arab countries, and in Islam there is no separation of church and state; a certain amount of religious participation is obligatory. Many Muslims believe in combining spiritual medicine, performing daily prayers, and reading or listening to the Qur'an with conventional medical treatment. The devout client may request that his or her chair or bed be turned to face Mecca and that a basin of water be provided for ritual washing or ablution before praying. Sometimes illness is considered punishment for one's sins.

Mental illness is a major social stigma. Psychiatric symptoms may be denied or attributed to "bad nerves" or evil spirits. When individuals suffering from mental distress seek medical care, they are likely to present with a variety of vague complaints such as abdominal pain, lassitude, anorexia, and shortness of breath. Clients often expect and may insist on somatic treatment, at least vitamins and tonics. When mental illness is accepted as a diagnosis, treatment with medications, rather than counseling, is preferred.

Jewish Americans

To be Jewish is to belong to a specific group of people and a specific religion. The term *Jewish* does not refer to a race. The Jewish people came to the United States mostly from Spain, Portugal, Germany, and Eastern Europe (Schwartz, 2013). There are more than 5 million Jewish Americans living in the United States, and they live primarily in the larger urban areas.

Four main Jewish religious groups exist today: Orthodox, Reform, Conservative, and Reconstructionist. Orthodox Jews adhere to strict interpretation and application of Jewish laws and ethics. They believe that the laws outlined in the Torah (the five books of Moses) are divine, eternal, and unalterable. Reform Judaism is the largest Jewish religious group in the United States. The Reform group believes in the autonomy of the individual in interpreting the Jewish code of law, and a more liberal interpretation is followed. Conservative Jews also accept a less strict interpretation. They believe that the code of laws comes from God, but accept flexibility and adaptation of those laws to absorb aspects of the culture while remaining true to Judaism's values. The Reconstructionists have modern views that generally override traditional Jewish laws. They do not believe that Jews are God's chosen people and they reject the notion of divine intervention. Reconstructionists are generally accepting of interfaith marriage.

The primary language of Jewish Americans is English. Hebrew, the official language of Israel and the Torah, is used for prayers and is taught in Jewish religious education. Early Jewish immigrants spoke a Judeo-German dialect called Yiddish, and some of those words have become part of American English (e.g., *klutz, kosher, tush, chutzpah, mazel tov*).

Although traditional Jewish law is clearly male oriented, with acculturation little difference is seen today with regard to gender roles. Formal education is a highly respected value among the Jewish people. More than half of all Jewish adults have received a college degree, and a quarter have earned a graduate degree (Chiswick, 2009). Jewish people hold a proportionately higher percentage of professional and executive positions when compared to the total U.S. population (United Jewish Communities, 2003).

While most Jewish people live for today and plan for and worry about tomorrow, they are raised with stories of their past, especially of the Holocaust. They are warned to "never forget," lest history be repeated. Therefore, their time orientation is simultaneously to the past, the present, and the future (Selekman, 2013).

Children are considered blessings and valued treasures, treated with respect, and deeply loved. They play an active role in most holiday celebrations and services. Respecting and honoring one's parents is one of the Ten Commandments. Children are expected to be forever grateful to their parents for giving them the gift of life (Selekman, 2013). The rite of passage into adulthood occurs during a religious ceremony called a *bar* or *bat mitzvah* (son or daughter of the commandment) and is usually commemorated by a family celebration.

Because of the respect afforded physicians and the emphasis on keeping the body and mind healthy, Jewish Americans tend to be health conscious. In general, they practice preventive health care, with routine physical, dental, and vision screening. Circumcision for male infants is both a medical procedure and a religious rite and is performed on the eighth day of life. The procedure is usually performed at home and is considered a family festivity.

A number of genetic diseases are more common in the Jewish population, including Tay-Sachs disease, Gaucher's disease, and familial dysautonomia. Other conditions that occur with increased incidence in the Jewish population include inflammatory bowel disease (ulcerative colitis and Crohn's disease), colorectal cancer, and breast and ovarian cancer. Jewish people have a higher rate of side effects from the antipsychotic clozapine. About 20 percent develop agranulocytosis, the cause of which has been attributed to a specific genetic haplotype (Selekman, 2013).

Alcohol, especially wine, is an essential part of religious holidays and festive occasions. It is viewed as appropriate and acceptable as long as it is used in moderation. For Jewish people who follow the dietary laws, a tremendous amount of attention is given to the slaughter of livestock and the preparation and consumption of food. Religious laws dictate which foods are permissible. The term *kosher* means "fit to eat," and following these guidelines is considered a commandment of God. Meat may be eaten only if the permitted animal has been slaughtered, cooked, or served following kosher guidelines. Pigs are considered unclean, and pork and pork products are forbidden. Dairy products and meat may not be mixed together in cooking, serving, or eating.

Judaism opposes discrimination against people with physical, mental, and developmental conditions. The maintenance of one's mental health is considered just as important as the maintenance of one's physical health. Mental incapacity has always been recognized as grounds for exemption from all obligations under Jewish law (Selekman, 2013).

A summary of information related to the six cultural phenomena as they apply to the cultural groups discussed here is presented in Table 6-1.

Culture-Bound Syndromes

Culture-bound syndromes are "unique patterns of aberrant behavior and troubling experiences, [that occur] in various parts of the world, whose clinical descriptions do not readily fit into the Western conventional diagnostic categories" (Gaw, 2008, p. 1537). It is important for nurses to understand that individuals from diverse cultural groups may exhibit these physical and behavioral manifestations. The syndromes are viewed within these cultural groups as folk, diagnostic categories with specific sets of experiences and observations. Examples of culture-bound syndromes are presented in Table 6-2.

Diagnosis/Outcome Identification

Nursing diagnoses are selected based on the information gathered during the assessment process. With background knowledge of cultural variables and information uniquely related to the individual, the following nursing diagnoses may be appropriate:

■ Impaired verbal communication related to cultural differences evidenced by inability to speak the dominant language
■ Anxiety (moderate to severe) related to entry into an unfamiliar health-care system and separation from support systems evidenced by apprehension and suspicion, restlessness, and trembling
■ Imbalanced nutrition, less than body requirements, related to refusal to eat unfamiliar foods provided in the health-care setting, evidenced by loss of weight
■ Spiritual distress related to inability to participate in usual religious practices because of hospitalization, evidenced by alterations in mood (e.g., anger, crying, withdrawal, preoccupation, anxiety, hostility, apathy)

Outcome criteria related to these nursing diagnoses may include the following:

The client has:

1. Had all basic needs fulfilled.
2. Communicated with staff through an interpreter.
3. Maintained anxiety at a manageable level by having family members stay with him or her during hospitalization.

TABLE 6–1 Summary of Six Cultural Phenomena in Comparison of Various Cultural Groups

CULTURAL GROUP AND COUNTRIES OF ORIGIN	COMMUNICATION	SPACE	SOCIAL ORGANIZATION	TIME	ENVIRONMENTAL CONTROL	BIOLOGICAL VARIATIONS
Northern European Americans (England, Ireland, Germany, others)	National languages (although many learn English very quickly) Dialects (often regional) English More verbal than nonverbal	Territory valued Personal space: 18 inches to 3 feet Uncomfortable with personal contact and touch	Families: nuclear and extended Religions: Jewish and Christian Organizations: social community	Future-oriented	Most value preventive medicine and primary health care through traditional health-care delivery system Alternative methods on the increase	Health concerns: Cardiovascular disease Cancer Diabetes mellitus
African Americans (Africa, West Indian Islands, Dominican Republic, Haiti, Jamaica)	National languages Dialects (pidgin, Creole, Gullah, French, Spanish) Highly verbal and nonverbal	Close personal space Comfortable with touch	Large, extended families Many female-headed households Strong religious orientation, mostly Protestant Community social organizations	Present-time oriented	Traditional health-care delivery system Some individuals prefer to use folk practitioner ("granny" or voodoo healer) Home remedies	Health concerns: Cardiovascular disease Hypertension Sickle cell disease Diabetes mellitus Lactose intolerance
Native Americans (North America, Alaska, Aleutian Islands)	200 tribal languages recognized Comfortable with silence Direct eye contact considered rude	Large, extended space important Uncomfortable with touch	Families: nuclear and extended Children taught importance of tradition Social organizations: tribe and family most important	Present-time oriented	Religion and health practices intertwined Nontraditional healer (shaman) uses folk practices to heal Shaman may work with modern medical practitioner	Health concerns: Alcoholism Tuberculosis Accidents Diabetes mellitus Heart disease
Asian/Pacific Islander Americans (Japan, China, Korea, Vietnam, Philippines, Thailand, Cambodia, Laos, Pacific Islands, others)	More than 30 different languages spoken Comfortable with silence Uncomfortable with eye-to-eye contact Nonverbal connotations may be misunderstood	Large personal space Uncomfortable with touch	Families: nuclear and extended Children taught importance of family loyalty and tradition Many religions: Taoism, Buddhism, Islam, Hinduism, Christianity Community social organizations	Present-time oriented Past is important and valued	Traditional health-care delivery system Some prefer to use folk practices (e.g., yin and yang, herbal medicine, and moxibustion)	Health concerns: Hypertension Cancer Diabetes mellitus Thalassemia Lactose intolerance

Group	Language	Personal space/touch	Family/social organization	Time orientation	Traditional health care	Health concerns
Latino Americans (Mexico, Spain, Cuba, Puerto Rico, other countries of Central and South America)	Spanish, with many dialects	Close personal space. Lots of touching and embracing. Very group oriented	Families: nuclear and large extended families. Strong ties to Roman Catholicism. Community social organizations	Present-time oriented	Traditional health-care delivery system. Some prefer to use folk practitioner, called *curandero* or *curandera*. Folk practices include "hot and cold" herbal remedies	Heart disease, Cancer, Diabetes mellitus, Accidents, Lactose intolerance
Western European Americans (France, Italy, Greece)	National languages. Dialects	Close personal space. Lots of touching and embracing. Very group oriented	Families: nuclear and large extended families. France and Italy: Roman Catholic. Greece: Greek Orthodox	Present-time oriented	Traditional health-care delivery system. Lots of home remedies and practices based on superstition	Heart disease, Cancer, Diabetes mellitus, Thalassemia
Arab Americans (Algeria, Bahrain, Comoros, Djibouti, Egypt, Iraq, Jordan, Kuwait, Lebanon, Libya, Mauritania, Morocco, Oman, Palestine, Qatar, Saudi Arabia, Somalia, Sudan, Syria, Tunisia, United Arab Emirates, Yemen)	Arabic, English	Large personal space between members of the opposite gender outside of the family. Touching common between members of same gender	Families: nuclear and extended. Religion: Muslim and Christianity	Past and present-time oriented	Traditional health-care delivery system. Some superstitious beliefs. Authority of physician is seldom challenged or questioned. Adverse outcomes are attributed to God's will. Mental illness viewed as a social stigma	Sickle cell disease, Thalassemia, Cardiovascular disease, Cancer
Jewish Americans (Spain, Portugal, Germany, Eastern Europe)	English, Hebrew, Yiddish	Touch forbidden between opposite genders in the Orthodox tradition. Closer personal space common among non-orthodox Jews	Families: nuclear and extended. Community social organizations	Past, present-time, and future oriented	Great respect for physicians. Emphasis on keeping body and mind healthy. Practice preventive health care	Tay-Sachs disease, Gaucher's disease, Familial dysautonomia, Ulcerative colitis, Crohn's disease, Colorectal cancer, Breast cancer, Ovarian cancer

SOURCES: Giger (2013); Murray, Zentner, & Yakimo (2009); Purnell (2013); and Spector (2013).

TABLE 6–2 Examples of Culture-Bound Syndromes

SYNDROME	CULTURE	SYMPTOMS
Amok	Malaysia; Philippines	Violent or homicidal behavior preceded by a state of brooding and ending with a period of somnolence and amnesia.
Ataque de nervios	Latin America; Latin Mediterranean	Uncontrollable shouting, crying, trembling, verbal or physical aggression, sometimes accompanied by dissociative experiences, seizure-like or fainting episodes, and suicidal gestures.
Brain fag	West Africa	Difficulty concentrating; poor memory retention; pain and pressure around head and neck; blurred vision. Students often complain of "brain fatigue."
Ghost sickness	American Indian tribes	Preoccupation with death and the deceased. Symptoms include anxiety, confusion, weakness, feelings of danger, anorexia, and bad dreams. Sometimes associated with witchcraft.
Hwa-byung	Korea	Attributed to the suppression of anger. Symptoms closely related to those of depression, including insomnia, fatigue, indigestion, dysphoria, anorexia, bodily aches, and loss of interest.
Koro	Southern and Eastern Asia	Intense anxiety associated with the fear that the penis (in males) or the vulva and nipples (in females) will retract into the body and cause the person to die.
Pibloktoq	Eskimo cultures	Sometimes called *arctic hysteria*. An abrupt episode of extreme excitement, preceded by withdrawal or mild irritability, and followed by seizure activity and coma. During the attack the individual engages in aberrant and bizarre verbal and motor behavior. Afterward, usually reports complete amnesia for the attack.
Susto	Latin America	Symptoms include appetite and sleep disturbances, sadness, pains, headache, stomachache, and diarrhea. The soul is thought to leave the body (during dreams or following a traumatic event), resulting in unhappiness and illness.
Taijin kyofusho	Japan	Intense anxiety and fear about possibly offending others, particularly with their body functions, appearance, or odor.

SOURCES: Gaw (2008); Giger (2013); Purnell (2013); and Spector (2013).

4. Maintained weight by eating foods that he or she likes brought to the hospital by family members.
5. Restored spiritual strength through use of cultural rituals and beliefs and visits from a spiritual leader.

Planning/Implementation

The following interventions have special cultural implications for nursing:

1. Use an interpreter if necessary to ensure that there are no barriers to communication. Be careful with nonverbal communication because it may be interpreted differently by different cultures (e.g., Asians and Native Americans may be uncomfortable with touch and direct eye contact, whereas Latinos and Western Europeans perceive touch as a sign of caring).

2. Make allowances for individuals from other cultures to have family members around them and even participate in their care. Large numbers of extended family members are very important to African Americans, Native Americans, Asian Americans, Latino Americans, and Western European Americans. To deny access to these family support systems could interfere with the healing process.

3. Ensure that the individual's spiritual needs are being met. Religion is an important source of support for many individuals, and the nurse must be tolerant of various rituals that may be connected

with different cultural beliefs about health and illness.

4. Be aware of the differences in concept of time among the various cultures. Most members of the dominant American culture are future oriented and place a high value on punctuality and efficiency. Other cultures such as African Americans, Native Americans, Asian Americans, Latino Americans, Arab Americans and Western European Americans are more present-time oriented. Nurses must be aware that such individuals may not share the value of punctuality. They may be late to appointments and appear to be indifferent to some aspects of their therapy. Nurses must be accepting of these differences and refrain from allowing existing attitudes to interfere with delivery of care.

5. Be aware of different beliefs about health care among the various cultures, and recognize the importance of these beliefs to the healing process. If an individual from another culture has been receiving health care from a spiritualist, granny, curandero, or other nontraditional healer, it is important for the nurse to listen to what has been done in the past and even to consult with these cultural healers about the care being given to the client.

6. Follow the health-care practices that the client views as essential, provided they do no harm or do not interfere with the healing process of the client. For example, the concepts of yin and yang and the "hot and cold" theory of disease are very important to the well-being of some Asians and Latinos, respectively. Try to ensure that a balance of these foods is included in the diet as an important reinforcement for traditional medical care.

7. Be aware of favorite foods of individuals from different cultures. The health-care setting may seem strange and somewhat isolated, and for some individuals it feels good to have anything around them that is familiar. They may even refuse to eat foods that are unfamiliar to them. If it does not interfere with his or her care, allow family members to provide favorite foods for the client.

8. The nurse working in psychiatry must realize that psychiatric illness is stigmatized in some cultures. Individuals who believe that expressing emotions is unacceptable (e.g., Asian Americans and Native Americans) will present unique problems when they are clients in a psychiatric setting. Nurses must have patience and work slowly to establish trust in order to provide these individuals with the assistance they require.

Evaluation

Evaluation of nursing actions is directed at achievement of the established outcomes. Part of the evaluation process is continuous reassessment to ensure that the selected actions are appropriate and the goals and outcomes are realistic. Including the family and extended support systems in the evaluation process is essential if cultural implications of nursing care are to be measured. Modifications to the plan of care are made as the need is determined.

Spiritual Concepts

CORE CONCEPT
Spirituality
The human quality that gives meaning and sense of purpose to an individual's existence. Spirituality exists within each individual regardless of belief system and serves as a force for interconnectedness between the self and others, the environment, and a higher power.

Spirituality is difficult to describe. Historically, it has had distinctly religious connections, with a spiritual person being described as "someone with whom the Spirit of God dwelt." More recently, however, it has been considered "something people define for themselves that is largely free of the rules, regulations and responsibilities associated with religion" (Koenig, 2009, p. 284).

In the treatment of mental illness, some of the earliest practices focused on including spiritual treatment, because insanity was considered a disruption of mind and spirit (Reeves & Reynolds, 2009). However, Freud (often described as a forefather of psychiatric treatment) believed that religion had a negative effect on mental health, and that it was linked to a host of psychiatric symptoms. Thus religion and spiritually have been avoided rather than embraced as a valuable aspect of treatment. More recently, the focus is changing once again. Reeves and Reynolds (2009) note that the large volume of contemporary research (more than 60 studies) demonstrating the value of spirituality for both medical and psychiatric patients is influencing this change. Nursing has embraced this new focus by the inclusion of nursing responsibility for spiritual care in the International Council of Nurses *Code of Ethics* and in the American Holistic Nurses Association *Standards for Holistic Nursing Practice*. The inclusion of spiritual care is also evidenced by the development of the nursing diagnosis category "Spiritual Distress" by NANDA International (Wright, 2005).

Smucker (2001) stated:

Spirituality is the recognition or experience of a dimension of life that is invisible, and both within us and yet beyond our material world, providing a sense of connectedness and interrelatedness with the universe. (p. 5)

Smucker (2001) identified the following factors as types of spiritual needs associated with human beings:

1. Meaning and purpose in life
2. Faith or trust in someone or something beyond ourselves
3. Hope
4. Love
5. Forgiveness

Spiritual Needs

Meaning and Purpose in Life

Humans by nature appreciate order and structure in their lives. Having a purpose in life gives one a sense of control and the feeling that life is worth living. Indeed, Burkhardt and Nagai-Jacobson (2002) describe the essence of spirituality as the developing awareness of who we are, what is our purpose in being, and the understanding of our connectedness with ourselves as well as beyond ourselves. Each nurse's exploration of his or her own spirituality and efforts to grow spiritually are foundational to being responsive to those needs in others. Walsh (1999) describes "seven perennial practices" that he believes promote enlightenment, aid in transformation, and encourage spiritual growth. He identified the seven perennial practices as follows:

1. **Transform your motivation:** Reduce craving and find your soul's desire.
2. **Cultivate emotional wisdom:** Heal your heart and learn to love.
3. **Live ethically:** Feel good by doing good.
4. **Concentrate and calm your mind:** Accept the challenge of mastering attention and mindfulness.
5. **Awaken your spiritual vision:** See clearly and recognize the sacred in all things.
6. **Cultivate spiritual intelligence:** Develop wisdom and understand life.
7. **Express spirit in action:** Embrace generosity and the joy of service. (p. 14)

In the final analysis, each individual must determine his or her own perception of what is important and what gives meaning to life. Throughout one's existence, the meaning of life will undoubtedly be challenged many times. A solid spiritual foundation may help an individual confront the challenges that result from life's experiences.

Faith

Faith is often thought of as the acceptance of a belief in the absence of physical or empirical evidence. Smucker (2001) stated:

> For all people, faith is an important concept. From childhood on, our psychological health depends on having faith or trust in something or someone to help meet our needs. (p. 7)

Having faith requires that individuals rise above that which they can only experience through the five senses. Indeed, faith transcends the appearance of the physical world. An increasing amount of medical and scientific research is showing that what individuals believe exists can have as powerful an impact as what actually exists. Karren, Hafen, Smith, and Jenkins (2010) stated:

> [There is a] growing appreciation of the healing power of faith among members of the medical community. Belief strongly impacts health outcomes, and belief of a large majority of Americans is connected to their religious commitments. Seventy-five percent of Americans say that their religious faith forms the foundation for their approach to life. Seventy-three percent of Americans say that prayer is an important part of their daily life. Religious belief provides power for an individual. With such beliefs so prevalent, it is no surprise that religious faith plays a significant role in healing. (p. 360)

Evidence suggests that faith, combined with conventional treatment and an optimistic attitude, can be a very powerful element in the healing process.

Hope

Hope has been defined as a special kind of positive expectation (Karren et al., 2010). With hope, individuals look at a situation, and no matter how negative, find something positive on which to focus. Hope functions as an energizing force. In addition, research indicates that hope may promote healing, facilitate coping, and enhance quality of life (Nekolaichuk, Jevne, & Maguire, 1999).

Kübler-Ross (1969), in her classic study of dying patients, stressed the importance of hope. She suggested that, even though these patients could not hope for a cure, they could hope for additional time to live, to be with loved ones, for freedom from pain, or for a peaceful death with dignity. She found hope to be a satisfaction unto itself, whether or not it was fulfilled. She stated, "If a patient stops expressing hope, it is usually a sign of imminent death" (p. 140).

Researchers in the field of psychoneuroimmunology have found that the attitudes we have and the emotions we experience have a definite effect on the body. An optimistic feeling of hope is not just a mental state. Hope and optimism produce positive physical changes in the body that can influence the immune system and the functioning of specific body organs. The medical literature abounds with countless examples of individuals with terminal conditions who suddenly improve when they find something to live for. Conversely, there are also many accounts of patients whose conditions deteriorate when they lose hope.

Love

Love may be identified as a projection of one's own good feelings onto others. To love others, one must first experience love of self, and then be able and willing to project that warmth and affectionate concern for others (Karren et al., 2010).

Smucker (2001) stated:

> Love, in its purest unconditional form, is probably life's most powerful force and our greatest spiritual need. Not only is it important to receive love, but equally important to give love to others. Thinking about and caring for the needs of others keeps us from being too absorbed with ourselves and our needs to the exclusion of others. We all have experienced the good feelings that come from caring for and loving others. (p. 10)

Love may be a very important key in the healing process. Karren and associates (2010) stated:

> People who become more loving and less fearful, who replace negative thoughts with the emotion of love, are often able to achieve physical healing. Most of us are familiar with the emotional effects of love, the way love makes us feel inside. But . . . true love— a love that is patient, trusting, protecting, optimistic, and kind—has actual physical effects on the body, too. (p. 406)

Some researchers suggest that love has a positive effect on the immune system. This has been shown to be true in adults and children, and also in animals (Fox & Fox, 1988; Ornish, 1998). The giving and receiving of love may also result in higher levels of endorphins, thereby contributing to a sense of euphoria and helping to reduce pain.

In one long-term study, researchers Werner and Smith (1992) studied children who were reared in impoverished environments. Their homes were troubled by discord, desertion, or divorce, or marred by parental alcoholism or mental illness. The subjects were studied at birth, childhood, adolescence, and adulthood. Two out of three of these high-risk children had developed serious learning and/or behavioral problems by age 10, or had a record of delinquencies, mental health problems, or pregnancies by age 18. One-fourth of them had developed "very serious" physical and psychosocial problems. By the time they reached adulthood, more than three-fourths of them suffered from profound psychological and behavioral problems and even more were in poor physical health. But of particular interest to the researchers were the 15 to 20 percent who remained resilient and well despite their impoverished and difficult existence. The children who remained resilient and well had experienced a warm and loving relationship with another person during their first year of life, whereas the children who developed serious psychological and physical problems had not. This research indicates that the earlier people have the benefit of a strong, loving relationship, the better they seem able to resist the effects of a deleterious lifestyle.

Forgiveness

Karren and associates (2010) stated, "Essential to a spiritual nature is forgiveness—the ability to release from the mind all the past hurts and failures, all sense of guilt and loss" (p. 377). Feelings of bitterness and resentment take a physical toll on an individual by generating stress hormones, which maintained for long periods can have a detrimental effect on a person's health. Forgiveness enables a person to cast off resentment and begin the pathway to healing.

Forgiveness is not easy. Individuals often have great difficulty when called upon to forgive others and even greater difficulty in attempting to forgive themselves. Many people carry throughout their lives a sense of guilt for having committed a mistake for which they do not believe they have been forgiven or for which they have not forgiven themselves.

To forgive is not necessarily to condone or excuse one's own or someone else's inappropriate behavior. Karren and associates (2010) have suggested that forgiveness is:

> . . . an attitude that implies that you are willing to accept responsibility for your perceptions, realizing that your perceptions are a choice and not an objective fact; a decision to see beyond the limits of another's personality, and to gradually transform yourself from being a helpless victim of your circumstances to being a powerful and loving co-creator of your reality. (p. 378)

Holding on to grievances causes pain, suffering, and conflict. Forgiveness (of self and others) is a gift to oneself. It offers freedom and peace of mind.

It is important for nurses to be able to assess the spiritual needs of their clients. Nurses need not serve the role of professional counselor or spiritual guide, but because of the closeness of their relationship with clients, nurses may be the part of the health-care team to whom clients may reveal the most intimate details of their lives. Smucker (2001) stated:

> Just as answering a patient's question honestly and with accurate information and responding to his needs in a timely and sensitive manner communicates caring, so also does high-quality professional nursing care reach beyond the physical body or the illness to that part of the person where identity, self-worth, and spirit lie. In this sense, good nursing care is also good spiritual care. (pp. 11-12)

Religion

Religion is one way in which an individual's spirituality may be expressed. There are more than 6500 religions in the world (Bronson, 2005). Some individuals seek out various religions in an attempt to find answers to fundamental questions that they have about life, and indeed, about their very existence. Others, although they may regard themselves as spiritual, choose not to affiliate with an organized religious group. In either situation, however, it is inevitable that questions related to life and the human condition arise during the progression of spiritual maturation.

Brodd (2009) suggested that all religious traditions manifest seven dimensions: experiential, mythic, doctrinal, ethical, ritual, social, and material. He explains that these seven dimensions are intertwined and complementary and, depending on the particular religion, certain dimensions are emphasized more than others. For example, Zen Buddhism has a strong experiential dimension, but says little about doctrines. Roman Catholicism is strong in both ritual and doctrine. The social dimension is a significant aspect of religion, as it provides a sense of community, of belonging to a group such as a parish or a congregation, which is empowering for some individuals.

Affiliation with a religious group has been shown to be a health-enhancing endeavor (Karren et al., 2010). A number of studies have been conducted that indicate a correlation between religious faith/church attendance and increased chance of survival following serious illness, less depression and other mental illness, longer life, and overall better physical and mental health. In an extensive review of the literature, Maryland psychologist John Gartner (1996) found that individuals with a religious commitment had lower suicide rates, lower drug use and abuse, less juvenile delinquency, lower divorce rates, and improved mental illness outcomes.

It is not known how religious participation protects health and promotes well-being. Some churches actively promote healthy lifestyles and discourage behavior that would be harmful to health or interfere with treatment of disease. But some researchers believe that the strong social support network found in churches may be the most important force in boosting the health and well-being of their members. More so than merely an affiliation, however, it is regular church attendance and participation that appear to be the key factors.

Addressing Spiritual and Religious Needs Through the Nursing Process

Assessment

It is important for nurses to consider spiritual and religious needs when planning care for their clients. The Joint Commission requires that nurses address the psychosocial, spiritual, and cultural variables that influence the perception of illness. Dossey (1998) has developed a spiritual assessment tool (Box 6-4) about which she stated,

> The Spiritual Assessment Tool provides reflective questions for assessing, evaluating, and increasing awareness of spirituality in patients and their significant others. The tool's reflective questions can facilitate healing because they stimulate spontaneous, independent, meaningful initiatives to improve the patient's capacity for recovery and healing (p. 45)

Assessing the spiritual needs of a client with a psychotic disorder can pose some additional challenges. Approximately 25 percent of people with schizophrenia and 15 to 22 percent of people with bipolar disorder have religious delusions (Koenig, 2009). Sometimes these delusions can be difficult to differentiate from general religious or cultural beliefs but "longitudinal studies suggest that nonpsychotic religious activity may actually improve long-term prognosis in patients with psychotic disorders" (Koenig, 2009, p. 288). Engaging family members and significant others in the assessment process can be a great help in determining which religious beliefs and activities have been beneficial to the patient versus those that have been detrimental to his or her progress.

Diagnoses/Outcome Identification

Nursing diagnoses that may be used when addressing spiritual and religious needs of clients include:

■ Risk for spiritual distress
■ Spiritual distress
■ Readiness for enhanced spiritual well-being
■ Risk for impaired religiosity
■ Impaired religiosity
■ Readiness for enhanced religiosity

The following outcomes may be used as guidelines for care and to evaluate effectiveness of the nursing interventions.

The client will:

1. Identify meaning and purpose in life that reinforce hope, peace, and contentment.

BOX 6-4 **Spiritual Assessment Tool**

The following reflective questions may assist you in assessing, evaluating, and increasing awareness of spirituality in yourself and others.

MEANING AND PURPOSE

These questions assess a person's ability to seek meaning and fulfillment in life, manifest hope, and accept ambiguity and uncertainty.

- What gives your life meaning?
- Do you have a sense of purpose in life?
- Does your illness interfere with your life goals?
- Why do you want to get well?
- How hopeful are you about obtaining a better degree of health?
- Do you feel that you have a responsibility in maintaining your health?
- Will you be able to make changes in your life to maintain your health?
- Are you motivated to get well?
- What is the most important or powerful thing in your life?

INNER STRENGTHS

These questions assess a person's ability to manifest joy and recognize strengths, choices, goals, and faith.

- What brings you joy and peace in your life?
- What can you do to feel alive and full of spirit?
- What traits do you like about yourself?
- What are your personal strengths?
- What choices are available to you to enhance your healing?
- What life goals have you set for yourself?
- Do you think that stress in any way caused your illness?
- How aware were you of your body before you became sick?
- What do you believe in?
- Is faith important in your life?
- How has your illness influenced your faith?
- Does faith play a role in recognizing your health?

INTERCONNECTIONS

These questions assess a person's positive self-concept, self-esteem, and sense of self; sense of belonging in the world with others; capacity to pursue personal interests; and ability to demonstrate love of self and self-forgiveness.

- How do you feel about yourself right now?
- How do you feel when you have a true sense of yourself?
- Do you pursue things of personal interest?
- What do you do to show love for yourself?
- Can you forgive yourself?
- What do you do to heal your spirit?

These questions assess a person's ability to connect in life-giving ways with family, friends, and social groups and to engage in the forgiveness of others.

- Who are the significant people in your life?
- Do you have friends or family in town who are available to help you?
- Who are the people to whom you are closest?
- Do you belong to any groups?
- Can you ask people for help when you need it?
- Can you share your feelings with others?
- What are some of the most loving things that others have done for you?
- What are the loving things that you do for other people?
- Are you able to forgive others?

These questions assess a person's capacity for finding meaning in worship or religious activities, and a connectedness with a divinity.

- Is worship important to you?
- What do you consider the most significant act of worship in your life?
- Do you participate in any religious activities?
- Do you believe in God or a higher power?
- Do you think that prayer is powerful?
- Have you ever tried to empty your mind of all thoughts to see what the experience might be?
- Do you use relaxation or imagery skills?
- Do you meditate?
- Do you pray?
- What is your prayer?
- How are your prayers answered?
- Do you have a sense of belonging in this world?

These questions assess a person's ability to experience a sense of connection with life and nature, an awareness of the effects of the environment on life and well-being, and a capacity or concern for the health of the environment.

- Do you ever feel a connection with the world or universe?
- How does your environment have an impact on your state of well-being?
- What are your environmental stressors at work and at home?
- What strategies reduce your environmental stressors?
- Do you have any concerns for the state of your immediate environment?
- Are you involved with environmental issues such as recycling environmental resources at home, work, or in your community?
- Are you concerned about the survival of the planet?

SOURCES: Burkhardt, M.A. (1989). Spirituality: An analysis of the concept. *Holistic Nursing Practice, 3*(3), 69-77; Dossey, B.M. et al., (Eds.), (1995). *Holistic nursing: A handbook for practice* (2nd ed.). Gaithersburg, MD: Aspen. From Dossey, B.M. (1998). Holistic modalities and healing moments. *American Journal of Nursing, 98*(6), 44-47, with permission.

2. Verbalize acceptance of self as a worthwhile human being.
3. Accept and incorporate change into life in a healthy manner.
4. Express understanding of relationship between difficulties in current life situation and interruption in previous religious beliefs and activities.
5. Discuss beliefs and values about spiritual and religious issues.
6. Express desire and ability to participate in beliefs and activities of desired religion.

Planning/Implementation

NANDA International (NANDA-I, 2012) information related to the diagnoses Risk for Spiritual Distress and Risk for Impaired Religiosity is provided in the subsections that follow.

Risk for Spiritual Distress

Definition: At risk for an impaired ability to experience and integrate meaning and purpose in life through a connectedness with self, others, art, music, literature, nature, and/or a power greater than oneself (NANDA-I, 2012, p. 412).

Risk Factors

Physical: Physical/chronic illness; substance abuse
Psychosocial: Low self-esteem; depression; anxiety; stress; poor relationships; separate from support systems; blocks to experiencing love; inability to forgive; loss; racial/cultural conflict; change in religious rituals; change in spiritual practices
Developmental: Life changes

Environmental: Environmental changes; natural disasters

Risk for Impaired Religiosity

Definition: At risk for an impaired ability to exercise reliance on religious beliefs and/or participate in rituals of a particular faith tradition (NANDA-I, 2012, p. 407).

Risk Factors

Physical: Illness/hospitalization; pain
Psychological: Ineffective support/coping/caregiving; depression; lack of security
Sociocultural: Lack of social interaction; cultural barrier to practicing religion; social isolation
Spiritual: Suffering
Environmental: Lack of transportation; environmental barriers to practicing religion
Developmental: Life transitions

A plan of care addressing client's spiritual/religious needs is presented in Table 6-3. Selected nursing diagnoses are presented, along with appropriate nursing interventions and rationales for each.

Evaluation

Evaluation of nursing actions is directed at achievement of the established outcomes. Part of the evaluation process is continuous reassessment to ensure that the selected actions are appropriate and the goals and outcomes are realistic. Including the family and extended support systems in the evaluation process is essential if spiritual and religious implications of nursing care are to be measured. Modifications to the plan of care are made as the need is determined.

Table 6-3 | CARE PLAN FOR THE CLIENT WITH SPIRITUAL AND RELIGIOUS NEEDS*

NURSING DIAGNOSIS: RISK FOR SPIRITUAL DISTRESS
RELATED TO: Life changes; environmental changes; stress; anxiety; depression

OUTCOME CRITERIA	NURSING INTERVENTIONS	RATIONALE
Client will identify meaning and purpose in life that reinforce hope, peace, contentment, and self-satisfaction.	1. Assess current situation. 2. Listen to client's expressions of anger, concern, self-blame. 3. Note reason for living and whether it is directly related to situation. 4. Determine client's religious/spiritual orientation, current involvement, and presence of conflicts, especially in current circumstances. 5. Assess sense of self-concept, worth, ability to enter into loving relationships.	1–8. Thorough assessment is necessary to develop an accurate care plan for the client.

Table 6-3 | CARE PLAN FOR THE CLIENT WITH SPIRITUAL AND RELIGIOUS NEEDS*—cont'd

OUTCOME CRITERIA	NURSING INTERVENTIONS	RATIONALE
	6. Observe behavior indicative of poor relationships with others.	
	7. Determine support systems available to and used by client and significant others.	
	8. Assess substance use/abuse.	
	9. Establish an environment that promotes free expression of feelings and concerns.	9. Trust is the basis of a therapeutic nurse-client relationship.
	10. Have client identify and prioritize current/immediate needs.	10. Helps client focus on what needs to be done and identify manageable steps to take.
	11. Discuss philosophical issues related to impact of current situation on spiritual beliefs and values.	11. Helps client to understand that certain life experiences can cause individuals to question personal values and that this response is not uncommon.
	12. Use therapeutic communication skills of reflection and active listening.	12. Helps client find own solutions to concerns.
	13. Review coping skills used and their effectiveness in current situation.	13. Identifies strengths to incorporate into plan and techniques that need revision.
	14. Provide a role model (e.g., nurse, individual experiencing similar situation).	14. Sharing of experiences and hope assists client to deal with reality.
	15. Suggest use of journaling.	15. Journaling can assist in clarifying beliefs and values and in recognizing and resolving feelings about current life situation.
	16. Discuss client's interest in the arts, music, and literature.	16. Provides insight into meaning of these issues and how they are integrated into an individual's life.
	17. Role-play new coping techniques. Discuss possibilities of taking classes, becoming involved in discussion groups, or cultural activities of their choice.	17. These activities will help to enhance integration of new skills and necessary changes in client's lifestyle.
	18. Refer client to appropriate resources for help.	18. Client may require additional assistance with an individual who specializes in these types of concerns.

Continued

Table 6-3 | CARE PLAN FOR THE CLIENT WITH SPIRITUAL AND RELIGIOUS NEEDS*–cont'd

NURSING DIAGNOSIS: RISK FOR IMPAIRED RELIGIOSITY

RELATED TO: Suffering; depression; illness; life transitions

OUTCOME CRITERIA	NURSING INTERVENTIONS	RATIONALE
Client will express achievement of support and personal satisfaction from spiritual/religious practices.	1. Assess current situation (e.g., illness, hospitalization, prognosis of death, presence of support systems, financial concerns).	1. This information identifies problems client is dealing with in the moment that is affecting desire to be involved with religious activities.
	2. Listen nonjudgmentally to client's expressions of anger and possible belief that illness/condition may be a result of lack of faith.	2. Individuals often blame themselves for what has happened and reject previous religious beliefs and/or God.
	3. Determine client's usual religious/spiritual beliefs, current involvement in specific church activities.	3. This is important background for establishing a database.
	4. Note quality of relationships with significant others and friends.	4. Individual may withdraw from others in relation to the stress of illness, pain, and suffering.
	5. Assess substance use/abuse.	5. When in distress, individuals often turn to use of various substances, and this can affect the ability to deal with problems in a positive manner.
	6. Develop nurse-client relationship in which individual can express feelings and concerns freely.	6. Trust is the basis for a therapeutic nurse-client relationship.
	7. Use therapeutic communication skills of active listening, reflection, and "I" messages.	7. Helps client to find own solutions to problems and concerns and promotes sense of control.
	8. Be accepting and nonjudgmental when client expresses anger and bitterness toward God. Stay with the client.	8. The nurse's presence and nonjudgmental attitude increase the client's feelings of self-worth and promote trust in the relationship.
	9. Encourage client to discuss previous religious practices and how these practices provided support in the past.	9. A nonjudgmental discussion of previous sources of support may help the client work through current rejection of them as potential sources of support.
	10. Allow the client to take the lead in initiating participation in religious activities, such as prayer.	10. Client may be vulnerable in current situation and needs to be allowed to decide own resumption of these actions.
	11. Contact spiritual leader of client's choice, if he or she requests.	11. These individuals serve to provide relief from spiritual distress and often can do so when other support persons cannot.

*The interventions for this care plan were adapted from Doenges, Moorhouse, & Murr (2013).

Summary and Key Points

- Culture encompasses shared patterns of belief, feeling, and knowledge that guide people's conduct and are passed down from generation to generation.
- Ethnic groups are tied together by a shared heritage.
- Cultural groups differ in terms of communication, space, social organization, time, environmental control, and biological variations.
- Northern European Americans are the descendants of the first immigrants to the United States and make up the current dominant cultural group. They value punctuality, work responsibility, and a healthy lifestyle.
- African Americans trace their roots in the United States to the days of slavery.
- Most African Americans have large support systems and a strong religious orientation. Many have assimilated into and have many of the same characteristics as the dominant culture. Some African Americans from the rural South may receive health care from a folk practitioner.
- Many Native Americans still live on reservations. They speak many different languages and dialects. They often appear silent and reserved and many are uncomfortable with touch and expressing emotions. Health care may be delivered by a healer called a *shaman*.
- Asian American languages are very diverse. Touching during communication has historically been considered unacceptable. Asian Americans may have difficulty expressing emotions and appear cold and aloof. Family loyalty is emphasized. Psychiatric illness is viewed as behavior that is out of control and brings shame on the family.
- The common language of Latino Americans is Spanish. Large family groups are important, and touch is a common form of communication. The predominant religion is Roman Catholicism and the church is often a source of strength in times of crisis. Health care may be delivered by a folk healer called a *curandero*, who uses various forms of treatment to restore the body to a balanced state.
- Western European Americans have their origins in Italy, France, and Greece. They are warm and expressive and use touch as a common form of communication. The dominant religion is Roman Catholicism for the Italians and French and Greek Orthodoxy for the Greeks. Most Western European Americans follow the health practices of the dominant culture, but some folk beliefs and superstitions endure.
- Arab Americans trace their ancestry and traditions to the nomadic desert tribes of the Arabian Peninsula. Arabic is the official language of the Arab world and the dominant religion is Islam. Mental illness is considered a social stigma, and symptoms are often somaticized.
- The Jewish people came to the United States predominantly from Spain, Portugal, Germany, and Eastern Europe. Four main Jewish religious groups exist today: Orthodox, Reform, Conservative, and Reconstructionist. The primary language is English. A high value is placed on education. Jewish Americans are very health conscious and practice preventive health care. The maintenance of one's mental health is considered just as important as the maintenance of one's physical health.
- Culture-bound syndromes are clusters of physical and behavioral symptoms that are considered as illnesses or "afflictions" by specific cultures, but do not readily fit into the Western conventional diagnostic categories.
- Spirituality is the human quality that gives meaning and sense of purpose to an individual's existence.
- Individuals possess a number of spiritual needs that include meaning and purpose in life, faith or trust in someone or something beyond themselves, hope, love, and forgiveness.
- Religion is a set of beliefs, values, rites, and rituals adopted by a group of people.
- Religion is one way in which an individual's spirituality may be expressed.
- Affiliation with a religious group has been shown to be a health-enhancing endeavor.
- Nurses must consider cultural, spiritual, and religious needs when planning care for their clients.

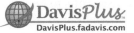 DavisPlus.fadavis.com   Additional info available at www.davisplus.com

Review Questions
Self-Examination/Learning Exercise

*Select the answer that is **most** appropriate for each of the following questions:*

1. Miss Lee is an Asian American on the psychiatric unit. She tells the nurse, "I must have the hot ginger root for my headache. It is the only thing that will help." What meaning does the nurse attach to this statement by Miss Lee?
   a. She is being obstinate and wants control over her care.
   b. She believes that ginger root has magical qualities.
   c. She subscribes to the restoration of health through the balance of yin and yang.
   d. Asian Americans refuse to take traditional medicine for pain.

2. Miss Lee, an Asian American on the psychiatric unit, says she is afraid that no one from her family will visit her. On what belief does Miss Lee base her statement?
   a. Many Asian Americans do not believe in hospitals.
   b. Many Asian Americans do not have close family support systems.
   c. Many Asian Americans believe the body will heal itself if left alone.
   d. Many Asian Americans view psychiatric problems as bringing shame to the family.

3. Joe, a Native American, appears at the community health clinic with an oozing stasis ulcer on his lower right leg. It is obviously infected, and he tells the nurse that the shaman has been treating it with herbs. The nurse determines that Joe needs emergency care, but Joe states he will not go to the emergency department (ED) unless the shaman is allowed to help treat him. How should the nurse handle this situation?
   a. Contact the shaman and have him meet them at the ED to consult with the attending physician.
   b. Tell Joe that the shaman is not allowed in the ED.
   c. Explain to Joe that the shaman is at fault for his leg being in the condition it is in now.
   d. Have the shaman try to talk Joe into going to the ED without him.

4. Joe, a Native American, goes to the emergency department (ED) because he has an oozing stasis ulcer on his leg. He is accompanied by the tribal shaman, who has been treating Joe on the reservation. As a greeting, the physician extends his hand to the shaman, who lightly touches the physician's hand, then quickly moves away. How should the physician interpret this gesture?
   a. The shaman is snubbing the physician.
   b. The shaman is angry at Joe for wanting to go to the ED.
   c. The shaman does not believe in traditional medicine.
   d. The shaman does not feel comfortable with touch.

5. Sarah is an African American woman who receives a visit from the psychiatric home health nurse. A referral for a mental health assessment was made by the public health nurse, who noticed that Sarah was becoming exceedingly withdrawn. When the psychiatric nurse arrives, Sarah says to her, "No one can help me. I was an evil person in my youth, and now I must pay." How might the nurse assess this statement?
   a. Sarah is having delusions of persecution.
   b. Some African Americans believe illness is God's punishment for their sins.
   c. Sarah is depressed and just wants to be left alone.
   d. African Americans do not believe in psychiatric help.

6. Sarah is an African American woman who lives in the rural South. She receives a visit from the public health nurse. Sarah says to the nurse, "Granny told me to eat a lot of poke greens and I would feel better." How should the nurse interpret this statement?
   a. Sarah's grandmother believes in the healing power of poke greens.
   b. Sarah believes everything her grandmother tells her.
   c. Sarah has been receiving health care from a "folk practitioner."
   d. Sarah is trying to determine if the nurse agrees with her grandmother.

Review Questions—cont'd
Self-Examination/Learning Exercise

7. Frank is a Latino American who has an appointment at the community health center for 1 p.m. The nurse is angry when Frank shows up at 3:30 p.m. stating, "I was visiting with my brother." How might the nurse best interpret this behavior?
   a. Frank is being passive-aggressive by showing up late.
   b. This is Frank's way of defying authority.
   c. Frank is a member of a cultural group that is present-time oriented.
   d. Frank is a member of a cultural group that rejects traditional medicine.

8. The nurse must give Frank, a Latino American, a physical examination. She tells him to remove his clothing and put on an examination gown. Frank refuses. How should the nurse interpret this behavior?
   a. Frank does not believe in taking orders from a woman.
   b. Frank is modest and embarrassed to remove his clothes.
   c. Frank doesn't understand why he must remove his clothes.
   d. Frank does not think he needs a physical examination.

9. Maria is an Italian American who is in the hospital after having suffered a miscarriage at 5 months' gestation. Her room is filled with relatives who have brought a variety of foods and gifts for Maria. They are all talking, seemingly at the same time, and some, including Maria, are crying. They repeatedly touch and hug Maria and each other. How should the nurse handle this situation?
   a. Explain to the family that Maria needs her rest and they must all leave.
   b. Allow the family to remain and continue their activity as described, as long as they do not disturb other clients.
   c. Explain that Maria will not get over her loss if they keep bringing it up and causing her to cry so much.
   d. Call the family priest to come and take charge of this family situation.

10. Maria is an Italian American who is in the hospital after having suffered a miscarriage at 5 months' gestation. Maria's mother says to the nurse, "If only Maria had told me she wanted the biscotti. I would have made them for her." What is the meaning behind Maria's mother's statement?
    a. Some Italian Americans believe a miscarriage can occur if a woman does not eat a food she craves.
    b. Some Italian Americans think biscotti can prevent miscarriage.
    c. Maria's mother is taking the blame for Maria's miscarriage.
    d. Maria's mother believes the physician should have told Maria to eat biscotti.

11. Joe, who has come to the mental health clinic with symptoms of depression, says to the nurse, "My father is dying. I have always hated my father. He physically abused me when I was a child. We haven't spoken for many years. He wants to see me now, but I don't know if I want to see him." With which spiritual need is Joe struggling?
    a. Forgiveness
    b. Faith
    c. Hope
    d. Meaning and purpose in life

12. As a child, Joe was physically abused by his father. The father is now dying and has expressed a desire to see his son before he dies. Joe is depressed and says to the mental health nurse, "I'm so angry! Why did God have to give me a father like this? I feel cheated of a father! I've always been a good person. I deserved better. I hate God!" From this subjective data, which nursing diagnosis might the nurse apply to Joe?
    a. Readiness for enhanced religiosity
    b. Risk for impaired religiosity
    c. Readiness for enhanced spiritual well-being
    d. Spiritual distress

References

Alegria, M., Mulvaney-Day, N., Torres, M., Polo, A., Cao, Z., & Canino, G. (2007). Prevalence of psychiatric disorders across Latino subgroups in the United States. *American Journal of Public Health, 97*(1), 68–75.

Brodd, J. (2009). *World religions: A voyage of discovery* (3rd ed.). Winona, MN: Saint Mary's Press.

Bronson, M. (2005). *Why are there so many religions?* Retrieved from http://www.biblehelp.org/relig.htm

Bureau of Indian Affairs (BIA). (2012). *Frequently asked questions.* Retrieved from http://www.bia.gov/FAQs/index.htm

Burkhardt, M., & Nagai-Jacobson, M.G. (2002). *Spirituality: Living our connectedness.* Albany, NY: Delmar Thomson Learning.

Centers for Disease Control (CDC). (2012). First marriages in the United States: Data from the 2006-2010 National Survey of Family Growth. U.S. Department of Health and Human Services. *National Health Statistics Reports, 49 (March 22, 2012).*

Chiswick, C.U. (2009). *Occupation and gender: American Jews at the Millennium.* Association of Religious Data Archives. http://www.thearda.com.

Cherry, B., & Giger, J.N. (2013). African-Americans. In J.N. Giger (Ed.), *Transcultural nursing: Assessment and intervention* (6th ed., pp. 162–206). St. Louis, MO: Mosby.

Doenges, M.E., Moorhouse, M.F., & Murr, A.C. (2013). *Nursing diagnosis manual: Planning, individualizing, and documenting client care* (4th ed.). Philadelphia, PA: F.A. Davis.

Dossey, B.M. (1998). Holistic modalities and healing moments. *American Journal of Nursing, 98*(6), 44–47.

Fox, A., & Fox, B. (1988). *Wake up! You're alive.* Deerfield Beach, FL: Health Communications.

Gallup. (2008). *No evidence bad times are boosting church attendance.* Retrieved from http://www.gallup.com/poll/113452/evidence-bad-times-boosting-church-attendance.aspx

Gallup (2012). *Americans' church attendance inches up in 2010.* Retrieved from http://www.gallup.com/poll/141044/Americans-Church-Attendance-Inches-2010.aspx?version

Gartner, J. (1996). Religious commitment, mental health, and prosocial behavior: A review of the empirical literature. In E. Shafranske (Ed.), *Religion and the clinical practice of psychology* (pp. 187–214). Washington, DC: American Psychological Association.

Gaw, A.C. (2008). Cultural issues. In R.E. Hales, S.C. Yudofsky, & G.O. Gabbard (Eds.), *Textbook of psychiatry* (5th ed., pp. 1529–1547). Washington, DC: American Psychiatric Publishing.

Giger, J.N. (2013). *Transcultural nursing: Assessment and intervention* (6th ed.). St. Louis, MO: Mosby.

Griffith, E.E.H., Gonzalez, C.A., & Blue, H.C. (2003). Introduction to cultural psychiatry. In R.E. Hales & S.C. Yudofsky (Eds.), *Textbook of clinical psychiatry* (4th ed., pp. 1551–1583). Washington, DC: American Psychiatric Publishing.

Hanley, C.E. (2013). Navajos. In J.N. Giger (Ed.), *Transcultural nursing: Assessment and intervention* (6th ed., pp. 240–259). St. Louis, MO: Mosby.

Indian Health Service (IHS). (2013). *Indian health disparities.* Retrieved from http://www.ihs.gov/PublicAffairs/IHSBrochure/Disparities.asp

Kaplan, A. (2007). Mental illness in U.S. Latinos addressed in survey, outreach efforts. *Psychiatric Times, 24*(3), 1-2.

Karren, K.J., Hafen, B.Q., Smith, N.L., & Jenkins, K.J. (2010). *Mind/body health: The effects of attitudes, emotions, and relationships* (4th ed.). San Francisco, CA: Benjamin Cummings.

Koenig, H.G. (2009). Research on religion, spirituality, and mental health: A review. *The Canadian Journal of Psychiatry, 54*(5), 283–291.

Kulwicki, A.D., & Ballout, S. (2013). People of Arab heritage. In L.D. Purnell (Ed.), *Transcultural health care: A culturally competent approach* (4th ed., pp. 159-177). Philadelphia, PA: F.A. Davis.

Kuo, P.Y., & Roysircar-Sodowsky, G. (2000). Political ethnic identity versus cultural ethnic identity: An understanding of research on Asian Americans. In D.S. Sandhu (Ed.), *Asian and Pacific Islander Americans: Issues and concerns for counseling and psychotherapy* (pp. 71–90). Hauppauge, NY: Nova Science Publishers.

Murray, R.B., Zentner, J.P., & Yakimo, R. (2009). *Health promotion strategies through the life span* (8th ed.). Upper Saddle River, NJ: Prentice Hall.

NANDA International (NANDA-I). (2012). *Nursing diagnoses: Definitions & classification 2012– 2014.* Hoboken, NJ: Wiley-Blackwell.

Nekolaichuk, C.L., Jevne, R.F., & Maguire, T.O. (1999). Structuring the meaning of hope in health and illness. *Social Science and Medicine, 48*(5), 591–605.

Ornish, D. (1998). *Love and survival: Eight pathways to intimacy and health.* New York, NY: Harper Perennial.

Owen, D.C., Gonzalez, E.W., & Esperat, M.C. (2013). Mexican Americans. In J.N. Giger (Ed.). *Transcultural nursing: Assessment and intervention* (6th ed., pp. 207–239). St. Louis, MO: Mosby.

Pew Forum on Religion and Public Life. (2009). *A religious portrait of African Americans.* Retrieved from http://www.pewforum.org/A-Religious-Portrait-of-African-Americans.aspx

Purnell, L.D. (2009). *Guide to culturally competent health care* (2nd ed.). Philadelphia, PA: F.A. Davis.

Purnell, L.D. (2013). *Transcultural health care: A culturally competent approach* (4th ed.). Philadelphia, PA: F.A. Davis.

Reeves, R., & Reynolds, M. (2009). What is the role of spirituality in mental health treatment. *Journal of Psychosocial Nursing, 54*(5), 8–9.

Schwartz, E.A. (2013). Jewish Americans. In J.N. Giger (Ed.), *Transcultural nursing: Assessment & intervention* (6th ed., pp. 508–530). St. Louis, MO: Mosby.

Selekman, J. (2013). People of Jewish heritage. In L.D. Purnell (Ed.), *Transcultural health care: A culturally competent approach* (4th ed., pp. 339–356). Philadelphia, PA: F.A. Davis.

Smucker, C.J. (2001). Overview of nursing the spirit. In D.L. Wilt & C.J. Smucker (Eds.), *Nursing the spirit: The art and science of applying spiritual care* (pp. 1–18). Washington, DC: American Nurses Publishing.

Spector, R.E. (2013). *Cultural diversity in health and illness* (8th ed.). Upper Saddle River, NJ: Pearson Prentice Hall.

United Jewish Communities. (2003). *The national Jewish population survey: Strength, challenge and diversity in the American Jewish population.* New York, NY: United Jewish Communities.

U.S. Census Bureau. (2012). *2011 American Community Survey.* Retrieved from http://www.census.gov/acs/www/

U.S. Department of Agriculture. (2012). *Food distribution program on Indian reservations.* Retrieved from http://www.fns.usda.gov/fdd/programs/fdpir/about_fdpir.htm

Wall, T.L., Peterson, C.M., Peterson, K.P., Johnson, M.L., Thomasson, H.R., Cole, M., and Ehlers, C.L. (1997). Alcohol metabolism in Asian-American men with genetic polymorphisms of aldehyde dehydrogenase. *Annals of Internal Medicine, 127,* 376–379.

Walsh, R. (1999). *Essential spirituality.* New York, NY: John Wiley & Sons.

Werner, E.E., & Smith, R.S. (1992). *Overcoming the odds: High risk children from birth to adulthood.* Ithaca, NY: Cornell University Press.

Wright, L.M. (2005). *Spirituality, suffering, and illness.* Philadelphia, PA: F.A. Davis.

Xu, Y., & Chang, K. (2013). Chinese Americans. In J.N. Giger (Ed.), *Transcultural nursing: Assessment and intervention* (6th ed., pp. 383–402). St. Louis, MO: Mosby.

Classical References

Hall, E.T. (1966). *The hidden dimension.* Garden City, NY: Doubleday.

Kübler-Ross, E. (1969). *On death and dying.* New York, NY: Macmillan.

3

Therapeutic Approaches in Psychiatric Nursing Care

7

Relationship Development

CORE CONCEPT

therapeutic relationship

KEY TERMS

attitude

belief

concrete thinking

confidentiality

countertransference

empathy

genuineness

rapport

sympathy

transference

unconditional positive regard

values

OBJECTIVES

After reading this chapter, the student will be able to:

1. Describe the relevance of a therapeutic nurse-client relationship.
2. Discuss the dynamics of a therapeutic nurse-client relationship.
3. Discuss the importance of self-awareness in the nurse-client relationship.
4. Identify goals of the nurse-client relationship.
5. Identify and discuss essential conditions for a therapeutic relationship to occur.
6. Describe the phases of relationship development and the tasks associated with each phase.

HOMEWORK ASSIGNMENT

Please read the chapter and answer the following questions:

1. When the nurse's verbal and nonverbal interactions are congruent, he or she is thought to be expressing which characteristic of a therapeutic relationship?
2. During which phase of the nurse-client relationship do each of the following occur:
   a. The nurse may become angry and anxious in the presence of the client.
   b. A plan of action for dealing with stress is established.
   c. The nurse examines personal feelings about working with the client.
   d. Nurse and client establish goals of care.
3. What is the goal of using the Johari Window?
4. How do sympathy and empathy differ?

The nurse-client relationship is the foundation on which psychiatric nursing is established. It is a relationship in which both participants must recognize each other as unique and important human beings. It is also a relationship in which mutual learning occurs. Peplau (1991) states:

> Shall a nurse do things *for* a patient or can participant relationships be emphasized so that a nurse comes to do things *with* a patient as her share of an agenda of work to be accomplished in reaching a goal—health. It is likely that the nursing process is educative and therapeutic when nurse and patient can come to know and to respect each other, as persons who are alike, and yet, different, as persons who share in the solution of problems. (p. 9)

This chapter examines the role of the psychiatric nurse and the use of self as the therapeutic tool in the nursing of clients with emotional illness. Phases of the therapeutic relationship are explored and conditions essential to the development of a therapeutic relationship are discussed. The importance of values clarification in the development of self-awareness is emphasized.

CORE CONCEPT

Therapeutic Relationship

An interaction between two people (usually a caregiver and a care receiver) in which input from both participants contributes to a climate of healing, growth promotion, and/or illness prevention.

Role of the Psychiatric Nurse

What is a nurse? Undoubtedly, this question would elicit as many different answers as the number of people to whom it was presented. Nursing as a *concept* has probably existed since the beginning of the civilized world, with the provision of "care" to the ill or infirm by anyone in the environment who took the time to administer to those in need. However, the emergence of nursing as a *profession* only began in the late 1800s with the graduation of Linda Richards from the New England Hospital for Women and Children in Boston upon achievement of the diploma in nursing. Since that time, the nurse's role has evolved from that of custodial caregiver and physician's handmaiden to recognition as a unique, independent member of the professional health-care team.

Peplau (1991) identified several subroles within the role of the nurse:

1. **The Stranger.** A nurse is at first a stranger to the client. The client is also a stranger to the nurse. Peplau (1991) stated:

> Respect and positive interest accorded a stranger is at first nonpersonal and includes the same ordinary courtesies that are accorded to a new guest who has been brought into any situation. This principle implies: (1) accepting the patient as he is; (2) treating the patient as an emotionally able stranger and relating to him on this basis until evidence shows him to be otherwise. (p. 44)

2. **The Resource Person.** According to Peplau, "a resource person provides specific answers to questions usually formulated with relation to a larger problem" (p. 47). In the role of resource person, the nurse explains, in language that the client can understand, information related to the client's health care.

3. **The Teacher.** In this subrole the nurse identifies learning needs and provides information required by the client or family to improve the health situation.

4. **The Leader.** According to Peplau, "democratic leadership in nursing situations implies that the patient will be permitted to be an active participant in designing nursing plans for him" (p. 49). Autocratic leadership promotes overvaluation of the nurse and clients' substitution of the nurse's goals for their own. Laissez-faire leaders convey a lack of personal interest in the client.

5. **The Surrogate.** Outside of their awareness, clients often perceive nurses as symbols of other individuals. They may view the nurse as a mother figure, a sibling, a former teacher, or another nurse who has provided care in the past. This occurs when a client is placed in a situation that generates feelings similar to ones he or she has experienced previously. Peplau (1991) explained that the nurse-client relationship progresses along a continuum. When a client is acutely ill, he or she may incur the role of infant or child, while the nurse is perceived as the mother surrogate. Peplau (1991) stated, "Each nurse has the responsibility for exercising her professional skill in aiding the relationship to move forward on the continuum, so that person to person relations compatible with chronological age levels can develop" (p. 55).

6. **The Technical Expert.** The nurse understands various professional devices and possesses the clinical skills necessary to perform the interventions that are in the best interest of the client.

7. **The Counselor.** The nurse uses "interpersonal techniques" to assist clients to learn to adapt to difficulties or changes in life experiences. Peplau (1991) stated, "Counseling in nursing has to do with helping the patient to remember and to understand fully what is happening to him in the present situation, so that the experience can be integrated with, rather than dissociated from, other experiences in life" (p. 64).

Peplau (1962) believed that the emphasis in psychiatric nursing is on the counseling subrole. How then does this emphasis influence the role of the nurse in the psychiatric setting? Many sources define the *nurse therapist* as having graduate preparation in psychiatric/mental health nursing. He or she has developed skills through intensive supervised educational experiences to provide helpful individual, group, or family therapy.

Peplau suggested that it is essential for the *staff nurse working in psychiatry* to have a general knowledge of basic counseling techniques. A therapeutic or "helping" relationship is established through use of these interpersonal techniques and is based on a sound knowledge of theories of personality development and human behavior.

Sullivan (1953) believed that emotional problems stem from difficulties with interpersonal relationships. Interpersonal theorists, such as Peplau and Sullivan, emphasize the importance of relationship development in the provision of emotional care. Through establishment of a satisfactory nurse-client relationship, individuals learn to generalize the ability to achieve satisfactory interpersonal relationships to other aspects of their lives.

Dynamics of a Therapeutic Nurse-Client Relationship

Travelbee (1971), who expanded on Peplau's theory of interpersonal relations in nursing, has stated that it is only when each individual in the interaction perceives the other as a unique human being that a relationship is possible. She refers not to a nurse-client relationship, but rather to a human-to-human relationship, which she describes as a "mutually significant experience." That is, both the nurse and the recipient of care have needs met when each views the other as a unique human being, not as "an illness," as "a room number," or as "all nurses" in general.

Therapeutic relationships are goal oriented. Ideally, the nurse and client decide together what the goal of the relationship will be. Most often the goal is directed at learning and growth promotion, in an effort to bring about some type of change in the client's life. In general, the goal of a therapeutic relationship may be based on a problem-solving model.

EXAMPLE

Goal

The client will demonstrate more adaptive coping strategies for dealing with (specific life situation).

Interventions

- Identify what is troubling the client at the present time.
- Encourage the client to discuss changes he or she would like to make.

- Discuss with the client which changes are possible and which are not possible.
- Have the client explore feelings about aspects that cannot be changed and alternative ways of coping more adaptively.
- Discuss alternative strategies for creating changes the client desires to make.
- Weigh the benefits and consequences of each alternative.
- Assist the client to select an alternative.
- Encourage the client to implement the change.
- Provide positive feedback for the client's attempts to create change.
- Assist the client to evaluate outcomes of the change and make modifications as required.

Therapeutic Use of Self

Travelbee (1971) described the instrument for delivery of the process of interpersonal nursing as the *therapeutic use of self*, which she defined as "the ability to use one's personality consciously and in full awareness in an attempt to establish relatedness and to structure nursing intervention" (p. 19).

Use of the self in a therapeutic manner requires that the nurse have a great deal of self-awareness and self-understanding, having arrived at a philosophical belief about life, death, and the overall human condition. The nurse must understand that the ability and extent to which one can effectively help others in time of need is strongly influenced by this internal value system—a combination of intellect and emotions.

Gaining Self-Awareness

Values Clarification

Knowing and understanding oneself enhances the ability to form satisfactory interpersonal relationships. Self-awareness requires that an individual recognize and accept what he or she values and learn to accept the uniqueness and differences in others. This concept is important in everyday life and in the nursing profession in general; but it is *essential* in psychiatric nursing.

An individual's value system is established very early in life and has its foundations in the value system held by the primary caregivers. It is culturally oriented; it may change many times over the course of a lifetime; and it consists of beliefs, attitudes, and values. Values clarification is one process by which an individual may gain self-awareness.

Beliefs

A **belief** is an idea that one holds to be true, and it can take any of several forms:

- *Rational beliefs*. Ideas for which objective evidence exists to substantiate their truth.

EXAMPLE

Alcoholism is a disease.

■ *Irrational beliefs.* Ideas that an individual holds as true despite the existence of objective contradictory evidence. Delusions can be a form of irrational beliefs.

EXAMPLE

Once an alcoholic has been through detox and rehab, he or she can drink socially if desired.

■ *Faith (sometimes called "blind beliefs").* An ideal that an individual holds as true for which no objective evidence exists.

EXAMPLE

Belief in a higher power can help an alcoholic stop drinking.

■ *Stereotype.* A socially shared belief that describes a concept in an oversimplified or undifferentiated matter.

EXAMPLE

All alcoholics are skid-row bums.

Attitudes

An **attitude** is a frame of reference around which an individual organizes knowledge about his or her world. An attitude also has an emotional component. It can be a prejudgment and may be selective and biased. Attitudes fulfill the need to find meaning in life and to provide clarity and consistency for the individual. The prevailing stigma attached to mental illness is an example of a negative attitude. An associated belief might be that "all people with mental illness are dangerous."

Values

Values are abstract standards, positive or negative, that represent an individual's ideal mode of conduct and ideal goals. Some examples of ideal modes of conduct include seeking truth and beauty; being clean and orderly; and behaving with sincerity, justice, reason, compassion, humility, respect, honor, and loyalty. Examples of ideal goals are security, happiness, freedom, equality, ecstasy, fame, and power.

Values differ from attitudes and beliefs in that they are action oriented or action producing. One may hold many attitudes and beliefs without behaving in a way that shows they hold those attitudes and beliefs. For example, a nurse may believe that all clients have the right to be told the truth about their diagnosis; however, he or she may not always act on the belief and tell all clients the complete truth about their condition. Only when the belief is acted on does it become a value.

Attitudes and beliefs flow out of one's set of values. An individual may have thousands of beliefs and hundreds of attitudes, but his or her values probably only number in the dozens. Values may be viewed as a kind of core concept or basic standards that determine one's attitudes and beliefs, and ultimately, one's behavior. Raths, Harmin, and Simon (1978) identified a seven-step process of valuing that can be used to help clarify personal values. This process is presented in Table 7-1. The process can be used by applying these seven steps to an attitude or belief that one holds. When an attitude or belief has met each of the seven criteria, it can be considered a value.

The Johari Window

The self arises out of self-appraisal and the appraisal of others and represents each individual's unique pattern of values, attitudes, beliefs, behaviors, emotions, and needs. Self-awareness is the recognition of these aspects and understanding about their impact on the self and others. The Johari Window is a representation of the self and a tool that can be used to increase

TABLE 7–1 **The Process of Values Clarification**			
LEVEL OF OPERATIONS	CATEGORY	CRITERIA	EXPLANATION
Cognitive	Choosing	1. Freely 2. From alternatives 3. After careful consideration of the consequences	"This value is mine. No one forced me to choose it. I understand and accept the consequences of holding this value."
Emotional	Prizing	4. Satisfied; pleased with the choice 5. Making public affirmation of the choice, if necessary	"I am proud that I hold this value, and I am willing to tell others about it."
Behavioral	Acting	6. Taking action to demonstrate the value behaviorally 7. Demonstrating this pattern of behavior consistently and repeatedly	The value is reflected in the individual's behavior for as long as he or she holds it.

self-awareness (Luft, 1970). The Johari Window is presented in Figure 7-1 and is divided into four quadrants.

The Open or Public Self

The upper left quadrant of the window represents the part of the self that is public; that is, aspects of the self about which both the individual and others are aware.

EXAMPLE

Susan, a nurse who is the adult child of an alcoholic, has strong feelings about helping alcoholics to achieve sobriety. She volunteers her time to be a support person on call to help recovering alcoholics. She is aware of her feelings and her desire to help others. Members of the Alcoholics Anonymous group in which she volunteers her time are also aware of Susan's feelings and they feel comfortable calling her when they need help refraining from drinking.

The Unknowing Self

The upper right quadrant of the window represents the part of the self that is known to others but remains hidden from the awareness of the individual.

EXAMPLE

When Susan takes care of patients in detox, she does so without emotion, tending to the technical aspects of the task in a way that the clients perceive as cold and judgmental. She is unaware that she comes across to the clients in this way.

The Private Self

The lower left quadrant of the window represents the part of the self that is known to the individual, but which the individual deliberately and consciously conceals from others.

EXAMPLE

Susan would prefer not to take care of the clients in detox because doing so provokes painful memories from her childhood. However, because she does not want the other staff members to know about these feelings, she volunteers to take care of the detox clients whenever they are assigned to her unit.

The Unknown Self

The lower right quadrant of the window represents the part of the self that is unknown to both the individual and to others.

EXAMPLE

Susan felt very powerless as a child growing up with an alcoholic father. She seldom knew in what condition she would find her father or what his behavior would be. She learned over the years to find small ways to maintain control over her life situation, and left home as soon as she graduated from high school. The need to stay in control has always been very important to Susan, and she is unaware that working with recovering alcoholics helps to fulfill this need in her. The people she is helping are also unaware that Susan is satisfying an unfulfilled personal need as she provides them with assistance.

The goal of increasing self-awareness by using the Johari Window is to increase the size of the quadrant that represents the open or public self. The individual who is open to self and others has the ability to be spontaneous and to share emotions and experiences with others. This individual also has a greater understanding of personal behavior and of others' responses to him or her. Increased self-awareness allows an individual to interact with others comfortably, to accept the differences in others, and to observe each person's right to respect and dignity.

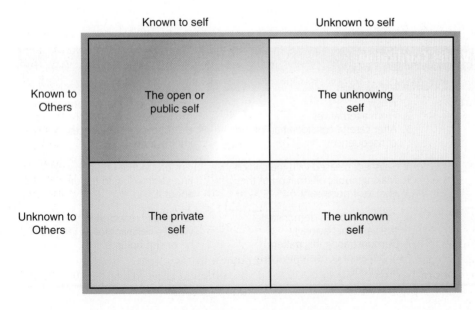

FIGURE 7–1 The Johari Window. (From Luft, J. [1970]. *Group processes: An introduction to group dynamics*, 3rd ed. Mayfield Publishing: Palo Alto, CA. 1984, with permission.)

Conditions Essential to Development of a Therapeutic Relationship

Several characteristics that enhance the achievement of a therapeutic relationship have been identified. These concepts are highly significant to the use of self as the therapeutic tool in interpersonal relationship development.

Rapport

Getting acquainted and establishing **rapport** is the primary task in relationship development. Rapport implies special feelings on the part of both the client and the nurse based on acceptance, warmth, friendliness, common interest, a sense of trust, and a nonjudgmental attitude. Establishing rapport may be accomplished by discussing non-health-related topics. Travelbee (1971) states:

> [To establish rapport] is to create a sense of harmony based on knowledge and appreciation of each individual's uniqueness. It is the ability to be still and experience the other as a human being—to appreciate the unfolding of each personality one to the other. The ability to truly care for and about others is the core of rapport. (pp. 152; 155)

Trust

To trust another, one must feel confidence in that person's presence, reliability, integrity, veracity, and sincere desire to provide assistance when requested. As discussed in Chapter 3, trust is the initial developmental task described by Erikson. If the task has not been achieved, this component of relationship development becomes more difficult. That is not to say that trust cannot be established, but only that additional time and patience may be required on the part of the nurse.

> **CLINICAL PEARL** The nurse must convey an aura of trustworthiness, which requires that he or she possess a sense of self-confidence. Confidence in the self is derived out of knowledge gained through achievement of personal and professional goals, as well as the ability to integrate these roles and to function as a unified whole.

Trust cannot be presumed; it must be earned. Trustworthiness is demonstrated through nursing interventions that convey a sense of warmth and caring to the client. These interventions are initiated simply and concretely and directed toward activities that address the client's basic needs for physiological and psychological safety and security. Many psychiatric clients experience **concrete thinking**, which focuses their thought processes on specifics rather than generalities, and immediate issues rather than eventual outcomes. Examples of nursing interventions that would promote trust in an individual who is thinking concretely include the following:

- Providing a blanket when the client is cold
- Providing food when the client is hungry
- Keeping promises
- Being honest (e.g., saying "I don't know the answer to your question, but I'll try to find out") and then following through
- Simply and clearly providing reasons for certain policies, procedures, and rules
- Providing a written, structured schedule of activities
- Attending activities with the client if he or she is reluctant to go alone
- Being consistent in adhering to unit guidelines
- Taking the client's preferences, requests, and opinions into consideration when possible in decisions concerning his or her care
- Ensuring **confidentiality**; providing reassurance that what is discussed will not be repeated outside the boundaries of the health-care team

Trust is the basis of a therapeutic relationship. The nurse working in psychiatry must perfect the skills that foster the development of trust. Trust must be established in order for the nurse-client relationship to progress beyond the superficial level of tending to the client's immediate needs.

Respect

To show respect is to believe in the dignity and worth of an individual regardless of his or her unacceptable behavior. The psychologist Carl Rogers called this **unconditional positive regard** (Raskin, Rogers, & Witty, 2011). The attitude is nonjudgmental, and the respect is unconditional in that it does not depend on the behavior of the client to meet certain standards. The nurse, in fact, may not approve of the client's lifestyle or pattern of behaving. However, with unconditional positive regard, the client is accepted and respected for no other reason than that he or she is considered to be a worthwhile and unique human being.

Many psychiatric clients have very little self-respect because, as a result of their behavior, they have been rejected by others in the past. Recognition that they are being accepted and respected as unique individuals on an unconditional basis can serve to elevate feelings of self-worth and self-respect. The nurse can convey an attitude of respect by:

- Calling the client by name (and title, if he or she prefers)
- Spending time with the client
- Allowing for sufficient time to answer the client's questions and concerns

■ Promoting an atmosphere of privacy during therapeutic interactions with the client or when the client may be undergoing physical examination or therapy
■ Always being open and honest with the client, even when the truth may be difficult to discuss
■ Taking the client's ideas, preferences, and opinions into consideration when planning care
■ Striving to understand the motivation behind the client's behavior, regardless of how unacceptable it may seem

Genuineness

The concept of **genuineness** refers to the nurse's ability to be open, honest, and "real" in interactions with the client. To be "real" is to be aware of what one is experiencing internally and to allow the quality of this inner experiencing to be apparent in the therapeutic relationship. When one is genuine, there is *congruence* between what is felt and what is being expressed (Raskin, Rogers, & Witty, 2011). The nurse who possesses the quality of genuineness responds to the client with truth and honesty, rather than with responses he or she may consider more "professional" or ones that merely reflect the "nursing role."

Genuineness may call for a degree of *self-disclosure* on the part of the nurse. This is not to say that the nurse must disclose to the client *everything* he or she is feeling or *all* personal experiences that may relate to what the client is going through. Indeed, care must be taken when using self-disclosure, to avoid reversing the roles of nurse and client.

When the nurse uses self-disclosure, a quality of "humanness" is revealed to the client, creating a role for the client to model in similar situations. The client may then feel more comfortable revealing personal information to the nurse.

Most individuals have an uncanny ability to detect other peoples' artificiality. When the nurse does not bring the quality of genuineness to the relationship, a reality base for trust cannot be established. These qualities are essential if the actualizing potential of the client is to be realized and for change and growth to occur (Raskin, Rogers, & Witty, 2011).

Empathy

Empathy is the ability to see beyond outward behavior and to understand the situation from the client's point of view. With empathy, the nurse can accurately perceive and comprehend the meaning and relevance of the client's thoughts and feelings. The nurse must also be able to communicate this perception to the client by attempting to translate words and behaviors into feelings.

It is not uncommon for the concept of empathy to be confused with that of **sympathy**. The major difference is that with *empathy* the nurse "accurately perceives or understands" what the client is feeling and encourages the client to explore these feelings. With *sympathy* the nurse actually "shares" what the client is feeling, and experiences a need to alleviate distress. Schuster (2000) stated:

> Empathy means that you remain emotionally separate from the other person, even though you can see the patient's viewpoint clearly. This is different from sympathy. Sympathy implies taking on the other's needs and problems as if they were your own and becoming emotionally involved to the point of losing your objectivity. To empathize rather than sympathize, you must show feelings but not get caught up in feelings or overly identify with the patient's and family's concerns. (p. 102)

Empathy is considered to be one of the most important characteristics of a therapeutic relationship. Accurate empathetic perceptions on the part of the nurse assist the client to identify feelings that may have been suppressed or denied. Positive emotions are generated as the client realizes that he or she is truly understood by another. As the feelings surface and are explored, the client learns aspects about self of which he or she may have been unaware. This contributes to the process of personal identification and the promotion of positive self-concept.

With empathy, while understanding the client's thoughts and feelings, the nurse is able to maintain sufficient objectivity to allow the client to achieve problem resolution with minimal assistance. With sympathy, the nurse actually feels what the client is feeling, objectivity is lost, and the nurse may become focused on relief of personal distress rather than on helping the client resolve the problem at hand. The following is an example of an empathetic and sympathetic response to the same situation.

EXAMPLE

Situation: BJ is a client on the psychiatric unit with a diagnosis of persistent depressive disorder (dysthymia). She is 5'5" tall and weighs 295 lb. BJ has been overweight all her life. She is single, has no close friends, and has never had an intimate relationship with another person. It is her first day on the unit, and she is refusing to come out of her room. When she appeared for lunch in the dining room following admission, she was embarrassed when several of the other clients laughed out loud and called her "fatso."

Sympathetic response: Nurse: "I can certainly identify with what you are feeling. I've been overweight most of my life, too. I just get so angry when people act like that. They are so insensitive! It's just so typical of skinny people to act that way. You have a right to want to stay away from them. We'll just see how loud they laugh when *you* get to choose what movie is shown on the unit after dinner tonight."

Empathetic response: Nurse: "You feel angry and embarrassed by what happened at lunch today." As tears fill BJ's eyes, the nurse encourages her to cry if she feels like it and to express her anger at the situation. She stays with BJ but does not dwell on her *own* feelings about what happened. Instead she focuses on BJ and what the client perceives are her most immediate needs at this time.

Phases of a Therapeutic Nurse-Client Relationship

Psychiatric nurses use interpersonal relationship development as the primary intervention with clients in various psychiatric/mental health settings. This is congruent with Peplau's (1962) identification of *counseling* as the major subrole of nursing in psychiatry. Sullivan (1953), from whom Peplau patterned her own interpersonal theory of nursing, strongly believed that many emotional problems were closely related to difficulties with interpersonal relationships. With this concept in mind, this role of the nurse in psychiatry becomes especially meaningful and purposeful. It becomes an integral part of the total therapeutic regimen.

The therapeutic interpersonal relationship is the means by which the nursing process is implemented. Through the relationship, problems are identified and resolution is sought. Tasks of the relationship have been categorized into four phases: (1) the preinteraction phase, (2) the orientation (introductory) phase, (3) the working phase, and (4) the termination phase. Although each phase is presented as specific and distinct from the others, there may be some overlapping of tasks, particularly when the interaction is limited. The major nursing goals during each phase of the nurse-client relationship are listed in Table 7-2.

TABLE 7–2	**Phases of Relationship Development and Major Nursing Goals**
PHASE	GOALS
1. Preinteraction	Explore self-perceptions
2. Orientation (introductory)	Establish trust Formulate contract for intervention
3. Working	Promote client change
4. Termination	Evaluate goal attainment Ensure therapeutic closure

The Preinteraction Phase

The preinteraction phase involves preparation for the first encounter with the client. Tasks include the following:

■ Obtaining available information about the client from his or her chart, significant others, or other health-team members. From this information, the initial assessment is begun. This initial information may also allow the nurse to become aware of personal responses to knowledge about the client.

■ Examining one's feelings, fears, and anxieties about working with a particular client. For example, the nurse may have been reared in an alcoholic family and have ambivalent feelings about caring for a client who is alcohol dependent. All individuals bring attitudes and feelings from prior experiences to the clinical setting. The nurse needs to be aware of how these preconceptions may affect his or her ability to care for individual clients.

The Orientation (Introductory) Phase

During the orientation phase, the nurse and client become acquainted. Tasks include:

■ Creating an environment for the establishment of trust and rapport

■ Establishing a contract for intervention that details the expectations and responsibilities of both nurse and client

■ Gathering assessment information to build a strong client database

■ Identifying the client's strengths and limitations

■ Formulating nursing diagnoses

■ Setting goals that are mutually agreeable to the nurse and client

■ Developing a plan of action that is realistic for meeting the established goals

■ Exploring feelings of both the client and nurse in terms of the introductory phase

Introductions are often uncomfortable, and the participants may experience some anxiety until a degree of rapport has been established. Interactions may remain on a superficial level until anxiety subsides. Several interactions may be required to fulfill the tasks associated with this phase.

The Working Phase

The therapeutic work of the relationship is accomplished during this phase. Tasks include:

■ Maintaining the trust and rapport that was established during the orientation phase

■ Promoting the client's insight and perception of reality

■ Problem-solving using the model presented earlier in this chapter

■ Overcoming resistance behaviors on the part of the client as the level of anxiety rises in response to discussion of painful issues

■ Continuously evaluating progress toward goal attainment

Transference and Countertransference

Transference and countertransference are common phenomena that often arise during the course of a therapeutic relationship.

Transference

Transference occurs when the client unconsciously displaces (or "transfers") to the nurse feelings formed toward a person from his or her past (Sadock & Sadock, 2007). These feelings toward the nurse may be triggered by something about the nurse's appearance or personality characteristics that reminds the client of the person. Transference can interfere with the therapeutic interaction when the feelings being expressed include anger and hostility. Anger toward the nurse can be manifested by uncooperativeness and resistance to the therapy.

Transference can also take the form of overwhelming affection for the nurse or excessive dependency on the nurse. The nurse is overvalued and the client forms unrealistic expectations of the nurse. When the nurse is unable to fulfill those expectations or meet the excessive dependency needs, the client becomes angry and hostile.

Interventions for Transference Hilz (2012) states:

> In cases of transference, the relationship does not usually need to be terminated, except when the transference poses a serious barrier to therapy or safety. The nurse should work with the patient in sorting out the past from the present, and assist the patient into identifying the transference and reassign a new and more appropriate meaning to the current nurse-patient relationship. The goal is to guide patients toward independence by teaching them to assume responsibility for their own behaviors, feelings, and thoughts, and to assign the correct meanings to the relationships based on present circumstances instead of the past.

Countertransference

Countertransference refers to the nurse's behavioral and emotional response to the client. These responses may be related to unresolved feelings toward significant others from the nurse's past, or they may be generated in response to transference feelings on the part of the client. It is not easy to refrain from becoming angry when the client is consistently antagonistic, to feel flattered when showered with affection and attention by the client, or even to feel quite powerful when the client exhibits excessive dependency

on the nurse. These feelings can interfere with the therapeutic relationship when they initiate the following types of behaviors:

■ The nurse overidentifies with the client's feelings, as they remind him or her of problems from the nurse's past or present.

■ The nurse and client develop a social or personal relationship.

■ The nurse begins to give advice or attempts to "rescue" the client.

■ The nurse encourages and promotes the client's dependence.

■ The nurse's anger engenders feelings of disgust toward the client.

■ The nurse feels anxious and uneasy in the presence of the client.

■ The nurse is bored and apathetic in sessions with the client.

■ The nurse has difficulty setting limits on the client's behavior.

■ The nurse defends the client's behavior to other staff members.

The nurse may be completely unaware or only minimally aware of the countertransference as it is occurring (Hilz, 2012).

Interventions for Countertransference Hilz (2012) states:

> The relationship usually should not be terminated in the presence of countertransference. Rather, the nurse or staff member experiencing the countertransference should be supportively assisted by other staff members to identify his or her feelings and behaviors and recognize the occurrence of the phenomenon. It may be helpful to have evaluative sessions with the nurse after his or her encounter with the patient, in which both the nurse and other staff members (who are observing the interactions) discuss and compare the exhibited behaviors in the relationship.

The Termination Phase

Termination of the relationship may occur for a variety of reasons: the mutually agreed-on goals may have been reached; the client may be discharged from the hospital; or, in the case of a student nurse, it may be the end of a clinical rotation. Termination can be a difficult phase for both the client and nurse. The main task involves bringing a therapeutic conclusion to the relationship. This occurs when:

■ Progress has been made toward attainment of mutually set goals.

■ A plan for continuing care or for assistance during stressful life experiences is mutually established by the nurse and client.

■ Feelings about termination of the relationship are recognized and explored. Both the nurse and client may experience feelings of sadness and loss. The nurse should share his or her feelings with the client. Through these interactions, the client learns that it is acceptable to have these kinds of feelings at a time of separation. With this knowledge, the client experiences growth during the process of termination.

> **CLINICAL PEARL** When the client feels sadness and loss, behaviors to delay termination may become evident. If the nurse experiences the same feelings, he or she may allow the client's behaviors to delay termination. For therapeutic closure, the nurse must establish the reality of the separation and resist being manipulated into repeated delays by the client.

Boundaries in the Nurse-Client Relationship

A boundary indicates a border or a limit. It determines the extent of acceptable limits. Many types of boundaries exist. Examples include the following:

- **Material boundaries.** These are physical property that can be seen, such as fences that border land.
- **Social boundaries.** These are established within a culture and define how individuals are expected to behave in social situations.
- **Personal boundaries.** These are boundaries that individuals define for themselves. They include *physical distance boundaries,* or just how close individuals will allow others to invade their physical space; and *emotional boundaries,* or how much individuals choose to disclose of their most private and intimate selves to others.
- **Professional boundaries.** These boundaries limit and outline expectations for appropriate professional relationships with clients. They separate therapeutic behavior from any other behavior that, well intentioned or not, could lessen the benefit of care to clients (College and Association of Registered Nurses of Alberta [CARNA], 2005).

Concerns regarding professional boundaries are commonly related to the following issues:

- **Self-disclosure.** Self-disclosure on the part of the nurse may be appropriate when it is judged that the information may therapeutically benefit the client. It should never be undertaken for the purpose of meeting the nurse's needs.
- **Gift-giving.** Individuals who are receiving care often feel indebted toward health-care providers. And, indeed, gift-giving may be part of the therapeutic process for people who receive care (CARNA, 2005). Cultural beliefs and values may also enter into the decision of whether to accept a gift from a client. In some cultures, failure to do so would be interpreted as an insult (Pies, 2012). Accepting financial gifts is never appropriate, but in some instances nurses may be permitted to suggest instead a donation to a charity of the client's choice. If acceptance of a small gift of gratitude is deemed appropriate, the nurse may choose to share it with other staff members who have been involved in the client's care. In all instances, nurses should exercise professional judgment when deciding whether to accept a gift from a client. Attention should be given to what the gift-giving means to the client, as well as to institutional policy, the American Nurses Association (ANA) *Code of Ethics for Nurses,* and the ANA *Scope and Standards of Practice.*
- **Touch.** Nursing by its very nature involves touching clients. Touching is required to perform the many therapeutic procedures involved in the physical care of clients. Caring touch is the touching of clients when there is no physical need (Registered Nurses Association of British Columbia [RNABC], 2003). Caring touch often provides comfort or encouragement and, when it is used appropriately, it can have a therapeutic effect on the client. However, certain vulnerable clients may misinterpret the meaning of touch. Certain cultures, such as Native Americans and Asian Americans, are often uncomfortable with touch. The nurse must be sensitive to these cultural nuances and aware when touch is crossing a personal boundary. Additionally, clients who are experiencing high levels of anxiety or exhibiting suspicious or psychotic behaviors may interpret touch as aggressive. These are times when touch should be avoided or considered with extreme caution.
- **Friendship or romantic association.** When a nurse is acquainted with a client, the relationship must move from one of a personal nature to professional. If the nurse is unable to accomplish this separation, he or she should withdraw from the nurse-client relationship. Likewise, nurses must guard against personal relationships developing as a result of the nurse-client relationship. Romantic, sexual, or similar personal relationships are never appropriate between nurse and client.

Certain warning signs exist that indicate that professional boundaries of the nurse-client relationship may be in jeopardy. Some of these include the following (Coltrane & Pugh, 1978):

- Favoring one client's care over that of another
- Keeping secrets with a client
- Changing dress style for working with a particular client
- Swapping client assignments to care for a particular client
- Giving special attention or treatment to one client over others

- Spending free time with a client
- Frequently thinking about the client when away from work
- Sharing personal information or work concerns with the client
- Receiving of gifts or continued contact/communication with the client after discharge

Boundary crossings can threaten the integrity of the nurse-client relationship. Nurses must gain self-awareness and insight to be able to recognize when professional integrity is being compromised. Peternelj-Taylor and Yonge (2003) stated:

> The nursing profession needs nurses who have the ability to make decisions about boundaries based on the best interests of the clients in their care. This requires nurses to reflect on their knowledge and experiences, on how they think and how they feel, and not simply to buy blindly into a framework that says, "do this," "don't do that." (p. 65)

Summary and Key Points

- Nurses who work in the psychiatric/mental health field use special skills, or "interpersonal techniques," to assist clients in adapting to difficulties or changes in life experiences.
- Therapeutic nurse-client relationships are goal oriented, and the problem-solving model is used to try to bring about some type of change in the client's life.
- The instrument for delivery of the process of interpersonal nursing is the therapeutic use of self, which requires that the nurse possess a strong sense of self-awareness and self-understanding.
- Hildegard Peplau identified seven subroles within the role of nurse: stranger, resource person, teacher, leader, surrogate, technical expert, and counselor.
- Characteristics that enhance the achievement of a therapeutic relationship include rapport, trust, respect, genuineness, and empathy.
- Phases of a therapeutic nurse-client relationship include the preinteraction phase, the orientation (introductory) phase, the working phase, and the termination phase.
- Transference occurs when the client unconsciously displaces (or "transfers") to the nurse feelings formed toward a person from the past.
- Countertransference refers to the nurse's behavioral and emotional response to the client. These responses may be related to unresolved feelings toward significant others from the nurse's past, or they may be generated in response to transference feelings on the part of the client.
- Types of boundaries include material, social, personal, and professional.
- Concerns associated with professional boundaries include self-disclosure, gift-giving, touch, and developing a friendship or romantic association.
- Boundary crossings can threaten the integrity of the nurse-client relationship.

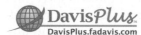 Additional info available at
DavisPlus.fadavis.com   www.davisplus.com

Review Questions
Self-Examination/Learning Exercise

*Select the answer that is **most** appropriate for each of the following questions.*

1. Nurse Mary has been providing care for Tom during his hospital stay. On Tom's day of discharge, his wife brings a bouquet of flowers and box of chocolates to his room. He presents these gifts to Nurse Mary saying, "Thank you for taking care of me." What is a correct response by the nurse?
   a. "I don't accept gifts from patients."
   b. "Thank you so much! It is so nice to be appreciated."
   c. "Thank you. I will share these with the rest of the staff."
   d. "Hospital policy forbids me to accept gifts from patients."

2. Nancy says to the nurse, "I worked as a secretary to put my husband through college, and as soon as he graduated, he left me. I hate him! I hate all men!" Which of the following is an empathetic response by the nurse?
   a. "You are very angry now. This is a normal response to your loss."
   b. "I know what you mean. Men can be very insensitive."
   c. "I understand completely. My husband divorced me, too."
   d. "You are depressed now, but you will feel better in time."

Review Questions—cont'd
Self-Examination/Learning Exercise

3. Which of the following behaviors suggest a possible breach of professional boundaries? (Select all that apply.)
   a. The nurse repeatedly requests to be assigned to a specific client.
   b. The nurse shares the details of her divorce with the client.
   c. The nurse makes arrangements to meet the client outside of the therapeutic environment.
   d. The nurse shares how she dealt with a similar difficult situation.

4. Which of the following tasks are associated with the orientation phase of relationship development? (Select all that apply.)
   a. Promoting the client's insight and perception of reality.
   b. Creating an environment for the establishment of trust and rapport.
   c. Using the problem-solving model toward goal fulfillment.
   d. Obtaining available information about the client from various sources.
   e. Formulating nursing diagnoses and setting goals.

5. Nurse Carol, who is the adult child of an alcoholic, is working with John, a client who abuses alcohol. John has experienced a successful detoxification process and is beginning a program of rehabilitation. He says to Carol, "I'm not going to go to those stupid AA meetings. They don't help anything." Carol, whose father died of complications from alcoholism, responds with anger: "Don't you even care what happens to your children?" Carol's response is an example of which of the following?
   a. Transference
   b. Countertransference
   c. Self-disclosure
   d. A breach of professional boundaries

6. Nurse Jones is working with Kim, a client in the anger-management program. Which of the following identifies actions associated with the working phase of the therapeutic relationship?
   a. Kim tells Nurse Jones she wants to learn more adaptive ways to handle her anger. Together, they set some goals.
   b. The goals of therapy have been met, but Kim cries and says she has to keep coming to therapy in order to be able to handle her anger appropriately.
   c. Nurse Jones reads Kim's previous medical records. She explores her feelings about working with a woman who has abused her child.
   d. Nurse Jones helps Kim practice various techniques to control her angry outbursts. She gives Kim positive feedback for attempting to improve maladaptive behaviors.

7. When there is congruence between what is felt and what is being expressed, the nurse is exhibiting which of the following characteristics?
   a. Trust
   b. Respect
   c. Genuineness
   d. Empathy

8. When the nurse shows unconditional acceptance of an individual as a worthwhile and unique human being, he or she is exhibiting which of the following characteristics?
   a. Trust
   b. Respect
   c. Genuineness
   d. Empathy

Continued

Review Questions—cont'd
Self-Examination/Learning Exercise

9. Hildegard Peplau identified seven subroles within the role of the nurse. She believed the emphasis in psychiatric nursing was on which of the subroles?
   a. The resource person
   b. The teacher
   c. The surrogate
   d. The counselor

10. Which of the following behaviors are associated with the phenomenon of *transference?* (Select all that apply.)
    a. The client attributes toward the nurse feelings associated with a person from the client's past.
    b. The nurse attributes toward the client feelings associated with a person from the nurse's past.
    c. The client forms an overwhelming affection for the nurse.
    d. The client becomes excessively dependent on the nurse and forms unrealistic expectations of him or her.

References

College and Association of Registered Nurses of Alberta (CARNA). (2005). *Professional boundaries for registered nurses: Guidelines for the nurse-client relationship.* Edmonton, AB: CARNA.

Hilz, L.M. (2012). Transference and countertransference. *Kathi's mental health review.* Retrieved from http://www.toddlertime .com/mh/terms/countertransference-transference-3.htm

Peplau, H.E. (1991). *Interpersonal relations in nursing.* New York, NY: Springer.

Peternelj-Taylor, C.A., & Yonge, O. (2003). Exploring boundaries in the nurse-client relationship: Professional roles and responsibilities. *Perspectives in Psychiatric Care, 39*(2), 55–66.

Pies, R.W. (2012). The patient gift conundrum. *Medscape Psychiatry & Mental Health.* Retrieved from http://www.medscape.com/ viewarticle/775575

Raskin, N.J., Rogers, C.R., & Witty, M.C. (2011). Client-centered therapy. In R.J. Corsini & D. Wedding (Eds.), *Current psychotherapies* (9th ed.). Belmont, CA: Brooks/Cole.

Registered Nurses' Association of British Columbia (RNABC). (2003). *Nurse-client relationships.* Vancouver, BC: RNABC.

Sadock, B.J., & Sadock, V.A. (2007). *Synopsis of psychiatry: Behavioral sciences/clinical psychiatry* (10th ed.). Philadelphia, PA: Lippincott Williams & Wilkins.

Schuster, P.M. (2000). *Communication: The key to the therapeutic relationship.* Philadelphia, PA: F.A. Davis.

Classical References

Coltrane, F., & Pugh, C. (1978). Danger signals in staff/patient relationships. *Journal of Psychiatric Nursing & Mental Health Services, 16*(6), 34–36.

Luft, J. (1970). *Group processes: An introduction to group dynamics* (3rd ed.). Palo Alto, CA: Mayfield Publishing.

Peplau, H.E. (1962). Interpersonal techniques: The crux of psychiatric nursing. *American Journal of Nursing, 62*(6), 50–54.

Raths, L., Harmin, M., & Simon, S. (1978). *Values and teaching: Working with values in the classroom* (2nd ed.). Columbus, OH: Merrill.

Sullivan, H.S. (1953). *The interpersonal theory of psychiatry.* New York, NY: W.W. Norton.

Travelbee, J. (1971). *Interpersonal aspects of nursing* (2nd ed.). Philadelphia, PA: F.A. Davis.

Therapeutic Communication 8

CORE CONCEPTS
communication
therapeutic
communication

KEY TERMS

density
distance
intimate distance

paralanguage
personal distance
public distance

social distance
territoriality

OBJECTIVES
After reading this chapter, the student will be able to:

1. Discuss the transactional model of communication.
2. Identify types of preexisting conditions that influence the outcome of the communication process.
3. Define territoriality, density, and distance as components of the environment.
4. Identify components of nonverbal expression.
5. Describe therapeutic and nontherapeutic verbal communication techniques.
6. Describe active listening.
7. Discuss therapeutic feedback.

HOMEWORK ASSIGNMENT
Please read the chapter and answer the following questions:

1. A client asks the nurse for advice about what to do regarding a personal situation and the nurse responds, "What do *you* think you should do?" This is an example of what technique? Is it therapeutic or nontherapeutic?
2. "Just hang in there. Everything will be all right." If the nurse makes this statement to a client, it is an example of what technique? Is it therapeutic or nontherapeutic?
3. Why might it be more appropriate to conduct a client interview in a conference room or interview room rather than in the client's room or nurse's office?
4. Name the five elements of constructive feedback.

Development of the *therapeutic interpersonal relationship* was described in Chapter 7 as the process by which nurses provide care for clients in need of psychosocial intervention. *Therapeutic use of self* was identified as the instrument for delivery of care. The focus of this chapter is on *techniques*—or, more specifically, *interpersonal communication techniques*—to facilitate the delivery of that care.

Hays and Larson (1963) stated, "To relate therapeutically with a patient it is necessary for the nurse to understand his or her role and its relationship to the patient's illness" (p. 1). They describe the role of the nurse as providing the client with the opportunity to accomplish the following:

1. Identify and explore problems in relating to others.
2. Discover healthy ways of meeting emotional needs.
3. Experience a satisfying interpersonal relationship.

These goals are achieved through use of interpersonal communication techniques (both verbal and nonverbal). The nurse must be aware of the therapeutic or nontherapeutic value of the communication techniques used with the client because they are the "tools" of psychosocial intervention.

CORE CONCEPT

Communication

An interactive process of transmitting information between two or more entities.

What Is Communication?

It has been said that individuals "cannot *not* communicate." Every word that is spoken, every movement that is made, and every action that is taken or failed to be taken gives a message to someone. Interpersonal communication is a *transaction* between the sender and the receiver. In the transactional model of communication, both participants simultaneously perceive each other, listen to each other, and are mutually involved in creating meaning in a relationship. The transactional model is illustrated in Figure 8-1.

The Impact of Preexisting Conditions

In all interpersonal transactions, both the sender and receiver bring certain preexisting conditions to the exchange that influence both the intended message and the way in which it is interpreted. Examples of

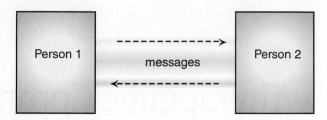

FIGURE 8–1 The Transactional Model of Communication.

these conditions include one's value system, internalized attitudes and beliefs, culture or religion, social status, gender, background knowledge and experience, and age or developmental level. The type of environment in which the communication takes place may also influence the outcome of the transaction. Figure 8-2 shows how these influencing factors are positioned on the transactional model.

Values, Attitudes, and Beliefs

Values, attitudes, and beliefs are learned ways of thinking. Children generally adopt the value systems and internalize the attitudes and beliefs of their parents. Children may retain this way of thinking into adulthood or develop a different set of attitudes and values as they mature.

Values, attitudes, and beliefs can influence communication in numerous ways. For example, prejudice is expressed verbally through negative stereotyping.

One's value system may be communicated with behaviors that are more symbolic in nature. For example, an individual who values youth may dress and behave in a manner that is characteristic of one who is much younger. Persons who value freedom and the American way of life may fly the U.S. flag in front of their homes each day. In each of these situations, a message is being communicated.

Culture or Religion

Communication has its roots in culture. Cultural mores, norms, ideas, and customs provide the basis

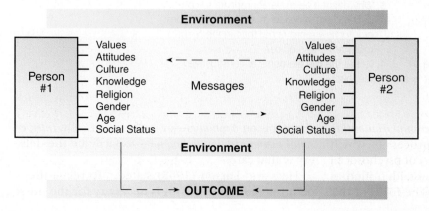

FIGURE 8–2 Factors influencing the Transactional Model of Communication.

for our way of thinking. Cultural values are learned and differ from society to society. For example, in some European countries (e.g., Italy, Spain, and France), men may greet each other with hugs and kisses. These behaviors are appropriate in those cultures but may communicate a different message in the United States or England.

Religion can influence communication as well. Priests and ministers who wear clerical collars publicly communicate their mission in life. The collar may also influence the way in which others relate to them, either positively or negatively. Other symbolic gestures, such as wearing a cross around the neck or hanging a crucifix on the wall, also communicate an individual's religious beliefs.

Social Status

Studies of nonverbal indicators of social status or power have suggested that high-status persons are associated with gestures that communicate their higher-power position. For example, they use less eye contact, have a more relaxed posture, use louder voice pitch, place hands on hips more frequently, are "power dressers," have greater height, and maintain more distance when communicating with individuals considered to be of lower social status.

Gender

Gender influences the manner in which individuals communicate. Most cultures have *gender signals* that are recognized as either masculine or feminine and provide a basis for distinguishing between members of each gender. Examples include differences in posture, both standing and sitting, between many men and women in the United States. Men usually stand with thighs 10 to 15 degrees apart, the pelvis rolled back, and the arms slightly away from the body. Women often are seen with legs close together, the pelvis tipped forward, and the arms close to the body. When sitting, men may lean back in the chair with legs apart or may rest the ankle of one leg over the knee of the other. Women tend to sit more upright in the chair with legs together, perhaps crossed at the ankles, or one leg crossed over the other at thigh level.

Roles have historically been identified as either male or female. For example, in the United States masculinity typically was communicated through such roles as husband, father, breadwinner, doctor, lawyer, or engineer. Traditional female roles included those of wife, mother, homemaker, nurse, teacher, or secretary.

Gender signals are changing in U.S. society as sexual roles become less distinct. Behaviors that had been considered typically masculine or feminine in the past may now be generally accepted in members of both genders. Words such as "unisex" communicate a desire by some individuals to diminish the distinction between genders and minimize the discrimination of either. Gender roles are changing as both women and men enter professions that were once dominated by members of the opposite gender.

Age or Developmental Level

Age influences communication and it is never more evident than during adolescence. In their struggle to separate from parental confines and establish their own identity, adolescents generate a unique pattern of communication that changes from generation to generation. Words such as *dude, groovy, clueless, awesome, cool,* and *wasted* have had special meaning for certain generations of adolescents. The technological age has produced a whole new language for today's adolescents. Communication by text messaging includes such acronyms as BRB ("be right back"), BFF ("best friends forever"), and MOS ("mom over shoulder").

Developmental influences on communication may relate to physiological alterations. One example is American Sign Language, the system of unique gestures used by many people who are deaf or hearing impaired. Individuals who are blind at birth never learn the subtle nonverbal gesticulations that accompany language and can totally change the meaning of the spoken word.

Environment in Which the Transaction Takes Place

The place where the communication occurs influences the outcome of the interaction. Some individuals who feel uncomfortable and refuse to speak during a group therapy session may be open and willing to discuss problems privately on a one-to-one basis with the nurse.

Territoriality, **density**, and **distance** are aspects of environment that communicate messages. *Territoriality* is the innate tendency to own space. Individuals lay claim to areas around them as their own. This influences communication when an interaction takes place in the territory "owned" by one or the other. Interpersonal communication can be more successful if the interaction takes place in a "neutral" area. For example, with the concept of territoriality in mind, the nurse may choose to conduct the psychosocial assessment in an interview room rather than in his or her office or in the client's room.

Density refers to the number of people within a given environmental space. It has been shown to influence interpersonal interaction. Some studies indicate that a correlation exists between prolonged high-density situations and certain behaviors, such as aggression, stress, criminal activity, hostility toward others, and a deterioration of mental and physical health.

Distance is the means by which various cultures use space to communicate. Hall (1966) identified four kinds of spatial interaction, or distances, that people maintain from each other in their interpersonal interactions and the kinds of activities in which people engage at these various distances. **Intimate distance** is the closest distance that individuals will allow between themselves and others. In the United States, this distance, which is restricted to interactions of an intimate nature, is 0 to 18 inches. **Personal distance** is approximately 18 to 40 inches and reserved for interactions that are personal in nature, such as close conversations with friends or colleagues. **Social distance** is about 4 to 12 feet away from the body. Interactions at this distance include conversations with strangers or acquaintances, such as at a cocktail party or in a public building. A **public distance** is one that exceeds 12 feet. Examples include speaking in public or yelling to someone some distance away. This distance is considered public space, and communicants are free to move about in it during the interaction.

Nonverbal Communication

It has been estimated that about 70 to 80 percent of all effective communication is nonverbal (Khan, 2009). Some aspects of nonverbal expression have been discussed in the previous section on preexisting conditions that influence communication. Other components of nonverbal communication include physical appearance and dress, body movement and posture, touch, facial expressions, eye behavior, and vocal cues or paralanguage. These nonverbal messages vary from culture to culture.

Physical Appearance and Dress

Physical appearance and dress are part of the total nonverbal stimuli that influence interpersonal responses and, under some conditions, they are the primary determinants of such responses. Body coverings—both dress and hair—are manipulated by the wearer in a manner that conveys a distinct message to the receiver. Dress can be formal or casual, stylish or unkempt. Hair can be long or short, and even the presence or absence of hair conveys a message about the person. Other body adornments that are also considered potential communicative stimuli include tattoos, masks, cosmetics, badges, jewelry, and eyeglasses. Some jewelry worn in specific ways can give special messages (e.g., a gold band or diamond ring worn on the third finger of the left hand, a pin bearing Greek letters worn on the lapel, or the wearing of a ring that is inscribed with the insignia of a college or university). Some individuals convey a specific message with the total absence of any type of body adornment.

Body Movement and Posture

The way in which an individual positions his or her body communicates messages regarding self-esteem, gender identity, status, and interpersonal warmth or coldness. The individual whose posture is slumped, with head and eyes pointed downward, conveys a message of low self-esteem. Specific ways of standing or sitting are considered to be either feminine or masculine within a defined culture. In the United States, to stand straight and tall with head high and hands on hips indicates a superior status over the person being addressed.

Reece and Whitman (1962) identified response behaviors that were used to designate individuals as either "warm" or "cold" persons. Individuals who were perceived as warm responded to others with a shift of posture toward the other person, a smile, direct eye contact, and hands that remained still. Individuals who responded to others with a slumped posture, by looking around the room, drumming fingers on the desk, and not smiling were perceived as cold.

Touch

Touch is a powerful communication tool. It can elicit both negative and positive reactions, depending on the people involved and the circumstances of the interaction. It is a very basic and primitive form of communication, and the appropriateness of its use is culturally determined.

Touch can be categorized according to the message communicated (Knapp & Hall, 2010):

- **Functional-Professional.** This type of touch is impersonal and businesslike. It is used to accomplish a task.

  EXAMPLE
  A tailor measuring a customer for a suit or a physician examining a client.

- **Social-Polite.** This type of touch is still rather impersonal, but it conveys an affirmation or acceptance of the other person.

  EXAMPLE
  A handshake.

- **Friendship-Warmth.** Touch at this level indicates a strong liking for the other person, a feeling that he or she is a friend.

  EXAMPLE
  Laying one's hand on the shoulder of another.

- **Love-Intimacy.** This type of touch conveys an emotional attachment or attraction for another person.

  EXAMPLE
  Engaging in a strong, mutual embrace.

■ **Sexual Arousal.** Touch at this level is an expression of physical attraction only.

EXAMPLE

Touching another in the genital region.

Some cultures encourage more touching of various types than others. "Contact cultures" (e.g., France, Latin America, Italy) use a greater frequency of touch cues than do those in "noncontact cultures" (e.g., Germany, United States, Canada) (Givens, 2010a). The nurse should understand the cultural meaning of touch before using this method of communication in specific situations.

Facial Expressions

Next to human speech, facial expression is the primary source of communication. Facial expressions primarily reveal an individual's emotional states, such as happiness, sadness, anger, surprise, and fear. The face is a complex multimessage system. Facial expressions serve to complement and qualify other communication behaviors, and at times even take the place of verbal messages. A summary of feelings associated with various facial expressions is presented in Table 8-1.

Eye Behavior

Eyes have been called the "windows of the soul." It is through eye contact that individuals view and are viewed by others in a revealing way. An interpersonal connectedness occurs through eye contact. In American culture, eye contact conveys a personal interest in the other person. Eye contact indicates that the communication channel is open, and it is often the initiating factor in verbal interaction between two people.

Eye behavior is regulated by social rules. These rules dictate where, when, for how long, and at whom we can look. Staring is often used to register disapproval of the behavior of another. People are extremely sensitive to being looked at, and if the gazing or staring behavior violates social rules, they often assign meaning to it, such as the following statement implies: "He kept staring at me, and I began to wonder if I was dressed inappropriately or had mustard on my face!"

Gazing at another's eyes arouses strong emotions. Thus, eye contact rarely lasts longer than 3 seconds before one or both viewers experience a powerful urge to glance away. Breaking eye contact lowers stress levels (Givens, 2010c).

Vocal Cues or Paralanguage

Paralanguage is the gestural component of the spoken word. It consists of pitch, tone, and loudness of

TABLE 8–1 Summary of Facial Expressions

FACIAL EXPRESSION	ASSOCIATED FEELINGS
Nose:	
Nostril flare	Anger; arousal
Wrinkling up	Dislike; disgust
Lips:	
Grin; smile	Happiness; contentment
Grimace	Fear; pain
Compressed	Anger; frustration
Canine-type snarl	Disgust
Pouted; frown	Unhappiness; discontented; disapproval
Pursing	Disagreement
Sneer	Contempt; disdain
Brows:	
Frown	Anger; unhappiness; concentration
Raised	Surprise; enthusiasm
Tongue:	
Stick out	Dislike; disagree
Eyes:	
Widened	Surprise; excitement
Narrowed; lids squeezed shut	Threat; fear
Stare	Threat
Stare/blink/look away	Dislike; disinterest
Eyes downcast; lack of eye contact	Submission; low self-esteem
Eye contact (generally intermittent, as opposed to a stare)	Self-confidence; interest

SOURCES: Adapted from Givens (2010b); Hughey (1990); and Simon (2005).

spoken messages; the rate of speaking; expressively placed pauses; and emphasis assigned to certain words. These vocal cues greatly influence the way individuals interpret verbal messages. A normally soft-spoken individual whose pitch and rate of speaking increases may be perceived as being anxious or tense.

Different vocal emphases can alter interpretation of the message. Three examples follow:

1. "I felt **SURE** you would notice the change."
   Interpretation: I was **SURE** you would, but you didn't.

2. "I felt sure **YOU** would notice the change."
   Interpretation: I thought **YOU** would, even if nobody else did.

3. "I felt sure you would notice the **CHANGE**."
   Interpretation: Even if you didn't notice anything else, I thought you would notice the **CHANGE**.

Verbal cues play a major role in determining responses in human communication situations. *How* a message is verbalized can be as important as *what* is verbalized.

CORE CONCEPT

Therapeutic Communication

Caregiver verbal and nonverbal techniques that focus on the care receiver's needs and advance the promotion of healing and change. Therapeutic communication encourages exploration of feelings and fosters understanding of behavioral motivation. It is nonjudgmental, discourages defensiveness, and promotes trust.

Therapeutic Communication Techniques

Hays and Larson (1963) identified a number of techniques to assist the nurse in interacting more therapeutically with clients. These are important "technical procedures" carried out by the nurse working in psychiatry, and they should serve to enhance development of a therapeutic nurse-client relationship. Table 8-2 includes a list of these techniques, a short explanation of their usefulness, and examples of each.

Nontherapeutic Communication Techniques

Several approaches are considered to be barriers to open communication between the nurse and client. Hays and Larson (1963) identified a number of these techniques, which are presented in Table 8-3. Nurses should recognize and eliminate the use of these patterns in their relationships with clients. Avoiding these communication barriers will maximize the

TABLE 8–2 Therapeutic Communication Techniques

TECHNIQUE	EXPLANATION/RATIONALE	EXAMPLES
Using silence	Gives the client the opportunity to collect and organize thoughts, to think through a point, or to consider introducing a topic of greater concern than the one being discussed.	
Accepting	Conveys an attitude of reception and regard.	"Yes, I understand what you said." Eye contact; nodding.
Giving recognition	Acknowledging and indicating awareness; better than complimenting, which reflects the nurse's judgment.	"Hello, Mr. J. I notice that you made a ceramic ash tray in OT." "I see you made your bed."
Offering self	Making oneself available on an unconditional basis, increasing client's feelings of self-worth.	"I'll stay with you awhile." "We can eat our lunch together." "I'm interested in you."
Giving broad openings	Allows the client to take the initiative in introducing the topic; emphasizes the importance of the client's role in the interaction.	"What would you like to talk about today?" "Tell me what you are thinking."
Offering general leads	Offers the client encouragement to continue.	"Yes, I see." "Go on." "And after that?"
Placing the event in time or sequence	Clarifies the relationship of events in time so that the nurse and client can view them in perspective.	"What seemed to lead up to . . .?" "Was this before or after . . .?" "When did this happen?"
Making observations	Verbalizing what is observed or perceived. This encourages the client to recognize specific behaviors and compare perceptions with the nurse.	"You seem tense." "I notice you are pacing a lot." "You seem uncomfortable when you . . ."

TABLE 8–2 **Therapeutic Communication Techniques–cont'd**

TECHNIQUE	EXPLANATION/RATIONALE	EXAMPLES
Encouraging description of perceptions	Asking the client to verbalize what is being perceived; often used with clients experiencing hallucinations.	"Tell me what is happening now." "Are you hearing the voices again?" "What do the voices seem to be saying?"
Encouraging comparison	Asking the client to compare similarities and differences in ideas, experiences, or interpersonal relationships. This helps the client recognize life experiences that tend to recur as well as those aspects of life that are changeable.	"Was this something like . . .?" "How does this compare with the time when . . .?" "What was your response the last time this situation occurred?"
Restating	Repeating the main idea of what the client has said. This lets the client know whether or not an expressed statement has been understood and gives him or her the chance to continue, or to clarify if necessary.	Cl: "I can't study. My mind keeps wandering." Ns: "You have trouble concentrating." Cl: "I can't take that new job. What if I can't do it?" Ns: "You're afraid you will fail in this new position."
Reflecting	Questions and feelings are referred back to the client so that they may be recognized and accepted, and so that the client may recognize that his or her point of view has value—a good technique to use when the client asks the nurse for advice.	Cl: "What do you think I should do about my wife's drinking problem?" Ns: "What do *you* think you should do?" Cl: "My sister won't help a bit toward my mother's care. I have to do it all!" Ns: "You feel angry when she doesn't help."
Focusing	Taking notice of a single idea or even a single word; works especially well with a client who is moving rapidly from one thought to another. This technique is *not* therapeutic, however, with the client who is very anxious. Focusing should not be pursued until the anxiety level has subsided.	"This point seems worth looking at more closely. Perhaps you and I can discuss it together."
Exploring	Delving further into a subject, idea, experience, or relationship; especially helpful with clients who tend to remain on a superficial level of communication. However, if the client chooses not to disclose further information, the nurse should refrain from pushing or probing in an area that obviously creates discomfort.	"Please explain that situation in more detail." "Tell me more about that particular situation."
Seeking clarification and validation	Striving to explain that which is vague or incomprehensible and searching for mutual understanding. Clarifying the meaning of what has been said facilitates and increases understanding for both client and nurse.	"I'm not sure that I understand. Would you please explain?" "Tell me if my understanding agrees with yours." "Do I understand correctly that you said . . .?"
Presenting reality	When the client has a misperception of the environment, the nurse defines reality or indicates his or her perception of the situation for the client.	"I understand that the voices seem real to you, but I do not hear any voices." "There is no one else in the room but you and me."

Continued

TABLE 8–2 Therapeutic Communication Techniques—cont'd

TECHNIQUE	EXPLANATION/RATIONALE	EXAMPLES
Voicing doubt	Expressing uncertainty as to the reality of the client's perceptions; often used with clients experiencing delusional thinking.	"I understand that you believe that to be true, but I see the situation differently." "I find that hard to believe (or accept)." "That seems rather doubtful to me."
Verbalizing the implied	Putting into words what the client has only implied or said indirectly; can also be used with the client who is mute or is otherwise experiencing impaired verbal communication. This clarifies that which is *implicit* rather than *explicit*.	Cl: "It's a waste of time to be here. I can't talk to you or anyone." Ns: "Are you feeling that no one understands?" Cl: (Mute) Ns: "It must have been very difficult for you when your husband died in the fire."
Attempting to translate words into feelings	When feelings are expressed indirectly, the nurse tries to "desymbolize" what has been said and to find clues to the underlying true feelings.	Cl: "I'm way out in the ocean." Ns: "You must be feeling very lonely right now."
Formulating a plan of action	When a client has a plan in mind for dealing with what is considered to be a stressful situation, it may serve to prevent anger or anxiety from escalating to an unmanageable level.	"What could you do to let your anger out harmlessly?" "Next time this comes up, what might you do to handle it more appropriately?"

SOURCE: Adapted from Hays & Larson (1963).

TABLE 8–3 Nontherapeutic Communication Techniques

TECHNIQUE	EXPLANATION/RATIONALE	EXAMPLES
Giving reassurance	Indicates to the client that there is no cause for anxiety, thereby devaluing the client's feelings; may discourage the client from further expression of feelings if he or she believes they will only be downplayed or ridiculed.	"I wouldn't worry about that if I were you." "Everything will be all right." **Better to say:** "We will work on that together."
Rejecting	Refusing to consider or showing contempt for the client's ideas or behavior. This may cause the client to discontinue interaction with the nurse for fear of further rejection.	"Let's not discuss . . ." "I don't want to hear about . . ." **Better to say:** "Let's look at that a little closer."
Approving or disapproving	Sanctioning or denouncing the client's ideas or behavior; implies that the nurse has the right to pass judgment on whether the client's ideas or behaviors are "good" or "bad," and that the client is expected to please the nurse. The nurse's acceptance of the client is then seen as conditional depending on the client's behavior.	"That's good. I'm glad that you . . ." "That's bad. I'd rather you wouldn't . . ." **Better to say:** "Let's talk about how your behavior invoked anger in the other clients at dinner."

TABLE 8-3 Nontherapeutic Communication Techniques—cont'd

TECHNIQUE	EXPLANATION/RATIONALE	EXAMPLES
Agreeing or disagreeing	Indicating accord with or opposition to the client's ideas or opinions; implies that the nurse has the right to pass judgment on whether the client's ideas or opinions are "right" or "wrong." Agreement prevents the client from later modifying his or her point of view without admitting error. Disagreement implies inaccuracy, provoking the need for defensiveness on the part of the client.	"That's right. I agree." "That's wrong. I disagree." "I don't believe that." **Better to say:** "Let's discuss what you feel is unfair about the new community rules."
Giving advice	Telling the client what to do or how to behave implies that the nurse knows what is best and that the client is incapable of any self-direction. It nurtures the client in the dependent role by discouraging independent thinking.	"I think you should . . ." "Why don't you . . ." **Better to say:** "What do *you* think you should do?" or "What do *you* think would be the best way to solve this problem?
Probing	Persistent questioning of the client; pushing for answers to issues the client does not wish to discuss. This causes the client to feel used and valued only for what is shared with the nurse and places the client on the defensive.	"Tell me how your mother abused you when you were a child." "Tell me how you feel toward your mother now that she is dead." "Now tell me about . . ." **Better technique:** The nurse should be aware of the client's response and discontinue the interaction at the first sign of discomfort.
Defending	Attempting to protect someone or something from verbal attack. To defend what the client has criticized is to imply that he or she has no right to express ideas, opinions, or feelings. Defending does not change the client's feelings and may cause the client to think the nurse is taking sides against the client.	"No one here would lie to you." "You have a very capable physician. I'm sure he only has your best interests in mind." **Better to say:** "I will try to answer your questions and clarify some issues regarding your treatment."
Requesting an explanation	Asking the client to provide the reasons for thoughts, feelings, behavior, and events. Asking "why" a client did something or feels a certain way can be very intimidating, and implies that the client must defend his or her behavior or feelings.	"Why do you think that?" "Why do you feel this way?" "Why did you do that?" **Better to say:** "Describe what you were feeling just before that happened."
Indicating the existence of an external source of power	Attributing the source of thoughts, feelings, and behavior to others or to outside influences. This encourages the client to project blame for his or her thoughts or behaviors on others rather than accepting the responsibility personally.	"What makes you say that?" "What made you do that?" "What made you so angry last night?" **Better to say:** "You became angry when your brother insulted your wife."

Continued

TABLE 8–3 Nontherapeutic Communication Techniques–cont'd

TECHNIQUE	EXPLANATION/RATIONALE	EXAMPLES
Belittling feelings expressed	When the nurse misjudges the degree of the client's discomfort, a lack of empathy and understanding may be conveyed. The nurse may tell the client to "perk up" or "snap out of it." This causes the client to feel insignificant or unimportant. When one is experiencing discomfort, it is no relief to hear that others are or have been in similar situations.	Cl: "I have nothing to live for. I wish I were dead." Ns: "Everybody gets down in the dumps at times. I feel that way myself sometimes." **Better to say:** "You must be very upset. Tell me what you are feeling right now."
Making stereotyped comments	Clichés and trite expressions are meaningless in a nurse-client relationship. When the nurse makes empty conversation, it encourages a like response from the client.	"I'm fine, and how are you?" "Hang in there. It's for your own good." "Keep your chin up." **Better to say:** "The therapy must be difficult for you at times. How do you feel about your progress at this point?"
Using denial	Denying that a problem exists blocks discussion with the client and avoids helping the client identify and explore areas of difficulty.	Cl: "I'm nothing." Ns: "Of course you're something. Everybody is somebody." **Better to say:** "You're feeling like no one cares about you right now."
Interpreting	With this technique the therapist seeks to make conscious that which is unconscious, to tell the client the meaning of his or her experience.	"What you really mean is . . ." "Unconsciously you're saying . . ." **Better technique:** The nurse must leave interpretation of the client's behavior to the psychiatrist. The nurse has not been prepared to perform this technique, and in attempting to do so, may endanger other nursing roles with the client.
Introducing an unrelated topic	Changing the subject causes the nurse to take over the direction of the discussion. This may occur in order to get to something that the nurse wants to discuss with the client or to get away from a topic that he or she would prefer not to discuss.	Cl: "I don't have anything to live for." Ns: "Did you have visitors this weekend?" **Better technique:** The nurse must remain open and free to hear the client and to take in all that is being conveyed, both verbally and nonverbally.

SOURCE: Adapted from Hays & Larson (1963).

effectiveness of communication and enhance the nurse-client relationship.

Active Listening

To listen actively is to be attentive to what the client is saying, both verbally and nonverbally. Attentive listening creates a climate in which the client can communicate. With active listening the nurse communicates acceptance and respect for the client, and trust is enhanced. A climate is established within the relationship that promotes openness and honest expression.

Several nonverbal behaviors have been designated as facilitative skills for attentive listening. Those listed here can be identified by the acronym SOLER:

S—Sit squarely facing the client. This gives the message that the nurse is there to listen and is interested in what the client has to say.

O—Observe an open posture. Posture is considered "open" when arms and legs remain uncrossed. This suggests that the nurse is "open" to what the client has to say. With a "closed" position, the nurse can convey a somewhat defensive stance, possibly invoking a similar response in the client.

L—Lean forward toward the client. This conveys to the client that you are involved in the interaction, interested in what is being said, and making a sincere effort to be attentive.

E—Establish eye contact. Eye contact, intermittently directed, is another behavior that conveys the nurse's involvement and willingness to listen to what the client has to say. The absence of eye contact or the constant shifting of eye contact elsewhere in the environment gives the message that the nurse is not really interested in what is being said.

> **CLINICAL PEARL** Ensure that eye contact conveys warmth and is accompanied by smiling and intermittent nodding of the head, and does not come across as staring or glaring, which can create intense discomfort in the client.

R—Relax. Whether sitting or standing during the interaction, the nurse should communicate a sense of being relaxed and comfortable with the client. Restlessness and fidgetiness communicate a lack of interest and may convey a feeling of discomfort that is likely to be transferred to the client.

Process Recordings

Process recordings are written reports of verbal interactions with clients. They are verbatim (to the extent that this is possible) accounts, written by the nurse or student as a tool for improving interpersonal communication techniques. The process recording can take many forms, but usually includes the verbal and nonverbal communication of both nurse and client. The exercise provides a means for the nurse to analyze both the content and the pattern of the interaction. The process recording, which is not considered documentation, is intended to be used as a learning tool for professional development. An example of one type of process recording is presented in Table 8-4.

Feedback

Feedback is a method of communication for helping the client consider a modification of behavior. Feedback gives information to clients about how they are being perceived by others. It should be presented in a manner that discourages defensiveness

TABLE 8–4 Sample Process Recording

NURSE VERBAL (NONVERBAL)	CLIENT VERBAL (NONVERBAL)	NURSE'S THOUGHTS AND FEELINGS CONCERNING THE INTERACTION	ANALYSIS OF THE INTERACTION
Do you still have thoughts about harming yourself? (Sitting facing the client; looking directly at client.)	Not really. I still feel sad, but I don't want to die. (Looking at hands in lap.)	Felt a little uncomfortable. Always a hard question to ask.	**Therapeutic.** Asking a direct question about suicidal intent.
Tell me what you were feeling before you took all the pills the other night. (Still using SOLER techniques of active listening.)	I was just so angry! To think that my husband wants a divorce now that he has a good job. I worked hard to put him through college. (Fists clenched. Face and neck reddened.)	Beginning to feel more comfortable. Client seems willing to talk and I think she trusts me.	**Therapeutic.** Exploring. Delving further into the experience.
You wanted to hurt him because you felt betrayed. (SOLER)	Yes! If I died, maybe he'd realize that he loved me more than that other woman. (Tears starting to well up in her eyes.)	Starting to feel sorry for her.	**Therapeutic.** Attempting to translate words into feelings.
Seems like a pretty drastic way to get your point across. (Small frown.)	I know. It was a stupid thing to do. (Wiping eyes.)	Trying hard to remain objective.	**Nontherapeutic.** Sounds disapproving. Better to have pursued her feelings.
How are you feeling about the situation now? (SOLER)	I don't know. I still love him. I want him to come home. I don't want him to marry her. (Starting to cry again.)	Wishing there was an easy way to help relieve some of her pain.	**Therapeutic.** Focusing on her feelings.

Continued

TABLE 8–4	**Sample Process Recording—cont'd**		
NURSE VERBAL (NONVERBAL)	**CLIENT VERBAL (NONVERBAL)**	**NURSE'S THOUGHTS AND FEELINGS CONCERNING THE INTERACTION**	**ANALYSIS OF THE INTERACTION**
Yes, I can understand that you would like things to be the way they were before. (Offer client a tissue.)	(Silence. Continues to cry softly.)	I'm starting to feel some anger toward her husband. Sometimes it's so hard to remain objective!	**Therapeutic.** Conveying empathy.
What do you think are the chances of your getting back together? (SOLER)	None. He's refused marriage counseling. He's already moved in with her. He says it's over. (Wipes tears. Looks directly at nurse.)	Relieved to know that she isn't using denial about the reality of the situation.	**Therapeutic.** Reflecting. Seeking client's perception of the situation.
So how are you preparing to deal with this inevitable outcome? (SOLER)	I'm going to do the things we talked about: join a divorced women's support group; increase my job hours to full-time; do some volunteer work; and call the suicide hotline if I feel like taking pills again. (Looks directly at nurse. Smiles.)	Positive feeling to know that she remembers what we discussed earlier and plans to follow through.	**Therapeutic.** Formulating a plan of action.
It won't be easy. But you have come a long way, and I feel you have gained strength in your ability to cope. (Standing. Looking at client. Smiling.)	Yes, I know I will have hard times. But I also know I have support, and I want to go on with my life and be happy again. (Standing, smiling at nurse.)	Feeling confident that the session has gone well; hopeful that the client will succeed in what she wants to do with her life.	**Therapeutic.** Presenting reality.

on the part of the client. Feedback can be useful to the client if presented with objectivity by a trusted individual.

Some criteria about useful feedback include the following:

■ Feedback is descriptive rather than evaluative and focuses on the behavior rather than on the client. Avoiding evaluative language reduces the need for the client to react defensively. Objective descriptions allow clients to take the information and use it in whatever way they choose. When the focus is on the client, the nurse makes judgments about the client.

EXAMPLE

Descriptive and on behavior	"Jane was very upset in group today when you called her 'fatty' and laughed at her in front of the others."
Evaluative	"You were very rude and inconsiderate to Jane in group today."
Focus on client	"You are a very insensitive person."

■ Feedback should be specific rather than general. Information that gives details about the client's behavior can be used more easily than a generalized description for modifying the behavior.

EXAMPLE

| Specific | "You were talking to Joe when we were deciding on the issue. Now you want to argue about the outcome." |
| General | "You just don't pay attention." |

■ Feedback should be directed toward behavior that the client has the capacity to modify. To provide feedback about a characteristic or situation that the client cannot change only provokes frustration.

EXAMPLE

| Can modify | "I noticed that you did not want to hold your baby when the nurse brought her to you." |
| Cannot modify | "Your baby daughter is mentally retarded because you took drugs when you were pregnant." |

■ Feedback should impart information rather than offer advice. Giving advice fosters dependence and may convey the message to the client that he or she is not capable of making decisions and solving problems independently. It is the client's right and privilege to be as self-sufficient as possible.

EXAMPLE

Imparting information	"There are various methods of assistance for people who want to lose weight, such as Overeaters Anonymous, Weight Watchers, regular visits to a dietitian, and the Physician's Weight Loss Program. You can decide what is best for you."
Giving advice	"You obviously need to lose a great deal of weight. I think the Physician's Weight Loss Program would be best for you."

■ Feedback should be well timed. Feedback is most useful when given at the earliest appropriate opportunity following the specific behavior.

EXAMPLE

Prompt response	"I saw you hit the wall with your fist just now when you hung up the phone after talking to your mother."
Delayed response	"You need to learn some more appropriate ways of dealing with your anger. Last week after group I saw you pounding your fist against the wall."

Summary and Key Points

■ Interpersonal communication is a transaction between the sender and the receiver.

■ In all interpersonal transactions, both the sender and receiver bring certain preexisting conditions to the exchange that influence both the intended message and the way in which it is interpreted.

■ Examples of these preexisting conditions include one's value system, internalized attitudes and beliefs, culture or religion, social status, gender, background knowledge and experience, age or developmental level, and the type of environment in which the communication takes place.

■ Nonverbal expression is a primary communication system in which meaning is assigned to various gestures and patterns of behavior.

■ Some components of nonverbal communication include physical appearance and dress, body movement and posture, touch, facial expressions, eye behavior, and vocal cues or paralanguage.

■ Meaning of the nonverbal components of communication is culturally determined.

■ Therapeutic communication includes verbal and nonverbal techniques that focus on the care receiver's needs and advance the promotion of healing and change.

■ Nurses must also be aware of and avoid a number of techniques that are considered to be barriers to effective communication.

■ Active listening is described as being attentive to what the client is saying, through both verbal and nonverbal cues. Skills associated with active listening include sitting squarely facing the client, observing an open posture, leaning forward toward the client, establishing eye contact, and being relaxed.

■ Process recordings are written reports of verbal interactions with clients. They are used as learning tools for professional development.

■ Feedback is a method of communication for helping the client consider a modification of behavior.

■ The nurse must be aware of the therapeutic or nontherapeutic value of the communication techniques used with the client because they are the "tools" of psychosocial intervention.

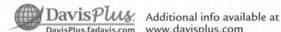
DavisPlus   Additional info available at
DavisPlus.fadavis.com   www.davisplus.com

Review Questions
Self-Examination/Learning Exercise

*Select the answer that is **most** appropriate for each of the following questions.*

1. A client states: "I refuse to shower in this room. I must be very cautious. The FBI has placed a camera in here to monitor my every move." Which of the following is the therapeutic response?
   a. "That's not true."
   b. "I have a hard time believing that is true."
   c. "Surely you don't really believe that."
   d. "I will help you search this room so that you can see there is no camera."

2. Nancy, a depressed client who has been unkept and untidy for weeks, today comes to group therapy wearing makeup and a clean dress and having washed and combed her hair. Which of the following responses by the nurse is most appropriate?
   a. "Nancy, I see you have put on a clean dress and combed your hair."
   b. "Nancy, you look wonderful today!"
   c. "Nancy, I'm sure everyone will appreciate that you have cleaned up for the group today."
   d. "Now that you see how important it is, I hope you will do this every day."

3. Dorothy was involved in an automobile accident while under the influence of alcohol. She swerved her car into a tree and narrowly missed hitting a child on a bicycle. She is in the hospital with multiple abrasions and contusions. She is talking about the accident with the nurse. Which of the following statements by the nurse is most appropriate?
   a. "Now that you know what can happen when you drink and drive, I'm sure you won't let it happen again."
   b. "You know that was a terrible thing you did. That child could have been killed."
   c. "I'm sure everything is going to be okay now that you understand the possible consequences of such behavior."
   d. "How are you feeling about what happened?"

4. Judy has been in the hospital for 3 weeks. She has used Valium "to settle my nerves" for the past 15 years. She was admitted by her psychiatrist for safe withdrawal from the drug. She has passed the physical symptoms of withdrawal at this time, but states to the nurse, "I don't know if I will be able to make it without Valium after I go home. I'm already starting to feel nervous. I have so many personal problems." Which is the most appropriate response by the nurse?
   a. "Why do you think you have to have drugs to deal with your problems?"
   b. "Everybody has problems, but not everybody uses drugs to deal with them. You'll just have to do the best that you can."
   c. "We will just have to think about some things that you can do to decrease your anxiety without resorting to drugs."
   d. "Just hang in there. I'm sure everything is going to be okay."

5. Mrs. S. asks the nurse, "Do you think I should tell my husband about my affair with my boss?" Which is the most appropriate response by the nurse?
   a. "What do you think would be best for you to do?"
   b. "Of course you should. Marriage has to be based on truth."
   c. "Of course not. That would only make things worse."
   d. "I can't tell you what to do. You have to decide for yourself."

6. Carol, an adolescent, just returned from group therapy and is crying. She says to the nurse, "All the other kids laughed at me! I try to fit in, but I always seem to say the wrong thing. I've never had a close friend. I guess I never will." Which is the most appropriate response by the nurse?
   a. "What makes you think you will never have any friends?"
   b. "You're feeling pretty down on yourself right now."
   c. "I'm sure they didn't mean to hurt your feelings."
   d. "Why do you feel this way about yourself?"

Review Questions—cont'd
Self-Examination/Learning Exercise

7. Walter is angry with his psychiatrist and says to the nurse, "He doesn't know what he is doing. That medication isn't helping a thing!" The nurse responds, "He has been a doctor for many years and has helped many people." This is an example of what nontherapeutic technique?
   a. Rejecting
   b. Disapproving
   c. Probing
   d. Defending

8. The client says to the nurse, "I've been offered a promotion, but I don't know if I can handle it." The nurse replies, "You're afraid you may fail in the new position." This is an example of which therapeutic technique?
   a. Restating
   b. Making observations
   c. Focusing
   d. Verbalizing the implied

9. The environment in which the communication takes place influences the outcome of the interaction. Which of the following are aspects of the environment that influence communication? (Select all that apply.)
   a. Territoriality
   b. Density
   c. Dimension
   d. Distance
   e. Intensity

10. The nurse says to a client, "You are being readmitted to the hospital. Why did you stop taking your medication?" What communication technique does this represent?
    a. Disapproving
    b. Requesting an explanation
    c. Disagreeing
    d. Probing

References

Givens, D.B. (2010a). *The nonverbal dictionary.* Center for Nonverbal Studies. Retrieved from http://web.archive.org/web/20060627081330/members.aol.com/doder1/touch1.htm

Givens, D.B. (2010b). *The nonverbal dictionary.* Center for Nonverbal Studies. Retrieved from http://web.archive.org/web/20060617171011/members.aol.com/nonverbal3/facialx.htm

Givens, D.B. (2010c). *The nonverbal dictionary.* Center for Nonverbal Studies. Retrieved from http://web.archive.org/web/20060619132216/members.aol.com/nonverbal3/eyecon.htm

Hughey, J.D. (1990). *Speech communication.* Stillwater, OK: Oklahoma State University.

Khan, A. (2009). *Principles for personal growth.* Bellevue, WA: YouMe Works.

Knapp, M.L., & Hall, J.A. (2010). *Nonverbal communication in human interaction* (7th ed.). Belmont, CA: Wadsworth.

Simon, M. (2005). *Facial expressions: A visual reference for artists.* New York, NY: Watson-Guptill.

Classical References

Hall, E.T. (1966). *The hidden dimension.* Garden City, NY: Doubleday.

Hays, J.S., & Larson, K.H. (1963). *Interacting with patients.* New York, NY: Macmillan.

Reece, M., & Whitman, R. (1962). Expressive movements, warmth, and verbal reinforcement. *Journal of Abnormal and Social Psychology, 64,* 234–236.

9

The Nursing Process in Psychiatric/Mental Health Nursing

CHAPTER OUTLINE

KEY TERMS

case management

case manager

concept mapping

critical pathways of care

Focus Charting®

interdisciplinary

managed care

Nursing Interventions
  Classification (NIC)

Nursing Outcomes
  Classification (NOC)

nursing process

PIE charting

problem-oriented recording

OBJECTIVES

After reading this chapter, the student will be able to:

1. Define *nursing process*.
2. Identify six steps of the nursing process and describe nursing actions associated with each.
3. Describe the benefits of using nursing diagnosis.
4. Discuss the list of nursing diagnoses approved by NANDA International for clinical use and testing.
5. Define and discuss the use of case management and critical pathways of care in the clinical setting.
6. Apply the six steps of the nursing process in the care of a client within the psychiatric setting.
7. Document client care that validates use of the nursing process.

HOMEWORK ASSIGNMENT

Please read the chapter and answer the following questions:

1. Nursing outcomes (sometimes referred to as goals) are derived from the nursing diagnosis. Name two essential aspects of an acceptable outcome or goal.
2. Define *managed care*.
3. The ANA identifies certain interventions that may be performed only by psychiatric nurses in advanced practice. What are they?
4. In Focus Charting®, one item cannot be used as the focus for documentation. What is this item?

For many years the **nursing process** has provided a systematic framework for the delivery of nursing care. It is nursing's means of fulfilling the requirement for a *scientific methodology* in order to be considered a profession.

This chapter examines the steps of the nursing process as they are set forth by the American Nurses Association (ANA) in *Nursing: Scope and Standards of Practice* (ANA, 2010a). An explanation is provided for the implementation of case management and the tool used in the delivery of care with this methodology, critical pathways of care. A description of concept mapping is included, and documentation that validates the use of the nursing process is discussed.

The Nursing Process

Definition

The nursing process consists of six steps and uses a problem-solving approach that has come to be accepted as nursing's scientific methodology. It is goal-directed, with the objective being delivery of quality client care.

The nursing process is dynamic, not static. It is an ongoing process that continues for as long as the nurse and client have interactions directed toward change in the client's physical or behavioral responses. Figure 9-1 presents a schematic of the ongoing nursing process.

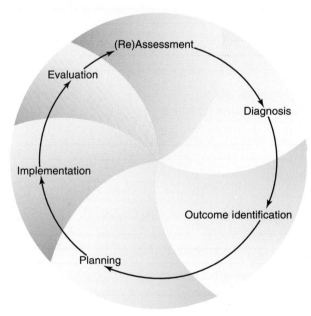

FIGURE 9-1   The ongoing nursing process.

Standards of Practice

The ANA, in collaboration with the American Psychiatric Nurses Association (APNA) and the International Society of Psychiatric-Mental Health Nurses (ISPN), has delineated a set of standards that psychiatric nurses are expected to follow as they provide care for their clients. The ANA (2010a) states:

> The Standards of Practice describe a competent level of nursing care as demonstrated by the critical thinking model known as the nursing process. The nursing process includes the components of assessment, diagnosis, outcomes identification, planning, implementation, and evaluation. Accordingly, the nursing process encompasses significant actions taken by registered nurses, and forms the foundation of the nurse's decision-making. (p. 9)

Following are the standards of practice for psychiatric/mental health nurses as set forth by the ANA, APNA, and ISPN (2007).

CORE CONCEPT

Assessment

A systematic, dynamic process by which the registered nurse, through interaction with the patient, family, groups, communities, populations, and health-care providers, collects and analyzes data. Assessment may include the following dimensions: physical, psychological, sociocultural, spiritual, cognitive, functional abilities, developmental, economic, and lifestyle (ANA, 2010a, p. 63).

Standard 1: Assessment

The Psychiatric-Mental Health Registered Nurse collects comprehensive health data that is pertinent to the patient's health or situation.

In this first step, information is gathered from which to establish a database for determining the best possible care for the client. Information for this database is gathered from a variety of sources including interviews with the client or family, observation of the client and his or her environment, consultation with other health-team members, review of the client's records, and a nursing physical examination. A biopsychosocial assessment tool based on the stress-adaptation framework is included in Box 9-1.

An example of a simple and quick mental status evaluation is presented in Table 9-1. Its focus is on the
(text continues on page 158)

BOX 9-1 **Nursing History and Assessment Tool**

I. General Information
Client name:_____ Allergies: _____
Room number:_____ Diet: _____
Doctor: _____ Height/weight: _____
Age: _____ Vital signs: TPR/BP _____
Sex: _____ Name and phone no. of significant other: _____
Race: _____
Dominant language: _____ City of residence: _____
Marital status: _____ Diagnosis (admitting & current): _____
Chief complaint: _____
_____

Conditions of admission:
Date: _____ Time: _____
Accompanied by: _____
Route of admission (wheelchair; ambulatory; cart): _____
Admitted from: _____

II. Predisposing Factors
A. *Genetic Influences*
1. Family configuration (use genograms):
　　　Family of origin:　　　　　Present family:

Family dynamics (describe significant relationships between family members): _____
_____
_____
_____
_____

2. Medical/psychiatric history: _____
a. Client: _____
_____
_____

b. Family members: _____
_____
_____

3. Other genetic influences affecting present adaptation. This might include effects specific to gender, race, appearance, such as genetic physical defects, or any other factor related to genetics that is affecting the client's adaptation that has not been mentioned elsewhere in this assessment.
_____
_____

B. *Past Experiences*
1. Cultural and social history:
a. Environmental factors (family living arrangements, type of neighborhood, special working conditions):
_____
_____
_____

b. Health beliefs and practices (personal responsibility for health; special self-care practices):
_____
_____

c. Religious beliefs and practices: _____
_____

d. Educational background: _____
_____
_____

BOX 9-1 **Nursing History and Assessment Tool–cont'd**

e. Significant losses/changes (include dates): _____

_____

_____

f. Peer/friendship relationships: _____

_____

_____

g. Occupational history: _____

_____

_____

h. Previous pattern of coping with stress: _____

_____

_____

i. Other lifestyle factors contributing to present adaptation: _____

_____

_____

C. *Existing Conditions*
1. Stage of development (Erikson):
    a. Theoretically: _____
    b. Behaviorally: _____
    c. Rationale: _____

    _____

    _____

2. Support systems: _____

_____

3. Economic security: _____

_____

4. Avenues of productivity/contribution:
    a. Current job status: _____

    _____

    b. Role contributions and responsibility for others: _____

    _____

III. Precipitating Event
Describe the situation or events that precipitated this illness/hospitalization: _____

_____

_____

IV. Client's Perception of the Stressor
Client's or family member's understanding or description of stressor/illness and expectations of hospitalization:

_____

_____

_____

_____

V. Adaptation Responses
A. *Psychosocial*
1. Anxiety level (circle one of the 4 levels and check the behaviors that apply):   Mild   Moderate Severe Panic
    calm _____ friendly_____ passive _____ alert _____ perceives environment correctly _____ cooperative _____
    impaired attention _____ "jittery" _____ unable to concentrate _____ hypervigilant _____ tremors _____ rapid
    speech _____ withdrawn _____ confused _____ disoriented _____ fearful _____ hyperventilating _____ misinterpreting
    the environment (hallucinations or delusions) _____ depersonalization _____ obsessions _____ compulsions _____
    somatic complaints _____ excessive hyperactivity _____ other _____

    _____

2. Mood/affect (circle as many as apply): happiness   sadness   dejection   despair   elation   euphoria
    suspiciousness   apathy (little emotional tone)   anger/hostility

Continued

BOX 9-1 Nursing History and Assessment Tool–cont'd

3. Ego defense mechanisms (describe how used by client):
   Projection _____
   Suppression _____
   Undoing _____
   Displacement _____
   Intellectualization _____
   Rationalization _____
   Denial _____
   Repression _____
   Isolation _____
   Regression _____
   Reaction Formation _____
   Splitting _____
   Religiosity _____
   Sublimation _____
   Compensation _____

4. Level of self-esteem (circle one):   low   moderate   high
   Things client likes about self _____
   _____
   Things client would like to change about self _____
   _____
   Objective assessment of self-esteem: _____
   Eye contact _____
   General appearance _____
   _____
   Personal hygiene _____
   Participation in group activities and interactions with others _____
   _____

5. Stage and manifestations of grief (circle one):
               Denial   Anger   Bargaining   Depression   Acceptance
   Describe the client's behaviors that are associated with this stage of grieving in response to loss or change.
   _____
   _____
   _____

6. Thought processes (circle as many as apply): clear logical easy to follow relevant confused blocking delusional
   rapid flow of thoughts   slowness in thought suspicious
   Recent memory (circle one): loss intact Remote memory (circle one): loss intact
   Other: _____
   _____

7. Communication patterns (circle as many as apply): clear coherent slurred speech incoherent neologisms
   loose associations flight of ideas aphasic perseveration rumination tangential speech loquaciousness slow,
   impoverished speech speech impediment (describe) _____
   Other _____
   _____

8. Interaction patterns (describe client's pattern of interpersonal interactions with staff and peers on the unit, e.g.,
   manipulative, withdrawn, isolated, verbally or physically hostile, argumentative, passive, assertive, aggressive, passive-
   aggressive, other): _____
   _____
   _____
   _____

9. Reality orientation (check those that apply):
   Oriented to: Time _____ Person _____
               Place _____ Situation _____

BOX 9-1 Nursing History and Assessment Tool–cont'd

10. Ideas of destruction to self/others?   Yes   No
     If yes, consider plan; available means _____
     _____
     _____
     _____

B. *Physiological*
1. Psychosomatic manifestations (describe any somatic complaints that may be stress-related): _____
   _____
   _____
   _____

2. Drug history and assessment:
   Use of prescribed drugs:

Name	Dosage	Prescribed For	Results

   Use of over-the-counter drugs:

Name	Dosage	Prescribed For	Results

   Use of street drugs or alcohol:

Name	Amount Used	How Often Used	When Last Used	Effects Produced

3. Pertinent physical assessments:
   a. Respirations: normal_____ labored _____
      Rate _____ Rhythm _____
   b. Skin: warm _____ dry _____ moist _____ cool _____ clammy _____ pink _____
      cyanotic _____ poor turgor _____ edematous _____
      Evidence of: rash _____ bruising _____ needle tracts _____ hirsutism _____
      loss of hair _____ other _____
      _____
   c. Musculoskeletal status: weakness _____ tremors _____
      Degree of range of motion (describe limitations) _____
      _____
      Pain (describe) _____
      _____
      Skeletal deformities (describe) _____
      Coordination (describe limitations) _____
   d. Neurological status:
      History of (check all that apply): seizures _____ (describe method of control) _____
      _____
      headaches (describe location and frequency) _____
      fainting spells _____ dizziness _____
      tingling/numbness (describe location) _____

Continued

BOX 9-1 **Nursing History and Assessment Tool—cont'd**

e. Cardiovascular: B/P _____ Pulse _____
   History of (check all that apply):
   hypertension _____ palpitations _____
   heart murmur _____ chest pain _____
   shortness of breath _____ pain in legs _____
   phlebitis _____ ankle/leg edema _____
   numbness/tingling in extremities _____
   varicose veins_____

f. Gastrointestinal:
   Usual diet pattern: _____
   Food allergies: _____
   Dentures? Upper _____ Lower _____
   Any problems with chewing or swallowing? _____
   Any recent change in weight? _____
   Any problems with:
   Indigestion/heartburn? _____
    Relieved by _____
   Nausea/vomiting? _____
    Relieved by _____
   History of ulcers? _____
   Usual bowel pattern _____
    Constipation? _____ Diarrhea? _____
    Type of self-care assistance provided for either of the above problems _____
   _____

g. Genitourinary/Reproductive:
   Usual voiding pattern _____
   Urinary hesitancy? _____ Frequency? _____
   Nocturia? _____ Pain/burning? _____
   Incontinence? _____
   Any genital lesions? _____
    Discharge?_____ Odor? _____
   History of sexually transmitted disease? _____
    If yes, please explain: _____
   _____
   Any concerns about sexuality/sexual activity? _____
   _____
   Method of birth control used _____
   Females:
    Date of last menstrual cycle _____
    Length of cycle _____
    Problems associated with menstruation? _____
   _____
   Breasts: Pain/tenderness? _____
    Swelling? _____ Discharge? _____
    Lumps? _____ Dimpling? _____
   Practice breast self-examination? _____
    Frequency? _____
   Males:
    Penile discharge? _____
    Prostate problems? _____

h. Eyes:

	Yes	No	Explain
Glasses?			
Contacts?			
Swelling?			
Discharge?			

BOX 9-1 **Nursing History and Assessment Tool–cont'd**

Itching? _____ _____ _____
Blurring? _____ _____ _____
Double vision? _____ _____ _____

i. Ears   **Yes**   **No**   **Explain**
   Pain? _____ _____ _____
   Drainage? _____ _____ _____
   Difficulty hearing? _____ _____ _____
   Hearing aid? _____ _____ _____
   Tinnitus? _____ _____ _____

j. Medication side effects:
   What symptoms is the client experiencing that may be attributed to current medication usage?
   _____
   _____

k. Altered lab values and possible significance: _____
   _____
   _____

l. Activity/rest patterns:
   Exercise (amount, type, frequency) _____
   _____
   Leisure time activities: _____
   _____
   Patterns of sleep: Number of hours per night _____
   Use of sleep aids? _____
   Pattern of awakening during the night? _____
   _____
   Feel rested upon awakening? _____

m. Personal hygiene/activities of daily living:
   Patterns of self-care: independent _____
   Requires assistance with: mobility _____
                              hygiene _____
                              toileting _____
                              feeding _____
                              dressing _____
                              other _____
   Statement describing personal hygiene and general appearance _____
   _____
   _____
   _____

n. Other pertinent physical assessments: _____
   _____
   _____

VI. Summary of Initial Psychosocial/Physical Assessment:

Knowledge Deficits Identified:

Nursing Diagnoses Indicated:

TABLE 9–1 **Brief Mental Status Evaluation**	
AREA OF MENTAL FUNCTION EVALUATED	EVALUATION ACTIVITY
Orientation to time	"What year is it? What month is it? What day is it? (3 points)
Orientation to place	"Where are you now?" (1 point)
Attention and immediate recall	"Repeat these words now: bell, book, & candle" (3 points) "Remember these words and I will ask you to repeat them in a few minutes."
Abstract thinking	"What does this mean: No use crying over spilled milk." (3 points)
Recent memory	"Say the 3 words I asked you to remember earlier." (3 points)
Naming objects	Point to eyeglasses and ask, "What is this?" Repeat with 1 other item (e.g., calendar, watch, pencil). (2 points possible)
Ability to follow simple verbal command	"Tear this piece of paper in half and put it in the trash container." (2 points)
Ability to follow simple written command	Write a command on a piece of paper (e.g., TOUCH YOUR NOSE), give the paper to the patient and say, "Do what it says on this paper. (1 point for correct action)
Ability to use language correctly	Ask the patient to write a sentence. (3 points if sentence has a subject, a verb, and has valid meaning).
Ability to concentrate	"Say the months of the year in reverse, starting with December." (1 point each for correct answer from November through August. 4 points possible.)
Understanding spatial relationships	Instruct client to draw a clock; put in all the numbers; and set the hands on 3 o'clock. (clock circle = 1 pt; numbers in correct sequence = 1 pt; numbers placed on clock correctly = 1 pt; two hands on the clock = 1 pt; hands set at correct time = 1 pt.) (5 points possible)

Scoring: 30-21 = normal; 20-11 = mild cognitive impairment; 10-0 = severe cognitive impairment. (Scores are not absolute and must be considered within the comprehensive diagnostic assessment.)
SOURCES: *Merck Manual of Health & Aging* (2005); Folstein, Folstein, & McHugh (1975); Kaufman & Zun (1995); Kokman et al. (1991); and Pfeiffer (1975).

cognitive aspects of mental functioning. Areas such as mood, affect, thought content, judgment, and insight are not evaluated. A number of these types of tests are available, but they must be considered only a part of the comprehensive diagnostic assessment. A mental status assessment guide, with explanations and selected sample interview questions, is provided in Appendix C.

CORE CONCEPT

Nursing Diagnosis

Clinical judgments about individual, family, or community experiences/responses to actual or potential health problems/life processes. A nursing diagnosis provides the basis for selection of nursing interventions to achieve outcomes for which the nurse has accountability. (NANDA, 2012).

Standard 2: Diagnosis

The Psychiatric-Mental Health Registered Nurse analyzes the assessment data to determine diagnoses or problems, including level of risk.

In the second step, data gathered during the assessment are analyzed. Diagnoses and potential problem statements are formulated and prioritized. Diagnoses are congruent with available and accepted classification systems (e.g., NANDA International Nursing Diagnosis Classification [see Appendix E]).

CORE CONCEPT

Outcomes

End results that are measurable, desirable, and observable, and translate into observable behaviors (ANA, 2010a, p. 65).

Standard 3: Outcomes Identification

The Psychiatric-Mental Health Registered Nurse identifies expected outcomes for a plan individualized to the patient or to the situation.

Expected outcomes are derived from the diagnosis. They must be measurable and include a time estimate for attainment. They must be realistic for the client's capabilities, and are most effective when formulated cooperatively by the interdisciplinary team members, the client, and significant others.

Nursing Outcomes Classification (NOC)

The **Nursing Outcomes Classification (NOC)** is a comprehensive, standardized classification of patient/client outcomes developed to evaluate the effects of nursing interventions (Moorhead, Johnson, Maas, & Swanson, 2013). The outcomes have been linked to NANDA International diagnoses and to the **Nursing Interventions Classification (NIC)**. NANDA-I, NIC, and NOC represent all domains of nursing and can be used together or separately (Moorhead & Dochterman, 2012). Each of the NOC outcomes has a label name, a definition, a list of indicators to evaluate client status in relation to the outcome, and a five-point Likert scale to measure client status (Moorhead et al., 2013).

Standard 4: Planning

The Psychiatric-Mental Health Registered Nurse develops a plan that prescribes strategies and alternatives to attain expected outcomes.

The care plan is individualized to the client's mental health problems, condition, or needs and is developed in collaboration with the client, significant others, and interdisciplinary team members, if possible. For each diagnosis identified, the most appropriate interventions, based on current psychiatric/mental health nursing practice and research, are selected. Client education and necessary referrals are included. Priorities for delivery of nursing care are determined.

Nursing Interventions Classification (NIC)

NIC is a comprehensive, standardized language describing treatments that nurses perform in all settings and in all specialties. NIC includes both physiological and psychosocial interventions, as well as those for illness treatment, illness prevention, and health promotion. NIC interventions are comprehensive, based on research, and reflect current clinical practice. They were developed inductively based on existing practice.

Each NIC intervention has a definition and a detailed set of activities that describe what a nurse does to implement the intervention. The use of a standardized language is thought to enhance continuity of care and facilitate communication among nurses and between nurses and other providers.

Standard 5: Implementation

The Psychiatric-Mental Health Registered Nurse implements the identified plan.

Interventions selected during the planning stage are executed, taking into consideration the nurse's level of practice, education, and certification. The care plan serves as a blueprint for delivery of safe, ethical, and appropriate interventions. Documentation of interventions also occurs at this step in the nursing process.

Several specific interventions are included among the standards of psychiatric/mental health clinical nursing practice (ANA, APNA, & ISPN, 2007):

Standard 5A: Coordination of Care

The Psychiatric-Mental Health Registered Nurse coordinates care delivery.

Standard 5B: Health Teaching and Health Promotion

The Psychiatric-Mental Health Registered Nurse employs strategies to promote health and a safe environment.

Standard 5C: Milieu Therapy

The Psychiatric-Mental Health Registered Nurse provides, structures, and maintains a safe and therapeutic environment in collaboration with patients, families, and other healthcare clinicians.

Standard 5D: Pharmacological, Biological, and Integrative Therapies

The Psychiatric-Mental Health Registered Nurse incorporates knowledge of pharmacological, biological, and complementary interventions with applied clinical skills to restore the patient's health and prevent further disability.

Standard 5E: Prescriptive Authority and Treatment

The Psychiatric-Mental Health Advanced Practice Registered Nurse uses prescriptive authority, procedures, referrals, treatments, and therapies in accordance with state and federal laws and regulations.

Standard 5F: Psychotherapy

The Psychiatric-Mental Health Advanced Practice Registered Nurse conducts individual, couples, group, and family psychotherapy using evidence-based psychotherapeutic frameworks and nurse-patient therapeutic relationships.

Standard 5G: Consultation

The Psychiatric-Mental Health Advanced Practice Registered Nurse provides consultation to influence the identified plan, enhance the abilities of other clinicians to provide services for patients, and effect change.

CORE CONCEPT

Evaluation

The process of determining the progress toward attainment of expected outcomes, including the effectiveness of care (ANA, 2010a, p. 65).

Standard 6: Evaluation

The Psychiatric-Mental Health Registered Nurse evaluates progress toward attainment of expected outcomes.

During the evaluation step, the nurse measures the success of the interventions in meeting the outcome criteria. The client's response to treatment is documented, validating use of the nursing process in the delivery of care. The diagnoses, outcomes, and plan of care are reviewed and revised as need is determined by the evaluation.

Why Nursing Diagnosis?

The concept of nursing diagnosis is not new. For centuries, nurses have identified specific client responses for which nursing interventions were used in an effort to improve quality of life. Historically, however, the autonomy of practice to which nurses were entitled by virtue of their licensure was lacking in the provision of nursing care. Nurses assisted physicians as required, and performed a group of specific tasks that were considered within their scope of responsibility.

The term *diagnosis* in relation to nursing first began to appear in the literature in the early 1950s. The formalized organization of the concept, however, was initiated only in 1973 with the convening of the First Task Force to Name and Classify Nursing Diagnoses. The Task Force of the National Conference Group on the Classification of Nursing Diagnoses was developed during this conference. These individuals were charged with the task of identifying and classifying nursing diagnoses.

Also in the 1970s, the ANA began to write standards of practice around the steps of the nursing process, of which nursing diagnosis is an inherent part. This format encompassed both the general and specialty standards outlined by the ANA. The standards of psychiatric/mental health nursing practice are summarized in Box 9-2.

BOX 9-2 Standards of Psychiatric-Mental Health Clinical Nursing Practice

Standard 1. Assessment
The Psychiatric-Mental Health Registered Nurse collects comprehensive health data that is pertinent to the patient's health or situation.

Standard 2. Diagnosis
The Psychiatric-Mental Health Registered Nurse analyzes the assessment data to determine diagnoses or problems, including level of risk.

Standard 3. Outcomes Identification
The Psychiatric-Mental Health Registered Nurse identifies expected outcomes for a plan individualized to the patient or to the situation.

Standard 4. Planning
The Psychiatric-Mental Health Registered Nurse develops a plan that prescribes strategies and alternatives to attain expected outcomes.

Standard 5. Implementation
The Psychiatric-Mental Health Registered Nurse implements the identified plan.

Standard 5A. Coordination of Care
The Psychiatric-Mental Health Registered Nurse coordinates care delivery.

Standard 5B. Health Teaching and Health Promotion
The Psychiatric-Mental Health Registered Nurse employs strategies to promote health and a safe environment.

Standard 5C. Milieu Therapy
The Psychiatric-Mental Health Registered Nurse provides, structures, and maintains a safe and therapeutic environment in collaboration with patients, families, and other health-care clinicians.

Standard 5D. Pharmacological, Biological, and Integrative Therapies
The Psychiatric-Mental Health Registered Nurse incorporates knowledge of pharmacological, biological, and complementary interventions with applied clinical skills to restore the patient's health and prevent further disability.

BOX 9-2 **Standards of Psychiatric-Mental Health Clinical Nursing Practice—cont'd**

Standard 5E. Prescriptive Authority and Treatment

The Psychiatric-Mental Health *Advanced Practice* Registered Nurse uses prescriptive authority, procedures, referrals, treatments, and therapies in accordance with state and federal laws and regulations.

Standard 5F. Psychotherapy

The Psychiatric-Mental Health *Advanced Practice* Registered Nurse conducts individual, couples, group, and family psychotherapy using evidence-based psychotherapeutic frameworks and nurse-patient therapeutic relationships.

Standard 5G. Consultation

The Psychiatric-Mental Health *Advanced Practice* Registered Nurse provides consultation to influence the identified plan, enhance the abilities of other clinicians to provide services for patients, and effect change.

Standard 6. Evaluation

The Psychiatric-Mental Health Registered Nurse evaluates progress toward attainment of expected outcomes.

SOURCE: © 2007 By American Nurses Association, American Psychiatric Association, and International Society of Psychiatric-Mental Health. Reprinted with permission. All Rights Reserred.

From this progression a statement of policy was published in 1980 and included a definition of nursing. The ANA defined nursing as "the diagnosis and treatment of human responses to actual or potential health problems" (ANA, 2010b). This definition has been expanded to describe more appropriately nursing's commitment to society and to the profession itself. The ANA (2010b) defines nursing as follows:

Nursing is the protection, promotion, and optimization of health and abilities, prevention of illness and injury, alleviation of suffering through the diagnosis and treatment of human response, and advocacy in the care of individuals, families, communities, and populations. (p. 10)

Nursing diagnosis is an inherent component of both the original and expanded definitions.

Decisions regarding professional negligence are made based on the standards of practice defined by the ANA and the individual state nursing practice acts. A number of states have incorporated the steps of the nursing process, including nursing diagnosis, into the scope of nursing practice described in their nursing practice acts. When this is the case, it is the legal duty of the nurse to show that nursing process and nursing diagnosis were accurately implemented in the delivery of nursing care.

NANDA International (NANDA-I) evolved from the original task force that was convened in 1973 to name and classify nursing diagnoses. The major purpose of NANDA-I is to "to develop, refine and promote terminology that accurately reflects nurses' clinical judgments. NANDA-I will be a global force for the development and use of nursing's standardized terminology to ensure patient safety through evidence-based care, thereby improving the health care of all people" (NANDA-I, 2013). A list of nursing diagnoses approved by NANDA-I for use and testing is presented in Appendix E. This list is by no means exhaustive or all-inclusive. In an effort to maintain a common language within nursing and to encourage clinical testing of what is available, most of the nursing diagnoses used in this text will come from the 2012-2014 list approved by NANDA-I. However, in a few instances, nursing diagnoses that have been retired by NANDA-I for various reasons will continue to be used because of their appropriateness and suitability in describing specific behaviors.

The use of nursing diagnosis affords a degree of autonomy that historically has been lacking in the practice of nursing. Nursing diagnosis describes the client's condition, facilitating the prescription of interventions and establishment of parameters for outcome criteria based on what is uniquely nursing. The ultimate benefit is to the client, who receives effective and consistent nursing care based on knowledge of the problems that he or she is experiencing and of the most beneficial nursing interventions to resolve them.

Nursing Case Management

The concept of **case management** evolved with the advent of diagnosis-related groups (DRGs) and shorter hospital stays. Case management is an innovative model of care delivery that can result in improved client care. Within this model, clients are assigned a manager who negotiates with multiple providers to obtain diverse services. This type of health-care delivery process serves to decrease fragmentation of care while striving to contain cost of services.

Case management in the acute care setting strives to organize client care through an episode of illness so that specific clinical and financial outcomes are achieved within an allotted time frame. Commonly, the allotted time frame is determined by the established protocols for length of stay as defined by the DRGs.

Case management has been shown to be an effective method of treatment for individuals with a severe and persistent mental illness. This type of care strives to improve functioning by assisting the individual to solve problems, improve work and socialization skills, promote leisure-time activities, and enhance overall independence.

Ideally, case management incorporates concepts of care at the primary, secondary, and tertiary levels of prevention. Various definitions have emerged and should be clarified, as follows.

Managed care refers to a strategy employed by purchasers of health services who make determinations about various types of services in order to maintain quality and control costs. In a managed care program, individuals receive health care based on need, as assessed by coordinators of the providership. Managed care exists in many settings, including (but not limited to) the following:

■ Insurance-based programs
■ Employer-based medical providerships
■ Social service programs
■ The public health sector

Managed care may exist in virtually any setting in which medical providership is a part of the service; that is, in any setting in which an organization (whether private or government-based) is responsible for payment of health-care services for a group of people. Examples of managed care are health maintenance organizations (HMOs) and preferred provider organizations (PPOs).

Case management is the method used to achieve managed care. It is the actual coordination of services required to meet the needs of a client within the fragmented health-care system. Case management strives to help at-risk clients prevent avoidable episodes of illness. Its goal is to provide these services while attempting to control health-care costs to the consumer and third-party payers.

Types of clients who benefit from case management include (but are not limited to) the following:

■ The frail elderly
■ Individuals with developmental disabilities
■ Individuals with physical disabilities
■ Individuals with mental disabilities
■ Individuals with long-term medically complex problems that require multifaceted, costly care (e.g., high-risk infants, those with human immunodeficiency virus [HIV] or acquired immunodeficiency syndrome [AIDS], and transplant clients)
■ Individuals who are severely compromised by an acute episode of illness or an acute exacerbation of a severe and persistent illness (e.g., schizophrenia)

The **case manager** is responsible for negotiating with multiple health-care providers to obtain a variety of services for the client. Nurses are exceptionally qualified to serve as case managers. The very nature of nursing, which incorporates knowledge about the biological, psychological, and sociocultural aspects related to human functioning, makes nurses highly appropriate as case managers. Several years of experience as a registered nurse is usually required for employment as a case manager. Some case management programs prefer advanced practice registered nurses who have experience working with the specific populations for whom the case management service will be rendered. The American Nurses Credentialing Center (ANCC) offers an examination for nurses to become board certified in nursing case management.

Critical Pathways of Care

Critical pathways of care (CPCs) may be used as the tools for provision of care in a case management system. A critical pathway is a type of abbreviated plan of care that provides outcome-based guidelines for goal achievement within a designated length of stay. A sample CPC is presented in Table 9-2. Only one nursing diagnosis is used in this sample. A CPC may have nursing diagnoses for several individual problems.

CPCs are intended to be used by the entire interdisciplinary team, which may include a nurse case manager, clinical nurse specialist, social worker, psychiatrist, psychologist, dietitian, occupational therapist, recreational therapist, chaplain, and others. The team decides what categories of care are to be performed, by what date, and by whom. Each member of the team is then expected to carry out his or her functions according to the time line designated on the CPC. The nurse, as case manager, is ultimately responsible for ensuring that each of the assignments is carried out. If variations occur at any time in any of the categories of care, rationale must be documented in the progress notes.

For example, with the sample CPC presented, the nurse case manager may admit the client into the detoxification center. The nurse contacts the psychiatrist to inform him or her of the admission. The psychiatrist performs additional assessments to determine if other consultations are required. The psychiatrist also writes the orders for the initial diagnostic work-up and medication regimen. Within 24 hours, the interdisciplinary team meets to decide on other categories of care, to complete the CPC, and to make individual care assignments from the CPC. This particular sample CPC relies heavily on nursing care of the client through the critical withdrawal period. However, other problems for the same client, such as imbalanced nutrition, impaired physical mobility, or spiritual distress, may involve other members of the team to a greater degree. Each member of the team stays in contact with the nurse case manager regarding individual assignments. Ideally, team meetings are held daily or every other day to review progress and modify the plan as required.

TABLE 9–2 Sample Critical Pathway of Care for Client in Alcohol Withdrawal

Estimated Length of Stay: 7 Days–Variations from Designated Pathway Should Be Documented in Progress Notes

NURSING DIAGNOSES AND CATEGORIES OF CARE	TIME DIMENSION	GOALS AND/ OR ACTIONS	TIME DIMENSION	GOALS AND/ OR ACTIONS	TIME DIMENSION	DISCHARGE OUTCOME
Risk for injury related to CNS agitation					Day 7	Client shows no evidence of injury obtained during ETOH withdrawal
Referrals	Day 1	Psychiatrist Assess need for: Neurologist Cardiologist Internist			Day 7	Discharge with follow-up appointments as required
Diagnostic studies	Day 1	Blood alcohol level Drug screen (urine and blood) Chemistry Profile Urinalysis Chest X-ray ECG	Day 4	Repeat of selected diagnostic studies as necessary		
Additional assessments	Day 1 Day 1-5 Ongoing Ongoing	VS q4h I&O Restraints p.r.n. for client safety Assess withdrawal symptoms: tremors, nausea/vomiting, tachycardia, sweating, high blood pressure, seizures, insomnia, hallucinations	Day 2-3 Day 6 Day 4	VS q8h if stable DC I&O Marked decrease in objective withdrawal symptoms	Day 4-7 Day 7	VS bid; remain stable Discharge; absence of objective withdrawal symptoms
Medications	Day 1 Day 2 Day 1-6 Day 1-7	Librium* 200 mg in divided doses Librium 160 mg in divided doses Librium p.r.n. Maalox pc & hs *Note: Some physicians may elect to use Serax or Tegretol in the detoxification process	Day 3 Day 4	Librium 120 mg in divided doses Librium 80 mg in divided doses	Day 5 Day 6 Day 7	Librium 40 mg Discontinue librium Discharge; no withdrawal symptoms
Client education			Day 5	Discuss goals of AA and need for outpatient therapy	Day 7	Discharge with information regarding AA attendance or outpatient treatment

AA, Alcoholics Anonymous; bid, twice a day; DC, discontinue; ECT, electrocardiogram; ETOH, alcohol; hs, bedtime; I&O, intake and output; pc, after meals; q4h, every 4 hours; q8h, every 8 hours; VS, vital signs.

CPCs can be standardized, as they are intended to be used with uncomplicated cases. A CPC can be viewed as protocol for various clients with problems for which a designated outcome can be predicted.

Applying the Nursing Process in the Psychiatric Setting

Based on the definition of *mental health* set forth in Chapter 2, the role of the nurse in psychiatry focuses on helping the client successfully adapt to stressors within the environment. Goals are directed toward changes in thoughts, feelings, and behaviors that are age appropriate and congruent with local and cultural norms.

Therapy within the psychiatric setting is very often team, or **interdisciplinary**, oriented. Therefore, it is important to delineate nursing's involvement in the treatment regimen. Nurses are indeed valuable members of the team. Having progressed beyond the role of custodial caregiver in the psychiatric setting, nurses now provide services that are defined within the scope of nursing practice. Nursing diagnosis is helping to define these nursing boundaries, providing the degree of autonomy and professionalism that has for so long been unrealized.

For example, a newly admitted client with the medical diagnosis of schizophrenia may be demonstrating the following behaviors:

■ Inability to trust others
■ Verbalizing hearing voices
■ Refusing to interact with staff and peers
■ Expressing a fear of failure
■ Poor personal hygiene

From these assessments, the treatment team may determine that the client has the following problems:

■ Paranoid delusions
■ Auditory hallucinations
■ Social withdrawal
■ Developmental regression

Team goals would be directed toward the following:

■ Reducing suspiciousness
■ Terminating auditory hallucinations
■ Increasing feelings of self-worth

From this team treatment plan, nursing may identify the following nursing diagnoses:

■ Disturbed sensory perception,* auditory (evidenced by hearing voices)
■ Disturbed thought processes* (evidenced by delusions)

■ Low self-esteem (evidenced by fear of failure and social withdrawal)
■ Self-care deficit (evidenced by poor personal hygiene)

Nursing diagnoses are prioritized according to life-threatening potential. Maslow's hierarchy of needs is a good model to follow in prioritizing nursing diagnoses. In this instance, disturbed sensory perception (auditory) is identified as the priority nursing diagnosis, because the client may be hearing voices that command him or her to harm self or others. Psychiatric nursing, regardless of the setting—hospital (inpatient or outpatient), office, home, community—is goal-directed care. The goals (or expected outcomes) are client oriented, are measurable, and focus on resolution of the problem (if this is realistic) or on a more short-term outcome (if resolution is unrealistic). For example, in the previous situation, expected outcomes for the identified nursing diagnoses might be as follows:

The client will:

■ Demonstrate trust in one staff member within 3 days.
■ Verbalize understanding that the voices are not real (not heard by others) within 5 days.
■ Complete one simple craft project within 5 days.
■ Take responsibility for own self-care and perform activities of daily living independently by time of discharge.

Nursing's contribution to the interdisciplinary treatment regimen will focus on establishing trust on a one-to-one basis (thus reducing the level of anxiety that may be promoting hallucinations), giving positive feedback for small day-to-day accomplishments in an effort to build self-esteem, and assisting with and encouraging independent self-care. These interventions describe *independent nursing* actions and goals that are evaluated apart from, while also being directed toward achievement of, the *team's* treatment goals.

In this manner of collaboration with other team members, nursing provides a service that is unique and based on sound knowledge of psychopathology, scope of practice, and legal implications of the role. Although there is no dispute that "following doctor's orders" continues to be accepted as a priority of care, nursing intervention that enhances achievement of the overall goals of treatment is being recognized for its important contribution. The nurse who administers a medication prescribed by the physician to decrease anxiety may also choose to stay with the anxious client and offer reassurance of safety and security, thereby providing an independent nursing action that is distinct from, yet complementary to, the medical treatment.

---

*Disturbed Sensory Perception and Disturbed Thought Processes have been resigned from the NANDA-I list of approved nursing diagnoses (NANDA-I, 2012). However, they will continue to be used in this textbook because of their appropriateness to certain behaviors.

Concept Mapping*

Concept mapping is a diagrammatic teaching and learning strategy that allows students and faculty to visualize interrelationships between medical diagnoses, nursing diagnoses, assessment data, and treatments. The concept map care plan is an innovative approach to planning and organizing nursing care. Basically, it is a diagram of client problems and interventions. Compared to the commonly used column format care plans, concept map care plans are more succinct. They are practical, realistic, and time saving, and they serve to enhance critical-thinking skills and clinical reasoning ability.

The nursing process is foundational to developing and using the concept map care plan, just as it is with all types of nursing care plans. Client data are collected and analyzed, nursing diagnoses are formulated, outcome criteria are identified, nursing actions are planned and implemented, and the success of the interventions in meeting the outcome criteria is evaluated.

The concept map care plan may be presented in its entirety on one page, or the assessment data and nursing diagnoses may appear in diagram format on one page, with outcomes, interventions, and evaluation written on a second page. Alternatively, the diagram may appear in circular format, with nursing diagnoses and interventions branching off the "client" in the center of the diagram. Or, it may begin with the "client" at the top of the diagram, with branches emanating in a linear fashion downward.

As stated previously, the concept map care plan is based on the components of the nursing process. Accordingly, the diagram is assembled in the nursing process stepwise fashion, beginning with the client and his or her reason for needing care, nursing diagnoses with subjective and objective clinical evidence for each, nursing interventions, and outcome criteria for evaluation.

Figure 9-2 presents one example of a concept map care plan. It is assembled for the hypothetical client with schizophrenia discussed in the previous section, "Applying the Nursing Process in the Psychiatric Setting." Different colors may be used in the diagram to designate various components of the care plan. Connecting lines are drawn between components to indicate any relationships that exist. For example, there may be a relationship between two nursing diagnoses (e.g., between the nursing diagnoses of pain or anxiety and disturbed sleep pattern). A line between these nursing diagnoses should be drawn to show the relationship.

---

*Content in this section is adapted from Doenges, Moorhouse, & Murr (2010) and Schuster (2012).

Concept map care plans allow for a great deal of creativity on the part of the user, and permit viewing the "whole picture" without generating a great deal of paperwork. Because they reflect the steps of the nursing process, concept map care plans also are valuable guides for documentation of client care. Doenges, Moorhouse, & Murr (2010) have stated:

> As students, you are asked to develop plans of care that often contain more detail than what you see in the hospital plans of care. This is to help you learn how to apply the nursing process and create individualized client care plans. However, even though much time and energy may be spent focusing on filling the columns of traditional clinical care plan forms, some students never develop a holistic view of their clients and fail to visualize how each client need interacts with other identified needs. A new technique or learning tool [concept mapping] has been developed to assist you in visualizing the linkages, to enhance your critical thinking skills, and to facilitate the creative process of planning client care. (p. 32)

Documentation of the Nursing Process

Equally important as using the nursing process in the delivery of care is the written documentation that it has been used. Some contemporary nursing leaders are advocating that with solid standards of practice and procedures in place within the institution, nurses need only chart when there has been a deviation in the care as outlined by that standard. This method of documentation, known as charting by exception, is not widely accepted, as many legal decisions are still based on the precept that "if it was not charted, it was not done."

Because nursing process and nursing diagnosis are mandated by nursing practice acts in some states, documentation of their use is being considered in those states as evidence in determining certain cases of negligence by nurses. Some health-care organization accrediting agencies also require that nursing process be reflected in the delivery of care. Therefore, documentation must bear written testament to the use of the nursing process.

A variety of documentation methods can be used to reflect use of the nursing process in the delivery of nursing care. Three examples are presented here: problem-oriented recording (POR); Focus Charting®; and the problem, intervention, evaluation (PIE) system of documentation.

Problem-Oriented Recording

Problem-oriented recording follows the subjective, objective, assessment, plan, implementation, and evaluation (SOAPIE) format. It has as its basis a list of problems. When it is used in nursing, the problems

Clinical Vignette: Harry has been admitted to the psychiatric unit with a diagnosis of schizophrenia. He is socially isolated and stays in his room unless strongly encouraged by the nurse to come out. He says to the nurse, "You have to be your own boss. You can't trust anybody." He refuses to eat any food from his tray, stating that the voice of his deceased grandfather is telling him it is poisoned. His clothes are dirty, and he has an objectionable body odor. The nurse develops the following concept map care plan for Harry.

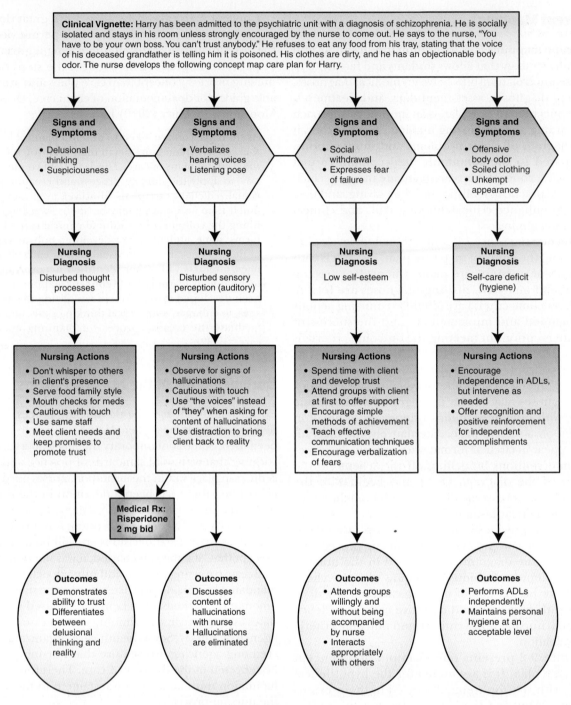

Signs and Symptoms
- Delusional thinking
- Suspiciousness

Signs and Symptoms
- Verbalizes hearing voices
- Listening pose

Signs and Symptoms
- Social withdrawal
- Expresses fear of failure

Signs and Symptoms
- Offensive body odor
- Soiled clothing
- Unkempt appearance

Nursing Diagnosis

Disturbed thought processes

Nursing Diagnosis

Disturbed sensory perception (auditory)

Nursing Diagnosis

Low self-esteem

Nursing Diagnosis

Self-care deficit (hygiene)

Nursing Actions
- Don't whisper to others in client's presence
- Serve food family style
- Mouth checks for meds
- Cautious with touch
- Use same staff
- Meet client needs and keep promises to promote trust

Nursing Actions
- Observe for signs of hallucinations
- Cautious with touch
- Use "the voices" instead of "they" when asking for content of hallucinations
- Use distraction to bring client back to reality

Nursing Actions
- Spend time with client and develop trust
- Attend groups with client at first to offer support
- Encourage simple methods of achievement
- Teach effective communication techniques
- Encourage verbalization of fears

Nursing Actions
- Encourage independence in ADLs, but intervene as needed
- Offer recognition and positive reinforcement for independent accomplishments

Medical Rx: Risperidone 2 mg bid

Outcomes
- Demonstrates ability to trust
- Differentiates between delusional thinking and reality

Outcomes
- Discusses content of hallucinations with nurse
- Hallucinations are eliminated

Outcomes
- Attends groups willingly and without being accompanied by nurse
- Interacts appropriately with others

Outcomes
- Performs ADLs independently
- Maintains personal hygiene at an acceptable level

FIGURE 9–2 Example: Concept map care plan for a client with schizophrenia.

(nursing diagnoses) are identified on a written plan of care, with appropriate nursing interventions described for each. Documentation written in the SOAPIE format includes the following:

S = Subjective data: Information gathered from what the client, family, or other source has said or reported.

O = Objective data: Information gathered through direct observation by the person performing the assessment; may include a physiological measurement such as blood pressure or a behavioral response such as affect.

A = Assessment: The nurse's interpretation of the subjective and objective data.

P = Plan: The actions or treatments to be carried out (may be omitted in daily charting if the plan is clearly explained in the written nursing care plan and no changes are expected).

I = Intervention: Those nursing actions that were actually carried out.

E = Evaluation of the problem following nursing intervention (some nursing interventions cannot be evaluated immediately, so this section may be optional).

Table 9-3 shows how POR corresponds to the steps of the nursing process.

Following is an example of a three-column documentation in the POR format.

EXAMPLE

DATE/TIME	PROBLEM	PROGRESS NOTES
9-12-13 1000	Social isolation	**S:** States he does not want to sit with or talk to others; "they frighten me." **O:** Stays in room alone unless strongly encouraged to come out; no group involvement; at times listens to group conversations from a distance but does not interact; some hypervigilance and scanning noted. **A:** Inability to trust; panic level of anxiety; delusional thinking **I:** Initiated trusting relationship by spending time alone with the client; discussed his feelings regarding interactions with others; accompanied client to group activities; provided positive feedback for voluntarily participating in assertiveness training.

TABLE 9–3 Validation of the Nursing Process with Problem-Oriented Recording

PROBLEM-ORIENTED RECORDING	WHAT IS RECORDED	NURSING PROCESS
S and O (Subjective and Objective data)	Verbal reports to, and direct observation and examination by, the nurse	Assessment
A (Assessment)	Nurse's interpretation of S and O	Diagnosis and outcome identification
P (Plan) (Omitted in charting if written plan describes care to be given)	Description of appropriate nursing actions to resolve the identified problem	Planning
I (Intervention)	Description of nursing actions actually carried out	Implementation
E (Evaluation)	A reassessment of the situation to determine results of nursing actions implemented	Evaluation

Focus Charting

Another type of documentation that reflects use of the nursing process is **Focus Charting®**. Focus Charting differs from POR in that the main perspective has been changed from "problem" to "focus," and a data, action, and response (DAR) format has replaced SOAPIE.

Lampe (1985) suggested that a focus for documentation can be any of the following:

■ Nursing diagnosis
■ Current client concern or behavior

■ Significant change in the client status or behavior
■ Significant event in the client's therapy

The focus cannot be a medical diagnosis. The documentation is organized in the format of DAR. These categories are defined as follows:

D = Data: Information that supports the stated focus or describes pertinent observations about the client

A = Action: Immediate or future nursing actions that address the focus, and evaluation of the present care plan along with any changes required

R = Response: Description of client's responses to any part of the medical or nursing care

Table 9-4 shows how Focus Charting corresponds to the steps of the nursing process. Following is an example of a three-column documentation in the DAR format.

EXAMPLE

DATE/TIME	FOCUS	PROGRESS NOTES
9-12-13 1000	Social isolation related to mistrust, panic anxiety, delusions	**D:** States he does not want to sit with or talk to others; they "frighten" him; stays in room alone unless strongly encouraged to come out; no group involvement; at times listens to group conversations from a distance, but does not interact; some hypervigilance and scanning noted. **A:** Initiated trusting relationship by spending time alone with client; discussed his feelings regarding interactions with others; accompanied client to group activities; provided positive feedback for voluntarily participating in assertiveness training. **R:** Cooperative with therapy; still acts uncomfortable in the presence of a group of people; accepted positive feedback from nurse.

TABLE 9–4 Validation of the Nursing Process with Focus Charting

FOCUS CHARTING	WHAT IS RECORDED	NURSING PROCESS
D (Data)	Information that supports the stated focus or describes pertinent observations about the client.	Assessment
Focus	A nursing diagnosis; current client concern or behavior; significant change in client status; significant event in the client's therapy. (*Note:* If outcome appears on written care plan, it need not be repeated in daily documentation unless a change occurs.)	Diagnosis and outcome identification
A (Action)	Immediate or future nursing actions that address the focus; appraisal of the care plan along with any changes required.	Plan and implementation
R (Response)	Description of client responses to any part of the medical or nursing care.	Evaluation

The PIE Method

The PIE method, or more specifically "APIE" (assessment, problem, intervention, evaluation), is a systematic approach of documenting to nursing process and nursing diagnosis. A problem-oriented system, **PIE charting** uses accompanying flow sheets that are individualized by each institution. Criteria for documentation are organized in the following manner:

A = Assessment: A complete client assessment is conducted at the beginning of each shift. Results are documented under this section in the progress notes. Some institutions elect instead to use a daily client assessment sheet designed to meet specific needs of the unit. Explanation of any deviation from the norm is included in the progress notes.

P = Problem: A problem list, or list of nursing diagnoses, is an important part of the APIE method of charting. The name or number of the problem being addressed is documented in this section.

I = Intervention: Nursing actions are performed, directed at resolution of the problem.

E = Evaluation: Outcomes of the implemented interventions are documented, including an evaluation of client responses to determine the effectiveness of nursing interventions and the presence or absence of progress toward resolution of a problem.

Table 9-5 shows how APIE charting corresponds to the steps of the nursing process. Following is an example of a three-column documentation in the APIE format.

EXAMPLE

DATE/TIME	PROBLEM	PROGRESS NOTES
9-12-13 1000	Social Isolation	**A:** States he does not want to sit with or talk to others; they "frighten" him; stays in room alone unless strongly encouraged to come out; no group involvement; at times listens to group conversations from a distance but does not interact; some hypervigilance and scanning noted. **P:** Social isolation related to inability to trust, panic level of anxiety, and delusional thinking. **I:** Initiated trusting relationship by spending time alone with client; discussed his feelings regarding interactions with others; accompanied client to group activities; provided positive feedback for voluntarily participating in assertiveness training. **E:** Cooperative with therapy; still uncomfortable in the presence of a group of people; accepted positive feedback from nurse.

TABLE 9–5 Validation of the Nursing Process with APIE Method

APIE CHARTING	WHAT IS RECORDED	NURSING PROCESS
A (Assessment)	Subjective and objective data about the client that are gathered at the beginning of each shift.	Assessment
P (Problem)	Name (or number) of nursing diagnosis being addressed from written problem list, and identified outcome for that problem. (*Note:* If outcome appears on written care plan, it need not be repeated in daily documentation unless a change occurs.)	Diagnosis and outcome identification
I (Intervention)	Nursing actions performed, directed at problem resolution.	Plan and implementation
E (Evaluation)	Appraisal of client responses to determine effectiveness of nursing interventions.	Evaluation

Electronic Documentation

Most health-care facilities have implemented—or are in the process of implementing—some type of electronic health records (EHRs) or electronic documentation system. EHRs have been shown to improve both the quality of client care and the efficiency of the health-care system (U.S. Government Accountability Office, 2010). In 2003, the U.S. Department of Health and Human Services commissioned the Institute of Medicine (IOM) to study the capabilities of an EHR system. The IOM identified a set of eight core functions that EHR systems should perform in the delivery of safer, higher quality, and more efficient health care. These eight core capabilities include the following (Tang, 2003):

■ **Health Information and Data.** EHRs would provide more rapid access to important patient information (e.g., allergies, lab test results, a medication list, demographic information, and clinical narratives) thereby improving care providers' ability to make sound clinical decisions in a timely manner.

■ **Results Management.** Computerized results of all types (e.g., laboratory test results, radiology procedure result reports) can be accessed more easily by the provider at the time and place they are needed.

■ **Order Entry/Order Management.** Computer-based order entries improve workflow processes by eliminating lost orders and ambiguities caused by illegible handwriting, generating related orders automatically, monitoring for duplicate orders, and improving the speed with which orders are executed.

■ **Decision Support.** Computerized decision support systems enhance clinical performance for many aspects of health care. Using reminders and prompts, improvement in regular screenings and other preventive practices can be accomplished. Other aspects of health-care support include identifying possible drug interactions and facilitating diagnosis and treatment.

■ **Electronic Communication and Connectivity.** Improved communication among care associates, such as medicine, nursing, laboratory, pharmacy, and radiology, can enhance client safety and quality of care. Efficient communication among providers improves continuity of care, allows for more timely interventions, and reduces the risk of adverse events.

■ **Patient Support.** Computer-based interactive client education, self-testing, and self-monitoring have been shown to improve control of chronic illnesses.

■ **Administrative Processes.** Electronic scheduling systems (e.g., for hospital admissions and outpatient procedures) increase the efficiency of health-care organizations and provide more timely service to patients.

■ **Reporting and Population Health Management.** Health-care organizations are required to report health-care data to government and private sectors for patient safety and public health. Uniform electronic data standards facilitate this process at the provider level, reduce the associated costs, and increase the speed and accuracy of the data reported.

Table 9-6 lists some of the advantages and disadvantages of paper records and EHRs.

Summary and Key Points

■ The nursing process provides a methodology by which nurses may deliver care using a systematic, scientific approach.

■ The focus of nursing process is goal directed and based on a decision-making or problem-solving model, consisting of six steps: assessment, diagnosis, outcome identification, planning, implementation, and evaluation.

■ Assessment is a systematic, dynamic process by which the nurse, through interaction with the client, significant others, and health-care providers, collects and analyzes data about the client.

■ Nursing diagnoses are clinical judgments about individual, family, or community responses to actual or potential health problems/life processes.

■ Outcomes are measurable, expected, patient-focused goals that translate into observable behaviors.

■ Evaluation is the process of determining both the client's progress toward the attainment of expected outcomes and the effectiveness of nursing care.

TABLE 9–6 Advantages and Disadvantages of Paper Records and EHRs

PAPER*	EHR
ADVANTAGES ■ People know how to use it. ■ It is fast for current practice. ■ It is portable. ■ It is nonbreakable. ■ It accepts multiple data types, such as graphs, photographs, drawings, and text. ■ Legal issues and costs are understood. **DISADVANTAGES** ■ It can be lost. ■ It is often illegible and incomplete. ■ It has no remote access. ■ It can be accessed by only one person at a time. ■ It is often disorganized. ■ Information is duplicated. ■ It is hard to store. ■ It is difficult to research, and continuous quality improvement is laborious. ■ Same client has separate records at each facility (physician's office, hospital, home care). ■ Records are shared only through hard copy	**ADVANTAGES** ■ Can be accessed by multiple providers from remote sites. ■ Facilitates communication between disciplines. ■ Provides reminders about completing information. ■ Provides warnings about incompatibilities of medications or variances from normal standards. ■ Reduces redundancy of information. ■ Requires less storage space and more difficult to lose. ■ Easier to research for audits, quality assurance, and epidemiological surveillance. ■ Provides immediate retrieval of information (e.g., test results). ■ Provides links to multiple databases of health-care knowledge, thus providing diagnostic support. ■ Decreases charting time. ■ Reduces errors due to illegible handwriting. ■ Facilitates billing and claims procedures. **DISADVANTAGES** ■ Excessive expense to initiate the system. ■ Substantial learning curve involved for new users; training and retraining required. ■ Stringent requirements to maintain security and confidentiality. ■ Technical difficulties are possible. ■ Legal and ethical issues involving privacy and access to client information. ■ Requires consistent use of standardized terminology to support information sharing across wide networks.

*From Young, K.M. (2012). Nursing informatics. In J.T. Catalano (Ed.), *Nursing Now! Today's issues, tomorrow's trends* (6th ed.). Philadelphia, PA: F.A. Davis. With permission.

■ The psychiatric nurse uses the nursing process to assist clients to adapt successfully to stressors within the environment.

■ The nurse serves as a valuable member of the interdisciplinary treatment team, working both independently and cooperatively with other team members.

■ Case management is an innovative model of care delivery that serves to provide quality client care while controlling health-care costs. Critical pathways of care (CPCs) serve as the tools for provision of care in a case management system.

■ Nurses may serve as case managers, who are responsible for negotiating with multiple health-care providers to obtain a variety of services for the client.

■ Concept mapping is a diagrammatic teaching and learning strategy that allows students and faculty to visualize interrelationships between medical diagnoses, nursing diagnoses, assessment data, and treatments. The concept map care plan is an innovative approach to planning and organizing nursing care.

■ Nurses must document that the nursing process has been used in the delivery of care. Three methods of documentation that reflect use of the nursing process include POR, Focus Charting, and the PIE method.

■ Many health-care facilities have implemented the use of electronic health records (EHRs) or electronic documentation systems. EHRs have been shown to improve both the quality of client care and the efficiency of the health-care system.

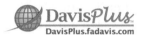 **DavisPlus** Additional info available at
DavisPlus.fadavis.com www.davisplus.com

Review Questions
Self-Examination/Learning Exercise

*Select the answer that is **most** appropriate for each of the following questions.*

1. The nurse is using nursing process to care for a suicidal client. Which of the following nursing actions is a part of the assessment step of the nursing process?
   a. Identifies nursing diagnosis: Risk for suicide.
   b. Notes that client's family reports recent suicide attempt.
   c. Prioritizes the necessity for maintaining a safe environment for the client.
   d. Obtains a short-term contract from the client to seek out staff if feeling suicidal.

2. The nurse is using nursing process to care for a suicidal client. Which of the following nursing actions is a part of the diagnosis step of the nursing process?
   a. Identifies nursing diagnosis: Risk for suicide.
   b. Notes that client's family reports recent suicide attempt.
   c. Prioritizes the necessity for maintaining a safe environment for the client.
   d. Obtains a short-term contract from the client to seek out staff if feeling suicidal.

3. The nurse is using nursing process to care for a suicidal client. Which of the following nursing actions is a part of the outcome identification step of the nursing process?
   a. Prioritizes the necessity for maintaining a safe environment for the client.
   b. Determines if nursing interventions have been appropriate to achieve desired results.
   c. Obtains a short-term contract from the client to seek out staff if feeling suicidal.
   d. Establishes goal of care: Client will not harm self during hospitalization.

4. The nurse is using nursing process to care for a suicidal client. Which of the following nursing actions is a part of the planning step of the nursing process?
   a. Prioritizes the necessity for maintaining a safe environment for the client.
   b. Determines if nursing interventions have been appropriate to achieve desired results.
   c. Obtains a short-term contract from the client to seek out staff if feeling suicidal.
   d. Establishes goal of care: Client will not harm self during hospitalization.

Continued

Review Questions—cont'd
Self-Examination/Learning Exercise

5. The nurse is using nursing process to care for a suicidal client. Which of the following nursing actions is a part of the implementation step of the nursing process?
   a. Prioritizes the necessity for maintaining a safe environment for the client.
   b. Determines if nursing interventions have been appropriate to achieve desired results.
   c. Obtains a short-term contract from the client to seek out staff if feeling suicidal.
   d. Establishes goal of care: Client will not harm self during hospitalization.

6. The nurse is using nursing process to care for a suicidal client. Which of the following nursing actions is a part of the evaluation step of the nursing process?
   a. Prioritizes the necessity for maintaining a safe environment for the client.
   b. Determines if nursing interventions have been appropriate to achieve desired results.
   c. Obtains a short-term contract from the client to seek out staff if feeling suicidal.
   d. Establishes goal of care: Client will not harm self during hospitalization.

7. S.T. is a 15-year-old girl who has just been admitted to the adolescent psychiatric unit with a diagnosis of anorexia nervosa. She is 5 ft. 5 in. tall and weighs 82 lb. She was elected to the cheerleading squad for the fall but states that she is not as good as the others on the squad. The treatment team has identified the following problems: refusal to eat, occasional purging, refusing to interact with staff and peers, and fear of failure. Which of the following nursing diagnoses would be appropriate for S.T.? (Select all that apply.)
   a. Social Isolation
   b. Disturbed Body Image
   c. Low Self-Esteem
   d. Imbalanced Nutrition: Less than body requirements

8. S.T. is a 15-year-old girl who has just been admitted to the adolescent psychiatric unit with a diagnosis of anorexia nervosa. She is 5 ft. 5 in. tall and weighs 82 lb. She was elected to the cheerleading squad for the fall but states that she is not as good as the others on the squad. The treatment team has identified the following problems: refusal to eat, occasional purging, refusing to interact with staff and peers, and fear of failure. Which of the following nursing diagnoses would be the priority diagnosis for S.T.?
   a. Social Isolation
   b. Disturbed Body Image
   c. Low Self-Esteem
   d. Imbalanced Nutrition: Less than body requirements

9. Nursing diagnoses are prioritized according to:
   a. Degree of potential for resolution
   b. Legal implications associated with nursing intervention
   c. Life-threatening potential
   d. Client and family requests

10. Which of the following describe advantages to electronic health records (EHRs)? (Select all that apply.)
   a. They reduce redundancy of information.
   b. They reduce issues regarding privacy.
   c. They decrease charting time.
   d. They facilitate communication between disciplines.

References

American Nurses Association (ANA). (2010a). *Nursing: Scope and standards of practice* (2nd ed.). Silver Spring, MD: ANA.

American Nurses Association. (2010b). *Nursing's social policy statement: The essence of the profession.* Silver Spring, MD: ANA.

American Nurses Association (ANA), American Psychiatric Nurses Association (APNA), & International Society of Psychiatric-Mental Health Nurses (ISPN). (2007). *Psychiatric-mental health nursing: Scope and standards of practice.* Silver Spring, MD: ANA.

Doenges, M.E., Moorhouse, M.F., & Murr, A.C. (2010). *Nursing diagnosis manual: Planning, individualizing, and documenting client care* (3rd ed.). Philadelphia, PA: F.A. Davis.

Folstein, M.F., Folstein, S.E., & McHugh, P.R. (1975). Mini-mental state: A practical method for grading the cognitive state of patients for the clinician. *Journal of Psychiatric Research, 12*(3), 189-198.

Kaufman, D.M., & Zun, L. (1995). A quantifiable, brief mental status examination for emergency patients. *Journal of Emergency Medicine, 13*(4), 440-456.

Kokman, E., Smith, G.E., Petersen, R.C., Tangalos, E., & Ivnik, R.C. (1991). The short test of mental status: Correlations with standardized psychometric testing. *Archives of Neurology, 48*(7), 725-728.

Lampe, S.S. (1985). Focus charting: Streamlining documentation. *Nursing Management, 16*(7), 43-46.

Merck manual of health & aging. (2005). New York, NY: Random House.

Moorhead, S., & Dochterman, J.M. (2012). Languages and development of the linkages. In M. Johnson, S. Moorhead, G. Bulechek, M. Butcher, M. Maas, & E. Swanson (Eds.), *NOC and NIC linkages to NANDA-I and clinical conditions: Supporting critical reasoning and quality care* (3rd ed., pp. 1–10). Maryland Heights, MO: Mosby.

Moorhead, S., Johnson, M., Maas, M., & Swanson, E. (2013). *Nursing outcomes classification (NOC)* (5th ed.). St. Louis, MO: Mosby Elsevier.

NANDA International. (2012). *Nursing diagnoses: Definitions and classification, 2012-2014.* Hoboken, NJ: Wiley-Blackwell.

NANDA International. (2013). *About NANDA international.* Retrieved from http://www.nanda.org/AboutUs.aspx

Pfeiffer, E. (1975). A short portable mental status questionnaire for the assessment of organic brain deficit in elderly patients. *Journal of the American Geriatric Society, 23*(10), 433-441.

Schuster, P.M. (2012). *Concept mapping: A critical-thinking approach to care planning* (3rd ed.). Philadelphia, PA: F.A. Davis.

Tang, P. (2003). *Key capabilities of an electronic health record system.* Institute of Medicine Committee on Data Standards for Patient Safety. Board on Health Care Services. Washington, DC: National Academies Press.

U.S. Government Accountability Office. (2010). *Features of integrated systems support patient care strategies and access to care, but systems face challenges.* Washington, DC: U.S. Government Accountability Office.

Young, K.M. (2012). Nursing informatics. In J.T. Catalano (Ed.), *Nursing now! Today's issues, tomorrow's trends* (6th ed., pp. 366–385). Philadelphia, PA: F.A. Davis.

10 Therapeutic Groups

CORE CONCEPTS

group

group therapy

KEY TERMS

altruism

autocratic

catharsis

democratic

laissez-faire

psychodrama

universality

OBJECTIVES
After reading this chapter, the student will be able to:

1. Define a *group*.
2. Discuss eight functions of a group.
3. Identify various types of groups.
4. Describe physical conditions that influence groups.
5. Discuss "curative factors" that occur in groups.
6. Describe the phases of group development.
7. Identify various leadership styles in groups.
8. Identify various roles that members assume within a group.
9. Discuss psychodrama as a specialized form of group therapy.
10. Describe the role of the nurse in group therapy.

HOMEWORK ASSIGNMENT
Please read the chapter and answer the following questions:

1. What is the difference between therapeutic groups and group therapy?
2. What are the expectations of the leader in the initial or orientation phase of group development?
3. How does an autocratic leadership style affect member enthusiasm and morale?
4. How does size of the group influence group dynamics?

Human beings are complex creatures who share their activities of daily living with various *groups* of people. Sampson and Marthas (1990) have stated:

> We are *biological* organisms possessing qualities shared with all living systems and with others of our species. We are *psychological* beings with distinctly human capabilities for thought, feeling, and action. We are also *social* beings, who function as part of the complex webs that link us with other people. (p. 3)

Health-care professionals not only share their personal lives with groups of people but also encounter multiple group situations in their professional operations. Team conferences, committee meetings, grand rounds, and in-service sessions are but a few.

In psychiatry, work with clients and families often takes the form of groups. With group work, not only does the nurse have the opportunity to reach out to a greater number of people at one time, but those individuals also assist each other by bringing to the group and sharing their feelings, opinions, ideas, and behaviors. Clients learn from each other in a group setting.

This chapter explores various types and methods of therapeutic groups that can be used with psychiatric clients, and the role of the nurse in group intervention.

CORE CONCEPT
Group
A *group* is a collection of individuals whose association is founded on shared commonalities of interest, values, norms, or purpose. Membership in a group is generally by chance (born into the group), by choice (voluntary affiliation), or by circumstance (the result of life-cycle events over which an individual may or may not have control).

Functions of a Group

Sampson and Marthas (1990) outlined eight functions that groups serve for their members. They contend that groups may serve more than one function and usually serve different functions for different members of the group. The eight functions are as follows:

1. **Socialization.** The cultural group into which we are born begins the process of teaching social norms. This is continued throughout our lives by members of other groups with which we become affiliated.
2. **Support.** One's fellow group members are available in time of need. Individuals derive a feeling of security from group involvement.
3. **Task completion.** Group members provide assistance in endeavors that are beyond the capacity of one individual alone or when results can be achieved more effectively as a team.
4. **Camaraderie.** Members of a group provide the joy and pleasure that individuals seek from interactions with significant others.
5. **Informational.** Learning takes place within groups. Knowledge is gained when individual members learn how others in the group have resolved situations similar to those with which they are currently struggling.
6. **Normative.** This function relates to the ways in which groups enforce the established norms.

7. **Empowerment.** Groups help to bring about improvement in existing conditions by providing support to individual members who seek to bring about change. Groups have power that individuals alone do not.
8. **Governance.** An example of the governing function is that of rules being made by committees within a larger organization.

Types of Groups

The functions of a group vary depending on the reason the group was formed. Clark (2003) identified three types of groups in which nurses most often participate: task, teaching, and supportive/therapeutic groups.

Task Groups

The function of a task group is to accomplish a specific outcome or task. The focus is on solving problems and making decisions to achieve this outcome. Often a deadline is placed on completion of the task, and such importance is placed on a satisfactory outcome that conflict in the group may be smoothed over or ignored in order to focus on the priority at hand.

Teaching Groups

Teaching, or educational, groups exist to convey knowledge and information to a number of individuals. Nurses can be involved in teaching groups of many varieties, such as medication education, childbirth education, breast self-examination, and effective parenting classes. These groups usually have a set time frame or a set number of meetings. Members learn from each other as well as from the designated instructor. The objective of teaching groups is verbalization or demonstration by the learner of the material presented by the end of the designated period.

Supportive/Therapeutic Groups

The primary concern of support groups is to prevent future upsets by teaching participants effective ways of dealing with emotional stress arising from situational or developmental crises.

CORE CONCEPT
Group Therapy
A form of psychosocial treatment in which a number of clients meet together with a therapist for purposes of sharing, gaining personal insight, and improving interpersonal coping strategies.

For the purposes of this text, it is important to differentiate between *therapeutic groups* and *group therapy*. Leaders of group therapy generally have advanced degrees in psychology, social work, nursing, or medicine. They often have additional training or experience under the supervision of an accomplished professional in conducting group psychotherapy based on various theoretical frameworks such as psychoanalytic, psychodynamic, interpersonal, or family dynamics. Approaches based on these theories are used by the group therapy leaders to encourage improvement in the ability of group members to function on an interpersonal level.

Therapeutic groups, on the other hand, are based to a lesser degree in theory. Focus is more on group relations, interactions among group members, and the consideration of a selected issue. Like group therapists, individuals who lead therapeutic groups must be knowledgeable in *group process*, that is, the *way* in which group members interact with each other. Interruptions, silences, judgments, glares, and scapegoating are examples of group processes (Clark, 2003). They must also have thorough knowledge of *group content*, the topic or issue being discussed within the group, and the ability to present the topic in language that can be understood by all group members. Many nurses who work in psychiatry lead supportive/ therapeutic groups.

Self-Help Groups

An additional type of group, in which nurses may or may not be involved, is the self-help group. Self-help groups have grown in numbers and in credibility in recent years. They allow clients to talk about their fears and relieve feelings of isolation, while receiving comfort and advice from others undergoing similar experiences. Examples of self-help groups are Alzheimer's Disease and Related Disorders, Anorexia Nervosa and Associated Disorders, Weight Watchers, Alcoholics Anonymous, Reach to Recovery, Parents Without Partners, Overeaters Anonymous, Adult Children of Alcoholics, and many others related to specific needs or illnesses. These groups may or may not have a professional leader or consultant. They are run by the members, and leadership often rotates from member to member.

Nurses may become involved with self-help groups either voluntarily or because their advice or participation has been requested by the members. The nurse may function as a referral agent, resource person, member of an advisory board, or leader of the group. Self-help groups are a valuable source of referral for clients with specific problems. However, nurses must be knowledgeable about the purposes of the group, membership, leadership, benefits, and problems that might threaten the success of the group before making referrals to their clients for a specific self-help group. The nurse may find it necessary to attend several meetings of a particular group, if possible, to assess its effectiveness of purpose and appropriateness for client referral.

Physical Conditions That Influence Group Dynamics

Seating

The physical conditions for the group should be set up so that there is no barrier between the members. For example, a circle of chairs is better than chairs set around a table. Members should be encouraged to sit in different chairs each meeting. This openness and change creates a feeling of discomfort that encourages anxious and unsettled behaviors that can then be explored within the group.

Size

Various authors have suggested different ranges of size as ideal for group interaction: 5 to 10 (Yalom & Leszcz, 2005), 2 to 15 (Sampson & Marthas, 1990), and 4 to 12 (Clark, 2003). Group size does make a difference in the interaction among members. The larger the group, the less time is available to devote to individual members. In fact, in larger groups, those more aggressive individuals are most likely to be heard, whereas quieter members may be left out of the discussions altogether. On the other hand, larger groups provide more opportunities for individuals to learn from other members. The wider range of life experiences and knowledge provides a greater potential for effective group problem solving. Studies have indicated that a composition of 7 or 8 members provides a favorable climate for optimal group interaction and relationship development.

Membership

Whether the group is open or closed ended is another condition that influences the dynamics of group process. Open-ended groups are those in which members leave and others join at any time while the group is active. The continuous movement of members in and out of the group creates the type of discomfort described previously that encourages unsettled behaviors in individual members and fosters the exploration of feelings. These are the most common types of groups held on short-term inpatient units, although they are used in outpatient and long-term care facilities as well. Closed-ended groups usually have a predetermined, fixed time frame. All members join at the time the group is organized and terminate at the end of the designated time period. Closed-ended groups are often composed of individuals with common issues or problems they wish to address.

Curative Factors

Why are therapeutic groups helpful? Yalom and Leszcz (2005) have described 11 curative factors that individuals can achieve through interpersonal interactions within the group, some of which are present in most groups in varying degrees:

1. **The Instillation of Hope.** By observing the progress of others in the group with similar problems, a group member garners hope that his or her problems can also be resolved.
2. **Universality.** Through **universality**, individuals come to realize that they are not alone in the problems, thoughts, and feelings they are experiencing. Anxiety is relieved by the support and understanding of others in the group who share similar (universal) experiences.
3. **The Imparting of Information.** Knowledge is gained through formal instruction as well as the sharing of advice and suggestions among group members.
4. **Altruism. Altruism** is assimilated by group members through mutual sharing and concern for each other. Providing assistance and support to others creates a positive self-image and promotes self-growth.
5. **The Corrective Recapitulation of the Primary Family Group.** Group members are able to re-experience early family conflicts that remain unresolved. Attempts at resolution are promoted through feedback and exploration.
6. **The Development of Socializing Techniques.** Through interaction with and feedback from other members within the group, individuals are able to correct maladaptive social behaviors and learn and develop new social skills.
7. **Imitative Behavior.** In this setting, one who has mastered a particular psychosocial skill or developmental task can be a valuable role model for others. Individuals may imitate selected behaviors that they wish to develop in themselves.
8. **Interpersonal Learning.** The group offers many and varied opportunities for interacting with other people. Insight is gained regarding how one perceives and is being perceived by others.
9. **Group Cohesiveness.** Members develop a sense of belonging that separates the individual ("I am") from the group ("we are"). Out of this alliance emerges a common feeling that both individual members and the total group are of value to each other.
10. **Catharsis.** Within the group, members are able to express both positive and negative feelings—perhaps feelings that have never been expressed before—in a nonthreatening atmosphere. This **catharsis**, or open expression of feelings, is beneficial for the individual within the group.
11. **Existential Factors.** The group is able to help individual members take direction of their own lives and to accept responsibility for the quality of their existence.

It may be helpful for a group leader to explain these curative factors to members of the group. Positive responses are experienced by individuals who understand and are able to recognize curative factors as they occur within the group.

Phases of Group Development

Groups, like individuals, move through phases of life-cycle development. Ideally, groups will progress from the phase of infancy to advanced maturity in an effort to fulfill the objectives set forth by the membership. Unfortunately, as with individuals, some groups become fixed in early developmental levels and never progress, or experience periods of regression in the developmental process. Three phases of group development are discussed here.

Phase I: Initial or Orientation Phase
Group Activities

Leader and members work together to establish the rules that will govern the group (e.g., when and where meetings will occur, the importance of confidentiality, how meetings will be structured). Goals of the group are established. Members are introduced to each other.

Leader Expectations

The leader is expected to orient members to specific group processes, encourage members to participate without disclosing too much too soon, promote an environment of trust, and ensure that rules established by the group do not interfere with fulfillment of the goals.

Member Behaviors

In phase I, members have not yet established trust and will respond to this lack of trust by being overly polite. There is a fear of not being accepted by the group. They may try to "get on the good side" of the leader with compliments and conforming behaviors. A power struggle may ensue as members compete for their position in the "pecking order" of the group.

Phase II: Middle or Working Phase

Group Activities

Ideally, during the working phase, cohesiveness has been established within the group. This is when the productive work toward completion of the task is undertaken. Problem solving and decision making occur within the group. In the mature group, cooperation prevails, and differences and disagreements are confronted and resolved.

Leader Expectations

The role of leader diminishes and becomes more one of facilitator during the working phase. Some leadership functions are shared by certain members of the group as they progress toward resolution. The leader helps to resolve conflict and continues to foster cohesiveness among the members while ensuring that they do not deviate from the intended task or purpose for which the group was organized.

Member Behaviors

At this point trust has been established among the members. They turn more often to each other and less often to the leader for guidance. They accept criticism from each other, using it in a constructive manner to create change. Occasionally, subgroups will form in which two or more members conspire with each other to the exclusion of the rest of the group. To maintain group cohesion, these subgroups must be confronted and discussed by the entire membership. Conflict is managed by the group with minimal assistance from the leader.

Phase III: Final or Termination Phase

Group Activities

The longer a group has been in existence, the more difficult termination is likely to be for the members. Termination should be mentioned from the outset of group formation. It should be discussed in depth for several meetings prior to the final session. A sense of loss that precipitates the grief process may be in evidence, particularly in groups that have been successful in their stated purpose.

Leader Expectations

In the termination phase, the leader encourages the group members to reminisce about what has occurred within the group, to review the goals and discuss the actual outcomes, and to encourage members to provide feedback to each other about individual progress within the group. The leader encourages members to discuss feelings of loss associated with termination of the group.

Member Behaviors

Members may express surprise over the actual materialization of the end. This represents the grief response of denial, which may then progress to anger. Anger toward other group members or toward the leader may reflect feelings of abandonment (Sampson & Marthas, 1990). These feelings may lead to individual members' discussions of previous losses for which similar emotions were experienced. Successful termination of the group may help members develop the skills needed when losses occur in other dimensions of their lives.

Leadership Styles

Lippitt and White (1958) identified three of the most common group leadership styles: autocratic, democratic, and laissez-faire. Table 10-1 shows an outline of various similarities and differences among the three leadership styles.

Autocratic

Autocratic leaders have personal goals for the group. They withhold information from group members, particularly issues that may interfere with achievement of their own objectives. The message that is conveyed to the group is: "We will do it my way. My way is best." The focus in this style of leadership is on the leader. Members are dependent on the leader for problem solving, decision making, and permission to perform. The approach of the autocratic leader is one of persuasion, striving to persuade others in the group that his or her ideas and methods are superior. Productivity is high with this type of leadership, but often morale within the group is low because of lack of member input and creativity.

Democratic

The **democratic** leadership style focuses on the members of the group. Information is shared with members in an effort to allow them to make decisions regarding achieving the goals for the group. Members are encouraged to participate fully in problem solving of issues that relate to the group, including taking action to effect change. The message that is conveyed to the group is: "Decide what must be done, consider the alternatives, make a selection, and proceed with the actions required to complete the task." The leader provides guidance and expertise as needed. Productivity is lower than it is with autocratic leadership, but morale is much higher because of the extent of input allowed all members of the group and the potential for individual creativity.

TABLE 10–1	**Leadership Styles–Similarities and Differences**		
CHARACTERISTICS	AUTOCRATIC	DEMOCRATIC	LAISSEZ-FAIRE
1. Focus	Leader	Members	Undetermined
2. Task strategy	Members are persuaded to adopt leader ideas	Members engage in group problem solving	No defined strategy exists
3. Member participation	Limited	Unlimited	Inconsistent
4. Individual creativity	Stifled	Encouraged	Not addressed
5. Member enthusiasm and morale	Low	High	Low
6. Group cohesiveness	Low	High	Low
7. Productivity	High	High (may not be as high as autocratic)	Low
8. Individual motivation and commitment	Low (tend to work only when leader is present to urge them to do so)	High (satisfaction derived from personal input and participation)	Low (feelings of frustration from lack of direction or guidance)

Laissez-Faire

This leadership style allows people to do as they please. There is no direction from the leader. In fact, the **laissez-faire** leader's approach is noninvolvement. Goals for the group are undefined. No decisions are made, no problems are solved, and no action is taken. Members become frustrated and confused, and productivity and morale are low.

Member Roles

Benne and Sheats (1948) identified three major types of roles that individuals play within the membership of the group. These are roles that serve to:

1. Complete the task of the group.
2. Maintain or enhance group processes.
3. Fulfill personal or individual needs.

Task roles and maintenance roles contribute to the success or effectiveness of the group. Personal roles satisfy needs of the individual members, sometimes to the extent of interfering with the effectiveness of the group.

Table 10-2 presents an outline of specific roles within these three major types and the behaviors associated with each.

Psychodrama

A specialized type of therapeutic group, called **psychodrama**, was introduced by J. L. Moreno, a Viennese psychiatrist. Moreno's method employs a dramatic approach in which clients become "actors" in life-situation scenarios.

The group leader is called the *director*, group members are the *audience*, and the *set*, or *stage*, may be specially designed or may just be any room or part of a room selected for this purpose. Actors are members from the audience who agree to take part in the "drama" by role-playing a situation about which they have been informed by the director. Usually the situation is an issue with which one individual client has been struggling. The client plays the role of himself or herself and is called the *protagonist*. In this role, the client is able to express true feelings toward individuals (represented by group members) with whom he or she has unresolved conflicts.

In some instances, the group leader may ask for a client to volunteer to be the protagonist for that session. The client may choose a situation he or she wishes to enact and select the audience members to portray the roles of others in the life situation. The psychodrama setting provides the client with a safer and less threatening atmosphere than the real situation in which to express true feelings. Resolution of interpersonal conflicts is facilitated.

When the drama has been completed, group members from the audience discuss the situation they have observed, offer feedback, express their feelings, and relate their own similar experiences. In this way, all group members benefit from the session, either directly or indirectly.

Nurses often serve as actors, or role players, in psychodrama sessions. Leaders of psychodrama have

TABLE 10–2 Member Roles Within Groups

ROLE	BEHAVIORS
TASK ROLES	
Coordinator	Clarifies ideas and suggestions that have been made within the group; brings relationships together to pursue common goals
Evaluator	Examines group plans and performance, measuring against group standards and goals
Elaborator	Explains and expands upon group plans and ideas
Energizer	Encourages and motivates group to perform at its maximum potential
Initiator	Outlines the task at hand for the group and proposes methods for solution
Orienter	Maintains direction within the group
MAINTENANCE ROLES	
Compromiser	Relieves conflict within the group by assisting members to reach a compromise agreeable to all
Encourager	Offers recognition and acceptance of others' ideas and contributions
Follower	Listens attentively to group interaction; is a passive participant
Gatekeeper	Encourages acceptance of and participation by all members of the group
Harmonizer	Minimizes tension within the group by intervening when disagreements produce conflict
INDIVIDUAL (PERSONAL) ROLES	
Aggressor	Expresses negativism and hostility toward other members; may use sarcasm in effort to degrade the status of others
Blocker	Resists group efforts; demonstrates rigid and sometimes irrational behaviors that impede group progress
Dominator	Manipulates others to gain control; behaves in authoritarian manner
Help-seeker	Uses the group to gain sympathy from others; seeks to increase self-confidence from group feedback; lacks concern for others or for the group as a whole
Monopolizer	Maintains control of the group by dominating the conversation
Mute or silent member	Does not participate verbally; remains silent for a variety of reasons—may feel uncomfortable with self-disclosure or may be seeking attention through silence
Recognition seeker	Talks about personal accomplishments in an effort to gain attention for self
Seducer	Shares intimate details about self with group; is the least reluctant of the group to do so; may frighten others in the group and inhibit group progress with excessive premature self-disclosure

SOURCES: Benne & Sheats, 1948; Hobbs & Powers, 1981; Larson & Williams, 1978.

graduate degrees in psychology, social work, nursing, or medicine with additional training in group therapy and specialty preparation to become a psychodramatist.

The Role of the Nurse in Group Therapy

Nurses participate in group situations on a daily basis. In health-care settings, nurses serve on or lead task groups that create policy, describe procedures, and plan client care. They are also involved in a variety of other groups aimed at the institutional effort of serving the consumer. Nurses are encouraged to use the steps of the nursing process as a framework for task group leadership.

In psychiatry, nurses may lead various types of therapeutic groups, such as client education, assertiveness training, support, parent, and transition to discharge groups, among others. To function effectively in the leadership capacity for these groups, nurses need to be able to recognize various processes that occur in groups, such as the phases of group development, the various roles that people play within group situations, and the motivation behind the behavior. They also need to be able to select the most appropriate leadership style for the type of group being led. Generalist nurses may develop these skills as part of their undergraduate education, or they may pursue additional study while serving and learning as the co-leader of a group with a more experienced nurse leader.

Generalist nurses in psychiatry rarely serve as leaders of psychotherapy groups. The *Psychiatric-Mental Health Nursing Scope and Standards of Practice* (American Nurses Association, 2007) specifies that nurses who serve as group psychotherapists should have a minimum of a master's degree in psychiatric nursing. Other criteria that have been suggested are educational preparation in group theory, extended practice as a group co-leader or leader under the supervision of an experienced psychotherapist, and participation in group therapy on an experiential level. Additional specialist training is required beyond the master's level to prepare nurses to become family therapists or psychodramatists.

Leading therapeutic groups is within the realm of nursing practice. Because group work is such a common therapeutic approach in the discipline of psychiatry, nurses working in this field must continually strive to expand their knowledge and use of group process as a significant psychiatric nursing intervention.

> **CLINICAL PEARL** Knowledge of human behavior in general and the group process in particular is essential to effective group leadership.

Summary and Key Points

- A group has been defined as a collection of individuals whose association is founded on shared commonalities of interest, values, norms, or purpose.
- Eight group functions have been identified: socialization, support, task completion, camaraderie, informational, normative, empowerment, and governance.
- There are three major types of groups: task groups, teaching groups, and supportive/therapeutic groups.
- The function of task groups is to solve problems, make decisions, and achieve a specific outcome.

- In teaching groups, knowledge and information are conveyed to a number of individuals.
- The function of supportive/therapeutic groups is to educate people to deal effectively with emotional stress in their lives.
- In self-help groups, individuals share a common problem. Members of the group provide each other with mutual support as they deal with, or possibly try to recover from, the problem.
- Therapeutic groups differ from group therapy in that group therapy is more theory based and the leaders generally have advanced degrees in psychology, social work, nursing, or medicine.
- Placement of the seating and size of the group can influence group interaction.
- Groups can be open-ended (when members leave and others join at any time while the group is active) or closed-ended (when groups have a predetermined, fixed time frame and all members join at the same time and leave when the group disbands).
- Yalom and Leszcz (2005) describe the following curative factors that individuals derive from participation in therapeutic groups: the instillation of hope, universality, the imparting of information, altruism, the corrective recapitulation of the primary family group, the development of socializing techniques, imitative behavior, interpersonal learning, group cohesiveness, catharsis, and existential factors.
- Groups progress through three phases: the initial (orientation) phase, the working phase, and the termination phase.
- Group leadership styles include autocratic, democratic, and laissez-faire.
- Members play various roles within groups. These roles are categorized according to task roles, maintenance roles, and personal roles.
- Psychodrama is a specialized type of group therapy that uses a dramatic approach in which clients become "actors" in life-situation scenarios.
- The psychodrama setting provides the client with a safer and less threatening atmosphere than the real situation in which to express and work through unresolved conflicts.
- Nurses lead various types of therapeutic groups in the psychiatric setting. Knowledge of human behavior in general and the group process in particular is essential to effective group leadership.
- Specialized training, in addition to a master's degree, is required for nurses to serve as group psychotherapists or psychodramatists.

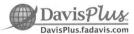 Additional info available at
DavisPlus.fadavis.com   www.davisplus.com

Review Questions
Self-Examination/Learning Exercise

*Select the answer that is **most** appropriate for each of the following questions.*

1. N.J. is the nurse leader of a childbirth preparation group. Each week she shows various films and sets out various reading materials. She expects the participants to utilize their time on a topic of their choice or practice skills they have observed on the films. Two couples have dropped out of the group, stating, "This is a big waste of time." Which type of group and style of leadership is described in this situation?
   a. Task/democratic
   b. Teaching/laissez-faire
   c. Self-help/democratic
   d. Supportive-therapeutic/autocratic

2. M.K. is a psychiatric nurse who has been selected to lead a group for women who desire to lose weight. The criterion for membership is that they must be at least 20 lb. overweight. All have tried to lose weight on their own many times in the past without success. At their first meeting, M.K. provides suggestions as the members determine what their goals will be and how they plan to go about achieving those goals. They decided how often they wanted to meet, and what they planned to do at each meeting. Which type of group and style of leadership is described in this situation?
   a. Task/autocratic
   b. Teaching/democratic
   c. Self-help/laissez-faire
   d. Supportive-therapeutic/democratic

3. J.J. is a staff nurse on a surgical unit. He has been selected as leader of a newly established group of staff nurses organized to determine ways to decrease the number of medication errors occurring on the unit. J.J. has definite ideas about how to bring this about. He has also applied for the position of Head Nurse on the unit and believes that if he is successful in leading the group toward achievement of its goals, he can also facilitate his chances for promotion. At each meeting he addresses the group in an effort to convince the members to adopt his ideas. Which type of group and style of leadership is described in this situation?
   a. Task/autocratic
   b. Teaching/autocratic
   c. Self-help/democratic
   d. Supportive-therapeutic/laissez-faire

4. The nurse leader is explaining about group "curative factors" to members of the group. She tells the group that group situations are beneficial because members can see that they are not alone in their experiences. This is an example of which curative factor?
   a. Altruism
   b. Imitative behavior
   c. Universality
   d. Imparting of information

5. Nurse Jones is the leader of a bereavement group for widows. Nancy is a new member. She listens to the group and sees that one member, Jane, has been a widow for 5 years now. Jane has adjusted well and Nancy thinks maybe she can too. This is an example of which curative factor?
   a. Universality
   b. Imitative behavior
   c. Installation of hope
   d. Imparting of information

Review Questions—cont'd
Self-Examination/Learning Exercise

6. Paul is a member of an anger management group. He knew that people did not want to be his friend because of his violent temper. In the group, he has learned to control his temper and form satisfactory interpersonal relationships with others. This is an example of which curative factor?
   a. Catharsis
   b. Altruism
   c. Imparting of information
   d. Development of socializing techniques

7. Henry is a member of an Alcoholics Anonymous group. He learned about the effects of alcohol on the body when a nurse from the chemical dependency unit spoke to the group. This is an example of which curative factor?
   a. Catharsis
   b. Altruism
   c. Imparting of information
   d. Universality

8. Sandra is the nurse leader of a supportive-therapeutic group for individuals with anxiety disorders. In this group, Helen talks incessantly. When someone else tries to make a comment, she refuses to allow him or her to speak. What type of member role is Helen assuming in this group?
   a. Aggressor
   b. Monopolizer
   c. Blocker
   d. Seducer

9. Sandra is the nurse leader of a supportive-therapeutic group for individuals with anxiety disorders. On the first day the group meets, Valerie speaks first and begins by sharing the intimate details of her incestuous relationship with her father. What type of member role is Valerie assuming in this group?
   a. Aggressor
   b. Monopolizer
   c. Blocker
   d. Seducer

10. Sandra is the nurse leader of a supportive-therapeutic group for individuals with anxiety disorders. Violet, who is beautiful but lacks self-confidence, states to the group, "Maybe if I became a blond my boyfriend would love me more." Larry responds, "Listen, dummy, you need more than blond hair to keep the guy around. A bit more in the brains department would help!" What type of member role is Larry assuming in this group?
   a. Aggressor
   b. Monopolizer
   c. Blocker
   d. Seducer

References

American Nurses Association (ANA). (2007). *Psychiatric-Mental Health Nursing: Scope and Standards of Practice.* Silver Spring, MD: ANA.

Clark, C.C. (2003). *Group leadership skills* (4th ed.). New York, NY: Springer.

Sampson, E.E., & Marthas, M. (1990). *Group process for the health professions* (3rd ed.). Albany, NY: Delmar Publishers.

Yalom, I.D., & Leszcz, M. (2005). *The theory and practice of group psychotherapy* (5th ed.). New York, NY: Basic Books.

Classical References

Benne, K.D., & Sheats, P. (1948, Spring). Functional roles of group members. *Journal of Social Issues, 4*(2), 41–49.

Hobbs, D.J., & Powers, R.C. (1981). *Group member roles: For group effectiveness.* Ames, IA: Iowa State University, Cooperative Extension Service.

Larson, M.L., & Williams, R.A. (1978). How to become a better group leader? *Nursing, 78*(August), 65–72.

Lippitt, R., & White, R.K. (1958). An experimental study of leadership and group life. In E.E. Maccoby, T.M. Newcomb, & E.L. Hartley (Eds.), *Readings in social psychology* (3rd ed.). New York, NY: Holt, Rinehart, & Winston.

11 Intervention With Families

OBJECTIVES

After reading this chapter, the student will be able to:

1. Define the term *family*.
2. Identify stages of family development.
3. Describe major variations to the American middle-class family life cycle.
4. Discuss characteristics of adaptive family functioning.
5. Describe behaviors that interfere with adaptive family functioning.
6. Discuss the essential components of family systems, structural, and strategic therapies.
7. Construct a family genogram.
8. Apply the steps of the nursing process in therapeutic intervention with families.

HOMEWORK ASSIGNMENT

Please read the chapter and answer the following questions:

1. Describe the concept of "reframing."
2. Describe the process of triangulation in a dysfunctional family pattern.
3. How are genograms helpful in family therapy?
4. What behaviors are indicative of a positive family climate?

What is a family? Wright and Leahey (2013) propose the following definition: a family is who they say they are. Many family forms exist within society today, such as the biological family of procreation, the nuclear family that incorporates one or more members of the extended family (family of origin), the sole-parent family, the stepfamily, the communal family, and the homosexual couple or family. Labeling individuals as "families" based on their group composition may not be the best way, however. Instead, family consideration may be more appropriately determined based on attributes of affection, strong emotional ties, a sense of belonging, and durability of membership (Wright & Leahey, 2013).

Many nurses have interactions with family members on a daily basis. A client's illness or hospitalization affects all members of the family, and nurses must understand how to work with the family as a unit, knowing that family members can have a profound effect on the client's healing process.

Nurse generalists should be familiar with the tasks associated with adaptive family functioning. With this knowledge, they are able to assess family interaction and recognize problems when they arise. They can provide support to families with an ill member and make referrals to other professionals when assistance is required to restore adaptive functioning.

Nurse specialists usually possess an advanced degree in nursing. Some nurse specialists have education or experience that qualifies them to perform family therapy. Family therapy is broadly defined as "a form of intervention in which members of a family are assisted in identifying and changing problematic, maladaptive, repetitive relationship patterns, as well as self-defeating or self-limiting belief systems" (Goldenberg, Goldenberg, & Pelavin, 2011, p. 417). Family therapy has a strong theoretical focus, and a number of conceptual approaches have been introduced and suggested as frameworks for this intervention.

This chapter explores the stages of family development and compares the "typical" family within various subcultures. Characteristics of adaptive family functioning and behaviors that interfere with this adaptation are discussed. Theoretical components of selected therapeutic approaches are described. Instructions for construction of a family genogram are included. Nursing process provides the framework for nursing intervention with families.

CORE CONCEPTS

Family

Two or more individuals who depend on one another for emotional, physical, and economical support. The members of the family are self-defined (Kaakinen, Hanson, & Denham, 2010, p. 5).

Stages of Family Development

McGoldrick, Carter, and Garcia-Preto (2011) identified stages and developmental tasks that describe the family life cycle. It is acknowledged that these tasks would vary greatly among diverse cultural groups, as well as the various forms of families previously described. These stages, however, provide a valuable framework from which the nurse may study families, emphasizing expansion (the addition of members), contraction (the loss of members), and realignment of relationships as members experience developmental changes. These stages of family development are described in the following paragraphs, and are summarized in Table 11-1.

The Single Young Adult

This model begins with the launching of the young adult from the family of origin. This is a difficult stage because young adults must decide what social standards from the family of origin will be preserved and what they will change for themselves to be incorporated into a new family. Tasks of this stage include forming an identity separate from the parents, establishing intimate peer relationships, and advancing

TABLE 11–1	**Stages of the Family Life Cycle**	
FAMILY LIFE-CYCLE STAGES	**EMOTIONAL PROCESS OF TRANSITION: KEY PRINCIPLES**	**CHANGES REQUIRED IN FAMILY STATUS TO PROCEED DEVELOPMENTALLY**
The Single Young Adult	Accepting separation from parents and emotional and financial responsibility for self	■ Differentiation of self in relation to family of origin ■ Development of intimate peer relationships ■ Establishment of self in respect to work and financial independence ■ Establishment of self in community and larger society
The Family Joined Through Marriage/ Union	Commitment to new system	■ Formation of partner systems ■ Realignment of relationships with extended family, friends, and larger community and social system to include new partners
The Family With Young Children	Accepting new members into the system	■ Adjustment of couple system to make space for children ■ Collaboration in child rearing, financial and housekeeping tasks ■ Realignment of relationships with extended family to include parenting and grandparenting roles ■ Realignment of relationships with community and larger social system to include new family structure and relationships

Continued

TABLE 11–1 Stages of the Family Life Cycle—cont'd

FAMILY LIFE-CYCLE STAGES	EMOTIONAL PROCESS OF TRANSITION: KEY PRINCIPLES	CHANGES REQUIRED IN FAMILY STATUS TO PROCEED DEVELOPMENTALLY
The Family With Adolescents	Increasing flexibility of family boundaries to permit children's independence and grandparents' frailties	■ Shifting of parent/child relationships to permit adolescents to move in and out of system ■ Refocus on midlife couple and career issues ■ Beginning shift toward caring for older generation ■ Realignment with community and larger social system to include shifting family of emerging adolescent and parents in new formation patterns of relating
The Family Launching Children and Moving On in Midlife	Accepting a multitude of exits from and entries into the family system	■ Renegotiation of couple system as a dyad ■ Development of adult-to-adult relationships between parents and grown children ■ Realignment of relationships to include in-laws and grandchildren ■ Realignment of relationships with community and larger social system to include new structure and constellation of family relationships ■ Exploration of new interests/career given the freedom from child-care responsibilities ■ Dealing with care needs, disabilities and death of parents (grandparents)
The Family in Later Life (late middle age to end of life)	■ Accepting the shifting of generational roles ■ Accepting the realities of limitations and death	■ Maintaining own and/or couple functioning and interests in face of physiological decline; exploration of new familial and social role options ■ Supporting more central role of middle generations ■ Realignment of the system in relation to community and larger social system to acknowledge changed pattern of family relationships of this stage ■ Making room in the system for the wisdom and experience of the elders; supporting the older generation without overfunctioning for them ■ Dealing with loss of spouse, siblings, and other peers, and preparation for own death; life review and integration ■ Managing reversed roles in caretaking between middle and older generations

Adapted from McGoldrick, M., Carter, B., & Garcia-Preto, N. (2011). Overview: The life cycle in its changing context. In M. McGoldrick, B. Carter, & N. Garcia-Preto (Eds.), *The expanded family life cycle* (4th ed., pp. 1-19). Boston, MA: Allyn & Bacon. Reprinted by permission.

toward financial independence. Problems can arise when either the young adults or the parents encounter difficulty terminating the interdependent relationship that has existed in the family of origin.

The Family Joined Through Marriage/Union

Uniting as a couple is a difficult transition because renegotiation must include the integration of contrasting issues that each partner brings to the relationship and issues they may have redefined for themselves as a couple. In addition, the new couple must renegotiate relationships with parents, siblings, and other relatives in view of the new partnership. Tasks of this stage include establishing a new identity as a couple, realigning relationships with members of extended

family, and making decisions about having children. Problems can arise if either partner remains too enmeshed with their family of origin or when the couple chooses to cut themselves off completely from extended family.

The Family With Young Children

Adjustments in relationships must occur with the arrival of children. The entire family system is affected and role realignments are necessary for both new parents and new grandparents. Tasks of this stage include making adjustments within the marital system to meet the responsibilities associated with parenthood while maintaining the integrity of the couple relationship, sharing equally in the tasks of child rearing, and integrating the roles of extended family members into the newly expanded family organization. Problems can arise when parents lack knowledge about normal childhood development and adequate patience to allow children to express themselves through behavior.

The Family With Adolescents

This stage of family development is characterized by a great deal of turmoil and transition. Parents are approaching a midlife stage and adolescents are undergoing biological, emotional, and sociocultural changes that place demands on each individual and on the family unit. Grandparents, too, may require assistance with the tasks of later life. These developments can create a "sandwich" effect for the parents, who must deal with issues confronting three generations. Tasks of this stage include redefining the level of dependence so that adolescents are provided with greater autonomy while parents remain responsive to the teenager's dependency needs. Midlife issues related to marriage, career, and aging parents must also be resolved during this period. Problems can arise when parents are unable to relinquish control and allow the adolescent greater autonomy and freedom to make independent decisions or when parents are unable to agree and support each other in this effort.

The Family Launching Children and Moving On in Midlife

A great deal of realignment of family roles occurs during this stage. This stage is characterized by the intermittent exiting and entering of various family members. Children leave home for further education and careers; marriages occur, and new spouses, in-laws, and children enter the system; and new grandparent roles are established. Adult-to-adult relationships among grown children and their parents are renegotiated. Tasks associated with this stage include reestablishing the bond of the dyadic marital relationship; realigning relationships to include grown children, in-laws, and new grandchildren; and accepting the additional caretaking responsibilities and eventual death of elderly parents. Problems can arise when feelings of loss and depression become overwhelming in response to the departure of children from the home, when parents are unable to accept their children as adults or cope with the disability or death of their own parents, and when the marital bond has deteriorated.

The Family in Later Life (Late Middle Age to End of Life)

This stage can begin with retirement and last until the death of both spouses (Wright & Leahey, 2013). However, many older people who have the opportunity to do so are choosing to retire early, while large numbers of those over age 65 are remaining in the workforce and delaying their retirement. Thus, the beginning of this stage varies widely. Most adults in their later years are still a prominent part of the family system, and many are able to offer support to their grown children in the middle generation. Tasks associated with this stage include exploring new social roles related to retirement and possible change in socioeconomic status; accepting some decline in physiological functioning; dealing with the deaths of spouse, siblings, and friends; and confronting and preparing for one's own death. Problems may arise when older adults have failed to fulfill the tasks associated with earlier levels of development and are dissatisfied with the way their lives have gone. They are unable to find happiness in retirement or emotional satisfaction with children and grandchildren, and they are unable to accept the deaths of loved ones or to prepare for their own impending death.

Major Variations

Divorce

McGoldrick, Carter, and Garcia-Preto (2011) also discuss stages and tasks of families experiencing divorce and remarriage. Data on marriage, divorce, and remarriage in the United States show that about half of first marriages end in divorce (Centers for Disease Control [CDC], 2012). Some statistics indicate that the divorce rate may be on the decline since the 1970s. In 2009, however, almost 30 percent of all families in the United States were headed by solo parents (U.S. Census Bureau, 2013). Stages in the family life cycle of divorce include deciding to divorce, planning the breakup of the system, separation, and divorce. Tasks include accepting one's own part in the failure of the marriage, working cooperatively on problems related to custody and visitation of children and finances, realigning relationships with extended family, and mourning the loss of the marriage relationship and the intact family.

After the divorce, the custodial parent must adjust to functioning as the single leader of an ongoing family while working to rebuild a new social network. The noncustodial parent must find ways to continue to be an effective parent while remaining outside the normal parenting role.

Remarriage

A large percentage of people who divorce eventually remarry. In 2009, 16 percent (11.7 million) of all children in the United States lived in blended families (those that contain stepchildren and their stepparents, half siblings, or stepsiblings) (Kreider & Ellis, 2011). The challenges that face the joining of two established families are immense, and statistics reveal that the rate of divorce for remarried couples is even higher than the divorce rate following first marriages (Cory, 2013). Stages in the remarried family life cycle include entering the new relationship, planning the new marriage and family, and remarriage and reestablishment of family. Tasks include making a firm commitment to confronting the complexities of combining two families, maintaining open communication, facing fears, realigning relationships with extended family to include new spouse and children, and encouraging healthy relationships with biological (noncustodial) parents and grandparents.

Problems can arise when there is a blurring of boundaries between the custodial and noncustodial families. Children may contemplate, "Who is the boss now? Who is most important, the child or the new spouse? Mom loves her new husband more than she loves me. Dad lets me do more than my new stepdad does. I don't have to mind him; he's not my real dad." Confusion and distress for both the children and the parents can be avoided with the establishment of clear boundaries.

Goldenberg and Goldenberg (2013) state:

> Successful adaptation to stepfamily life calls for the ability to recognize and cope with a variety of problems: stepparents assuming a parental role, rule changes, jealousy and competition between stepsiblings as well as between birth parents and stepparents, loyalty conflicts in children between the absent parent and the stepparent, and financial obligations for child support while entering into a new marriage, to name but a few. Remarriage itself may resurrect old, unresolved feelings, such as anger and hurt left over from a previous marriage. (p. 435)

Cultural Variations

It is difficult to generalize about variations in family life-cycle development according to culture. Most families have become acculturated to the U.S. society and conform to the life-cycle stages previously described. However, cultural diversity does exist and nurses must be aware of possible differences in family expectations related to sociocultural beliefs. They must also be aware of a great deal of variation within ethnic groups as well as among them. Some variations that may be considered follow.

Marriage

A number of U.S. subcultures maintain traditional values in terms of marriage. Traditional views about family life and Roman Catholicism exert important influences on attitudes toward marriage in many Italian American and Latino American families. Although the tradition of arranged marriages is disappearing in Asian American families, there is still frequently a strong influence by the family on mate selection in this culture. In most of these subcultures, the father is considered the authority figure and head of the household and the mother assumes the role of homemaker and caretaker. Family loyalty is intense and a breach of this loyalty brings considerable shame to the family.

Valley (2005) makes the following statement about Jewish families:

> The Jewish family today encompasses a wide variety of textures and forms. Decades of high intermarriage have diversified the customs and complexions of the family. High divorce rates, meanwhile, have altered the very definition of what is "normal." Whereas single-parent households were once a rare exception, they now account for an increasing proportion of American Jewish families. Some in the community have interpreted the changing family in strident and judgmental terms: it is a sign of rampant assimilation, loss of tradition or moral permissiveness. But such scolding does nothing to respond to the new realities and to the changing needs of Jews today. (p. 2)

Children

In traditional Latino American and Italian American cultures, children are central to the family system. Many of these individuals have strong ties to Roman Catholicism, which historically has promoted marital relations for procreation only, and encouraged families to have large numbers of children. Regarding birth control, the Catechism of the Catholic Church pronounces as immoral any means that interferes with or hinders procreation (U.S. Catholic Church, 2006).

In the traditional Jewish community, having children is seen as a scriptural and social obligation. "You shall be fruitful and multiply" is a commandment of the Torah.

In some traditional Asian American cultures, sons are more highly valued than are daughters, and there is a strong preference for sons over daughters (Earp, 2013; Xu & Chang, 2013). Younger siblings are expected to follow the guidance of the oldest son throughout their lives, and when the father dies, the oldest son takes over the leadership of the family.

In all of these cultures, children are expected to be respectful of their parents and not bring shame to the family. Especially in the Asian culture, children learn a sense of obligation to their parents for bringing them into this world and caring for them when they were helpless. This is viewed as a debt that can never be truly repaid, and no matter what the parents may do, the child is still obligated to give respect and obedience.

Extended Family

The concept of extended family varies among societies (Purnell, 2013). The extended family is extremely important in the Western European, Latino, and Asian cultures, playing a central role in all aspects of life, including decision making.

In some U.S. subcultures, such as Asian, Latino, Italian, and Iranian, it is not uncommon to find several generations living together. Older family members are valued for their experience and wisdom. Because extended families often share living quarters, or at least live nearby, tasks of child rearing may be shared by several generations.

Divorce

In the Jewish community, divorce is often seen as a violation of family togetherness. Some Jewish parents take their child's divorce personally, with a response that reflects, "How could you possibly do this to me?"

Because Roman Catholicism has traditionally opposed divorce, those cultures that are largely Catholic have followed this dictate. Historically, a low divorce rate has existed among Italian Americans, Irish Americans, and Latino Americans. The number of divorces among these subcultures is on the rise, however, particularly in successive generations that have become more acculturated into a society where divorce is more acceptable.

Family Functioning

Boyer and Jeffrey (1994) describe six elements on which families are assessed to be either functional or dysfunctional. Each can be viewed on a continuum, although families rarely fall at extreme ends of the continuum. Rather, they tend to be dynamic and fluctuate from one point to another within the different areas. These six elements of assessment are described below and summarized in Table 11-2.

Communication

Functional communication patterns are those in which verbal and nonverbal messages are clear, direct, and congruent between sender and intended receiver. Family members are encouraged to express honest feelings and opinions, and all members participate in decisions that affect the family system. Each member is an active listener to the other members of the family.

Behaviors that interfere with functional communication include the following.

Making Assumptions

With this behavior, one assumes that others will know what is meant by an action or an expression (or sometimes even what one is thinking); or, on the other hand, assumes to know what another member is thinking or feeling without checking to make certain.

> **EXAMPLE**
>
> A mother says to her teenaged daughter, "You should have known that I expected you to clean up the kitchen while I was gone!"

Belittling Feelings

This action involves ignoring or minimizing another's feelings when they are expressed. This encourages the individual to withhold honest feelings to avoid being hurt by the negative response.

TABLE 11–2 **Family Functioning: Elements of Assessment**		
ELEMENTS OF ASSESSMENT	CONTINUUM	
	FUNCTIONAL	**DYSFUNCTIONAL**
Communication	Clear, direct, open, and honest, with congruence between verbal and nonverbal	Indirect, vague, controlled, with many double-bind messages
Self-concept reinforcement	Supportive, loving, praising, approving, with behaviors that instill confidence	Unsupportive, blaming, "put-downs," refusing to allow self-responsibility
Family members' expectations	Flexible, realistic, individualized	Judgmental, rigid, controlling, ignoring individuality
Handling differences	Tolerant, dynamic, negotiating	Attacking, avoiding, surrendering
Family interactional patterns	Workable, constructive, flexible, and promoting the needs of all members	Contradictory, rigid, self-defeating, and destructive
Family climate	Trusting, growth-promoting, caring, general feeling of well-being	Distrusting, emotionally painful, with absence of hope for improvement

SOURCE: Adapted from Boyer & Jeffery (1994).

EXAMPLE

When the young woman confides to her mother that she is angry because the grandfather has touched her breast, the mother responds, "Oh, don't be angry. He doesn't mean anything by that."

Failing to Listen

With this behavior, one does not hear what the other individual is saying. This can mean not hearing the words by "tuning out" what is being said, or it can be "selective" listening, in which a person hears only a selective part of the message or interprets it in a selective manner.

EXAMPLE

The father explains to Johnny, "If the contract comes through and I get this new job, we'll have a little extra money and we will consider sending you to State U." Johnny relays the message to his friend, "Dad says I can go to State U!"

Communicating Indirectly

This usually means that an individual does not or cannot present a message to a receiver directly, so seeks to communicate through a third person.

EXAMPLE

A father does not want his teenage daughter to see a certain boyfriend, but wants to avoid the angry response he expects from his daughter if he tells her so. He expresses his feelings to his wife, hoping she will share them with their daughter.

Presenting Double-Bind Messages

Double-bind communication conveys a "damned if I do and damned if I don't" message. A family member may respond to a direct request by another family member, only to be rebuked when the request is fulfilled.

EXAMPLE

The father tells his son he is spending too much time playing football, and as a result, his grades are falling. He is expected to bring his grades up over the next 9 weeks or his car will be taken away. When the son tells the father he has quit the football team so he can study more, Dad responds angrily, "I won't allow any son of mine to be a quitter!"

Self-Concept Reinforcement

Functional families strive to reinforce and strengthen each member's self-concept, with the positive results being that family members feel loved and valued. Boyer and Jeffrey (1994) stated:

> The manner in which children see and value themselves is influenced most significantly by the messages they receive concerning their value to other members of the family. Messages that convey praise, approval, appreciation, trust, and confidence in decisions and

that allow family members to pursue individual needs and ultimately to become independent are the foundation blocks of a child's feelings of self-worth. Adults also need and depend heavily on this kind of reinforcement for their own emotional well-being. (p. 27)

Behaviors that interfere with self-concept reinforcement follow.

Expressing Denigrating Remarks

These remarks are commonly called "put-downs." Individuals receive messages that they are worthless or unloved.

EXAMPLE

A child spills a glass of milk at the table. The mother responds, "You are hopeless! How could anybody be so clumsy?!"

Withholding Supportive Messages

Some family members find it very difficult to provide others with reinforcing and supportive messages. This may be because they themselves have not been the recipients of reinforcement from significant others and have not learned how to provide support to others.

EXAMPLE

A 10-year-old boy playing Little League baseball retrieves the ball and throws it to second base for an out. After the game he says to his Dad, "Did you see my play on second base?" Dad responds, "Yes, I did, son, but if you had been paying better attention, you could have caught the ball for a direct and immediate out."

Taking Over

This occurs when one family member fails to permit another member to develop a sense of responsibility and self-worth, by doing things for the individual instead of allowing him or her to manage the situation independently.

EXAMPLE

Twelve-year-old Eric has a job delivering the evening paper, which he usually begins right after school. Today he must serve a 1-hour detention after school for being late to class yesterday. He tells his Mom, "Tommy said he would throw my papers for me today if I help him wash his Dad's car on Saturday." Mom responds, "Never mind. Tell Tommy to forget it. I'll take care of your paper route today."

Family Members' Expectations

All individuals have some expectations about the outcomes of the life situations they experience. These expectations are related to and significantly influenced by earlier life experiences. In functional families, expectations are realistic, thereby avoiding setting up family members for failure. In functional families, expectations are also flexible. Life situations are full of extraneous and unexpected interferences. Flexibility allows for changes and interruptions to occur without creating conflict. Finally, in functional families, expectations are individualized. Each family member is different, with different strengths and limitations. The outcome of a life situation for one family member may not be realistic for another. Each member must be valued independently, and comparison among members avoided.

Behaviors that interfere with adaptive functioning in terms of member expectations include the following.

Ignoring Individuality

This occurs when family members are expected to perform or behave in ways that undermine their individuality or that do not suit their current life situation. This sometimes happens when parents expect their children to fulfill the hopes and dreams the parents have failed to achieve, yet the children have their own, different hopes and dreams.

EXAMPLE

Bob, an only child, leaves for college next year. Bob's father, Robert, inherited a hardware store that was founded by Bob's great-grandfather and has been in the family for three generations. Robert expects Bob to major in business, work in the store after college, and take over the business when Robert retires. Bob, however, has a talent for writing, wants to major in communication, and wants to work in TV news when he graduates. Robert sees this as a betrayal of the family.

Demanding Proof of Love

Boyer and Jeffrey (1994) state:

> Family members place expectations on others' behavior that are used as standards by which the expecting member determines how much the other members care for him or her. The message attached to these expectations is: "If you will not be as I wish you to be, you don't love me." (p. 32)

EXAMPLE

This is the message that Bob receives from his father in the example cited in the previous paragraph.

Handling Differences

It is difficult to conceive of two or more individuals living together who agree on everything all of the time. Serious problems in a family's functioning appear when differences become equated with disapproval or when disagreement is perceived as offensive. Members of a functional family understand that it is acceptable to disagree and deal with differences in an open, nonattacking manner. Members are willing to hear the other person's position, respect the other person's right to hold an opposing position, and work to modify the expectations on both sides of the issue in order to negotiate a workable solution.

Behaviors that interfere with successful family negotiations follow.

Attacking

Personal attacks can occur when a difference of opinion deteriorates. One person may blame the other with insulting remarks, reminders of past transgressions may occur, and the situation intensifies with destructive expressions of anger and hurt.

EXAMPLE

When Nancy's husband, John, buys an expensive set of golf clubs, Nancy responds, "How could you do such a thing? You know we can't afford those! No wonder we don't have a nice house like all our friends. You spend all our money before we can save for a down payment. You're so selfish! We'll never have anything nice and it's all your fault!"

Avoiding

With this tactic, differences are never acknowledged openly. The individual who disagrees avoids discussing it for fear that the other person will withdraw love or approval or become angry in response to the disagreement. Avoidance also occurs when an individual fears loss of control of his or her temper if the disagreement is brought out into the open.

EXAMPLE

Vicki and Clint have been married 6 months. This is Vicki's second marriage and she has a 4-year-old son from her first marriage, Derek, who lives with her and Clint. Both Vicki and Clint work, and Derek goes to day care. Since the marriage 6 months ago, Derek cries every night continuously unless Vicki spends all her time with him, which she does in order to keep him quiet. Clint resents this but says nothing for fear he will come across as interfering; however, he has started going back to work in his office in the evenings to avoid the family situation.

Surrendering

The person who surrenders in the face of disagreement does so at the expense of denying his or her own needs or rights. The individual avoids expressing a difference of opinion for fear of angering another person or of losing approval and support.

EXAMPLE

Elaine is the only child of wealthy parents. She attends an exclusive private college in a small New England town, where she met Andrew, the son of a farming couple from the area. Andrew attended the local community college for 2 years but chose to work on his parents' farm rather than continue college. Elaine and Andrew love each other and want to be married, but Elaine's parents say they will disown her if she marries Andrew, who they believe is below her social status. Elaine breaks off her relationship with Andrew rather than challenge her parents' wishes.

Family Interactional Patterns

Interactional patterns have to do with the ways in which families "behave." All families develop recurring, predictable patterns of interaction over time. These are often thought of as "family rules." The mentality conveys, "This is the way we have always done it" and provides a sense of security and stability for family members that comes from predictability. These interactions may have to do with communication, self-concept reinforcement, expressing expectations, and handling differences (all of the behaviors that were discussed previously), but because they are repetitive, and recur over time, they become the "rules" that govern patterns of interaction among family members.

Family rules are functional when they are workable, are constructive, and promote the needs of all family members. They are dysfunctional when they become contradictory, self-defeating, and destructive. Family therapists often find that individuals are unaware that dysfunctional family rules exist and may vehemently deny their existence even when confronted with a specific behavioral interaction. The development of dysfunctional interactional patterns occurs through a habituation process and out of fear of change or reprisal or a lack of knowledge as to how a given situation might be handled differently. Many are derived out of the parents' own growing-up experiences.

Patterns of interaction that interfere with adaptive family functioning include the following.

Patterns That Cause Emotional Discomfort

Interactions can promote hurt and anger in family members. This is particularly true of emotions that individuals feel uncomfortable expressing or are not permitted (according to "family rules") to express openly. These interactional patterns include behaviors such as never apologizing or never admitting that one has made a mistake, forbidding flexibility in life situations ("you must do it my way, or you will not do it at all"), making statements that devalue the worth of others, or withholding statements that promote increased self-worth.

EXAMPLE

Priscilla and Bill had been discussing buying a new car but could not agree on the make or model to buy. One day, Bill appeared at Priscilla's office over the lunch hour and said, "Come outside and see our new car." In front of the building, Bill had parked a brand new sports car that he explained he had purchased with their combined savings. Priscilla was furious, but kept quiet and proceeded to finish her workday. At home she expressed her anger to Bill for making the purchase without consulting her. Bill refused to apologize or admit to making a mistake. They both remained cool and hardly spoke to each other for weeks.

Patterns That Perpetuate or Intensify Problems Rather Than Solve Them

When problems go unresolved over a long period of time, it sometimes appears to be easier just to ignore them. If problems of the same nature occur, the tendency to ignore them then becomes the safe and predictable pattern of interaction for dealing with this type of situation. This may occur until the problem intensifies to a point when it can no longer be ignored.

EXAMPLE

Dan works hard in the automobile factory and demands peace and quiet from his family when he comes home from work. His children have learned over the years not to share their problems with him because they fear his explosive temper. Their mother attempts to handle unpleasant situations alone as best she can. When son Ron was expelled from school for being caught smoking pot for the third time, Dan yelled, "Why wasn't I told about this before?"

Patterns That Are in Conflict With Each Other

Some family rules may appear to be functional—very workable and constructive—on the surface, but in practice may serve to destroy healthy interactional patterns. Boyer and Jeffrey (1994) describe the following scenario as an example.

EXAMPLE

Dad insists that all members of the family eat dinner together every evening. No one may leave the table until everyone is finished because dinnertime is one of the few times left when the family can be together. Yet Dad frequently uses the time to reprimand Bobby about his poor grades in math, to scold Ann for her sloppy room, or to make not-so-subtle gibes at Mom for "spending all day on the telephone and never getting anything accomplished."

Family Climate

The atmosphere or climate of a family is composed of a blend of the feelings and experiences that are the result of family members' verbal and nonverbal sharing and interacting. A positive family climate is founded on trust and is reflected in open communication, joyfulness and laughter, expressions of caring and mutual respect, the valuing of each individual as unique, and a general feeling of security and well-being. In a dysfunctional family, the climate is evidenced by tension, frustration, guilt, anger and resentment, depression, and despair.

Therapeutic Modalities With Families

The Family as a System

General systems theory is a way of organizing thought according to the holistic perspective. A system is considered greater than the sum of its parts. A system is considered dynamic and ever changing. A change in one part of the system causes a change in the other parts of the system and in the system as a whole. When studying families, it is helpful to conceptualize a hierarchy of systems.

The family can be viewed as a system composed of various **subsystems**, such as the marital subsystem, parent-child subsystems, and sibling subsystems. Each of these subsystems is further divided into subsystems of individuals. The family system is also a subsystem of a larger suprasystem, such as the neighborhood or community. A schematic of a hierarchy of systems is presented in Figure 11-1.

Major Concepts

Bowen (1978) did a great deal of work with families using a systems approach. Bowen's theoretical approach

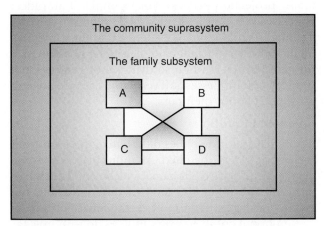

Key:

A = Father subsystem	CD = Sibling subsystem
B = Mother subsystem	AD = Parent-child subsystem
C = Child subsystem	BC = Parent-child subsystem
D = Child subsystem	AC = Parent-child subsystem
AB =Marital subsystem	BD = Parent-child subsystem

FIGURE 11-1 A hierarchy of systems.

to family therapy is composed of eight major concepts: (1) differentiation of self, (2) triangles, (3) nuclear family emotional process, (4) family projection process, (5) multigenerational transmission process, (6) sibling position, (7) emotional cutoff, and (8) societal emotional process.

Differentiation of Self

Differentiation of self is the ability to define oneself as a separate being. The Bowen theory suggests that "a person with a well-differentiated self recognizes his [or her] realistic dependence on others, but can stay calm and clear headed enough in the face of conflict, criticism, and rejection to distinguish thinking rooted in a careful assessment of the facts from thinking clouded by emotionality" (Georgetown Family Center, 2013a).

The degree of differentiation of self can be viewed on a continuum from high levels, in which an individual manifests a clearly defined sense of self, to low levels, or undifferentiated, in which emotional fusion exists and the individual is unable to function separately from a relationship system. Healthy families encourage differentiation, and the process of separation from the family ego mass is most pronounced during the ages of 2 to 5 and again between the ages of 13 and 15. Families that do not understand the child's need to be different during these times may perceive their behavior as objectionable.

Bowen (1971) used the term *stuck-togetherness* to describe the family with the fused ego mass. When family fusion occurs, none of the members has a true sense of self as an independent individual. Boundaries between members are blurred, and the family becomes enmeshed without individual distinguishing characteristics. In this situation, family members can neither gain true intimacy nor separate and become individuals.

Triangles

The concept of **triangles** refers to a three-person emotional configuration that is considered the basic building block of the family system. Bowen (1978) offers the following description of triangles:

> The basic building block of any emotional system is the triangle. When emotional tension in a two-person system exceeds a certain level, it triangles in a third person, permitting the tension to shift about within the triangle. Any two in the original triangle can add a new triangle. An emotional system is composed of a series of interlocking triangles. (p. 306)

Triangles are dysfunctional in that they offer relief from anxiety through diversion rather than through resolution of the issue. When stress develops in a two-person relationship, "one or both partners will turn to someone else for sympathy or the conflict will draw in a third person to try to help" (Nichols, 2010, p. 115). When the dynamics within a triangle stabilize, a fourth person may be brought in to form additional triangles, in an effort to reduce tension. This triangulation can continue almost indefinitely as extended family and people outside the family, including the family therapist, can become entangled in the process. The therapist working with families must strive to remain "de-triangled" from this emotional system.

Nuclear Family Emotional Process

The nuclear family emotional process describes the patterns of emotional functioning in a single generation. The nuclear family begins with a relationship between two people who form a couple. The most open relationship usually occurs during courtship, when most individuals choose partners with similar levels of differentiation. The lower the level of differentiation, the greater the possibility of problems in the future. A degree of fusion occurs with permanent commitment. This fusion results in anxiety and must be dealt with by each partner in an effort to maintain a healthy degree of differentiation.

Family Projection Process

Spouses who are unable to work through the undifferentiation or fusion that occurs with permanent commitment may, when they become parents, project the resulting anxiety onto the children. This occurrence is manifested as a father-mother-child triangle. These triangles are common and exist in various gradations of intensity in most families with children.

The child who becomes the target of the projection may be selected for various reasons:

■ A particular child reminds one of the parents of an unresolved childhood issue.

■ The child is of a particular gender or position in the family.

■ The child is born with special needs.

■ The parent has a negative attitude about the pregnancy.

This behavior is called **scapegoating**. It is harmful to both the child's emotional stability and his or her ability to function outside the family. Goldenberg, Goldenberg, & Pelavin (2011) have stated:

> Scapegoated family members not only assume the role assigned them, but they may become so entrenched in that role that they are unable to act otherwise. Particularly in dysfunctional families, individuals may be repeatedly labeled as the 'bad child'—incorrigible, destructive, unmanageable, troublesome—and they proceed to act accordingly. Scapegoated children are inducted into specific family roles, which over time become fixed and serve as the basis for chronic behavioral disturbance. (p. 432)

Multigenerational Transmission Process

Bowen (1978) described the multigenerational transmission process as the manner in which interactional patterns are transferred from one generation to another. Attitudes, values, beliefs, behaviors, and patterns of interaction are passed along from parents to children over many lifetimes, so that it becomes possible to show in a family assessment that a certain behavior has existed within a family through multiple generations.

Genograms. A convenient way to plot a multigenerational assessment is with the use of **genograms**. Genograms offer the convenience of a great deal of information in a small amount of space. They can also be used as teaching tools with the family itself. An overall picture of the life of the family over several generations can be conveyed, including roles that various family members play as well as emotional distance between specific individuals. Areas for change can be easily identified. A sample genogram is presented in Figure 11-2.

Sibling Position

The view regarding sibling position profiles is that the position one holds in a family influences the development of predictable personality characteristics. For example, firstborn children are thought to be perfectionistic, reliable, and conscientious; middle children are described as independent, loyal, and intolerant of conflict; and youngest children tend to be charming, precocious, and gregarious (Leman, 2009). Bowen used this thesis to help determine levels of differentiation within a family and the possible direction of the family projection process. For example, if an oldest child exhibits characteristics more representative of a youngest child, there is evidence that this child may be the product of triangulation. Sibling position profiles are also used when studying multigenerational transmission processes and verifiable data are missing for certain family members.

Emotional Cutoff

Emotional cutoff describes differentiation of self from the perception of the child. All individuals have some degree of unresolved emotional attachment to their parents and the lower the level of differentiation, the greater the degree of unresolved emotional attachment.

Emotional cutoff has very little to do with how far away one lives from the family of origin. Individuals who live great distances from their parents can still be undifferentiated, whereas some individuals are emotionally cut off from their parents who live in the same town or even the same neighborhood.

Bowen (1976) suggests that emotional cutoff is the result of dysfunction within the family of origin in

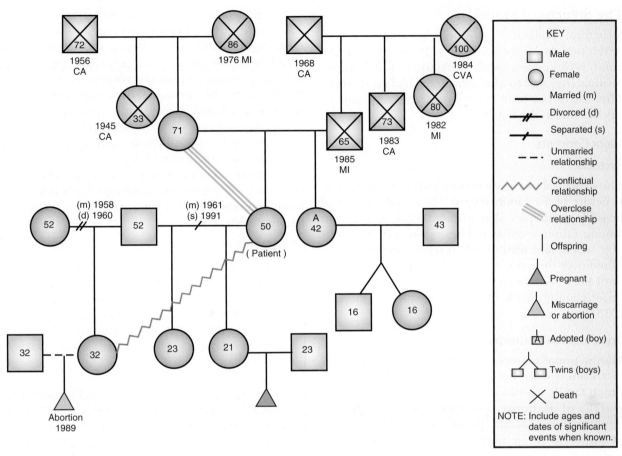

FIGURE 11-2 Sample genogram.

which fusion has occurred and that emotional cutoff promotes the same type of dysfunction in the new nuclear family. He contends that maintaining some emotional contact with the family of origin promotes healthy differentiation.

Societal Emotional Process

The Bowen theory views society as an emotional system. The concept of societal emotional process compares society's response to stress to the same type of response seen in individuals and families in response to emotional crisis: stress creates uncomfortable levels of anxiety, that leads to hasty solutions, which add to the problems, and the cycle continues. This concept of Bowen's theory is explained as follows (Georgetown Family Center, 2013b):

> Human societies undergo periods of regression and progression in their history. The current regression seems related to factors such as the population explosion, a sense of diminishing frontiers, and the depletion of natural resources. The "symptoms" of societal regression include a growth of crime and violence, an increasing divorce rate, a more litigious attitude, a greater polarization between racial groups, less principled decision-making by leaders, the drug

abuse epidemic, an increase in bankruptcy, and a focus on rights over responsibilities.

Goal and Techniques of Therapy

The goal of Bowen's systems approach to family therapy is to increase the level of differentiation of self, while remaining in touch with the family system. The premise is that intense emotional problems within the nuclear family can be resolved only by resolving undifferentiated relationships with the family of origin. Emphasis is given to the understanding of past relationships.

The therapeutic role is that of "coach" or supervisor, and emotional involvement with the family is minimized. Therapist techniques include:

1. Defining and clarifying the relationship between the family members.
2. Helping family members develop one-to-one relationships with each other and minimizing triangles within the system.
3. Teaching family members about the functioning of emotional systems.
4. Promoting differentiation by encouraging members to speak as individuals rather than as a family unit.

The Structural Model

Structural family therapy is associated with a model developed by Minuchin (1974). In this model, the family is viewed as a social system within which the individual lives and to which the individual must adapt. The individual both contributes and responds to stresses within the family.

Major Concepts

Systems

The structural model views the family as a system. The structure of the **family system** is founded on a set of invisible principles that influence the interaction among family members. These principles concern how, when, and with whom to relate, and are established over time and through repeated transactions, until they become rules that govern the conduct of various family members (Goldenberg & Goldenberg, 2013).

Transactional Patterns

Transactional patterns are the rules that have been established over time that organize the ways in which family members relate to one another. A hierarchy of authority is one example of a transactional pattern. Usually, parents have a higher level of authority in a family than the children, so parental behavior reflects this role. A balance of authority may exist between husband and wife, or one may reflect a higher level than the other. These patterns of behavioral expectations differ from family to family and may trace their origin over generations of family negotiations.

Subsystems

Minuchin (1974) describes subsystems as smaller elements that make up the larger family system. Subsystems can be individuals or can consist of two or more persons united by gender, relationship, generation, interest, or purpose. A family member may belong to several subsystems at the same time, in which he or she may experience different levels of power and require different types of skills. For example, a young man has a different level of power and a different set of expectations in his father-son subsystem than in a subsystem with his younger brother.

Boundaries

Boundaries define the level of participation and interaction among subsystems. Boundaries are appropriate when they permit appropriate contact with others while preventing excessive interference. Clearly defined boundaries promote adaptive functioning. Maladaptive functioning can occur when boundaries are *rigid* or *diffuse.*

A rigid boundary is characterized by decreased communication and lack of support and responsiveness. Rigid boundaries prevent a subsystem (family member or subgroup) from achieving appropriate closeness or interaction with others in the system. Rigid boundaries promote **disengagement**, or extreme separateness, among family members.

A diffuse boundary is characterized by dependency and overinvolvement. Diffuse boundaries interfere with adaptive functioning because of the overinvestment, overinvolvement, and lack of differentiation between certain subsystems. Diffuse boundaries promote **enmeshment**, or exaggerated connectedness, among family members.

EXAMPLE

Sally and Jim have been married for 12 years, during which time they have tried without success to have children. Six months ago they were thrilled to have the opportunity to adopt a 5-year-old girl, Annie. Since both Sally and Jim have full-time teaching jobs, Annie stays with her maternal grandmother, Krista, during the day after she gets home from half-day kindergarten.

At first, Annie was a polite and obedient child. However, in the last few months, she has become insolent and oppositional, and has temper tantrums when she cannot have her way. Sally and Krista agree that Annie should have whatever she desires and should not be punished for her behavior. Jim believes that discipline is necessary, but Sally and Krista refuse to enforce any guidelines he tries to establish. Annie is aware of this discordance and manipulates it to her full advantage.

In this situation, diffuse boundaries exist among the Sally-Krista-Annie subsystems. They have become enmeshed. They have also established a rigid boundary against Jim, disengaging him from the system.

Goal and Techniques of Therapy

The goal of structural family therapy is to facilitate change in the **family structure**. Family structure is changed with modification of the family "principles" or transactional patterns that are contributing to dysfunction within the family. The family is viewed as the unit of therapy, and all members are counseled together. Little, if any, time is spent exploring past experiences. The focus of structural therapy is on the present. Therapist techniques include the following:

■ **Joining the Family.** The therapist must become a part of the family if restructuring is to occur. The therapist joins the family but maintains a leadership position. He or she may at different times join various subsystems within the family, but ultimately includes the entire family system as the target of intervention.

- ■ **Evaluating the Family Structure.** Even though a family may come for therapy because of the behavior of one family member (the identified patient), the family as a unit is considered problematic. The family structure is evaluated by assessing transactional patterns, system flexibility and potential for change, boundaries, family developmental stage, and role of the identified patient within the system.
- ■ **Restructuring the Family.** An alliance or contract for therapy is established with the family. By becoming an actual part of the family, the therapist is able to manipulate the system and facilitate the circumstances and experiences that can lead to structural change.

The Strategic Model

The strategic model of family therapy uses the interactional or communications approach. Communication theory is viewed as the foundation for this model. Communication is the actual transmission of information among individuals. All behavior sends a message, so all behavior in the presence of two or more individuals is communication. In this model, families considered to be functional are open systems where clear and precise messages, congruent with the situation, are sent and received. Healthy communication patterns promote nurturance and individual self-worth. Dysfunctional families are viewed as partially closed systems in which communication is vague, and messages are often inconsistent and incongruent with the situation. Destructive patterns of communication tend to inhibit healthful nurturing and decrease individual feelings of self-worth.

Major Concepts

Double-Bind Communication

Double-bind communication occurs when a statement is made and succeeded by a contradictory statement. It also occurs when a statement is made accompanied by nonverbal expression that is inconsistent with the verbal communication. These incompatible communications can interfere with ego development in an individual and promote mistrust of all communications. Double-bind communication often results in a "damned if I do and damned if I don't" situation.

EXAMPLE

A mother freely gives and receives hugs and kisses from her 6-year-old son some of the time, while at other times she pushes him away saying, "Big boys don't act like that." The little boy receives a conflicting message and is presented with an impossible dilemma: "To please my mother I must not show her that I love her, but if I do not show her that I love her, I'm afraid I will lose her."

Pseudomutuality and Pseudohostility

A healthy functioning individual is able to relate to other people while still maintaining a sense of separate identity. In a dysfunctional family, patterns of interaction may be reflected in the remoteness or closeness of relationships. These relationships may reflect erratic interaction (i.e., sometimes remote and sometimes close) or inappropriate interaction (i.e., excessive closeness or remoteness).

Pseudomutuality and pseudohostility are seen as collective defenses against the reality of the underlying meaning of the relationships in a dysfunctional family system. **Pseudomutuality** is characterized by a facade of mutual regard. Emotional investment is directed at maintaining outward representation of reciprocal fulfillment rather than in the relationship itself. The style of relating is fixed and rigid, and pseudomutuality allows family members to deny underlying fears of separation and hostility.

EXAMPLE

Janet, age 16, is the only child of State Senator J. and his wife. Janet was recently involved in a joyriding experience with a group of teenagers her parents call "the wrong crowd." In family therapy, Mrs. J. says, "We have always been a close family. I can't imagine why she is doing these things." Senator J. states, "I don't know another colleague who has a family that is as close as mine." Janet responds, "Yes, we are close. I just don't see my parents very much. Dad has been in politics since I was a baby, and Mom is always with him. I wish I could spend more time with them. But we are a close family."

Pseudohostility is also a fixed and rigid style of relating, but the facade being maintained is that of a state of chronic conflict and alienation among family members. This relationship pattern allows family members to deny underlying fears of tenderness and intimacy.

EXAMPLE

Jack, 14, and his sister Jill, 15, will have nothing to do with each other. When they are together they can agree on nothing, and the barrage of "put-downs" is constant. This behavior reflects pseudohostility used by individuals who are afraid to reveal feelings of intimacy.

Schism and Skew

Lidz, Cornelison, Fleck, and Terry (1957) observed two patterns within families that relate to a dysfunctional marital dyad. A **marital schism** is defined as "a state of severe chronic disequilibrium and discord, with recurrent threats of separation." Each partner undermines the other, mutual trust is absent, and a competition exists for closeness with the children. Often a partner establishes an alliance with his or her parent against the spouse. Children lack appropriate role models. **Marital skew** describes a relationship in which there is lack of equal partnership. One partner dominates the relationship and the other partner. The marriage remains intact as long as the passive partner allows the domination to continue. Children also lack role models when a marital skew exists.

Goal and Techniques of Therapy

The goal of strategic family therapy is to create change in destructive behavior and communication patterns among family members. The identified family *problem* is the unit of therapy, and all family members need not be counseled together. In fact, strategic therapists may prefer to see subgroups or individuals separately in an effort to achieve problem resolution. Therapy is oriented in the present and the therapist assumes full responsibility for devising an effective strategy for family change. Therapeutic techniques include the following:

■ **Paradoxical Intervention.** A paradox can be called a contradiction in therapy, or "prescribing the symptom." With **paradoxical intervention**, the therapist requests that the family continue to engage in the behavior that they are trying to change. Alternatively, specific directions may be given for continuing the defeating behavior. For example, a couple that regularly engages in insulting shouting matches is instructed to have one of these encounters on Tuesdays and Thursdays from 8:30 to 9 p.m. Boyer and Jeffrey (1994) explained this technique in the following manner:

> A family using its maladaptive behavior to control or punish other people loses control of the situation when it finds itself continuing the behavior under a therapist's direction and being praised for following instructions. If the family disobeys the therapist's instruction, the price it pays is sacrificing the old behavior pattern and experiencing more satisfying ways of interacting with one another. A family that maintains it has no control over its behavior, or whose members contend that others must change before they can themselves, suddenly finds itself unable to defend such statements. (p. 125)

■ **Reframing.** Goldenberg and associates (2011) describe **reframing** as "relabeling problematic behavior by viewing it in a new, more positive light that emphasizes its good intention." Therefore, with reframing, the *behavior* may not actually change, but the *consequences* of the behavior may change, because of a change in the meaning attached to the behavior. This technique is sometimes referred to as *positive reframing*.

EXAMPLE

Tom has a construction job and makes a comfortable living for his wife, Sue, and their two children. Tom and Sue have been arguing a lot and came to the therapist for counseling. Sue says Tom frequently drinks too much and is often late getting home from work. Tom counters, "I never used to drink on my way home from work, but Sue started complaining to me the minute I walked in the door about being so dirty and about tracking dirt and mud on 'her nice, clean floors.' It was the last straw when she made me undress before I came in the house and leave my dirty clothes and shoes in the garage. I thought a man's home was his castle. Well, I sure don't feel like a king. I need a few stiff drinks to face her nagging!"

The therapist used reframing to attempt change by helping Sue to view the situation in a more positive light. He suggested to Sue that she try to change her thinking by focusing on how much her husband must love her and her children to work as hard as he does. He asked her to focus on the dirty clothes and shoes as symbols of his love for them and to respond to his "dirty" arrivals home with greater affection. This positive reframing set the tone for healing and for increased intimacy within the marital relationship.

The Evolution of Family Therapy

Bowen's family theory and the structural and strategic models are sometimes referred to as basic models of family therapy. Goldenberg and Goldenberg (2013) state:

> While noteworthy differences continue to exist in the theoretical assumptions each school of thought makes about the nature and origin of psychological dysfunction, in what precisely they look for in understanding family patterns, and in their strategies for therapeutic intervention, in practice the trend today is toward eclecticism and integration in family therapy. (p. 165)

Nichols (2010) suggested that contemporary family therapists "borrow from each other's arsenal of techniques." The basic models described here have provided a foundation for the progression and growth of the discipline of family therapy. Examples of newer models include the following:

■ **Narrative therapy:** Narrative therapy is an approach to treatment that emphasizes the role of the stories people construct about their experience. (Nichols, 2010, p. 463)
■ **Feminist family therapy:** This form of family therapy employs a collaborative, egalitarian, nonsexist intervention, applicable to both men and women, addressing family gender roles, patriarchal attitudes,

and social and economic inequalities in male-female relationships. (Goldenberg & Goldenberg, 2013, p. 518)

■ **Social constructionist therapy:** Social constructionist therapy shifts attention away from an inspection of the origin or the exact nature of a family's presenting problems to an examination of the stories (interpretations, explanations, theories about relationships) family members have told themselves that account for how they have lived their lives. Social constructionist therapists are particularly interested in expanding clients' rigid and inflexible views of the world (Goldenberg & Goldenberg, 2013, p. 375).

■ **Psychoeducational family therapy:** This type of family therapy emphasizes educating family members to help them understand and cope with a seriously disturbed family member (Nichols, 2010, p. 464).

The goal of most family therapy models is to provide the opportunity for change based on family members' perceptions of available options. The basic differences among models arise in how they go about achieving this goal. Goldenberg & Goldenberg (2013) stated:

> Regardless of procedures, all attempt to create a therapeutic environment conducive to self-examination, to reduce discomfort and conflict, to mobilize family resilience and empowerment, and to help the family members improve their overall functioning. (p. 483)

The Nursing Process—A Case Study

Assessment

Wright and Leahey (2013) have developed the Calgary Family Assessment Model (CFAM), a multidimensional model originally adapted from a framework developed by Tomm and Sanders (1983). The CFAM consists of three major categories: structural, developmental, and functional. Wright and Leahey (2013) state:

> Each category contains several subcategories. It is important for each nurse to decide which subcategories are relevant and appropriate to explore and assess with each family at each point in time—that is, not all subcategories need to be assessed at a first meeting with a family, and some subcategories need never be assessed. If the nurse uses too many subcategories, he or she may become overwhelmed by all the data. If the nurse and the family discuss too few subcategories, each may have a distorted view of the family's strengths or problems and the family situation. (pp. 51–52)

A diagram of the CFAM is presented in Figure 11-3. The three major categories are listed, along with the subcategories for assessment under each. This diagram is used to assess the Marino family, a case study presented in Box 11-1.

Structural Assessment

A graphic representation of the Marino family structure is presented in the genogram in Figure 11-4.

Internal Structure

The Marino family consists of a husband, wife, and their biological son and daughter who live together in the same home. They conform to the traditional gender roles. John is the eldest child from a rather large family, and Nancy has no siblings. In this family, their son, Peter, is the firstborn and his sister, Anna, is 2 years younger. Neither spousal, sibling, nor spousal-sibling subsystems appear to be close in this family, and some are clearly conflictual. Problematic subsystems include John-Nancy, John-Nancy-children, and Nancy-Ethyl. The subsystem boundaries are quite rigid, and the family members appear to be emotionally disengaged from one another.

External Structure

This family has ties to extended family, although the availability of support is questionable. Nancy's parents offered little emotional support to her as a developing child. They never approved of her marriage to John and still remain distant and cold. John's family consists of a father, mother, two brothers, and two sisters. They are warm and supportive most of the time, but cultural influences interfere with their understanding of this current situation. At this time, the Marino family is probably receiving the most support from healthcare professionals who have intervened during Anna's hospitalization.

Context

John is a second-generation Italian American. His family of origin is large, warm, and supportive. However, John's parents believe that family problems should be dealt with in the family, and disapprove of bringing "strangers" in to hear what they consider to be private information. They believe that Anna's physical condition should be stabilized, and then she should be discharged to deal with family problems at home.

John and Nancy were reared in different social classes. In John's family, money was not available to seek out professional help for every problem that arose. Italian cultural beliefs promote the provision of help within the nuclear and extended family network. If outside counseling is sought, it is often with the family priest. John and Nancy did not seek this type of counseling because they no longer attend church regularly.

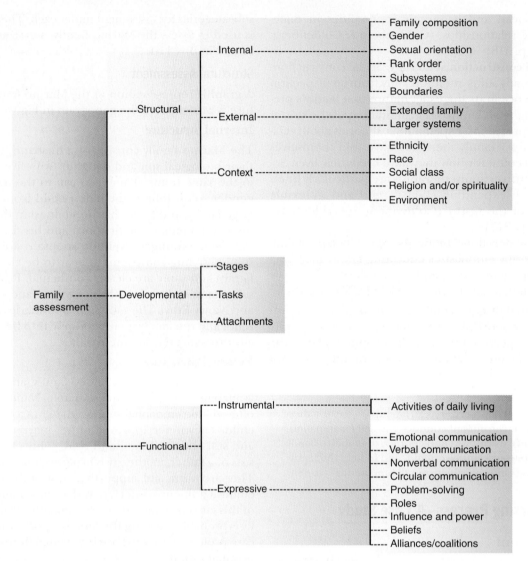

FIGURE 11–3 Branching diagram of the Calgary Family Assessment Model (CFAM). (From Wright, L. M., & Leahey, M. [2013]. *Nurses and families: A guide to family assessment and intervention* [6th ed.]. Philadelphia, PA: F.A. Davis Company, with permission.)

BOX 11-1 The Marino Family—A Case Study

John and Nancy Marino have been married for 19 years. They have a 17-year-old son, Peter, and a 15-year-old daughter, Anna. Anna was recently hospitalized for taking an overdose of fluoxetine, her mother's prescription antidepressant. The family is attending family therapy sessions while Anna is in the hospital. Anna states, "I just couldn't take the fighting anymore! Our house is an awful place to be. Everyone hates each other, and everyone is unhappy. Dad drinks too much and Mom is always sick! Peter stays away as much as he can and I don't blame him. I would too if I had someplace to stay. I just thought I'd be better off dead."

John Marino, age 44, is the oldest of five children. His father, Paulo, age 66, is a first-generation Italian American whose parents emigrated from Italy in the early 1900s. Paulo retired last year after 32 years as a cutter in a meatpacking plant. His wife, Carla, age 64, has never worked outside the home. John and his siblings all worked at minimum-wage jobs during high school, and John and his two brothers worked their way through college. His two sisters married young, and both are housewives and mothers. John was able to go to law school with the help of loans, grants, and scholarships. He has held several positions since graduation and is currently employed as a corporate attorney for a large aircraft company.

Nancy, age 43, is the only child of Sam and Ethyl Jones. Sam, age 67, inherited a great deal of money from his family who had been in the shipping business. He is currently the chief executive officer of this business. Ethyl, also 67, was an aspiring concert pianist when she met Sam. She chose to give up her career for marriage and family, although Nancy

BOX 11-1 The Marino Family—A Case Study—cont'd

believes her mother always resented doing so. Nancy was reared in an affluent lifestyle. She attended private boarding schools as she was growing up and chose an exclusive college in the East to pursue her interest in art. She studied in Paris during her junior year. Nancy states that she was never emotionally close to her parents. They traveled a great deal, and she spent much of her time under the supervision of a nanny.

Nancy's parents were opposed to her marrying John. They perceived John's family to be below their social status. Nancy, on the other hand, loved John's family. She felt them to be very warm and loving, so unlike what she was used to in her own family. Her family is Protestant and also disapproved of her marrying in the Roman Catholic Church.

FAMILY DYNAMICS

As their marriage progressed, Nancy's health became very fragile. She had continued her artistic pursuits but seemed to achieve little satisfaction from it. She tried to keep in touch with her parents but often felt spurned by them. They traveled a great deal and often did not even inform her of their whereabouts. They were not present at the birth of her children. She experiences many aches and pains and spends many days in bed. She sees several physicians, who have prescribed various pain medications, antianxiety agents, and antidepressants but can find nothing organically wrong. Five years ago she learned that John had been having an affair with his secretary. He promised to break it off and fired the

secretary, but Nancy has had difficulty trusting him since that time. She brings up his infidelity whenever they have an argument, which is more and more often lately. When he is home, John drinks, usually until he falls asleep. Peter frequently comes home smelling of alcohol and a number of times has been clearly intoxicated.

When Nancy called her parents to tell them that Anna was in the hospital, Ethyl replied, "I'm sorry to hear that, dear. We certainly never had any of those kinds of problems on our side of the family. But I'm sure everything will be okay now that you are getting help. Please give our love to your family. Your father and I are leaving for Europe on Saturday and will be gone for 6 weeks."

Although more supportive, John's parents view this situation as somewhat shameful for the family. John's dad responded, "We had hard times when you were growing up, but never like this. We always took care of our own problems. We never had to tell a bunch of strangers about them. It's not right to air your dirty laundry in public. Bring Anna home. Give her your love and she will be okay."

In therapy, Nancy blames John's drinking and his admitted affair for all their problems. John states that he drinks because it is the only way he can tolerate his wife's complaining about his behavior and her many illnesses. Peter is very quiet most of the time but says he will be glad when he graduates in 4 months and can leave "this looney bunch of people." Anna cries as she listens to her family in therapy and says, "Nothing's ever going to change."

In Nancy's family, money was available to obtain the very best professional help at the first sign of trouble. However, Nancy's parents refused to acknowledge, both then and now, that any difficulty ever existed in their family situation.

The Marino family lives comfortably on John's salary as a corporate attorney. They have health insurance and access to any referrals that are deemed necessary. They are well educated but have been attempting to deny the dysfunctional dynamics that exist in their family.

Developmental Assessment

The Marino family falls within the "family with adolescents" stage of McGoldrick and associates' family life cycle. In this stage, parents are expected to respond to adolescents' requests for increasing independence, while being available to continue to fulfill dependency needs. They may also be required to provide additional support to aging grandparents. This may be a time when parents may also begin to reexamine their own marital and career issues.

The Marino family is not fulfilling the dependency needs of its adolescents; in fact, they may be

establishing premature independence. The parents are absorbed in their own personal problems to the exclusion of their children. Peter responds to this neglect by staying away as much as possible, drinking with his friends, and planning to leave home at the first opportunity. Anna's attempted suicide is a cry for help. She has needs that are unfulfilled by her parents, and this crisis situation may be required for them to recognize that a problem exists. This may be the time when they begin to reexamine their unresolved marital issues. Extended family are still self-supporting and do not require assistance from John and Nancy at this time.

Functional Assessment

Instrumental Functioning

This family has managed to adjust to the maladaptive functioning in an effort to meet physical activities of daily living. They subsist on fast food, or sometimes Nancy or Anna will prepare a meal. Seldom do they sit down at table to eat together. Nancy must take pain medication or sedatives to sleep. John usually drinks himself to sleep. Anna and Peter take care of their own needs independently. Often they do not even see

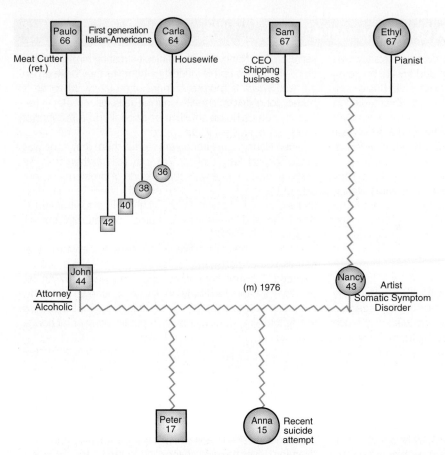

FIGURE 11-4 Genogram of the Marino family.

their parents in the evenings. Each manages to do fairly well in school. Peter says, "I don't intend to ruin my chances of getting out of this hell hole as soon as I can!"

Expressive Functioning

John and Nancy Marino argue a great deal about many topics. This family seldom shows affection to one another. Nancy and Anna express sadness with tears, whereas John and Peter have a tendency to withdraw or turn to alcohol when experiencing unhappiness. Nancy somaticizes her internal pain, and numbs this pain with medication. Anna internalized her emotional pain until it became unbearable. A notable lack of constructive communication is evident.

This family is unable to solve its problems effectively. In fact, it is unlikely that it has even identified its problems, which undoubtedly have been in existence for a long while. These problems have only recently been revealed in light of Anna's suicide attempt.

Diagnosis

The following nursing diagnoses were identified for the Marino family:

■ **Interrupted family processes** related to unsuccessful achievement of family developmental tasks and dysfunctional coping strategies evidenced by inability of family members to relate to each other in an adaptive manner; adolescents' unmet dependency needs; inability of family members to express a wide range of feelings and to send and receive clear messages.

■ **Disabled family coping** related to highly ambivalent family relationships and lack of support evidenced by inability to problem-solve; each member copes in response to dysfunctional family processes with destructive behavior (John drinks, Nancy somaticizes, Peter drinks and withdraws, and Anna attempts suicide).

Outcome Identification

The following criteria were identified as measurement of outcomes in counseling of the Marino family:

■ Family members will demonstrate effective communication patterns.

■ Family members will express feelings openly and honestly.

■ Family members will establish more adaptive coping strategies.

■ Family members will be able to identify destructive patterns of functioning and problem-solve them effectively.

■ Boundaries between spousal subsystems and spousal-children subsystems will become more clearly defined.

■ Family members will establish stronger bonds with extended family.

Planning/Implementation

The Marino family will undoubtedly require many months of outpatient therapy. It is even likely that each member will need individual psychotherapy in addition to the family therapy. Once Anna has been stabilized physiologically and is discharged from the hospital, family/individual therapy will begin.

Several strategies for family therapy have been discussed in this chapter. As mentioned previously, family therapy has a strong theoretical framework and is performed by individuals with specialized education in family theory and process. Some advanced practice nurses possess the credentials required to perform family therapy. It is important, however, for all nurses to have some knowledge about working with families, to be able to assess family interaction, and to recognize when problems exist.

Some interventions with the Marino family might include the following:

1. Create a therapeutic environment that fosters trust, and in which the family members can feel safe and comfortable. The nurse can promote this type of environment by being empathetic, listening actively (see Chapter 8), accepting feelings and attitudes, and being nonjudgmental.

2. Promote effective communication by
   a. Seeking clarification when vague and generalized statements are made (e.g., Anna states, "I just want my family to be like my friends' families." Nurse: "Anna, would you please explain to the group exactly what you mean by that?").
   b. Setting clear limits (e.g., "Peter, it is okay to state when you are angry about something that has been said. It is not okay to throw the chair against the wall.").
   c. Being consistent and fair (e.g., "I encourage each of you to contribute to the group process and to respect one another's opportunity to contribute equally.").
   d. Addressing each individual clearly and directly and encouraging family members to do the same (e.g., "Nancy, I think it would be more appropriate if you directed that statement to John instead of to me.").

3. Identify patterns of interaction that interfere with successful problem resolution. For example, John asks Nancy many "Why?" questions that keep her on the defensive. He criticizes her for "always being sick." Nancy responds by frequently reminding John of his infidelity. Peter and Anna interrupt each other and their parents when the level of conflict reaches a certain point. Provide examples of more appropriate ways to communicate that can improve interpersonal relations and lead to more effective patterns of interaction.

4. Help the Marino family to identify problems that may necessitate change. Encourage each member to discuss a family process that he or she would like to change. As a group, promote discussion of what must take place for change to occur and allow each member to explore whether he or she could realistically cooperate with the necessary requirements for change.

5. As the problem-solving process progresses, encourage all family members to express honest feelings. Address each one directly, "John (Nancy, Peter, Anna), how do you feel about what the others are suggesting?" Ensure that all participants understand that each member may express honest feelings (e.g., anger, sadness, fear, anxiety, guilt, disgust, helplessness) without criticism, judgment, or fear of personal reprisal.

6. Avoid becoming triangled in the family emotional system. Remain neutral and objective. Do not take sides in family disagreements; instead, provide alternative explanations and suggestions (e.g., "Perhaps we can look at that situation in a different light . . .").

7. Reframe vague problem descriptions into ones for which resolution is more realistic. For example, rather than defining the problem as "We don't love each other any more," the problem could be defined as "We do not spend time together in family activities any more." This definition evolves from the family members' description of what they mean by the more general problem description.

8. Discuss present coping strategies. Encourage each family member to describe how he or she copes with stress and with the adversity within the family. Explore each member's possible contribution to the family's problems. Encourage family members to discuss possible solutions among themselves.

9. Identify community resources that may assist individual family members and provide support for establishing more adaptive coping mechanisms. For example, Alcoholics Anonymous for John; Al-Anon for Nancy; and Alateen for Peter and Anna. Other groups that may be of assistance to this family include Emotions Anonymous, Parent's Support Group, Families Helping Families, Marriage Enrichment, Parents of Teenagers, and We Saved Our Marriage (WESOM). Local self-help networks often provide a directory of resources within specific communities.

10. Discuss with the family the possible need for psychotherapy for individual members. Provide names of therapists who would perform assessments to determine individual needs. Encourage follow-through with appointments.

11. Assist family members in planning leisure time activities together. This could include time to play together, exercise together, or engage in a shared project.

Evaluation

Evaluation is the final step in the nursing process. In this step, progress toward attainment of outcomes is measured.

1. Do family members demonstrate effective patterns of communication?

2. Can family members express feelings openly and honestly without fear of reprisal?

3. Can family members accept their own personal contribution to the family's problems?

4. Can individual members identify maladaptive coping methods and express a desire to improve?

5. Do family members work together to solve problems?

6. Can family members identify resources in the community from which they can seek assistance and support?

7. Do family members express a desire to form stronger bonds with the extended family?

8. Are family members willing to seek individual psychotherapy?

9. Are family members pursuing shared activities?

Summary and Key Points

■ Nurses must have sufficient knowledge of family functioning to assess family interaction and recognize when problems exist.

■ McGoldrick, Carter, and Garcia-Preto (2011) identify stages that describe the family life cycle. They include the following:
  ■ The single young adult
  ■ The family joined through marriage/union
  ■ The family with young children

■ The family with adolescents
■ The family launching children and moving on in midlife
■ The family in later life (late middle age to end of life)

■ Tasks of families experiencing divorce and remarriage, and those that vary according to cultural norms were also presented.

■ Families are assessed as functional or dysfunctional based on the following six elements: communication, self-concept reinforcement, family members' expectations, handling differences, family interactional patterns, and family climate.

■ Bowen viewed the family as a system that was composed of various subsystems. His theoretical approach to family therapy includes eight major concepts: differentiation of self, triangles, nuclear family emotional process, family projection process, multigenerational transmission process, sibling position, emotional cutoff, and societal emotional process.

■ In the structural model of family therapy, the family is viewed as a social system within which the individual lives and to which the individual must adapt.

■ In the strategic model of family therapy, communication is viewed as the foundation of functioning. Functional families are open systems where clear and precise messages are sent and received. Dysfunctional families are viewed as partially closed systems in which communication is vague, and messages are often inconsistent and incongruent with the situation.

■ Many family therapists today follow an eclectic approach and incorporate concepts from several models into their practices.

■ The nursing process is used as a framework for assessing, diagnosing, planning, implementing, and evaluating care to families who require assistance to maintain or regain adaptive functioning.

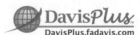 **DavisPlus** DavisPlus.fadavis.com Additional info available at www.davisplus.com

Review Questions
Self-Examination/Learning Exercise

*Select the answer that is **most** appropriate for each of the following questions.*

1. The nurse-therapist is counseling the Smith family: Mr. and Mrs. Smith, 10-year-old Rob, and 8-year-old Lisa. When Mr. and Mrs. Smith start to argue, Rob hits Lisa and Lisa starts to cry. The Smiths then turn their attention to comforting Lisa and scolding Rob, complaining that he is "out of control and we don't know what to do about his behavior." These dynamics are an example of which of the following?
   a. Double-bind messages
   b. Triangulation
   c. Pseudohostility
   d. Multigenerational transmission

2. Using Bowen's systems approach with a family in therapy, the therapist would:
   a. Try to change family principles that may be promoting dysfunctional behavior patterns.
   b. Strive to create change in destructive behavior through improvement in communication and interaction patterns.
   c. Encourage increase in the differentiation of individual family members.
   d. Promote change in dysfunctional behavior by encouraging the formation of more diffuse boundaries between family members.

3. Using the structural approach with a family in therapy, the therapist would:
   a. Try to change family principles that may be promoting dysfunctional behavior patterns.
   b. Strive to create change in destructive behavior through improvement in communications and interaction patterns.
   c. Encourage increase in the differentiation of individual family members.
   d. Promote change in dysfunctional behavior by encouraging the formation of more diffuse boundaries between family members.

4. Using the strategic approach with a family in therapy, the therapist would:
   a. Try to change family principles that may be promoting dysfunctional behavior patterns.
   b. Strive to create change in destructive behavior through improvement in communication and interaction patterns.
   c. Encourage increase in the differentiation of individual family members.
   d. Promote change in dysfunctional behavior by encouraging the formation of more diffuse boundaries between family members.

5. Carol, a nurse in a family medicine outpatient clinic, conducts initial interviews when new families are referred. She has just finished interviewing a mother who has come to the clinic with her three children, ages 5, 7, and 11. The mother says to the oldest child, "You have been such a help to me, playing with your brothers while I talk to the nurse." In assessing family interaction, the nurse recognizes this statement as a direct indicator of which of the following?
   a. Family climate
   b. Family members' expectations
   c. Handling differences
   d. Self-concept reinforcement

6. The intermittent exiting and entering of various family members and reestablishing of the bond of the dyadic marital relationship are characteristics associated with which stage of family development?
   a. The newly married couple
   b. The family with adolescents
   c. The family launching grown children
   d. The family in later life

Continued

Review Questions—cont'd
Self-Examination/Learning Exercise

7. The nurse psychotherapist is working with the Jones family in the outpatient mental health clinic. The husband says, "We can't agree on anything! And it seems like every time we disagree on something it ends up in a screaming match." Which of the following prescriptions by the nurse represents a paradoxical intervention for the Jones family?
   a. Mr. and Mrs. Jones must not have a disagreement for one full day.
   b. Mr. and Mrs. Jones will yell at each other on Tuesdays and Thursdays from 8 p.m. until 8:10 p.m.
   c. Mr. and Mrs. Jones must refrain from yelling at each other until the next counseling session.
   d. Mr. and Mrs. Jones must not discuss serious issues until they can do so without yelling at each other.

8. Mr. and Mrs. Jones have been married for 21 years. Mr. Jones is the family breadwinner, and Mrs. Jones has never worked outside the home. Mr. Jones has always made all the decisions for the family and Mrs. Jones has always been compliant. According to the strategic model of family therapy, this is an example of which of the following?
   a. Marital schism
   b. Pseudomutuality
   c. Marital skew
   d. Pseudohostility

9. Jack and Ann have come to the clinic for family therapy. They have been married for 18 years. Jack had an affair with his secretary 5 years ago. He fired the secretary and assures Ann and the nurse that he has been faithful ever since. Jack tells the nurse, "We have never been able to get along with each other. We can't talk about anything . . . all we do is shout at each other. And every time she gets angry with me, she brings up my infidelity. I can't even imagine how many times each of us has threatened divorce over the years. Our kids don't have any idea what it is like to have parents who get along with each other. I've really had enough!" The nurse would most likely document which of the following in her assessment of this couple?
   a. Marital skew
   b. Pseudohostility
   c. Double-bind communication
   d. Marital schism

10. Mr. and Mrs. Smith and their three children (ages 5, 8, and 10) are in therapy with the nurse psychotherapist. Mrs. Smith tells the nurse that their marriage has been "falling apart" since the birth of their youngest child, Tom. She explains that they "did not want a third child, and I became pregnant even after my husband had undergone a vasectomy. We were very angry, the pregnancy was a problematic one, and the child has been difficult since birth. We had problems before he was born, but since Tom was born, things have gone from bad to worse. No one can control him, and he is wrecking our family!" The nurse assesses that which of the following may be occurring in this family?
   a. Scapegoating
   b. Triangling
   c. Disengagement
   d. Enmeshment

References

Boyer, P.A., & Jeffrey, R.J. (1994). *A guide for the family therapist.* Northvale, NJ: Jason Aronson.

Centers for Disease Control (CDC). (2012). First marriages in the United States: Data from the 2006-2010 National Survey of Family Growth. U.S. Department of Health and Human Services. *National Health Statistics Reports, 49* (March 22, 2012).

Cory, T.L. (2013). Second marriages—think before you leap. *Health-Scope Magazine.* Retrieved from http://www.healthscopemag.com/Second_Marriages.aspx

Earp, J.B.K. (2013). Korean Americans. In J.N. Giger (Ed.), *Transcultural nursing: Assessment and Intervention* (6th ed., pp. 531-550). St. Louis, MO: Mosby.

Georgetown Family Center. (2013a). Bowen theory: Differentiation of self. Retrieved from http://www.thebowencenter.org/pages/conceptds.html

Georgetown Family Center. (2013b). Bowen theory: Societal emotional process. Retrieved from http://www.thebowencenter.org/pages/conceptsep.html

Goldenberg, I., & Goldenberg, H. (2013). *Family therapy: An overview* (8th ed.). Belmont, CA: Brooks/Cole.

Goldenberg, I., Goldenberg, H., & Pelavin, E.G. (2011). Family therapy. In R.J. Corsini & D. Wedding (Eds.), *Current Psychotherapies* (9th ed., 417–453). Belmont, CA: Brooks/Cole.

Kaakinen, J.R., Hanson, S.M.H., & Denham, S.A. (2010). Family health care nursing: An introduction. In J.R. Kaakinen, V. Gedaly-Duff, D.P. Coehlo, & S.M.H. Hanson (Eds.), *Family health care nursing* (4th ed., pp. 3–33). Philadelphia, PA: F.A. Davis.

Kreider, R.M., & Ellis, R. (2011). *Living arrangements of children: 2009.* Current Population Reports, p. 70–126. Washington, DC: U.S. Census Bureau.

Leman, K. (2009). *The birth order book: Why you are the way you are.* Grand Rapids, MI: Revell.

McGoldrick, M., Carter, B., & Garcia-Preto, N. (2011). *The expanded family life cycle: Individual, family, and social perspectives* (4th ed.). Boston, MA: Allyn & Bacon.

Nichols, M.P. (2010). *Family therapy: Concepts and methods* (9th ed.). Boston, MA: Allyn and Bacon.

Purnell, L.D. (2013). The Purnell model for cultural competence. In L.D. Purnell (Ed.), *Transcultural health care: A culturally competent approach* (4th ed., pp. 15–44). Philadelphia, PA: F.A. Davis.

Tomm, K., & Sanders, G. (1983). Family assessment in a problem oriented record. In J.C. Hansen & B.F. Keeney (Eds.), *Diagnosis and assessment in family therapy.* London: Aspen Systems.

U.S. Catholic Church. (2006). *Compendium of the Catechism of the Catholic Church.* Washington, DC: USCCB Publishing.

U.S. Census Bureau. (2013). *Statistical abstract of the United States: 2012.* Retrieved from http://www.census.gov/compendia/statab/2012/tables/12s1337.pdf

Valley, E. (2005). The changing nature of the Jewish family. *Contact: The Journal of Jewish Life Network, 7*(3), 1–16.

Wright, L.M., and Leahey, M. (2013). *Nurses and families: A guide to family assessment and intervention* (6th ed.). Philadelphia, PA: F.A. Davis.

Xu, Y., & Chang, K. (2013). Chinese Americans. In J.N. Giger (Ed.), *Transcultural nursing: Assessment and Intervention* (6th ed., pp. 383–402). St. Louis, MO: Mosby.

Classical References

Bowen, M. (1971). The use of family theory in clinical practice. In J. Haley (Ed.), *Changing families.* New York, NY: Grune & Stratton.

Bowen, M. (1976). Theory in the practice of psychotherapy. In P. Guerin (Ed.), *Family therapy: Theory and practice.* New York, NY: Gardner Press.

Bowen, M. (1978). *Family therapy in clinical practice.* New York, NY: Jason Aronson.

Lidz, T., Cornelison, A., Fleck, S., & Terry, D. (1957). The intrafamilial environment of schizophrenic patients: II. Marital schism and marital skew. *American Journal of Psychiatry, 114,* 241–248.

Minuchin, S. (1974). *Families and family therapy.* Cambridge, MA: Harvard University Press.

12 Milieu Therapy—The Therapeutic Community

OBJECTIVES
After reading this chapter, the student will be able to:

1. Define *milieu therapy*.
2. Explain the goal of therapeutic community/milieu therapy.
3. Identify seven basic assumptions of a therapeutic community.
4. Discuss conditions that characterize a therapeutic community.
5. Identify the various therapies that may be included within the program of the therapeutic community and the health-care workers that make up the interdisciplinary treatment team.
6. Describe the role of the nurse on the interdisciplinary treatment team.

HOMEWORK ASSIGNMENT
Please read the chapter and answer the following questions:

1. How are unit rules established in a therapeutic community setting?
2. Which member of the interdisciplinary treatment team has a focus on rehabilitation and vocational training?
3. How are client responsibilities assigned in the therapeutic community setting?
4. Which member of the interdisciplinary treatment team serves as leader?

Standard 5c of the *Psychiatric-Mental Health Nursing: Scope and Standards of Practice* (American Nurses Association [ANA], 2007) states: "The psychiatric-mental health nurse provides, structures, and maintains a safe and therapeutic environment in collaboration with patients, families, and other health care clinicians" (p. 39).

This chapter defines and explains the goal of milieu therapy. The conditions necessary for a therapeutic environment are discussed, and the roles of the various health-care workers within the interdisciplinary team are delineated. An interpretation of the nurse's role in milieu therapy is included.

Milieu, Defined

The word **milieu** is French for "middle." The English translation of the word is "surroundings, or environment." In psychiatry, therapy involving the milieu, or environment, may be called milieu therapy, **therapeutic community**, or the therapeutic environment. The goal of milieu therapy is to manipulate the environment so that all aspects of the client's hospital experience are considered therapeutic. Within this therapeutic community setting the client is expected to learn adaptive coping, interaction, and relationship skills that can be generalized to other aspects of his or her life.

▌ CORE CONCEPTS

Milieu Therapy
A scientific structuring of the environment in order to effect behavioral changes and to improve the psychological health and functioning of the individual (Skinner, 1979).

Current Status of the Therapeutic Community

Milieu therapy came into its own during the 1960s through early 1980s. During this period, psychiatric inpatient treatment provided sufficient time to implement programs of therapy that were aimed at social rehabilitation. Nursing's focus of establishing interpersonal relationships with clients fit well within this concept of therapy. Patients were encouraged to be active participants in their therapy, and individual autonomy was emphasized.

The current focus of inpatient psychiatric care has changed. Hall (1995) stated:

> Care in inpatient psychiatric facilities can now be characterized as short and biologically based. By the time patients have stabilized enough to benefit from the socialization that would take place in a milieu as treatment program, they [often] have been discharged. (p. 51)

Although strategies for milieu therapy are still used, they have been modified to conform to the short-term approach to care or to outpatient treatment programs. Some programs (e.g., those for children and adolescents, clients with substance addictions, and geriatric clients) have successfully adapted the concepts of milieu treatment to their specialty needs (Bowler, 1991; DeSocio, Bowllan, & Staschak, 1997; Jani & Fishman, 2004; Menninger Clinic, 2012; Whall, 1991).

Echternacht (2001) suggested that more emphasis should be placed on unstructured components of milieu therapy. She described the unstructured components as a multitude of complex interactions between clients, staff, and visitors that occur around the clock. Echternacht called these interactions "fluid group work." They involve spontaneous opportunities within the milieu environment for the psychiatric nurse to provide "on-the-spot therapeutic interventions designed to enhance socialization competency and interpersonal relationship awareness. Emphasis is on social skills and activities in the context of interpersonal interactions" (p. 40). With fluid group work, the nurse applies psychotherapeutic knowledge and skills to brief clinical encounters that occur spontaneously in the therapeutic milieu setting. Echternacht (2001) believes that by using these techniques, nurses can "reclaim their milieu therapy functions in the midst of a changing health care environment" (p. 40).

Many of the original concepts of milieu therapy are presented in this chapter. It is important to remember that a number of modifications to these concepts have been applied in practice for use in a variety of settings.

Basic Assumptions

Skinner (1979) outlined seven basic assumptions on which a therapeutic community is based:

1. **The Health in Each Individual Is to be Realized and Encouraged to Grow.** All individuals are considered to have strengths as well as limitations. These healthy aspects of the individual are identified and serve as a foundation for growth in the personality and in the ability to function more adaptively and productively in all aspects of life.
2. **Every Interaction Is an Opportunity for Therapeutic Intervention.** Within this structured setting, it is virtually impossible to avoid interpersonal interaction. The ideal situation exists for clients to improve communication and relationship development skills. Learning occurs from immediate feedback of personal perceptions.
3. **The Client Owns His or Her Own Environment.** Clients make decisions and solve problems related to government of the unit. In this way, personal needs for autonomy as well as needs that pertain to the group as a whole are fulfilled.
4. **Each Client Owns His or Her Behavior.** Each individual within the therapeutic community is expected to take responsibility for his or her own behavior.
5. **Peer Pressure is a Useful and a Powerful Tool.** Behavioral group norms are established through peer pressure. Feedback is direct and frequent, so

that behaving in a manner acceptable to the other members of the community becomes essential.

6. **Inappropriate Behaviors Are Dealt With as They Occur.** Individuals examine the significance of their behavior, look at how it affects other people, and discuss more appropriate ways of behaving in certain situations.

7. **Restrictions and Punishment Are to Be Avoided.** Destructive behaviors can usually be controlled with group discussion. However, if an individual requires external controls, temporary isolation is preferred over lengthy restriction or other harsh consequences.

Conditions That Promote a Therapeutic Community

In a therapeutic community setting, everything that happens to the client, or within the client's environment, is considered to be part of the treatment program. The community setting is the foundation for the program of treatment. Community factors—such as social interactions, the physical structure of the treatment setting, and schedule of activities—may generate negative responses from some clients. These stressful experiences are used as examples to help the client learn how to manage stress more adaptively in real-life situations.

Under what conditions, then, is a hospital environment considered therapeutic? A number of criteria have been identified:

1. **Basic Physiological Needs Are Fulfilled.** As Maslow (1968) suggested, individuals do not move to higher levels of functioning until the basic biological needs for food, water, air, sleep, exercise, elimination, shelter, and sexual expression have been met.

2. **The Physical Facilities Are Conducive to Achievement of the Goals of Therapy.** Space is provided so that each client has sufficient privacy, as well as physical space, for therapeutic interaction with others. Furnishings are arranged to present a homelike atmosphere—usually in spaces that accommodate communal living, dining, and activity areas—for facilitation of interpersonal interaction and communication.

3. **A Democratic Form of Self-Government Exists.** In the therapeutic community, clients participate in the decision-making and problem-solving that affect the management of the treatment setting. This is accomplished through regularly scheduled community meetings. These meetings are attended by staff and clients, and all individuals have equal input into the discussions. At these meetings, the norms and rules and behavioral limits of the treatment setting are set forth. This reinforces the democratic posture of the

treatment setting, because these are expectations that affect all clients on an equal basis. An example might be the rule that no client may enter a room being occupied by a client of the opposite gender. Consequences of violating the rules are explained.

Other issues that may be discussed at the community meetings include those with which certain clients have some disagreements. A decision is then made by the entire group in a democratic manner. For example, several clients in an inpatient unit may disagree with the hours that have been designated for watching television on a weekend night. They may elect to bring up this issue at a community meeting and suggest an extension in television-viewing time. After discussion by the group, a vote will be taken, and clients and staff agree to abide by the expressed preference of the majority. Some therapeutic communities elect officers (usually a president and a secretary) who serve for a specified time. The president calls the meeting to order, conducts the business of discussing old and new issues, and asks for volunteers (or makes appointments, alternately, so that all clients have a turn) to accomplish the daily tasks associated with community living; for example, cleaning the tables after each meal and watering plants in the treatment facility. New assignments are made at each meeting. The secretary reads the minutes of the previous meeting and takes minutes of the current meeting. Minutes are important in the event that clients have a disagreement about issues that were discussed at various meetings. Minutes provide written evidence of decisions made by the group. In treatment settings where clients have short attention spans or disorganized thinking, meetings are brief. Business is generally limited to introductions and expectations of the here and now. Discussions also may include comments about a recent occurrence in the group or something that has been bothering a person and about which he or she has some questions. These meetings are usually conducted by staff, although all clients have equal input into the discussions.

All clients are expected to attend the meetings. Exceptions are made when aspects of an individual's therapy interfere or take precedence. An explanation is made to clients present so that false perceptions of danger are not generated by another person's absence. All staff members are expected to attend the meetings, unless client care precludes their attendance.

4. **Responsibilities Are Assigned According to Client Capabilities.** Increasing self-esteem is an ultimate goal of the therapeutic community. Therefore, a client should not be set up for failure by being assigned a responsibility that is beyond his or her level of ability. By assigning clients responsibilities that promote achievement, self-esteem is enhanced. Consideration must also be given to times

during which the client will show some regression in the treatment regimen. Adjustments in assignments should be made in a way that preserves self-esteem and provides for progression to greater degrees of responsibility as the client returns to previous level of functioning.

5. **A Structured Program of Social and Work-Related Activities Is Scheduled as Part of the Treatment Program.** Each client's therapeutic program consists of group activities in which interpersonal interaction and communication with other individuals are emphasized. Time is also devoted to personal problems. Various group activities may be selected for clients with specific needs (e.g., an exercise group for a person who expresses anger inappropriately, an assertiveness group for a person who is passive-aggressive, or a stress-management group for a person who is anxious). A structured schedule of activities is the major focus of a therapeutic community. Through these activities, change in the client's personality and behavior can be achieved. New coping strategies are learned and social skills are developed. In the group situation, the client is able to practice what he or she has learned to prepare for transition to the general community.

6. **Community and Family Are Included in the Program of Therapy in an Effort to Facilitate Discharge from Treatment.** An attempt is made to include family members, as well as certain aspects of the community that affect the client, in the treatment program. It is important to keep as many links to the client's life outside of therapy as possible. Family members are invited to participate in specific therapy groups and, in some instances, to share meals with the client in the communal dining room. Connection with community life may be maintained through client group activities, such as shopping, picnicking, attending movies, bowling, and visiting the zoo. Inpatient clients may be awarded passes to visit family or may participate in work-related activities, the length of time being determined by the activity and the client's condition. These connections with family and community facilitate the discharge process and may help to prevent the client from becoming too dependent on the therapy.

The Program of Therapeutic Community

Care for clients in the therapeutic community is directed by an interdisciplinary treatment (IDT) team. An initial assessment is made by the admitting psychiatrist, nurse, or other designated admitting agent who establishes a priority of care. The IDT team determines a comprehensive treatment plan and goals of therapy and assigns intervention responsibilities. All members sign the treatment plan and meet regularly to update the plan as needed. Depending on the size of the treatment facility and scope of the therapy program, members representing a variety of disciplines may participate in the promotion of a therapeutic community. For example, an IDT team may include a psychiatrist, clinical psychologist, psychiatric clinical nurse specialist, psychiatric nurse, mental health technician, psychiatric social worker, occupational therapist, recreational therapist, art therapist, music therapist, psychodramatist, dietitian, and chaplain. Table 12-1 provides an explanation of responsibilities and educational preparation required for these members of the IDT team.

TABLE 12–1	**The Interdisciplinary Treatment Team in Psychiatry**	
TEAM MEMBER	**RESPONSIBILITIES**	**CREDENTIALS**
Psychiatrist	Serves as the leader of the team. Responsible for diagnosis and treatment of mental disorders. Performs psychotherapy; prescribes medication and other somatic therapies.	Medical degree with residency in psychiatry and license to practice medicine.
Clinical psychologist	Conducts individual, group, and family therapy. Administers, interprets, and evaluates psychological tests that assist in the diagnostic process.	Doctorate in clinical psychology with 2- to 3-year internship supervised by a licensed clinical psychologist. State license is required to practice.
Psychiatric clinical nurse specialist	Conducts individual, group, and family therapy. Presents educational programs for nursing staff. Provides consultation services to nurses who require assistance in the planning and implementation of care for individual clients.	Registered nurse with minimum of a master's degree in psychiatric nursing. Some institutions require certification by national credentialing association.
Psychiatric nurse	Provides ongoing assessment of client condition, both mentally and physically. Manages the therapeutic milieu on a 24-hour basis. Administers medications. Assists clients with all therapeutic activities as required. Focus is on one-to-one relationship development.	Registered nurse with hospital diploma, associate degree, or baccalaureate degree. Some psychiatric nurses have national certification.

Continued

TABLE 12–1 The Interdisciplinary Treatment Team in Psychiatry–cont'd

TEAM MEMBER	RESPONSIBILITIES	CREDENTIALS
Mental health technician (also called psychiatric aide or assistant or psychiatric technician)	Functions under the supervision of the psychiatric nurse. Provides assistance to clients in the fulfillment of their activities of daily living. Assists activity therapists as required in conducting their groups. May also participate in one-to-one relationship development.	Varies from state to state. Requirements include high school education, with additional vocational education or on-the-job training. Some hospitals hire individuals with a baccalaureate degree in psychology in this capacity. Some states require a licensure examination to practice.
Psychiatric social worker	Conducts individual, group, and family therapy. Is concerned with client's social needs, such as placement, financial support, and community requirements. Conducts in-depth psychosocial history on which the needs assessment is based. Works with client and family to ensure that requirements for discharge are fulfilled and needs can be met by appropriate community resources.	Minimum of a master's degree in social work. Some states require additional supervision and subsequent licensure by examination.
Occupational therapist	Works with clients to help develop (or redevelop) independence in performance of activities of daily living. Focus is on rehabilitation and vocational training in which clients learn to be productive, thereby enhancing self-esteem. Creative activities and therapeutic relationship skills are used.	Baccalaureate or master's degree in occupational therapy.
Recreational therapist	Uses recreational activities to promote clients to redirect their thinking or to rechannel destructive energy in an appropriate manner. Clients learn skills that can be used during leisure time and during times of stress following discharge from treatment. Examples include bowling, volleyball, exercises, and jogging. Some programs include activities such as picnics, swimming, and even group attendance at the state fair when it is in session.	Baccalaureate or master's degree in recreational therapy.
Music therapist	Encourages clients in self-expression through music. Clients listen to music, play instruments, sing, dance, and compose songs that help them get in touch with feelings and emotions that they may not be able to experience in any other way.	Graduate degree with specialty in music therapy.
Art therapist	Uses the client's creative abilities to encourage expression of emotions and feelings through artwork. Helps clients to analyze their own work in an effort to recognize and resolve underlying conflict.	Graduate degree with specialty in art therapy.
Psychodramatist	Directs clients in the creation of a "drama" that portrays real-life situations. Individuals select problems they wish to enact, and other clients play the roles of significant others in the situations. Some clients are able to "act out" problems that they are unable to work through in a more traditional manner. All members benefit through intensive discussion that follows.	Graduate degree in psychology, social work, nursing, or medicine with additional training in group therapy and specialty preparation to become a psychodramatist.
Dietitian	Plans nutritious meals for all clients. Consults with clients with specific eating disorders, such as anorexia nervosa, bulimia nervosa, obesity, and pica.	Baccalaureate or master's degree with specialty in dietetics.
Chaplain	Assesses, identifies, and attends to the spiritual needs of clients and their family members. Provides spiritual support and comfort as requested by client or family. May provide counseling if educational background includes this type of preparation.	College degree with advanced education in theology, seminary, or rabbinical studies.

The Role of the Nurse in Milieu Therapy

Milieu therapy can take place in a variety of inpatient and outpatient settings. In the hospital, nurses are generally the only members of the IDT team who spend time with the clients on a 24-hour basis, and they assume responsibility for management of the therapeutic milieu. In all settings, the nursing process is used for the delivery of nursing care. Ongoing assessment, diagnosis, outcome identification, planning, implementation, and evaluation of the environment are necessary for the successful management of a therapeutic milieu. Nurses are involved in all day-to-day activities that pertain to client care. Suggestions and opinions of nursing staff are given serious consideration in the planning of care for individual clients. Information from the initial nursing assessment is used to create the IDT plan. Nurses have input into therapy goals and participate in the regular updates and modification of treatment plans.

In some treatment facilities, a separate nursing care plan is required in addition to the IDT plan. When this is the case, the nursing care plan must reflect diagnoses that are specific to nursing and include problems and interventions from the IDT plan that have been assigned specifically to the discipline of nursing.

In the therapeutic milieu, nurses are responsible for ensuring that clients' physiological needs are met. Clients must be encouraged to perform as independently as possible in fulfilling activities of daily living. However, the nurse must make ongoing assessments to provide assistance for those who require it. Assessing physical status is an important nursing responsibility that must not be overlooked in a psychiatric setting that emphasizes holistic care.

Reality orientation for clients who have disorganized thinking or who are disoriented or confused is important in the therapeutic milieu. Clocks with large hands and numbers, calendars that give the day and date in large print, and orientation boards that discuss daily activities and news happenings can help keep clients oriented to reality. Nurses should ensure that clients have written schedules of activities to which they are assigned and that they arrive at those activities on schedule. Some clients may require an identification sign on their door to remind them which room is theirs. On short-term units, nurses who are dealing with psychotic clients usually rely on a basic activity or topic that helps keep people oriented: for example, showing pictures of the hospital where they are housed, introducing people who were admitted during the night, and providing name badges with their first name.

Nurses are responsible for the management of medication administration on inpatient psychiatric units. In some treatment programs, clients are expected to accept the responsibility and request their medication at the appropriate time. Although ultimate responsibility lies with the nurse, he or she must encourage clients to be self-reliant. Nurses must work with the clients to determine methods that result in achievement and provide positive feedback for successes.

A major focus of nursing in the therapeutic milieu is the one-to-one relationship that grows out of a developing trust between client and nurse. Many clients with psychiatric disorders have never achieved the ability to trust. If this can be accomplished in a relationship with the nurse, the trust may be generalized to other relationships in the client's life. Within an atmosphere of trust, the client is encouraged to express feelings and emotions and to discuss unresolved issues that are creating problems in his or her life.

CLINICAL PEARL

Developing trust means keeping promises that have been made. It means total acceptance of the individual as a person, separate from behavior that is unacceptable. It means responding to the client with concrete behaviors that are understandable to him or her (e.g., "If you are frightened, I will stay with you"; "If you are cold, I will bring you a blanket"; "If you are thirsty, I will bring you a drink of water").

The nurse is responsible for setting limits on unacceptable behavior in the therapeutic milieu. This requires stating to the client in understandable terminology what behaviors are not acceptable and what the consequences will be should the limits be violated. These limits must be established, written, and carried out by all staff. Consistency in carrying out the consequences of violation of the established limits is essential if the learning is to be reinforced.

The role of client teacher is important in the psychiatric area, as it is in all areas of nursing. Nurses must be able to assess learning readiness in individual clients. Do they want to learn? What is their level of anxiety? What is their level of ability to understand the information being presented? Topics for client education in psychiatry include information about medical diagnoses, side effects of medications, the importance of continuing to take medications, and stress management, among others. Some topics must be individualized for specific clients, whereas others may be taught in group situations. Table 12-2 outlines various topics of nursing concern for client education in psychiatry. (Sample client teaching guides may be found at www.DavisPlus.com.)

Echternacht (2001) stated:

Milieu therapy interventions are recognized as one of the basic-level functions of psychiatric-mental health nurses as addressed [in the *Psychiatric-Mental Health*

TABLE 12-2 The Therapeutic Milieu—Topics for Client Education

1. Ways to increase self-esteem

2. Ways to deal with anger appropriately

3. Stress-management techniques

4. How to recognize signs of increasing anxiety and intervene to stop progression

5. Normal stages of grieving and behaviors associated with each stage

6. Assertiveness techniques

7. Relaxation techniques
   a. Progressive relaxation
   b. Tense and relax
   c. Deep breathing
   d. Mental imagery

8. Medications (specify)
   a. Reason for taking
   b. Harmless side effects
   c. Side effects to report to physician
   d. Importance of taking regularly
   e. Importance of not stopping abruptly

9. Effects of (substance) on the body
   a. Alcohol
   b. Other depressants
   c. Stimulants
   d. Hallucinogens
   e. Narcotics
   f. Cannabinoids

10. Problem-solving skills

11. Thought-stopping/thought-switching techniques

12. Sex education
    a. Structure and function of reproductive system
    b. Contraceptives
    c. Sexually transmitted diseases

13. The essentials of good nutrition

14. (For parents/guardians)
    a. Signs and symptoms of substance abuse
    b. Effective parenting techniques

Nursing: Scope and Standards of Practice, (ANA, 2007)]. Milieu therapy has been described as an excellent framework for operationalizing [Hildegard] Peplau's interpretation and extension of Harry Stack Sullivan's Interpersonal Theory for use in nursing practice. (p. 39)

Now is the time to rekindle interest in the therapeutic milieu concept and to reclaim nursing's traditional milieu intervention functions. Nurses need to identify the number of registered nurses necessary to carry out structured and unstructured milieu functions consistent with their Standards of Practice. (p. 43)

Summary and Key Points

■ In psychiatry, milieu therapy (or a therapeutic community) constitutes a manipulation of the environment in an effort to create behavioral changes and to improve the psychological health and functioning of the individual.

■ The goal of therapeutic community is for the client to learn adaptive coping, interaction, and relationship skills that can be generalized to other aspects of his or her life.

■ The community environment itself serves as the primary tool of therapy.

■ According to Skinner (1979), a therapeutic community is based on seven basic assumptions:
   ■ The health in each individual is to be realized and encouraged to grow.
   ■ Every interaction is an opportunity for therapeutic intervention.
   ■ The client owns his or her own environment.
   ■ Each client owns his or her behavior.
   ■ Peer pressure is a useful and a powerful tool.
   ■ Inappropriate behaviors are dealt with as they occur.
   ■ Restrictions and punishment are to be avoided.

■ Because the goals of milieu therapy relate to helping the client learn to generalize that which is learned to other aspects of his or her life, the conditions that promote a therapeutic community in the psychiatric setting are similar to the types of conditions that exist in real-life situations.

■ Conditions that promote a therapeutic community include the following:
   ■ The fulfillment of basic physiological needs.
   ■ Physical facilities that are conducive to achievement of the goals of therapy.
   ■ The existence of a democratic form of self-government.
   ■ The assignment of responsibilities according to client capabilities.
   ■ A structured program of social and work-related activities.
   ■ The inclusion of community and family in the program of therapy in an effort to facilitate discharge from treatment.

■ The program of therapy on the milieu unit is conducted by the IDT team.

■ The team includes some, or all, of the following disciplines and may include others that are not specified here: psychiatrist, clinical psychologist, psychiatric clinical nurse specialist, psychiatric nurse, mental health technician, psychiatric social worker, occupational therapist, recreational therapist, art therapist, music therapist, psychodramatist, dietitian, and chaplain.

■ Nurses play a crucial role in the management of a therapeutic milieu. They are involved in the assessment, diagnosis, outcome identification, planning, implementation, and evaluation of all treatment programs.

■ Nurses have significant input into the IDT plans, which are developed for all clients. They are responsible for ensuring that clients' basic needs are fulfilled; assessing physical and psychosocial status; administering medication; helping the client develop trusting relationships; setting limits on unacceptable behaviors; educating clients; and ultimately, helping clients, within the limits of their capability, to become productive members of society.

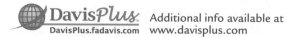

DavisPlus. Additional info available at
DavisPlus.fadavis.com   www.davisplus.com

Review Questions
Self-Examination/Learning Exercise

*Select the answer that is **most** appropriate for each of the following questions.*

1. Which of the following are basic assumptions of milieu therapy? (Select all that apply.)
   a. The client owns his or her own environment.
   b. Each client owns his or her behavior.
   c. Peer pressure is a useful and powerful tool.
   d. Inappropriate behaviors are punished immediately.

2. John tells the nurse, "I think lights out at 10 o'clock on a weekend is stupid. We should be able to watch TV until midnight!" Which of the following is the most appropriate response from the nurse on the milieu unit?
   a. "John, you were told the rules when you were admitted."
   b. "You may bring it up before the others at the community meeting, John."
   c. "Some people want to go to bed early, John."
   d. "You are not the only person on this unit, John. You must think of others besides yourself."

3. In prioritizing care within the therapeutic environment, which of the following nursing interventions would receive the highest priority?
   a. Ensuring that the physical facilities are conducive to achievement of the goals of therapy.
   b. Scheduling a community meeting for 8:30 each morning.
   c. Attending to the nutritional and comfort needs of all clients.
   d. Establishing contacts with community resources.

4. In the community meeting, which of the following actions is most important for reinforcing the democratic posture of the therapy setting?
   a. Allowing each person a specific and equal amount of time to talk.
   b. Reviewing group rules and behavioral limits that apply to all clients.
   c. Reading the minutes from yesterday's meeting.
   d. Waiting until all clients are present before initiating the meeting.

5. One of the goals of therapeutic community is for clients to become more independent and accept self-responsibility. Which of the following approaches by staff best encourages fulfillment of this goal?
   a. Including client input and decisions into the treatment plan.
   b. Insisting that each client take a turn as "president" of the community meeting.
   c. Making decisions for the client regarding plans for treatment.
   d. Requiring that the client be bathed, dressed and attend breakfast on time each morning.

6. Client teaching is an important nursing function in milieu therapy. Which of the following statements by the client indicates the need for knowledge and a readiness to learn?
   a. "Get away from me with that medicine! I'm not sick!"
   b. "I don't need psychiatric treatment. It's my migraine headaches that I need help with."
   c. "I've taken Valium every day of my life for the last 20 years. I'll stop when I'm good and ready!"
   d. "The doctor says I have bipolar disorder. What does that really mean?"

Continued

Review Questions—cont'd
Self-Examination/Learning Exercise

7. Which of the following activities would be a responsibility of the clinical psychologist member of the IDT?
   a. Locates halfway house and arranges living conditions for client being discharged from the hospital.
   b. Manages the therapeutic milieu on a 24-hour basis.
   c. Administers and evaluates psychological tests that assist in diagnosis.
   d. Conducts psychotherapy and administers electroconvulsive therapy treatments.

8. Which of the following activities would be a responsibility of the psychiatric clinical nurse specialist on the IDT team?
   a. Manages the therapeutic milieu on a 24-hour basis.
   b. Conducts group therapies and provides consultation and education to staff nurses.
   c. Directs a group of clients in acting out a situation that is otherwise too painful for a client to discuss openly.
   d. Locates halfway house and arranges living conditions for client being discharged from the hospital.

9. On the milieu unit, duties of the staff psychiatric nurse include which of the following? (Select all that apply.)
   a. Medication administration
   b. Client teaching
   c. Medical diagnosis
   d. Reality orientation
   e. Relationship development
   f. Group therapy

10. Sally was sexually abused as a child. She is a client on the milieu unit with a diagnosis of borderline personality disorder. She has refused to talk to anyone. Which of the following therapies might the IDT team choose for Sally? (Select all that apply.)
    a. Music therapy
    b. Art therapy
    c. Psychodrama
    d. Electroconvulsive therapy

References

American Nurses Association (2007). *Psychiatric-mental health nursing: Scope and standards of practice.* Silver Spring, MD: American Nurses Association.

Bowler, J.B. (1991). Transformation into a healing healthcare environment: Recovering the possibilities of psychiatric/mental health nursing. *Perspectives in Psychiatric Care, 27*(2), 21-25.

DeSocio, J., Bowllan, N., & Staschak, S. (1997). Lessons learned in creating a safe and therapeutic milieu for children, adolescents, and families: Developmental considerations. *Journal of Child and Adolescent Psychiatric Nursing 10*(4), 18-26.

Echternacht, M.R. (2001). Fluid group: Concept and clinical application in the therapeutic milieu. *Journal of the American Psychiatric Nurses Association, 7*(2), 39-44.

Hall, B.A. (1995). Use of milieu therapy: The context and environment as therapeutic practice for psychiatric-mental health nurses. In C.A. Anderson (Ed.), *Psychiatric nursing 1974 to 1994: A report on the state of the art* (pp. 46-56). St. Louis, MO: Mosby-Year Book.

Jani, S., & Fishman, M. (2004). *Advances in milieu therapy for adolescent residential treatment.* Program presented at the American Academy of Child and Adolescent Psychiatry 2004 Annual National Meeting. Retrieved from http://www.milieu-therapy.com/Presentations.en.html

Menninger Clinic. (2012). *Professionals in crisis program.* Retrieved from http://www.menningerclinic.com/patient-care/inpatient-treatment/professionals-in-crisis-program/milieu-therapy

Whall, A.L. (1991). Using the environment to improve the mental health of the elderly. *Journal of Gerontological Nursing, 17*(7), 39.

Classical References

Maslow, A. (1968). *Towards a psychology of being* (2nd ed.). New York, NY: D. Van Nostrand.

Skinner, K. (1979, August). The therapeutic milieu: Making it work. *Journal of Psychiatric Nursing and Mental Health Services,* 38-44.

Crisis Intervention 13

CORE CONCEPT
crisis

KEY TERMS

crisis intervention   disaster

OBJECTIVES
After reading this chapter, the student will be able to:

1. Define *crisis*.
2. Describe four phases in the development of a crisis.
3. Identify types of crises that occur in people's lives.
4. Discuss the goal of crisis intervention.
5. Describe the steps in crisis intervention.
6. Identify the role of the nurse in crisis intervention.
7. Apply the nursing process to care of victims of disasters.

HOMEWORK ASSIGNMENT
Please read the chapter and answer the following questions:

1. Name the three factors that determine whether or not a person experiences a crisis in response to a stressful situation.
2. What is the goal of crisis intervention?
3. Individuals in crisis need to develop more adaptive coping strategies. How does the nurse provide assistance with this process?
4. Describe behaviors common to preschool children following a traumatic event.

Stressful situations are a part of everyday life. Any stressful situation can precipitate a crisis. Crises result in a disequilibrium from which many individuals require assistance to recover. **Crisis intervention** requires problem-solving skills that are often diminished by the level of anxiety accompanying disequilibrium. Assistance with problem solving during the crisis period preserves self-esteem and promotes growth with resolution.

In recent years, individuals in the United States have been faced with a number of catastrophic events, including natural disasters such as tornados, earthquakes, hurricanes, and floods. Also, man-made disasters, such as the Oklahoma City and Boston Marathon bombings and the attacks on the World Trade Center and the Pentagon, have created psychological stress of astronomical proportions in populations around the world.

This chapter examines the phases in the development of a crisis and the types of crises that occur in people's lives. The methodology of crisis intervention, including the role of the nurse, is explored. A discussion of disaster nursing is also presented.

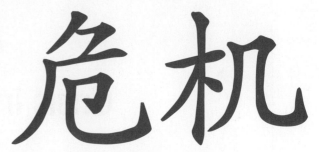

FIGURE 13–1   Chinese symbol for crisis.

> ## CORE CONCEPT
> **Crisis**
> A sudden event in one's life that disturbs homeostasis, during which usual coping mechanisms cannot resolve the problem (Lagerquist, 2006, p. 393)

Characteristics of a Crisis

A number of characteristics have been identified that can be viewed as assumptions upon which the concept of crisis is based (Aguilera, 1998; Caplan, 1964; Winston, 2008). They include the following:

1. Crisis occurs in all individuals at one time or another and is not necessarily equated with psychopathology.
2. Crises are precipitated by specific identifiable events.
3. Crises are personal by nature. What may be considered a crisis situation by one individual may not be so for another.
4. Crises are acute, not chronic, and will be resolved in one way or another within a brief period.
5. A crisis situation contains the potential for psychological growth or deterioration.

Individuals who are in crisis feel helpless to change. They do not believe they have the resources to deal with the precipitating stressor. Levels of anxiety rise to the point that the individual becomes nonfunctional, thoughts become obsessional, and all behavior is aimed at relief of the anxiety being experienced. The feeling is overwhelming and may affect the individual physically as well as psychologically.

Bateman and Peternelj-Taylor (1998) stated:

> Outside Western culture, a crisis is often viewed as a time for movement and growth. The Chinese symbol for crisis [Figure 13-1] consists of the characters for *danger* and *opportunity*. When a crisis is viewed as an opportunity for growth, those involved are much more capable of resolving related issues and more able to move toward positive changes. When the crisis experience is overwhelming because of its scope and nature or when there has not been adequate preparation for the necessary changes, the dangers seem paramount and overshadow any potential growth. The results are maladaptive coping and dysfunctional behavior. (pp. 144-145)

Phases in the Development of a Crisis

The development of a crisis situation follows a relatively predictable course. Caplan (1964) outlined four specific phases through which individuals progress in response to a precipitating stressor and that culminate in the state of acute crisis.

1. **Phase 1.** *The individual is exposed to a precipitating stressor.* Anxiety increases; previous problem-solving techniques are employed.
2. **Phase 2.** *When previous problem-solving techniques do not relieve the stressor, anxiety increases further.* The individual begins to feel a great deal of discomfort at this point. Coping techniques that have worked in the past are attempted, only to create feelings of helplessness when they are not successful. Feelings of confusion and disorganization prevail.
3. **Phase 3.** *All possible resources, both internal and external, are called on to resolve the problem and relieve the discomfort.* The individual may try to view the problem from a different perspective, or even to overlook certain aspects of it. New problem-solving techniques may be used, and, if effectual, resolution may occur at this phase, with the individual returning to a higher, a lower, or the previous level of premorbid functioning.
4. **Phase 4.** *If resolution does not occur in previous phases, Caplan states that "the tension mounts beyond a further threshold or its burden increases over time to a breaking point. Major disorganization of the individual with drastic results often occurs"* (p. 41). Anxiety may reach panic levels. Cognitive functions are disordered, emotions are labile, and behavior may reflect the presence of psychotic thinking.

These phases are congruent with the Transactional Model of Stress/Adaptation outlined in Chapter 1. The relationship between the two perspectives is presented in Figure 13-2. Similarly, Aguilera (1998) spoke of "balancing factors" that affect the way in which an individual perceives and responds to a precipitating stressor. A schematic of these balancing factors is illustrated in Figure 13-3.

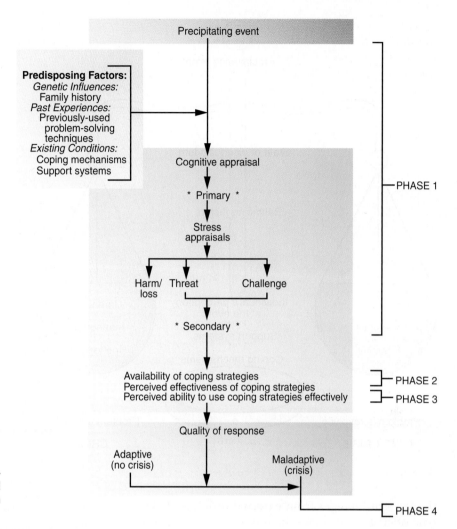

FIGURE 13–2 Relationship between Transactional Model of Stress/Adaptation and Caplan's phases in the development of a crisis.

The paradigm set forth by Aguilera suggests that whether or not an individual experiences a crisis in response to a stressful situation depends upon the following three factors:

1. **The individual's perception of the event.** If the event is perceived realistically, the individual is more likely to draw upon adequate resources to restore equilibrium. If the perception of the event is distorted, attempts at problem solving are likely to be ineffective, and restoration of equilibrium goes unresolved.

2. **The availability of situational supports.** Aguilera stated, "Situational supports are those persons who are available in the environment and who can be depended on to help solve the problem" (p. 37). Without adequate situational supports during a stressful situation, an individual is most likely to feel overwhelmed and alone.

3. **The availability of adequate coping mechanisms.** When a stressful situation occurs, individuals draw upon behavioral strategies that have been successful for them in the past. If these coping strategies work, a crisis may be diverted. If not, disequilibrium may continue and tension and anxiety increase.

As previously set forth, it is assumed that crises are acute, not chronic, situations that will be resolved in one way or another within a brief period. Winston (2008) stated, "Crises tend to be time limited, generally lasting no more than a few months; the duration depends on the stressor and on the individual's perception of and response to the stressor" (p. 1270). Crises can become growth opportunities when individuals learn new methods of coping that can be preserved and used when similar stressors recur.

Types of Crises

Baldwin (1978) identified six classes of emotional crises, which progress by degree of severity. As the measure of psychopathology increases, the source of

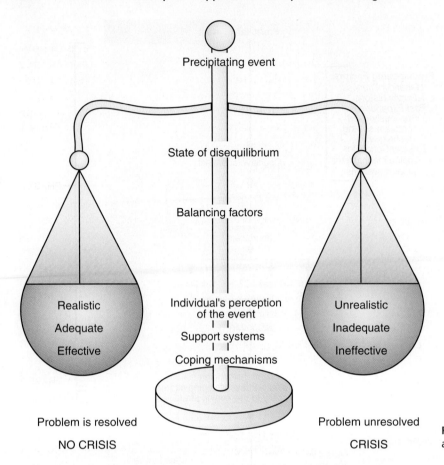

FIGURE 13–3 The effects of balancing factors in a stressful event.

the stressor changes from external to internal. The type of crisis determines the method of intervention selected.

Class 1: Dispositional Crises

Definition An acute response to an external situational stressor.

EXAMPLE

Nancy and Ted have been married for 3 years and have a 1-year-old daughter. Ted has been having difficulty with his boss at work. Twice during the past 6 months he has exploded in anger at home and become abusive with Nancy. Last night he became angry that dinner was not ready when he expected. He grabbed the baby from Nancy and tossed her, screaming, into her crib. He hit and punched Nancy until she feared for her life. This morning when he left for work, she took the baby and went to the emergency department of the city hospital, not having anywhere else to go.

Intervention Nancy's physical wounds were cared for in the emergency department. The mental health counselor provided support and guidance in terms of presenting alternatives to her. Needs and issues were clarified, and referrals for agency assistance were made.

Class 2: Crises of Anticipated Life Transitions

Definition Normal life-cycle transitions that may be anticipated but over which the individual may feel a lack of control.

EXAMPLE

College student J.T. is placed on probationary status because of low grades this semester. His wife had a baby and had to quit her job. He increased his working hours from part time to full time to compensate, and therefore had little time for studies. He presents himself to the student-health nurse practitioner complaining of numerous vague physical complaints.

Intervention Physical examination should be performed (physical symptoms could be caused by depression) and ventilation of feelings encouraged. Reassurance and support should be provided as needed. J.T. should be referred to services that can provide financial and other types of needed assistance. Problematic areas should be identified and approaches to change discussed.

Class 3: Crises Resulting From Traumatic Stress

Definition Crisis precipitated by an unexpected external stressor over which the individual has little or no control and as a result of which he or she feels emotionally overwhelmed and defeated.

EXAMPLE

Sally is a waitperson whose shift ended at midnight. Two weeks ago, while walking to her car in the deserted parking lot, she was abducted by two men with guns, taken to an abandoned building, and raped and beaten. Since that time, her physical wounds have nearly healed. However, Sally cannot be alone, is constantly fearful, relives the experience in flashbacks and dreams, and is unable to eat, sleep, or work at her job in the restaurant. Her friend offers to accompany her to the mental health clinic.

Intervention The nurse should encourage Sally to talk about the experience and to express her feelings associated with it. The nurse should offer reassurance and support; discuss stages of grief and how rape causes a loss of self-worth, triggering the grief response; identify support systems that can help Sally to resume her normal activities; and explore new methods of coping with emotions arising from a situation with which she has had no previous experience.

Class 4: Maturational/Developmental Crises

Definition Crises that occur in response to situations that trigger emotions related to unresolved conflicts in one's life. These crises are of internal origin and reflect underlying developmental issues that involve dependency, value conflicts, sexual identity, control, and capacity for emotional intimacy.

EXAMPLE

Bob is 40 years old. He has just been passed over for a job promotion for the third time. He has moved many times within the large company for which he works, usually after angering and alienating himself from the supervisor. His father was domineering and became abusive when Bob did not comply with his every command. Over the years, Bob's behavioral response became one of passive-aggressiveness—first with his father, then with his supervisors. This third rejection has created feelings of depression and intense anxiety in Bob. At his wife's insistence, he has sought help at the mental health clinic.

Intervention The primary intervention is to help Bob identify the unresolved developmental issue that is creating the conflict. Support and guidance are offered during the initial crisis period, then assistance is given to help Bob work through the underlying conflict in an effort to change response patterns that are creating problems in his current life situation.

Class 5: Crises Reflecting Psychopathology

Definition Emotional crises in which preexisting psychopathology has been instrumental in precipitating the crisis or in which psychopathology significantly impairs or complicates adaptive resolution. Examples of psychopathology that may precipitate crises include personality disorders, anxiety disorders, bipolar disorder, and schizophrenia.

EXAMPLE

Sonja, age 29, was diagnosed with borderline personality disorder at age 18. She has been in therapy on a weekly basis for 10 years, with several hospitalizations for suicide attempts during that time. She has had the same therapist for the past 6 years. This therapist told Sonja today that she is to be married in 1 month and will be moving across the country with her new husband. Sonja is distraught and experiencing intense feelings of abandonment. She is found wandering in and out of traffic on a busy expressway, oblivious to her surroundings. Police bring her to the emergency department of the hospital.

Intervention The initial intervention is to help bring down the level of anxiety in Sonja that has created feelings of unreality in her. She requires that someone stay with her and reassure her of her safety and security. After the feelings of panic anxiety have subsided, she should be encouraged to verbalize her feelings of abandonment. Regressive behaviors should be discouraged. Positive reinforcement should be given for independent activities and accomplishments. The primary therapist will need to pursue this issue of termination with Sonja at length. Referral to a long-term care facility may be required.

Class 6: Psychiatric Emergencies

Definition Crisis situations in which general functioning has been severely impaired and the individual rendered incompetent or unable to assume personal responsibility. Examples include acutely suicidal individuals, drug overdoses, reactions to hallucinogenic drugs, acute psychoses, uncontrollable anger, and alcohol intoxication.

EXAMPLE

Jennifer, age 16, had been dating Joe, the star high school football player, for 6 months. After the game on Friday night, Jennifer and Joe went to Jackie's house, where a number of high school students had gathered for an after-game party. No adults were present. About midnight, Joe told Jennifer that he did not want to date her anymore. Jennifer became hysterical, and Jackie was frightened by her behavior. She took Jennifer to her parent's bedroom and gave her a Valium from a bottle in her mother's medicine cabinet. She left Jennifer lying on her parent's bed and returned to the party downstairs. About an hour later, she returned to her parent's bedroom and found that Jennifer had removed the bottle of Valium from the cabinet and swallowed all of the tablets. Jennifer was unconscious and Jackie could not awaken her. An ambulance was called and Jennifer was transported to the local hospital.

Intervention The crisis team monitored vital signs, ensured maintenance of adequate airway, initiated gastric lavage, and administered activated charcoal to minimize absorption. Jennifer's parents were notified and rushed to the hospital. The situation was explained to them, and they were encouraged to stay by her side. When the physical crisis was resolved, Jennifer was transferred to the psychiatric unit. In therapy, she was encouraged to ventilate her feelings regarding the rejection and subsequent overdose. Family therapy sessions were conducted in an effort to clarify interpersonal issues and to identify areas for change. On an individual level, Jennifer's therapist worked with her to establish more adaptive methods of coping with stressful situations.

Crisis Intervention

Individuals experiencing crises have an urgent need for assistance. In **crisis intervention** the therapist, or other intervener, becomes a part of the individual's life situation. Because of the individual's emotional state, he or she is unable to problem-solve, so requires guidance and support from another to help mobilize the resources needed to resolve the crisis.

Lengthy psychological interpretations are not appropriate for crisis intervention. It is a time for doing what is needed to help the individual get relief and for calling into action all the people and other resources required to do so. Aguilera (1998) stated:

> The goal of crisis intervention is the resolution of an immediate crisis. Its focus is on the supportive,

with the restoration of the individual to his precrisis level of functioning or possibly to a higher level of functioning. The therapist's role is direct, supportive, and that of an active participant. (p. 24)

Crisis intervention takes place in both inpatient and outpatient settings. The basic methodology relies heavily on orderly problem-solving techniques and structured activities that are focused on change. Through adaptive change, crises are resolved and growth occurs. Because of the time limitation of crisis intervention, the individual must experience some degree of relief almost from the first interaction. Crisis intervention, then, is not aimed at major personality change or reconstruction (as may be the case in long-term psychotherapy), but rather at using a given crisis situation, at the very least, to restore functioning and, at most, to enhance personal growth.

Phases of Crisis Intervention: The Role of the Nurse

Nurses respond to crisis situations on a daily basis. Crises can occur on every unit in the general hospital, in the home setting, in the community health care setting, in schools and offices, and in private practice. Indeed, nurses may be called on to function as crisis helpers in virtually any setting committed to the practice of nursing.

Roberts and Ottens (2005) provided a seven-stage model of crisis intervention. This model is summarized in Table 13-1. Aguilera (1998) described four specific phases in the technique of crisis intervention that are clearly comparable to the steps of the nursing process. These phases are discussed in the following paragraphs.

Phase 1. Assessment

In this phase, the crisis helper gathers information regarding the precipitating stressor and the resulting

TABLE 13–1 **Roberts' Seven-Stage Crisis Intervention Model**	
STAGE	INTERVENTIONS
Stage I. Psychosocial and Lethality Assessment	■ Conduct a rapid but thorough biopsychosocial assessment.
Stage II. Rapidly Establish Rapport	■ The counselor uses genuineness, respect, and unconditional acceptance to establish rapport with the client. ■ Skills such as good eye contact, a nonjudgmental attitude, flexibility, and maintaining a positive mental attitude are important.

TABLE 13–1 **Roberts' Seven-Stage Crisis Intervention Model—cont'd**	
STAGE	INTERVENTIONS
Stage III. Identify the Major Problems or Crisis Precipitants	■ Identify the precipitating event that has led the client to seek help at the present time. ■ Identify other situations that led up to the precipitating event. ■ Prioritize major problems with which the client needs help. ■ Discuss client's current style of coping, and offer assistance in areas where modification would be helpful in resolving the present crisis and preventing future crises.
Stage IV. Deal With Feelings and Emotions	■ Encourage the client to vent feelings. Provide validation. ■ Use therapeutic communication techniques to help the client explain his or her story about the current crisis situation. ■ Eventually, and cautiously, begin to challenge maladaptive beliefs and behaviors, and help the client adopt more rational and adaptive options.
Stage V. Generate and Explore Alternatives	■ Collaboratively explore options with the client. ■ Identify coping strategies that have been successful for the client in the past. ■ Help the client problem-solve strategies for confronting current crisis adaptively.
Stage VI. Implement an Action Plan	■ There is a shift at this stage from crisis to resolution. ■ Develop a concrete plan of action to deal directly with the current crisis. ■ Having a concrete plan restores the client's equilibrium and psychological balance. ■ Work through the meaning of the event that precipitated the crisis. How could it have been prevented? What responses may have aggravated the situation?
Stage VII. Follow-Up	■ Plan a follow-up visit with the client to evaluate the post-crisis status of the client. ■ Beneficial scheduling of follow-up visits include 1-month and 1-year anniversaries of the crisis event.

Adapted from Roberts, A.R., & Ottens, A.J. (2005). The seven-stage crisis intervention model: A road map to goal attainment, problem solving, and crisis resolution. *Brief Treatment and Crisis Intervention, 5*(4), 329-339.

crisis that prompted the individual to seek professional help. A nurse in crisis intervention might perform some of the following assessments:

■ Ask the individual to describe the event that precipitated this crisis.
■ Determine when it occurred.
■ Assess the individual's physical and mental status.
■ Determine if the individual has experienced this stressor before. If so, what method of coping was used? Have these methods been tried this time?
  ■ If previous coping methods were tried, what was the result?
  ■ If new coping methods were tried, what was the result?
■ Assess suicide or homicide potential, plan, and means.
■ Assess the adequacy of support systems.

■ Determine level of precrisis functioning. Assess the usual coping methods, available support systems, and ability to problem-solve.
■ Assess the individual's perception of personal strengths and limitations.
■ Assess the individual's use of substances.

Information from the comprehensive assessment is then analyzed, and appropriate nursing diagnoses reflecting the immediacy of the crisis situation are identified. Some nursing diagnoses that may be relevant include:

■ Ineffective coping
■ Anxiety (severe to panic)
■ Disturbed thought processes (has been removed from the NANDA-I list of approved diagnoses, but is used for purposes of this textbook)
■ Risk for self- or other-directed violence
■ Rape-trauma syndrome

■ Post-trauma syndrome
■ Fear

Phase 2. Planning of Therapeutic Intervention

In the planning phase of crisis intervention, the nurse selects the appropriate nursing actions for the identified nursing diagnoses. In planning the interventions, the type of crisis, as well as the individual's strengths and available resources for support, are taken into consideration. Goals are established for crisis resolution and a return to, or increase in, the precrisis level of functioning.

Phase 3. Intervention

During phase 3, the actions that were identified in phase 2 are implemented. The following interventions are the focus of nursing in crisis intervention:

■ Use a reality-oriented approach. The focus of the problem is on the here and now.
■ Remain with the individual who is experiencing panic anxiety.
■ Establish a rapid working relationship by showing unconditional acceptance, by active listening, and by attending to immediate needs.
■ Discourage lengthy explanations or rationalizations of the situation; promote an atmosphere for verbalization of true feelings.
■ Set firm limits on aggressive, destructive behaviors. At high levels of anxiety, behavior is likely to be impulsive and regressive. Establish at the outset what is acceptable and what is not, and maintain consistency.
■ Clarify the problem that the individual is facing. The nurse does this by describing his or her perception of the problem and comparing it with the individual's perception of the problem.
■ Help the individual determine what he or she believes precipitated the crisis.
■ Acknowledge feelings of anger, guilt, helplessness, and powerlessness, while taking care not to provide positive feedback for these feelings.
■ Guide the individual through a problem-solving process by which he or she may move in the direction of positive life change:
  ■ Help the individual confront the source of the problem that is creating the crisis response.
  ■ Encourage the individual to discuss changes he or she would like to make. Jointly determine whether or not desired changes are realistic.
  ■ Encourage exploration of feelings about aspects that cannot be changed, and explore alternative ways of coping more adaptively in these situations.
  ■ Discuss alternative strategies for creating changes that are realistically possible.
  ■ Weigh benefits and consequences of each alternative.
  ■ Assist the individual to select alternative coping strategies that will help alleviate future crisis situations.

> **CLINICAL PEARL** Coping mechanisms are highly individual and the choice ultimately must be made by the client. The nurse may offer suggestions and provide guidance to help the client identify coping mechanisms that are realistic for him or her, and that can promote positive outcomes in a crisis situation.

■ Identify external support systems and new social networks from which the individual may seek assistance in times of stress.

Phase 4. Evaluation of Crisis Resolution and Anticipatory Planning

To evaluate the outcome of crisis intervention, a reassessment is made to determine if the stated objective was achieved:

■ Have positive behavioral changes occurred?
■ Has the individual developed more adaptive coping strategies? Have they been effective?
■ Has the individual grown from the experience by gaining insight into his or her responses to crisis situations?
■ Does the individual believe that he or she could respond with healthy adaptation in future stressful situations to prevent crisis development?
■ Can the individual describe a plan of action for dealing with stressors similar to the one that precipitated this crisis?

During the evaluation period, the nurse and client summarize what has occurred during the intervention. They review what the individual has learned and "anticipate" how he or she will respond in the future. A determination is made regarding follow-up therapy; if needed, the nurse provides referral information.

Disaster Nursing

Although there are many definitions of **disaster**, a common feature is that the event overwhelms local resources and threatens the function and safety of the community (Norwood, Ursano, & Fullerton, 2000). A violent disaster, whether natural or man-made, may leave devastation of property or life. Such tragedies also leave victims with a damaged sense of safety and well-being, and varying degrees of emotional trauma. Children, who lack life experiences and coping skills, are particularly vulnerable. Their sense of order and security has been seriously disrupted, and they are unable to understand that the disruption is time-limited and that their world will eventually return to normal.

Application of the Nursing Process to Disaster Nursing

Background Assessment Data

Individuals respond to traumatic events in many ways. Grieving is a natural response following any loss, and it may be more extreme if the disaster is directly experienced or witnessed. The emotional effects of loss and disruption may show up immediately or may appear weeks or months later.

Psychological and behavioral responses common in adults following trauma and disaster include anger; disbelief; sadness; anxiety; fear; irritability; arousal; numbing; sleep disturbance; and increases in alcohol, caffeine, and tobacco use (Norwood et al., 2000). Preschool children commonly experience separation anxiety, regressive behaviors, nightmares, and hyperactive or withdrawn behaviors. Older children may have difficulty concentrating, somatic complaints, sleep disturbances, and concerns about safety. Adolescents' responses are often similar to those of adults.

Norwood and associates (2000) stated:

> Traumatic bereavement is recognized as posing special challenges to survivors. While the death of loved ones is always painful, an unexpected and violent death can be more difficult to assimilate. Family members may develop intrusive images of the death based on information gleaned from authorities or the media. Witnessing or learning of violence to a loved one also increases vulnerability to psychiatric disorders. The knowledge that one has been exposed to toxins is a potent traumatic stressor . . . and the focus of much concern in the medical community preparing for responses to terrorist attacks using biological, chemical, or nuclear agents. (p. 214)

Nursing Diagnoses/Outcome Identification

Information from the assessment is analyzed, and appropriate nursing diagnoses reflecting the immediacy of the situation are identified. Some nursing diagnoses that may be relevant include:

■ Risk for injury (trauma, suffocation, poisoning)
■ Risk for infection
■ Anxiety (panic)
■ Fear
■ Spiritual distress
■ Risk for post-trauma syndrome
■ Ineffective community coping

The following criteria may be used for measurement of outcomes in the care of the client having experienced a traumatic event. Timelines are individually determined.

The client:

■ Experiences minimal/no injury to self.
■ Demonstrates behaviors necessary to protect self from further injury.
■ Identifies interventions to prevent/reduce risk of infection.
■ Is free of infection.
■ Maintains anxiety at manageable level.
■ Expresses beliefs and values about spiritual issues.
■ Demonstrates ability to deal with emotional reactions in an individually appropriate manner.
■ Demonstrates an increase in activities to improve community functioning.

Planning/Implementation

Table 13-2 provides a plan of care for the client who has experienced a traumatic event. Selected nursing diagnoses are presented, along with outcome criteria, appropriate nursing interventions, and rationales for each.

Evaluation

In the final step of the nursing process, a reassessment is conducted to determine if the nursing actions have been successful in achieving the objectives of care. Evaluation of the nursing actions for the client who has experienced a traumatic event may be facilitated by gathering information utilizing the following types of questions:

■ Has the client escaped serious injury, or have injuries been resolved?
■ Have infections been prevented or resolved?
■ Is the client able to maintain anxiety at manageable level?
■ Does he or she demonstrate appropriate problem-solving skills?
■ Is the client able to discuss his or her beliefs about spiritual issues?
■ Does the client demonstrate the ability to deal with emotional reactions in an individually appropriate manner?
■ Does he or she verbalize a subsiding of the physical manifestations (e.g., pain, nightmares, flashbacks, fatigue) associated with the traumatic event?
■ Has there been recognition of factors affecting the community's ability to meet its own demands or needs?
■ Has there been a demonstration of increased activities to improve community functioning?
■ Has a plan been established and put in place to deal with future contingencies?

(Text continued on page 232)

Table 13-2 | CARE PLAN FOR THE CLIENT WHO HAS EXPERIENCED A TRAUMATIC EVENT

NURSING DIAGNOSIS: ANXIETY (PANIC)/FEAR

RELATED TO: Real or perceived threat to physical well-being; threat of death; situational crisis; exposure to toxins; unmet needs

EVIDENCED BY: Persistent feelings of apprehension and uneasiness; sense of impending doom; impaired functioning; verbal expressions of having no control or influence over situation, outcome, or self-care; sympathetic stimulation; extraneous physical movements

OUTCOME CRITERIA	NURSING INTERVENTIONS	RATIONALE
Client will maintain anxiety at manageable level.	1. Determine degree of anxiety/ fear present, associated behaviors (e.g., laughter, crying, calm or agitation, excited/hysterical behavior, expressions of disbelief and/ or self-blame), and reality of perceived threat.	1. Clearly understanding client's perception is pivotal to providing appropriate assistance in overcoming the fear. Individual may be agitated or totally overwhelmed. Panic state increases risk for client's own safety as well as the safety of others in the environment.
	2. Note degree of disorganization.	2. Client may be unable to handle ADLs or work requirements and need more intensive intervention.
	3. Create as quiet an area as possible. Maintain a calm, confident manner. Speak in even tone using short simple sentences.	3. Decreases sense of confusion or overstimulation; enhances sense of safety. Helps client focus on what is said and reduces transmission of anxiety.
	4. Develop trusting relationship with the client.	4. Trust is the basis of a therapeutic nurse-client relationship and enables them to work effectively together.
	5. Identify whether incident has reactivated preexisting or coexisting situations (physical or psychological).	5. Concerns and psychological issues will be recycled every time trauma is re-experienced and affect how the client views the current situation.
	6. Determine presence of physical symptoms (e.g., numbness, headache, tightness in chest, nausea, and pounding heart).	6. Physical problems need to be differentiated from anxiety symptoms so appropriate treatment can be given.
	7. Identify psychological responses (e.g., anger, shock, acute anxiety, panic, confusion, denial). Record emotional changes.	7. Although these are normal responses at the time of the trauma, they will recycle again and again until they are dealt with adequately.
	8. Discuss with client the perception of what is causing the anxiety.	8. Increases the ability to connect symptoms to subjective feeling of anxiety, providing opportunity to gain insight/control and make desired changes.
	9. Assist client to correct any distortions being experienced. Share perceptions with client.	9. Perceptions based on reality will help to decrease fearfulness. How the nurse views the situation may help client to see it differently.

Table 13-2 | CARE PLAN FOR THE CLIENT WHO HAS EXPERIENCED A TRAUMATIC EVENT—cont'd

OUTCOME CRITERIA	NURSING INTERVENTIONS	RATIONALE
	10. Explore with client or significant other the manner in which client has previously coped with anxiety-producing events.	10. May help client regain sense of control and recognize significance of trauma.
	11. Engage client in learning new coping behaviors (e.g., progressive muscle relaxation, thought-stopping).	11. Replacing maladaptive behaviors can enhance ability to manage and deal with stress. Interrupting obsessive thinking allows client to use energy to address underlying anxiety, whereas continued rumination about the incident can retard recovery.
	12. Encourage use of techniques to manage stress and vent emotions such as anger and hostility.	12. Reduces the likelihood of eruptions that can result in abusive behavior.
	13. Give positive feedback when client demonstrates better ways to manage anxiety and is able to calmly and realistically appraise the situation.	13. Provides acknowledgement and reinforcement, encouraging use of new coping strategies. Enhances ability to deal with fearful feelings and gain control over situation, promoting future successes.
	14. Administer medications as indicated: Antianxiety: diazepam, alprazolam, oxazepam; or Antidepressants: fluoxetine, paroxetine, bupropion.	14. Antianxiety medication provides temporary relief of anxiety symptoms, enhancing ability to cope with situation. Antidepressants lift mood and help suppress intrusive thoughts and explosive anger.

NURSING DIAGNOSIS: SPIRITUAL DISTRESS

RELATED TO: Physical or psychological stress; energy-consuming anxiety; loss(es), intense suffering; separation from religious or cultural ties; challenged belief and value system

EVIDENCED BY: Expressions of concern about disaster and the meaning of life and death or belief systems; inner conflict about current loss of normality and effects of the disaster; anger directed at deity; engaging in self-blame; seeking spiritual assistance

OUTCOME CRITERIA	NURSING INTERVENTIONS	RATIONALE
Client expresses beliefs and values about spiritual issues.	1. Determine client's religious/spiritual orientation, current involvement, and presence of conflicts.	1. Provides baseline for planning care and accessing appropriate resources.
	2. Establish environment that promotes free expression of feelings and concerns. Provide calm, peaceful setting when possible.	2. Promotes awareness and identification of feelings so they can be dealt with.
	3. Listen to client's and significant others' expressions of anger, concern, alienation from God, belief that situation is a punishment for wrongdoing, etc.	3. It is helpful to understand the client's and significant others' points of view and how they are questioning their faith in the face of tragedy.

Continued

Table 13-2 | CARE PLAN FOR THE CLIENT WHO HAS EXPERIENCED A TRAUMATIC EVENT–cont'd

OUTCOME CRITERIA	NURSING INTERVENTIONS	RATIONALE
	4. Note sense of futility, feelings of hopelessness and helplessness, lack of motivation to help self.	4. These thoughts and feelings can result in the client feeling paralyzed and unable to move forward to resolve the situation.
	5. Listen to expressions of inability to find meaning in life and reason for living. Evaluate for suicidal ideation.	5. May indicate need for further intervention to prevent suicide attempt.
	6. Determine support systems available to client.	6. Presence or lack of support systems can affect client's recovery.
	7. Ask how you can be most helpful. Convey acceptance of client's spiritual beliefs and concerns.	7. Promotes trust and comfort, encouraging client to be open about sensitive matters.
	8. Make time for nonjudgmental discussion of philosophic issues and questions about spiritual impact of current situation.	8. Helps client to begin to look at basis for spiritual confusion. *Note:* There is a potential for care provider's belief system to interfere with client finding own way. Therefore, it is most beneficial to remain neutral and not espouse own beliefs.
	9. Discuss difference between grief and guilt and help client to identify and deal with each, assuming responsibility for own actions, expressing awareness of the consequences of acting out of false guilt.	9. Blaming self for what has happened impedes dealing with the grief process and needs to be discussed and dealt with.
	10. Use therapeutic communication skills of reflection and active listening.	10. Helps client find own solutions to concerns.
	11. Encourage client to experience meditation, prayer, and forgiveness. Provide information that anger with God is a normal part of the grieving process.	11. This can help to heal past and present pain.
	12. Assist client to develop goals for dealing with life situation.	12. Enhances commitment to goal, optimizing outcomes and promoting sense of hope.
	13. Identify and refer to resources that can be helpful, e.g., pastoral/ parish nurse or religious counselor, crisis counselor, psychotherapy, Alcoholics/ Narcotics Anonymous.	13. Specific assistance may be helpful to recovery (e.g., relationship problems, substance abuse, suicidal ideation).
	14. Encourage participation in support groups.	14. Discussing concerns and questions with others can help client resolve feelings.

Table 13-2 | CARE PLAN FOR THE CLIENT WHO HAS EXPERIENCED A TRAUMATIC EVENT–cont'd

NURSING DIAGNOSIS: RISK FOR POST-TRAUMA SYNDROME

RELATED TO: Events outside the range of usual human experience; serious threat or injury to self or loved ones; witnessing horrors or tragic events; exaggerated sense of responsibility; survivor's guilt or role in the event; inadequate social support

OUTCOME CRITERIA	NURSING INTERVENTIONS	RATIONALE
Client demonstrates ability to deal with emotional reactions in an individually appropriate manner.	1. Determine involvement in event (e.g., survivor, significant other, rescue/aid worker, health-care provider, family member).	1. All those concerned with a traumatic event are at risk for emotional trauma and have needs related to their involvement in the event. *Note:* Close involvement with victims affects individual responses and may prolong emotional suffering.
	2. Evaluate current factors associated with the event, such as displacement from home due to illness/injury, natural disaster, or terrorist attack. Identify how client's past experiences may affect current situation.	2. Affects client's reaction to current event and is basis for planning care and identifying appropriate support systems and resources.
	3. Listen for comments of taking on responsibility (e.g., "I should have been more careful or gone back to get her.")	3. Statements such as these are indicators of "survivor's guilt" and blaming self for actions.
	4. Identify client's current coping mechanisms.	4. Noting positive or negative coping skills provides direction for care.
	5. Determine availability and usefulness of client's support systems, family, social contacts, and community resources.	5. Family and others close to the client may also be at risk and require assistance to cope with the trauma.
	6. Provide information about signs and symptoms of post-trauma response, especially if individual is involved in a high-risk occupation.	6. Awareness of these factors helps individual identify need for assistance when signs and symptoms occur.
	7. Identify and discuss client's strengths as well as vulnerabilities.	7. Provides information to build on for coping with traumatic experience.
	8. Evaluate individual's perceptions of events and personal significance (e.g., rescue worker trained to provide lifesaving assistance but recovering only dead bodies).	8. Events that trigger feelings of despair and hopelessness may be more difficult to deal with, and require long-term interventions.
	9. Provide emotional and physical presence by sitting with client/significant other and offering solace.	9. Strengthens coping abilities.
	10. Encourage expression of feelings. Note whether feelings expressed appear congruent with events experienced.	10. It is important to talk about the incident repeatedly. Incongruencies may indicate deeper conflict and can impede resolution.

Continued

Table 13-2 | CARE PLAN FOR THE CLIENT WHO HAS EXPERIENCED A TRAUMATIC EVENT—cont'd

OUTCOME CRITERIA	NURSING INTERVENTIONS	RATIONALE
	11. Note presence of nightmares, reliving the incident, loss of appetite, irritability, numbness and crying, and family or relationship disruption.	11. These responses are normal in the early post-incident time frame. If prolonged and persistent, they may indicate need for more intensive therapy.
	12. Provide a calm, safe environment.	12. Helps client deal with the disruption in his or her life.
	13. Encourage and assist client in learning stress-management techniques.	13. Promotes relaxation and helps individual exercise control over self and what has happened.
	14. Recommend participation in debriefing sessions that may be provided following major disaster events.	14. Dealing with the stresses promptly may facilitate recovery from the event or prevent exacerbation.
	15. Identify employment, community resource groups.	15. Provides opportunity for ongoing support to deal with recurrent feelings related to the trauma.
	16. Administer medications as indicated, such as antipsychotics (e.g., chlorpromazine, haloperidol, olanzapine, or quetiapine) or carbamazepine (Tegretol).	16. Low doses of antipsychotics may be used for reduction of psychotic symptoms when loss of contact with reality occurs, usually for clients with especially disturbing flashbacks. Carbamazepine may be used to alleviate intrusive recollections or flashbacks, impulsivity, and violent behavior.

NURSING DIAGNOSIS: INEFFECTIVE COMMUNITY COPING

RELATED TO: Natural or man-made disasters (earthquakes, tornados, floods, reemerging infectious agents, terrorist activity); ineffective or nonexistent community systems (e.g., lack of or inadequate emergency medical system, transportation system, or disaster planning systems)

EVIDENCED BY: Deficits of community participation; community does not meet its own expectations; expressed vulnerability; community powerlessness; stressors perceived as excessive; excessive community conflicts; high illness rates

OUTCOME CRITERIA	NURSING INTERVENTIONS	RATIONALE
Client demonstrates an increase in activities to improve community functioning.	1. Evaluate community activities that are related to meeting collective needs within the community itself and between the community and the larger society. Note immediate needs, such as health care, food, shelter, funds.	1. Provides a baseline to determine community needs in relation to current concerns or threats.
	2. Note community reports of functioning including areas of weakness or conflict.	2. Provides a view of how the community itself sees these areas.

Table 13-2 | CARE PLAN FOR THE CLIENT WHO HAS EXPERIENCED A TRAUMATIC EVENT—cont'd

OUTCOME CRITERIA	NURSING INTERVENTIONS	RATIONALE
	3. Identify effects of related factors on community activities.	3. In the face of a current threat, local or national, community resources need to be evaluated, updated, and given priority to meet the identified need.
	4. Determine availability and use of resources. Identify unmet demands or needs of the community.	4. Information necessary to identify what else is needed to meet the current situation.
	5. Determine community strengths.	5. Promotes understanding of the ways in which the community is already meeting the identified needs.
	6. Encourage community members/ groups to engage in problem-solving activities.	6. Promotes a sense of working together to meet the needs.
	7. Develop a plan jointly with the members of the community to address immediate needs.	7. Deals with deficits in support of identified goals.
	8. Create plans managing interactions within the community itself and between the community and the larger society.	8. Meets collective needs when the concerns/threats are shared beyond a local community.
	9. Make information accessible to the public. Provide channels for dissemination of information to the community as a whole (e.g., print media, radio/television reports and community bulletin boards, Internet sites, speaker's bureau, reports to committees/ councils/advisory boards).	9. Readily available accurate information can help citizens deal with the situation.
	10. Make information available in different modalities and geared to differing educational levels/ cultures of the community.	10. Using languages other than English and making written materials accessible to all members of the community will promote understanding.
	11. Seek out and evaluate needs of underserved populations.	11. Homeless and those residing in lower income areas may have special requirements that need to be addressed with additional resources.

SOURCE: Doenges, Moorhouse, & Murr (2010). With permission.

Summary and Key Points

■ A *crisis* is defined as "a sudden event in one's life that disturbs homeostasis, during which usual coping mechanisms cannot resolve the problem" (Lagerquist, 2006, p. 393).

■ All individuals experience crises at one time or another. This does not necessarily indicate psychopathology.

■ Crises are precipitated by specific identifiable events and are determined by an individual's personal perception of the situation.

■ Crises are acute rather than chronic and generally last no more than a few weeks to a few months.

■ Crises occur when an individual is exposed to a stressor and previous problem-solving techniques are ineffective. This causes the level of anxiety to rise. Panic may ensue when new techniques are tried and resolution fails to occur.

■ Six types of crises have been identified. They include dispositional crises, crises of anticipated life transitions, crises resulting from traumatic stress, maturation/developmental crises, crises reflecting psychopathology, and psychiatric emergencies. The type of crisis determines the method of intervention selected.

■ Crisis intervention is designed to provide rapid assistance for individuals who have an urgent need.

■ The minimum therapeutic goal of crisis intervention is psychological resolution of the individual's immediate crisis and restoration to at least the level of functioning that existed before the crisis period. A maximum goal is improvement in functioning above the precrisis level.

■ Nurses regularly respond to individuals in crisis in all types of settings. Nursing process is the vehicle by which nurses assist individuals in crisis with a short-term problem-solving approach to change.

■ A four-phase technique of crisis intervention includes assessment/analysis, planning of therapeutic intervention, intervention, and evaluation of crisis resolution and anticipatory planning.

■ Through this structured method of assistance, nurses help individuals in crisis to develop more adaptive coping strategies for dealing with stressful situations in the future.

■ Nurses have many important skills that can assist individuals and communities in the wake of traumatic events. Nursing interventions presented in this chapter were developed for the nursing diagnoses of panic anxiety/fear, spiritual distress, risk for post-trauma syndrome, and ineffective community coping.

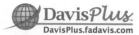 **DavisPlus**™ Additional info available at
DavisPlus.fadavis.com www.davisplus.com

Review Questions
Self-Examination/Learning Exercise

*Select the answer that is **most** appropriate for each of the following questions.*

1. Which of the following is a correct assumption regarding the concept of crisis?
   a. Crises occur only in individuals with psychopathology.
   b. The stressful event that precipitates crisis is seldom identifiable.
   c. A crisis situation contains the potential for psychological growth or deterioration.
   d. Crises are chronic situations that recur many times during an individual's life.

2. Crises occur when an individual:
   a. Is exposed to a precipitating stressor
   b. Perceives a stressor to be threatening
   c. Has no support systems
   d. Experiences a stressor and perceives coping strategies to be ineffective

3. Amanda's mobile home was destroyed by a tornado. Amanda received only minor injuries, but is experiencing disabling anxiety in the aftermath of the event. This type of crisis is called:
   a. Crisis resulting from traumatic stress
   b. Maturational/developmental crisis
   c. Dispositional crisis
   d. Crisis of anticipated life transitions

4. The most appropriate crisis intervention with Amanda (from question 3) would be to:
   a. Encourage her to recognize how lucky she is to be alive.
   b. Discuss stages of grief and feelings associated with each.
   c. Identify community resources that can help Amanda.
   d. Suggest that she find a place to live that provides a storm shelter.

5. Jenny reported to the high school nurse that her mother drinks too much. She is drunk every afternoon when Jenny gets home from school. Jenny is afraid to invite friends over because of her mother's behavior. This type of crisis is called:
   a. Crisis resulting from traumatic stress
   b. Maturational/developmental crisis
   c. Dispositional crisis
   d. Crisis reflecting psychopathology

6. The most appropriate nursing intervention with Jenny (from question 5) would be to:
   a. Make arrangements for her to start attending Alateen meetings.
   b. Help her identify the positive things in her life and recognize that her situation could be a lot worse than it is.
   c. Teach her about the effects of alcohol on the body and that it can be hereditary.
   d. Refer her to a psychiatrist for private therapy to learn to deal with her home situation.

7. Ginger, age 19 and an only child, left 3 months ago to attend a college of her choice 500 miles away from her parents. It is Ginger's first time away from home. She has difficulty making decisions and will not undertake anything new without first consulting her mother. They talk on the phone almost every day. Ginger has recently started having anxiety attacks. She consults the nurse practitioner in the student health center. This type of crisis is called:
   a. Crisis resulting from traumatic stress
   b. Dispositional crisis
   c. Psychiatric emergency
   d. Maturational/developmental crisis

8. The most appropriate nursing intervention with Ginger (from question 7) would be to:
   a. Suggest she move to a college closer to home.
   b. Work with Ginger on unresolved dependency issues.
   c. Help her find someone in the college town from whom she could seek assistance rather than calling her mother regularly.
   d. Recommend that the college physician prescribe an antianxiety medication for Ginger.

9. Marie, age 56, is the mother of five children. Her youngest child, who had been living at home and attending the local college, recently graduated and accepted a job in another state. Marie has never worked outside the home and has devoted her life to satisfying the needs of her husband and children. Since the departure of her last child from home, Marie has become more and more despondent. Her husband has become very concerned, and takes her to the local mental health center. This type of crisis is called:
   a. Dispositional crisis
   b. Crisis of anticipated life transitions
   c. Psychiatric emergency
   d. Crisis resulting from traumatic stress

10. The most appropriate nursing intervention with Marie (from question 9) would be to:
    a. Refer her to her family physician for a complete physical examination.
    b. Suggest she seek outside employment now that her children have left home.
    c. Identify convenient support systems for times when she is feeling particularly despondent.
    d. Begin grief work and assist her to recognize areas of self-worth separate and apart from her children.

Continued

Review Questions—cont'd
Self-Examination/Learning Exercise

11. The desired outcome of working with an individual who has witnessed a traumatic event and is now experiencing panic anxiety is:
    a. The individual will experience no anxiety.
    b. The individual will demonstrate hope for the future.
    c. The individual will maintain anxiety at manageable level.
    d. The individual will verbalize acceptance of self as worthy.

12. Andrew, a New York City firefighter, and his entire unit responded to the terrorist attacks at the World Trade Center. Working as a team, he and his best friend, Carlo, entered the area together. Carlo was killed when the building collapsed. Andrew was injured, but survived. Since that time, Andrew has had frequent nightmares and anxiety attacks. He says to the mental health worker, "I don't know why Carlo had to die and I didn't!" This statement by Andrew suggests that he is experiencing:
    a. Spiritual distress
    b. Night terrors
    c. Survivor's guilt
    d. Suicidal ideation

13. Intervention with Andrew (from question 12) would include:
    a. Encouraging expression of feelings
    b. Antianxiety medications
    c. Participation in a support group
    d. a and c
    e. All of the above

References

Aguilera, D.C. (1998). *Crisis intervention: Theory and methodology* (8th ed.). St. Louis, MO: C.V. Mosby.

Bateman, A., & Peternelj-Taylor, C. (1998). Crisis intervention. In C.A. Glod (Ed.), *Contemporary psychiatric-mental health nursing: The brain-behavior connection.* Philadelphia, PA: F.A. Davis.

Doenges, M.E., Moorhouse, M.F., & Murr, A.C. (2010). *Nursing care plans: Guidelines for individualizing client care across the life span* (8th ed.). Philadelphia, PA: F.A. Davis.

Lagerquist, S.L. (2006). *Davis's NCLEX-RN Success* (2nd ed.). Philadelphia, PA: F.A. Davis.

Norwood, A.E., Ursano, R.J., & Fullerton, C.S. (2000). Disaster psychiatry: Principles and practice. *Psychiatric Quarterly, 71*(3), 207-226.

Roberts, A.R., & Ottens, A.J. (2005). The seven-stage crisis intervention model: A road map to goal attainment, problem solving, and crisis resolution. *Brief treatment and crisis intervention, 5*(4), 329-339.

Winston, A. (2008). Supportive psychotherapy. In R.E. Hales, S.C. Yudofsky, & G.O. Gabbard (Eds.), *Textbook of psychiatry* (5th ed., pp. 1257-1277). Washington, DC: American Psychiatric Publishing.

Classical References

Baldwin, B.A. (1978, July). A paradigm for the classification of emotional crises: Implications for crisis intervention. *American Journal of Orthopsychiatry, 48*(3), 538-551.

Caplan, G. (1964). *Principles of preventive psychiatry.* New York, NY: Basic Books.

Assertiveness Training

14

CORE CONCEPT
assertive behavior

CHAPTER OUTLINE

Objectives

Homework Assignment

Assertive Communication

Basic Human Rights

Response Patterns

Behavioral Components of Assertive Behavior

Techniques That Promote Assertive Behavior

Thought-Stopping Techniques

Role of the Nurse in Assertiveness Training

Summary and Key Points

Review Questions

KEY TERMS

aggressive

assertive

nonassertive

passive-aggressive

thought-stopping

OBJECTIVES
After reading this chapter, the student will be able to:

1. Define *assertive behavior*.
2. Discuss basic human rights.
3. Differentiate among nonassertive, assertive, aggressive, and passive-aggressive behaviors.
4. Describe techniques that promote assertive behavior.
5. Demonstrate thought-stopping techniques.
6. Discuss the role of the nurse in assertiveness training.

HOMEWORK ASSIGNMENT
Please read the chapter and answer the following questions:

1. What is the goal of assertive behavior?
2. Assertive individuals accept negative aspects about themselves, and admit when they have made a mistake. What is this technique called?
3. What technique may be used to rid the mind of negative thoughts with which an individual may be obsessed? Give an example.
4. Why are "I" statements an effective communication technique?

Alberti and Emmons (2008) have proposed the following questions:

> Are you able to express warm, positive feelings to another person? Are you comfortable starting a conversation with strangers at a party? Do you sometimes feel ineffective in making your desires clear to others? Do you have difficulty saying no to persuasive people? Are you often at the bottom of the "pecking order," pushed around by others? Or maybe you're the one who pushes others around to get your way? (p. 5)

Assertive behavior promotes a feeling of personal power and self-confidence. These two components are commonly lacking in clients with emotional disorders. Becoming more assertive empowers individuals by promoting self-esteem, without diminishing the esteem of others.

This chapter describes a number of rights that are considered basic to human beings. Various kinds of behaviors are explored, including assertive, nonassertive, aggressive, and passive-aggressive. Techniques that promote assertive behavior and the nurse's role in assertiveness training are presented.

CORE CONCEPT

Assertive Behavior

Assertive behavior promotes equality in human relationships, enabling us to act in our own best interests, to stand up for ourselves without undue anxiety, to express honest feelings comfortably, to exercise personal rights without denying the rights of others (Alberti & Emmons, 2008, p. 8).

Assertive Communication

Assertive behavior helps us feel good about ourselves and increases our self-esteem. It helps us feel good about other people and increases our ability to develop satisfying relationships with others. This is accomplished out of honesty, directness, appropriateness, and respecting one's own basic rights as well as the rights of others.

Honesty is basic to assertive behavior. Assertive honesty is not an outspoken declaration of everything that is on one's mind. It is instead an accurate representation of feelings, opinions, or preferences expressed in a manner that promotes self-respect and respect for others.

Direct communication is stating what one wants to convey with clarity and candor. Hinting and "beating around the bush" are indirect forms of communication.

Communication must occur in an appropriate context to be considered assertive. The location and timing, as well as the manner (tone of voice, nonverbal gestures) in which the communication is presented, must be correct for the situation.

Basic Human Rights

A number of authors have identified a variety of "assertive rights" (Bishop, 2013; Davis, Eshelman, & McKay, 2008; Lloyd, 2002; Schuster, 2000; Sobel & Ornstein, 1996). Following is a composite of 10 basic assertive human rights adapted from the aggregation of sources.

1. The right to be treated with respect.
2. The right to express feelings, opinions, and beliefs.
3. The right to say "no" without feeling guilty.
4. The right to make mistakes and accept the responsibility for them.
5. The right to be listened to and taken seriously.
6. The right to change your mind.
7. The right to ask for what you want.
8. The right to put yourself first, sometimes.
9. The right to set your own priorities.
10. The right to refuse justification for your feelings or behavior.

In accepting these rights, an individual also accepts the responsibilities that accompany them. Rights and responsibilities are reciprocal entities. To experience one without the other is inherently destructive to an individual. Some responsibilities associated with basic assertive human rights are presented in Table 14-1.

Response Patterns

Individuals develop patterns of responding to others. Some of these patterns that have been identified include:

1. Watching other people (role modeling).
2. Being positively reinforced or punished for a certain response.
3. Inventing a response.
4. Not being able to think of a better way to respond.
5. Not developing the proper skills for a better response.
6. Consciously choosing a response style.

The nurse should be able to recognize his or her own pattern of responding, as well as that of others. Four response patterns will be discussed here: nonassertive, assertive, aggressive, and passive-aggressive.

Nonassertive Behavior

Individuals who are **nonassertive** (sometimes called *passive*) seek to please others at the expense of denying their own basic human rights. They seldom let their true feelings show and often feel hurt and anxious because they allow others to choose for them. They seldom achieve their own desired goals. They come across as being very apologetic and tend to be self-deprecating. They use actions instead of words and hope someone will "guess" what they want. Their voices are hesitant, weak, and expressed in a monotone. Their eyes are usually downcast. They feel uncomfortable in interpersonal interactions. All they want is to please and to be liked by others. Their behavior helps them avoid unpleasant situations and confrontations with others; however, they often harbor anger and resentment.

Assertive Behavior

Assertive individuals stand up for their own rights while protecting the rights of others. Feelings are expressed openly and honestly. They assume responsibility for

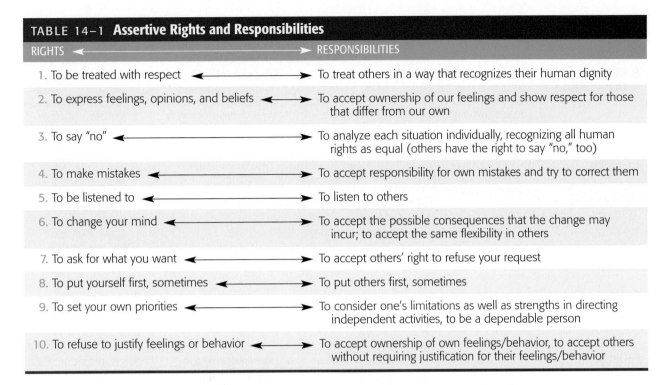

TABLE 14–1 Assertive Rights and Responsibilities

RIGHTS ←	→ RESPONSIBILITIES
1. To be treated with respect	To treat others in a way that recognizes their human dignity
2. To express feelings, opinions, and beliefs	To accept ownership of our feelings and show respect for those that differ from our own
3. To say "no"	To analyze each situation individually, recognizing all human rights as equal (others have the right to say "no," too)
4. To make mistakes	To accept responsibility for own mistakes and try to correct them
5. To be listened to	To listen to others
6. To change your mind	To accept the possible consequences that the change may incur; to accept the same flexibility in others
7. To ask for what you want	To accept others' right to refuse your request
8. To put yourself first, sometimes	To put others first, sometimes
9. To set your own priorities	To consider one's limitations as well as strengths in directing independent activities, to be a dependable person
10. To refuse to justify feelings or behavior	To accept ownership of own feelings/behavior, to accept others without requiring justification for their feelings/behavior

their own choices and allow others to choose for themselves. They maintain self-respect and respect for others by treating everyone equally and with human dignity. They communicate tactfully, using lots of "I" statements. Their voices are warm and expressive, and eye contact is intermittent but direct. These individuals desire to communicate effectively with, and be respected by, others. They are self-confident and experience satisfactory and pleasurable relationships with others.

Aggressive Behavior

Individuals who are **aggressive** defend their own basic rights by violating the basic rights of others. Feelings are often expressed dishonestly and inappropriately. They say what is on their mind, often at the expense of others. Aggressive behavior commonly results in *"put-downs,"* leaving the receiver feeling hurt, defensive, and humiliated. Aggressive individuals devalue the self-worth of others on whom they impose their choices. They express an air of superiority, and their voices are often loud, demanding, angry, or cold, without emotion. Eye contact may be "to intimidate others by staring them down." They want to increase their feeling of power by dominating or humiliating others. Aggressive behavior hinders interpersonal relationships.

Passive-Aggressive Behavior

Passive-aggressive individuals defend their own rights by expressing resistance and general obstructiveness in response to the expectations of others (Black &

Andreasen, 2011). This kind of behavior is sometimes referred to as *indirect, or covert, aggression,* and takes the form of passive, nonconfrontative action. These individuals are devious, manipulative, and sly, and they undermine others with behavior that expresses the opposite of what they are feeling. They are highly critical and sarcastic. They allow others to make choices for them, then resist by using passive behaviors, such as procrastination, dawdling, stubbornness, and "forgetfulness." They use actions instead of words to convey their message, and the actions express covert aggression. They become sulky, irritable, or argumentative when asked to do something they do not want to do. They may protest to others about the demand but will not confront the person who is making the demand. Instead, they may deal with the demand by "forgetting" to do it. The goal is domination through retaliation. This behavior offers a feeling of control and power, although passive-aggressive individuals actually feel resentment and that they are being taken advantage of. They possess extremely low self-confidence.

A comparison of these four behavior patterns is presented in Table 14-2.

Behavioral Components of Assertive Behavior

Alberti and Emmons (2008) have identified several defining characteristics of assertive behavior:

■ **Eye contact.** Eye contact is considered appropriate when it is intermittent (i.e., looking directly at the

TABLE 14–2 Comparison of Behavioral Response Patterns

	NONASSERTIVE	ASSERTIVE	AGGRESSIVE	PASSIVE-AGGRESSIVE
Behavioral characteristics	Passive, does not express true feelings, self-deprecating, denies own rights	Stands up for own rights, protects rights of others, honest, direct, appropriate	Violates rights of others, expresses feelings dishonestly and inappropriately	Defends own rights with passive resistance, is critical and sarcastic; often expresses opposite of true feelings
Examples	"Uh, well, uh, sure, I'll be glad to stay and work an extra shift."	"I don't want to stay and work an extra shift today. I stayed over yesterday. It's someone else's turn today."	"You've got to be kidding!"	"Okay, I'll stay and work an extra shift." (Then to peer: "How dare she ask me to work over again! Well, we'll just see how much work she gets out of me!")
Goals	To please others; to be liked by others	To communicate effectively; to be respected by others	To dominate or humiliate others	To dominate through retaliation
Feelings	Anxious, hurt, disappointed with self, angry, resentful	Confident, successful, proud, self-respecting	Self-righteous, controlling, superior	Anger, resentment, manipulated, controlled
Compensation	Is able to avoid unpleasant situations and confrontations with others	Increased self-confidence, self-respect, respect for others, satisfying interpersonal relationships	Anger is released, increasing feeling of power and superiority	Feels self-righteous and in control
Outcomes	Goals not met; others meet *their* goals at nonassertive person's expense; anger and resentment grow; feels violated and manipulated	Goals met; desires most often fulfilled while defending own rights as well as rights of others	Goals may be met but at the expense of others; they feel hurt and vengeful	Goals not met, nor are the goals of others met due to retaliatory nature of the interaction

SOURCES: Alberti & Emmons, 2008; Bishop, 2013; Davis, Eshelman, & McKay, 2008; Lloyd, 2002; and Powell & Enright, 1990.

person to whom one is speaking but looking away now and then). Individuals feel uncomfortable when someone stares at them continuously and intently. Intermittent eye contact conveys the message that one is interested in what is being said.
■ **Body posture.** Sitting and leaning slightly toward the other person in a conversation suggests an active interest in what is being said. Emphasis on an assertive stance can be achieved by standing with an erect posture, squarely facing the other person. A slumped posture conveys passivity or nonassertiveness.
■ **Distance/physical contact.** The distance between two individuals in an interaction or the physical contact between them has a strong cultural influence. For example, in the United States, intimate distance is

considered approximately 18 inches from the body. We are very careful about whom we allow to enter this intimate space. Invasion of this space may be interpreted by some individuals as very aggressive.
■ **Gestures.** Nonverbal gestures may also be culturally related. Gesturing can add emphasis, warmth, depth, or power to the spoken word.
■ **Facial expression.** Various facial expressions convey different messages (e.g., frown, smile, surprise, anger, fear). It is difficult to "fake" these messages. In assertive communication, the facial expression is congruent with the verbal message.
■ **Voice.** The voice conveys a message by its loudness, softness, degree and placement of emphasis, and evidence of emotional tone.

■ **Fluency.** Being able to discuss a subject with ease and with obvious knowledge conveys assertiveness and self-confidence. This message is impeded by numerous pauses or filler words such as "and, uh . . ." or "you know . . ."

■ **Timing.** Assertive responses are most effective when they are spontaneous and immediate. However, most people have experienced times when it was not appropriate to respond (e.g., in front of a group of people) or times when an appropriate response is generated only after the fact ("If only I had said . . ."). Alberti and Emmons (2008, p. 77) stated that "it is never too late to be assertive!" It is correct and worthwhile to seek out the individual at a later time and express the assertive response.

■ **Listening.** Assertive listening means giving the other individual full attention by making eye contact, nodding to indicate acceptance of what is being said, and taking time to understand what is being said before giving a response.

■ **Thoughts.** Cognitive processes affect one's assertive behavior. Two such processes are (1) an individual's attitudes about the appropriateness of assertive behavior in general and (2) the appropriateness of assertive behavior for himself or herself specifically.

■ **Content.** Many times individuals do not respond to an unpleasant situation because "I just didn't know what to say." Perhaps *what* is being said is not as important as *how* it is said. Emotions should be expressed when they are experienced. It is also important to accept ownership of those emotions and not devalue the worth of another individual to assert oneself.

■ **Persistence.** This element of assertive behavior speaks to not giving up; that is, to refrain from concluding that the individual is not worth whatever it is he or she is pursuing. Alberti and Emmons (2008) suggest that all of the components of assertive behavior are important; "the element of persistence simply means applying them again, and again, and again, as needed." (p. 81)

Techniques That Promote Assertive Behavior

The following techniques have been shown to be effective in responding to criticism and avoiding manipulation by others.

1. **Standing up for one's basic human rights.**

EXAMPLE

"I have the right to express my opinion."

2. **Assuming responsibility for one's own statements.**

EXAMPLE

"I *don't want* to go out with you tonight," instead of "I *can't* go out with you tonight." The latter implies a lack of power or ability.

3. **Responding as a "broken record."** Persistently repeating in a calm voice what is wanted.

EXAMPLE

Telephone salesperson: "I want to help you save money by changing long-distance services."
Assertive response: "I don't want to change my long-distance service."
Telephone salesperson: "I can't believe you don't want to save money!"
Assertive response: "I don't want to change my long-distance service."

4. **Agreeing assertively.** Assertively accepting negative aspects about oneself; admitting when an error has been made.

EXAMPLE

Ms. Jones: "You sure let that meeting get out of hand. What a waste of time."
Ms. Smith: "Yes, I didn't do a very good job of conducting the meeting today."

5. **Inquiring assertively.** Seeking additional information about critical statements.

EXAMPLE

Male board member: "You made a real fool of yourself at the board meeting last night."
Female board member: "Oh, really? Just what about my behavior offended you?"
Male board member: "You were so damned pushy!"
Female board member: "Were you offended that I spoke up for my beliefs, or was it because my beliefs are in direct opposition to yours?"

6. **Shifting from content to process.** Changing the focus of the communication from discussing the topic at hand to analyzing what is actually going on in the interaction.

EXAMPLE

Wife: "Would you please call me if you will be late for dinner?"
Husband: "Why don't you just get off my back! I always have to account for every minute of my time with you!"
Wife: "Sounds to me like we need to discuss some other things here. What are you *really* angry about?"

7. **Clouding/fogging.** Concurring with the critic's argument without becoming defensive and without agreeing to change.

EXAMPLE

Nurse 1: "You never come to the Nurses' Association meetings. I don't know why you even belong!"

Nurse 2: "You're right. I haven't attended very many of the meetings."

8. **Defusing.** Putting off further discussion with an angry individual until he or she is calmer.

EXAMPLE

"You are very angry right now. I don't want to discuss this matter with you while you are so upset. I will discuss it with you in my office at 3 o'clock this afternoon."

9. **Delaying assertively.** Putting off further discussion with another individual until one is calmer.

EXAMPLE

"That's a very challenging position you have taken, Mr. Brown. I'll need time to give it some thought. I'll call you later this afternoon."

10. **Responding assertively with irony.**

EXAMPLE

Man: "I bet you're one of them so-called 'women's libbers,' aren't you?"
Woman: "Why, yes. Thank you for noticing."

11. **Using "I" statements.** "I" statements allow an individual to take ownership for his or her feelings rather than saying they are caused by another person.

"I" statements are sometimes called "feeling" statements. They express directly what an individual is feeling. "You" statements are accusatory and put the receiver on the defensive. "I" statements have four parts:

1. How I feel: *these are my feelings and I accept ownership of them.*
2. When: *describe in a neutral manner the behavior that is the problem.*
3. Why: *describe what it is about the behavior that is objectionable.*
4. Suggest change: *offering a preferred alternative to the behavior.*

EXAMPLE

John has just returned from a hunting trip and walked into the living room in his muddy boots leaving a trail of mud on the carpet. His wife, Mary, may respond as follows:

With a "you" statement: "You are such a jerk! Can't you see the trail of mud you are leaving on the carpet? I just cleaned this carpet. You make me so angry!"
With an "I" statement: "I feel so angry when you walk on the carpet in your muddy boots. I just cleaned it, and now I will have to clean it again. I would appreciate it if you would remove your boots on the porch before you come in the house."

"You" statements are negative and focus on what the person has done wrong. They don't explain what is being requested of the person. "I" statements are more positive. They explain *how* one is feeling, *why* he or she is feeling that way, and *what* the individual wants instead. Hopkins (2013) stated the following about the importance of "I" statements:

> Part of being assertive involves the ability to appropriately express your needs and feelings. You can accomplish this by using "I" statements. These [statements] indicate ownership, do not attribute blame, focus on behavior, identify the effect of the behavior, are direct and honest, and contribute to the growth of your relationship with each other. (p. 2)

Thought-Stopping Techniques

Assertive thinking is sometimes inhibited by repetitive, negative thoughts of which the mind refuses to let go. Individuals with low self-worth may be obsessed with thoughts such as, "I know he'd never want to go out with me. I'm too ugly (or plain, or fat, or dumb)" or "I just know I'll never be able to do this job well" or "I just can't seem to do anything right." This type of thinking fosters the belief that one's individual rights do not deserve the same consideration as those of others, and reflects nonassertive communication and behavioral response patterns.

Thought-stopping techniques, as described here, were developed by psychiatrist Joseph Wolpe (1990) and are intended to eliminate intrusive, unwanted thoughts.

Method

In a practice setting, with eyes closed, the individual concentrates on an unwanted recurring thought. Once the thought is clearly established in the mind, he or she shouts aloud: "STOP!" This action will interrupt the thought, and it is actually removed from one's awareness. The individual then immediately shifts his or her thoughts to one that is considered pleasant and desirable.

It is possible that the unwanted thought may soon recur, but with practice, the length of time between recurrences will increase until the unwanted thought is no longer intrusive.

Obviously, one cannot go about his or her daily life shouting, "STOP!" in public places. After a number of practice sessions, the technique is equally effective if the word "stop!" is used silently in the mind.

Role of the Nurse in Assertiveness Training

It is important for nurses to become aware of and recognize their own behavioral responses. Are they mostly nonassertive? Assertive? Aggressive? Passive-aggressive? Do they consider their behavioral responses effective? Do they wish to change? Remember, all individuals have the right to choose whether or not they want to be assertive. A self-assessment of assertiveness is found in Box 14-1.

The ability to respond assertively is especially important to nurses who are committed to further development of the profession. Assertive skills facilitate the implementation of change—change that is required if the image of nursing is to be upgraded to the level of professionalism that most nurses desire. Assertive communication is useful in the political arena for nurses who choose to become involved at both state and national levels in striving to influence legislation and, ultimately, to improve the system of health-care provision in our country.

Nurses who understand and use assertiveness skills themselves can in turn assist clients who wish to effect behavioral change in an effort to increase self-esteem and improve interpersonal relationships. The nursing process is a useful tool for nurses who are involved in helping clients increase their assertiveness.

Assessment

Nurses can help clients become more aware of their behavioral responses. Many tools for assessing the level of assertiveness have been attempted over the years. None have been very effective. Perhaps this is because it is so difficult to *generalize* when attempting to measure assertive behaviors. Box 14-2 and Figure 14-1 represent examples of assertiveness inventories that could be personalized to describe life situations of individual clients more specifically. Obviously, "everyday situations that may require assertiveness" are not the same for all individuals.

Diagnosis

Possible nursing diagnoses for individuals needing assistance with assertiveness include:

1. Coping, defensive
2. Coping, ineffective
3. Decisional conflict
4. Denial, ineffective
5. Personal identity, disturbed
6. Powerlessness
7. Rape-trauma syndrome
8. Self-esteem, low
9. Social interaction, impaired
10. Social isolation

Outcome Identification/Implementation

The goal for nurses working with individuals needing assistance with assertiveness is to help them develop

---

BOX 14-1 **An Assertiveness Quiz**

Assign a number to each item using the following scale: 1 = Never; 3 = Sometimes; 5 = Always

_____ 1. I ask others to do things without feeling guilty or anxious.
_____ 2. When someone asks me to do something I don't want to do, I say no without feeling guilty or anxious.
_____ 3. I am comfortable when speaking to a large group of people.
_____ 4. I confidently express my honest opinions to authority figures (such as my boss).
_____ 5. When I experience powerful feelings (anger, frustration, disappointment, and so on), I verbalize them easily.
_____ 6. When I express anger, I do so without blaming others for "making me mad."
_____ 7. I am comfortable speaking up in a group situation.
_____ 8. If I disagree with the majority opinion in a meeting, I can "stick to my guns" without feeling uncomfortable or being abrasive.
_____ 9. When I make a mistake, I acknowledge it.
_____10. I tell others when their behavior creates a problem for me.
_____11. Meeting new people in social situations is something I do with ease and comfort.
_____12. When discussing my beliefs, I do so without labeling the opinions of others as "crazy," "stupid," "ridiculous," or "irrational."
_____13. I assume that most people are competent and trustworthy, and I do not have difficulty delegating tasks to others.
_____14. When considering doing something I have never done, I feel confident I can learn to do it.
_____15. I believe that my needs are as important as those of others, and I am entitled to have my needs satisfied.
_____   TOTAL SCORE

SCORING:
1. If your total score is 60 or higher, you have a consistently assertive philosophy and probably handle most situations well.
2. If your total score is 45-59, you have a fairly assertive outlook but may benefit from some assertiveness training.
3. If your total score is 30-44, you may be assertive in some situations, but your natural response is either nonassertive or aggressive. Assertiveness training is suggested.
4. If your total score is 15-29, you have considerable difficulty being assertive. Assertiveness training is recommended.

SOURCE: Lloyd, S.R. (2002). *Developing positive assertiveness* (3rd ed.). Menlo Park, CA: Crisp Publications. With permission.

BOX 14-2 Everyday Situations That May Require Assertiveness

AT WORK

How do you respond when:

1. You receive a compliment on your appearance or someone praises your work?
2. You are criticized unfairly?
3. You are criticized legitimately by a superior?
4. You have to confront a subordinate for continual lateness or sloppy work?
5. Your boss makes a sexual innuendo or makes a pass at you?

IN PUBLIC

How do you respond when:

1. In a restaurant, the food you ordered arrives cold or overcooked?
2. A fellow passenger in a no-smoking compartment lights a cigarette?
3. You are faced with an unhelpful shop assistant?
4. Somebody barges in front of you in a waiting line?
5. You take an inferior article back to a shop?

AMONG FRIENDS

How do you respond when:

1. You feel angry with the way a friend has treated you?
2. A friend makes what you consider to be an unreasonable request?
3. You want to ask a friend for a favor?
4. You ask a friend for repayment of a loan of money?
5. You have to negotiate with a friend on which film to see or where to meet?

AT HOME

How do you respond when:

1. One of your parents criticizes you?
2. You are irritated by a persistent habit in someone you love?
3. Everybody leaves the cleaning-up chores to you?
4. You want to say "no" to a proposed visit to a relative?
5. Your partner feels amorous but you are not in the mood?

SOURCE: From Powell, T. J., & Enright, S. J. (1990). *Anxiety and stress management.* London: Routledge. With permission.

---

more satisfying interpersonal relationships. Individuals who do not feel good about themselves either allow others to violate their rights or cover up their low self-esteem by being overtly or covertly aggressive. Individuals should be given information regarding their individual human rights. They must know what these rights are before they can stand up for them.

Outcome criteria would be derived from specific nursing diagnoses. Some examples include the following. Timelines are individually determined.

■ The client verbalizes and accepts responsibility for his or her own behavior.
■ The client is able to express opinions and disagree with the opinions of others in a socially acceptable manner and without feeling guilty.
■ The client is able to verbalize positive aspects about self.
■ The client verbalizes choices made in a plan to maintain control over his or her life situation.
■ The client approaches others in an appropriate manner for one-to-one interaction.

In a clinical setting, nurses can teach clients the techniques to use to increase their assertive responses. This can be done on a one-to-one basis or in group situations. Once these techniques have been discussed, nurses can assist clients to practice them through role-playing. Each client should compose a list of specific personal examples of situations that create difficulties for him or her. These situations will then be simulated in the therapy setting so that the client may practice assertive responses in a nonthreatening environment. In a group situation, feedback from peers can provide valuable insight about the effectiveness of the response.

> **CLINICAL PEARL** An important part of this type of intervention is to ensure that clients are aware of the differences among assertive, nonassertive, aggressive, and passive-aggressive behaviors in the same situation. When discussion is held about what the best (assertive) response would be, it is also important to discuss the other types of responses as well, so that clients can begin to recognize their pattern of response and make changes accordingly.

CLINICAL EXAMPLE

Linda comes to day hospital once a week to attend group therapy and assertiveness training. She has had problems with depression and low self-esteem. She is married to a man who is verbally abusive. He is highly critical, is seldom satisfied with anything Linda does, and blames her for negative consequences that occur in their lives, whether or not she is involved.

Since the group began, the nurse who leads the assertiveness training group has taught the participants about basic human rights and the various types of response patterns. When the nurse asks for client situations to be presented in group, Linda volunteers to discuss an incident that occurred in her home this week. She related that she had just put some chicken on the stove to cook for supper when her 7-year-old son came running in the house yelling that he had been hurt. Linda went to him and observed that he had blood

DIRECTIONS: Fill in each block with a rating of your assertiveness on a 5-point scale. A rating of 0 means you have no difficulty asserting yourself. A rating of 5 means that you are completely unable to assert yourself. Evaluation can be made by analyzing the scores:

1. totally by activity, including all of the different people categories
2. totally by people, including all of the different activity categories
3. on an individual basis, considering specific people and specific activities

PEOPLE / ACTIVITY	Friends of the same sex	Friends of the opposite sex	Intimate relations or spouse	Authority figures	Relatives/ family members	Colleagues and sub-ordinates	Strangers	Service workers; waiters; shop assistants, etc.
Giving and receiving compliments								
Asking for favors/help								
Initiating and maintaining conversation								
Refusing requests								
Expressing personal opinions								
Expressing anger/dis-pleasure								
Expressing liking, love, affection								
Stating your rights and needs								

FIGURE 14–1 Rating your assertiveness. (From Powell, T. J., & Enright, S. J. [1990]. *Anxiety and stress management.* London: Routledge, with permission.)

dripping down the side of his head from his forehead. He said he and some friends had been playing on the jungle gym in the schoolyard down the street, and he had fallen and hit his head. Linda went with him to the bathroom to clean the wound and apply some medication. Her husband, Joe, was reading the newspaper in the living room. By the time she got back to the chicken on the stove, it was burned and inedible. Her husband shouted, "You stupid woman! You can't do anything right!" Linda did not respond but burst into tears.

The nurse asked the other members in the group to present some ideas about how Linda could have responded to Joe's criticism. After some discussion, they agreed that Linda might have stated, "I made a mistake. I am not stupid and I do lots of things right." They also discussed other types of responses and why they were less acceptable. They recognized that Linda's lack of verbal response and bursting into tears was a nonassertive response. They also agreed on other examples, such as:

1. An aggressive response might be, "Cook your own supper!" and toss the skillet out the back door.
2. A passive-aggressive response might be to fix sandwiches for supper and not speak to Joe for 3 days.

Practice on the assertive response began, with the nurse and various members of the group playing the role of Joe so that Linda could practice until she felt comfortable with the response. She participated in the group for 6 months, regularly submitting situations with which she needed help. She also learned from the situations presented by other members of the group. These weekly sessions gave Linda the self-confidence that she needed to stand up to Joe's criticism. She was aware of her basic human rights and, with practice, was able to stand up for them in an assertive manner. She was happy to report to the group after a few months that Joe seemed to be less critical and that their relationship was improving.

Evaluation

Evaluation requires that the nurse and client assess whether or not these techniques are achieving the desired outcomes. Reassessment might include the following questions:

■ Is the client able to accept criticism without becoming defensive?

■ Can the client express true feelings to (spouse, friend, boss, and others) when his or her basic human rights are violated?

■ Is the client able to decline a request without feeling guilty?

■ Can the client verbalize positive qualities about himself or herself?

■ Does the client verbalize improvement in interpersonal relationships?

Assertiveness training serves to extend and create more flexibility in an individual's communication style so that he or she has a greater choice of responses in various situations. Although change does not come easily, assertiveness training can be an effective way of changing behavior. Nurses can assist individuals to become more assertive, thereby encouraging them to become what they want to be, promoting an improvement in self-esteem, and fostering a respect for their own rights and the rights of others.

Summary and Key Points

■ Assertive behavior helps individuals feel better about themselves by encouraging them to stand up for their own basic human rights.

■ Basic human rights have equal representation for all individuals.

■ Along with rights comes an equal number of responsibilities. Part of being assertive includes living up to these responsibilities.

■ Assertive behavior increases self-esteem and the ability to develop satisfying interpersonal relationships. This is accomplished through honesty, directness, appropriateness, and respecting one's own rights, and the rights of others.

■ Individuals develop patterns of responding in various ways, such as role modeling, by receiving positive or negative reinforcement, or by conscious choice.

■ Patterns of responding can take the form of nonassertiveness, assertiveness, aggressiveness, or passive-aggressiveness.

■ *Nonassertive* individuals seek to please others at the expense of denying their own basic human rights.

■ *Assertive* individuals stand up for their own rights while protecting the rights of others.

■ Those who respond *aggressively* defend their own rights by violating the basic rights of others.

■ Individuals who respond in a *passive-aggressive* manner defend their own rights by expressing resistance to social and occupational demands.

■ Some important behavioral considerations of assertive behavior include eye contact, body posture, distance/physical contact, gestures, facial expression, voice, fluency, timing, listening, thoughts, content, and persistence.

■ A discussion of techniques that have been developed to assist individuals in the process of becoming more assertive was presented.

■ Negative thinking can sometimes interfere with one's ability to respond assertively. Thought-stopping techniques help individuals remove negative, unwanted thoughts from awareness and promote the development of a more assertive attitude.

■ Nurses can assist individuals to learn and practice assertiveness techniques.

■ The nursing process is an effective vehicle for providing the information and support to clients as they strive to create positive change in their lives.

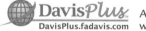 Additional info available at
DavisPlus.fadavis.com   www.davisplus.com

Review Questions
Self-Examination/Learning Exercise

*Select the answer that is **most** appropriate for each of the following questions.*

1. Your husband says, "You're crazy to think about going to college! You're not smart enough to handle the studies and the housework, too." Which of the following is an example of a nonassertive response?
   a. "I will do what I can, and the best that I can."
   b. (Thinking to yourself): "We'll see how *he* likes cooking dinner for a change."
   c. "You're probably right. Maybe I should reconsider."
   d. "I'm going to do what I want to do, when I want to do it, and you can't stop me!"

Review Questions—cont'd
Self-Examination/Learning Exercise

2. You are having company for dinner and they are due to arrive in 20 minutes. You are about to finish cooking and still have to shower and dress. The doorbell rings and it is a man selling a new product for cleaning windows. Which of the following is an example of an aggressive response?

   a. "I don't do windows!" and slam the door in his face.

   b. "I'll take a case," and write him a check.

   c. "Sure, I'll take three bottles." Then to yourself you think: "I'm calling this company tomorrow and complaining to the manager about their salespeople coming around at dinnertime!"

   d. "I'm very busy at the moment. I don't wish to purchase any of your product. Thank you."

3. You are in a movie theater that prohibits smoking. The person in the seat next to you just lit a cigarette and the smoke is very irritating. Which of the following is an example of an assertive response?

   a. You say nothing.

   b. "Please put your cigarette out. Smoking is prohibited."

   c. You say nothing, but begin to frantically fan the air in front of you and cough loudly and convulsively.

   d. "Put your cigarette out, you slob! Can't you read the 'no smoking' sign?"

4. You have been studying for a nursing exam all afternoon and lost track of time. Your husband expects dinner on the table when he gets home from work. You have not started cooking yet when he walks in the door and shouts, "Why the heck isn't dinner ready?" Which of the following is an example of a passive-aggressive response?

   a. "I'm sorry. I'll have it done in no time, honey." But then you move very slowly and take a long time to cook the meal.

   b. "I'm tired from studying all afternoon. Make your own dinner, you bum! I'm tired of being your slave!"

   c. "I haven't started dinner yet. I'd like some help from you."

   d. "I'm so sorry. I know you're tired and hungry. It's all my fault. I'm such a terrible wife!"

5. You and your best friend, Jill, have had plans for 6 months to go on vacation together to Hawaii. You have saved your money and have plane tickets to leave in 3 weeks. She has just called you and reported that she is not going. She has a new boyfriend, they are moving in together, and she does not want to leave him. You are very angry with Jill for changing your plans. Which of the following is an example of an assertive response?

   a. "I'm very disappointed and very angry. I'd like to talk to you about this later. I'll call you."

   b. "I'm very happy for you, Jill. I think it's wonderful that you and Jack are moving in together."

   c. You tell Jill that you are very happy for her, but then say to another friend, "Well, that's the end of my friendship with Jill!"

   d. "What? You can't do that to me! We've had plans! You're acting like a real slut!"

6. A typewritten report for your psychiatric nursing class is due tomorrow at 8 a.m. The assignment was made 4 weeks ago, and yours is ready to turn in. Your roommate says, "I finally finished writing my report, but now I have to go to work, and I don't have time to type it. Please be a dear and type it for me, otherwise I'll fail!" You have a date with your boyfriend. Which of the following is an example of an aggressive response?

   a. "Okay, I'll call Ken and cancel our date."

   b. "I don't want to stay here and type your report. I'm going out with Ken."

   c. "You've got to be kidding! What kind of a fool do you take me for, anyway?"

   d. "Okay, I'll do it." However, when your roommate returns from work at midnight, you are asleep and the report has not been typed.

Continued

Review Questions—cont'd
Self-Examination/Learning Exercise

7. You are asked to serve on a committee on which you do not wish to serve. Which of the following is an example of a nonassertive response?
   a. "Thank you, but I don't wish to be a member of that committee."
   b. "I'll be happy to serve." But then you don't show up for any of the meetings.
   c. "I'd rather have my teeth pulled!"
   d. "Okay, if I'm really needed, I'll serve."

8. You're on your way to the laundry room when you encounter a fellow dorm tenant who often asks you to "throw a few of my things in with yours." You view this as an imposition. He asks you where you're going. Which of the following is an example of a passive-aggressive response?
   a. "I'm on my way to the Celtics game. Where do you think I'm going?"
   b. "I'm on my way to do some laundry. Do you have anything you want me to wash with mine?"
   c. "It's none of your damn business!"
   d. "I'm going to the laundry room. Please don't ask me to do some of yours. I resent being taken advantage of in that way."

9. At a hospital committee meeting, a fellow nurse who is the chairperson has interrupted you each time you have tried to make a statement. The next time it happens, you intend to respond assertively. Which of the following is an example of an assertive response?
   a. "You make a lousy leader! You won't even let me finish what I'm trying to say!"
   b. You say nothing.
   c. "Excuse me. I would like to finish my statement."
   d. You say nothing, but you fail to complete your assignment and do not show up for the next meeting.

10. A fellow worker often borrows small amounts of money from you with the promise that she will pay you back "tomorrow." She currently owes you $15, and has not yet paid back any that she has borrowed. She asks if she can borrow a couple of dollars for lunch. Which of the following is an example of a nonassertive response?
    a. "I've decided not to loan you any more money until you pay me back what you already borrowed."
    b. "I'm so sorry. I only have enough to pay for my own lunch today."
    c. "Get a life, will you? I'm tired of you sponging off me all the time!"
    d. "Sure, here's two dollars." Then to the other workers in the office: "Be sure you never lend Cindy any money. She never pays her debts. I'd be sure never to go to lunch with her if I were you!"

References

Alberti, R.E., & Emmons, M.L. (2008). *Your perfect right* (9th ed.). Atascadero, CA: Impact Publishers.

Bishop, S. (2013). *Develop your assertiveness.* Philadelphia, PA: Kogan Page.

Black, D.W., & Andreasen, N.C. (2011). *Introductory textbook of psychiatry* (5th ed.). Washington, DC: American Psychiatric Publishing.

Davis, M., Eshelman, E.R., & McKay, M. (2008). *The relaxation and stress reduction workbook* (6th ed). Oakland, CA: New Harbinger Publications.

Hopkins, L. (2013). Assertive communication: Six tips for effective use. *EzineArticles.* Retrieved from http://ezinearticles. com/?Assertive-Communication—6-Tips-For-Effective-Use &id=10259

Lloyd, S.R. (2002). *Developing positive assertiveness* (3rd ed.). Menlo Park, CA: Crisp Publications.

Powell, T.J., & Enright, S.J. (1990). *Anxiety and stress management.* London: Routledge.

Schuster, P.M. (2000). *Communication: The key to the therapeutic relationship.* Philadelphia, PA: F.A. Davis.

Sobel, D.S., & Ornstein, R. (1996). *The healthy mind/healthy body handbook.* New York, NY: Patient Education Media.

Wolpe, J. (1990). *The practice of behavior therapy* (4th ed.) Elmsford, NY: Pergamon Press.

Promoting Self-Esteem 15

CORE CONCEPTS

self-concept
self-esteem

KEY TERMS

body image
boundaries
contextual stimuli
enmeshed boundaries
flexible boundaries

focal stimuli
moral-ethical self
physical self
residual stimuli
rigid boundaries

self-consistency
self-expectancy
self-ideal

OBJECTIVES
After reading this chapter, the student will be able to:

1. Identify and define components of the self-concept.
2. Discuss influencing factors in the development of self-esteem and its progression through the life span.
3. Describe the verbal and nonverbal manifestations of low self-esteem.
4. Discuss the concept of boundaries and its relationship to self-esteem.
5. Apply the nursing process with clients who are experiencing disturbances in self-esteem.

HOMEWORK ASSIGNMENT
Please read the chapter and answer the following questions:

1. Children need unconditional love to promote positive self-esteem. How do parents demonstrate unconditional love?
2. Since her parents' divorce, 10-year-old Nancy and her mother have become inseparable. They spend all their spare time together, and Nancy has become her mother's confidant. This is an example of what type of boundary?
3. How does fulfillment of the developmental tasks described by Erikson promote a healthy self-esteem?
4. Name the three components of the self-concept and the meaning that individuals attach to each.

McKay and Fanning (2000) described **self-esteem** as an emotional *sine qua non*, a component that is essential for psychological survival. They state, "Without some measure of self-worth, life can be enormously painful, with many basic needs going unmet" (p. 1).

The awareness of self (i.e., the ability to form an identity and then attach a value to it) is an important differentiating factor between humans and other animals. This capacity for judgment, then, becomes a contributing factor in disturbances of self-esteem.

The promotion of self-esteem is about stopping self-judgments. It is about helping individuals change how they perceive and feel about themselves. This chapter describes the developmental progression and the verbal and behavioral manifestations of self-esteem. The concept of **boundaries** and its relationship to self-esteem is explored. Nursing care of clients with disturbances in self-esteem is described in the context of the nursing process.

CORE CONCEPT

Self-Concept

Self-concept is the cognitive or thinking component of the self, and generally refers to the totality of a complex, organized, and dynamic system of learned beliefs, attitudes and opinions that each person holds to be true about his or her personal existence (Huitt, 2011).

Components of Self-Concept

Physical Self or Body Image

An individual's **body image** is a subjective perception of one's physical appearance based on self-evaluation and on reactions and feedback from others. Gorman and Sultan (2008) state:

> Body image is the mental picture a person has of his or her own body. It significantly influences the way a person thinks and feels about his or her body as a whole, about its functions, and about the internal and external sensations associated with it. It also includes perceptions of the way others see the person's body and is central to self-concept and self-esteem. (p. 9)

An individual's body image may not necessarily coincide with his or her actual appearance. For example, individuals who have been overweight for many years and then lose weight often have difficulty perceiving of themselves as thin. They may even continue to choose clothing in the size they were before they lost weight.

A disturbance in one's body image may occur with changes in structure or function. Examples of changes in bodily structure include amputations, mastectomy,

and facial disfigurements. Functional alterations are conditions such as colostomy, paralysis, and impotence. Alterations in body image are often experienced as losses.

Personal Identity

This component of the self-concept is composed of the moral-ethical self, the self-consistency, and the self-ideal/self-expectancy.

The **moral-ethical self** is that aspect of the personal identity that evaluates who the individual says he or she is. This component of the personal self observes, compares, sets standards, and makes judgments that influence an individual's self-evaluation.

Self-consistency is the component of the personal identity that strives to maintain a stable self-image. Even if the self-image is negative, because of this need for stability and self-consistency, the individual resists letting go of the image from which he or she has achieved a measure of constancy.

Self-ideal/self-expectancy relates to an individual's perception of what he or she wants to be, to do, or to become. The concept of the ideal self arises out of the perception one has of the expectations of others. Disturbances in self-concept can occur when individuals are unable to achieve their ideals and expectancies.

CORE CONCEPT

Self-Esteem

Self-esteem refers to the degree of regard or respect that individuals have for themselves and is a measure of worth that they place on their abilities and judgments.

Self-Esteem

Warren (1991) stated:

> Self-esteem breaks down into two components: (1) the ability to say that "I am important," "I matter," and (2) the ability to say "I am competent," "I have something to offer to others and the world. (p. 1)

Maslow (1970) postulated that individuals must achieve a positive self-esteem before they can achieve self-actualization (see Chapter 2). On a day-to-day basis, one's self-value is challenged by changes within the environment. With a positive self-worth, individuals are able to adapt successfully to the demands associated with situational and maturational crises that occur. The ability to adapt to these environmental changes is impaired when individuals hold themselves in low esteem.

Self-esteem is very closely related to the other components of the self-concept. Just as with body image and personal identity, the development of self-esteem is largely influenced by the perceptions of how one is viewed by significant others. It begins in early childhood and vacillates throughout the life span.

Development of Self-Esteem

How self-esteem is established has been the topic of investigation for a number of theorists and clinicians. From a review of personality theories, Coopersmith (1981) identified the following antecedent conditions of positive self-esteem:

■ **Power.** It is important for individuals to have a feeling of control over their own life situation and an ability to claim some measure of influence over the behaviors of others.

■ **Significance.** Self-esteem is enhanced when individuals feel loved, respected, and cared for by significant others.

■ **Virtue.** Individuals feel good about themselves when their actions reflect a set of personal, moral, and ethical values.

■ **Competence.** Positive self-esteem develops out of one's ability to perform successfully or achieve self-expectations and the expectations of others.

■ **Consistently set limits.** A structured lifestyle demonstrates acceptance and caring and provides a feeling of security.

Warren (1991) outlined the following focus areas to be emphasized by parents and others who work with children when encouraging the growth and development of positive self-esteem:

■ **A sense of competence.** Everyone needs to feel skilled at something. Warren (1991) stated, "Children do not necessarily need to be THE best at a skill in order to have positive self-esteem; what they need to feel is that they have accomplished their PERSONAL best effort" (p. 1).

■ **Unconditional love.** Children need to know that they are loved and accepted by family and friends regardless of success or failure. This is demonstrated by expressive touch, realistic praise, and separation of criticism of the person from criticism of the behavior.

■ **A sense of survival.** Everyone fails at something from time to time. Self-esteem is enhanced when individuals learn from failure and grow in the knowledge that they are stronger for having experienced it.

■ **Realistic goals.** Low self-esteem can be the result of not being able to achieve established goals. Individuals may "set themselves up" for failure by setting goals that are unattainable. Goals can be unrealistic when they are beyond a child's capability to achieve, require an inordinate amount of effort to accomplish, and are based on exaggerated fantasy.

■ **A sense of responsibility.** Children gain positive self-worth when they are assigned areas of responsibility or are expected to complete tasks that they perceive are valued by others.

■ **Reality orientation.** Personal limitations abound within our world, and it is important for children to recognize and achieve a healthy balance between what they can possess and achieve, and what is beyond their capability or control.

Other factors that have been found to be influential in the development of self-esteem include the following:

■ **The responses of others.** The development of self-esteem can be positively or negatively influenced by the responses of others, particularly significant others, and by how individuals perceive those responses.

■ **Hereditary factors.** Factors that are genetically determined, such as physical appearance, size, or inherited infirmity, can have an effect on the development of self-esteem.

■ **Environmental conditions.** The development of self-esteem can be influenced by demands from the environment. For example, intellectual prowess may be incorporated into the self-worth of an individual who is reared in an academic environment.

Developmental Progression of Self-Esteem Through the Life Span

The development of self-esteem progresses throughout the life span. Erikson's (1963) theory of personality development provides a useful framework for illustration (see Chapter 3). Erikson describes eight transitional or maturational crises, the resolution of which can have a profound influence on self-esteem. If a crisis is successfully resolved at one stage, the individual develops healthy coping strategies that he or she can draw on to help fulfill tasks of subsequent stages. When an individual fails to achieve the tasks associated with a developmental stage, emotional growth is inhibited, and he or she is less able to cope with subsequent maturational or situational crises.

Trust versus Mistrust (Birth to 18 Months)

The development of trust results in a feeling of confidence in the predictability of the environment. Achievement of trust results in positive self-esteem through the instillation of self-confidence, optimism, and faith in the gratification of needs.

Unsuccessful resolution results in the individual experiencing emotional dissatisfaction with the self and suspiciousness of others, thereby promoting negative self-esteem.

Autonomy versus Shame and Doubt (18 Months to 3 Years)

With motor and mental development come greater movement and independence within the environment. The child begins active exploration and experimentation. Achievement of the task results in a sense of self-control and the ability to delay gratification, as well as a feeling of self-confidence in one's ability to perform.

This task remains unresolved when the child's independent behaviors are restricted or when the child fails because of unrealistic expectations. Negative self-esteem is promoted by a lack of self-confidence, a lack of pride in the ability to perform, and a sense of being controlled by others.

Initiative versus Guilt (3 to 6 Years)

Positive self-esteem is gained through initiative when creativity is encouraged and performance is recognized and positively reinforced. In this stage, children strive to develop a sense of purpose and the ability to initiate and direct their own activities.

This is the stage during which the child begins to develop a conscience. He or she becomes vulnerable to the labeling of behaviors as "good" or "bad." Guidance and discipline that rely heavily on shaming the child creates guilt and results in a decrease in self-esteem.

Industry versus Inferiority (6 to 12 Years)

Self-confidence is gained at this stage through learning, competing, performing successfully, and receiving recognition from significant others, peers, and acquaintances.

Negative self-esteem is the result of nonachievement, unrealistic expectations, or when accomplishments are consistently met with negative feedback. The child develops a sense of personal inadequacy.

Identity versus Role Confusion (12 to 20 Years)

During adolescence, the individual is striving to redefine the sense of self. Positive self-esteem occurs when individuals are allowed to experience independence by making decisions that influence their lives.

Failure to develop a new self-definition results in a sense of self-consciousness, doubt, and confusion about one's role in life. This can occur when adolescents are encouraged to remain in the dependent position; when discipline in the home has been overly harsh, inconsistent, or absent; and when parental support has been lacking. These conditions are influential in the development of low self-esteem.

Intimacy versus Isolation (20 to 30 Years)

Intimacy is achieved when one is able to form a lasting relationship or a commitment to another person, a cause, an institution, or a creative effort (Murray, Zentner, & Yakimo, 2009). Positive self-esteem is promoted through this capacity for giving of oneself to another.

Failure to achieve intimacy results in behaviors such as withdrawal, social isolation, aloneness, and the inability to form lasting intimate relationships. Isolation occurs when love in the home has been deprived or distorted through the younger years, causing a severe impairment in self-esteem.

Generativity versus Stagnation (30 to 65 Years)

Generativity promotes positive self-esteem through gratification from personal and professional achievements, and from meaningful contributions to others.

Failure to achieve generativity occurs when earlier developmental tasks are not fulfilled and the individual does not achieve the degree of maturity required to derive gratification out of a personal concern for the welfare of others. He or she lacks self-worth and becomes withdrawn and isolated.

Ego Integrity versus Despair (65 Years to Death)

Ego integrity results in a sense of self-worth and self-acceptance as one reviews life goals, accepting that some were achieved and some were not. The individual has little desire to make major changes in how his or her life has progressed. Positive self-esteem is evident.

Individuals in despair possess a sense of self-contempt and disgust with how life has progressed. They feel worthless and helpless, and they would like to have a second chance at life. Earlier developmental tasks of self-confidence, self-identity, and concern for others remain unfulfilled. Negative self-esteem prevails.

Manifestations of Low Self-Esteem

Individuals with low self-esteem perceive themselves to be incompetent, unlovable, insecure, and unworthy. The number of manifestations exhibited is influenced by the degree to which an individual experiences low self-esteem. Roy (1976, 2009) categorized behaviors according to the type of stimuli that give rise to these behaviors and affirmed the importance of including this type of information in the nursing assessment. Stimulus categories are identified as *focal, contextual,* and *residual.* A summary of these types of influencing factors is presented in Table 15-1.

Focal Stimuli

A **focal stimulus** is the immediate concern that is causing the threat to self-esteem and the stimulus that is engendering the current behavior. Examples of focal stimuli include termination of a significant relationship, loss of employment, and failure to pass the nursing state board examination.

TABLE 15–1 Factors That Influence Manifestations of Low Self-Esteem

FOCAL	CONTEXTUAL	RESIDUAL
1. Any experience or situation causing the individual to question or decrease his or her value of self; experiences of loss are particularly significant.	1. Body changes experienced because of growth or illness.	1. Age and coping mechanisms one has developed.
	2. Maturational crises associated with developmental stages.	2. Stressful situations previously experienced and how well one coped with them.
	3. Situational crises and the individual's ability to cope.	3. Previous feedback from significant others that contributed to self-worth.
	4. The individual's perceptions of feedback from significant others.	4. Coping strategies developed through experiences with previous developmental crises.
	5. Ability to meet expectations of self and others.	5. Previous experiences with powerlessness and hopelessness and how one coped with them.
	6. The feeling of control one has over life situation.	6. Coping with previous losses.
	7. One's self-definition and the use of it to measure self-worth.	7. Coping with previous failures.
	8. How one copes with feelings of guilt, shame, and powerlessness.	8. Previous experiences meeting expectations of self and others.
	9. How one copes with the required changes in self-perception.	9. Previous experiences with control of self and the environment and quality of coping response.
	10. Awareness of what affects self-concept and the manner with which these stimuli are dealt.	10. Previous experience with decision making and subsequent consequences.
	11. The number of failures experienced before judging self as worthless.	11. Previous experience with childhood limits, and whether or not those limits were clear, defined, and enforced.
	12. The degree of self-esteem one possesses.	
	13. How one copes with limits within the environment.	
	14. The type of support from significant others and how one responds to it.	
	15. One's awareness of and ability to express feelings.	
	16. One's current feeling of hope and comfort with the self.	

From Driever, M.J. (1976). Problem of low self-esteem. In C. Roy (Ed.), *Introduction to nursing: An adaptation model* (pp. 232-242). Englewood Cliffs, NJ: Prentice-Hall, with permission.

Contextual Stimuli

Contextual stimuli are all of the other stimuli present in the person's environment that *contribute* to the behavior being caused by the focal stimulus. Examples of contextual stimuli related to the previously mentioned focal stimuli might be a child of the relationship becoming emotionally disabled in response to the divorce, advanced age interfering with obtaining employment, or a significant other who states, "I knew you weren't smart enough to pass state boards."

Residual Stimuli

Residual stimuli are factors that may influence one's maladaptive behavior in response to focal and contextual stimuli. An individual conducting a self-esteem assessment might presume from previous knowledge that certain beliefs, attitudes, experiences, or traits have an effect on client behavior, even though it cannot be clearly substantiated. For example, being reared in an atmosphere of ridicule and deprecation may be affecting current adaptation to failure on the state board examination.

Symptoms of Low Self-Esteem

Driever (1976) identified a number of behaviors manifested by the individual with low self-esteem. These behaviors are presented in Box 15-1.

Boundaries

The word *boundary* is used to denote the personal space, both physical and psychological, that individuals identify as their own. Boundaries are sometimes referred to as limits: the limit or degree to which individuals feel comfortable in a relationship. Boundaries define and differentiate an individual's physical and psychological space from the physical and psychological space of others.

Boundaries help individuals define the self and are part of the individuation process. Individuals who are aware of their boundaries have a healthy self-esteem because they must know and accept their inner selves. The inner self includes beliefs, thoughts, feelings, decisions, choices, experiences, wants, needs, sensations, and intuitions.

Types of physical boundaries include physical closeness, touching, sexual behavior, eye contact, privacy (e.g., mail, diary, doors, nudity, bathroom, telephone), and pollution (e.g., noise and smoke), among others. Examples of invasions of physical boundaries are reading someone else's diary, smoking in a nonsmoking public area, and touching someone who does not wish to be touched.

Types of psychological boundaries include beliefs, feelings, choices, needs, time alone, interests, confidences, individual differences, and spirituality, among others. Examples of invasions of psychological boundaries are being criticized for doing something differently than others; having personal information shared in confidence told to others; and being told one "should" believe, feel, decide, choose, or think in a certain way.

Boundary Pliancy

Boundaries can be rigid, flexible, or enmeshed. The behavior of dogs and cats can be a good illustration of **rigid boundaries** and **flexible boundaries**. Most dogs want to be as close to people as possible. When "their people" walk into the room, the dog is likely to be all over them. They want to be where their people are and do what they are doing. Dogs have very flexible boundaries.

Cats, on the other hand, have very distinct boundaries. They do what they want, when they want. They decide how close they will be to their people, and when. Cats take notice when their people enter a room but may not even acknowledge their presence (until the cat decides the time is right). Their boundaries are less flexible than those of dogs.

BOX 15-1 Manifestations of Low Self-Esteem

1. Loss of appetite/weight loss
2. Overeating
3. Constipation or diarrhea
4. Sleep disturbances (insomnia or difficulty falling or staying asleep)
5. Hypersomnia
6. Complaints of fatigue
7. Poor posture
8. Withdrawal from activities
9. Difficulty initiating new activities
10. Decreased libido
11. Decrease in spontaneous behavior
12. Expression of sadness, anxiety, or discouragement
13. Expression of feeling of isolation, being unlovable, unable to express or defend oneself, and too weak to confront or overcome difficulties
14. Fearful of angering others
15. Avoidance of situations of self-disclosure or public exposure
16. Tendency to stay in background; be a listener rather than a participant
17. Sensitivity to criticism; self-conscious
18. Expression of feelings of helplessness
19. Various complaints of aches and pains
20. Expression of being unable to do anything "good" or productive; expression of feelings of worthlessness and inadequacy
21. Expressions of self-deprecation, self-dislike, and unhappiness with self
22. Denial of past successes/accomplishments and of possibility for success with current activities
23. Feeling that anything one does will fail or be meaningless
24. Rumination about problems
25. Seeking reinforcement from others; making efforts to gain favors, but failing to reciprocate such behavior
26. Seeing self as a burden to others
27. Alienation from others by clinging and self-preoccupation
28. Self-accusatory
29. Demanding reassurance but not accepting it
30. Hostile behavior
31. Angry at self and others but unable to express these feelings directly
32. Decreased ability to meet responsibilities
33. Decreased interest, motivation, concentration
34. Decrease in self-care, hygiene

Adapted from *Developing Positive Assertiveness,* Third Edition, a Crisp series book by Sam R. Lloyd, available from Axzo Press (axzopress.com).

Rigid Boundaries

Individuals who have rigid boundaries often have a hard time trusting others. They keep others at a distance and are difficult to communicate with. They reject new ideas or experiences, and often withdraw, both emotionally and physically.

EXAMPLE

Fred and Alice were seeing a marriage counselor because they were unable to agree on many aspects of raising their children and it was beginning to interfere with their relationship. Alice runs a day-care service out of their home, and Fred is an accountant. Alice states, "He never once changed a diaper or got up at night with a child. Now that they are older, he refuses to discipline them in any way." Fred responds, "In my family, my Mom took care of the house and kids and my Dad kept us clothed and fed. That's the way it should be. It's Alice's job to raise the kids. It's my job to make the money." Fred's boundaries are considered rigid because he refuses to consider the ideas of others, or to experience alternative ways of doing things.

Flexible Boundaries

Healthy boundaries are flexible. That is, individuals must be able to let go of their boundaries and limits when appropriate. In order to have flexible boundaries, one must be aware of who is considered safe and when it is safe to let others invade our personal space.

EXAMPLE

Nancy always takes the hour from 4 to 5 p.m. for her own. She takes no phone calls and tells the children that she is not to be disturbed during that hour. She reads or takes a long leisurely bath and relaxes before it is time to start dinner. Today her private time was interrupted when her 15-year-old daughter came home from school crying because she had not made the cheerleading squad. Nancy used her private time to comfort her daughter who was experiencing a traumatic response to the failure.

Sometimes boundaries can be too flexible. Individuals with boundaries that are too loose are like chameleons. They take their "colors" from whomever they happen to be with at the time. That is, they allow others to make their choices and direct their behavior.

EXAMPLE

At a cocktail party Diane agreed with one person that the winter had been so unbearable she had hardly been out of the house. Later at the same party, she agreed with another person that the winter had seemed milder than usual.

Enmeshed Boundaries

Enmeshed boundaries occur when two people's boundaries are so blended together that neither can be sure where one stops and the other begins, or one individual's boundaries may be blurred with another's. The individual with the enmeshed boundaries may be unable to differentiate his or her feelings, wants, and needs from the other person's.

EXAMPLES

1. Fran's parents are in town for a visit. They say to Fran, "Dear, we want to take you and Dave out to dinner tonight. What is your favorite restaurant?" Fran automatically responds, "Villa Roma," knowing that the Italian restaurant is Dave's favorite.
2. If a mother has difficulty allowing her daughter to individuate, the mother may perceive the daughter's experiences as happening to her. For example, Aileen got her hair cut without her mother's knowledge. It was styled with spikes across the top of her head. When her mother saw it, she said, "How dare you go around looking like that! What will people think of me?"

Establishing Boundaries

Boundaries are established in childhood. Unhealthy boundaries are the products of unhealthy, troubled, or dysfunctional families. The boundaries enclose painful feelings that have their origin in the dysfunctional family and that have not been dealt with. McKay and Fanning (2000) explain the correlation between unhealthy boundaries and self-esteem disturbances and how they can arise out of negative role models:

> Modeling self-esteem means valuing oneself enough to take care of one's own basic needs. When parents put themselves last, or chronically sacrifice for their kids, they teach them that a person is only worthy insofar as he or she is of service to others. When parents set consistent, supportive limits and protect themselves from overbearing demands, they send a message to their children that both are important and both have legitimate needs. (p. 312)

In addition to the lack of positive role models, unhealthy boundaries may also be the result of abuse or neglect. These circumstances can cause a delay in psychosocial development. The individual must then resume the grief process as an adult in order to continue the developmental progression. They learn to recognize feelings, work through core issues, and learn to tolerate emotional pain as their own. They complete the individuation process, go on to develop healthy boundaries, and learn to appreciate their self-worth.

The Nursing Process

Assessment

Clients with self-esteem problems may manifest any of the symptoms presented in Box 15-1. Some clients with disturbances in self-esteem will make direct statements that reflect guilt, shame, or negative self-appraisal, but often it is necessary for the nurse to ask specific questions to obtain this type of information. In particular, clients who have experienced abuse or other severe trauma often have kept feelings and fears buried for years, and behavioral manifestations of low self-esteem may not be readily evident.

Various tools for measuring self-esteem exist. One is presented in Box 15-2. This particular tool can be used as a self-inventory by the client, or it can be adapted and used by the nurse to format questions for assessing level of self-esteem in the client.

Diagnosis/Outcome Identification

NANDA International has accepted, for use and testing, four nursing diagnoses that relate to self-esteem. These diagnoses are chronic low self-esteem, situational low self-esteem, risk for chronic low self-esteem, and risk for situational low self-esteem (NANDA International, 2012). Each is described here with its definitions and defining characteristics.

Chronic Low Self-Esteem

Definition: Long-standing negative self-evaluating/feelings about self or self-capabilities.

Defining Characteristics

■ Dependent on others' opinions
■ Hesitant to try new situations
■ Evaluation of self as unable to deal with events
■ Hesitant to try new things
■ Indecisive behavior
■ Exaggerates negative feedback about self
■ Lack of eye contact
■ Nonassertive behavior
■ Excessively seeks reassurance
■ Overly conforming
■ Expressions of guilt and shame
■ Passive
■ Frequent lack of success in life events
■ Rejects positive feedback about self

Situational Low Self-Esteem

Definition: Development of a negative perception of self-worth in response to a current situation.

BOX 15-2 **Self-Esteem Inventory**

Place a check mark in the column that most closely describes your answer to each statement. Each check is worth the number of points listed above each column.

	3 Often or A Great Deal	2 Sometimes	1 Seldom or Occasionally	0 Never or Not at All
1. I become angry or hurt when criticized.				
2. I am afraid to try new things.				
3. I feel stupid when I make a mistake.				
4. I have difficulty looking people in the eye.				
5. I have difficulty making small talk.				
6. I feel uncomfortable in the presence of strangers.				
7. I am embarrassed when people compliment me.				
8. I am dissatisfied with the way I look.				
9. I am afraid to express my opinions in a group.				
10. I prefer staying home alone than participating in group social situations.				
11. I have trouble accepting teasing.				
12. I feel guilty when I say "no" to people.				
13. I am afraid to make a commitment to a relationship for fear of rejection.				
14. I believe that most people are more competent than I.				
15. I feel resentment toward people who are attractive and successful.				
16. I have trouble thinking of any positive aspects about my life.				
17. I feel inadequate in the presence of authority figures.				
18. I have trouble making decisions.				
19. I fear the disapproval of others.				
20. I feel tense, stressed out, or "uptight."				

Problems with low self-esteem are indicated by items scored with a "3" or by a total score higher than 46.

Defining Characteristics

- Reports current situational challenge to self-worth
- Self-negating verbalizations
- Indecisive, nonassertive behavior
- Evaluation of self as unable to deal with situations or events
- Expressions of helplessness and uselessness

Risk for Chronic Low Self-Esteem

Definition: At risk for long-standing negative self-evaluating/feelings about self or self-capabilities.

Risk Factors

- Ineffective adaptation to loss
- Perceived lack of belonging
- Lack of affection
- Perceived lack of respect from others
- Lack of membership in group
- Psychiatric disorder
- Perceived discrepancy between self and cultural or spiritual norms
- Repeated failures
- Repeated negative reinforcement
- Traumatic event or situation

Risk for Situational Low Self-Esteem

Definition: At risk for developing negative perception of self-worth in response to a current situation.

Risk Factors

- Behavior inconsistent with values
- History of learned helplessness
- Decreased control over environment
- History of neglect
- Developmental changes
- Lack of recognition
- Failures
- Physical illness
- Functional impairment
- Rejections
- History of abandonment
- Social role changes
- History of abuse
- Disturbed body image
- Loss
- Unrealistic self-expectations

Outcome Criteria

Outcome criteria include short- and long-term goals. Timelines for achievement are individually determined. The following criteria may be used for measurement of outcomes in the care of the client with disturbances of self-esteem.

The client:

- Is able to express positive aspects about self and life situation
- Is able to accept positive feedback from others
- Is able to attempt new experiences
- Is able to accept personal responsibility for own problems
- Is able to accept constructive criticism without becoming defensive
- Is able to make independent decisions about life situation
- Uses good eye contact
- Is able to develop positive interpersonal relationships
- Is able to communicate needs and wants to others assertively

Planning/Implementation

In Table 15-2, a plan of care using selected self-esteem diagnoses accepted by NANDA International is presented. Outcome criteria, appropriate nursing interventions, and rationales are included for each diagnosis.

> **CLINICAL PEARL** Ensure that client goals are realistic. Unrealistic goals set up the client for failure. Provide encouragement and positive reinforcement for attempts at change. Give recognition of accomplishments, however small.

Table 15-2 | CARE PLAN FOR THE CLIENT WITH PROBLEMS RELATED TO SELF-ESTEEM

NURSING DIAGNOSIS: CHRONIC LOW SELF-ESTEEM

RELATED TO: Lack of affection/approval; repeated failures; repeated negative reinforcement

EVIDENCED BY: Exaggerates negative feedback about self and expressions of shame and guilt

OUTCOME CRITERIA	NURSING INTERVENTIONS	RATIONALE
Client will verbalize positive aspects of self and abandon judgmental self-perceptions.	1. Be supportive, accepting, and respectful without invading the client's personal space.	1. Individuals who have had long-standing feelings of low self-worth may be uncomfortable with personal attentiveness.
	2. Discuss inaccuracies in self-perception with client.	2. Client may not see positive aspects of self that others see, and bringing it to awareness may help change perception.

Continued

Table 15-2 | CARE PLAN FOR THE CLIENT WITH PROBLEMS RELATED TO SELF-ESTEEM—cont'd

OUTCOME CRITERIA	NURSING INTERVENTIONS	RATIONALE
	3. Have client list successes and strengths. Provide positive feedback.	3. Helps client to develop internal self-worth and new coping behaviors.
	4. Assess content of negative self-talk.	4. Self-blame, shame, and guilt promote feelings of low self-worth. Depending on chronicity and severity of the problem, this is likely to be the focus of long-term psychotherapy with this client.

NURSING DIAGNOSIS: SITUATIONAL LOW SELF-ESTEEM

RELATED TO: Failure (either real or perceived) in a situation of importance to the individual or loss (either real or perceived) of a concept of value to the individual

EVIDENCED BY: Indecisive behavior and expressions of helplessness and uselessness

OUTCOME CRITERIA	NURSING INTERVENTIONS	RATIONALE
Client will identify source of threat to self-esteem and work through the stages of the grief process to resolve the loss or failure.	1. Convey an accepting attitude; encourage client to express self openly.	1. An accepting attitude enhances trust and communicates to the client that you believe he or she is a worthwhile person, regardless of what is expressed.
	2. Encourage client to express anger. Do not become defensive if initial expression of anger is displaced on nurse/therapist. Assist client to explore angry feelings and direct them toward the intended object/person or other loss.	2. Verbalization of feelings in a non-threatening environment may help client come to terms with unresolved issues related to the loss.
	3. Assist client to avoid ruminating about past failures. Withdraw attention if client persists.	3. Lack of attention to these undesirable behaviors may discourage their repetition.
	4. Client needs to focus on positive attributes if self-esteem is to be enhanced. Encourage discussion of past accomplishments and offer support in undertaking new tasks. Offer recognition of successful endeavors and positive reinforcement of attempts made.	4. Recognition and positive reinforcement enhance self-esteem and encourage repetition of desirable behaviors.

NURSING DIAGNOSIS: RISK FOR SITUATIONAL LOW SELF-ESTEEM

RISK FACTORS: Developmental changes; functional impairment; disturbed body image; loss; history of abuse or neglect; unrealistic self-expectations; physical illness; failures/rejections

OUTCOME CRITERIA	NURSING INTERVENTIONS	RATIONALE
Client's self-esteem will be preserved.	1. Provide an open environment and trusting relationship.	1. To facilitate client's ability to deal with current situation.

| Table 15-2 | CARE PLAN FOR THE CLIENT WITH PROBLEMS RELATED TO SELF-ESTEEM—cont'd |

OUTCOME CRITERIA	NURSING INTERVENTIONS	RATIONALE
	2. Determine client's perception of the loss/failure and the meaning of it to him or her.	2. Assessment of the cause or contributing factor is necessary to provide assistance to the client.
	3. Identify response of family or significant others to client's current situation.	3. This provides additional background assessment data with which to plan client's care.
	4. Permit appropriate expressions of anger.	4. Anger is a stage in the normal grieving process and must be dealt with for progression to occur.
	5. Provide information about normalcy of individual grief reaction.	5. Individuals who are unaware of normal feelings associated with grief may feel guilty and try to deny certain feelings.
	6. Discuss and assist with planning for the future. Provide hope, but avoid giving false reassurance.	6. In a state of anxiety and grief, individuals need assistance with decision making and problem solving. They may find it difficult or impossible to envision any hope for the future.

Evaluation

Reassessment is conducted to determine if the nursing actions have been successful in achieving the objectives of care. Evaluation of the nursing actions for the client with self-esteem disturbances may be facilitated by gathering information using the following types of questions:

- Is the client able to discuss past accomplishments and other positive aspects about his or her life?
- Does the client accept praise and recognition from others in a gracious manner?
- Is the client able to try new experiences without extreme fear of failure?
- Can he or she accept constructive criticism now without becoming overly defensive and shifting the blame to others?
- Does the client accept personal responsibility for problems, rather than attributing feelings and behaviors to others?
- Does the client participate in decisions that affect his or her life?
- Can the client make rational decisions independently?
- Has he or she become more assertive in interpersonal relations?
- Is improvement observed in the physical presentation of self-esteem, such as eye contact, posture, changes in eating and sleeping, fatigue, libido, elimination patterns, self-care, and complaints of aches and pains?

Summary and Key Points

- Emotional wellness requires that an individual have some degree of self-worth—a perception that he or she possesses a measure of value to self and others.
- Self-concept consists of body image, personal identity, and self-esteem.
- Body image encompasses one's appraisal of personal attributes, functioning, sexuality, wellness-illness state, and appearance.
- The personal identity component of self-concept is composed of the moral-ethical self, the self-consistency, and the self-ideal.
- The moral-ethical self functions as observer, standard setter, dreamer, comparer, and most of all evaluator of who the individual says he or she is.
- Self-consistency is the component of the personal identity that strives to maintain a stable self-image.
- Self-ideal relates to an individual's perception of what he or she wants to be, do, or become.
- Self-esteem refers to the degree of regard or respect that individuals have for themselves and is a measure of worth that they place on their abilities

and judgments. It is largely influenced by the perceptions of how one is viewed by significant others.

■ Predisposing factors to the development of positive self-esteem include a sense of competence, unconditional love, a sense of survival, realistic goals, a sense of responsibility, and reality orientation. Genetics and environmental conditions may also be influencing factors.

■ The development of self-esteem progresses throughout the life span. Erikson's theory of personality development was used in this chapter as a framework for illustration of this progression.

■ The behaviors associated with low self-esteem are numerous.

■ Stimuli that trigger behaviors associated with low self-esteem were presented according to focal, contextual, or residual types.

■ Boundaries, or personal limits, help individuals define the self and are part of the individuation process.

■ Boundaries are physical and psychological and may be rigid, flexible, or enmeshed.

■ Unhealthy boundaries are often the result of dysfunctional family systems.

■ The nursing process is the vehicle for delivery of care to clients needing assistance with self-esteem disturbances.

■ The four nursing diagnoses relating to self-esteem that have been accepted by NANDA International include: chronic low self-esteem, situational low self-esteem, risk for chronic low self-esteem, and risk for situational low self-esteem.

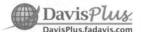 Additional info available at
DavisPlus.fadavis.com   www.davisplus.com

Review Questions
Self-Examination/Learning Exercise

*Select the answer that is **most** appropriate for each of the following questions.*

1. Karen, age 23, graduated from nursing school with a 3.2/4.0 grade point average. She recently took the NCLEX exam and did not pass. Because of this, she had to give up her graduate nursing job until she can pass the exam. She has become very depressed and has sought counseling at the mental health clinic. Karen says to the psychiatric nurse, "I am a complete failure. I'm so dumb, I can't do anything right." What is the most appropriate nursing diagnosis for Karen?
   a. Chronic low self-esteem
   b. Situational low self-esteem
   c. Defensive coping
   d. Risk for situational low self-esteem

2. Which of the following outcome criteria would be most appropriate for the client described in question 1?
   a. Karen is able to express positive aspects about herself and her life situation.
   b. Karen is able to accept constructive criticism without becoming defensive.
   c. Karen is able to develop positive interpersonal relationships.
   d. Karen is able to accept positive feedback from others.

3. Nancy tried out for the cheerleading squad in junior high, but was rejected. At age 15, she had looked forward to trying out for the cheerleading squad in high school. She took cheerleading classes and practiced for many hours every day. However, when tryouts were held, she was not selected. She has become despondent, and her mother takes her to the mental health clinic for counseling. Nancy tells the nurse, "What's the use of trying? I'm not good at anything!" Which of the following nursing interventions is best for Nancy's specific problem?
   a. Encourage Nancy to talk about her feeling of shame over the second failure.
   b. Assist Nancy to problem-solve her reasons for not making the team.
   c. Help Nancy understand the importance of good self-care and personal hygiene in the maintenance of self-esteem.
   d. Explore with Nancy her past successes and accomplishments.

Review Questions—cont'd
Self-Examination/Learning Exercise

4. The psychiatric nurse encourages Nancy (the client in question 3) to express her anger. Why is this an appropriate nursing intervention?
   a. Anger is the basis for self-esteem problems.
   b. The nurse suspects that Karen was abused as a child.
   c. The nurse is attempting to guide Karen through the grief process.
   d. The nurse recognizes that Karen has long-standing repressed anger.

5. A nursing school graduate failing the NCLEX exam and a 15-year-old high school girl not being selected for the cheerleading squad are examples of which of the following?
   a. Focal stimuli
   b. Contextual stimuli
   c. Residual stimuli
   d. Spatial stimuli

6. The husband says to the wife, "What do you want to do tonight?" and the wife responds, "Whatever you want to do." This is an example of which of the following?
   a. Rigid boundary
   b. A boundary violation
   c. Too flexible boundary
   d. Showing respect for the boundary of another

7. Twins Jan and Jean still dress alike even though they are grown and married. This is an example of which of the following?
   a. Rigid boundary
   b. Enmeshed boundary
   c. A boundary violation
   d. Boundary pliancy

8. Karen's counselor asked her if she would like a hug. This is an example of which of the following?
   a. Rigid boundary
   b. A boundary violation
   c. Enmeshed boundary
   d. Showing respect for the boundary of another

9. Velma told Betty a secret that Mary had told her. This is an example of which of the following?
   a. Too flexible boundary
   b. A boundary violation
   c. Rigid boundary
   d. Enmeshed boundary

10. Tommy says to his friend, "I can't ever talk to my Daddy until after he has read his newspaper." This is an example of which of the following?
   a. Rigid boundary
   b. A boundary violation
   c. Enmeshed boundary
   d. Too flexible boundary

References

Gorman, L.M., & Sultan, D.F. (2008). *Psychosocial nursing for general patient care* (3rd ed.). Philadelphia, PA: F.A. Davis.

Huitt, W. (2011). Self and self-views. *Educational Psychology Interactive.* Valdosta, GA: Valdosta State University. Retrieved from http://www.edpsycinteractive.org/topics/self/self.html

McKay, M., & Fanning, P. (2000). *Self-esteem: A proven program of cognitive techniques for assessing, improving, and maintaining your self-esteem* (3rd ed.). Oakland, CA: New Harbinger Publications.

Murray, R.B., Zentner, J.P., & Yakimo, R. (2009). *Health promotion strategies through the life span* (8th ed.). Upper Saddle River, NJ: Prentice Hall.

NANDA International. (2012). *Nursing diagnoses: Definitions and classification 2012-2014.* Hoboken, NJ: Wiley-Blackwell.

Roy, C. (2009). *The Roy adaptation model* (3rd ed.). Upper Saddle River, NJ: Pearson Education.

Warren, J. (1991). Your child and self-esteem. *The Prairie View, 30*(2), 1.

Classical References

Coopersmith, S. (1981). *The antecedents of self-esteem* (2nd ed.). Palo Alto, CA: Consulting Psychologists Press.

Driever, M.J. (1976). Problem of low self-esteem. In C. Roy (Ed.), *Introduction to nursing: An adaptation model* (pp. 232-242). Englewood Cliffs, N.J.: Prentice-Hall.

Erikson, E.H. (1963). *Childhood and society* (2nd ed.). New York, NY: W.W. Norton.

Maslow, A. (1970). *Motivation and personality* (2nd ed.). New York, NY: Harper & Row.

Roy, C. (1976). *Introduction to nursing: An adaptation model.* Englewood Cliffs, N.J.: Prentice Hall.

Anger/Aggression Management

16

CORE CONCEPTS

aggression

anger

anger management

KEY TERMS

modeling
operant conditioning
prodromal syndrome

OBJECTIVES
After reading this chapter, the student will be able to:

1. Define and differentiate between *anger* and *aggression*.
2. Identify when the expression of anger becomes a problem.
3. Discuss predisposing factors to the maladaptive expression of anger.
4. Apply the nursing process to clients expressing anger or aggression.
   a. **Assessment:** Describe physical and psychological responses to anger.
   b. **Diagnosis/Outcome Identification:** Formulate nursing diagnoses and

outcome criteria for clients expressing anger and aggression.
   c. **Planning/Intervention:** Describe nursing interventions for clients demonstrating maladaptive expressions of anger.
   d. **Evaluation:** Evaluate achievement of the projected outcomes in the intervention with clients demonstrating maladaptive expression of anger.

HOMEWORK ASSIGNMENT
Please read the chapter and answer the following questions:

1. What symptoms often precede violent behavior?
2. What is the goal of anger management?
3. What psychiatric diagnoses are correlated with increased risk of violence?
4. Under what conditions might a nurse determine that a client should be placed in restraints?

Anger need not be a negative expression. It is a normal human emotion that, when handled appropriately and expressed assertively, can provide an individual with a positive force to solve problems and make decisions concerning life situations. Anger becomes a problem when it is not expressed and when it is expressed aggressively. Violence occurs when individuals lose control of their anger. Violent acts are becoming commonplace in the United States. They are reported daily by the news media, and health-care workers see the results on a regular basis in the emergency departments of general hospitals.

This chapter addresses the concepts of anger and aggression. Predisposing factors to the maladaptive expression of anger are discussed, and the nursing process as a vehicle for delivery of care to assist clients in the management of anger and aggression is described.

Anger and Aggression, Defined

CORE CONCEPT

Anger

Anger is an emotional state that varies in intensity from mild irritation to intense fury and rage. It is accompanied by physiological and biological changes, such as increases in heart rate, blood pressure, and levels of the hormones epinephrine and norepinephrine (American Psychological Association, 2013).

Anger is a normal, healthy emotion that serves as a warning signal and alerts us to potential threat or trauma. It triggers energy that sets us up for a good fight or quick flight, and can range from mild irritation to hot, fiery energy (Butterfield, 2000). Warren (1999) outlines some fundamental points about anger:

■ Anger is not a primary emotion, but it is typically experienced as an almost automatic inner response to hurt, frustration, or fear.
■ Anger is physiological arousal. It instills feelings of power and generates preparedness.
■ Anger and aggression are significantly different.
■ The expression of anger is learned.
■ The expression of anger can come under personal control.

Anger is a very powerful emotion. When it is denied or buried, it can precipitate a number of physical problems such as migraine headaches, ulcers, colitis, and even coronary heart disease. When turned inward on oneself, anger can result in depression and low self-esteem. When it is expressed inappropriately, it commonly interferes with relationships. When suppressed, anger may turn into resentment, which often manifests itself in negative, passive-aggressive behavior.

Anger creates a state of preparedness by arousing the sympathetic nervous system. The activation of this system results in increased heart rate and blood pressure, increased secretion of epinephrine (resulting in additional physiological arousal), and increased levels of serum glucose, among others. Anger prepares the body, physiologically, to fight. When anger goes unresolved, this physiological arousal can be the predisposing factor to a number of health problems. Even if the situation that created the anger is removed by miles or years, it can be replayed through the memory, reactivating the sympathetic arousal when this occurs.

Table 16-1 lists positive and negative functions of anger.

CORE CONCEPT

Aggression

Aggression is a behavior intended to threaten or injure the victim's security or self-esteem. It means "to go against," "to assault," or "to attack." It is a response that aims at inflicting pain or injury on objects or persons. Whether the damage is caused by words, fists, or weapons, the behavior is virtually always designed to punish. It is frequently accompanied by bitterness, meanness, and ridicule. An aggressive person is often vengeful (Warren, 1999, pp. 119-120).

TABLE 16–1 **The Functions of Anger**	
POSITIVE FUNCTIONS OR CONSTRUCTIVE USES	NEGATIVE FUNCTIONS OR DESTRUCTIVE USES
Anger energizes and mobilizes the body for self-defense.	Without cognitive input, anger may result in impulsive behavior, disregarding possible negative consequences.
Communicated assertively, anger can promote conflict resolution.	Communicated passive-aggressively or aggressively, conflict escalates, and the problem that created the conflict goes unresolved.
Anger arousal is a personal signal of threat or injustice against the self. The signal elicits coping responses to deal with the distress.	Anger can lead to aggression when the coping response is displacement. Anger can be destructive if it is discharged against an object or person unrelated to the true target of the anger.
Anger is constructive when it provides a feeling of control over a situation and the individual is able to assertively take charge of a situation.	Anger can be destructive when the feeling of control is exaggerated and the individual uses the power to intimidate others.
Anger is constructive when it is expressed assertively, serves to increase self-esteem, and leads to mutual understanding and forgiveness.	Anger can be destructive when it masks honest feelings, weakens self-esteem, and leads to hostility and rage.

SOURCES: Adapted from Gorman & Sultan (2008) and Waughfield (2002).

The term *anger* often takes on a negative connotation because of its link with aggression. Aggression is one way individuals express anger. It is sometimes used to try to force someone into compliance with the aggressor's wishes, but at other times the only objective seems to be the infliction of punishment and pain. In virtually all instances, aggression is a negative function or destructive use of anger.

Predisposing Factors to Anger and Aggression

A number of factors have been implicated in the way individuals express anger. Some theorists view aggression as purely biological, and some suggest that it results from individuals' interactions with their environments. It is likely a combination of both.

Modeling

Role **modeling** is one of the strongest forms of learning. Children model their behavior at a very early age after their primary caregivers, usually parents. How parents or significant others express anger becomes the child's method of anger expression.

Whether role modeling is positive or negative depends on the behavior of the models. Much has been written about the abused child becoming physically abusive as an adult.

Role models are not always in the home, however. Evidence supports the role of television violence as a predisposing factor to later aggressive behavior (American Psychological Association, 2004). The American Academy of Pediatrics (2012) has suggested that monitoring what children view and regulation of violence in the media are necessary to prevent this type of violent modeling.

Operant Conditioning

Operant conditioning occurs when a specific behavior is reinforced. A positive reinforcement is a response to the specific behavior that is pleasurable or offers a reward. A negative reinforcement is a response to the specific behavior that prevents an undesirable result from occurring.

Anger responses can be learned through operant conditioning. For example, when a child wants something and has been told "no" by a parent, he or she might have a temper tantrum. If, when the temper tantrum begins, the parent lets the child have what is wanted, the anger has been positively reinforced (or rewarded).

An example of learning by negative reinforcement follows: A mother asks the child to pick up her toys and the child becomes angry and has a temper tantrum. If, when the temper tantrum begins, the

mother thinks, "Oh, it's not worth all this!" and picks up the toys herself, the anger has been negatively reinforced (the child was rewarded by not having to pick up her toys).

Neurophysiological Disorders

Some research has implicated epilepsy of temporal and frontal lobe origin in episodic aggression and violent behavior (Sadock & Sadock, 2007). Clients with episodic dyscontrol often respond to anticonvulsant medication.

Tumors in the brain, particularly in the areas of the limbic system and the temporal lobes; trauma to the brain, resulting in cerebral changes; and diseases, such as encephalitis (or medications that may effect this syndrome), have all been implicated in the predisposition to aggression and violent behavior. A study by Lee and associates (1998) showed that destruction of the amygdaloid body in patients with intractable aggression resulted in a reduction in autonomic arousal levels and in the number of aggressive outbursts.

Biochemical Factors

Violent behavior may be associated with hormonal dysfunction caused by Cushing's disease or hyperthyroidism (Tardiff, 2003). Studies have not supported a correlation between violence and increased levels of androgens or alterations in hormone levels associated with hypoglycemia or premenstrual syndrome.

Some research indicates that various neurotransmitters (e.g., epinephrine, norepinephrine, dopamine, acetylcholine, and serotonin) may play a role in the facilitation and inhibition of aggressive impulses (Sadock & Sadock, 2007).

Socioeconomic Factors

High rates of violence exist within the subculture of poverty in the United States. This has been attributed to lack of resources, breakup of families, alienation, discrimination, and frustration (Tardiff, 2003). An ongoing controversy exists as to whether economic inequality or absolute poverty is most responsible for violent behavior within this subculture. That is, does violence occur because individuals perceive themselves as disadvantaged relative to other persons, or does violence occur because of the deprivation itself? These concepts are not easily understood and are still under investigation.

Environmental Factors

Physical crowding may be related to violence through increased contact and decreased defensible space (Tardiff, 2003). A relationship between heat and aggression also has been indicated (Anderson,

2001). Moderately uncomfortable temperature appears to be associated with an increase in aggression, while extremely hot temperatures seem to decrease aggression.

A number of epidemiological studies have found a strong link between use of alcohol and violent behavior. Other substances, including cocaine, amphetamines, hallucinogens, and anabolic steroids, have also been associated with violent behavior (Tardiff, 2003).

The Nursing Process

CORE CONCEPT

Anger Management

The use of various techniques and strategies to control responses to anger-provoking situations. The goal of anger management is to reduce both the emotional feelings and the physiological arousal that anger engenders.

Assessment

Nurses must be aware of the symptoms associated with anger and aggression in order to make an accurate assessment. The best intervention is prevention, so risk factors for assessing violence potential are also presented.

Anger

Anger can be associated with a number of typical behaviors, including (but not limited to) the following:

- Frowning facial expression
- Clenched fists
- Low-pitched verbalizations forced through clenched teeth
- Yelling and shouting
- Intense eye contact or avoidance of eye contact
- Easily offended
- Defensive response to criticism
- Passive-aggressive behaviors
- Emotional overcontrol with flushing of the face
- Intense discomfort; continuous state of tension

Anger has been identified as a stage in the grieving process. Individuals who become fixed in this stage may become depressed. In this instance, the anger is turned inward as a way for the individual to maintain control over the pent-up anger. Because of the negative connotation to the word *anger*, some clients will not acknowledge that what they are feeling is anger. These individuals need assistance to recognize their true feelings and to understand that anger is a perfectly acceptable emotion when it is expressed appropriately.

Aggression

Aggression can arise from a number of feeling states, including anger, anxiety, guilt, frustration, or suspiciousness. Aggressive behaviors can be classified as mild (e.g., sarcasm), moderate (e.g., slamming doors), severe (e.g., threats of physical violence against others), or extreme (e.g., physical acts of violence against others). Aggression may be associated with (but not limited to) the following defining characteristics:

- Pacing, restlessness
- Tense facial expression and body language
- Verbal or physical threats
- Loud voice, shouting, use of obscenities, argumentative
- Threats of homicide or suicide
- Increase in agitation, with overreaction to environmental stimuli
- Panic anxiety, leading to misinterpretation of the environment
- Disturbed thought processes; suspiciousness
- Angry mood, often disproportionate to the situation

Kassinove & Tafrate (2002) stated, "In contrast to anger, aggression is almost always goal directed and has the aim of harm to a specific person or object. Aggression is one of the negative outcomes that may emerge from general arousal and anger" (pp. 40; 50)

Intent is a requisite in the definition of aggression. It refers to behavior that is *intended* to inflict harm or destruction. Accidents that lead to *unintentional* harm or destruction are not considered aggression.

Assessing Risk Factors

Prevention is the key issue in the management of aggressive or violent behavior. The individual who becomes violent usually feels an underlying helplessness. Three factors that have been identified as important considerations in assessing for potential violence include the following:

1. Past history of violence
2. Client diagnosis
3. Current behavior

Past history of violence is widely recognized as a major risk factor for violence in a treatment setting. Also highly correlated with assaultive behavior is diagnosis. Diagnoses that have a strong association with violent behavior are schizophrenia, major depression, bipolar disorder, and substance use disorders (Friedman, 2006). Substance abuse, in addition to mental illness, compounds the increased risk of violence. Neurocognitive disorders and antisocial, borderline, and intermittent explosive personality disorders have also been associated with a risk for violent behavior.

Novitsky, Julius, and Dubin (2009) state:

> The successful management of violence is predicated on an understanding of the dynamics of violence. A patient's threatening behavior is commonly an over-reaction to feelings of impotence, helplessness, and perceived or actual humiliation. Aggression rarely occurs suddenly and unexpectedly. (p. 50)

They describe a **"prodromal syndrome"** that is characterized by anxiety and tension, verbal abuse and profanity, and increasing hyperactivity. These escalating behaviors usually do not occur in stages but most often overlap and sometimes occur simultaneously. Behaviors associated with this prodromal stage include rigid posture; clenched fists and jaws; grim, defiant affect; talking in a rapid, raised voice; arguing and demanding; using profanity and threatening verbalizations; agitation and pacing; and pounding and slamming.

Most assaultive behavior is preceded by a period of increasing hyperactivity. Behaviors associated with the prodromal syndrome should be considered emergent and demand immediate attention. Keen observation skills and background knowledge for accurate assessment are critical factors in predicting potential for violent behavior. The Brøset Violence Checklist (BVC) is presented in Box 16-1. It is a quick, simple, and reliable checklist that can be used as a risk assessment for potential violence. Testing has shown a 63 percent accuracy for prediction of violence at a score of 2 and above (Almvik, Woods, & Rasmussen, 2000). De-escalation techniques are also included.

Diagnosis/Outcome Identification

NANDA International does not include a separate nursing diagnosis for anger. The nursing diagnosis of complicated grieving may be used when anger is expressed inappropriately and the etiology is related to a loss.

The following nursing diagnoses may be considered for clients demonstrating inappropriate expression of anger or aggression:

- Ineffective coping related to negative role modeling and dysfunctional family system evidenced by yelling, name calling, hitting others, and temper tantrums as expressions of anger
- Risk for self-directed or other-directed violence related to having been nurtured in an atmosphere of violence; history of violence

Outcome Criteria

Outcome criteria include short- and long-term goals. Timelines are individually determined. The following criteria may be used for measurement of outcomes in

---

BOX 16-1 **The Brøset Violence Checklist**

Behaviors	**Score** (Score 1 point for each behavior observed. At a score of ≥ 2, begin de-escalation techniques.)
Confusion	
Irritability	
Boisterousness	
Physical threats	
Verbal threats	
Attacks on objects	
TOTAL SCORE	

De-escalation techniques:

Calm voice	Helpful attitude
Walk outdoors or fresh air	Reduction in demands
Identify consequences	Decrease waiting times and request refusals
Group participation	
Open hands and non-threatening posture	Verbal redirection and limit setting
Relaxation techniques	Distract with a more positive activity (e.g., soft music or a quiet room)
Allow phone call	
Express concern	
Offer food or drink	Time-out/quiet time/open seclusion
Reduce stimulation and loud noise	Offer prn medication

If de-escalation techniques fail:

1. Suggest prn medications
2. Time-out or unlocked seclusion, which can progress to locked seclusion

From Almvik, R., Woods, P., & Rasmussen, K. (2000). The Brøset violence checklist: Sensitivity, specificity, and interrater reliability. *Journal of Interpersonal Violence*, 15(12), 1284-1296, with permission. De-escalation techniques reprinted with permission from Barbara Barnes, Milwaukee County Behavioral Health Division.

---

the care of the client needing assistance with management of anger and aggression.

The client:

- Is able to recognize when he or she is angry, and seeks out staff/support person to talk about his or her feelings
- Is able to take responsibility for own feelings of anger
- Demonstrates the ability to exert internal control over feelings of anger
- Is able to diffuse anger before losing control
- Uses the tension generated by the anger in a constructive manner
- Does not cause harm to self or others

■ Is able to use steps of the problem-solving process rather than becoming violent as a means of seeking solutions

Planning/Implementation

In Table 16-2, a plan of care is presented for the client who expresses anger inappropriately. Outcome criteria, appropriate nursing interventions, and rationales are included for each diagnosis.

Evaluation

Evaluation consists of reassessment to determine if the nursing interventions have been successful in achieving the objectives of care. The following type of information may be gathered to determine the success of working with a client exhibiting inappropriate expression of anger.

■ Is the client able to recognize when he or she is angry now?
■ Can the client take responsibility for these feelings and keep them in check without losing control?
■ Does the client seek out staff/support person to talk about feelings of anger when they occur?
■ Is the client able to transfer tension generated by the anger into constructive activities?
■ Has harm to client and others been avoided?
■ Is the client able to solve problems adaptively without undue frustration and without becoming violent?

Table 16-2 | CARE PLAN FOR THE INDIVIDUAL WHO EXPRESSES ANGER INAPPROPRIATELY

NURSING DIAGNOSIS: INEFFECTIVE COPING

RELATED TO: Negative role modeling and dysfunctional family system

EVIDENCED BY: Yelling, name calling, hitting others, and temper tantrums as expressions of anger

OUTCOME CRITERIA	NURSING INTERVENTIONS	RATIONALE
Client will be able to recognize anger in self and take responsibility before losing control.	1. Remain calm when dealing with an angry client.	1. Anger expressed by the nurse will most likely incite increased anger in the client.
	2. Set verbal limits on behavior. Clearly delineate the consequences of inappropriate expression of anger and always follow through.	2. Consistency in enforcing the consequences is essential if positive outcomes are to be achieved. Inconsistency creates confusion and encourages testing of limits.
	3. Have the client keep a diary of angry feelings, what triggered them, and how they were handled.	3. This provides a more objective measure of the problem.
	4. Avoid touching the client when he or she becomes angry.	4. The client may view touch as threatening and could become violent.
	5. Help the client determine the true source of the anger.	5. Many times anger is being displaced onto a safer object or person. If resolution is to occur, the first step is to identify the source of the problem.
	6. It may be constructive to ignore initial derogatory remarks by the client.	6. Lack of feedback often extinguishes an undesirable behavior.
	7. Help the client find alternate ways of releasing tension, such as physical outlets, and more appropriate ways of expressing anger, such as seeking out staff when feelings emerge.	7. Client will likely need assistance to problem-solve more appropriate ways of behaving.

Table 16-2 | CARE PLAN FOR THE INDIVIDUAL WHO EXPRESSES ANGER INAPPROPRIATELY—cont'd

OUTCOME CRITERIA	NURSING INTERVENTIONS	RATIONALE
	8. Role-model appropriate ways of expressing anger assertively, such as, "I dislike being called names. I get angry when I hear you saying those things about me."	8. Role modeling is one of the strongest methods of learning.

NURSING DIAGNOSIS: RISK FOR SELF-DIRECTED OR OTHER-DIRECTED VIOLENCE

RISK FACTORS: Having been nurtured in an atmosphere of violence; history of violence

OUTCOME CRITERIA	NURSING INTERVENTIONS	RATIONALE
The client will not harm self or others. The client will verbalize anger rather than hit others.	1. Observe client for escalation of anger (called the prodromal syndrome): increased motor activity, pounding, slamming, tense posture, defiant affect, clenched teeth and fists, arguing, demanding, and challenging or threatening staff.	1. Violence may be prevented if risks are identified in time.
	2. When these behaviors are observed, first ensure that sufficient staff are available to help with a potentially violent situation. Attempt to defuse the anger beginning with the least restrictive means.	2. The initial consideration must be having enough help to diffuse a potentially violent situation. Client rights must be honored, while preventing harm to client and others.
	3. Techniques for dealing with aggression include:	3. Aggression control techniques promote safety and reduce risk of harm to client and others:
	a. Talking down. Say, "John, you seem very angry. Let's go to your room and talk about it." (Ensure that client does not position self between door and nurse.)	a. Promotes a trusting relationship and may prevent the client's anxiety from escalating.
	b. Physical outlets. "Maybe it would help if you punched your pillow or the punching bag for a while." "I'll stay here with you if you want."	b. Provides effective way for client to release tension associated with high levels of anger.
	c. Medication. If agitation continues to escalate, offer client choice of taking medication voluntarily. If he or she refuses, reassess the situation to determine if harm to self or others is imminent.	c. Tranquilizing medication may calm client and prevent violence from escalating.
	d. Call for assistance. Remove self and other clients from the immediate area. Call violence code, push "panic" button, call	d. Client and staff safety are of primary concern.

Continued

Table 16-2 | CARE PLAN FOR THE INDIVIDUAL WHO EXPRESSES ANGER INAPPROPRIATELY—cont'd

OUTCOME CRITERIA	NURSING INTERVENTIONS	RATIONALE
	for assault team, or institute measures established by the institution. Sufficient staff to indicate a show of strength may be enough to de-escalate the situation, and client may agree to take the medication.	
	e. Restraints. If client is not calmed by "talking down" or by medication, use of mechanical restraints and/or seclusion may be necessary. Be sure to have sufficient staff available to assist. Figures 16-1, 16-2, and 16-3 illustrate ways in which staff can safely and appropriately deal with an out-of-control client. Follow protocol for restraints/ seclusion established by the institution. The Joint Commission (formerly the Joint Commission	e. Clients who do not have internal control over their own behavior may require external controls, such as mechanical restraints, in order to prevent harm to self or others.

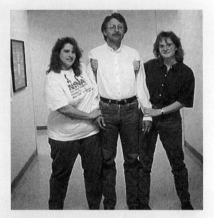

FIGURE 16–1 Walking a client to the seclusion room.

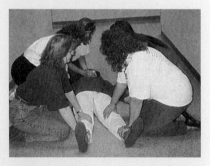

FIGURE 16–2 Staff restraint of a client in supine position. The client's head is controlled to prevent biting.

Table 16-2 | CARE PLAN FOR THE INDIVIDUAL WHO EXPRESSES ANGER INAPPROPRIATELY—cont'd

OUTCOME CRITERIA	NURSING INTERVENTIONS	RATIONALE

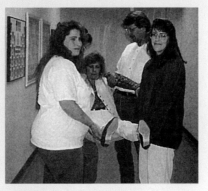

FIGURE 16–3 Transporting a client to the seclusion room.

	on Accreditation of Healthcare Organizations [JCAHO]) requires that an in-person evaluation by a physician or other licensed independent practitioner (LIP) be conducted within 1 hour of the initiation of the restraint or seclusion (The Joint Commission, 2010). The physician or LIP must reissue a new order for restraints every 4 hours for adults and every 1-2 hours for children and adolescents. Restraints should be used as a last resort, after all other interventions have been unsuccessful, and the client is clearly at risk of harm to self or others.	
	f. Observation and documentation. The client in restraints should be observed on a one-to-one basis for the first hour. This in-person observation can progress to audio and visual monitoring after the first hour. Every 15 minutes the client should be monitored to ensure that circulation to extremities is not compromised (check temperature, color, pulses). Assist client with needs related to nutrition, hydration, and elimination. Position client so that comfort is facilitated and aspiration can be prevented. Document all observations.	f. Client well-being is a nursing priority.

Continued

Table 16-2 | CARE PLAN FOR THE INDIVIDUAL WHO EXPRESSES ANGER INAPPROPRIATELY–cont'd

OUTCOME CRITERIA	NURSING INTERVENTIONS	RATIONALE
	g. Ongoing assessment. As agitation decreases, assess client's readiness for restraint removal or reduction. With assistance from other staff members, remove one restraint at a time, while assessing client's response. This minimizes the risk of injury to client and staff.	g. Gradual removal of the restraints allows for testing of the client's self-control. Client and staff safety are of primary concern.
	h. Staff debriefing. It is important when a client loses control for staff to follow up with a discussion about the situation. Tardiff (2003) states, "The violent episode should be discussed in terms of what happened, what would have prevented it, why seclusion or restraint was used (if it was), and how the patient or the staff felt in terms of using seclusion and restraint." (p. 1495). It is also important to discuss the situation with other clients who witnessed the episode. It is important that they understand what happened. Some clients may fear that they could be secluded or restrained at some time for no apparent reason.	h. Debriefing helps to diminish the emotional impact of the intervention. Mutual feedback is shared, and staff has an opportunity to process and learn from the event.

Summary and Key Points

■ Statistics show that violence is rampant in the United States.

■ The precursor to violence is anger, which is a normal human emotion, and need not necessarily be a negative response.

■ When used appropriately, anger can provide positive assistance with problem solving and decision-making in everyday life situations.

■ Violence occurs when individuals lose control of their anger.

■ Anger is viewed as the emotional response to one's perception of a situation.

■ Anger is a very powerful emotion and, when denied or buried, can precipitate a number of psychophysiological disorders.

■ When anger is turned inward on the self, it can result in depression.

■ When expressed inappropriately, anger commonly interferes with interpersonal relationships.

■ When anger is suppressed, it often turns to resentment.

■ Anger generates a physiological arousal comparable to the stress response discussed in Chapter 1.

■ Aggression is one way in which individuals express anger.

■ Aggression is behavior intended to threaten or injure the victim's security or self-esteem.

■ Aggression can be physical or verbal, but it is virtually always designed to punish.

■ Aggression is a negative function or destructive use of anger.

■ Various predisposing factors to the way individuals express anger have been implicated. Some theorists suggest that the etiology is purely biological, whereas others believe it depends on psychological and environmental factors.

■ Some possible predisposing factors include role modeling, operant conditioning, neurophysiological disorders (e.g., brain tumors, trauma, or diseases), biochemical factors (e.g., increased levels of androgens or other alterations in hormone levels and neurotransmitter involvement), socioeconomic factors (e.g., living in poverty), and environmental factors (e.g., physical crowding, uncomfortable temperature, use of alcohol or drugs, and availability of firearms).

■ Nurses must be aware of the symptoms associated with anger and aggression in order to make an accurate assessment.

■ Prevention is the key issue in the management of aggressive or violent behavior.

■ Three elements have been identified as key risk factors in the potential for violence: (1) past history of violence, (2) client diagnosis, and (3) current behaviors.

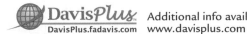

DavisPlus.fadavis.com   Additional info available at www.davisplus.com

Review Questions
Self-Examination/Learning Exercise

*Select the answer that is **most** appropriate for each of the following questions.*

1. John, age 27, was brought to the emergency department by two police officers. He smelled strongly of alcohol and was combative. His blood alcohol level was measured at 293 mg/dL. His girlfriend reports that he drinks excessively every day and is verbally and physically abusive. The nurses give John the nursing diagnosis of Risk for Other-Directed Violence. What would be appropriate outcome objectives for this diagnosis? (Select all that apply.)
   a. The client will not verbalize anger or hit anyone.
   b. The client will verbalize anger rather than hit others.
   c. The client will not harm self or others.
   d. The client will be restrained if he becomes verbally or physically abusive.

2. John, who was hospitalized with alcohol intoxication and violent behavior, is sitting in the dayroom watching TV with the other clients when the nurse approaches with his 5 p.m. dose of haloperidol. John says, "I feel in control now. I don't need any drugs." The nurse's best response is based on which of the following statements?
   a. John must have the medication, or he will become violent.
   b. John knows that if he will not take the medication orally, he will be restrained and given an intramuscular injection.
   c. John has the right to refuse the medication provided there is no immediate danger to self or others.
   d. John must take the medication at this time in order to maintain adequate blood levels.

3. The nurse hears John, a client with a history of violence, yelling in the dayroom. The nurse observes his increased agitation, clenched fists, and loud, demanding voice. He is challenging and threatening staff and the other clients. The nurse's *priority* intervention would be to:
   a. Call for assistance.
   b. Draw up a syringe of prn haloperidol.
   c. Ask John if he would like to talk about his anger.
   d. Tell John if he does not calm down he will have to be restrained.

Continued

Review Questions—cont'd
Self-Examination/Learning Exercise

4. John, a client with a history of violence, has been hospitalized on the psychiatric unit. He becomes agitated and begins to threaten the staff and other clients. When all other interventions fail, John is placed in restraints in the seclusion room for his and others' protection. Which of the following are interventions for the client in restraints? (Select all that apply.)
   a. Check temperature and pulse of extremities.
   b. Document all observations.
   c. Explain to the client that restraint is his punishment for violent behavior
   d. Provide ongoing assessment and observation.
   e. Withhold food and fluid until client is calm and can be released from restraints.

5. When it has been assessed that a client is in control and no longer requires restraining, how does the nurse proceed?
   a. The nurse removes the restraints.
   b. The nurse calls for assistance to remove the restraints.
   c. With assistance, the nurse removes one restraint.
   d. The nurse tells the client he will have to wait until the doctor comes in.

6. Which of these procedures is important in following up an episode of violence on the unit? (Select all that apply.)
   a. Document all observations and occurrences.
   b. Conduct a debriefing with staff.
   c. Discuss what occurred with other clients who witnessed the incident.
   d. Warn the client that it could happen again if he becomes violent.

7. A client who has been in restraints is now calm. He apologizes to the nurse and says, "I hope I didn't hurt anyone." The nurse's best response is:
   a. "This is our job. We know how to handle violent clients."
   b. "We understand you were out of control and didn't really mean to hurt anyone."
   c. "It is fortunate that no one was hurt. You will not be placed in restraints as long as you can control your behavior."
   d. "It is an unpleasant situation to have to restrain someone, but we have to think of the other clients. We can't have you causing injury to others. I just hope it won't happen again."

8. John and his girlfriend had an argument during her visit. Which behavior by John would indicate he is learning to adaptively problem-solve his frustrations?
   a. John says to the nurse, "Give me some of that medication before I end up in restraints!"
   b. When his girlfriend leaves, John goes to the exercise room and punches on the punching bag.
   c. John says to the nurse, "I guess I'm going to have to dump that broad!"
   d. John says to his girlfriend, "You'd better leave before I do something I'm sorry for."

9. Which of the following assessment data would the nurse consider as risk factors for possible violence in a client? (Select all that apply.)
   a. A diagnosis of somatization disorder
   b. A diagnosis of bipolar disorder
   c. Substance intoxication
   d. Argumentative and demanding behavior
   e. Past history of violence

10. Which of the following is true about *aggression*? (Select all that apply.)
    a. It is goal directed.
    b. Its aim is to do harm to a person or object.
    c. It has a requisite of *intent*.
    d. It energizes and mobilizes the body for self-defense.

References

Almvik, R., Woods, P. & Rasmussen, K. (2000). The Brøset violence checklist: Sensitivity, specificity, and interrater reliability. *Journal of Interpersonal Violence, 15*(12), 1284-1296.

American Academy of Pediatrics. (2012). *Pulling the plug on TV violence.* Retrieved from http://www.healthychildren.org/English/family- life/Media/pages/Pulling-the-Plug-on-TV-Violence.aspx

American Psychological Association. (2004). *Violence in the media—Psychologists help protect children from harmful effects.* Retrieved from http://www.apa.org/research/action/protect.aspx

American Psychological Association. (2013). *Controlling anger before it controls you.* Retrieved from http://www.apa.org/topics/anger/control.aspx

Anderson, C.A. (2001). Heat and violence. *Current Directions in Psychological Science 10*(1), 33-38.

Butterfield, P. (2000). *Understanding and managing anger: Diagnosis, treatment, and prevention.* Sunnyvale, CA: CorText Mind Matters Educational Seminars.

Friedman, R.A. (2006). Violence and mental illness—How strong is the link? *New England Journal of Medicine, 355*(20), 2064-2066.

Gorman, L.M., & Sultan, D.F. (2008). *Psychosocial nursing for general patient care* (3rd ed.). Philadelphia, PA: F.A. Davis.

Kassinove, H., & Tafrate, R.C. (2002). *Anger management.* Atascadero, CA: Impact Publishers.

Lee, G.P., Bechara, A., Adolphs, R., Arena, J., Meador, K.J., Loring, D.W., & Smith, J.R. (1998). Clinical and physiological effects of stereotaxic bilateral amygdalotomy for intractable aggression. *Journal of Neuropsychiatry and Clinical Neurosciences 10*(4), 413-420.

Novitsky, M.A., Julius, R.J., & Dubin, W.R. (2009). Non-pharmacologic management of violence in psychiatric emergencies. *Primary Psychiatry, 16*(9), 49-53.

Sadock, B.J., & Sadock, V.A. (2007). *Synopsis of psychiatry: Behavioral sciences/clinical psychiatry* (10th ed.). Philadelphia, PA: Lippincott Williams & Wilkins.

Tardiff, K.J. (2003). Violence. In R.E. Hales & S.C. Yudofsky (Eds.), *Textbook of clinical psychiatry* (4th ed., 1485-1509). Washington, DC: American Psychiatric Publishing.

The Joint Commission. (2010). *The comprehensive accreditation manual for hospitals: The official handbook* (January, 2010). Oakbrook Terrace, IL: Joint Commission Resources.

Turgut, T., Lagace, D., Izmir, M., & Dursun, S. (2006). Assessment of violence and aggression in psychiatric settings: Descriptive approaches. *Bulletin of Clinical Psychopharmacology, 16*(3), 179-194.

Warren, N.C. (1999). *Make anger your ally* (3rd ed.). Wheaton, IL: Tyndale House Publishers.

Waughfield, C.G. (2002). *Mental health concepts* (5th ed.). Albany, NY: Delmar.

17

The Suicidal Client

CHAPTER OUTLINE

KEY TERMS

altruistic suicide   anomic suicide   egoistic suicide

OBJECTIVES

After reading this chapter, the student will be able to:

1. Discuss epidemiological statistics and risk factors related to suicide.
2. Describe predisposing factors implicated in the etiology of suicide.
3. Differentiate between facts and fables regarding suicide.
4. Apply the nursing process to individuals exhibiting suicidal behavior.

HOMEWORK ASSIGNMENT

Please read the chapter and answer the following questions:

1. How do age, race, and gender affect suicide risk?
2. Your neighbor tells you he is going to visit his sister-in-law in the hospital. The sister-in-law has been hospitalized after attempting suicide. Your neighbor asks, "What should I say when I go to visit Jane?" What suggestions might you give him?
3. John's father committed suicide when John was a teenager. John's wife, Mary, tells the mental health nurse that she is afraid John "inherited" that predisposition from his father. How should the nurse respond to Mary?
4. The nurse notes that the mood of a client being treated for depression and suicidal ideation suddenly brightens and the client states, "I feel fine now. I don't feel depressed anymore." Why would this statement alert the nurse of a potential problem?

Suicide is not a diagnosis or a disorder; it is a behavior. The Judeo-Christian belief has been that life is a gift from God and that taking it is strictly forbidden (Carroll-Ghosh, Victor, & Bourgeois, 2003). A recent, and more secular, view has influenced how some individuals view suicide in our society. Growing support for an individual's right to choose death over pain has been evidenced. Some individuals are striving to advance the cause of physician-assisted suicides for the terminally ill. Can suicide be a rational act? Most people in our society do not yet believe that it can.

More than 90 percent of all persons who commit or attempt suicide have a diagnosed mental disorder (National Institute of Mental Health [NIMH], 2013). This chapter explores suicide from an epidemiological and etiological perspective. Care of the suicidal client is presented in the context of the nursing process.

Historical Perspectives

In ancient Greece, suicide was an offense against the state and individuals who committed suicide were denied burial in community sites (Minois, 2001). In the culture of the imperial Roman army, individuals sometimes resorted to suicide to escape humiliation or abuse.

In the Middle Ages, suicide was viewed as a selfish or criminal act (Minois, 2001). Individuals who committed suicide were often denied cemetery burial and their property was confiscated and shared by the crown and the courts (MacDonald & Murphy, 1991). The issue of suicide changed during the period of the Renaissance. Although condemnation was still expected, the view became more philosophical, and intellectuals could discuss the issue more freely.

Most philosophers of the 17th and 18th centuries condemned suicide, but some writers recognized a connection between suicide and melancholy or other severe mental disturbances (Minois, 2001). Suicide was illegal in England until 1961, and only in 1993 was it decriminalized in Ireland.

Most religions consider suicide as a sin against God. Judaism, Christianity, Islam, Hinduism, and Buddhism all condemn suicide. In 1995, Pope John II restated Church opposition to suicide, euthanasia, and abortion as crimes against life, not unlike homicide and genocide (Tondo & Baldessarini, 2001).

Epidemiological Factors

More than 38,000 people committed suicide in 2010, the latest year for which statistics have been recorded (American Foundation for Suicide Prevention [AFSP], 2013). This is the highest rate of suicide in 15 years. These statistics have established suicide as the third leading cause of death (behind accidents and homicide) among young Americans ages 15 to 24 years, the fourth leading cause of death for ages 25 to 44, the eighth leading cause of death for individuals ages 45 to 64, and the tenth leading cause of death overall (Centers for Disease Control and Prevention [CDC], 2013). Many more people attempt suicide than succeed, and countless others seriously contemplate the act without carrying it out. Suicide has become a major health-care problem in the United States today.

Over the years confusion has existed over the reality of various notions regarding suicide. Some facts and fables relating to suicide are presented in Table 17-1.

Risk Factors

Marital Status

The suicide rate for single persons is twice that of married persons. Divorced, separated, or widowed persons have rates four to five times greater than those of the married (Jacobs et al., 2006).

TABLE 17–1 **Facts and Fables About Suicide**	
FABLES	FACTS
People who talk about suicide do not commit suicide. Suicide happens without warning.	Eight out of 10 people who kill themselves have given definite clues and warnings about their suicidal intentions. Very subtle clues may be ignored or disregarded by others.
You cannot stop a suicidal person. He or she is fully intent on dying.	Most suicidal people are very ambivalent about their feelings regarding living or dying. Most are "gambling with death" and see it as a cry for someone to save them.
Once a person is suicidal, he or she is suicidal forever.	People who want to kill themselves are only suicidal for a limited time. If they are saved from feelings of self-destruction, they can go on to lead normal lives.
Improvement after severe depression means that the suicidal risk is over.	Most suicides occur within about 3 months after the beginning of "improvement," when the individual has the energy to carry out suicidal intentions.
Suicide is inherited, or "runs in families."	Suicide is not inherited. It is an individual matter and can be prevented. However, suicide by a close family member increases an individual's risk factor for suicide.
All suicidal individuals are mentally ill, and suicide is the act of a psychotic person.	Although suicidal persons are extremely unhappy, they are not necessarily psychotic. They are merely unable at that point in time to see an alternative solution to what they consider an unbearable problem.

Continued

TABLE 17–1 **Facts and Fables About Suicide—cont'd**	
FABLES	FACTS
Suicidal threats and gestures should be considered manipulative or attention-seeking behavior, and should not be taken seriously.	All suicidal behavior must be approached with the gravity of the potential act in mind. Attention should be given to the possibility that the individual is issuing a cry for help.
People usually commit suicide by taking an overdose of drugs.	Gunshot wounds are the leading cause of death among suicide victims.
If an individual has attempted suicide, he or she will not do it again.	Between 50% and 80% of all people who ultimately kill themselves have a history of a previous attempt.

SOURCES: Corr & Corr (2013); Friends for Survival, Inc. (2013); and The Samaritans (2013).

Gender

Women attempt suicide more, but men succeed more often. Successful suicides number about 70 percent for men and 30 percent for women. This has to do with the lethality of the means. Women tend to overdose; men use more lethal means such as firearms. In the United States, from 1970 to 2008, annual suicide rates per 100,000 rose from 16.8 to 19.0 in men, but decreased from 6.6 to 4.9 in women (National Center for Health Statistics [NCHS], 2012). These differences between men and women may also reflect a tendency for women to seek and accept help from friends or professionals, whereas men often view help-seeking as a sign of weakness.

Age

Suicide risk and age are positively correlated. This is particularly true with men. Although rates among women remain fairly constant throughout life, rates among men show a higher age correlation. The rates rise sharply during adolescence, peak between 40 and 50, and level off until age 65, when rates rise again for the remaining years (NCHS, 2012).

The suicide rate among young people ages 15 to 19 peaked in 1990 at 11.1 per 100,000 and declined to 7.5 per 100,000 in 2008 (NCHS, 2012). Several factors put adolescents at risk for suicide, including impulsive and high-risk behaviors, untreated mood disorders (e.g., major depression and bipolar disorder), access to lethal means (e.g., firearms), and substance abuse. The latest statistics from the Centers for Disease Control and Prevention indicate that the most common method of completed suicide for adolescent males is firearm; for adolescent females it is suffocation (CDC, 2012).

The suicide rate for the elderly peaked in 1990 at 20.5 per 100,000 and declined to 14.8 per 100,000 in 2008 (NCHS, 2012). While the elderly make up just over 13 percent of the population, they account for almost 15 percent of all suicides. White males over the age of 80 are at the greatest risk of all age/gender/race groups. Eighty-four percent of elderly suicides are male, which is 5.25 times greater than for females, and firearms are the most common means of committing suicide (American Association of Suicidology, 2013). The overall rate of suicide for females declines after age 65.

Religion

Historically, suicide rates among Roman Catholic populations have been lower than rates among Protestants and Jews (Sadock & Sadock, 2007). A study published in the *Journal of Affective Disorders* revealed that men and women who consider themselves affiliated with a religion are less likely to attempt suicide than their nonreligious counterparts (Rasic et al., 2009). The authors found that religious attendance is associated with decreased suicide attempts in both the general population and in those with a mental illness, independent of the availability of social support systems.

Socioeconomic Status

Individuals in the very highest and lowest social classes have higher suicide rates than those in the middle classes (Sadock & Sadock, 2007). With regard to occupation, suicide rates are higher among physicians, artists, dentists, law enforcement officers, lawyers, and insurance agents.

Ethnicity

With regard to ethnicity, statistics show that whites are at highest risk for suicide, followed by Native Americans, African Americans, Hispanic Americans, and Asian Americans (NCHS, 2012).

Other Risk Factors

As previously stated, more than 90 percent of people who kill themselves have a diagnosable mental disorder, most commonly a mood disorder or a substance abuse disorder (NIMH, 2013). Suicide risk may increase early during treatment with antidepressants, as the return of energy brings about an increased ability to act out self-destructive wishes. Other psychiatric disorders that may account for suicidal behavior include schizophrenia, personality disorders, and anxiety disorders (Jacobs et al., 2006).

Severe insomnia is associated with increased suicide risk, even in the absence of depression. Use of alcohol, and particularly a combination of alcohol and barbiturates, increases the risk of suicide. Psychosis, especially with command hallucinations, poses a higher than normal risk. Affliction with a chronic painful or disabling illness also increases the risk of suicide.

Several studies have indicated a higher risk factor for suicide among gay men and lesbians (Cochran & Mays, 2000; Eisenberg & Resnick, 2006; King et al., 2008; Medscape Psychiatry, 2011). It is thought that this increased risk may be a function of the social stigma and discrimination associated with the gay and lesbian orientation. Additional personal stressors, including isolation, victimization, and stressful interpersonal relationships with family, peers, and community, are not uncommon. A report by the Suicide Prevention Resource Center (2008) states:

> Research indicates that lesbian, gay, and bisexual (LGB) youth have significantly higher rates of suicide attempts and suicidal ideation than their heterosexual peers. Data limitations make it difficult to draw conclusions about higher rates of death by suicide among LGB youth; however, the higher number of suicide attempts, as well as the seriousness of attempts among LGB youth, make it probable that this group of youth has a higher rate of suicide deaths than their heterosexual counterparts. (p. 19)

Higher risk is also associated with a family history of suicide, especially in a same-gender parent. Persons who have made prior suicide attempts are at higher risk for suicide. About half of individuals who kill themselves have previously attempted suicide. Loss of a loved one through death or separation and lack of employment or increased financial burden also increase risk.

In recent years, a number of suicides have been reported in the media among young people who are the victims of bullying. Klomek, Sourander, and Gould (2011) report:

> Studies among middle school and high school students show an increased risk of suicidal behavior among bullies and victims. Both perpetrators and victims are at the highest risk for suicidal ideation.

Being bullied via the Internet or e-mail (called *cyberbullying*) has also been associated with increased risk of depression and suicidal behavior among young people. Researchers found that both perpetrators and victims of cyberbullying had more suicidal ideation and were more likely to attempt suicide than those who had not experienced such forms of peer aggression (Hinduja & Patchin, 2010).

Predisposing Factors: Theories of Suicide

Psychological Theories

Anger Turned Inward

Freud (1957) believed that suicide was a response to the intense self-hatred that an individual possessed. The anger had originated toward a love object but was ultimately turned inward against the self. Freud believed that suicide occurred as a result of an earlier repressed desire to kill someone else. He interpreted suicide to be an aggressive act toward the self that often was really directed toward others.

Hopelessness

Carroll-Ghosh and associates (2003) identified hopelessness as a central underlying factor in the predisposition to suicide. Beck, Brown, and Berchick (1990) also found a high correlation between hopelessness and suicide.

Desperation and Guilt

Hendin (1991) identified desperation as another important factor in suicide. With desperation, an individual feels helpless to change, but he or she also feels that life is impossible without such change. Guilt and self-recrimination are other aspects of desperation. These affective components were found to be prominent in Vietnam veterans with post-traumatic stress disorder exhibiting suicidal behaviors (Carroll-Ghosh et al., 2003).

History of Aggression and Violence

Some studies have indicated that violent behavior often goes hand-in-hand with suicidal behavior (Carroll-Ghosh et al., 2003). These studies correlate the suicidal behavior in violent individuals to conscious rage, therefore citing rage as an important psychological factor underlying the suicidal behavior (Hendin, 1991).

Shame and Humiliation

Some individuals have viewed suicide as a "face-saving" mechanism—a way to prevent public humiliation following a social defeat such as a sudden loss of status or income. Often these individuals are too embarrassed to seek treatment or other support systems.

Developmental Stressors

Rich, Warsradt, and Nemiroff (1991) have associated developmental level with certain life stressors and their correlation to suicide. The stressors of conflict, separation, and rejection are associated with suicidal behavior in adolescence and early adulthood. The principal stressor associated with suicidal behavior in the 40- to 60-year-old group is economic problems. Medical illness plays an increasingly significant role after age 60 and becomes the leading predisposing factor to suicidal behavior in individuals older than age 80.

Sociological Theory

Durkheim (1951) studied the individual's interaction with the society in which he or she lived. He believed that the more cohesive the society, and the more that the individual felt an integrated part of the society, the less likely he or she was to commit suicide. Durkheim described three social categories of suicide:

Egoistic suicide is the response of the individual who feels separate and apart from the mainstream of society. Integration is lacking and the individual does not feel a part of any cohesive group (such as a family or a church).

Altruistic suicide is the opposite of egoistic suicide. The individual who is prone to altruistic suicide is excessively integrated into the group. The group is often governed by cultural, religious, or political ties, and allegiance is so strong that the individual will sacrifice his or her life for the group.

Anomic suicide occurs in response to changes that occur in an individual's life (e.g., divorce, loss of job) that disrupt feelings of relatedness to the group. An interruption in the customary norms of behavior instills feelings of "separateness," and fears of being without support from the formerly cohesive group.

Biological Theories

Genetics

Twin studies have shown a much higher concordance rate for monozygotic twins than for dizygotic twins. Some studies with suicide attempters have focused on the genotypic variations in the gene for tryptophan hydroxylase, with results indicating significant association to suicidality (Abbar et al., 2001). These results suggest a possible existence of genetic predisposition toward suicidal behavior.

Neurochemical Factors

A number of studies have been conducted to determine if there is a correlation between neurochemical functioning in the central nervous system (CNS) and suicidal behavior. Some studies have revealed a deficiency of serotonin (measured as a decrease in the levels of 5-hydroxyindole acetic acid [5-HIAA] of the cerebrospinal fluid) in depressed clients who attempted suicide (Sadock & Sadock, 2007). Some

changes in the noradrenergic system of suicide victims have also been reported.

Application of the Nursing Process With the Suicidal Client

Assessment

The following items should be considered when conducting a suicidal assessment: demographics, presenting symptoms/medical-psychiatric diagnosis, suicidal ideas or acts, interpersonal support system, analysis of the suicidal crisis, psychiatric/medical/family history, and coping strategies. Dr. David Satcher, as Surgeon General of the United States, in his "Call to Action to Prevent Suicide," spoke of risk factors and protective factors (U.S. Public Health Service, 1999). Risk factors are associated with a greater potential for suicide and suicidal behavior, whereas protective factors are associated with reduced potential for suicide. These risk and protective factors are outlined in Box 17-1. Table 17-2 presents some additional guidelines for determining the degree of suicide potential.

Demographics

The following demographics are assessed:

■ **Age.** Suicide is highest in persons older than 50. Adolescents are also at high risk.

■ **Gender.** Males are at higher risk than females.

■ **Ethnicity.** Caucasians are at higher risk than are Native Americans, who are at higher risk than African Americans.

■ **Marital status.** Single, divorced, and widowed are at higher risk than married.

■ **Socioeconomic status.** Individuals in the highest and lowest socioeconomic classes are at higher risk than those in the middle classes.

■ **Occupation.** Professional health-care personnel and business executives are at highest risk.

■ **Method.** Use of firearms presents a significantly higher risk than overdose of substances.

■ **Religion.** Individuals who are not affiliated with any religious group are at higher risk than those who have this type of affiliation.

■ **Family history.** Higher risk if individual has family history of suicide.

Presenting Symptoms/Medical-Psychiatric Diagnosis

Assessment data must be gathered regarding any psychiatric or physical condition for which the client is being treated. Mood disorders (major depression and bipolar disorders) are the most common disorders that precede suicide. Individuals with substance use disorders are also at high risk. Other psychiatric disorders in which suicide may be a risk include anxiety disorders, schizophrenia, and borderline and

BOX 17-1 **Suicide Risk Factors and Protective Factors**

RISK FACTORS

- Previous suicide attempt
- Mental disorders—particularly mood disorders such as depression and bipolar disorder
- Co-occurring mental and alcohol and substance abuse disorders
- Family history of suicide
- Hopelessness
- Impulsive and/or aggressive tendencies
- Barriers to accessing mental health treatment
- Relational, social, work, or financial loss
- Physical illness
- Easy access to lethal methods, especially guns
- Unwillingness to seek help because of stigma attached to mental and substance abuse disorders and/or suicidal thoughts
- Influence of significant people—family members, celebrities, peers who have died by suicide—both through direct personal contact or inappropriate media representations
- Cultural and religious beliefs—for instance, the belief that suicide is a noble resolution of a personal dilemma
- Local epidemics of suicide that have a contagious influence
- Isolation, a feeling of being cut off from other people

PROTECTIVE FACTORS

- Effective and appropriate clinical care for mental, physical, and substance abuse disorders
- Easy access to a variety of clinical interventions and support for help seeking
- Restricted access to highly lethal methods of suicide
- Family and community support
- Support from ongoing medical and mental health care relationships
- Learned skills in problem solving, conflict resolution, and nonviolent handling of disputes
- Cultural and religious beliefs that discourage suicide and support self-preservation instincts

From U.S. Public Health Service (1999). *The Surgeon General's call to action to prevent suicide.* Washington, DC: U.S. Government Printing Office.

TABLE 17–2 **Assessing the Degree of Suicidal Risk**

BEHAVIOR	INTENSITY OF RISK		
	LOW	MODERATE	HIGH
Anxiety	Mild	Moderate	High or panic
Depression	Mild	Moderate	Severe
Isolation; withdrawal	Some feelings of isolation; no withdrawal	Some feelings of helplessness, hopelessness, and withdrawal	Hopeless, helpless, withdrawn, and self-deprecating
Daily functioning	Fairly good in most activities	Moderately good in some activities	Not good in any activities
Resources	Several	Some	Few or none
Coping strategies being used	Generally constructive	Some that are constructive	Predominantly destructive
Significant others	Several who are available	Few or only one available	Only one or none available
Psychiatric help in past	None, or positive attitude toward	Yes, and moderately satisfied with results	Negative view of help received
Lifestyle	Stable	Moderately stable	Unstable
Alcohol or drug use	Infrequently to excess	Frequently to excess	Continual abuse
Previous suicide attempts	None, or of low lethality	One or more of moderate lethality	Multiple attempts of high lethality
Disorientation; disorganization	None	Some	Marked

Continued

TABLE 17–2 Assessing the Degree of Suicidal Risk—cont'd

BEHAVIOR	INTENSITY OF RISK		
	LOW	**MODERATE**	**HIGH**
Hostility	Little or none	Some	Marked
Suicidal plan	Vague, fleeting thoughts but no plan	Frequent thoughts, occasional ideas about a plan	Frequent or constant thought with a specific plan

From Hatton, C.L., Valente, S.M., & Rink, A. (1984). *Suicide: Assessment and intervention* (2nd ed.) Norwalk, CT: Appleton & Lange, with permission.

antisocial personality disorders (Jacobs et al., 2006). Other chronic and terminal physical illnesses have also precipitated suicidal acts.

Suicidal Ideas or Acts

How serious is the intent? Does the person have a plan? If so, does he or she have the means? How lethal are the means? Has the individual ever attempted suicide before? These are all questions that must be answered by the person conducting the suicidal client assessment.

Individuals may leave both behavioral and verbal clues as to the intent of their act. Examples of behavioral clues include giving away prized possessions, getting financial affairs in order, writing suicide notes, or sudden lifts in mood (may indicate a decision to carry out the intent).

Verbal clues may be both direct and indirect. Examples of direct statements include "I want to die" or "I'm going to kill myself." Examples of indirect statements include "This is the last time you'll see me," "I won't be around much longer for the doctor to have to worry about," or "I don't have anything worth living for anymore."

Other assessments include determining whether the individual has a plan, and if so, whether he or she has the means to carry out that plan. If the person states the suicide will be carried out with a gun, does he or she have access to a gun? Bullets? If pills are planned, what kind of pills? Are they accessible?

Interpersonal Support System

Does the individual have support persons on whom he or she can rely during a crisis situation? Lack of a meaningful network of satisfactory relationships may implicate an individual as a high risk for suicide during an emotional crisis.

Analysis of the Suicidal Crisis

■ **The precipitating stressor:** Adverse life events in combination with other risk factors such as depression may lead to suicide. Life stresses accompanied by an increase in emotional disturbance include the loss of a loved person either by death

or by divorce, problems in major relationships, changes in roles, or serious physical illness.

■ **Relevant history:** Has the individual experienced numerous failures or rejections that would increase his or her vulnerability for a dysfunctional response to the current situation?

■ **Life-stage issues:** The ability to tolerate losses and disappointments is often compromised if those losses and disappointments occur during various stages of life in which the individual struggles with developmental issues (e.g., adolescence, midlife).

Psychiatric/Medical/Family History

The individual should be assessed with regard to previous psychiatric treatment for depression, alcoholism, or for previous suicide attempts. Medical history should be obtained to determine presence of chronic, debilitating, or terminal illness. Is there a history of depressive disorder in the family, and has a close relative committed suicide in the past?

Coping Strategies

How has the individual handled previous crisis situations? How does this situation differ from previous ones?

Diagnosis/Outcome Identification

Nursing diagnoses for the suicidal client may include the following:

■ Risk for suicide related to feelings of hopelessness and desperation.

■ Hopelessness related to absence of support systems and perception of worthlessness.

Outcome Criteria

Outcome criteria include short- and long-term goals. Timelines are individually determined. The following criteria may be used for measurement of outcomes in the care of the suicidal client.

The client:

1. Has experienced no physical harm to self
2. Sets realistic goals for self
3. Expresses some optimism and hope for the future

Planning/Implementation

Table 17-3 provides a plan of care for the hospitalized suicidal client. Nursing diagnoses are presented, along with outcome criteria, appropriate nursing interventions, and rationales for each.

Intervention With the Suicidal Client Following Discharge (or Outpatient Suicidal Client)

In some instances, it may be determined that suicidal intent is low and that hospitalization is not required. Instead, the client with suicidal ideation may be

Table 17-3 | CARE PLAN FOR THE SUICIDAL CLIENT		
NURSING DIAGNOSIS: RISK FOR SUICIDE		
RELATED TO: Feelings of hopelessness and desperation		
OUTCOME CRITERIA	**NURSING INTERVENTIONS**	**RATIONALE**
Client will not harm self.	1. Ask client directly: "Have you thought about harming yourself in any way? If so, what do you plan to do? Do you have the means to carry out this plan?"	1. The risk of suicide is greatly increased if the client has developed a plan and particularly if means exist for the client to execute the plan.
	2. Create a safe environment for the client. Remove all potentially harmful objects from client's access (sharp objects, straps, belts, ties, glass items, alcohol). Supervise closely during meals and medication administration. Perform room searches as deemed necessary.	2. Client safety is a nursing priority.
	3. Formulate a short-term verbal or written contract that the client will not harm self. When time is up, make another, and so forth. Secure a promise that the client will seek out staff when feeling suicidal.	3. A degree of the responsibility for his or her safety is given to the client. Increased feelings of self-worth may be experienced when client feels accepted unconditionally regardless of thoughts or behavior.
	4. Maintain close observation of client. Depending on level of suicide precaution, provide one-to-one contact, constant visual observation, or every-15-minute checks. Place in room close to nurse's station; do not assign to private room. Accompany to off-unit activities if attendance is indicated. May need to accompany to bathroom.	4. Close observation is necessary to ensure that client does not harm self in any way. Being alert for suicidal and escape attempts facilitates being able to prevent or interrupt harmful behavior.
	5. Maintain special care in administration of medications.	5. Prevents saving up to overdose or discarding and not taking.
	6. Make rounds at frequent, *irregular* intervals (especially at night, toward early morning, at change of shift, or other predictably busy times for staff).	6. Prevents staff surveillance from becoming predictable. To be aware of client's location is important, especially when staff is busy and least available and observable.

Continued

Table 17-3 | CARE PLAN FOR THE SUICIDAL CLIENT—cont'd

OUTCOME CRITERIA	NURSING INTERVENTIONS	RATIONALE
	7. Encourage client to express honest feelings, including anger. Provide hostility release if needed.	7. Depression and suicidal behaviors may be viewed as anger turned inward on the self. If this anger can be verbalized in a nonthreatening environment, the client may be able to eventually resolve these feelings.

NURSING DIAGNOSIS: HOPELESSNESS

RELATED TO: Absence of support systems and perception of worthlessness

EVIDENCED BY: Verbal cues (despondent content, "I can't"); decreased affect; lack of initiative; suicidal ideas or attempts

OUTCOME CRITERIA	NURSING INTERVENTIONS	RATIONALE
Client will verbalize a measure of hope and acceptance of life and situations over which he or she has no control.	1. Identify stressors in client's life that precipitated current crisis.	1. Important to identify causative or contributing factors in order to plan appropriate assistance.
	2. Determine coping behaviors previously used and client's perception of effectiveness then and now.	2. It is important to identify client's strengths and encourage their use in current crisis situation.
	3. Encourage client to explore and verbalize feelings and perceptions.	3. Identification of feelings underlying behaviors helps client to begin process of taking control of own life.
	4. Provide expressions of hope to client in positive, low-key manner (e.g., "I know you feel you cannot go on, but I believe that things can get better for you. What you are feeling is temporary. It is okay if you don't see it just now." "You are very important to the people who care about you.").	4. Even though the client feels hopeless, it is helpful to hear positive expressions from others. The client's current state of mind may prevent him or her from identifying anything positive in life. It is important to accept the client's feelings nonjudgmentally and to affirm the individual's personal worth and value.
	5. Help client identify areas of life situation that are under own control.	5. The client's emotional condition may interfere with ability to problem-solve. Assistance may be required to perceive the benefits and consequences of available alternatives accurately.
	6. Identify sources that client may use after discharge when crises occur or feelings of hopelessness and possible suicidal ideation prevail.	6. Client should be made aware of local suicide hotlines or other local support services from which he or she may seek assistance following discharge from the hospital. A concrete plan provides hope in the face of a crisis situation.

treated in an outpatient setting. Guidelines for treatment of the suicidal client on an outpatient basis include the following:

■ The person should not be left alone. Arrangements must be made for the client to stay with family or friends. If this is not possible, hospitalization should be reconsidered.

■ Establish a no-suicide contract with the client. Formulate a written contract that the client will not harm himself or herself in a stated period of time. For example, the client writes, "I will not harm myself in any way between now and the time of our next counseling session," or "I will call the suicide hotline (or go to the emergency room) if I start to feel like harming myself." When the time period of this short-term contract has lapsed, a new contract is negotiated. **NOTE:** Some clinicians believe that suicide prevention contracting is not helpful (Knoll, 2011). Obviously, the contract for safety comes with no guarantee, and it holds no legal credibility. It should never be used as a single intervention, but can be viewed as one among many that serve to ensure the client's safety. Garvey and associates (2009) stated:

> Contracts should be considered for use only in patients who are deemed capable of giving informed consent and, even in these circumstances, should be used with caution. A contract should never replace a thorough assessment of a patient's suicide risk factors. (p. 363)

■ Enlist the help of family or friends to ensure that the home environment is safe from dangerous items, such as firearms or stockpiled drugs. Give support persons the telephone number of the counselor, or an emergency contact person in the event that the counselor is not available.

■ Appointments may need to be scheduled daily or every other day at first until the immediate suicidal crisis has subsided.

■ Establish rapport and promote a trusting relationship. It is important for the suicide counselor to become a key person in the client's support system at this time.

■ Accept the client's feelings in a nonjudgmental manner.

> **CLINICAL PEARL** Be direct. Talk openly and matter-of-factly about suicide. Listen actively and encourage expression of feelings, including anger.

■ Discuss the current crisis situation in the client's life. Use the problem-solving approach (see Chapter 13). Offer alternatives to suicide. Macnab (1993) suggested the following statements:

 [It is my belief that] you are incorrect in your belief that suicide is the only and the best solution to your problem. There are alternatives, and they are good. What is more, you will be alive to test them. (p. 265)

■ Help the client identify areas of the life situation that are within his or her control and those that the client does not have the ability to control. Discuss feelings associated with these control issues. It is important for the client to feel some control over his or her life situation in order to perceive a measure of self-worth.

■ The physician may prescribe antidepressants for an individual who is experiencing suicidal depression. It is wise to prescribe no more than a 3-day supply of the medication with no refills. The prescription can then be renewed at the client's next counseling session.

NOTE: Sadock and Sadock (2007) stated:

> As the depression lifts, patients become energized and are thus able to put their suicidal plans into action. Sometimes, depressed patients, with or without treatment, suddenly appear to be at peace with themselves because they have reached a secret decision to commit suicide. Clinicians should be especially suspicious of such a dramatic clinical change, which may portend a suicidal attempt. (p. 905)

■ Macnab (1993) suggests the following steps in crisis counseling with the suicidal client:

  ■ Focus on the current crisis and how it can be alleviated. Identify the client's appraisals of how things are, and how things will be. Note how these appraisals change in changing contexts.

  ■ Note the client's reactivity to the crisis and how this can be changed. Discuss strategies and procedures for the management of anxiety, anger, and frustration.

  ■ Work toward restoration of the client's self-worth, status, morale, and control. Introduce alternatives to suicide.

  ■ Rehearse cognitive reconstruction—more positive ways of thinking about the self, events, the past, the present, and the future.

  ■ Identify experiences and actions that affirm self-worth and self-efficacy.

  ■ Encourage movement toward the new reality, with the coping skills required to manage adaptively.

  ■ Be available for ongoing therapeutic support and growth.

Information for Family and Friends of the Suicidal Client

The following suggestions are made for family and friends of an individual who is suicidal:

■ Take any hint of suicide seriously. Anyone expressing suicidal feelings needs immediate attention.

■ Do not keep secrets. If a suicidal person says, "Promise you won't tell anyone," do not make that promise. Suicidal individuals are ambivalent about dying, and suicidal behavior is a cry for help. It is that ambivalence that leads the person to confide to you the suicidal thoughts. Get help for the person and for you. 1-800-SUICIDE is a national hotline that is available 24 hours a day.

■ Be a good listener. If people express suicidal thoughts or feel depressed, hopeless, or worthless, be supportive. Let them know you are there for them and are willing to help them seek professional help.

■ Many people find it awkward to put into words how another person's life is important for their own well-being, but it is important to stress that the person's life is important to you and to others. Emphasize in specific terms the ways in which the person's suicide would be devastating to you and to others.

■ Express concern for individuals who express thoughts about committing suicide. The individual may be withdrawn and reluctant to discuss what he or she is thinking. Acknowledge the person's pain and feelings of hopelessness, and encourage the individual to talk to someone else if he or she does not feel comfortable talking with you.

■ Familiarize yourself with suicide intervention sources, such as mental health centers and suicide hotlines.

■ Ensure that access to firearms or other means of self-harm is restricted.

■ Fleener (2013) offers the following suggestions:
  ■ Acknowledge and accept their feelings and be an active listener.
  ■ Try to give them hope and remind them that what they are feeling is temporary.
  ■ Stay with them. Do not leave them alone. Go to where they are, if necessary.
  ■ Show love and encouragement. Hold them, hug them, touch them. Allow them to cry and express anger.
  ■ Help them seek professional help.
  ■ Remove any items from the home with which the person may harm himself or herself.
  ■ If there are children present, try to remove them from the home. Perhaps another friend or relative can assist by taking them to their home. This type of situation can be extremely traumatic for children.
  ■ DO NOT: judge suicidal people, show anger toward them, provoke guilt in them, discount their feelings, or tell them to "snap out of it." This is a very real and serious situation to suicidal individuals. They are in real pain. They feel the situation is hopeless and that there is no other way to resolve it aside from taking their own life.

Intervention With Families and Friends of Suicide Victims

Cvinar (2005) stated:

> Suicide has a profound effect on the family, friends, and associates of the victim that transcends the immediate loss. As those close to the victim suffer through bereavement, a variety of reactions and coping mechanisms are engaged as each individual sorts through individual reactions to the difficult loss. Bereavement following suicide is complicated by the complex psychological impact of the act on those close to the victim. It is further complicated by the societal perception that the act of suicide is a failure by the victim and the family to deal with some emotional issue and ultimately society affixes blame for the loss on the survivors. This individual or societal stigma introduces a unique stress on the bereavement process that in some cases requires clinical intervention. (p. 14)

Suicide of a family member can induce a whole gamut of feelings in the survivors. Macnab (1993) identified the following symptoms, which may be evident following the suicide of a loved one:

■ A sense of guilt and responsibility
■ Anger, resentment, and rage that can never find its "object"
■ A heightened sense of emotionality, helplessness, failure, and despair
■ A recurring self-searching: "If only I had done something," "If only I had not done something," "If only . . ."
■ A sense of confusion and search for an explanation: "Why did this happen?" "What does it mean?" "What could have stopped it?" "What will people think?"
■ A sense of inner injury. The family feels wounded. They do not know how they will ever get over it and get on with life
■ A severe strain is placed on relationships. A sense of impatience, irritability, and anger exists between family members
■ A heightened vulnerability to illness and disease exists with this added burden of emotional stress

Strategies for assisting survivors of suicide victims include:

■ Encourage the clients to talk about the suicide, each responding to the others' viewpoints and reconstructing of events. Share memories.
■ Be aware of any blaming or scapegoating of specific family members. Discuss how each person fits into the family situation, both before and after the suicide.
■ Listen to feelings of guilt and self-persecution. Gently move the individuals toward the reality of the situation.

■ Encourage the family members to discuss individual relationships with the lost loved one. Focus on both positive and negative aspects of the relationships. Gradually, point out the irrationality of any idealized concepts of the deceased person. The family must be able to recognize both positive and negative aspects about the person before grief can be resolved.

■ No two people grieve in the same way. It may appear that some family members are "getting over" the grief faster than others. All family members must be made to understand that if this occurs, it is not because they "care less," just that they "grieve differently." Variables that enter into this phenomenon include individual past experiences, personal relationship with the deceased person, and individual temperament and coping abilities.

■ Recognize how the suicide has caused disorganization in family coping. Reassess interpersonal relationships in the context of the event. Discuss coping strategies that have been successful in times of stress in the past, and work to reestablish these within the family. Identify new adaptive coping strategies that can be incorporated.

■ Identify resources that provide support: religious beliefs and spiritual counselors, close friends and relatives, support groups for survivors of suicide. One online connection that puts individuals in contact with survivors groups specific to each state is the American Foundation for Suicide Prevention at http://www.afsp.org. A list of resources that provide information and help for issues regarding suicide is presented in Box 17-2.

Evaluation

Evaluation of the suicidal client is an ongoing process accomplished through continuous reassessment of the client, as well as determination of goal achievement. Once the immediate crisis has been resolved, extended psychotherapy may be indicated. The long-term goals of individual or group psychotherapy for the suicidal client would be for him or her to:

■ Develop and maintain a more positive self-concept.
■ Learn more effective ways to express feelings to others.
■ Achieve successful interpersonal relationships.
■ Feel accepted by others and achieve a sense of belonging.

BOX 17-2 Sources for Information Related to Issues of Suicide

National Suicide Hotline
1-800-SUICIDE (24/7)
National Suicide Prevention Lifeline
www.suicidepreventionlifeline.org
1-800-273-TALK (24/7)
American Association of Suicidology
www.suicidology.org
1-202-237-2280
Depression and Bipolar Support Alliance (DBSA)
www.dbsalliance.org/
1-800-826-3632
American Foundation for Suicide Prevention
www.afsp.org
1-888-333-AFSP
National Institute of Mental Health
www.nimh.nih.gov
1-866-615-6464
American Psychiatric Association
www.psych.org
1-703-907-7300
Mental Health America
www.nmha.org
1-703-684-7722
1-800-969-6642

American Psychological Association
www.apa.org
1-800-374-2721
Screening for Mental Health
Stop a Suicide Today!
www.stopasuicide.org
1-781-239-0071
Boys Town
Cares for troubled boys and girls and families in crisis.
Staff is trained to handle calls related to violence and suicide.
www.boystown.org
1-800-448-3000 (24/7 National hotline)
Centre for Suicide Prevention
www.suicideinfo.ca
1-403-245-3900
Centers for Disease Control and Prevention
National Center for Injury Prevention and Control
Division of Violence Prevention
www.cdc.gov/injury/index.html
1-800-CDC-INFO
National Alliance on Mental Illness
www.nami.org
1-800-950-NAMI

A suicidal person feels worthless and hopeless. These goals serve to instill a sense of self-worth, while offering a measure of hope and a meaning for living.

Summary and Key Points

- More than 90 percent of all persons who commit or attempt suicide have a diagnosed mental disorder.
- Suicide is the third leading cause of death among young Americans ages 15 to 24 years, the fourth leading cause of death for ages 25 to 44, and the eighth leading cause of death for individuals ages 45 to 64.
- Single people are at greater risk for suicide than married people.
- Women attempt suicide more, but men succeed more often.
- Suicide and age are positively correlated.
- Depressed men and women who consider themselves affiliated with a religion are less likely to attempt suicide than their nonreligious counterparts.
- Individuals in the very highest and lowest social classes have higher suicide rates than those in the middle classes.
- Whites are at highest risk for suicide, followed by Native Americans, African Americans, Hispanic Americans, and Asian Americans.

- Psychiatric disorders that predispose individuals to suicide include mood disorders, substance use disorders, schizophrenia, personality disorders, and anxiety disorders.
- Predisposing factors include internalized anger, hopelessness, desperation and guilt, history of aggression and violence, shame and humiliation, developmental stressors, sociological influences, genetics, and neurochemical factors.
- It is important for the nurse to determine the seriousness of the intent, the existence of a plan, and the availability and lethality of the method.
- The suicidal person should not be left alone.
- Once the crisis intervention is complete, the individual may require long-term psychotherapy, during which he or she works to:
  - Develop and maintain a more positive self-concept
  - Learn more effective ways to express feelings
  - Improve interpersonal relationships
  - Achieve a sense of belonging and a measure of hope for living

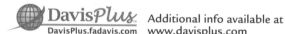
DavisPlus Additional info available at
DavisPlus.fadavis.com   www.davisplus.com

Review Questions
Self-Examination/Learning Exercise

*Select the answer that is **most** appropriate for each of the following questions.*

1. Which of the following individuals is at highest risk for suicide?
   a. Nancy, age 33, Asian American, Catholic, middle socioeconomic group, alcoholic
   b. John, age 72, white, Methodist, low socioeconomic group, diagnosis of metastatic cancer of the pancreas
   c. Carol, age 15, African American, Baptist, high socioeconomic group, no physical or mental health problems
   d. Mike, age 55, Jewish, middle socioeconomic group, suffered myocardial infarction a year ago

2. Some biological factors may be associated with the predisposition to suicide. Which of the following biological factors have been implicated?
   a. Genetics and decreased levels of serotonin
   b. Heredity and increased levels of norepinephrine
   c. Temporal lobe atrophy and decreased levels of acetylcholine
   d. Structural alterations of the brain and increased levels of dopamine

3. Theresa, age 27, was admitted to the psychiatric unit from the medical intensive care unit where she was treated for taking a deliberate overdose of her antidepressant medication, trazodone (Desyrel). She says to the nurse, "My boyfriend broke up with me. We had been together for 6 years. I love him so much. I know I'll never get over him." Which is the best response by the nurse?
   a. "You'll get over him in time, Theresa."
   b. "Forget him. There are other fish in the sea."
   c. "You must be feeling very sad about your loss."
   d. "Why do you think he broke up with you, Theresa?"

Review Questions—cont'd
Self-Examination/Learning Exercise

4. The nurse identifies the primary nursing diagnosis for Theresa as Risk for Suicide related to feelings of hopelessness from loss of relationship. Which is the outcome criterion that would most accurately measure achievement of this diagnosis?
   a. The client has experienced no physical harm to herself.
   b. The client sets realistic goals for herself.
   c. The client expresses some optimism and hope for the future.
   d. The client has reached a stage of acceptance in the loss of the relationship with her boyfriend.

5. Theresa is hospitalized following a suicide attempt after breaking up with her boyfriend. Freudian psychoanalytic theory would explain Theresa's suicide attempt in which of the following ways?
   a. She feels hopeless about her future without her boyfriend.
   b. Without her boyfriend, she feels like an outsider with her peers.
   c. She is feeling intense guilt because her boyfriend broke up with her.
   d. She is angry at her boyfriend for breaking up with her and has turned the anger inward on herself.

6. Theresa is hospitalized following a suicide attempt after breaking up with her boyfriend. Theresa says to the nurse, "When I get out of here, I'm going to try this again, and next time I'll choose a no-fail method." Which is the best response by the nurse?
   a. "You are safe here. We will make sure nothing happens to you."
   b. "You're just lucky your roommate came home when she did."
   c. "What exactly do you plan to do?"
   d. "I don't understand. You have so much to live for."

7. In determining degree of suicidal risk with a suicidal client, the nurse assesses the following behavioral manifestations: severely depressed, withdrawn, statements of worthlessness, difficulty accomplishing activities of daily living, no close support systems. The nurse identifies the client's risk for suicide as:
   a. Low
   b. Moderate
   c. High
   d. Unable to determine

8. Theresa, who has been hospitalized following a suicide attempt, is placed on suicide precautions on the psychiatric unit. She admits that she is still feeling suicidal. Which of the following interventions is most appropriate in this instance?
   a. Obtain an order from the physician to place Theresa in restraints to prevent any attempts to harm herself.
   b. Check on Theresa every 15 minutes or assign a staff person to stay with her on a one-to-one basis.
   c. Obtain an order from the physician to give Theresa a sedative to calm her and reduce suicide ideas.
   d. Do not allow Theresa to participate in any unit activities while she is on suicide precautions.

9. Which of the following interventions are appropriate for a client on suicide precautions? (Select all that apply.)
   a. Remove all sharp objects, belts, and other potentially dangerous articles from the client's environment.
   b. Accompany the client to off-unit activities.
   c. Obtain a promise from the client that she will not do anything to harm herself for the next 12 hours.
   d. Put all of the client's possessions in storage and explain to her that she may have them back when she is off suicide precautions.

10. Success of long-term psychotherapy with Theresa (who attempted suicide following a breakup with her boyfriend) could be measured by which of the following behaviors?
    a. Theresa has a new boyfriend.
    b. Theresa has an increased sense of self-worth.
    c. Theresa does not take antidepressants anymore.
    d. Theresa told her old boyfriend how angry she was with him for breaking up with her.

References

Abbar, M., Courtet, P., Bellivier, F., Leboyer, M., Boulenger, J.P., Castelhau, D., Ferreira, M., Lambercy, C., Mouthon, D., Paoloni-Giacobino, A., Vessaz, M., Malafosse, A., & Buresi, C. (2001). Suicide attempters and the tryptophan hydroxylase gene. *Molecular Psychiatry, 6,* 268-273.

American Association of Suicidology. (2013). *Elderly suicide fact sheet.* Retrieved from http://www.suicidology.org

American Foundation for Suicide Prevention (AFSP). (2013). *Suicide facts and figures.* Retrieved from http://www.afsp.org/index.cfm?page_id=04ea1254-bd31-1fa3-c549d77e6ca6aa37

Beck, A.T., Brown, G., & Berchick, R.J. (1990). Relationship between hopelessness and ultimate suicide: A replication with psychiatric outpatients. *American Journal of Psychiatry, 147,* 190-195.

Carroll-Ghosh, T., Victor, B.S., & Bourgeois, J.A. (2003). Suicide. In R.E. Hales and S.C. Yudofsky (Eds.), *Textbook of clinical psychiatry* (4th ed., 1457-1483). Washington, DC: American Psychiatric Publishing.

Centers for Disease Control and Prevention (CDC). (2012). *National suicide statistics at a glance.* Retrieved from http://www.cdc.gov

Centers for Disease Control and Prevention (CDC). (2013). *20 leading causes of death, United States.* National Center for Injury Prevention and Control. Retrieved from http://webappa.cdc.gov/sasweb/ncipc/leadcaus10_us.html

Cochran, S.D., & Mays, V.M. (2000). Lifetime prevalence of suicide symptoms and affective disorders among men reporting same-sex sexual partners: Results from NHANES III. *American Journal of Public Health, 90*(4), 573-578.

Corr, C.A. & Corr, D.M. (2013). *Death & Dying, Life & Living.* Belmont, CA: Wadsworth.

Cvinar, J.G. (2005). Do suicide survivors suffer social stigma: A review of the literature. *Perspectives in Psychiatric Care, 41*(1), 14-21.

Eisenberg, M.E., & Resnick, M.D. (2006). Suicidality among gay, lesbian and bisexual youth: The role of protective factors. *Journal of Adolescent Health, 39*(5), 662-668.

Fleener, P. (2013). How to help a suicidal persona. *Mental Health Today.* Retrieved from http://www.mental-health-today.com/suicide/sui2.htm

Friends for Survival, Inc. (2013). *Facts and fables.* Retrieved from http://www.friendsforsurvival.org/facts-and-fables

Garvey, K.A., Penn, J.V., Campbell, A.L., Esposito-Smythers, C., & Spirito, A. (2009). Contracting for safety with patients: Clinical practice and forensic implications. *Journal of the American Academy of Psychiatry and the Law, 37,* 363-370.

Hatton, C.L., Valente, S.M., & Rink, A. (1984). *Suicide: Assessment and intervention* (2nd ed.). Norwalk, CT: Appleton & Lange.

Hendin, H. (1991). Psychodynamics of suicide, with particular reference to the young. *American Journal of Psychiatry, 148,* 1150-1158.

Hinduja, S., & Patchin, J.W. (2010). Bullying, cyberbullying, and suicide. *Archives of Suicide Research, 14,* 206-221.

Jacobs, D.G., Baldessarini, R.J., Conwell, Y., Fawcett, J.A., Horton, L., Meltzer, H., Pfeffer, C.R., & Simon, R.I. (2006). Practice guideline for the assessment and treatment of patients with suicidal behaviors. *American Psychiatric Association practice guidelines for the treatment of psychiatric disorders, Compendium 2006.* Arlington, VA: American Psychiatric Association.

King, M., Semlyen, J., Tai, S.S., Killaspy, H., Osborn, D., Popelyuk, D., & Nazareth, I. (2008). A systematic review of mental disorder, suicide, and deliberate self harm in lesbian, gay, and bisexual people. *BMC Psychiatry, 8*(70). Retrieved from http://www.biomedcentral.com/1471-244X/8/70

Klomek, A.B., Sourander, A., & Gould, M.S. (2011). Bullying and suicide: Detection and intervention. *Psychiatric Times, 28*(2). Retrieved from http://www.psychiatrictimes.com/suicide/content/article/10168/1795797#

Knoll, J. (2011, March 11). The suicide prevention contract: Contracting for comfort. *Psychiatric Times.* Retrieved from http://www.psychiatrictimes.com/blog/couchincrisis/content/article/10168/1811702

MacDonald, M., & Murphy, T.R. (1991). *Sleepless souls: Suicide in early modern England.* New York, NY: Oxford University Press.

Macnab, F. (1993). *Brief psychotherapy: An integrative approach in clinical practice.* West Sussex, England: John Wiley & Sons.

Medscape Psychiatry (2011). *Striking risk for suicidality, depression in gay teens.* Retrieved from http://www.medscape.com/viewarticle/740429

Minois, G. (2001). *History of suicide: Voluntary death in Western culture.* Baltimore, MD: Johns Hopkins University Press.

National Center for Health Statistics (NCHS). (2012). *Health, United States, 2011.* Library of Congress Catalog Number 76-641496. Washington, DC: U.S. Government Printing Office.

National Institute of Mental Health (NIMH). (2013). *The numbers count: Mental disorders in America.* Retrieved from http://www.nimh.nih.gov/health/publications/the-numbers-count-mental-disorders-in-america/index.shtml

Rasic, D.T., Belik, S.L., Elias, B., Katz, L.Y., Enns, M., & Sareen, J. (2009). Spirituality, religion, and suicidal behavior in a nationally representative sample. *Journal of Affective Disorders, 114*(1), 32-40.

Rich, C.L., Warsradt, G.M., & Nemiroff, R.A. (1991). Suicide, stressors, and the life cycle. *American Journal of Psychiatry, 148,* 524-527.

Sadock, B.J. & Sadock, V.A. (2007). *Synopsis of psychiatry: Behavioral sciences/clinical psychiatry* (10th ed.). Philadelphia, PA: Lippincott Williams & Wilkins.

Suicide Prevention Resource Center. (2008). *Suicide risk and prevention for lesbian, gay, bisexual, and transgender youth.* Newton, MA: Education Development Center.

The Samaritans. (2013). *Suicide myths and misconceptions.* Retrieved from http://www.samaritansnyc.org/myths.html

Tondo, L., & Baldessarini, R.J. (2001). *Suicide: Historical, descriptive, and epidemiological considerations.* Retrieved from http://www.medscape.com/viewarticle/413194

U.S. Public Health Service (USPHS). (1999). *The Surgeon General's call to action to prevent suicide.* Washington, DC: USPHS.

Classical References

Durkheim, E. (1951). *Suicide: A study of sociology.* Glencoe, IL: Free Press.

Freud, S. (1957). *Mourning and melancholia* (Vol. 14, Standard ed.) London: Hogarth Press. (Original work published 1917.)

Behavior Therapy

18

CORE CONCEPTS

behavior therapy

stimulus

KEY TERMS

aversive stimulus	flooding	shaping
classical conditioning	modeling	stimulus generalization
conditioned response	negative reinforcement	systematic desensitization
conditioned stimulus	operant conditioning	time-out
contingency contracting	overt sensitization	token economy
covert sensitization	positive reinforcement	unconditioned response
discriminative stimuli	Premack principle	unconditioned stimulus
extinction	reciprocal inhibition	

OBJECTIVES

After reading this chapter, the student will be able to:

1. Discuss the principles of classical and operant conditioning as foundations for behavior therapy.
2. Identify various techniques used in the modification of client behavior.
3. Implement the principles of behavior therapy using the steps of the nursing process.

HOMEWORK ASSIGNMENT

Please read the chapter and answer the following questions:

1. A mother is teaching her young child how to dress himself. Each time he makes an attempt, she praises him profusely, even though he has made several mistakes. She does this until he is able to dress himself appropriately. What is this technique called?
2. Flooding (implosive therapy) is used to desensitize individuals to phobic stimuli. When is this technique contraindicated?
3. A nurse is working with parents of a toddler whom they say falls to the ground, screams, and kicks his legs whenever he doesn't get his way. They usually just give in to his wishes to keep him from behaving this way. The nurse decides to teach the parents about the technique of extinction. What would this entail?

A behavior is considered to be maladaptive when it is age inappropriate, when it interferes with adaptive functioning, or when others misunderstand it in terms of cultural inappropriateness. The behavioral approach to therapy is that people have become what they are through learning processes or, more correctly, through the interaction of the environment with their genetic endowment. The basic assumption is that problematic behaviors occur when there has been inadequate learning and therefore can be corrected through the provision of appropriate learning experiences. The principles of behavior therapy as we know it today are based on the early studies of **classical conditioning** by Pavlov (1927) and **operant conditioning** by Skinner (1938). Although in this text the concepts are presented separately for reasons of clarification, behavioral change procedures are often combined with cognitive procedures, and many behavior therapies are referred to as *cognitive-behavioral* therapies. Concepts of cognitive therapy are presented in Chapter 19.

Classical Conditioning

Classical conditioning is a process of learning that was introduced by the Russian physiologist Ivan Pavlov. In his experiments with dogs, during which he hoped to learn more about the digestive process, he inadvertently discovered that organisms can learn to respond in specific ways if they are conditioned to do so.

In his trials he found that, as expected, the dogs salivated when they began to eat the food that was offered to them. This was a reflexive response that Pavlov called an **unconditioned response**. However, he also noticed that with time, the dogs began to salivate when the food came into their range of view, before it was even presented to them for consumption. Pavlov, concluding that this response was not reflexive but had been learned, called it a **conditioned response**. He carried the experiments even further by introducing an unrelated stimulus, one that had had no previous connection to the animal's food. He simultaneously presented the food with the sound of a bell. The animal responded with the expected reflexive salivation to the food. After a number of trials with the combined stimuli (food and bell), Pavlov found that the reflexive salivation began to occur when the dog was presented with the sound of the bell in the absence of food.

CORE CONCEPT
Stimulus
A stimulus is an environmental event that interacts with and influences an individual's behavior.

This was an important discovery in terms of how learning can occur. Pavlov found that unconditioned responses (salivation) occur in response to unconditioned stimuli (eating food). He also found that, over time, an unrelated stimulus (sound of the bell) introduced with the **unconditioned stimulus** can elicit the same response alone—that is, the conditioned response. The unrelated stimulus is called the **conditioned stimulus**. A graphic of Pavlov's classical conditioning model is presented in Figure 18-1. An example of the application of Pavlov's classical conditioning model to humans is shown in Figure 18-2. The process by which the fear response is elicited from similar stimuli (all individuals in white uniforms) is called **stimulus generalization**.

Sequence of Conditioning Operations:

1. UCS - ► UCR
   Unconditioned stimulus   Unconditioned response
   (eating food)   (salivation)

2. UCS - ► CR
   Unconditioned stimulus   Conditioned response
   (sight of food)   (salivation)

3. CS - ► NR
   Conditioned stimulus   No response or
   (bell)   response unrelated to salivation

4. UCS + CS - ► CR
   Unconditioned + Conditioned stimuli   Conditioned response
   (food)   (bell)   (salivation)

5. CS - ► CR
   Conditioned stimulus   Conditioned response
   (bell)   (salivation)

FIGURE 18–1   Pavlov's model of classic conditioning.

Classical Conditioning and Stimulus Generalization

Subject: 6-month-old baby
Sequence of Conditioning Operations:

1. CS - ► NR
   Conditioned stimulus   No response
   (Nurse A in white uniform walks into room)

2. UCS - ► UCR
   Unconditioned stimulus   Unconditioned response
   (Nurse A in white uniform gives shot)   (cries; clings to mother)

3. CS - ► CR
   Conditioned stimulus   Conditioned response
   (Nurse A in white uniform walks into room)   (cries; clings to mother)

4. CS - ► CR
   Conditioned stimulus   Conditioned response
   (Nurse B in white uniform walks into room)   (cries; clings to mother)
   or:
   (family friend comes to visit wearing a white dress)

FIGURE 18-2   Example: Classical conditioning and stimulus generalization.

Operant Conditioning

The focus of operant conditioning differs from that of classical conditioning. With classical conditioning, the focus is on behavioral responses that are elicited by specific objects or events. With operant conditioning, additional attention is given to the consequences of the behavioral response.

Operant conditioning was introduced by B. F. Skinner (1953), an American psychologist whose work was largely influenced by Edward Thorndike's (1911) law of effect—that is, that the connection between a stimulus and a response is strengthened or weakened by the consequences of the response. A number of terms must be defined in order to understand the concept of operant conditioning.

As defined previously, stimuli are environmental events that interact with and influence an individual's behavior. Stimuli may precede or follow a behavior. A stimulus that follows a behavior (or response) is called a reinforcing stimulus or *reinforcer*. The function is called *reinforcement*. When the reinforcing stimulus increases the probability that the behavior will recur, it is called a *positive reinforcer*, and the function is called **positive reinforcement**. **Negative reinforcement** is increasing the probability that a behavior will recur by removal of an undesirable reinforcing stimulus. A stimulus that follows a behavioral response and decreases the probability that the behavior will recur is called an **aversive stimulus** or *punisher*. Examples of these reinforcing stimuli are presented in Table 18-1.

Stimuli that precede a behavioral response and predict that a particular reinforcement will occur are called **discriminative stimuli**. Discriminative stimuli are under the control of the individual. The individual is said to be able to *discriminate* between stimuli and to *choose* according to the type of reinforcement he or she has come to associate with a specific stimulus. The following is an example of the concept of discrimination:

EXAMPLE

Mrs. M. was admitted to the hospital from a nursing home 2 weeks ago. She has no family, and no one visits her. She is very lonely. Nurse A and Nurse B have taken care of Mrs. M. on a regular basis during her hospital stay. When she is feeling particularly lonely, Mrs. M. calls Nurse A to her room, for she has learned that Nurse A will stay and talk to her for a while, but Nurse B only takes care of her physical needs and leaves. She no longer seeks out Nurse B for emotional support and comfort.

After several attempts, Mrs. M. is able to discriminate between stimuli. She can predict with assurance that calling Nurse A (and not Nurse B) will result in the reinforcement she desires.

CORE CONCEPT

Behavior Therapy

A form of psychotherapy, the goal of which is to modify maladaptive behavior patterns by reinforcing more adaptive behaviors.

Techniques for Modifying Client Behavior

Shaping

In **shaping** the behavior of another, reinforcements are given for increasingly closer approximations to the desired response. For example, in eliciting speech from an autistic child, the teacher may first reward the child for (a) watching the teacher's lips, then (b) for making any sound in imitation of the teacher, then (c) for forming sounds similar to the word uttered by the teacher. Shaping has been shown to be an effective way of modifying behavior for tasks that a child has not mastered on command or are not in the child's repertoire (Souders, DePaul, Freeman, & Levy, 2002).

Modeling

Modeling refers to the learning of new behaviors by imitating the behavior in others.

Role models are individuals who have qualities or skills that a person admires and wishes to imitate (Howard, 2000). Modeling occurs in various ways. Children imitate the behavior patterns of their parents, teachers, friends, and others. Adults and children

TABLE 18–1 **Examples of Reinforcing Stimuli**			
TYPE	STIMULUS	BEHAVIORAL RESPONSE	REINFORCING STIMULUS
Positive	Messy room	Child cleans her messy room.	Child gets allowance for cleaning room.
Negative	Messy room	Child cleans her messy room.	Child does not receive scolding from the mother.
Aversive	Messy room	Child does not clean her messy room.	Child receives scolding from the mother.

alike model many of their behaviors after individuals observed on television and in movies. Unfortunately, modeling can result in maladaptive behaviors, as well as adaptive ones.

In the practice setting clients may imitate the behaviors of practitioners who are charged with their care. This can occur naturally in the therapeutic community environment. It can also occur in a therapy session in which the client watches a model demonstrate appropriate behaviors in a role-play of the client's problem. The client is then instructed to imitate the model's behaviors in a similar role-play and is positively reinforced for appropriate imitation.

Premack Principle

This technique, named for its originator, states that a frequently occurring response (R_1) can serve as a positive reinforcement for a response (R_2) that occurs less frequently (Premack, 1959). This is accomplished by allowing R_1 to occur only after R_2 has been performed. For example, 13-year-old Jennie has been neglecting her homework for the past few weeks. She spends a lot of time on the telephone talking to her friends. Applying the **Premack principle**, being allowed to talk on the telephone to her friends could serve as a positive reinforcement for completing her homework. A schematic of the Premack principle for this situation is presented in Figure 18-3.

Extinction

Extinction is the gradual decrease in frequency or disappearance of a response when the positive reinforcement is withheld. A classic example of this technique is its use with children who have temper tantrums. The tantrum behaviors continue as long as the parent gives attention to them but decrease and often disappear when the parent simply walks away from the child and ignores the behavior.

Contingency Contracting

In **contingency contracting**, a contract is drawn up among all parties involved. The behavior change that is desired is stated explicitly in writing. The contract specifies the behavior change desired and the reinforcers to be given for performing the desired behaviors. The negative consequences or punishers that will be rendered for not fulfilling the terms of the contract are also delineated. The contract is specific about how reinforcers and punishment will be presented; however, flexibility is important so that renegotiations can occur if necessary.

Token Economy

Token economy is a type of contingency contracting (although there may or may not be a written and signed contract involved) in which the reinforcers for desired behaviors are presented in the form of *tokens*. Essential to this type of technique is the prior determination of items and situations of significance to the client that can be employed as reinforcements. With this therapy, tokens are awarded when desired behaviors are performed and may be exchanged for designated privileges. For example, a client may be able to "buy" a snack or cigarettes for 2 tokens, a trip to the coffee shop or library for 5 tokens, or even a trip outside the hospital (if that is a realistic possibility) for another designated number of tokens. The tokens themselves provide immediate positive feedback, and clients should be allowed to make the decision of whether to spend the token as soon as it is presented or to accumulate tokens that may be exchanged later for a more desirable reward.

Time-Out

Time-out is an aversive stimulus or punishment during which the client is removed from the environment where the unacceptable behavior is being exhibited. The client is usually isolated so that reinforcement from the attention of others is absent.

Reciprocal Inhibition

Also called counter-conditioning, **reciprocal inhibition** decreases or eliminates a behavior by introducing a more adaptive behavior, but one that is incompatible with the unacceptable behavior (Wolpe, 1958). An example is the introduction of relaxation exercises to an individual who is phobic. Relaxation is practiced in the presence of anxiety so that in time the individual is able to manage the anxiety in the presence of the phobic stimulus by engaging in relaxation exercises. Relaxation and anxiety are incompatible behaviors.

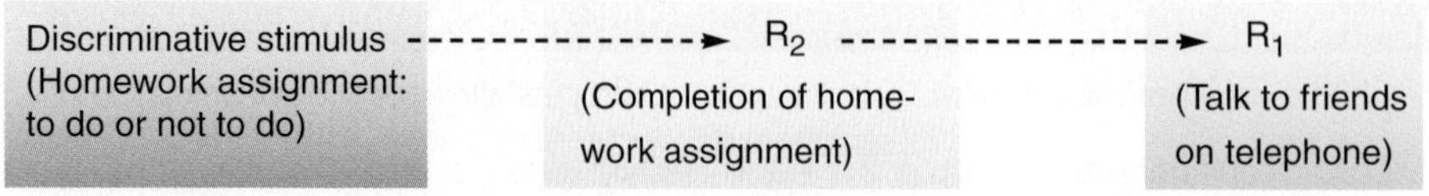

Discriminative stimulus (Homework assignment: to do or not to do) $---\rightarrow$ R_2 (Completion of homework assignment) $---\rightarrow$ R_1 (Talk to friends on telephone)

FIGURE 18-3 Example: Premack principle.

Overt Sensitization

Overt sensitization is a type of aversion therapy that produces unpleasant consequences for undesirable behavior. For example, disulfiram (Antabuse) is a drug that is given to individuals who wish to stop drinking alcohol. If an individual consumes alcohol while on Antabuse therapy, symptoms of severe nausea and vomiting, dyspnea, palpitations, and headache will occur. Instead of the euphoric feeling normally experienced from the alcohol (the positive reinforcement for drinking), the individual receives a severe punishment that is intended to extinguish the unacceptable behavior (drinking alcohol).

Covert Sensitization

Covert sensitization relies on the individual's imagination to produce unpleasant symptoms rather than on medication. The technique is under the client's control and can be used whenever and wherever it is required. The individual learns, through mental imagery, to visualize nauseating scenes and even to induce a mild feeling of nausea. This mental image is visualized when the individual is about to succumb to an attractive but undesirable behavior. It is most effective when paired with relaxation exercises that are performed instead of the undesirable behavior. The primary advantage of covert sensitization is that the individual does not have to perform the undesired behaviors but simply imagines them.

Systematic Desensitization

Systematic desensitization is a technique for assisting individuals to overcome their fear of a phobic stimulus. It is "systematic" in that there is a hierarchy of anxiety-producing events through which the individual progresses during therapy. An example of a hierarchy of events associated with a fear of elevators may be as follows:

1. Discuss riding an elevator with the therapist.
2. Look at a picture of an elevator.
3. Walk into the lobby of a building and see the elevators.
4. Push the button for the elevator.
5. Walk into an elevator with a trusted person; disembark before the doors close.
6. Walk into an elevator with a trusted person; allow doors to close; then open the doors and walk out.
7. Ride one floor with a trusted person, then walk back down the stairs.
8. Ride one floor with a trusted person and ride the elevator back down.
9. Ride the elevator alone.

As each of these steps is attempted, it is paired with relaxation exercises as an antagonistic behavior to anxiety. Generally, the desensitization procedures occur in the therapy setting by instructing the client to engage in relaxation exercises. When relaxation has been achieved, the client uses mental imagery to visualize the step in the hierarchy being described by the therapist. If the client becomes anxious, the therapist suggests relaxation exercises again, and presents a scene that is lower in the hierarchy. Therapy continues until the individual is able to progress through the entire hierarchy with manageable anxiety. The effects of relaxation in the presence of imagined anxiety-producing stimuli transfer to the real situation, once the client has achieved relaxation capable of suppressing or inhibiting anxiety responses (Ford-Martin, 2005). However, some clients are not successful in extinguishing phobic reactions through imagery. For these clients, *real-life desensitization* may be required. In these instances, the therapist may arrange for the client to be exposed to the hierarchy of steps in the desensitization process, but in real-life situations. Relaxation exercises may or may not be a part of real-life desensitization.

Flooding

This technique, sometimes called *implosive therapy*, is also used to desensitize individuals to phobic stimuli. It differs from systematic desensitization in that, instead of working up a hierarchy of anxiety-producing stimuli, the individual is "flooded" with a continuous presentation (through mental imagery) of the phobic stimulus until it no longer elicits anxiety. **Flooding** is believed to produce results faster than systematic desensitization; however, some therapists report more lasting behavioral changes with systematic desensitization. Some questions have also been raised in terms of the psychological discomfort that this therapy produces for the client. Flooding is contraindicated with clients for whom intense anxiety would be hazardous (e.g., individuals with heart disease or fragile psychological adaptation) (Sadock & Sadock, 2007).

Role of the Nurse in Behavior Therapy

The nursing process is the vehicle for delivery of nursing care with the client requiring assistance with behavior modification. The steps of the nursing process are illustrated in the following example case study.

CASE STUDY

(This example focuses on inpatient care, but these interventions can be modified and are applicable to various health-care settings, including partial hospitalization, community outpatient clinic, home health, and private practice.)

ASSESSMENT

Sammy, age 8, has been admitted to the child psychiatric unit of a university medical center following evaluation by a child psychiatrist. His parents, Tom and Nancy, are at an impasse, and their marriage is suffering because of constant conflict over their son's behavior at home and at school. Tom complains bitterly that Nancy is overly permissive with their son. Tom reports that Sammy argues and has temper tantrums and insists on continuing games, books, and TV, whenever Nancy puts him to bed, so that an 8:30 p.m. bedtime regularly is delayed until 10:30 or later every night. Also, Nancy often cooks four or five different meals for her son's dinner if Sammy stubbornly insists that he will not eat what has been prepared. At school, several teachers have complained that the child is stubborn and argumentative, is often disruptive in the classroom, and refuses to follow established rules.

When asked by the psychiatric nurse about other maladaptive behaviors, such as destruction of property, stealing, lying, or setting fires, the parents denied that these had been a problem. During the interview, Sammy sat quietly without interrupting. He answered questions that were directed to him with brief responses and made light of the problems described by his parents and reported by his teachers.

During his first 3 days on the unit, the following assessments were made:

1. Sammy loses his temper when he cannot have his way. He screams, stomps his feet, and sometimes kicks the furniture.
2. Sammy refuses to follow directions given by staff. He merely responds, "No, I won't."
3. Sammy likes to engage in behaviors that annoy the staff and other children: belching loudly, scraping his fingernails across the blackboard, making loud noises when the other children are trying to watch television, opening his mouth when it is full of food.
4. Sammy blames others when he makes a mistake. He spilled his milk at lunchtime while racing to get to a specific seat he knew Tony wanted. He blamed the accident on Tony saying, "He made me do it! He tripped me!"

Upon completion of the initial assessments, the psychiatrist diagnosed Sammy with oppositional defiant disorder.

DIAGNOSIS/OUTCOME IDENTIFICATION

Nursing diagnoses and outcome criteria for Sammy include:

NURSING DIAGNOSES	OUTCOME CRITERIA
Noncompliance with therapy	Sammy participates in and cooperates during therapeutic activities.
Defensive coping	Sammy accepts responsibility for own behaviors and interacts with others without becoming defensive.
Impaired social interaction	Sammy interacts with staff and peers using age-appropriate, acceptable behaviors.

PLANNING/IMPLEMENTATION

A contract for Sammy's care was drawn up by the admitting nurse and others on the treatment team. Sammy's contract was based on a system of token economies. He discussed with the nurse the kinds of privileges he would like to earn. They included:

- Getting to wear his own clothes (5 tokens)
- Having a can of pop for a snack (2 tokens)
- Getting to watch 30 minutes of TV (5 tokens)
- Getting to stay up later on Friday nights with the other clients (7 tokens)
- Getting to play the video games (3 tokens)
- Getting to walk with the nurse to the gift shop to spend some of his money (8 tokens)
- Getting to talk to his parents/grandparents on the phone (5 tokens)
- Getting to go on the outside therapeutic recreation activities such as movies, the zoo, and picnics (10 tokens)

Tokens were awarded for appropriate behaviors:

- Gets out of bed when the nurse calls him (1 token)
- Gets dressed for breakfast (1 token)
- Presents himself for *all* meals in an appropriate manner, that is, no screaming, no belching, no opening his mouth when it is full of food, no throwing of food, staying in his chair during the meal, putting his tray away in the appropriate place when he is finished (2 tokens × 3 meals = 6 tokens)
- Completes hygiene activities (1 token)
- Accepts blame for own mistakes (1 token)
- Does not fight; uses no obscene language; does not "sass" staff (1 token)
- Remains quiet while others are watching TV (1 token)
- Participates and is not disruptive in unit meetings and group therapy sessions (2 tokens)
- Displays no temper tantrums (1 token)

CASE STUDY—cont'd

■ Follows unit rules (1 token)
■ Goes to bed at designated hour without opposition (1 token)

Tokens are awarded at bedtime for absence of inappropriate behaviors during the day. For example, if Sammy has no temper tantrums during the day, he is awarded 1 token. Likewise, if Sammy has a temper tantrum (or exhibits other inappropriate behavior), he must pay back the token amount designated for that behavior. No other attention is given to inappropriate behaviors other than withholding and payback of tokens.

EXCEPTION: If Sammy is receiving reinforcement from peers for inappropriate behaviors, staff has the option of imposing time-out or isolation until the behavior is extinguished.

The contract may be renegotiated at any time between Sammy and staff. Additional privileges or responsibilities may be added as they develop and are deemed appropriate.

All staff members are consistent with the terms of the contract and do not allow Sammy to manipulate. There are no exceptions without renegotiation of the contract.

NOTE: Parents meet regularly with the case manager from the treatment team. Effective parenting techniques are discussed, as are other problems identified within the marriage relationship. Parenting instruction coordinates with the pattern of behavior modification Sammy is receiving on the psychiatric unit. The importance of follow-through is emphasized, along with strong encouragement that the parents maintain a united front in disciplining Sammy. Oppositional behaviors are nurtured by divided management.

EVALUATION

Reassessment is conducted to determine if the nursing actions have been successful in achieving the objectives of Sammy's care. Evaluation can be facilitated by gathering information using the following questions:

■ Does Sammy participate in and cooperate during therapeutic activities?
■ Does he follow the rules of the unit (including mealtimes, hygiene, and bedtime) without opposition?
■ Does Sammy accept responsibility for his own mistakes?
■ Is he able to complete a task without becoming defensive?
■ Does he refrain from interrupting when others are talking or making noise in situations where quiet is in order?
■ Does he attempt to manipulate the staff?
■ Is he able to express anger appropriately without tantrum behaviors?
■ Does he demonstrate acceptable behavior in interactions with peers?

Summary and Key Points

■ The basic assumption of behavior therapy is that problematic behaviors occur when there has been inadequate learning and, therefore, can be corrected through the provision of appropriate learning experiences.
■ The antecedents of today's principles of behavior therapy are largely the products of laboratory efforts by Pavlov and Skinner.
■ Pavlov introduced a process that came to be known as classical conditioning.
■ Pavlov demonstrated in his trials with laboratory animals that a neutral stimulus could acquire the ability to elicit a conditioned response through pairing with an unconditioned stimulus. He considered the conditioned response to be a new, learned response.
■ Skinner, in his model of operant conditioning, gave additional attention to the consequences of the response as an approach to learning new behaviors.
■ Skinner believed that the connection between a stimulus and a response is strengthened or weakened by the consequences of the response.

■ Various techniques for modifying client behavior include the following:
  ■ Shaping: a technique in which reinforcements are given for increasingly closer approximations to the desired response.
  ■ Modeling: refers to the learning of new behaviors by imitating the behavior of others.
  ■ Premack principle: this technique states that a frequently occurring response can serve as a positive reinforcement for a response that occurs less frequently.
  ■ Extinction: the gradual decrease in frequency or disappearance of a response when the positive reinforcement is withheld.
  ■ Contingency contracting: a contract is drawn up specifying a specific behavior change and the reinforcers to be given for performing the desired behaviors.
  ■ Token economy: a type of contingency contracting in which the reinforcers for desired behaviors are presented in the form of tokens.
  ■ Time-out: an aversive stimulus or punishment during which the client is removed from the environment where the unacceptable behavior is being exhibited.

■ Reciprocal inhibition: a technique that decreases or eliminates a behavior by introducing a more adaptive behavior, but one that is incompatible with the unacceptable behavior.

■ Overt sensitization: a type of aversion therapy that produces unpleasant consequences for undesirable behavior.

■ Covert sensitization: relies on an individual's imagination to produce unpleasant consequences for undesirable behaviors.

■ Systematic desensitization: a technique for overcoming phobias in which there is a hierarchy of anxiety-producing events through which the individual progresses.

■ Flooding (also called implosion therapy): desensitizes individuals to phobic stimuli by "flooding" them with a continuous presentation (through mental imagery) of the phobic stimulus until it no longer elicits anxiety.

■ Nurses can implement behavior therapy techniques to help clients modify maladaptive behavior patterns.

■ The nursing process is a systematic method of directing care for clients who require this type of assistance.

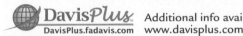

DavisPlus   Additional info available at
DavisPlus.fadavis.com   www.davisplus.com

Review Questions
Self-Examination/Learning Exercise

*Select the answer that is **most** appropriate for each of the following questions.*

1. A positive reinforcer:
   a. Increases the probability that a behavior will recur
   b. Decreases the probability that a behavior will recur
   c. Has nothing to do with modifying behavior
   d. Always results in positive behavior

2. A negative reinforcer:
   a. Increases the probability that a behavior will recur
   b. Decreases the probability that a behavior will recur
   c. Has nothing to do with modifying behavior
   d. Always results in unacceptable behavior

3. An aversive stimulus or punisher:
   a. Increases the probability that a behavior will recur
   b. Decreases the probability that a behavior will recur
   c. Has nothing to do with modifying behavior
   d. Always results in unacceptable behavior

Situation: B.J. has been out with his friends. He is late getting home. He knows his wife will be angry and will yell at him for being late. He stops at the florist's and buys a dozen red roses for her. Questions 4, 5, and 6 are related to this situation.

4. Which of the following behaviors represents positive reinforcement on the part of the wife?
   a. She meets him at the door, accepts the roses, and says nothing further about his being late.
   b. She meets him at the door, yelling that he is late, and makes him spend the night on the couch.
   c. She meets him at the door, expresses delight with the roses, and kisses him on the cheek.
   d. She meets him at the door and says, "How could you? You know I'm allergic to roses!"

5. Which of the following behaviors represents negative reinforcement on the part of the wife?
   a. She meets him at the door, accepts the roses, and says nothing further about his being late.
   b. She meets him at the door, yelling that he is late, and makes him spend the night on the couch.
   c. She meets him at the door, expresses delight with the roses, and kisses him on the cheek.
   d. She meets him at the door and says, "How could you? You know I'm allergic to roses!"

Review Questions—cont'd
Self-Examination/Learning Exercise

6. Which of the following behaviors represents an aversive stimulus on the part of the wife?
   a. She meets him at the door, accepts the roses, and says nothing further about his being late.
   b. She meets him at the door, yelling that he is late, and makes him spend the night on the couch.
   c. She meets him at the door, expresses delight with the roses, and kisses him on the cheek.
   d. She meets him at the door and says, "How could you? You know I'm allergic to roses!"

7. Fourteen-year-old Sally has been spending many hours after school watching TV. She has virtually stopped practicing her piano lessons. Sally's parents ask for advice about how to encourage Sally to practice more. The nurse believes the Premack principle may be helpful. Which of the following does she suggest to Sally's parents?
   a. She tells Sally's parents to reward Sally each time she practices the piano, even if it is only for 5 minutes.
   b. She tells Sally's parents to ignore this behavior and eventually she will start practicing on her own.
   c. She tells Sally's parents to draw up a contract with Sally stating what the consequences will be if she doesn't practice the piano.
   d. She tells Sally's parents to explain to Sally that she may watch TV only after she has practiced the piano for 1 hour.

8. Nancy has a fear of dogs. In helping her overcome this fear, the therapist is using systematic desensitization. List the following steps in the order in which the therapist would proceed.
   Having Nancy:
   a. Look at a real dog.
   b. Look at a stuffed toy dog.
   c. Pet a real dog.
   d. Pet the stuffed toy dog.
   e. Walk past a real dog.
   f. Look at a picture of a dog.

References

Ford-Martin, P.A. (2005). Behavioral therapy. *Gale Encyclopedia of Public Health*. Retrieved from http://www.healthline.com/galecontent/behavioral-therapy

Howard, D. (2000). *The effect of role modeling*. Retrieved from http://www.dianehoward.com/Effect_Role_Modeling.htm

Sadock, B.J., & Sadock, V.A. (2007). *Synopsis of psychiatry: Behavioral sciences/clinical psychiatry* (10th ed.). Philadelphia, PA: Lippincott Williams & Wilkins.

Souders, M.C., DePaul, D., Freeman, K.G., & Levy, S.E. (2002). Caring for children and adolescents with autism who require challenging procedures. *Pediatric Nursing, 28*(6), 555-564.

Classical References

Pavlov, I.P. (1927). *Conditioned reflexes*. London: Oxford University Press.

Premack, D. (1959). Toward empirical behavior laws: I. Positive reinforcement. *Psychological Review, 66*, 219-233.

Skinner, B.F. (1938). *The behavior of organisms*. New York, NY: Appleton-Century-Crofts.

Skinner, B.F. (1953). *Science and human behavior*. New York, NY: Macmillan.

Thorndike, E.L. (1911). *Animal intelligence*. New York, NY: Macmillan.

Wolpe, J. (1958). *Psychotherapy by reciprocal inhibition*. Stanford, CA: Stanford University Press.

19

Cognitive Therapy

CHAPTER OUTLINE

KEY TERMS

OBJECTIVES

After reading this chapter, the student will be able to:

1. Discuss historical perspectives associated with cognitive therapy.
2. Identify various indications for cognitive therapy.
3. Describe goals, principles, and basic concepts of cognitive therapy.
4. Discuss a variety of cognitive therapy techniques.
5. Apply techniques of cognitive therapy within the context of the nursing process.

HOMEWORK ASSIGNMENT

Please read the chapter and answer the following questions:

1. Define *automatic thoughts*.
2. Why are automatic thoughts problematic for some people?
3. What are the three major components of cognitive therapy?
4. John submits his design of a house to some prospective clients. They ask for a few changes to be made. John thinks, "I'm a terrible architect!" What automatic thought does this statement represent?

Wright, Thase, and Beck (2008) stated:

> The writing of Epictetus in the *Enchiridion*, *"Men are disturbed not by things, but by the views which they take of them,"* captures the essence of the perspective that our ideas or thoughts are a controlling factor in our emotional lives. (p. 1212)

This concept provides a foundation on which the cognitive model is established. In cognitive therapy, the therapist's objective is to use a variety of methods to create change in the client's thinking and belief system in an effort to bring about lasting emotional and behavioral change (Beck, 1995).

This chapter examines the historical development of the cognitive model, defines the goals of therapy, and describes various techniques of the cognitive approach. A discussion of the role of the nurse in the implementation of cognitive behavioral techniques with clients is presented.

NOTE: Although in this text the concepts are presented separately for reasons of clarification, cognitive therapy procedures are often combined with behavioral modification techniques and may be referred to as *cognitive-behavioral* therapy.

CORE CONCEPT

Cognitive
Relating to the mental processes of thinking and reasoning.

Historical Background

Cognitive therapy has its roots in the early 1960s research on depression conducted by Aaron Beck (1963, 1964). Beck had been trained in the Freudian psychoanalytic view of depression as "anger turned inward." In his clinical research, he began to observe a common theme of negative cognitive processing in the thoughts and dreams of his depressed clients (Beck & Weishaar, 2011).

A number of theorists have both taken from and expanded upon Beck's original concept. The common theme is the rejection of the passive listening of the psychoanalytic method in favor of active, direct dialogues with clients (Beck & Weishaar, 2011). The work of contemporary behavioral therapists has also influenced the evolution of cognitive therapy. Behavioral techniques such as expectancy of reinforcement and modeling are used within the cognitive domain.

Lazarus and Folkman (1984), upon whose premise of *personal appraisal* and *coping* the conceptual format of this book is founded, have also contributed a great deal to the cognitive approach to therapy. The model for cognitive therapy is based on an individual's cognition, or more specifically, an individual's personal cognitive appraisal of an event and the resulting emotions or behaviors. Personality—which undoubtedly influences our cognitive appraisal of an event—is viewed as having been shaped by the interaction between innate predisposition and environment (Beck, Freeman, & Davis, 2007). Whereas some therapies may be directed toward improvement in coping strategies or adaptiveness of behavioral response, cognitive therapy is aimed at modifying distorted cognitions about a situation.

CORE CONCEPT

Cognitive Therapy
Cognitive therapy is a type of psychotherapy based on the concept of pathological mental processing. The focus of treatment is on the modification of distorted cognitions and maladaptive behaviors.

Indications for Cognitive Therapy

Cognitive therapy was originally developed for use with depression. Today it is used for a broad range of emotional disorders. The proponents of cognitive therapy suggest that the emphasis of therapy must be varied and individualized for clients according to their specific diagnosis, symptoms, and level of functioning. In addition to depression, cognitive therapy may be used with the following clinical conditions: panic disorder, generalized anxiety disorder, social phobias, obsessive-compulsive disorder, post-traumatic stress disorder, eating disorders, substance abuse, personality disorders, schizophrenia, couples' problems, bipolar disorder, illness anxiety disorder, and somatic symptom disorder (Beck, 1995; Sadock & Sadock, 2007; Wright, Thase, & Beck, 2008).

Goals and Principles of Cognitive Therapy

Beck and associates (1987) defined the goals of cognitive therapy in the following way:

The client will:

1. Monitor his or her negative, automatic thoughts.
2. Recognize the connections between cognition, affect, and behavior.
3. Examine the evidence for and against distorted automatic thoughts.
4. Substitute more realistic interpretations for these biased cognitions.
5. Learn to identify and alter the dysfunctional beliefs that predispose him or her to distort experiences.

Cognitive therapy is highly structured and short-term, lasting from 12 to 16 weeks (Beck & Weishaar, 2011). Sadock & Sadock (2007) suggested that if a client does not improve within 25 weeks of therapy, a reevaluation of the diagnosis should be made. Although therapy must be tailored to the individual, the following principles underlie cognitive therapy for all clients (Beck, 1995).

Principle 1. Cognitive therapy is based on an ever-evolving formulation of the client and his or her problems in cognitive terms. The therapist identifies the event that precipitated the distorted cognition. Current thinking patterns that serve to maintain the problematic behaviors are reviewed. The therapist then hypothesizes about certain developmental events and enduring patterns of cognitive appraisal that may have predisposed the client to specific emotional and behavioral responses.

Principle 2. Cognitive therapy requires a sound therapeutic alliance. A trusting relationship between therapist and client must exist for cognitive therapy to succeed. The therapist must convey warmth, empathy, caring, and genuine positive regard. Development of a working relationship between therapist and client is an individual process, and clients with various disorders will require varying degrees of effort to achieve this therapeutic alliance.

Principle 3. Cognitive therapy emphasizes collaboration and active participation. Teamwork between therapist and client is emphasized. They decide together what to work on during each session, how often they should meet, and what homework assignments should be completed between sessions.

Principle 4. Cognitive therapy is goal oriented and problem focused. At the beginning of therapy, the client is encouraged to identify what he or she perceives to be the problem or problems. With guidance from the therapist, goals are established as outcomes of therapy. Assistance in problem solving is provided as required as the client comes to recognize and correct distortions in thinking.

Principle 5. Cognitive therapy initially emphasizes the present. Resolution of distressing situations that are based in the present usually lead to symptom reduction. It is therefore of more benefit to begin with current problems and delay shifting attention to the past until (1) the client expresses a desire to do so, (2) the work on current problems produces little or no change, or (3) the therapist decides it is important to determine how dysfunctional ideas affecting the client's current thinking originated.

Principle 6. Cognitive therapy is educative, aims to teach the client to be his or her own therapist, and emphasizes relapse prevention. From the beginning of therapy, the client is taught about the nature and course of his or her disorder, about the cognitive model (i.e., how thoughts influence emotions and behavior), and about the process of cognitive therapy. The client is taught how to set goals, plan behavioral change, and intervene on his or her own behalf.

Principle 7. Cognitive therapy aims to be time limited. Clients often are seen weekly for a couple of months, followed by a number of biweekly sessions, then possibly a few monthly sessions. Some clients will want periodic "booster" sessions every few months.

Principle 8. Cognitive therapy sessions are structured. Each session has a set structure which includes (1) reviewing the client's week, (2) collaboratively setting the agenda for this session, (3) reviewing the previous week's session, (4) reviewing the previous week's homework, (5) discussing this week's agenda items, (6) establishing homework for next week, and (7) summarizing this week's session. This format focuses attention on what is important and maximizes the use of therapy time.

Principle 9. Cognitive therapy teaches clients to identify, evaluate, and respond to their dysfunctional thoughts and beliefs. Through gentle questioning and review of data, the therapist helps the client identify his or her dysfunctional thinking, evaluate the validity of the thoughts, and devise a plan of action. This is done by helping the client to examine evidence that supports or contradicts the accuracy of the thought, rather than directly challenging or confronting the belief.

Principle 10. Cognitive therapy uses a variety of techniques to change thinking, mood, and behavior. Techniques from various therapies may be used within the cognitive framework. Emphasis in treatment is guided by the client's particular disorder and directed toward modification of the client's dysfunctional cognitions that are contributing to the maladaptive behavior associated with their disorder. Examples of disorders and the dysfunctional thinking for which cognitive therapy may be of benefit are discussed later in this chapter.

Basic Concepts

Wright and associates (2008) stated, "The general thrust of cognitive therapy is that emotional responses are largely dependent upon cognitive appraisals of the significance of environmental cues" (p. 1213). Basic concepts include **automatic thoughts** and **schemas** or core beliefs.

Automatic Thoughts

Automatic thoughts are those that occur rapidly in response to a situation and without rational analysis. These thoughts are often negative and based on erroneous logic. Beck and associates (1987) called these thoughts *cognitive errors.* Following are some examples of common cognitive errors:

Arbitrary Inference In a type of thinking error known as **arbitrary inference**, the individual automatically comes to a conclusion about an incident without the facts to support it, or even sometimes despite contradictory evidence to support it.

EXAMPLE

Two months ago, Mrs. B. sent a wedding gift to the daughter of an old friend. She has not yet received acknowledgment of the gift. Mrs. B. thinks, "They obviously think I have poor taste."

Overgeneralization (Absolutistic Thinking) Sweeping conclusions are **overgeneralizations** made based on one incident—a type of "all or nothing" kind of thinking.

EXAMPLE

Frank submitted an article to a nursing journal and it was rejected. Frank thinks, "No journal will ever be interested in anything I write."

Dichotomous Thinking An individual who is using **dichotomous thinking** views situations in terms of all-or-nothing, black-or-white, or good-or-bad.

EXAMPLE

Frank submits an article to a nursing journal and the editor returns it and asks Frank to rewrite parts of it. Frank thinks, "I'm a bad writer," instead of recognizing that revision is a common part of the publication process.

Selective Abstraction A **selective abstraction** (sometimes referred to as a "mental filter") is a conclusion that is based on only a selected portion of the evidence. The selected portion is usually the negative evidence or what the individual views as a failure, rather than any successes that have occurred.

EXAMPLE

Jackie just graduated from high school with a 3.98/4.00 grade point average. She won a scholarship to the large state university near her home. She was active in sports and activities in high school and well liked by all her peers. However, she is very depressed and dwells on the fact that she did not earn a scholarship to a prestigious Ivy League college to which she had applied.

Magnification Exaggerating the negative significance of an event is known as **magnification**.

EXAMPLE

Nancy hears that her colleague at work is having a cocktail party over the weekend and she is not invited. Nancy thinks, "She doesn't like me."

Minimization Undervaluing the positive significance of an event is called **minimization**.

EXAMPLE

Mrs. M. is feeling lonely. She telephones her granddaughter Amy, who lives in a nearby town, and invites her to visit. Amy apologizes that she must go out of town on business and would not be able to visit at that time. While Amy is out of town, she calls Mrs. M. twice, but Mrs. M. still feels unloved by her granddaughter.

Catastrophic Thinking Always thinking that the worst will occur without considering the possibility of more likely positive outcomes is considered **catastrophic thinking**.

EXAMPLE

On Janet's first day in her secretarial job, her boss asked her to write a letter to another firm and put it on his desk for his signature. She did so and left for lunch. When she returned, the letter was on her desk with a typographical error circled in red and a note from her boss to redo the letter. Janet thinks, "This is it! I will surely be fired now!"

Personalization With **personalization**, the person takes complete responsibility for situations without considering that other circumstances may have contributed to the outcome.

EXAMPLE

Jack, who sells vacuum cleaners door-to-door, has just given a 2-hour demonstration to Mrs. W. At the end of the demonstration, Mrs. W tells Jack that she appreciates his demonstration, but she won't be purchasing a vacuum cleaner from him. Jack thinks, "I'm a lousy salesman" (when in fact, Mrs. W's husband lost his job last week and they have no extra money to buy a new vacuum cleaner at this time).

Schemas (Core Beliefs)

Beck and Weishaar (2011) defined cognitive schemas as:

> Structures that contain the individual's fundamental beliefs and assumptions. Schemas develop early in life from personal experience and identification with significant others. These concepts are reinforced by further learning experiences and, in turn, influence the formation of beliefs, values, and attitudes. (p. 284)

These schemas, or core beliefs, may be adaptive or maladaptive. They may be general or specific, and they may be latent, becoming evident only when triggered by a specific stressful stimulus. Schemas differ from automatic thoughts in that they are deeper cognitive structures that serve to screen information from the environment. For this reason they are often more difficult to modify than automatic thoughts. However, the same techniques are used at the schema level as at the level of automatic thoughts. Schemas can be positive or negative, and generally fall into two broad categories: those associated with *helplessness* and those associated with *unlovability* (Beck, 1995). Some examples of types of schemas are presented in Table 19-1.

Techniques of Cognitive Therapy

The three major components of cognitive therapy are didactic or educational aspects, cognitive techniques, and behavioral interventions (Sadock & Sadock, 2007; Wright, Thase, & Beck, 2008).

TABLE 19–1 Examples of Schemas (or Core Beliefs)

SCHEMA CATEGORY	MALADAPTIVE/NEGATIVE	ADAPTIVE/POSITIVE
Helplessness	No matter what I do, I will fail.	If I try and work very hard, I will succeed.
	I must be perfect. If I make one mistake, I will lose everything.	I am not afraid of a challenge. If I make a mistake, I will try again.
Unloveability	I'm stupid. No one would love me.	I'm a loveable person.
	I'm nobody without a man.	People respect me for myself.

Didactic (Educational) Aspects

One of the basic principles of cognitive therapy is to prepare the client to eventually become his or her own cognitive therapist. The therapist provides information to the client about what cognitive therapy is, how it works, and the structure of the cognitive process. Explanation about expectations of both client and therapist is provided. Reading assignments are given in order to reinforce learning. Some therapists use audiotape or videotape sessions to teach clients about cognitive therapy. A full explanation about the relationship between depression (or anxiety, or whatever maladaptive response the client is experiencing) and distorted thinking patterns is an essential part of cognitive therapy.

Cognitive Techniques

Strategies used in cognitive therapy include recognizing and modifying automatic thoughts (cognitive errors) and recognizing and modifying schemas (core beliefs). Wright, Thase, and Beck (2008) identify the following techniques commonly used in cognitive therapy.

Recognizing Automatic Thoughts and Schemas

Socratic Questioning

In **Socratic questioning** (also called *guided discovery*), the therapist questions the client about his or her situation. With Socratic questioning, the client is asked to describe feelings associated with specific situations. Questions are stated in a way that may stimulate in the client recognition of possible dysfunctional thinking and produce dissonance about the validity of the thoughts.

Imagery and Role Play

When Socratic questioning does not produce the desired results, the therapist may choose to guide the client through imagery exercises or role-play in an effort to elicit automatic thoughts. Through guided imagery, the client is asked to "relive" the stressful situation by imagining the setting in which it occurred. Where did it occur? Who was there? What happened just prior to the stressful situation? What feelings did the client experience in association with the situation?

Role-play is not used as commonly as imagery. It is a technique that should be used only when the relationship between client and therapist is exceptionally strong and there is little likelihood of maladaptive transference occurring. With role-play, the therapist assumes the role of an individual within a situation that produces a maladaptive response in the client. The situation is played out in an effort to elicit recognition of automatic thinking on the part of the client.

Thought Recording

This technique, one of the most frequently used methods of recognizing automatic thoughts, is taught to and discussed with the client in the therapy session. Thought recording is assigned as homework for the client outside of therapy. In thought recording, the client is asked to keep a written record of situations that occur and the automatic thoughts that are elicited by the situation. This is called a "two-column" thought recording. Some therapists ask their clients to keep a "three-column" recording, which includes a description of the emotional response also associated with the situation, as illustrated in Table 19-2.

TABLE 19–2 Three-Column Thought Recording

SITUATION	AUTOMATIC THOUGHTS	EMOTIONAL RESPONSE
Girlfriend broke up with me.	I'm a stupid person. No one would ever want to marry me.	Sadness; depression.
I was turned down for a promotion.	Stupid boss!! He doesn't know how to manage people. It's not fair!	Anger

Modifying Automatic Thoughts and Schemas

Generating Alternatives

To help the client see a broader range of possibilities than had originally been considered, the therapist guides the client in generating alternatives.

Examining the Evidence

With this technique, the client and therapist set forth the automatic thought as the hypothesis, and they study the evidence both for and against the hypothesis.

Decatastrophizing

With the technique of **decatastrophizing**, the therapist assists the client to examine the validity of a negative automatic thought. Even if some validity exists, the client is then encouraged to review ways to cope adaptively, moving beyond the current crisis situation.

Reattribution

It is believed that depressed clients attribute life events in a negatively distorted manner; that is, they have a tendency "to blame themselves for adverse life events and to believe that these negative situations will last indefinitely" (Wright, Thase, & Beck, 2008, p. 1216). Through Socratic questioning and testing of automatic thoughts, this technique is aimed at reversing the negative attribution of depressed clients from internal and enduring to the more external and transient manner of nondepressed individuals.

Daily Record of Dysfunctional Thoughts (DRDT)

The DRDT is a tool commonly used in cognitive therapy to help clients identify and modify automatic thoughts. Two more columns are added to the three-column thought record presented earlier. Clients are then asked to rate the intensity of the thoughts and emotions on a 0- to 100-percent scale. The fourth column of the DRDT asks the client to describe a more rational cognition than the automatic thought identified in the second column and rate the intensity of the belief in the rational thought. In the fifth column, the client records any changes that have occurred as a result of modifying the automatic thought and the new rate of intensity associated with it. With this tool, the client is able to modify automatic thoughts by identifying them and actually formulating a more rational alternative. Table 19-3 presents an example of a DRDT as an extension to the three-column thought recording presented in Table 19-2.

Cognitive Rehearsal

This technique uses mental imagery to uncover potential automatic thoughts in advance of their occurrence in a stressful situation. A discussion is held to identify ways to modify these dysfunctional cognitions. The client is then given "homework" assignments to try these newly learned methods in real situations.

Behavioral Interventions

It is believed that in cognitive therapy, an interactive relationship exists between cognitions and behavior; that is, that cognitions affect behavior and behavior influences cognitions. With this concept in mind, a number of interventions are structured for the client to assist him or her to identify and modify maladaptive cognitions and behaviors.

The following procedures, which are behavior-oriented, are directed toward helping clients learn more adaptive behavioral strategies that will in turn

TABLE 19–3 **Daily Record of Dysfunctional Thoughts (DRDT)**				
SITUATION	AUTOMATIC THOUGHT	EMOTIONAL RESPONSE	RATIONAL RESPONSE	OUTCOME: EMOTIONAL RESPONSE
Girlfriend broke up with me.	I'm a stupid person. No one would ever want to marry me. (95%)	Sadness; depression (90%)	I'm not stupid. Lots of people like me. Just because one person doesn't want to date me doesn't mean that no one would want to. (75%)	Sadness; depression (50%)
I was turned down for a promotion.	Stupid boss!! He doesn't know how to manage people. It's not fair! (90%)	Anger (95%)	I guess I have to admit the other guy's education and experience fit the position better than mine. The boss was being fair because he filled the position based on qualifications. I'll try for the next promotion that fits my qualifications better. (70%)	Anger (20%) Disappointment (80%) Hope (80%)

have a more positive effect on cognitions (Basco, McDonald, Merlock, & Rush, 2004; Sadock & Sadock, 2007; Wright et al., 2008):

1. **Activity Scheduling.** With this intervention, clients are asked to keep a daily log of their activities on an hourly basis and rate each activity, for mastery and pleasure, on a zero-to-ten scale. The schedule is then shared with the therapist and used to identify important areas needing concentration during therapy.

2. **Graded Task Assignments.** This intervention is used with clients who are facing a situation that they perceive as overwhelming. The task is broken down into subtasks that clients can complete one step at a time. Each subtask will have a goal and a time interval attached to it. Successful completion of each subtask helps to increase self-esteem and decrease feelings of helplessness.

3. **Behavioral Rehearsal.** Somewhat akin to, and often used in conjunction with, cognitive rehearsal, this technique uses role-play to "rehearse" a modification of maladaptive behaviors that may be contributing to dysfunctional cognitions.

4. **Distraction.** When dysfunctional cognitions have been recognized, **distraction** can occur by engaging in activities that redirect the client's thinking and divert him or her from the intrusive thoughts or depressive ruminations that are contributing to the maladaptive responses.

5. **Miscellaneous Techniques.** Relaxation exercises, assertiveness training, role modeling, and social skills training are additional types of behavioral interventions that are used in cognitive therapy to assist clients to modify dysfunctional cognitions. Thought-stopping techniques (described in Chapter 14) may also be used to restructure dysfunctional thinking patterns.

Role of the Nurse in Cognitive Therapy

Many of the techniques used in cognitive therapy are well within the scope of nursing practice, from generalist through specialist levels. Cognitive therapy requires an understanding of educational principles and the ability to use problem-solving skills to guide clients' thinking through a reframing process. The scope of contemporary psychiatric nursing practice is expanding, and although psychiatric nurses have been using some of these techniques in various degrees within their practices for years, it is important that knowledge and skills related to this type of therapy be promoted further. The value of cognitive therapy as a useful and cost-effective tool has been observed in a number of inpatient and community outpatient mental health settings.

The following case study presents the role of the nurse in cognitive therapy in the context of the nursing process.

CASE STUDY

ASSESSMENT

Sam is a 45-year-old white male admitted to the psychiatric unit of a general medical center by his family physician, Dr. Jones, who reported that Sam had become increasingly despondent over the last month. His wife reported that he had made statements such as, "Life is not worth living," and "I think I could just take all those pills Dr. Jones prescribed at one time, then it would all be over." He was admitted at 6:40 p.m., via wheelchair from admissions, accompanied by his wife. He reports no known allergies. Vital signs upon admission were temperature, 97.9°F; pulse, 80; respirations, 16; and blood pressure, 132/77. He is 5 feet 11 inches tall and weighs 160 pounds. He was referred to the psychiatrist on call, Dr. Smith. Orders include suicide precautions, level I; regular diet; chemistry profile and routine urinalysis in a.m.; Desyrel, 200 mg tid; Dalmane, 30 mg hs prn for sleep.

FAMILY DYNAMICS

Sam says he loves his wife and children and does not want to hurt them, but feels they no longer need him. He states, "They would probably be better off without me."

His wife appears to be very concerned about his condition, although in his despondency, he seems oblivious to her feelings. His mother lives in a neighboring state, and he sees her infrequently. He admits that he is somewhat bitter toward her for allowing him and his siblings to "suffer from the physical and emotional brutality of their father." His siblings and their families live in distant states, and he sees them rarely, during holiday gatherings. He feels closest to the older of the two brothers.

MEDICAL/PSYCHIATRIC HISTORY

Sam's father died 5 years ago at age 65 of a myocardial infarction. Sam and both his brothers have a history of high cholesterol and triglycerides from approximately age 30. During his regular physical examination 1 month ago, Sam's family doctor recognized symptoms of depression and prescribed fluoxetine. Sam's mother has a history of depressive episodes. She was hospitalized once about 7 years ago for depression, and she has taken various antidepressant medications over the years. Her family physician has also prescribed Valium for her on numerous occasions for her "nerves." No other family members have a history of psychiatric problems.

CASE STUDY—cont'd

PAST EXPERIENCES

Sam was the first child in a family of four. He is 2 years older than his sister and 4 years older than the third child, a brother. He was 6 years old when his youngest sibling, also a boy, was born. Sam's father was a career Army man, who moved his family many times during their childhood years. Sam attended 15 schools from the time he entered kindergarten until he graduated from high school.

Sam reports that his father was very autocratic and had many rules that he expected his children to obey without question. Infraction resulted in harsh discipline. Because Sam was the oldest child, his father believed he should assume responsibility for the behavior of his siblings. Sam describes the severe physical punishment he received from his father when he or his siblings allegedly violated one of the rules. It was particularly intense when Sam's father had been drinking, which he did most evenings and weekends.

Sam's mother was very passive. Sam believes she was afraid of his father, particularly when he was drinking, so she quietly conformed to his lifestyle and offered no resistance, even though she did not agree with his disciplining of the children. Sam reports that he observed his father physically abusing his mother on a number of occasions, most often when he had been drinking.

Sam states that he had very few friends when he was growing up. With all the family moves, he gave up trying to make new friends because it became too painful to give them up when it was time to leave. He took a paper route when he was 13 years old and then worked in fast-food restaurants from age 15 on. He was a hard worker and never seemed to have difficulty finding work in any of the places where the family relocated. He states that he appreciated the independence and the opportunity of being away from home as much as his job would allow. "I guess I can honestly say I hated my father, and working was my way of getting away from all the stress that was going on in that house. I guess my dad hated me, too, because he never was satisfied with anything I did. I never did well enough for him in school, on the job, or even at home. When I think of my dad now, the memories I have are of being criticized and beaten with a belt."

On graduation from high school, Sam joined the Navy, where he learned a skill that he used after discharge to obtain a job in a large aircraft plant. He also attended the local university at night, where he earned his accounting degree. When he completed his degree, he was reassigned to the administration department of the aircraft company, and he has been in the same position for 12 years without a promotion.

PRECIPITATING EVENT

Over the last 12 years, Sam has watched while a number of his peers were promoted to management positions. Sam has been considered for several of these positions but has never been selected. Last month a management position became available for which Sam felt he was qualified. He applied for this position, believing he had a good chance of being promoted. However, when the announcement was made, the position had been given to a younger man who had been with the company only 5 years. Sam seemed to accept the decision, but over the last few weeks he has become more and more withdrawn. He speaks to very few people at the office and is becoming more and more behind in his work. At home, he eats very little, talks to family members only when they ask a direct question, withdraws to his bedroom very early in the evening, and does not come out until it is time to leave for work the next morning. Today, he refused to get out of bed or to go to work. His wife convinced him to talk to their family doctor, who admitted him to the hospital.

CLIENT'S PERCEPTION OF THE STRESSOR

Sam states that all his life he has "not been good enough at anything. I could never please my father. Now I can't seem to please my boss. What's the use of trying? I came to the hospital because my wife and my doctor are afraid I might try to kill myself. I must admit the thought has crossed my mind more than once. I seem to have very little motivation for living. I just don't care anymore."

DIAGNOSES/OUTCOME IDENTIFICATION

The following nursing diagnoses were formulated for Sam:

1. Risk for suicide related to depressed mood and expressions of having nothing to live for.
2. Chronic low self-esteem related to lack of positive feedback and learned helplessness evidenced by a sense of worthlessness, lack of eye contact, social isolation, and negative/pessimistic outlook.

The following may be used as criteria for measurement of outcomes in the planning of care for Sam:

The client will:

1. Not harm self
2. Acquire a feeling of hope for the future
3. Demonstrate increased self-esteem and perception of self as a worthwhile person

PLANNING/IMPLEMENTATION

Table 20-4 presents a nursing care plan for Sam employing some techniques associated with cognitive therapy that are within the scope of nursing practice. Rationales are presented for each intervention.

EVALUATION

Reassessment is conducted to determine if the nursing interventions have been successful in achieving the objectives of Sam's care. Evaluation can be facilitated by gathering information using the following questions:

1. Has self-harm to Sam been avoided?
2. Have Sam's suicidal ideations subsided?
3. Does Sam know where to seek help in a crisis situation?
4. Has Sam discussed the recent loss with staff and family?
5. Is Sam able to verbalize personal hope for the future?
6. Can Sam identify positive attributes about himself?
7. Does Sam demonstrate motivation to move on with his life without a fear of failure?

Table 19-4 | CARE PLAN FOR "SAM" (AN EXAMPLE OF INTERVENTION WITH COGNITIVE THERAPY)

NURSING DIAGNOSIS: RISK FOR SUICIDE

RELATED TO: Depressed mood

OUTCOME CRITERIA	NURSING INTERVENTIONS*	RATIONALE*
Sam will not harm himself.	1. Acknowledge Sam's feelings of despair.	1. Cognitive therapists actively pursue the client's point of view
	2. Convey warmth, accurate empathy, and genuineness.	2. Cognitive therapists use these skills to understand the client's personal view of the world and to establish rapport.
	3. Through Socratic questioning, challenge irrational pessimism. Ask Sam to discuss what problems suicide would solve. Then try to get him to think of reasons for *not* attempting suicide.	3. Cognitive therapists use problem-solving techniques to help the suicidal client think beyond the immediate future.
	4. Begin a serious discussion of alternatives.	4. Cognitive therapists use this strategy to decrease feelings of hopelessness in suicidal clients.

NURSING DIAGNOSIS: CHRONIC LOW SELF-ESTEEM

RELATED TO: Lack of positive feedback and learned helplessness

EVIDENCED BY: A sense of worthlessness, lack of eye contact, social isolation, and negative/pessimistic outlook

OUTCOME CRITERIA	NURSING INTERVENTIONS	RATIONALE
Sam will demonstrate increased self-esteem and perception of himself as a worthwhile person.	1. Ask Sam to keep a 3-column automatic thought recording.	1. Cognitive therapists use this tool to help clients identify automatic thoughts (cognitive errors).
	2. Help Sam to recognize that his worth as a person is not tied to his promotion at work. The world will go on and he can survive this loss.	2. Cognitive therapists use the technique of "decatastrophizing" to help clients get past a crisis situation.
	3. Help Sam to identify ways in which he could feel better about himself. For example, Sam states that he would like to update his computer skills, but he is afraid he is too old. Challenge his negative thinking about his age by using the cognitive therapy technique of "examining the evidence."	3. Cognitive therapists use the technique of "generating alternatives" to help clients recognize that a broader range of possibilities may exist than may be evident at the moment. "Examining the evidence" may help Sam understand that self-improvement is worthwhile at any age.
	4. Ask Sam to expand on his 3-column automatic thought recording and make a Daily Record of Dysfunctional Thoughts (DRDT).	4. Cognitive therapists use this tool to help clients identify their automatic thoughts and modify them by coming up with more rational responses.

Table 19-4 | CARE PLAN FOR "SAM" (AN EXAMPLE OF INTERVENTION WITH COGNITIVE THERAPY)—cont'd

OUTCOME CRITERIA	NURSING INTERVENTIONS	RATIONALE
	5. Discourage Sam's ruminating about his failures. May need to withdraw attention if he persists. Focus on past accomplishments and offer support in undertaking new tasks. Offer recognition of successful endeavors and positive reinforcement of attempts made.	5. Cognitive therapy employs some techniques of behavior therapy. Lack of attention to undesirable behavior may discourage its repetition. Recognition and positive reinforcement enhance self-esteem and encourage repetition of desirable behaviors.

*Interventions and rationale for the diagnosis Risk for Suicide are adapted from Harvard Medical School (2003) and Beck & Weishaar (2011).

Summary and Key Points

■ Cognitive therapy is founded on the premise that how people think significantly influences their feelings and behavior.

■ The concept was initiated in the 1960s by Aaron Beck in his work with depressed clients. Since that time, it has been expanded for use with a number of emotional illnesses.

■ Cognitive therapy is short-term, highly structured, and goal-oriented therapy that consists of three major components: didactic, or educational, aspects; cognitive techniques; and behavioral interventions.

■ The therapist teaches the client about the relationship between his or her illness and the distorted thinking patterns. Explanation about cognitive therapy and how it works is provided.

■ The therapist helps the client to recognize his or her negative automatic thoughts (sometimes called *cognitive errors*).

■ Once these automatic thoughts have been identified, various cognitive and behavioral techniques are used to assist the client to modify the dysfunctional thinking patterns.

■ Independent homework assignments are an important part of the cognitive therapist's strategy.

■ Many of the cognitive therapy techniques are within the scope of nursing practice.

■ As the role of the psychiatric nurse continues to expand, the knowledge and skills associated with a variety of therapies will need to be broadened. Cognitive therapy is likely to be one in which nurses will become more involved.

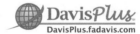 Additional info available at
DavisPlus.fadavis.com   www.davisplus.com

Review Questions
Self-Examination/Learning Exercise

*Select the answer that is **most** appropriate for each of the following questions.*

1. Janet failed her first test in nursing school. She thinks, "Well, that's it! I'll never be a nurse." What automatic thought does this statement represent?
   a. Overgeneralization
   b. Magnification
   c. Catastrophic thinking
   d. Personalization

Continued

Review Questions—cont'd
Self-Examination/Learning Exercise

2. When Jack is not accepted at the law school of his choice, he thinks, "I'm so stupid. No law school will ever accept me." What automatic thought does this statement represent?
   a. Overgeneralization
   b. Magnification
   c. Selective abstraction
   d. Minimization

3. Nancy's new in-laws came to dinner for the first time. When Nancy's mother-in-law left some food on her plate, Nancy thought, "I must be a lousy cook." What automatic thought does this statement represent?
   a. Dichotomous thinking
   b. Overgeneralization
   c. Minimization
   d. Personalization

4. Barbara burned the toast. She thinks, "I'm a totally incompetent person." What automatic thought does this statement represent?
   a. Selective abstraction
   b. Magnification
   c. Minimization
   d. Personalization

5. Opal is a 43-year-old woman who is suffering from depression and suicidal ideation. Opal says, "I'm such a worthless person. I don't deserve to live." The therapist responds, "I would like for you to think about what problems committing suicide would solve." The therapist is using which of the following cognitive therapy techniques?
   a. Imagery
   b. Role play
   c. Problem solving
   d. Thought recording

6. The thought recording (2-column and 3-column) cognitive therapy techniques help clients:
   a. Identify automatic thoughts.
   b. Modify automatic thoughts.
   c. Identify rational alternatives.
   d. All of the above.

7. The daily record of dysfunctional thoughts (DRDT) is used in cognitive therapy to help clients:
   a. Identify automatic thoughts.
   b. Modify automatic thoughts.
   c. Identify rational alternatives.
   d. All of the above.

8. A client tells the therapist, "I thought I would just die when my husband told me he was leaving me. If I had been a better wife, he wouldn't have fallen in love with another woman. It's all my fault." The therapist asks the client to think back to the day her husband told her he was leaving and to describe the situation and her feelings. What cognitive therapy technique is the therapist using?
   a. Imagery
   b. Role play
   c. Problem solving
   d. Thought recording

Review Questions—cont'd
Self-Examination/Learning Exercise

9. A client tells the therapist, "I thought I would just die when my husband told me he was leaving me. If I had been a better wife, he wouldn't have fallen in love with another woman. It's all my fault." The therapist wants to use the technique of "examining the evidence." Which of the following statements reflects this technique?
   a. "How do you think you could have been a better wife?"
   b. "Okay, you say it's all your fault. Let's discuss why it might be your fault and then we will look at why it may not be."
   c. "Let's talk about what would make you a happier person."
   d. "Would you have wanted him to stay if he didn't really want to?"

10. The therapist teaches a client that when the idea of herself as a worthless person starts to form in her mind, she should immediately start to whistle the tune of "Dixie." This is an example of the cognitive therapy technique of:
    a. Behavioral rehearsal
    b. Social skills training
    c. Distraction
    d. Generating alternatives

References

Basco, M.R., McDonald, N., Merlock, M., & Rush, A.J. (2004). A cognitive-behavioral approach to treatment of bipolar I disorder. In J.H. Wright (Ed.), *Cognitive-behavioral therapy* (pp. 25-53). Washington, DC: American Psychiatric Publishing.

Beck, A.T., Freeman, A., & Davis, D.D. (2007). *Cognitive therapy of personality disorders* (2nd ed.). New York, NY: Guilford Publications.

Beck, A.T., Rush, A.H., & Shaw, B.F., & Emery, G. (1987). *Cognitive therapy of depression*. New York, NY: Guilford Press.

Beck, A. T., & Weishaar, M.E. (2011). Cognitive therapy. In R.J. Corsini and D. Wedding (Eds.), *Current psychotherapies* (9th ed., pp. 276-309). Belmont, CA: Brooks/Cole.

Beck, J.S. (1995). *Cognitive therapy: Basics and beyond*. New York, NY: The Guilford Press.

Harvard Medical School (2003). Confronting suicide—part II. *Harvard Mental Health Letter, 19*(12), 1-5.

Sadock, B.J., & Sadock, V.A. (2007). *Synopsis of psychiatry: Behavioral sciences/clinical psychiatry* (10th ed.). Philadelphia, PA: Lippincott Williams & Wilkins.

Wright, J.H., Thase, M.E., & Beck, A.T. (2008). Cognitive therapy. In R.E. Hales, S.C. Yudofsky, & G.O. Gabbard (Eds.), *Textbook of psychiatry* (5th ed., pp. 1211-1256). Washington, DC: American Psychiatric Publishing.

Classical References

Beck, A.T. (1963). Thinking and depression, I. Idiosyncratic content and cognitive distortions. *Archives of General Psychiatry, 9*, 324-333.

Beck, A.T. (1964). Thinking and depression, II. Theory and therapy. *Archives of General Psychiatry, 10*, 561-571.

Lazarus, R.S., & Folkman, S. (1984). *Stress, appraisal, and coping*. New York, NY: Springer.

20

Electroconvulsive Therapy

CORE CONCEPT

electroconvulsive therapy

KEY TERMS

insulin coma therapy

pharmacoconvulsive therapy

OBJECTIVES

After reading this chapter, the student will be able to:

1. Define *electroconvulsive therapy*.
2. Discuss historical perspectives related to electroconvulsive therapy.
3. Discuss indications, contraindications, mechanism of action, and side effects of electroconvulsive therapy.
4. Identify risks associated with electroconvulsive therapy.
5. Describe the role of the nurse in the administration of electroconvulsive therapy.

HOMEWORK ASSIGNMENT

Please read the chapter and answer the following questions:

1. Mr. J. says to the nurse, "This consent form says there is a possibility of permanent memory loss with ECT. I don't want to lose my memory!" How should the nurse respond to Mr. J.?
2. What medication is commonly given before the ECT treatment to decrease secretions?
3. Why is the client given oxygen during the procedure?

Electroconvulsive therapy (ECT) has had very bad press. In the movie *One Flew Over the Cuckoo's Nest*, it is depicted as a physically and emotionally brutal procedure imposed on unwilling clients in order to calm them. Today, ECT remains one of the most controversial treatments for psychological disorders and continues to be the subject of impassioned debate among various factions of society, within both the professional and lay communities.

Despite its controversial image, ECT has been used continuously for more than 50 years, longer than any other physical treatment available for mental illness. It has achieved this longevity because when administered properly, for the right illness, it can help as much as or more than any other treatment (Kellner, 2010).

This chapter explores the historical perspectives, indications and contraindications, mechanism of action, side effects, and risks associated with ECT. The role of the nurse in the care of the client receiving ECT is presented in the context of the nursing process.

Electroconvulsive Therapy, Defined

CORE CONCEPT
Electroconvulsive Therapy
The induction of a grand mal (generalized) seizure through the application of electrical current to the brain.

The stimulus is applied through electrodes that are placed either bilaterally in the frontotemporal region or unilaterally on the same side as the dominant hand (Marangell, Silver, Goff, & Yudofsky, 2003). Controversy exists over optimal placement of the electrodes in terms of possible greater efficacy with bilateral placement versus the potential in some clients for less confusion and acute amnesia with unilateral placement.

The amount of electrical stimulus applied is another point of controversy among clinicians. Dose of stimulation is based on the client's seizure threshold, which is highly variable among individuals. The duration of the seizure should be at least 15 to 25 seconds (Karasu, Gelenberg, Merriam, & Wang, 2006). Movements are very minimal because of the administration of a muscle relaxant before the treatment. The tonic phase of the seizure usually lasts 10 to 15 seconds and may be identified by a rigid plantar extension of the feet. The clonic phase follows and is usually characterized by rhythmic movements of the muscles that decrease in frequency and finally disappear. Because of the muscle relaxant, movements may be observed merely as a rhythmic twitching of the toes.

Most clients require an average of 6 to 12 treatments, but some may require up to 20 treatments (Sadock & Sadock, 2007). Treatments are usually administered every other day, three times per week. Treatments are performed on an inpatient basis for those who require close observation and care (e.g., clients who are suicidal, agitated, delusional, catatonic, or acutely manic). Those at less risk may have the option of receiving therapy at an outpatient treatment facility.

Historical Perspectives

The first electroconvulsive therapy treatment was performed in April 1938 by Italian psychiatrists Ugo Cerletti and Lucio Bini in Rome. Other somatic therapies had been tried before that time, in particular **insulin coma therapy** and **pharmacoconvulsive therapy**.

Insulin coma therapy was introduced by the German psychiatrist Manfred Sakel in 1933. His therapy was used for clients with schizophrenia. The insulin injection treatments would induce a hypoglycemic coma, which Sakel claimed was effective in alleviating schizophrenic symptoms. This therapy required vigorous medical and nursing intervention through the stages of induced coma. Some fatalities occurred when clients failed to respond to efforts directed at termination of the coma. The efficacy of insulin coma therapy has been questioned, and its use has been discontinued in the treatment of mental illness.

Pharmacoconvulsive therapy was introduced in Budapest in 1934 by Ladislas Meduna (Fink, 2009). He induced convulsions with intramuscular injections of camphor in oil in clients with schizophrenia. He based his treatment on clinical observation and on his theory that there was a biological antagonism between schizophrenia and epilepsy. Thus, by inducing seizures he hoped to reduce schizophrenic symptoms. Because he discovered that camphor was unreliable for inducing seizures, he began using pentylenetetrazol (Metrazol). Some successes were reported in terms of reduction of psychotic symptoms, and, until the advent of ECT in 1938, pentylenetetrazol was the most frequently used procedure for producing seizures in psychotic clients. There was a brief resurgence of pharmacoconvulsive therapy in the late 1950s, when flurothyl (Indoklon), a potent inhalant convulsant, was introduced as an alternative for individuals who were unwilling to consent to ECT for the treatment of depression and schizophrenia. Pharmacoconvulsive therapy is no longer used in psychiatry.

Periodic recognition of the important contribution of ECT in the treatment of mental illness has been evident in the United States. An initial acceptance was observed from 1940 to 1960, followed by a 20-year period in which ECT was considered objectionable by both the psychiatric profession and the lay public. A second wave of acceptance began around 1980 and has been increasing to the present. The period of nonacceptability coincided with the introduction of tricyclic and monoamine oxidase inhibitor antidepressant drugs and ended with the realization among many psychiatrists that the widely heralded replacement of ECT with these chemical agents had failed to materialize (Abrams, 2002). Some individuals showed improvement with ECT after failing to respond to other forms of therapy.

Currently, an estimated 100,000 people in the United States and about 2 million people worldwide receive ECT treatments each year (Mathew, Amiel, & Sackeim, 2013). The typical client is white, female, middle-aged, and from a middle- to upper-income background, receiving treatment in a private or university hospital for major depression, usually after drug therapy has proved ineffective. Largely because of the expense involved, as well as the need for a team of highly skilled medical specialists, many public hospitals are not able to offer this service to their clients.

Indications

Major Depression

ECT has been shown to be effective in the treatment of severe depression. It appears to be particularly effective in depressed clients who are also experiencing psychotic symptoms and those with psychomotor retardation and neurovegetative changes, such as disturbances in sleep, appetite, and energy. These symptoms are associated with the diagnoses of major depressive disorder, major depressive disorder with psychotic or melancholic symptoms, and bipolar disorder depression (Fink, 2009). ECT is not often used as the treatment of choice for depressive disorders but is considered only after a trial of therapy with antidepressant medication has proved ineffective.

Mania

ECT is also indicated in the treatment of acute manic episodes of bipolar disorder (Black & Andreasen, 2011). At present it is rarely used for this purpose, having been superceded by the widespread use of antipsychotic drugs and/or lithium. However, ECT has been shown to be effective in the treatment of manic clients who do not tolerate or fail to respond to lithium or other drug treatment, or when life is threatened by dangerous behavior or exhaustion.

Schizophrenia

ECT can induce a remission in some clients who present with acute schizophrenia, particularly if it is accompanied by catatonic or affective (depression or mania) symptomatology (Black & Andreasen, 2011). It does not appear to be of value to individuals with chronic schizophrenic illness.

Other Conditions

ECT has also been tried with clients experiencing a variety of neuroses, obsessive-compulsive disorders, and personality disorders. Little evidence exists to support the efficacy of ECT in the treatment of these conditions.

Contraindications

The only absolute contraindication for ECT is increased intracranial pressure (from brain tumor, recent cardiovascular accident, or other cerebrovascular lesion). ECT is associated with a physiological rise in cerebrospinal fluid pressure during the treatment, resulting in increased intracranial pressure that could lead to brainstem herniation (Marangell et al., 2003).

Various other conditions, not considered absolute contraindications but rendering clients at high risk for the treatment, have been identified (Black & Andreasen, 2011; Eisendrath & Lichtmacher, 2013; Marangell et al., 2003). These conditions are largely cardiovascular in nature and include myocardial infarction or cerebrovascular accident within the preceding 3 to 6 months, aortic or cerebral aneurysm, severe underlying hypertension, and congestive heart failure. Clients with cardiovascular problems are placed at risk because of the response of the body to the seizure itself. The initial vagal response results in a sinus bradycardia and drop in blood pressure. This is followed immediately by tachycardia and a hypertensive response. These changes can be life threatening to an individual with an already compromised cardiovascular system. Other factors that place clients at risk for ECT include severe osteoporosis, acute and chronic pulmonary disorders, and high-risk or complicated pregnancy.

Mechanism of Action

The exact mechanism by which ECT effects a therapeutic response is unknown. Several theories exist, but the one to which the most credibility has been given is the biochemical theory. A number of researchers have demonstrated that electric stimulation results in significant increases in the circulating levels of several neurotransmitters (Wahlund & von Rosen, 2003). These neurotransmitters include serotonin, norepinephrine, and dopamine, the same biogenic amines that are affected by antidepressant drugs. Additional evidence suggests that ECT may also result in increases in glutamate and gamma-aminobutyric acid (Grover, Mattoo, & Gupta, 2005).

One recent study revealed that the therapeutic response from ECT may be related to the modulation of white matter microstructure in pathways connecting frontal and limbic areas, which are altered in major depression (Lyden, et al., 2014). The results of studies relating to the mechanism underlying the effectiveness of ECT are still ongoing and continue to be controversial.

Side Effects

The most common side effects of ECT are temporary memory loss and confusion. Critics of the therapy argue that these changes represent irreversible brain damage. Proponents insist they are temporary and reversible. Black and Andreasen (2011) state:

> Because ECT disrupts new memories that have not been incorporated into long-term memory stores,

ECT can cause anterograde and retrograde amnesia that is most dense around the time of treatment. The anterograde component usually clears quickly, but the retrograde amnesia can extend back to months before treatment. It is unclear if the memory loss is due to the ECT or to ongoing depressive symptoms. (p. 550)

The controversy continues regarding the choice of unilateral versus bilateral ECT. Studies have shown that unilateral placement of the electrodes decreases the amount of memory disturbance. However, unilateral ECT often requires a higher stimulus dose or a greater number of treatments to match the efficacy of bilateral ECT in the relief of depression (Geddes, 2003).

Risks Associated With Electroconvulsive Therapy

Mortality

Studies indicate that the mortality rate from ECT is about 2 per 100,000 treatments (Marangell et al., 2003; Sadock & Sadock, 2007). Although the occurrence is rare, the major cause of death with ECT is from cardiovascular complications (e.g., acute myocardial infarction or cerebrovascular accident), usually in individuals with previously compromised cardiac status. Assessment and management of cardiovascular disease *prior to* treatment is vital in the reduction of morbidity and mortality rates associated with ECT.

Permanent Memory Loss

Most individuals report no problems with their memory, aside from the time immediately surrounding the ECT treatments. However, some clients have reported retrograde amnesia extending back to months before treatment. In rare instances, more extensive amnesia has occurred, resulting in memory gaps dating back years (Joska & Stein, 2008). These clients report gaps in recollections of specific personal memories.

Sackeim and associates (2007) reported on the results of a longitudinal study of clinical and cognitive outcomes in patients with major depression treated with ECT at seven facilities in the New York City metropolitan area. Subjects were evaluated shortly following the ECT course and 6 months later. Data revealed that cognitive deficits at the 6-month interval were directly related to type of electrode placement and electrical waveform used. Bilateral electrode placement resulted in more severe and persisting (as evaluated at the 6-month follow-up) retrograde amnesia than unilateral placement. The extent of the amnesia was directly related to the number of ECT treatments received. The researchers also found that stimulation produced by sine wave (continuous) current resulted in greater short- and long-term deficits than that produced by short-pulse wave (intermittent) current.

Black and Andreasen (2011) suggested that all clients receiving ECT should be informed of the possibility for some degree of permanent memory loss. Although the potential for these effects appears to be minimal, the client must be made aware of the risks involved before consenting to treatment.

Brain Damage

Brain damage from ECT remains a concern for those who continue to believe in its usefulness and efficacy as a treatment for depression. Critics of the procedure remain adamant in their belief that ECT always results in some degree of immediate brain damage (Frank, 2002). However, evidence is based largely on animal studies in which the subjects received excessive electrical dosages, and the seizures were unmodified by muscle paralysis and oxygenation (Abrams, 2002). Although this is an area for continuing study, there is no evidence to substantiate that ECT produces any permanent changes in brain structure or functioning (McClintock & Husain, 2011).

The Role of the Nurse in Electroconvulsive Therapy

Nurses play an integral role in the teaching and preparation for and administration of ECT. They provide support before, during, and after the treatment to the client and family, and assist the medical professionals who are conducting the therapy. The nursing process provides a systematic approach to the provision of care for the client receiving ECT.

Assessment

A complete physical examination must be completed by the appropriate medical professional prior to the initiation of ECT. This evaluation should include a thorough assessment of cardiovascular and pulmonary status as well as laboratory blood and urine studies. A skeletal history and x-ray assessment should also be considered.

The nurse may be responsible for ensuring that informed consent has been obtained from the client. If the depression is severe and the client is clearly unable to consent to the procedure, permission may be obtained from family or other legally responsible individual. Consent is secured only after the client or responsible individual acknowledges understanding of the procedure, including possible side effects and potential risks involved. Client and family must also understand that ECT is voluntary, and that consent may be withdrawn at any time (American Psychiatric Association, 2001; Fetterman & Ying, 2011).

Nurses may also be required to assess:

- The client's mood and level of interaction with others
- Evidence of suicidal ideation, plan, and means
- Level of anxiety and fears associated with receiving ECT
- Thought and communication patterns
- Baseline memory for short- and long-term events
- Client and family knowledge of indications for, side effects of, and potential risks associated with ECT
- Current and past use of medications
- Baseline vital signs and history of allergies
- The client's ability to carry out activities of daily living

Diagnosis/Outcome Identification

Selection of appropriate nursing diagnoses for the client undergoing ECT is based on continual assessment before, during, and after treatment. Selected potential nursing diagnoses with outcome criteria for evaluation are presented in Table 20-1.

Planning/Implementation

ECT treatments are usually performed in the morning. The client is given nothing by mouth (NPO) for 6 to 8 hours before the treatment. Some institutional policies require that the client be placed on NPO status at midnight prior to the treatment day. The treatment team routinely consists of the psychiatrist, anesthesiologist, and two or more nurses.

Nursing interventions before the treatment include:

- Ensure that the physician has obtained informed consent and that a signed permission form is on the chart.
- Ensure that the most recent laboratory reports (complete blood count, urinalysis) and results of electrocardiogram (ECG) and x-ray examination are available.
- Approximately 1 hour before treatment is scheduled, take vital signs and record them. Have the client void and remove dentures, eyeglasses or contact lenses, jewelry, and hairpins. Following institutional requirements, the client should change into hospital gown or, if permitted, into own loose clothing or pajamas. At this point it is best for the client to remain in bed. Side rails may be raised unless prohibited by institutional policy or assessed as unsafe for the individual client.
- Approximately 30 minutes before treatment, administer the pretreatment medication as prescribed by the physician. The usual order is for atropine sulfate or glycopyrrolate (Robinul) given intramuscularly. Either of these medications may be ordered to decrease secretions (to prevent aspiration) and counteract the effects of vagal stimulation (bradycardia) induced by the ECT.
- Stay with the client to help allay fears and anxiety. Maintain a positive attitude about the procedure, and encourage the client to verbalize feelings.

In the treatment room the client is placed on the treatment table in a supine position, and the

TABLE 20–1 **Potential Nursing Diagnoses and Outcome Criteria for Client Receiving ECT**	
NURSING DIAGNOSES	OUTCOME CRITERIA
Anxiety (moderate to severe) related to impending therapy	Client verbalizes a decrease in anxiety following explanation of procedure and expression of fears.
Deficient knowledge related to necessity for and side effects or risks of ECT	Client verbalizes understanding of need for and side effects/risks of ECT following explanation.
Risk for injury related to risks associated with ECT	Client undergoes treatment without sustaining injury.
Risk for aspiration related to altered level of consciousness immediately following treatment	Client experiences no aspiration during ECT.
Decreased cardiac output related to vagal stimulation occurring during the ECT	Client demonstrates adequate tissue perfusion during and after treatment (absence of cyanosis or severe change in mental status).
Impaired memory/acute confusion related to side effects of ECT	Client maintains reality orientation following ECT treatment.
Self-care deficit related to incapacitation during postictal stage	Client's self-care needs are fulfilled at all times.
Risk for activity intolerance related to post-ECT confusion and memory loss	Client gradually increases participation in therapeutic activities to the highest level of personal capability.

anesthesiologist administers intravenously a short-acting anesthetic. The two most commonly used anesthetic agents for ECT in the United States are methohexital and propofol (Kellner & Bryson, 2012). A muscle relaxant, usually succinylcholine chloride, is given intravenously to prevent severe muscle contractions during the seizure, thereby reducing the possibility of fractured or dislocated bones. Because succinylcholine paralyzes respiratory muscles as well, the client is oxygenated with pure oxygen during and after the treatment, except for the brief interval of electrical stimulation, until spontaneous respirations return (Kellner & Bryson, 2012). A blood pressure cuff may be placed on the lower leg and inflated above systolic pressure prior to the injection of the succinylcholine. This is to ensure that the seizure activity can be observed in this one limb that is unaffected by the muscle relaxant.

An airway/bite block is placed in the client's mouth and he or she is positioned to facilitate airway patency. Electrodes are placed (either bilaterally or unilaterally) on the temples to deliver the electrical stimulation.

Nursing interventions during the treatment include:

■ Ensure patency of airway. Provide suctioning if needed.
■ Assist anesthesiologist with oxygenation as required.
■ Observe readouts on machines monitoring vital signs and cardiac functioning.
■ Provide support to the client's arms and legs during the seizure.
■ Observe and record the type and amount of movement induced by the seizure.

After the treatment the anesthesiologist continues to oxygenate the client with pure oxygen until spontaneous respirations return. Most clients awaken within 10 or 15 minutes of the treatment and are confused and disoriented; however, some clients will sleep for 1 to 2 hours following the treatment. All clients require close observation in this immediate post-treatment period.

Nursing interventions in the post-treatment period include:

■ Monitor pulse, respirations, and blood pressure every 15 minutes for the first hour, during which time the client should remain in bed.
■ Position the client on side to prevent aspiration.
■ Orient the client to time and place.
■ Describe what has occurred.
■ Provide reassurance that confusion and memory loss will subside, and memories should return following the course of ECT therapy.
■ Allow the client to verbalize fears and anxieties related to receiving ECT.
■ Stay with the client until he or she is fully awake, oriented, and able to perform self-care activities without assistance.

■ Provide the client with a highly structured schedule of routine activities in order to minimize confusion.

Evaluation

Evaluation of the effectiveness of nursing interventions is based on the achievement of the projected outcomes. Reassessment may be based on answers to the following questions:

■ Was the client's anxiety maintained at a manageable level?
■ Was the client/family teaching completed satisfactorily?
■ Did the client/family verbalize understanding of the procedure, its side effects, and risks involved?
■ Did the client undergo treatment without experiencing injury or aspiration?
■ Has the client maintained adequate tissue perfusion during and following treatment? Have vital signs remained stable?
■ With consideration to the individual client's condition and response to treatment, is the client reoriented to time, place, and situation?
■ Have all of the client's self-care needs been fulfilled?
■ Is the client participating in therapeutic activities to his or her maximum potential?
■ What is the client's level of social interaction?

Careful documentation is an important part of the evaluation process. Some routine observations may be evaluated on flow sheets specifically identified for ECT. However, progress notes with detailed descriptions of client behavioral changes are essential to evaluate improvement and help determine the number of treatments that will be administered. Continual reassessment, planning, and evaluation will ensure that the client receives adequate and appropriate nursing care throughout the course of therapy.

Summary and Key Points

■ Electroconvulsive therapy (ECT) is the induction of a grand mal seizure through the application of electrical current to the brain.
■ ECT is a safe and effective treatment alternative for individuals with depression, mania, or schizoaffective disorder who do not respond to other forms of therapy.
■ ECT is contraindicated for individuals with increased intracranial pressure.
■ Individuals with cardiovascular problems are at high risk for complications from ECT.
■ Other factors that place clients at risk include severe osteoporosis, acute and chronic pulmonary disorders, and high-risk or complicated pregnancy.

- The exact mechanism of action of ECT is unknown, but it is thought that the electrical stimulation results in significant increases in the circulating levels of the neurotransmitters serotonin, norepinephrine, and dopamine. Modulation of white matter microstructure in pathways connecting frontal and limbic areas of the brain may also be involved.
- The most common side effects with ECT are temporary memory loss and confusion.
- Although it is rare, death must be considered a risk associated with ECT. When it does occur, the most common cause is cardiovascular complications.
- There may be a risk for some degree of permanent long-term memory loss, and some opponents suggest that a risk for brain damage also exists (although there is little or no substantiating evidence).
- The nurse assists with ECT using the steps of the nursing process before, during, and after treatment.
- Important nursing interventions include ensuring client safety, managing client anxiety, and providing adequate client education.
- Nursing input into the ongoing evaluation of client behavior is an important factor in determining the therapeutic effectiveness of ECT.

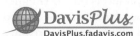 **DavisPlus**
DavisPlus.fadavis.com

Additional info available at
www.davisplus.com

Review Questions
Self-Examination/Learning Exercise

*Select the answer that is **most** appropriate for each of the following questions.*

1. Electroconvulsive therapy is most commonly prescribed for:
   a. Bipolar disorder, manic
   b. Paranoid schizophrenia
   c. Major depression
   d. Obsessive-compulsive disorder

2. Which of the following best describes the average number of ECT treatments given and the timing of administration?
   a. One treatment per month for 6 months
   b. One treatment every other day for a total of 6 to 12 treatments
   c. One treatment three times per week for a total of 20 to 30 treatments
   d. One treatment every day for a total of 10 to 15 treatments

3. Which of the following conditions is considered to be the only absolute contraindication for ECT?
   a. Increased intracranial pressure
   b. Recent myocardial infarction
   c. Severe underlying hypertension
   d. Congestive heart failure

4. Electroconvulsive therapy is thought to effect a therapeutic response by:
   a. Stimulation of the CNS
   b. Decreasing the levels of acetylcholine and monoamine oxidase
   c. Increasing the levels of serotonin, norepinephrine, and dopamine
   d. Altering sodium metabolism within nerve and muscle cells

5. The most common side effects of ECT are:
   a. Permanent memory loss and brain damage
   b. Fractured and dislocated bones
   c. Myocardial infarction and cardiac arrest
   d. Temporary memory loss and confusion

Review Questions—cont'd
Self-Examination/Learning Exercise

6. Sam has a diagnosis of major depression. After an unsuccessful trial of antidepressant medication, Sam's physician has hospitalized Sam for a course of ECT treatments. Sam says to the nurse on admission, "I don't want to end up like McMurphy in *One Flew Over the Cuckoo's Nest!* I'm scared!" Sam's priority nursing diagnosis at this time would be:
   a. Anxiety related to deficient knowledge about ECT
   b. Risk for injury related to risks associated with ECT
   c. Deficient knowledge related to negative media presentation of ECT
   d. Acute confusion related to side effects of ECT

7. Sam, who has been hospitalized for ECT treatments, says to the nurse on admission, "I don't want to end up like McMurphy in *One Flew Over the Cuckoo's Nest!* I'm scared!" Which of the following statements would be most appropriate by the nurse in response to Sam's expression of concern?
   a. "I guarantee you won't end up like McMurphy, Sam."
   b. "The doctor knows what he is doing. There's nothing to worry about."
   c. "I know you are scared, Sam, and we're going to talk about what you can expect from the therapy."
   d. "I'm going to stay with you as long as you are scared."

8. The priority nursing intervention before starting ECT therapy is to:
   a. Take vital signs and record.
   b. Have the patient void.
   c. Administer succinylcholine.
   d. Ensure that the consent form has been signed.

9. Atropine sulfate is administered to a client receiving ECT for what purpose?
   a. To alleviate anxiety
   b. To decrease secretions
   c. To relax muscles
   d. As a short-acting anesthetic

10. Succinylcholine is administered to a client receiving ECT for what purpose?
   a. To alleviate anxiety
   b. To decrease secretions
   c. To relax muscles
   d. As a short-acting anesthetic

References

Abrams, R. (2002). *Electroconvulsive therapy* (4th ed). New York, NY: Oxford University Press.

American Psychiatric Association (APA). (2001). *The practice of electroconvulsive therapy: Recommendations for treatment, training, and privileging* (2nd ed.). Washington, DC: American Psychiatric Publishing.

Black, D.W., & Andreasen, N.C. (2011). *Introductory textbook of psychiatry* (5th ed.). Washington, DC: American Psychiatric Publishing.

Eisendrath, S.J., & Lichtmacher, J.E. (2013). Psychiatric disorders. In M.A. Papadakis & S.J. McPhee (Eds.), *Current medical diagnosis & treatment* (52nd ed., pp. 1038-1092). New York, NY: McGraw-Hill.

Fetterman, T.C., & Ying, P. (2011). Informed consent and electroconvulsive therapy. *Journal of the American Psychiatric Nurses Association, 17*(3), 219-222.

Fink, M. (2009). *Electroconvulsive therapy.* New York, NY: Oxford University Press.

Frank, L.R. (2002). Electroshock: A crime against the spirit. *Ethical Human Sciences & Services, 4*(1), 63-71.

Geddes, J.R. (2003). Efficacy and safety of electroconvulsive therapy in depressive disorders: A systematic review and meta-analysis. *The Lancet, 361*(9360), 799-808.

Grover, S., Mattoo, S.K., & Gupta, N. (2005). Theories on mechanism of action of electroconvulsive therapy. *German Journal of Psychiatry, 8*(4), 70-84.

Joska, J.A., & Stein, D.J. (2008). Mood disorders. In R.E. Hales, S.C. Yudofsky, & G.O. Gabbard (Eds.), *Textbook of psychiatry* (5th ed., 457-503). Washington, DC: American Psychiatric Publishing.

Karasu, T.B., Gelenberg, A., Merriam, A., & Wang, P. (2006). Practice guideline for the treatment of patients with major depressive disorder. *Practice guidelines for the treatment of psychiatric disorders, Compendium 2006.* Washington, DC: American Psychiatric Publishing.

Kellner, C.H. (2010, May 11). Speed of response to ECT. *Psychiatric Times, 27*(5). Retrieved from http://www.psychiatrictimes.com/display/article/10168/1567001

Kellner, C.H., & Bryson, E.O. (2012). Anesthesia advances add to safety of ECT. *Psychiatric Times, 29*(1). Available from http://www.psychiatrictimes.com/display/article/10168/2013636

Lyden, H., Espinoza, R.T., Pirnia, T., Clark, K., Joshi, S.H., Leaver, A.M., Woods, R.P., and Narr, K.L. (2014). Electroconvulsive therapy mediates neuroplasticity of white matter microstructure in major depression. *Translational Psychiatry* 4, e380; doi: 10.1038/tp.2014.21; published online 8 April 2014.

Marangell, L.B., Silver, J.M., Goff, D.C., & Yudofsky, S.C. (2003). Psychopharmacology and electroconvulsive therapy. In R.E. Hales & S.C. Yudofsky (Eds.), *Textbook of clinical psychiatry* (pp. 1047-1149). Washington, DC: American Psychiatric Publishing.

Mathew, S.J., Amiel, J.M., & Sackeim, H.A. (2013). Electroconvulsive therapy in treatment-resistant depression. *Psychiatry Weekly.* Retrieved from http://www.psychweekly.com/aspx/article/article_pf.aspx?articleid=52

McClintock, S.M., & Husain, M.M. (2011). Electroconvulsive therapy does not damage the brain. *Journal of the American Psychiatric Nurses Association, 17*(3), 212-213.

Sackeim, H.A., Prudic, J., Fuller, R., Keilp, J., Lavori, P.W., & Olfson, M. (2007). The cognitive effects of electroconvulsive therapy in community settings. *Neuropsychopharmacology, 32*(1), 244-254.

Sadock, B.J., & Sadock, V.A. (2007). Synopsis of psychiatry: Behavioral sciences/clinical psychiatry (10th ed.). Philadelphia, PA: Lippincott Williams & Wilkins.

Wahlund, B., & von Rosen, D. (2003). ECT of major depressed patients in relation to biological and clinical variables: A brief overview. *Neuropsychopharmacology, 28*, S21-S26.

The Recovery Model 21

CORE CONCEPT

recovery

KEY TERMS

hope

purpose

Tidal Model

Wellness Recovery Action Plan (WRAP) Model

Psychological Recovery Model

OBJECTIVES
After reading this chapter, the student will be able to:

1. Define *recovery*.
2. Discuss the 10 guiding principles of recovery as delineated by the Substance Abuse and Mental Health Services Administration.
3. Describe three models of recovery: the Tidal Model, the WRAP Model, and the Psychological Recovery Model.
4. Identify nursing interventions to assist individuals with mental illness in the process of recovery.

HOMEWORK ASSIGNMENT
Please read the chapter and answer the following questions:

1. What is the basic concept of a recovery model?
2. How is recovery supported by peer groups?
3. What is the focus of the Tidal Model of Recovery?
4. What is the intended outcome in the Psychological Recovery Model?

For many years, the belief was that individuals with mental illnesses do not recover. Optimistically, the course of the illness was viewed in terms of maintenance, and pessimistically, with the expectation for deterioration. But research suggests that striving for and achieving recovery is in fact realistic for many individuals.

The concept of recovery is not new. It originally began in the addictions field, referring to a person recovering from a substance-related disorder. The term has recently been adopted by mental health professionals who believe that recovery from mental illness is also possible.

CORE CONCEPT

Recovery

Restoration to a former and/or better state or condition.

319

What Is Recovery?

A number of definitions of recovery as it applies to mental illness have been proposed. The Substance Abuse and Mental Health Services Administration (SAMHSA, 2011) suggests the following:

> Recovery from mental health disorders and substance use disorders is a process of change through which individuals improve their health and wellness, live a self-directed life, and strive to reach their full potential.

SAMHSA suggests that a life in recovery is supported by four major dimensions:

1. **Health:** overcoming or managing one's disease as well as living in a physically and emotionally healthy way.
2. **Home:** a stable and safe place to live.
3. **Purpose:** meaningful daily activities, such as a job, school, volunteerism, family caretaking, or creative endeavors, and the independence, income, and resources to participate in society.
4. **Community:** relationships and social networks that provide support, friendship, love, and **hope**.

William A. Anthony (1993), executive director of the Center for Psychiatric Rehabilitation at Boston University, offers this definition:

> Recovery is described as a deeply personal, unique process of changing one's attitudes, values, feelings, goals, skills, and/or roles. It is a way of living a satisfying, hopeful, and contributing life even with limitations caused by illness. Recovery involves the development of new meaning and purpose in one's life as one grows beyond the catastrophic effects of mental illness. (p. 13)

The President's New Freedom Commission on Mental Health (2003) proposes to transform the mental health system by shifting the paradigm of care of persons with serious mental illness from traditional medical psychiatric treatment toward the concept of recovery, and the American Psychiatric Association has endorsed a recovery model from a psychiatric services perspective (Sharfstein, 2005).

The basic concept of a recovery model is empowerment of the consumer. The recovery model is designed to allow consumers primary control over decisions about their own care. The National Association of Social Workers (NASW, 2006) suggests that this means, "Consumers need to be as fully informed as possible about the potential benefits and consequences of each decision. They also need to know the possible results if they become a danger to themselves or others."

Guiding Principles of Recovery

As part of its Recovery Support Strategic Initiative, a yearlong effort by SAMHSA and a wide range of partners in the behavioral health-care community and other fields, a working definition of recovery from mental health and substance use disorders (previously stated) was developed. In addition, a set of guiding principles that support the recovery definition were delineated. These guiding principles include the following (SAMHSA, 2011, for use in the public domain):

■ **Recovery emerges from hope.** The belief that recovery is real provides the essential and motivating message of a better future—that people can and do overcome the internal and external challenges, barriers, and obstacles that confront them. Hope is internalized and can be fostered by peers, families, providers, allies, and others. Hope is the catalyst of the recovery process.

■ **Recovery is person-driven.** Self-determination and self-direction are the foundations for recovery as individuals define their own life goals and design their unique path(s) toward those goals. Individuals optimize their autonomy and independence to the greatest extent possible by leading, controlling, and exercising choice over the services and supports that assist their recovery and resilience. In so doing, they are empowered and provided the resources to make informed decisions, initiate recovery, build on their strengths, and gain or regain control over their lives.

■ **Recovery occurs via many pathways.** Individuals are unique with distinct needs, strengths, preferences, goals, culture, and backgrounds (including trauma experiences) that affect and determine their pathway(s) to recovery. Recovery is built on the multiple capacities, strengths, talents, coping abilities, resources, and inherent value of each individual. Recovery pathways are highly personalized. They may include professional clinical treatment; use of medications; support from families and in schools; faith-based approaches; peer support; and other approaches. Recovery is nonlinear, characterized by continual growth and improved functioning that may involve setbacks. Because setbacks are a natural, though not inevitable, part of the recovery process, it is essential to foster resilience for all individuals and families. Abstinence is the safest approach for those with substance use disorders. Use of tobacco and nonprescribed or illicit drugs is not safe for anyone. In some cases, recovery pathways can be enabled by creating a supportive environment. This is especially true for children, who may not have the legal or developmental capacity to set their own course.

■ **Recovery is holistic.** Recovery encompasses an individual's whole life, including mind, body, spirit, and community. This includes addressing: self-care practices, family, housing, employment, education, clinical treatment for mental disorders and substance use disorders, services and supports, primary health care, dental care, complementary and alternative services, faith, spirituality, creativity, social networks, transportation, and community participation. The array of services and supports available should be integrated and coordinated.

■ **Recovery is supported by peers and allies.** Mutual support and mutual aid groups, including the sharing of experiential knowledge and skills, as well as social learning, play an invaluable role in recovery. Peers encourage and engage other peers and provide each other with a vital sense of belonging, supportive relationships, valued roles, and community. Through helping others and giving back to the community, one helps one's self. Peer-operated supports and services provide important resources to assist people along their journeys of recovery and wellness. Professionals can also play an important role in the recovery process by providing clinical treatment and other services that support individuals in their chosen recovery paths. While peers and allies play an important role for many in recovery, their role for children and youth may be slightly different. Peer supports for families are very important for children with behavioral health problems and can also play a supportive role for youth in recovery.

■ **Recovery is supported through relationship and social networks.** An important factor in the recovery process is the presence and involvement of people who believe in the person's ability to recover; who offer hope, support, and encouragement; and who also suggest strategies and resources for change. Family members, peers, providers, faith groups, community members, and other allies form vital support networks. Through these relationships, people leave unhealthy and/or unfulfilling life roles behind and engage in new roles (e.g., partner, caregiver, friend, student, employee) that lead to a greater sense of belonging, personhood, empowerment, autonomy, social inclusion, and community participation.

■ **Recovery is culturally-based and influenced.** Culture and cultural background in all of its diverse representations (including values, traditions, and beliefs) are keys in determining a person's journey and unique pathway to recovery. Services should be culturally grounded, attuned, sensitive, congruent, and competent, as well as personalized to meet each individual's unique needs.

■ **Recovery is supported by addressing trauma.** The experience of trauma (such as physical or sexual abuse, domestic violence, war, disaster, and others) is often a precursor to or associated with alcohol and drug use, mental health problems, and related issues. Services and supports should be trauma-informed to foster safety (physical and emotional) and trust, as well as promote choice, empowerment, and collaboration.

■ **Recovery involves individual, family, and community strengths and responsibility.** Individuals, families, and communities have strengths and resources that serve as a foundation for recovery. In addition, individuals have a personal responsibility for their own self-care and journeys of recovery. Individuals should be supported in speaking for themselves. Families and significant others have responsibilities to support their loved ones, especially for children and youth in recovery. Communities have responsibilities to provide opportunities and resources to address discrimination and to foster social inclusion and recovery. Individuals in recovery also have a social responsibility and should have the ability to join with peers to speak collectively about their strengths, needs, wants, desires, and aspirations.

■ **Recovery is based on respect.** Community, systems, and societal acceptance and appreciation for people affected by mental health and substance use problems—including protecting their rights and eliminating discrimination—are crucial in achieving recovery. There is a need to acknowledge that taking steps toward recovery may require great courage. Self-acceptance, developing a positive and meaningful sense of identity, and regaining belief in one's self are particularly important.

The recovery model integrates services provided by professionals (e.g., medication, therapy, case management), services provided by consumers (e.g., advocacy, peer support programs, hotlines, mentoring), and services provided in collaboration (e.g., recovery education, crisis planning, community integration, consumer rights education) (Jacobson & Greenley, 2001).

Jacobson and Greenley state:

Although many of these services may sound similar to services currently being offered in many mental health systems, it is important to recognize that no service is recovery-oriented unless it incorporates the attitude that recovery is possible and has the goal of promoting hope, healing, empowerment, and connection. (p. 485)

Models of Recovery

The Tidal Model

The **Tidal Model** was developed in the late 1990s by Phil Barker and Poppy Buchanan-Barker of Newcastle, United Kingdom. It is a mental health nursing recovery model that may be used as the basis for interdisciplinary mental health care (Barker & Buchanan-Barker, 2012). The authors use the power of metaphor to engage with the person in distress. The metaphor of *water* is used to describe how individuals in distress can become emotionally, physically, and spiritually *shipwrecked* (Barker & Buchanan-Barker, 2005). The Tidal Model was the first recovery model to be developed by nurses in practice, drawing largely on nursing research, and in collaboration with users and consumers of mental health services (Barker & Buchanan-Barker, 2005; Brookes, 2006).

The Tidal Model uses a person-centered approach to help people deal with their problems of human living. Focus is on the individual's personal story, which is where his or her problems first appeared and where any growth, benefit, or recovery will be found (Barker & Buchanan-Barker, 2000).

Barker and Buchanan-Barker (2005) developed a set of essential values upon which the model is based. These values, which they call the 10 Tidal Commitments, "provide practitioners with a philosophical focus for helping people make their own life changes, rather than trying to manage or control 'patient symptoms'" (Buchanan-Barker & Barker, 2008, p. 95). From these commitments, the authors developed Tidal Competencies, which reflect the way the commitments are practiced in the clinical setting. These commitments and competencies include the following:

1. **Value the voice.** The person is encouraged to tell his or her story. "The person's story represents the beginning and endpoint of the helping encounter, embracing not only an account of the person's distress, but also the hope for its resolution" (Buchanan-Barker & Barker, 2008, p. 95). Practitioner competencies include a capacity to actively listen to the person's story and to help the person record the story in his or her own words.

2. **Respect the language.** Individuals are encouraged to speak their own words in their own unique way. "The language of the story—complete with its unusual grammar and personal metaphors—is the ideal medium for illuminating the way to recovery. We encourage people to speak their own words in their distinctive voice" (Buchanan-Barker & Barker, 2008, pp. 95-96). Practitioner competencies include helping individuals express in their own language their understanding of personal experiences through use of stories, anecdotes, and metaphors.

3. **Develop genuine curiosity.** Nurses and other caregivers "need to express genuine interest in the story so that they can better understand the storyteller and the story. Genuine curiosity reflects an interest in the person and the person's unique experience" (Buchanan-Barker & Barker, 2008, p. 96). Practitioner competencies include showing interest in the person's story, asking for clarification of certain points, and assisting the person to unfold the story at his or her own rate.

4. **Become the apprentice.** The individual is the expert on his or her life story, and he or she must be the leader in deciding what needs to be done. "Professionals may learn something of the power of that story, but only if they apply themselves diligently and respectfully to the task by becoming apprentice-minded" (Buchanan-Barker & Barker, 2008, p. 96). Practitioner competencies include developing a plan of care for the individual, based on his or her expressed needs or wishes, and helping the individual identify specific problems and ways to address them.

5. **Use the available toolkit.** Concentration is given to the individual's strengths, which are the major tools in the recovery process. "The story contains examples of 'what has worked' for the person in the past or beliefs about 'what might work' for this person in the future. These represent the main tools that need to be used to unlock or build the story of recovery" (Buchanan-Barker & Barker, 2008, p. 96). Practitioner competencies include helping individuals identify what efforts may be successful in relation to solving identified problems and which persons in the individual's life may be able to provide assistance.

6. **Craft the step beyond.** The individual and the practitioner decide together what needs to be done immediately. "Any 'first step' is a crucial step, revealing the power of change and potentially pointing towards the ultimate goal of recovery" (Buchanan-Barker & Barker, 2008, p. 96). Practitioner competencies include helping the individual determine what kind of change would represent a step toward recovery and what he or she needs to do to take that "first step" in the progress toward that goal.

7. **Give the gift of time.** Change happens when the individual and practitioner spend quality time in a therapeutic relationship. "The challenge is using time for things that are important" (Young, 2010, p. 573). Practitioner competencies include acknowledging (and helping the individual understand) the importance of time dedicated to addressing the needs of the individual and the planning and implementing of care.

8. **Reveal personal wisdom.** People often do not realize their own personal wisdom, strengths, and

abilities. "A key task for the professional is to help the person reveal and come to value that wisdom, so that it might be used to sustain the person throughout the voyage of recovery" (Buchanan-Barker & Barker, 2008, p. 97). Practitioner competencies include helping individuals to identify personal strengths and weaknesses and to develop self-confidence in their ability to help themselves.

9. **Know that change is constant.** Because change is a constant in everyone's life, important decisions and choices must be made along the path to recovery in order for growth to occur. Professional competencies include helping the individual develop awareness of the changes that are occurring and how he or she has influenced these changes. "The task of the professional helper is to develop awareness of how change is happening and to support the person in making decisions regarding the course of the recovery voyage" (Buchanan-Barker & Barker, 2008, p. 97).

10. **Be transparent.** Transparency is important in the teambuilding process between the individual and the professional helper. "Professionals are in a privileged position and should model confidence by being transparent at all times, helping the person understand exactly what is being done and why" (Buchanan-Barker & Barker, 2008, p. 97). Professional competencies include ensuring that the individual is aware of the significance of all interventions and that he or she receives copies of all documents related to the plan of care.

Young (2010) states:

> The Tidal Model is not a typical boxes-and-arrows diagram to use and follow. Instead, it is way of thinking, a paradigm for giving person-centered care that is strength-based, empowering, and relational. (p. 574)

The Wellness Recovery Action Plan (WRAP)

The **Wellness Recovery Action Plan (WRAP) Model** was developed in 1997 by a group of 30 individuals who were attending a mental health recovery skills seminar conducted by Mary Ellen Copeland in Vermont. This group (which included persons with psychiatric symptoms, family members, and care providers) determined the need for a system to incorporate the skills and strategies they were learning in the seminar into their everyday lives. Copeland (2001) states:

> [WRAP] is a structured system for monitoring uncomfortable and distressing symptoms and, through planned responses, reducing, modifying or eliminating those symptoms. It also includes plans for responses from others when a person's symptoms have made it impossible to continue to make decisions, take care of him/herself and keep him/herself safe. (p. 129)

Copeland suggests that all a person needs to begin the program is a system for storing information (e.g., a notebook, computer, or tape recorder), and possibly a friend, health-care provider, or other supporter to give assistance and feedback. The program is a step-wise process through which an individual is able to monitor and manage distressing symptoms that occur in daily life. Individuals may be assisted in the process by others (e.g., health-care professionals, significant others, friends), "but to be effective and empowering, the person experiencing the symptoms must develop the plan for himself/herself" (p. 129). Steps of the WRAP process are described in the following paragraphs.

Step 1: Developing a Wellness Toolbox

In this first step, the individual creates a list of tools, strategies, and skills that he or she has used in the past (or has heard of in the past that he or she would like to try) to assist in relieving disturbing symptoms. Copeland (2001) offers a number of examples:

- Talking to a friend or health-care professional
- Peer counseling or exchange listening
- Relaxation and stress-reduction exercises
- Guided imagery
- Journaling
- Physical exercise
- Attending a support group
- Doing something special for someone else
- Listening to music

Step 2: Daily Maintenance List

This list is divided into three parts. In part 1, the individual writes a description of how he or she feels (or would like to feel) when experiencing wellness (e.g., bright, cheerful, talkative, happy, optimistic, capable). This information is used as a reference point. In part 2, using the wellness toolbox as a reference, the individual makes a list of things he or she needs to do every day to maintain wellness. This is an important part of the plan and must be realistic so as not to set up the individual for "failure" or create additional frustration. Example items for part 2 may include the following (Copeland, 2001):

- Eat three healthy meals and three healthy snacks.
- Drink at least six 8-ounce glasses of water.
- Avoid caffeine, sugar, junk foods, and alcohol.
- Exercise for at least 30 minutes.
- Have 20 minutes of relaxation or meditation time.
- Write in my journal for at least 15 minutes.
- Take medications and vitamin supplements.
- Spend at least 30 minutes enjoying a fun, affirming, and/or creative activity.

In part 3 of this step, the individual keeps a list of things that need to be done. The individual reads this list daily as a reminder, and items may be considered for accomplishment on any given day at the individual's discretion. For part 3, Copeland (2001) suggests items such as the following:

- Spend time with counselor or case manager.
- Make an appointment with health-care professional.
- Spend time with friend or partner.
- Be in touch with my family.
- Spend time with children or pets.
- Buy groceries.
- Do the laundry.
- Write some letters.
- Remember someone's birthday or anniversary.

Step 3: Triggers

This step is divided into two parts. In part 1, the individual lists events or circumstances that, should they occur, would cause distress or discomfort. These triggers are situations to which the individual is susceptible or that have triggered or increased symptoms in the past. Copeland (2001) lists the following examples:

- The anniversary dates of losses or trauma
- Being overtired or exhausted
- Work stress
- Family friction
- A relationship ending
- Being judged, criticized, or teased
- Financial problems
- Physical illness
- Sexual harassment or inappropriate sexual behavior
- Substance abuse

In part 2, the individual uses items from the wellness toolbox to develop a plan for "what to do" if triggers interfere with wellness.

Step 4: Early Warning Signs

This step is divided into two parts. Part 1 involves identification of subtle signs that indicate a possible worsening of the situation. Copeland (2001) states, "Recognizing early warning signs and reviewing them regularly will help the person to become more aware of these early warning signs, allowing the person to take action before the signs worsen" (p. 136). Some types of early warning signs include anxiety, forgetfulness, lack of motivation, avoiding others or isolating, increased irritability, increase in smoking, using substances, or feeling worthless and inadequate. In part 2, the individual develops a plan for responding to the early warning signs that result in relief or in preventing them from escalating. The plan may include items such as consulting a supporter or counselor, increasing focus on peer counseling, increasing time spent in relaxation exercises, or utilizing other interventions from the wellness toolbox until warning signs diminish.

Step 5: Things Are Breaking Down or Getting Worse

This step is divided into two parts. In part 1, the individual lists symptoms that are occurring that indicate that the situation has worsened. In this stage, the symptoms are producing great discomfort, but the individual is still able to take some action on his or her own behalf. Immediate action is required to prevent a crisis from developing. Symptoms at this stage differ greatly from person to person, and Copeland (2001) states, "What may mean 'things are breaking down' to one person may mean 'crisis' to another" (p. 137). She lists a number of examples of symptoms, which may include the following:

- Irrational responses to events and the actions of others
- Inability to sleep or sleeping all the time
- Headaches
- Not eating or overeating
- Social isolation
- Thoughts of self-harm
- Substance abuse or chain smoking
- Bizarre behaviors
- Seeing things that aren't there
- Paranoia

In part 2, the individual makes a plan that he or she thinks will help when the symptoms have worsened to this degree. The plan must be very specific and direct, with clear instructions. Some examples include the following (Copeland, 2001):

- Call my health care-professional; ask for and follow directions.
- Arrange for someone to stay with me around the clock until my symptoms subside.
- Take action so that I cannot hurt myself if my symptoms get worse, such as give my medication, checkbook, credit cards, and car keys to a previously designated friend for safe keeping.
- Make sure I do everything on my daily check list.
- Have at least two peer counseling sessions daily.
- Increase use of items from wellness toolbox (e.g., relaxation exercises, physical exercises, creative activities).

Step 6: Crisis Planning

This stage identifies symptoms indicating that individuals can no longer care for themselves, make independent decisions, or keep themselves safe. This stage is multifaceted and is meant for use by caregivers on behalf of the individual who developed the plan. It is composed of the following parts (Copeland, 2001):

- Part 1: Gathers information that describes what the person is like when well.
- Part 2: Identifies the symptoms that indicate when others need to take responsibility for the person's care.

■ Part 3: Provides names of supporters previously identified by the individual to speak on his or her behalf.

■ Part 4: Includes the name of health-care providers and phone numbers; medications currently using; allergies to medications; medications the individual would prefer to take, if additional medication is necessary; medications that the individual refuses to take.

■ Part 5: Includes the individual's preferred treatments and treatments that he or she wishes to be avoided.

■ Part 6: Identifies the individual's preferences in treatment facilities (e.g., home, community care, respite center).

■ Part 7: Identifies acceptable facilities if previous preferences cannot be executed. Facilities to be avoided are also indicated.

■ Part 8: Includes an extensive description of what the individual expects from identified supporters who are acting on his or her behalf during a crisis situation.

■ Part 9: Consists of a list of indicators, developed by the individual, that communicates to supporters when their services are no longer required. The individual should update this plan periodically when he or she learns new information or changes his or her mind about certain situations. Assurance of the use of the crisis plan may be increased if it is notarized and signed in the presence of two witnesses. To further increase its potential for use, the person may appoint a durable power of attorney, although because of the variability of the legality of these documents from state to state, there is no guarantee that the plan will be followed.

Copeland states:

WRAP is a systematic method for developing skills in self-management and empowerment. It provides a means for individuals with a mental illness to work more collaboratively with healthcare providers. It is highly individualized and addresses the unique needs of the person and his/her situation. It is applicable to most any long-term illness/disability or problem situation. These benefits suggest that it can be used more widely and should be introduced as an option for individuals in need of a self-management system. (p. 149)

The Psychological Recovery Model

Andresen, Oades, and Caputi (2011) define psychological recovery as "the establishment of a fulfilling, meaningful life and a positive sense of identity founded on hopefulness and self-determination. Psychological recovery is necessary whether mental illness is biologically based or the result of the exacerbation of emotional problems caused by stress"

(p. 40). The **Psychological Recovery Model** does not emphasize the absence of symptoms, but focuses on the person's self-determination in the course of his or her recovery process.

In examining a number of studies, Andresen and associates (2011) identified four components that were consistently evident in the recovery process:

■ **Hope**: finding and maintaining hope that recovery can occur

■ **Responsibility**: taking responsibility for one's life and well-being

■ **Self and identity**: renewing the sense of self and building a positive identity

■ **Meaning and purpose**: finding purpose and meaning in life

Andresen and associates (2011) conceptualized a five-stage model of recovery, which they define by integrating into each stage the four components of the recovery process. An explanation of these stages is presented in the following paragraphs.

Stage 1: Moratorium

This stage is identified by dark despair and confusion. "It is called moratorium, because it seems 'life is on hold'" (p. 47).

■ **Hope:** In the moratorium stage, hopelessness prevails. Clients may even perceive feelings of hopelessness from practitioners when treatment plans emphasize stabilization and maintenance, thereby conveying messages of no hope for recovery.

■ **Responsibility:** In the moratorium stage, the individual feels out of control and powerless to change.

■ **Self and identity:** In the moratorium stage, individuals feel "as though they no longer know who they are as a person" (p. 59). An individual's sense of identity as a valuable and functional member of society can be lost with a diagnosis of mental illness.

■ **Meaning and purpose:** The diagnosis of severe mental illness is a traumatic event that can challenge an individual's fundamental beliefs, creating a loss of meaning and purpose in life.

Stage 2: Awareness

In this stage, the individual comes to a realization that a possibility for recovery exists. Andresen and associates state, "It involves an awareness of a possible self other than that of 'sick person': a self that is capable of recovery" (p. 47).

■ **Hope:** In the awareness stage, there is a dawn of hope that indeed "life is not over." This feeling of hope may emanate from significant others, professionals, or family members. Individuals may also be inspired by others who have recovered. Hope may also be derived from strong inner determination and from personal faith and spirituality.

- **Responsibility:** In this stage, the individual develops an awareness of the need to take control of his or her life. Feelings of control and responsibility lead to a sense of personal empowerment that paves the way for recovery.
- **Self and identity:** In the awareness stage, the individual comes to realize that he or she is a person independent of the illness. "The person realizes that there still exists an 'intact self' capable of taking action on one's own behalf" (p. 72).
- **Meaning and purpose:** In the awareness stage, the individual strives for a personal comprehension of the illness, why it occurred, and what the implications of the illness are for his or her future. "Seeking a meaning of the illness can be explained by theories of cognitive control, in which one tries to understand unexplainable negative events by finding a reason for them" (p. 74).

Stage 3: Preparation

This stage begins with the individual's resolve to begin the work of recovery.

- **Hope:** In the preparation stage, hope is manifested in the mobilization of personal and external resources to foster self-care and find pathways to goals. This includes identifying strengths and weaknesses, gathering knowledge and information, and seeking out available support systems.
- **Responsibility:** Taking responsibility in the preparation stage involves learning about the effects of the illness and how to recognize, monitor, and manage symptoms. Taking charge of one's life also includes the ability to be independent and take care of basic needs.
- **Self and identity:** Andresen and associates state, "During the preparation stage, the person takes stock of his or her skills and strengths in order to build on them to rediscover a positive sense of identity" (p. 81). The person is willing to take risks and try new activities to reestablish a sense of self. Lost aspects of self are rediscovered, new aspects are identified, and both are incorporated into a new self-identity.
- **Meaning and purpose:** The basis for a meaningful life lies in solid core values. "Living according to one's valued directions gives meaning to the work of recovery, and for this reason, some people hold on tenaciously to their goals" (p. 83). Each individual must live by certain tenets that make life personally valuable and enriching. Individuals living with a severe mental illness may require a reordering of priorities and setting of new goals as part of their recovery.

Stage 4: Rebuilding

The hard work of recovery takes place in the rebuilding stage. The individual "takes the necessary steps to work towards his or her goals in rebuilding a meaningful life" (p. 87).

- **Hope:** In the rebuilding stage, the individual has hope for and looks forward to a more fulfilling life. Realistic goals are set, and the individual is encouraged to pursue the recovery process at his or her own pace. With each success, hope is renewed.
- **Responsibility:** "Through setting and working towards goals, the person begins to actively take control of his or her life; not only management of symptoms, but also enlisting social support, improvement of self-image, handling social pressures, and building social competence" (p. 90). Assuming control of treatment decisions and illness management is an essential part of the recovery process.
- **Self and identity:** The individual elaborates and enhances his or her sense of identity by having succeeded in previous stages in developing a positive self-identity separate from the illness and a new sense of self-confidence by succeeding at new activities. In the rebuilding stage, the work of examining core values and working toward value-congruent goals reinforce a positive sense of identity and a commitment to recovery.
- **Meaning and purpose:** Having realistic goals and a positive sense of identity provides a sense of purpose in life. Individuals need a reason to start each day. Andresen and associates state, "Finding meaning [in life] is more than finding a valued occupation, but rather is more akin to finding a way to live. This may include, but is not limited to, vocational goals. It includes examining one's spirituality or philosophy of life. The journey is, in itself, a source of meaning for many" (p. 99).

Stage 5: Growth

The outcome of the psychological recovery process is growth. Although it is called the *final* stage of the Psychological Recovery Model, it is important to remember that this is a dynamic stage and that personal growth is a continuing life process.

- **Hope:** In the growth stage, the individual feels a sense of optimism and hope of a rewarding future. Skills that have been nurtured in the previous stages are applied with confidence, and the individual strives for higher levels of well-being.
- **Responsibility:** "Achieving control requires sustained commitment in the face of set-backs" (p. 106). In the growth phase, individuals exhibit confidence in managing their illnesses and are resilient when relapses occur. They are empowered by personal input and decision-making regarding their treatment.
- **Self and identity:** The individual in the growth stage has developed a strong, positive sense of self and identity. Andresen and associates state, "Many

consumers have reported feeling that they are a better person as a result of their struggle with the illness. [In one research study] participants reported developing personal qualities, including strength and courage; more confidence in the self; resourcefulness and responsibility; a new philosophy of life; compassion and empathy; a sense of self-worth; and being happier and more carefree" (pp. 108-109).

■ **Meaning and purpose:** Individuals who have reached the growth stage often report a more profound sense of meaning. Some describe having achieved a sense of serenity and peace, and for others it takes the form of a spiritual awakening. Some individuals find reward in educating others about the experience of mental illness and recovery.

Andresen and associates (2011) state,

Recovery from serious mental illness is more than staying out of the hospital or a return to some arbitrary level of functioning. It is more than merely coping with the illness. In [the growth] stage, the notion of wellbeing replaces that of wellness. While wellness implies the absence of illness, wellbeing refers to a more holistic psychological experience of fulfilling life. Although we may not expect everyone (including those who do not have a mental illness) to reach the highest levels of self-actualization, we can expect that all people have the opportunity to develop a positive sense of self and identity and to live a meaningful life filled with purpose and hope for the future. (p. 113)

Nursing Interventions That Assist With Recovery

The President's New Freedom Commission on Mental Health (2003) proposes to transform the mental health system by shifting the paradigm of care of persons with serious mental illness from traditional medical psychiatric treatment toward the concept of recovery. It is within the scope of nursing to assist individuals in many aspects of the mental health recovery process. Caldwell, Sclafani, Swarbrick, and Piren (2010) state:

Professional nurses must play an active role in client recovery because they are employed in all aspects of service delivery systems, and most times professional nurses are responsible for the delivery and coordination of care. The professional nurse must be center stage in the development and implementation of any action plan involving client recovery. (p. 44)

Nurses have historically held as a primary goal the promotion of wellness within a collaborative nurse-client relationship. Peplau (1991) described nursing as "a human relationship between an individual who is sick, or in need of health services, and a nurse especially educated to recognize and to respond to the need for help" (pp. 5-6). As previously noted, recovery models are inherently collaborative in that services are provided by professionals, by clients, and cooperatively by both. Examples of interventions and activities in which nurses and clients may collaborate in the client's journey to recovery are outlined in Table 21-1.

If the proposals from the President's New Freedom Commission on Mental Health become reality, it would surely mean improvement in the promotion of mental health and the care of individuals with mental illness. Many nurse leaders see this period of health-care reform as an opportunity for nurses to expand their roles and assume key positions in education, prevention, assessment, and referral. Nurses are, and will continue to be, in key positions to assist

TABLE 21–1 **Nurse-Client Collaboration in the Mental Health Recovery Process**			
	THE TIDAL MODEL	THE WRAP MODEL	PSYCHOLOGICAL RECOVERY MODEL
Assessment	■ Client tells his or her personal story ■ Nurse actively listens and expresses interest in the story ■ Nurse helps client record story in client's own language ■ Client identifies specific problems he or she wishes to address ■ Nurse and client identify client's strengths and weaknesses	■ Client develops a wellness toolbox by creating a list of tools, strategies, and skills that have been helpful in the past ■ Client identifies strengths and weaknesses ■ Nurse provides assistance and feedback	■ Client is feeling hopeless and powerless ■ Client seeks meaning of the illness ■ Nurse helps by offering hope ■ Client begins to develop an awareness of the need to take control of and responsibility for his or her life

Continued

TABLE 21–1 Nurse-Client Collaboration in the Mental Health Recovery Process—cont'd		
	THE TIDAL MODEL	THE WRAP MODEL	PSYCHOLOGICAL RECOVERY MODEL
Interventions	■ Nurse and client determine what has worked in the past ■ Client suggests new tools he or she would like to try ■ Client decides what changes he or she would like to make and sets realistic goals ■ Nurse and client decide what must be done as the first step ■ Nurse gives positive feedback for client's efforts to make life changes and for successes achieved ■ Nurse encourages client to be as independent as possible, but offers assistance when required ■ Nurse gives the "gift of time"	■ Client creates a daily maintenance list 　■ How he or she feels at best 　■ What must be done daily to maintain wellness 　■ Reminder list of other things that need to be accomplished ■ Client identifies "triggers" that cause distress or discomfort and identifies what to do if triggers interfere with wellness ■ Client identifies signs of worsening of symptoms and develops a plan to prevent escalation ■ Client identifies when symptoms have worsened and help is needed ■ Client identifies when he or she can no longer care for self and makes decisions (in writing) about treatment issues (what type, who will provide, who will represent client's interests) ■ Nurse offers support, and provides feedback and assistance when needed	■ Client resolves to begin work of recovery ■ Client and nurse identify strengths and weaknesses ■ Nurse assists client to learn about effects of the illness and how to recognize, monitor, and manage symptoms ■ Client identifies changes he or she wishes to occur and sets realistic goals to rebuild a meaningful life ■ Client examines personal spirituality and philosophy of life in search of a meaning and purpose—one that gives him or her a "reason to start each day"
Outcomes	■ Client acknowledges that change has occurred and is ongoing ■ Client feels empowered to manage own self-care ■ Nurse is available for support	■ Client develops skills in self-management ■ Client develops self-confidence and hope for a brighter future	■ Client develops a positive self-identity separate from the illness ■ Client maintains commitment to recovery in the face of set-backs ■ Client feels a sense of optimism and hope of a rewarding future

individuals with mental illness to remain as independent as possible, to manage their illness within the community setting, and to strive to minimize the number of hospitalizations required. A vision of recovery from mental illness exists, and hope, trust, and self-determination should be incorporated into all treatment models.

Summary and Key Points

■ Recovery is the restoration to a former and/or better state or condition.
■ SAMHSA identifies four major dimensions that support a life in recovery: health, home, purpose, and community.

■ The President's New Freedom Commission on Mental Health proposes to transform the mental health system by shifting the paradigm of care of persons with serious mental illness from traditional medical psychiatric treatment toward the concept of recovery.
■ SAMHSA outlines 10 guiding principles that support recovery:
　■ Recovery emerges from hope.
　■ Recovery is person-driven.
　■ Recovery occurs via many pathways.
　■ Recovery is holistic.
　■ Recovery is supported by peers and allies.
　■ Recovery is supported through relationship and social networks.

■ Recovery is culturally-based and influenced.
■ Recovery is supported by addressing trauma.
■ Recovery involves individual, family, and community strengths and responsibility.
■ Recovery is based on respect.

■ Many models of recovery exist. Three models were discussed in this chapter: the Tidal Model, the Wellness Recovery Action Plan (WRAP) Model, and the Psychological Recovery Model.

■ Nurses work in key positions to assist individuals with mental illness in the recovery process. Interventions based on the three previously mentioned recovery models were included in this chapter.

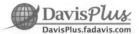 **DavisPlus** Additional info available at
DavisPlus.fadavis.com   www.davisplus.com

Review Questions
Self-Examination/Learning Exercise

*Select the answer that is **most** appropriate for each of the following questions.*

1. Which of the following is a true statement about mental health recovery? (Select all that apply.)
   a. Mental health recovery applies only to severe and persistent mental illnesses.
   b. Mental health recovery serves to provide empowerment to the client.
   c. Mental health recovery is based on the medical model.
   d. Mental health recovery is a collaborative process.

2. A nurse is assisting an individual with mental illness recovery using the Tidal Model. Which of the following is a component of this model?
   a. The wellness toolbox
   b. The daily maintenance list
   c. The individual's personal story
   d. Triggers

3. A nurse is assisting an individual with mental illness recovery using the Psychological Recovery Model. The client says to the nurse, "I have schizophrenia. Nothing can be done. I might as well die." In which stage of the Psychological Recovery Model would the nurse assess this individual to be?
   a. The awareness stage
   b. The preparation stage
   c. The rebuilding stage
   d. The moratorium stage

4. A nurse who is helping a client in the preparation stage of the Psychological Recovery Model might include which of the following interventions?
   a. Teach about effects of the illness and how to recognize, monitor, and manage symptoms.
   b. Help the client identify "triggers" that cause distress or discomfort.
   c. Help the client establish a daily maintenance list.
   d. Listen actively while the client composes his or her personal story.

5. A nurse who is helping a client with mental illness recovery using the WRAP Model says to the client, "First you must create a wellness toolbox." She explains to the client that a wellness toolbox is which of the following?
   a. A list of words that describe how the individual feels when he or she is feeling well
   b. A list of things the client needs to do every day to maintain wellness
   c. A list of strategies the client has used in the past that help relieve disturbing symptoms
   d. A list of the client's favorite health-care providers and phone numbers

References

Andresen, R., Oades, L.G., & Caputi, P. (2011). *Psychological recovery: Beyond mental illness*. West Sussex, UK: John Wiley & Sons.

Anthony, W.A. (1993). Recovery from mental illness: The guiding vision of the mental health service system in the 1990s. *Psychosocial Rehabilitation Journal, 16*(4), 11-23.

Barker, P.J., & Buchanan-Barker, P. (2000). *The Tidal Model: Reclaiming stories, recovering lives*. Retrieved from http://www.tidal-model.com

Barker, P.J., & Buchanan-Barker, P. (2005). *The tidal model: A guide for mental health professionals*. London: Brunner-Routledge.

Barker, P.J., & Buchanan-Barker, P. (2012). *Tidal Model of mental health nursing*. Retrieved from http://www.currentnursing.com/nursing_theory/Tidal_Model.html

Brookes, N. (2006). Phil Barker: The Tidal Model of mental health recovery. In A.M. Tomey & M.R. Alligood (Eds.), *Nursing theorists and their work* (6th ed., pp. 696-725). New York, NY: Elsevier.

Buchanan-Barker, P., & Barker, P.J. (2008). The Tidal commitments: Extending the value base of mental health recovery. *Journal of Psychiatric and Mental Health Nursing, 15*(2), 93-100.

Caldwell, B.A., Sclafani, M., Swarbrick, M., & Piren, K. (2010). Psychiatric nursing practice and the recovery model of care. *Journal of Psychosocial Nursing, 48*(7), 42-48.

Copeland, M.E. (2001). Wellness recovery action plan: A system for monitoring, reducing and eliminating uncomfortable or dangerous physical symptoms and emotional feelings. In C. Brown (Ed.), *Recovery and wellness: Models of hope and empowerment for people with mental illness* (pp. 127-150). New York, NY: The Haworth Press.

Jacobson, N., & Greenley, D. (2001). What is recovery? A conceptual model and explication. *Psychiatric Services, 52*(4), 482-485.

National Association of Social Workers (NASW). (2006). *NASW Practice snapshot: The mental health recovery model*. Retrieved from http://www.socialworkers.org/practice/behavioral_health/0206snapshot.asp?

Peplau, H.E. (1991). *Interpersonal relations in nursing: A conceptual frame of reference for psychodynamic nursing*. New York, NY: Springer.

President's New Freedom Commission on Mental Health. (2003). *Achieving the Promise: Transforming Mental Health Care in America*. Retrieved from http://govinfo.library.unt.edu/mentalhealthcommission/index.htm

Sharfstein, S. (2005). Recovery model will strengthen psychiatrist-patient relationship. *Psychiatric News, 40*(20), 3.

Substance Abuse and Mental Health Services Administration, Center for Mental Health Services. (2011). *SAMHSA's definition and guiding principles of recovery—Answering the call for feedback*. Retrieved from http://blog.samhsa.gov/2011/12/22/samhsa-definition-and-guiding-principles-of-recovery-answering-the-call-for-feedback/#.U4Y_Rnwo_cs

Young, B.B. (2010). Using the Tidal Model of mental health recovery to plan primary health care for women in residential substance abuse recovery. *Issues in Mental Health Nursing, 31*(9), 569-575.

4

Nursing Care of Clients With Alterations in Psychosocial Adaptation

22 Neurocognitive Disorders

CHAPTER OUTLINE

KEY TERMS

aphasia

apraxia

ataxia

confabulation

pseudodementia

sundowning

OBJECTIVES
After reading this chapter, the student will be able to:

1. Define and differentiate among various neurocognitive disorders (NCDs).
2. Discuss predisposing factors implicated in the etiology of NCDs.
3. Describe clinical symptoms and use the information to assess clients with NCDs.
4. Identify nursing diagnoses common to clients with NCDs, and select appropriate nursing interventions for each.
5. Identify topics for client and family teaching relevant to NCDs.
6. Discuss criteria for evaluating nursing care of clients with NCDs.
7. Describe various treatment modalities relevant to care of clients with NCDs.

HOMEWORK ASSIGNMENT
Please read the chapter and answer the following questions:

1. An alteration in which neurotransmitter is most closely associated with the etiology of Alzheimer's disease?
2. How does vascular neurocognitive disorder (NCD) differ from NCD due to Alzheimer's disease?
3. What is pseudodementia?
4. What is the primary concern for nurses working with clients with NCDs?

Neurocognitive disorders (NCDs) include those in which a clinically significant deficit in cognition or memory exists, representing a significant change from a previous level of functioning. These disorders were previously identified in the *Diagnostic and Statistical Manual of Mental Disorders, Fourth Edition, Text Revision (DSM-IV-TR)* (American Psychiatric Association [APA], 2000) as "Delirium, Dementia, and Amnestic Disorders." In the *DSM-5*, this category is entitled "Neurocognitive Disorders," and includes the disorders of delirium and mild and major NCDs.

This chapter presents predisposing factors, clinical symptoms, and nursing interventions for care of clients with neurocognitive disorders. The objective is to provide these individuals with the dignity and quality of life they deserve, while offering guidance and support to their families or primary caregivers.

CORE CONCEPT
Delirium
Delirium is a mental state characterized by a disturbance of cognition, which is manifested by confusion, excitement, disorientation, and a clouding of consciousness. Hallucinations and illusions are common.

Delirium

Clinical Findings and Course

A **delirium** is characterized by a disturbance in attention and awareness and a change in cognition that develop rapidly over a short period (APA, 2013). Symptoms of delirium include difficulty sustaining and shifting attention. The person is extremely distractible and must be repeatedly reminded to focus attention. Disorganized thinking prevails and is reflected by speech that is rambling, irrelevant, pressured, and incoherent, and that unpredictably switches from subject to subject. Reasoning ability and goal-directed behavior are impaired. Disorientation to time and place is common, and impairment of recent memory is invariably evident. Misperceptions of the environment, including illusions and hallucinations, prevail. Disturbances in the sleep-wake cycle occur.

The state of awareness may range from that of hypervigilance (heightened awareness to environmental stimuli) to stupor or semicoma. Sleep may fluctuate between hypersomnolence (excessive sleepiness) and insomnia. Vivid dreams and nightmares are common.

Psychomotor activity may fluctuate between agitated, purposeless movements (e.g., restlessness, hyperactivity, striking out at nonexistent objects) and a vegetative state resembling catatonic stupor. Various forms of tremor are frequently present.

Emotional instability may be manifested by fear, anxiety, depression, irritability, anger, euphoria, or apathy. These various emotions may be evidenced by crying, calls for help, cursing, muttering, moaning, acts of self-destruction, fearful attempts to flee, or attacks on others who are falsely viewed as threatening. Autonomic manifestations, such as tachycardia, sweating, flushed face, dilated pupils, and elevated blood pressure, are common.

The symptoms of delirium usually begin quite abruptly (e.g., following a head injury or seizure). At other times, they may be preceded by several hours or days of prodromal symptoms (e.g., restlessness, difficulty thinking clearly, insomnia or hypersomnolence, and nightmares). The slower onset is more common if the underlying cause is systemic illness or metabolic imbalance.

The duration of delirium is usually brief (e.g., 1 week; rarely more than 1 month) and, upon recovery from the underlying determinant, symptoms usually diminish over a 3- to 7-day period, but in some instances may take as long as 2 weeks (Sadock & Sadock, 2007). The age of the client and duration of the delirium influence rate of symptom resolution. Delirium may transition into a more permanent cognitive disorder (e.g., major neurocognitive disorder) and also is associated with a high mortality rate (Bourgeois, Seaman, & Servis, 2008).

Predisposing Factors
Delirium

Delirium most commonly occurs in individuals with serious medical, surgical, or neurological conditions. Some examples of conditions that have been known to precipitate delirium in some individuals include the following (Black & Andreasen, 2011; Bourgeois et al., 2008; Sadock & Sadock, 2007).

■ Systemic infections
■ Febrile illness
■ Metabolic disorders, such as hypoxia, hypercarbia, or hypoglycemia
■ Hepatic encephalopathy
■ Head trauma
■ Seizures
■ Migraine headaches
■ Brain abscess
■ Stroke
■ Postoperative states
■ Electrolyte imbalance

Other Etiological Implications
Substance Intoxication Delirium

In this subtype, the symptoms of delirium are attributed to intoxication from certain substances, such as alcohol; amphetamines; cannabis; cocaine; hallucinogens; inhalants; opioids; phencyclidine; sedative, hypnotic, and anxiolytics; or other (or unknown) substance (APA, 2013).

Substance Withdrawal Delirium

Withdrawal from certain substances can precipitate symptoms of delirium that are sufficiently severe to warrant clinical attention. These substances include alcohol; opioids; sedative, hypnotics, and anxiolytics; and others.

Medication-Induced Delirium

Medications that have been known to precipitate delirium include anticholinergics, antihypertensives, corticosteroids, anticonvulsants, cardiac glycosides, analgesics, anesthetics, antineoplastic agents, antiparkinson drugs, H$_2$-receptor antagonists (e.g., cimetidine), and others (Puri & Treasaden, 2012; Sadock & Sadock, 2007).

Delirium Due to Another Medical Condition or to Multiple Etiologies

There may be evidence from the history, physical examination, or laboratory findings that the symptoms of delirium are associated with another medical condition or can be attributable to more than one cause.

■ CORE CONCEPT

Neurocognitive

A term that is used to describe cognitive functions closely linked to particular areas of the brain that have to do with thinking, reasoning, memory, learning, and speaking.

Neurocognitive Disorder

Neurocognitive disorder (NCD) is classified in the *DSM-5* (APA, 2013) as either *mild* or *major*, with the distinction primarily being one of severity of symptomatology. Mild NCD has been known in some settings

as *mild cognitive impairment*, and is particularly critical because it can be a focus of early intervention to prevent or slow progression of the disorder. Major NCD constitutes what was previously described as *dementia* in the *DSM-IV-TR* (APA, 2000). In progressive neurodegenerative conditions, these two diagnoses may serve to identify earlier and later stages of the same disorder. Either diagnosis may be appropriate (depending on severity of symptoms) for certain other neurocognitive disorders that are the result of a reversible or temporary condition. Criteria for these disorders are presented in Box 22-1.

Clinical Findings, Epidemiology, and Course

NCD constitutes a large and growing public health problem. An estimated 5.4 million people in the United States currently have Alzheimer's disease (AD), the most common form of NCD, and the prevalence (the number of people with the disease at any one time) doubles for every 5-year age group beyond age 65 (National Institute on Aging [NIA], 2011). The Alzheimer's Association (2013a) reports that of those with AD, an estimated 4 percent are under age 65, 6 percent are age 65 to 74, 44 percent are age

---

BOX 22-1 **Comparison of Diagnostic Criteria**

MILD NEUROCOGNITIVE DISORDER

A. Evidence of modest cognitive decline from a previous level of performance in one or more cognitive domains (complex attention, executive function, learning and memory, language, perceptual-motor, or social cognition) based on:
  1. Concern of the individual, a knowledgeable informant, or the clinician that there has been a mild decline in cognitive function; and
  2. A modest impairment in cognitive performance, preferably documented by standardized neuropsychological testing, or, in its absence, another quantified clinical assessment.

B. The cognitive deficits do not interfere with capacity for independence in everyday activities (i.e., complex instrumental activities of daily living such as paying bills or managing medications are preserved, but greater effort, compensatory strategies or accommodation may be required).

C. The cognitive deficits do not occur exclusively in the context of a delirium.

D. The cognitive deficits are not better explained by another mental disorder (e.g., major depressive disorder, schizophrenia).

Specify whether due to:
Alzheimer's disease
Frontotemporal lobar degeneration

MAJOR NEUROCOGNITIVE DISORDER

A. Evidence of significant cognitive decline from a previous level of performance in one or more cognitive domains (complex attention, executive function, learning and memory, language, perceptual-motor, or social cognition) based on:
  1. Concern of the individual, a knowledgeable informant, or the clinician that there has been a significant decline in cognitive function; and
  2. A substantial impairment in cognitive performance, preferably documented by standardized neuropsychological testing, or, in its absence, another quantified clinical assessment.

B. The cognitive deficits interfere with independence in everyday activities (i.e., at a minimum, requiring assistance with complex instrumental activities of daily living such as paying bills or managing medications).

C. The cognitive deficits do not occur exclusively in the context of a delirium.

D. The cognitive deficits are not better explained by another mental disorder (e.g., major depressive disorder, schizophrenia).

Specify whether due to:
Alzheimer's disease
Frontotemporal lobar degeneration

BOX 22-1 **Comparison of Diagnostic Criteria—cont'd**

Lewy body disease
Vascular disease
Traumatic brain injury
Substance/medication use
HIV infection
Prion disease
Parkinson's disease
Huntington's disease
Another medical condition
Multiple etiologies
Unspecified

Specify:
   Without behavioral disturbance: If the cognitive disturbance is not accompanied by any clinically significant behavioral disturbance.
   With behavioral disturbance: *(specify disturbance):* If the cognitive disturbance is accompanied by a clinically significant behavioral disturbance (e.g., psychotic symptoms, mood disturbance, agitation, apathy, or other behavioral symptoms).

Lewy body disease
Vascular disease
Traumatic brain injury
Substance/medication use
HIV infection
Prion disease
Parkinson's disease
Huntington's disease
Another medical condition
Multiple etiologies
Unspecified

Specify:
   Without behavioral disturbance: If the cognitive disturbance is not accompanied by any clinically significant behavioral disturbance.
   With behavioral disturbance: *(specify disturbance):* If the cognitive disturbance is accompanied by a clinically significant behavioral disturbance (e.g., psychotic symptoms, mood disturbance, agitation, apathy, or other behavioral symptoms).
   Specify current severity:
   Mild: Difficulties with instrumental activities of daily living (e.g., housework, managing money)
   Moderate: Difficulties with basic activities of daily living (e.g., feeding, dressing)
   Severe: Fully dependent

Reprinted with permission from the Diagnostic and Statistical Manual of Mental Disorders, Fifth Edition *(Copyright 2013). American Psychiatric Association.*

75 to 84, and 46 percent are 85 or older. It is projected that by 2050, the number of individuals aged 65 and older with AD will number between 11 million and 16 million, if current population trends continue and no preventive treatments become available (Alzheimer's Association, 2013a). After heart disease and cancer, AD is the third most costly disease to society, accounting for $100 billion in yearly costs (NIA, 2011). This proliferation is not the result of an "epidemic." It has occurred because more people now survive into the high-risk period for neurocognitive disorder, which is age 65 and beyond.

NCDs can be classified as either primary or secondary. Primary NCDs are those, such as AD, in which the NCD itself is the major sign of some organic brain disease not directly related to any other organic illness. Secondary NCDs are caused by or related to another disease or condition, such as human immunodeficiency virus (HIV) disease or a cerebral trauma.

In NCD, impairment is evident in abstract thinking, judgment, and impulse control. The conventional rules of social conduct are often disregarded. Behavior may be uninhibited and inappropriate. Personal appearance and hygiene are often neglected.

Language may or may not be affected. Some individuals may have difficulty naming objects, or the language may seem vague and imprecise. In severe forms of NCD, the individual may not speak at all (**aphasia**). The client may know his or her needs, but may not know how to communicate those needs to a caregiver.

Personality change is common in NCD and may be manifested by either an alteration or accentuation of premorbid characteristics. For example, an individual who was previously very socially active may become apathetic and socially isolated. A previously neat person may become markedly untidy in his or her appearance. Conversely, an individual who may have had difficulty trusting others prior to the illness may exhibit extreme fear and paranoia as manifestations of the disorder.

The reversibility of NCD is dependent on the basic etiology of the disorder. Truly reversible NCD occurs in only a small percentage of cases and might be more appropriately termed *temporary*. Reversible NCD can occur as a result of cerebral lesions, depression, side effects of certain medications, normal pressure hydrocephalus, vitamin or nutritional deficiencies (especially B_{12} or folate), central nervous system infections, and metabolic disorders (Srikanth & Nagaraja, 2005). In most clients, NCD runs a progressive, irreversible course.

As the disease progresses, **apraxia**, which is the inability to carry out motor activities despite intact motor function, may develop. The individual may be irritable, moody, or exhibit sudden outbursts over trivial issues. The ability to work or care for personal needs independently will no longer be possible. These individuals can no longer be left alone because they do not comprehend their limitations and are therefore at serious risk for accidents. Wandering away from the home or care setting often becomes a problem.

Several causes have been described for NCD (see later "Predisposing Factors" section), but AD accounts for 50 to 60 percent of all cases (Black & Andreasen, 2011). The progressive nature of symptoms associated with AD has been described according to stages (Alzheimer's Association, 2013a; NIA, 2013; Stanley, Blair, & Beare, 2005):

Stage 1: No Apparent Symptoms

In the first stage of Alzheimer's disease, there is no apparent decline in memory.

Stage 2: Forgetfulness

The individual begins to lose things or forget names of people. Losses in short-term memory are common. The individual is aware of the intellectual decline and may feel ashamed, becoming anxious and depressed, which in turn may worsen the symptom. Maintaining organization with lists and a structured routine provide some compensation. These symptoms often are not observed by others.

Stage 3: Mild Cognitive Decline

In this stage, there is interference with work performance, which becomes noticeable to coworkers. The individual may get lost when driving his or her car. Concentration may be interrupted. There is difficulty recalling names or words, which becomes noticeable to family and close associates. A decline occurs in the ability to plan or organize.

Stage 4: Mild-to-Moderate Cognitive Decline

At this stage of AD, the individual may forget major events in personal history, such as his or her own child's birthday; experience declining ability to perform tasks, such as shopping and managing personal finances; or be unable to understand current news events. He or she may deny that a problem exists by covering up memory loss with **confabulation** (creating imaginary events to fill in memory gaps). Depression and social withdrawal are common.

Stage 5: Moderate Cognitive Decline

At this stage, individuals lose the ability to perform some activities of daily living (ADLs) independently, such as hygiene, dressing, and grooming, and require some assistance to manage these on an ongoing basis. They may forget addresses, phone numbers, and names of close relatives. They may become disoriented about place and time, but they maintain knowledge about themselves. Frustration, withdrawal, and self-absorption are common.

Stage 6: Moderate-to-Severe Cognitive Decline

At this stage, the individual with AD may be unable to recall recent major life events or even the name of his or her spouse. Disorientation to surroundings is common, and the person may be unable to recall the day, season, or year. The person is unable to manage ADLs without assistance. Urinary and fecal incontinence are common. Sleeping becomes a problem. Psychomotor symptoms include wandering, obsessiveness, agitation, and aggression. Symptoms seem to worsen in the late afternoon and evening—a phenomenon termed **sundowning**. Communication becomes more difficult, with increasing loss of language skills. Institutional care is usually required at this stage.

Stage 7: Severe Cognitive Decline

In the end stages of AD, the individual is unable to recognize family members. He or she most commonly is bedfast and aphasic. Problems of immobility, such as decubiti and contractures, may occur.

Stanley and associates (2005) described the late stages of neurocognitive disorders in the following manner:

> During late-stage [NCD], the person becomes more chairbound or bedbound. Muscles are rigid, contractures may develop, and primitive reflexes may be present. The person may have very active hands and repetitive movements, grunting, or other vocalizations. There is depressed immune system function, and this impairment coupled with immobility may lead to the development of pneumonia, urinary tract infections, sepsis, and pressure ulcers. Appetite decreases and dysphagia is present; aspiration is common. Weight loss generally occurs. Speech and language are severely impaired, with greatly decreased verbal communication. The person may no longer recognize any family members. Bowel and bladder incontinence are present and caregivers need to complete most ADLs for the person. The sleep-wake cycle is greatly altered, and the person spends a lot of time dozing and appears socially withdrawn and more unaware of the environment or surroundings. Death may be caused by infection, sepsis, or aspiration, although there are not many studies examining cause of death. (p. 358)

Predisposing Factors

Neurocognitive disorders are differentiated by their etiology, although they share a common symptom presentation. Categories include the following (APA, 2013):

■ Neurocognitive Disorder Due to Alzheimer's Disease
■ Vascular Neurocognitive Disorder

- Frontotemporal Neurocognitive Disorder
- Neurocognitive Disorder Due to Traumatic Brain Injury
- Neurocognitive Disorder With Lewy Bodies
- Neurocognitive Disorder Due to Parkinson's Disease
- Neurocognitive Disorder Due to HIV Infection
- Substance-Induced Neurocognitive Disorder
- Neurocognitive Disorder Due to Huntington's Disease
- Neurocognitive Disorder Due to Prion Disease
- Neurocognitive Disorder Due to Another Medical Condition
- Neurocognitive Disorder Due to Multiple Etiologies
- Unspecified Neurocognitive Disorder

Neurocognitive Disorder Due to Alzheimer's Disease

Alzheimer's disease is characterized by the syndrome of symptoms identified as *mild or major NCD* and in the seven stages described previously. The onset of symptoms is slow and insidious, and the course of the disorder is generally progressive and deteriorating. Memory impairment is an early and prominent feature.

Refinement of diagnostic criteria now enables clinicians to use specific clinical features to identify the disease with considerable accuracy. Examination by computerized tomography (CT) scan or magnetic resonance imagery (MRI) reveals a degenerative pathology of the brain that includes atrophy, widened cortical sulci, and enlarged cerebral ventricles (Figures 22-1 and 22-2). Microscopic examinations

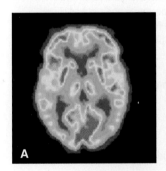
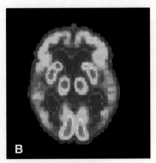
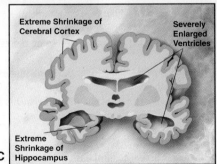

FIGURE 22-1 Changes in the Alzheimer's brain. *A.* Metabolic activity in a normal brain. *B.* Diminished metabolic activity in the Alzheimer's diseased brain. *C.* Late stage Alzheimer's disease with generalized atrophy and enlargement of the ventricles and sulci. (Source: Alzheimer's Disease Education & Referral Center, A Service of the National Institute on Aging.)

reveal numerous neurofibrillary tangles and senile plaques in the brains of clients with AD. These changes apparently occur as a part of the normal aging process. However, in clients with AD, they are found in dramatically increased numbers and their profusion is concentrated in the hippocampus and certain parts of the cerebral cortex.

Etiology

The exact cause of AD is unknown. Several hypotheses have been supported by varying amounts and quality of data. These hypotheses include:

- **Acetylcholine Alterations.** Research has indicated that in the brains of Alzheimer's clients, the enzyme required to produce acetylcholine is dramatically reduced. The reduction seems to be greatest in the nucleus basalis of the inferior medial forebrain area (Cummings & Mega, 2003). This decrease in production of acetylcholine reduces the amount of the neurotransmitter that is released to cells in the cortex and hippocampus, resulting in a disruption of the cognitive processes. Other neurotransmitters implicated in the pathology and clinical symptoms of AD include norepinephrine, serotonin, dopamine, and the amino acid glutamate. It has been proposed that in NCD, excess glutamate leads to overstimulation of the *N*-methyl-D-aspartate (NMDA) receptors, leading to increased intracellular calcium, and subsequent neuronal degeneration and cell death.

- **Plaques and Tangles.** As mentioned previously, an overabundance of structures called *plaques* and *tangles* appear in the brains of individuals with AD. The plaques are made of a protein called amyloid beta (Aβ), which are fragments of a larger protein called amyloid precursor protein (APP) (NIA, 2011). Plaques are formed when these fragments clump together and mix with molecules and other cellular matter. Tangles are formed from a special kind of cellular protein called *tau protein*, whose function it is to provide stability to the neuron. In AD, the tau protein is chemically altered (NIA, 2011). Strands of the protein become tangled together, interfering with the neuronal transport system. It is not known whether the plaques and tangles cause AD or are a consequence of the AD process. It is thought that the plaques and tangles contribute to the destruction and death of neurons, leading to memory failure, personality changes, inability to carry out ADLs, and other features of the disease.

- **Head Trauma.** Individuals who have a history of head trauma are at risk for AD (Black & Andreasen, 2011). Studies have shown that some individuals who had experienced head trauma had

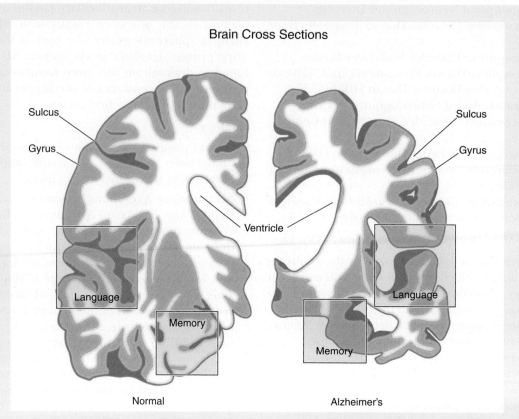

FIGURE 22–2 Neurobiology of Alzheimer's disease. (Source: American Health Assistance Foundation (2012). http://www.ahaf.org/alzdis/about/BrainAlzheimer.htm, with permission.)

NEUROTRANSMITTERS

A decrease in the neurotransmitter acetylcholine has been implicated in the etiology of Alzheimer's disease. Cholinergic sources arise from the brainstem and the basal forebrain to supply areas of the basal ganglia, thalamus, limbic structures, hippocampus, and cerebral cortex.

Cell bodies of origin for the serotonin pathways lie within the raphe nuclei located in the brainstem. Those for norepinepherine originate in the locus ceruleus. Projections for both neurotransmitters extend throughout the forebrain, prefrontal cortex, cerebellum, and limbic system. Dopamine pathways arise from areas in the midbrain and project to the frontal cortex, limbic system, basal ganglia, and thalamus. Dopamine neurons in the hypothalamus innervate the posterior pituitary.

Glutamate, an excitatory neurotransmitter, has largely descending pathways with highest concentrations in the cerebral cortex. It is also found in the hippocampus, thalamus, hypothalamus, cerebellum, and spinal cord.

AREAS OF THE BRAIN AFFECTED

Areas of the brain affected by Alzheimer's disease and associated symptoms include the following:
- Frontal lobe: Impaired reasoning ability; unable to solve problems and perform familiar tasks; poor judgment; inability to evaluate the appropriateness of behavior; aggressiveness.
- Parietal lobe: Impaired orientation ability; impaired visuospatial skills (unable to remain oriented within own environment).
- Occipital lobe: Impaired language interpretation; unable to recognize familiar objects.
- Temporal lobe: Inability to recall words; inability to use words correctly (language comprehension). In late stages, some clients experience delusions, and hallucinations.
- Hippocampus: Impaired memory. Short-term memory is affected initially. Later, the individual is unable to form new memories.
- Amygdala: Impaired emotions: depression, anxiety, fear, personality changes, apathy, paranoia.
- Neurotransmitters: Alterations in acetylcholine, dopamine, norepinephrine, serotonin and others may play a role in behaviors such as restlessness, sleep impairment, mood, and agitation.

MEDICATIONS AND THEIR EFFECTS ON THE BRAIN

1. Cholinesterase inhibitors (e.g., donepezil, rivastigmine, and galantamine) act by inhibiting acetylcholinesterase, which slows the degradation of acetylcholine, thereby increasing concentrations of the neurotransmitter in the brain. Most common side effects include dizziness, gastrointestinal upset, fatigue, and headache.
2. NMDA receptor antagonists (e.g., memantine) act by blocking NMDA receptors from excessive glutamate, preventing continuous influx of calcium into the cells, and ultimately slowing down neuronal degradation. Possible side effects include dizziness, headache, and constipation.

subsequently (after years) developed AD. This hypothesis is being investigated as a possible cause. Munoz and Feldman (2000) reported an increased risk for AD in individuals who are both genetically predisposed and who experience traumatic head injury.

■ **Genetic Factors.** There is clearly a familial pattern with some forms of AD. Some families exhibit a pattern of inheritance that suggests possible autosomal-dominant gene transmission (Sadock & Sadock, 2007). Some studies indicate that early-onset cases are more likely to be familial than late-onset cases, and that from one-third to one-half of all cases may be of the genetic form. Some research indicates that there is a link between AD and gene mutations found on chromosomes 21, 14, and 1 (Alzheimer's Disease Education & Referral [ADEAR], 2012). Mutations on chromosome 21 cause the formation of abnormal APP. Mutations on chromosome 14 cause abnormal presenilin 1 (*PS-1*) to be made, and mutations on chromosome 1 lead to the formation of abnormal presenilin 2 (*PS-2*). Each of these mutations results in an increased amount of the Aβ protein that is a major component of the plaques associated with AD. Individuals with Down syndrome (who carry an extra copy of chromosome 21) have been found to be unusually susceptible to AD (Blazer, 2008).

Two genetic variants have been identified as risk factors for late-onset AD. The apolipoprotein E epsilon4 (ApoE ε4) gene, found on chromosome 19, was identified in 1993. Its exact role in the development of AD is not yet clear (ADEAR, 2012). A second genetic variant, the SORL1 gene, was identified in 2007 (Rogaeva et al., 2007). The researchers believe that the altered gene function results in increasing production of the toxic Aβ protein and subsequently the plaques associated with AD.

Vascular Neurocognitive Disorder

In vascular NCD, the syndrome of cognitive symptoms is due to significant cerebrovascular disease. The blood vessels of the brain are affected, and progressive intellectual deterioration occurs. Vascular NCD is the second most common form of NCD, ranking after AD (Bourgeois et al., 2008).

Vascular NCD differs from AD in that it has a more abrupt onset and runs a highly variable course. Steckl (2008) states:

> Memory loss often occurs later in [Vascular NCD] compared to when it emerges in people with Alzheimer's. Typically, people with AD notice memory problems first. In contrast, people with Vascular [NCD] usually experience problems with reflexes, gait, and muscle weakness first.

In vascular NCD, progression of the symptoms occurs in "steps" rather than as a gradual deterioration; that is, at times the symptoms seem to clear up and the individual exhibits fairly lucid thinking. Memory may seem better, and the client may become optimistic that improvement is occurring, only to experience further decline of functioning in a fluctuating pattern of progression. This irregular pattern of decline appears to be an intense source of anxiety for the client with this disorder.

In vascular NCD, clients suffer the equivalent of small strokes that destroy many areas of the brain. The pattern of deficits is variable, depending on which regions of the brain have been affected. Certain focal neurological signs are commonly seen with vascular NCD, including weaknesses of the limbs, small-stepped gait, and difficulty with speech.

The disorder is more common in men than in women. Arvanitakis (2000) states:

> Prognosis for patients with vascular [NCD] is worse than that for Alzheimer's patients. The three-year mortality rate in cases over the age of 85 years old is quoted at 67 percent as compared to 42 percent in Alzheimer's disease, and 23 percent in individuals with no NCD. However, outcome is ultimately dependent on the underlying risk factors and mechanism of disease, and further studies taking these distinctions into account are warranted.

Etiology

The cause of vascular NCD is directly related to an interruption of blood flow to the brain. Symptoms result from death of nerve cells in regions nourished by diseased vessels. Various diseases and conditions that interfere with blood circulation have been implicated.

High blood pressure is thought to be one of the most significant factors in the etiology of multiple small strokes or cerebral infarcts. Hypertension leads to damage to the lining of blood vessels. This can result in rupture of the blood vessel with subsequent hemorrhage or an accumulation of fibrin in the vessel with intravascular clotting and inhibited blood flow. NCD also can result from infarcts related to occlusion of blood vessels by particulate matter that travels through the bloodstream to the brain. These emboli may be solid (e.g., clots, cellular debris, platelet aggregates), gaseous (e.g., air, nitrogen), or liquid (e.g., fat, following soft tissue trauma or fracture of long bones).

Cognitive impairment can occur with multiple small infarcts (sometimes called "silent strokes") over time or with a single cerebrovascular insult that occurs in a strategic area of the brain. An individual may have both vascular NCD and AD simultaneously. This is referred to as a *mixed* disorder, the prevalence of which is likely to increase as the population ages (Langa, Foster, & Larson, 2004).

Frontotemporal Neurocognitive Disorder

Symptoms from frontotemporal NCD occur as a result of shrinking of the frontal and temporal anterior lobes of the brain (National Institute of Neurological Disorders and Stroke [NINDS], 2012). This type of NCD was identified as Pick's disease in the *DSM-IV-TR*. The cause of frontotemporal NCD is unknown, but a genetic factor appears to be involved. Symptoms tend to fall into two clinical patterns: (1) behavioral and personality changes and (2) speech and language problems. Common behavioral changes include increasingly inappropriate actions, lack of judgment and inhibition, and repetitive compulsive behavior. There may be a marked impairment or loss of speech or increasing difficulty in using and understanding written and spoken language (Mayo Clinic, 2011). The disease progresses steadily and often rapidly, ranging from less than 2 years in some individuals to more than 10 years in others (NINDS, 2012).

Neurocognitive Disorder Due to Traumatic Brain Injury

DSM-5 criteria states that this disorder "is caused by an impact to the head or other mechanisms of rapid movement or displacement of the brain within the skull, with one or more of the following: loss of consciousness, posttraumatic amnesia, disorientation and confusion, or neurological signs (e.g., positive neuroimaging demonstrating injury, a new onset of seizures or a marked worsening of a preexisting seizure disorder, visual field cuts, anosmia, hemiparesis)" (APA, 2013, p. 625). Amnesia is the most common neurobehavioral symptom following head trauma (Bourgeois et al., 2008). Other symptoms may include confusion and changes in speech, vision, and personality. Depending on the severity of the injury, these symptoms may eventually subside or may become permanent (Smith, 2011). Repeated head trauma, such as the type experienced by boxers, can result in *dementia pugilistica*, a syndrome characterized by emotional lability, dysarthria, ataxia, and impulsivity (Sadock & Sadock, 2007).

Neurocognitive Disorder With Lewy Bodies

Clinically, Lewy body NCD is fairly similar to AD; however, it tends to progress more rapidly, and there is an earlier appearance of visual hallucinations and parkinsonian features (Rabins et al., 2006). This disorder is distinguished by the presence of Lewy bodies—eosinophilic inclusion bodies—seen in the cerebral cortex and brainstem (Black & Andreasen, 2011). These patients are highly sensitive to extrapyramidal effects of antipsychotic medications. The disease is progressive and irreversible, and may account for as many as 25 percent of all NCD cases.

Neurocognitive Disorder Due to Parkinson's Disease

NCD is observed in as many as 60 percent of clients with Parkinson's disease (Bourgeois et al., 2008). In this disease, there is a loss of nerve cells located in the substantia nigra, and dopamine activity is diminished, resulting in involuntary muscle movements, slowness, and rigidity. Tremor in the upper extremities is characteristic. In some instances, the cerebral changes that occur in NCD due to Parkinson's disease closely resemble those of AD.

Neurocognitive Disorder Due to HIV Infection

Infection with the human immunodeficiency virus-type 1 (HIV-1) can result in a NCD called *HIV-1-associated cognitive/motor complex*. A less severe form, known as *HIV-1-associated minor cognitive/motor disorder*, also occurs. The severity of symptoms is correlated to the extent of brain pathology. The immune dysfunction associated with HIV disease can lead to brain infections by other organisms, and the HIV-1 also appears to cause NCD directly. In the early stages, neuropsychiatric symptoms may be manifested by barely perceptible changes in a person's normal psychological presentation. Severe cognitive changes, particularly confusion, changes in behavior, and sometimes psychoses, are not uncommon in the later stages.

With the advent of the highly active antiretroviral therapies (HAART), incidence rates of NCD due to HIV infection have been on the decline. However, it is possible that the prolonged life span of HIV-infected patients taking medications may actually increase the numbers of individuals living with HIV-associated NCD.

Substance/Medication-Induced Neurocognitive Disorder

NCD can occur as the result of substance reactions, overuse, or abuse (Davis, 2012). Symptoms are consistent with major or mild neurocognitive disorder, and persist beyond the usual duration of intoxication and acute withdrawal (APA, 2013). Substances that have been associated with the development of NCDs include alcohol, sedatives, hypnotics, anxiolytics, and inhalants. Drugs that cause anticholinergic side effects, and toxins such as lead and mercury, have also been implicated.

Neurocognitive Disorder Due to Huntington's Disease

Huntington's disease is transmitted as a Mendelian dominant gene. Damage is seen in the areas of the basal ganglia and the cerebral cortex. The onset of symptoms (i.e., involuntary twitching of the limbs or facial muscles, mild cognitive changes, depression, and apathy) usually occurs between age 30 and 50 years. The client usually declines into a profound state of cognitive impairment and **ataxia** (muscular incoordination). The average duration of the disease is based on age at onset. One study concluded that juvenile-onset and late-onset clients have the shortest duration (Foroud, Gray, Ivashina, & Conneally, 1999). In this study, the median duration of the disease was 21.4 years.

Neurocognitive Disorder Due to Prion Disease

This disorder is identified by its insidious onset, rapid progression, and manifestations of motor features of prion disease, such as myoclonus or ataxia, or biomarker evidence (APA, 2013). Five to 15 percent of cases have a genetic component. The clinical presentation is typical of the syndrome of mild or major NCD, along with involuntary movements, muscle rigidity, and ataxia. Symptoms may develop at any age in adults, but typically occur between ages 40 and 60 years. The clinical course is extremely rapid, with the progression from diagnosis to death in less than 2 years (Rentz, 2008).

Neurocognitive Disorder Due to Another Medical Condition

A number of other general medical conditions can cause NCD. Some of these include hypothyroidism, hyperparathyroidism, pituitary insufficiency, uremia, encephalitis, brain tumor, pernicious anemia, thiamine deficiency, pellagra, uncontrolled epilepsy, cardiopulmonary insufficiency, fluid and electrolyte imbalances, CNS and systemic infections, systemic lupus erythematosus, and multiple sclerosis (Black & Andreasen, 2011; Puri & Treasaden, 2011).

The etiological factors associated with delirium and NCD are summarized in Box 22-2.

Application of the Nursing Process

Assessment

Nursing assessment of the client with delirium or mild or major NCD is based on knowledge of the symptomatology associated with the various disorders previously described in this chapter. Subjective and objective data are gathered by various members of the health-care team. Clinicians report use of a variety of methods for obtaining assessment information.

Client History

Nurses play a significant role in acquiring the client history, including the specific mental and physical changes that have occurred and the age at which the changes began. If the client is unable to relate information adequately, the data should be obtained from family members or others who would be aware of the client's physical and psychosocial history.

BOX 22-2 Etiological Factors Implicated in the Development of Delirium and/or Mild or Major Neurocognitive Disorder

BIOLOGICAL FACTORS

Hypoxia: any condition leading to a deficiency of oxygen to the brain

Nutritional deficiencies: vitamins (particularly B and C); protein; fluid and electrolyte imbalances

Metabolic disturbances: porphyria; encephalopathies related to hepatic, renal, pancreatic, or pulmonary insufficiencies; hypoglycemia

Endocrine dysfunction: thyroid, parathyroid, adrenal, pancreas, pituitary

Cardiovascular disease: stroke, cardiac insufficiency, atherosclerosis

Primary brain disorders: epilepsy, Alzheimer's disease, Huntington's disease, multiple sclerosis, Parkinson's disease

Infections: encephalitis, meningitis, pneumonia, septicemia, neurosyphilis (dementia paralytica), HIV disease, acute rheumatic fever, Creutzfeldt-Jakob disease

Intracranial neoplasms

Congenital defects: prenatal infections, such as first-trimester maternal rubella

EXOGENOUS FACTORS

Birth trauma: prolonged labor, damage from use of forceps, other obstetric complications

Cranial trauma: concussion, contusions, hemorrhage, hematomas

Volatile inhalant compounds: gasoline, glue, paint, paint thinners, spray paints, cleaning fluids, typewriter correction fluid, varnishes, and lacquers

Heavy metals: lead, mercury, manganese

Other metallic elements: aluminum

Organic phosphates: various insecticides

Substance abuse/dependence: alcohol, amphetamines, caffeine, cannabis, cocaine, hallucinogens, inhalants, nicotine, opioids, phencyclidine, sedatives, hypnotics, anxiolytics

Other medications: anticholinergics, antihistamines, antidepressants, antipsychotics, antiparkinsonians, antihypertensives, steroids, digitalis

From the client history, nurses should assess the following areas of concern: (1) type, frequency, and severity of mood swings, personality and behavioral changes, and catastrophic emotional reactions; (2) cognitive changes, such as problems with attention span, thinking process, problem solving, and memory (recent and remote); (3) language difficulties; (4) orientation to person, place, time, and situation; and (5) appropriateness of social behavior.

The nurse also should obtain information regarding current and past medication usage, history of other drug and alcohol use, and possible exposure to toxins. Knowledge regarding the history of related symptoms or specific illnesses (e.g., Huntington's disease, AD, or Parkinson's disease) in other family members might be useful.

Physical Assessment

Assessment of physical systems by both the nurse and the physician has two main emphases: (1) signs of damage to the nervous system and (2) evidence of diseases of other organs that could affect mental function. Diseases of various organ systems can induce confusion, loss of memory, and behavioral changes. These causes must be considered in diagnosing cognitive disorders. In the neurological examination, the client is asked to perform maneuvers or answer questions that are designed to elicit information about the condition of specific parts of the brain or peripheral nerves. Testing will assess mental status and alertness, muscle strength, reflexes, sensory perception, language skills, and coordination. An example of a mental status examination for a client with NCD is presented in Box 22-3.

A battery of psychological tests may be ordered as part of the diagnostic examination. The results of these tests may be used to make a differential diagnosis between NCD and **pseudodementia** (depression). Depression is the most common mental illness in the elderly, but it is often misdiagnosed and treated

---

BOX 22-3 Mental Status Examination for Neurocognitive Disorder

Patient Name_____ Date_____

Age_____ Sex_____ Diagnosis_____

	Maximum	Client's Score
1. VERBAL FLUENCY		
Ask client to name as many animals as he/she can. (Time: 60 seconds) (Score 1 point/2 animals)	10 points	_____
2. COMPREHENSION		
a. Point to the ceiling.	1 point	_____
b. Point to your nose and the window.	1 point	_____
c. Point to your foot, the door, and ceiling.	1 point	_____
d. Point to the window, your leg, the door, and your thumb.	1 point	_____
3. NAMING AND WORD FINDING		
Ask the client to name the following as you point to them:		
a. Watch stem (winder)	1 point	_____
b. Teeth	1 point	_____
c. Sole of shoe	1 point	_____
d. Buckle of belt	1 point	_____
e. Knuckles	1 point	_____
4. ORIENTATION		
a. Date	2 points	_____
b. Day of week	2 points	_____
c. Month	1 point	_____
d. Year	1 point	_____

5. NEW LEARNING ABILITY

Tell the client: "I'm going to tell you four words, which I want you to remember." Have the client repeat the four words after they are initially presented, and then say that you will ask him/her to remember the words later. Continue with the examination, and at intervals of 5 and 10 minutes, ask the client to recall the words. Three different sets of words are provided here.

		5 min.	10 min.
a. Brown (Fun) (Grape)	2 points each:	_____	_____
b. Honesty (Loyalty) (Happiness)	2 points each:	_____	_____
c. Tulip (Carrot) (Stocking)	2 points each:	_____	_____
d. Eyedropper (Ankle) (Toothbrush)	2 points each:	_____	_____

BOX 22-3 **Mental Status Examination for Neurocognitive Disorder–cont'd**

6. VERBAL STORY FOR IMMEDIATE RECALL

Tell the client: "I'm going to read you a short story, which I want you to remember. Listen closely to what I read because I will ask you to tell me the story when I finish." Read the story slowly and carefully, but without pausing at the slash marks. After completing the paragraph, tell the client to retell the story as accurately as possible. Record the number of correct memories (information within the slashes) and describe confabulation if it is present. (1 point = 1 remembered item [13 maximum points])
It was July / and the Rogers family, mom, dad, and four children / were packing up their station wagon / to go on vacation.
They were taking their yearly trip / to the beach at Gulf Shores.
This year they were making a special 1-day stop / at The Aquarium in New Orleans. After a long day's drive they arrived at the motel / only to discover that in their excitement / they had left the twins / and their suitcases / in the front yard.

13 points   _____

7. VISUAL MEMORY (HIDDEN OBJECTS)

Tell the client that you are going to hide some objects around the office (desk, bed) and that you want him/her to remember where they are. Hide four or five common objects (e.g., keys, pen, reflex hammer) in various places in the client's sight. After a delay of several minutes, ask the client to find the objects. (1 point per item found)

a. Coin	1 point	_____
b. Pen	1 point	_____
c. Comb	1 point	_____
d. Keys	1 point	_____
e. Fork	1 point	_____

8. PAIRED ASSOCIATE LEARNING

Tell the client that you are going to read a list of words two at a time. The client will be expected to remember the words that go together (e.g., big–little). When he/she is clear on the directions, read the first list of words at the rate of one pair per second. After reading the first list, test for recall by presenting the first recall list. Give the first word of a pair and ask for the word that was paired with it. Correct incorrect responses and proceed to the next pair. After the first recall has been completed, allow a 10-second delay and continue with the second presentation and recall lists.

Presentation Lists

1	2
a. High–Low	a. Good–Bad
b. House–Income	b. Book–Page
c. Good–Bad	c. High–Low
d. Book–Page	d. House–Income

Recall Lists

1	2		
a. House _____	a. High _____	2 points	_____
b. Book _____	b. Good _____	2 points	_____
c. High _____	c. House _____	2 points	_____
d. Good _____	d. Book _____	2 points	_____

9. CONSTRUCTIONAL ABILITY

Ask client to reconstruct this drawing and to draw the other 2 items:

3 points   _____

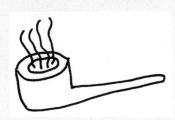

Continued

BOX 22-3 Mental Status Examination for Neurocognitive Disorder—cont'd

Draw a daisy in a flowerpot	3 points	_____
Draw a clock with all the numbers and set the clock at 2:30.	3 points	_____

10. WRITTEN COMPLEX CALCULATIONS

a. Addition	108 + 79	1 point	_____
b. Subtraction	605 − 86	1 point	_____
c. Multiplication	108 × 36	1 point	_____
d. Division	559 ÷ 43	1 point	_____

11. PROVERB INTERPRETATION
Tell the client to explain the following sayings. Record the answers.

a. Don't cry over spilled milk.	2 points	_____
b. Rome wasn't built in a day.	2 points	_____
c. A drowning man will clutch at a straw.	2 points	_____
d. A golden hammer can break down an iron door.	2 points	_____
e. The hot coal burns, the cold one blackens.	2 points	_____

12. SIMILARITIES
Ask the client to name the similarity or relationship between each of the two items.

a. Turnip... Cauliflower	2 points	_____
b. Car... Airplane	2 points	_____
c. Desk.. Bookcase	2 points	_____
d. Poem... Novel	2 points	_____
e. Horse.. Apple	2 points	_____
	Maximum: 100 points	_____

Normal Individuals		Clients with Alzheimer's Disease	
Age Group	**Mean Score (standard deviation)**	**Stage**	**Mean Score (standard deviation)**
40-49	80.9 (9.7)	I	57.2 (9.1)
50-59	82.3 (8.6)	II	37.0 (7.8)
60-69	75.5 (10.5)	III	13.4 (8.1)
70-79	66.9 (9.1)		
80-89	67.9 (11.0)		

Adapted from Strub, R.L., & Black, F.W. (2000). *The mental status examination in neurology* (4th ed.), Philadelphia, PA: F.A. Davis. With permission.

inadequately. Cognitive symptoms of depression may mimic NCD, and because of the prevalence of NCD in the elderly, diagnosticians are often too eager to make this diagnosis. A comparison of symptoms of NCD and pseudodementia (depression) is presented in Table 22-1. Nurses can assist in this assessment by carefully observing and documenting these sometimes subtle differences.

Diagnostic Laboratory Evaluations

The nurse also may be required to help the client fulfill the physician's orders for special diagnostic laboratory evaluations. Many of these tests are routinely included with the physical examination and may include evaluation of blood and urine samples to test for various infections; hepatic and renal dysfunction; diabetes or hypoglycemia; electrolyte imbalances; metabolic and endocrine disorders; nutritional deficiencies; and presence of toxic substances, including alcohol and other drugs.

Other diagnostic evaluations may be made by electroencephalogram (EEG), which measures and records the brain's electrical activity. With CT scanning, an image of the size and shape of the brain can be obtained. MRI is used to obtain a computerized image of soft tissue in the body. It provides a sharp detailed picture of the tissues of the brain. A lumbar puncture may be performed to examine the cerebrospinal fluid for evidence of CNS infection or hemorrhage. Positron emission tomography (PET) is used to reveal the metabolic activity of the brain, an evaluation some researchers believe is important in the diagnosis of AD. Researchers at the University of California Los Angeles used PET following injections of FDDNP (a molecule that binds to plaques and tangles in vitro) (Small et al., 2006). With this test, the researchers were able to distinguish between subjects with AD, those with mild cognitive impairment, and those with no cognitive impairment. With FDDNP-PET, researchers are able to accurately diagnose AD in its earlier stages and track disease progression noninvasively in a clinical setting. The researchers hope that this tool will help clinicians define therapeutic interventions before neuronal death occurs, thereby retarding the progression of the disease.

Nursing Diagnosis/Outcome Identification

Using information collected during the assessment, the nurse completes the client database, from which the selection of appropriate nursing diagnoses is determined. Table 22-2 presents a list of client behaviors and the NANDA nursing diagnoses that correspond to those behaviors, which may be used in planning care for the client with a neurocognitive disorder.

Outcome Criteria

The following criteria may be used for measurement of outcomes in the care of the client with a neurocognitive disorder.

The client:

■ Has not experienced physical injury
■ Has not harmed self or others
■ Has maintained reality orientation to the best of his or her capability
■ Is able to communicate with consistent caregiver

TABLE 22–1 A Comparison of Neurocognitive Disorder (NCD) and Pseudodementia (Depression)

SYMPTOM ELEMENT	NCD	PSEUDODEMENTIA (DEPRESSION)
Progression of symptoms	Slow	Rapid
Memory	Progressive deficits; recent memory loss greater than remote; may confabulate for memory "gaps"; no complaints of loss	More like forgetfulness; no evidence of progressive deficit; recent and remote loss equal; complaints of deficits; no confabulation (will more likely answer "I don't know")
Orientation	Disoriented to time and place; may wander in search of the familiar	Oriented to time and place; no wandering
Task performance	Consistently poor performance, but struggles to perform	Performance is variable; little effort is put forth
Symptom severity	Worse as the day progresses	Better as the day progresses
Affective distress	Appears unconcerned	Communicates severe distress
Appetite	Unchanged	Diminished
Attention and concentration	Impaired	Intact

TABLE 22–2 Assigning Nursing Diagnoses to Behaviors Commonly Associated with Neurocognitive Disorders

BEHAVIORS	NURSING DIAGNOSES
Falls, wandering, poor coordination, confusion, misinterpretation of the environment (illusions, hallucinations), lack of understanding of environmental hazards, memory deficits	Risk for trauma
Disorientation, confusion, memory deficits, inaccurate interpretation of the environment, suspiciousness, paranoia	Disturbed thought processes*; Impaired memory
Having hallucinations (hears voices, sees visions, feels crawling sensation on skin)	Disturbed sensory perception*
Aggressiveness, assaultiveness (hitting, scratching, or kicking)	Risk for other-directed violence
Inability to name objects/people, loss of memory for words, difficulty finding the right word, confabulation, incoherent, screaming and demanding verbalizations	Impaired verbal communication
Inability to perform activities of daily living (ADLs): feeding, dressing, hygiene, toileting	Self-care deficit (specify)
Expressions of shame and self-degradation, progressive social isolation, apathy, decreased activity, withdrawal, depressed mood	Situational low self-esteem; Grieving

*These nursing diagnoses have been retired from the NANDA-I list of approved diagnoses, but are used for purposes of this text.

■ Fulfills activities of daily living with assistance (or for client who is unable: has needs met, as anticipated by caregiver)
■ Discusses positive aspects about self and life

Planning/Implementation

Care for an individual with a NCD must focus on immediate needs and keeping the individual safe from harm.

Risk for Trauma

Because the individual has impairments in cognitive and psychomotor functioning, it is important to ensure that the environment be made as safe as possible to prevent injury. NANDA defines *risk for trauma* as "at risk of accidental tissue injury (e.g., wound, burn, fracture)" (NANDA International [NANDA-I], 2012, p. 444). Table 22-3 presents this nursing diagnosis in care plan format.

Client Goals

Outcome criteria include short- and long-term goals. Timelines are individually determined.

Short-Term Goals

■ Client will call for assistance when ambulating or carrying out other activities (if it is within his or her cognitive ability).
■ Client will maintain a calm demeanor, with minimal agitated behavior.
■ Client will not experience physical injury.

Long-Term Goal

■ Client will not experience physical injury.

Interventions

Interventions for preventing injury in the cognitively impaired client include the following:

■ Arrange the furniture and other items in the room to accommodate the client's disabilities. Ensure that frequently used items are stored within easy access.
■ Keep the bed in its lowest position. If allowed by hospital regulation or accrediting body, limited use of bedrails may provide a measure of safety.
■ A room near the nurse's station may be helpful to ensure that the client has close observation. In some instances, one-to-one observation may be necessary, particularly for the delirious client.
■ If the client is a smoker, ensure that cigarettes and lighter are kept at the nurses' station and dispensed only when someone is available to stay with the client while he or she is smoking.
■ Assist the client with ambulation. Provide cane or walker for balance, and instruct client in their proper use. Transport client in wheelchair when longer excursions are necessary.
■ Teach client to hold on to hand railing, if one is available, or to call for assistance when ambulating, if he or she is cognitively able.

For the Agitated Client

■ Maintain as low a level of stimuli as possible in the environment of an individual with disruptions in

Table 22-3 | CARE PLAN FOR THE CLIENT WITH A NEUROCOGNITIVE DISORDER

NURSING DIAGNOSIS: RISK FOR TRAUMA

RELATED TO: Impairments in cognitive and psychomotor functioning

OUTCOME CRITERIA	NURSING INTERVENTIONS	RATIONALE
Short-Term Goals • Client will call for assistance when ambulating or carrying out other activities (if it is within his or her cognitive ability). • Client will maintain a calm demeanor, with minimal agitated behavior. • Client will not experience physical injury. **Long-Term Goal** • Client will not experience physical injury.	The following measures may be instituted: a. Arrange furniture and other items in the room to accommodate client's disabilities. b. Store frequently used items within easy access. c. Do not keep bed in an elevated position. Pad siderails and headboard if client has history of seizures. Keep bedrails up when client is in bed (if regulations permit). d. Assign room near nurses' station; observe frequently. e. Assist client with ambulation. f. Keep a dim light on at night. g. If client is a smoker, cigarettes and lighter or matches should be kept at the nurses' station and dispensed only when someone is available to stay with client while he or she is smoking. h. Frequently orient client to place, time, and situation. i. If client is prone to wander, provide an area within which wandering can be carried out safely. j. Soft restraints may be required if client is very disoriented and hyperactive.	To ensure client safety.

cognitive processes. Irritability, hostility, aggression, and psychotic behaviors are troublesome problems that require management in individuals with cognitive disorders. It is often these behaviors that make it difficult for family to care for their loved one, and is a common cause for placement in an institution.

■ Antipsychotics have historically been used to help control behavioral problems in patients with NCD.

The conventional antipsychotics are problematic, however, because of their tendency to induce extrapyramidal side effects. The newer atypical antipsychotics have shown some effectiveness in controlling these behaviors. Although antipsychotic medications are still used for this purpose by some physicians, the U.S. Food and Drug Administration (FDA) has issued black box warnings against their use in elderly patients with NCD-related psychosis. They have been associated with increased mortality in this patient population.

■ Remain calm and undemanding, and avoid pressing the individual to perform activities that he or she is refusing. It may not be possible to reason with these clients; this may only increase the possibility for agitation. Practicing relaxation exercises and walking with the client may be of some help.

For the Client Who Wanders

A number of reasons have been proposed as to why individuals with NCD wander. Some clinicians associate wandering behavior with increased stress and anxiety or restless agitation. Others relate the behavior to stages of cognitive decline. When memory diminishes and fear sets in, individuals may wander in search of something that seems familiar to them. Increased walking at night corresponds with disruption of diurnal rhythm. In any event, wandering behavior in NCD can cause great problems for caregivers. Wandering is often a bigger problem in mid-stage NCD, and less so in later stages. Often patients new to a nursing home will wander in an attempt to become oriented to new surroundings. Wandering behavior can also be attributed to physical causes, such as hunger, thirst, and urinary or fecal urgency. When the wandering behavior begins after a long period of stability, it is likely that a new complication may be occurring—medical, psychiatric, or cognitive. Delirium may produce the abrupt onset of wandering behavior. The goals of wandering therapy are to keep the individual safe, to prevent intrusion into others' rooms, and to try to determine contributing factors to the behavior. When caring for a client who wanders, it is important to keep the following interventions in mind:

■ Keep the individual on a structured schedule of recreational activities and a strict feeding and toileting schedule.

■ Provide a safe, enclosed place for pacing and wandering.

■ Walk with the individual for a while and gently redirect him or her back to the care unit.

■ Ensure that outdoor exits are electronically controlled.

Disturbed Thought Processes/Impaired Memory and Disturbed Sensory Perception

Disturbed thought processes and sensory perception have been retired as nursing diagnoses by NANDA-I, but they are retained in this text because of their appropriateness in describing specific behaviors. In this instance, they are evidenced by disorientation, confusion, and inaccurate interpretation of the environment, including illusions, delusions, and hallucinations. *Disturbed thought processes* has been defined as

a disruption in cognitive operations and activities. *Disturbed sensory perception* is defined as a "change in the amount or patterning of incoming stimuli accompanied by a diminished, exaggerated, distorted, or impaired response to such stimuli" (NANDA-I, 2012, p. 490). *Impaired memory* is defined as the "inability to remember or recall bits of information or behavioral skills" (NANDA-I, 2012, p. 273).

Client Goals

Outcome criteria include short- and long-term goals. Timelines are individually determined.

Short-Term Goals

■ Client will utilize measures provided (e.g., clocks, calendars, room identification) to maintain reality orientation.

■ Client will experience fewer episodes of acute confusion.

Long-Term Goal

■ Client will maintain reality orientation to the best of his or her cognitive ability.

Interventions

For the Client Who Is Disoriented

■ Try to keep the client as oriented to reality as possible.

■ Use clocks and calendars with large numbers that are easy to read.

■ Place large colorful signs on the doors to identify clients' rooms, bathrooms, activity rooms, dining rooms, and chapel.

■ Allow the client to have as many of his or her personal items as possible. Even an old familiar chair in the room can provide a degree of comfort.

■ If at all possible, encourage family and close friends to be a part of the client's care, to promote feelings of security and orientation.

■ Provide the client with radio, television, and music if they are diversions the client enjoys; these may add a feeling of familiarity to the environment.

■ Ensure that noise level is controlled to prevent excess stimulation.

■ Allow the client to view old photograph albums and utilize reminiscence therapy. These are excellent ways to provide orientation to reality.

■ Maintain consistency of staff and caregivers to the best extent possible. Familiarity promotes comfort and feelings of security.

■ Continuously monitor for medication side effects. Physiological changes in the elderly can alter the body's response to certain medications. Toxic effects may intensify altered cognitive processes.

■ There has been some criticism in recent years about reality orientation of individuals with NCD (particularly those with moderate to severe disease process), suggesting that constant relearning of material contributes to problems with mood and self-esteem (Spector, Davies, Woods, & Orrell, 2000). (See Box 22-4, Validation Therapy.)

For the Client With Delusions and Hallucinations

■ Discourage rumination of delusional thinking. Do not disagree with made up stories. Instead, gently correct the client, and guide the conversation toward topics about real events and real people.

■ Never argue a point with the client; to do so only serves to increase his or her anxiety and agitation.

■ Do not ignore reports of hallucinations when it is clear that the client is experiencing them. It is important for the nurse to hear an explanation of the hallucination from the client. These perceptions are very real and often very frightening to the client. Unless they are appropriately managed, hallucinations can escalate into disturbing and even hostile behaviors. Visual and auditory hallucinations are the most common type in NCD. Often the

---

BOX 22-4 **Validation Therapy**

Some people believe it is not helpful (and sometimes even cruel) to try to insist that a person with moderate to severe NCD continually try to grasp what we know as the "real world." Allen (2000) states,

> There is no successful alternative but to accept whatever the dementia person claims as their reality, no matter how untrue it is to us. There is no successful way to 'force' a person with dementia to join the 'real' world. The most frustrated caregivers are the ones who do not accept this simple fact: the world of dementia is defined by the dementia victim.

Validation therapy (VT) was originated by Naomi Feil, a gerontological social worker, who describes the process as "communicating with a disoriented elderly person by validating and respecting their feelings in whatever time or place is real to them at the time, even though this may not correspond with our 'here and now' reality" (Day, 2013). Feil suggests that the validation principle is truthful to the person with NCD because people live on several levels of awareness (Feil, 2013). She suggests that if an individual asks to see his or her spouse, and the spouse has been dead for many years, that on some level of awareness, that person knows the truth. To keep reminding the person that the spouse is dead may only serve to cause repeated episodes of grief and distress, as he or she receives the information "anew" each time it is presented (Allen, 2000).

Validation therapy validates the feelings and emotions of a person with NCD. It often also integrates redirection techniques. Allen (2000) states, "The key is to 'agree' with what they want but by conversation and 'steering' get them to do something else without them realizing they are actually being redirected. This is both validation and redirection therapy."

EXAMPLES

💬 Mrs. W (agitated): "That old lady stole my watch! I know she did. She goes into people's rooms and takes our things. We call her 'sticky fingers'!"

Nurse: That watch is very important to you. Have you looked around the room for it?"

Mrs. W: "My husband gave it to me. He will be so upset that it is gone. I'm afraid to tell him."

Nurse: "I'm sure you miss your husband very much. Tell me what it was like when you were together. What kinds of things did you do for fun?"

Mrs. W: "We did a lot of traveling. To Italy, and England, and France. We ate wonderful food."

Nurse: "Speaking of food, it is lunch time, and I will walk with you to the dining room."

Mrs. W: "Yes, I'm getting really hungry."

In this situation, the nurse validated Mrs. W's feelings about not being able to find her watch. She did not deny that it had been stolen, nor did she remind Mrs. W that her husband was deceased. (*Remember: a concept of VT is that on some level, Mrs. W knows that her husband is dead.*) The nurse validated the emotions Mrs. W was feeling about missing her husband. She brought up special times that Mrs. W and her husband had spent together, which served to elevate her mood and self-esteem. And lastly, she redirected Mrs. W to the dining room to have her lunch. (The watch was eventually found in Mrs. W's medicine cabinet, where she had hidden it for safekeeping.)

Feil (2013) presents another example:

> When a resident asks for his wife who is dead, caregivers reply, "She'll be here to see you later." The resident may not remember much, but he clings to that statement. He continues to ask for his wife on a daily basis, and the caregivers continue to lie. Eventually he loses trust in the caregivers, knowing that what they say is not true. With VT, the caregivers would encourage the resident to talk about his wife. They would validate his emotions, and encourage him to express his needs, accepting the fact that there is a reason behind his behavior. He has not simply "forgotten that his wife died;" he needs to grieve for her. This is unfinished business. When the emotion is expressed and someone listens with empathy, it is relieved. The old man no longer needs to search for his wife. He feels safe with the caregiver, whom he trusts. He always knew on a deep level of awareness that his wife had died. (pp. 3, 4)

physician will treat these manifestations with antipsychotic medication.

■ Rule out the disturbed sensory perception as a possible side effect of certain physical conditions or medications.

■ Check to ensure that hearing aid is working properly and to ensure that faulty sounds are not being emitted.

■ Check eyeglasses to ensure that the individual is indeed wearing his or her own glasses.

■ Try to determine from where the visual hallucination is emanating. Clients often see faces in patterns on fabrics or in pictures on the wall. A mirror can also be the culprit of false perceptions. These may need to be moved or covered.

■ Provide reassurance that the client is safe. It may be necessary to stay with the client for a while until he or she is calm.

■ Never argue that the hallucination is not real. Try to let the client know that, although you are not sharing their experience, you understand how very distressing it is for him or her.

■ Distract the client. Hallucinations are less likely to occur when the person is occupied or involved in what is going on around them. Focus on real situations and real people.

■ Depending on the situation, it may be better to go along with the client rather than attempting to distract him or her (McShane, 2000). Not all hallucinations are upsetting.

EXAMPLE

An elderly woman approaches the nurses' station and says, "I'm so perturbed. The woman in my room refuses to turn down my bed so that I can go to sleep." The nurse may respond, "I'm sorry for the inconvenience, Mrs. G., but I will walk to your room with you and see that your bed is turned down." The nurse chats with Mrs. G. about something that occurred during the day, and by the time they arrive at her room, there is no further mention of a woman in her room.

Impaired Verbal Communication

When individuals who are cognitively impaired begin to lose their ability to process verbal communication, how words are expressed becomes as important as what is said. NANDA defines *impaired verbal communication* as "decreased, delayed, or absent ability to receive, process, transmit, and/or use a system of symbols" (NANDA-I, 2012, p. 275).

Client Goals

Outcome criteria include short- and long-term goals. Timelines are individually determined.

Short-Term Goals

■ Client will be able to make needs known to primary caregiver.

■ Client is able to understand basic communications in interactions with primary caregiver.

Long-Term Goal

■ (In later stages of the illness, when client is unable to communicate), needs are anticipated and fulfilled by primary caregiver.

Interventions

■ Keep interactions with the client calm and reassuring.

■ Use simple words, speak slowly and distinctly, and keep face-to-face contact with the client.

■ Always identify yourself to the client, and call the client by name at each meeting.

■ Use nonverbal gestures to help the client understand what you want him or her to accomplish, if appropriate.

■ Ask only one question (or give only one direction) at a time, and give the client plenty of time to process the information and respond. The question may need to be rephrased if it is clear that the client has not understood the meaning of the direction.

■ Always try to approach the client from the front. An unexpected approach or touch from behind may startle and upset the client, and may even promote aggressive behavior.

■ Maintain consistency of staff and caregivers to the best extent possible. This facilitates comfort and security and promotes an effective communication process with the client.

■ Should the client become verbally aggressive, remain calm, and provide validation for his or her feelings: "I know this is a hard time for you. You were always so busy and so active, and you took care of so many people. Maybe you could tell me about some of those people."

■ When it is clearly appropriate, use touch and affection to communicate. Sometimes clients will respond to a hug or to a hand reaching for theirs when they will respond to nothing else.

Self-Care Deficit

It is important for clients to remain as independent as possible for as long as possible. They should be encouraged to accomplish ADLs to the best of their ability. NANDA defines *self-care deficit* as "impaired ability to perform [activities of daily living] for self" (NANDA-I, 2012, pp. 250-253).

Client Goals

Outcome criteria include short- and long-term goals. Timelines are individually determined.

Short-Term Goal

■ Client will participate in ADLs with assistance from caregiver.

Long-Term Goals

■ Client will accomplish ADLs to the best of his or her ability.

■ Unfulfilled needs will be met by caregiver.

Interventions

■ Provide a simple, structured environment for the client, identify self-care deficits, and offer assistance as required.

■ Allow plenty of time for the client to complete tasks.

■ Provide guidance and support for independent actions by talking the client through the task one step at a time.

■ Provide a structured schedule of activities that does not change from day to day.

■ Ensure that ADLs follow the client's usual routine as closely as possible.

■ Minimize confusion by providing for consistency in assignment of daily caregivers.

■ Perform an ongoing assessment of the client's ability to fulfill his or her nutritional needs, ensure personal safety, follow the medication regimen, and communicate the need for assistance with activities that he or she cannot accomplish independently. Anticipate needs that are not verbally communicated.

■ If the client is to be discharged to family caregivers, assess those caregivers' ability to anticipate and fulfill client's unmet needs. Provide information to assist caregivers with this responsibility. Ensure that caregivers are aware of available community support systems from which they may seek assistance when required. Examples include adult day-care centers, housekeeping and homemaker services, respite care services, or the local chapter of a national support organization. Two of these include the following:

  ■ For Alzheimer's disease information:
  Alzheimer's Association
  225 N. Michigan Ave., Fl. 17
  Chicago, IL 60601-7633
  1-800-272-3900
  http://www.alz.org

  ■ For Parkinson's disease information:
  National Parkinson Foundation, Inc.
  1501 N.W. 9th Ave.
  Miami, FL 33136-1494
  1-800-272-3900
  http://www.parkinson.org

Concept Care Mapping

The concept map care plan is an innovative approach to planning and organizing nursing care (see Chapter 9). It is a diagrammatic teaching and learning strategy that allows visualization of interrelationships among medical diagnoses, nursing diagnoses, assessment data, and treatments. An example of a concept map care plan for a client with a neurocognitive disorder is presented in Figure 22-3.

Client/Family Education

The role of client teacher is important in the psychiatric area, as it is in all areas of nursing. A list of topics for client/family education relevant to neurocognitive disorders is presented in Box 22-5. Sample client teaching guides can be found online at davisplus.fadavis.com.

Evaluation

In the final step of the nursing process, reassessment occurs to determine if the nursing interventions have been effective in achieving the intended goals of care. Evaluation of the client with a NCD is based on a series of short-term goals rather than on long-term goals. Resolution of identified problems is unrealistic for this client. Instead, outcomes must be measured in terms of slowing down the process rather than stopping or curing the problem. Evaluation questions may include the following:

■ Has the client experienced injury?

■ Does the client maintain orientation to time, person, place, and situation to the best of his or her cognitive ability?

■ Is the client able to fulfill basic needs? Have those needs unmet by the client been fulfilled by caregivers?

■ Is confusion minimized by familiar objects and structured, routine schedule of activities?

■ Do the prospective caregivers have information regarding the progression of the client's illness?

■ Do caregivers have information regarding where to go for assistance and support in the care of their loved one?

■ Have the prospective caregivers received instruction in how to promote the client's safety, minimize confusion and disorientation, and cope with difficult client behaviors (e.g., hostility, anger, depression, agitation)?

Quality and Safety Education for Nurses (QSEN)

The Institute of Medicine (IOM), in its 2003 report, *Health Professions Education: A Bridge to Quality,* challenged faculties of medicine, nursing, and other health professions to ensure that their graduates have achieved a core set of competencies in order to meet the needs of the 21st-century health-care system. These competencies include *providing patient-centered care, working in interdisciplinary teams, employing evidence-based practice, applying quality improvement, ensuring safety,* and *utilizing informatics.* A QSEN teaching strategy is included in Box 22-6. The use of this type of activity is intended to arm the instructor and the student with guidelines for attaining the knowledge, skills, and attitudes necessary for achievement of quality and safety competencies in nursing.

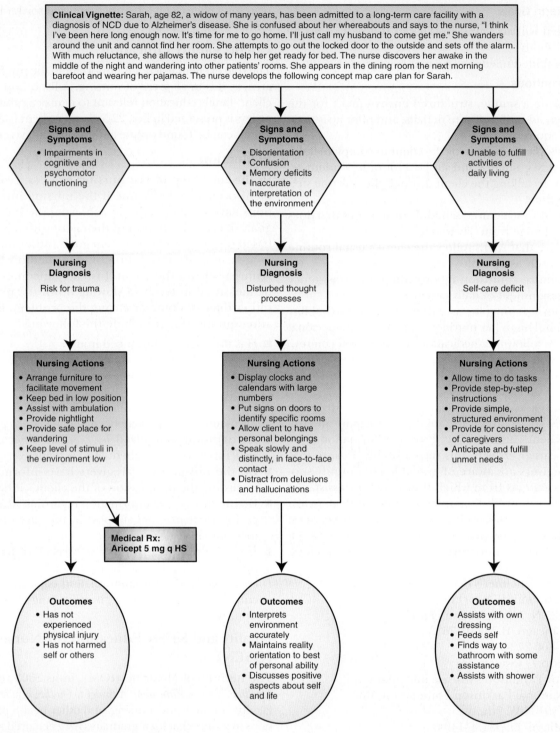

Clinical Vignette: Sarah, age 82, a widow of many years, has been admitted to a long-term care facility with a diagnosis of NCD due to Alzheimer's disease. She is confused about her whereabouts and says to the nurse, "I think I've been here long enough now. It's time for me to go home. I'll just call my husband to come get me." She wanders around the unit and cannot find her room. She attempts to go out the locked door to the outside and sets off the alarm. With much reluctance, she allows the nurse to help her get ready for bed. The nurse discovers her awake in the middle of the night and wandering into other patients' rooms. She appears in the dining room the next morning barefoot and wearing her pajamas. The nurse develops the following concept map care plan for Sarah.

Signs and Symptoms
- Impairments in cognitive and psychomotor functioning

Signs and Symptoms
- Disorientation
- Confusion
- Memory deficits
- Inaccurate interpretation of the environment

Signs and Symptoms
- Unable to fulfill activities of daily living

Nursing Diagnosis
Risk for trauma

Nursing Diagnosis
Disturbed thought processes

Nursing Diagnosis
Self-care deficit

Nursing Actions
- Arrange furniture to facilitate movement
- Keep bed in low position
- Assist with ambulation
- Provide nightlight
- Provide safe place for wandering
- Keep level of stimuli in the environment low

Nursing Actions
- Display clocks and calendars with large numbers
- Put signs on doors to identify specific rooms
- Allow client to have personal belongings
- Speak slowly and distinctly, in face-to-face contact
- Distract from delusions and hallucinations

Nursing Actions
- Allow time to do tasks
- Provide step-by-step instructions
- Provide simple, structured environment
- Provide for consistency of caregivers
- Anticipate and fulfill unmet needs

Medical Rx:
Aricept 5 mg q HS

Outcomes
- Has not experienced physical injury
- Has not harmed self or others

Outcomes
- Interprets environment accurately
- Maintains reality orientation to best of personal ability
- Discusses positive aspects about self and life

Outcomes
- Assists with own dressing
- Feeds self
- Finds way to bathroom with some assistance
- Assists with shower

FIGURE 22–3 Concept map care plan for client with major NCD.

Medical Treatment Modalities

Delirium

The first step in the treatment of delirium should be the determination and correction of the underlying causes. Additional attention must be given to fluid and electrolyte status, hypoxia, anoxia, and diabetic problems. Staff members should remain with the client at all times to monitor behavior and provide reorientation and assurance. The room should maintain a low level of stimuli.

Some physicians prefer not to prescribe medications for the client with delirium, reasoning that additional agents may only compound the syndrome of brain dysfunction. However, the agitation and aggression demonstrated by the client with delirium

<table>
<tr><td>

BOX 22-5 Topics for Client/Family Education Related to Neurocognitive Disorders

1. Nature of the illness
   a. Possible causes
   b What to expect
   c. Symptoms
2. Management of the illness
   a. Ways to ensure client safety
   b. How to maintain reality orientation
   c. Providing assistance with ADLs
   d. Nutritional information
   e. Difficult behaviors
   f. Medication administration
   g. Matters related to hygiene and toileting
3. Support services
   a. Financial assistance
   b. Legal assistance
   c. Caregiver support groups
   d. Respite care
   e. Home health care

</td></tr>
</table>

may require chemical and/or mechanical restraint for his or her personal safety. Choice of specific therapy is made with consideration for the client's clinical condition and the underlying cause of the delirium. Low-dose antipsychotics are the pharmacological treatment of choice in most cases (Schatzberg, Cole, & DeBattista, 2010). A benzodiazepine (e.g.,

lorazepam) is commonly used when the etiology is substance withdrawal (Eisendrath & Lichtmacher, 2012).

Neurocognitive Disorder

Once a definitive diagnosis of NCD has been made, a primary consideration in the treatment of the disorder is the etiology. Focus must be directed to the identification and resolution of potentially reversible processes. Sadock and Sadock (2007) stated:

> Once dementia is diagnosed, patients must undergo a complete medical and neurological workup, because 10 to 15 percent of all patients with dementia have a potentially reversible condition if treatment is initiated before permanent brain damage occurs. [Causes of potentially-reversible NCD include] hypothyroidism, normal pressure hydrocephalus, and brain tumors. (p. 340)

The need for general supportive care, with provisions for security, stimulation, patience, and nutrition, has been recognized and accepted. A number of pharmaceutical agents have been tried, with varying degrees of success, in the treatment of clients with NCD. Some of these drugs are described in the following sections according to symptomatology for which they are indicated. A summary of medications for clients with NCD is provided in Table 22-4.

Cognitive Impairment

The cholinesterase inhibitor physostigmine (Antilirium) has been shown to enhance cognitive functioning in individuals with mild to moderate AD, although

---

BOX 22-6 QSEN TEACHING STRATEGY

Assignment: Linking Evidence-Based Practice With a Nursing Procedure
Reality Orientation of Clients With Neurocognitive Disorder

Competency Domain: Evidence-Based Practice

Learning Objectives: Student will:
- Locate an evidence-based practice article on a hospital protocol, and compare and contrast this information with the facility's protocol.
- Identify whether evidence-based practice is utilized with this protocol, and identify barriers or challenges with implementing evidence-based practice in the clinical setting.

Strategy Overview:
1. Research the nursing intervention of reality orientation of clients with NCD. Identify the pros and cons and ethical issues associated with this intervention (particularly with clients who have advanced NCD).
2. Find an evidence-based practice journal article about the intervention.
3. Locate the facility's protocol for reality orientation of clients with NCD.
4. Compare and contrast the facility's protocol with how unit staff carry out this intervention. If there are deviations from the written protocol, what are they and why do they occur?
5. Compare and contrast the hospital's protocol with the information found in the evidence-based practice article.
6. At postconference, summarize the article on evidence-based practice to the clinical group, and report information gathered throughout the clinical day. Discuss any ethical dilemmas associated with the intervention.
7. Write a paper discussing personal reflections and feelings about this intervention.

Adapted from teaching strategy submitted by Chris Tesch, Instructor, University of South Dakota, Sioux Falls, SD. © 2009 QSEN; http://qsen.org. With permission.

TABLE 22–4	**Selected Medications Used in the Treatment of Clients with NCD**			
MEDICATION	CLASSIFICATION	FOR TREATMENT OF	DAILY DOSAGE RANGE (mg)	SIDE EFFECTS
Donepezil (Aricept)	Cholinesterase inhibitor	Cognitive impairment	5–10	Insomnia, dizziness, GI upset, headache
Rivastigmine (Exelon)	Cholinesterase inhibitor	Cognitive impairment	6–12	Dizziness, headache, GI upset, fatigue
Galantamine (Razadyne)	Cholinesterase inhibitor	Cognitive impairment	8–24	Dizziness, headache, GI upset
Memantine (Namenda)	NMDA receptor antagonist	Cognitive impairment	5–20	Dizziness, headache, constipation
Risperidone* (Risperdal)	Antipsychotic	Agitation, aggression, hallucinations, thought disturbances, wandering	1–4 (Increase dosage cautiously)	Agitation, insomnia, headache, extrapyramidal symptoms
Olanzapine* (Zyprexa)	Antipsychotic	Agitation, aggression, hallucinations, thought disturbances, wandering	5 (Increase dosage cautiously)	Hypotension, dizziness, sedation, constipation, weight gain, dry mouth
Quetiapine* (Seroquel)	Antipsychotic	Agitation, aggression, hallucinations, thought disturbances, wandering	Initial dose 25 (Titrate slowly)	Hypotension, tachycardia, dizziness, drowsiness, headache, constipation, dry mouth
Haloperidol* (Haldol)	Antipsychotic	Agitation, aggression, hallucinations, thought disturbances, wandering	1–4 (Increase dosage cautiously)	Dry mouth, blurred vision, orthostatic hypotension, extrapyramidal symptoms, sedation
Sertraline (Zoloft)	Antidepressant (SSRI)	Depression	50–100	Fatigue, insomnia, sedation, GI upset, headache, dizziness
Paroxetine (Paxil)	Antidepressant (SSRI)	Depression	10–40	Dizziness, headache, insomnia, somnolence, GI upset
Nortriptyline (Pamelor)	Antidepressant (Tricyclic)	Depression	30–50	Anticholinergic, orthostatic hypotension, sedation, arrhythmia
Lorazepam (Ativan)	Antianxiety (Benzodiazepine)	Anxiety	1–2	Drowsiness, dizziness, GI upset, hypotension, tolerance, dependence
Oxazepam (Serax)	Antianxiety (Benzodiazepine)	Anxiety	10–30	Drowsiness, dizziness, GI upset, hypotension, tolerance, dependence
Temazepam (Restoril)	Sedative/ Hypnotic (Benzodiazepine)	Insomnia	15	Drowsiness, dizziness, GI upset, hypotension, tolerance, dependence

Continued

TABLE 22–4	**Selected Medications Used in the Treatment of Clients with NCD—cont'd**			
MEDICATION	CLASSIFICATION	FOR TREATMENT OF	DAILY DOSAGE RANGE (mg)	SIDE EFFECTS
Zolpidem (Ambien)	Sedative/ Hypnotic (Nonbenzodiazepine)	Insomnia	5	Headache, drowsiness, dizziness, GI upset
Zaleplon (Sonata)	Sedative/ Hypnotic (Nonbenzodiazepine)	Insomnia	5	Headache, drowsiness, dizziness, GI upset
Eszopiclone (Lunesta)	Sedative- Hypnotic (Nonbenzodiazepine)	Insomnia	1–2	Headache, drowsiness, dizziness, GI upset, unpleasant taste
Ramelteon (Rozerem)	Sedative- Hypnotic (Nonbenzodiazepine)	Insomnia	8	Dizziness, fatigue, drowsiness, GI upset
Trazodone	Antidepressant (Heterocyclic)	Depression and Insomnia	50	Dizziness, drowsiness, dry mouth, blurred vision, GI upset
Mirtazapine (Remeron)	Antidepressant (Tetracyclic)	Depression and Insomnia	7.5–15	Somnolence, dry mouth, constipation, increased appetite

*Although clinicians may still prescribe these medications in low-risk patients, no antipsychotics have been approved by the FDA for the treatment of patients with NCD-related psychosis. All antipsychotics include black box warnings about increased risk of death in elderly patients with NCD.

its short half-life makes it less desirable than the newer medications (Coelho Filho & Birks, 2001).

Other cholinesterase inhibitors are also being used for treatment of mild to moderate cognitive impairment in AD. (Higher dose donepezil has also been approved for moderate to severe AD.) Some of the clinical manifestations of AD are thought to be the result of a deficiency of the neurotransmitter acetylcholine. In the brain, acetylcholine is inactivated by the enzyme acetylcholinesterase. Donepezil (Aricept), rivastigmine (Exelon), and galantamine (Razadyne) act by inhibiting acetylcholinesterase, which slows the degradation of acetylcholine, thereby increasing concentrations of the neurotransmitter in the cerebral cortex. Because their action relies on functionally intact cholinergic neurons, the effects of these medications may lessen as the disease process advances, and there is no evidence that these medications alter the course of the underlying degenerative process.

Another medication, an N-methyl-D-aspartate (NMDA) receptor antagonist, was approved by the FDA in 2003. The medication, memantine (Namenda), was approved for the treatment of moderate to severe AD. High levels of glutamate in the brains of AD patients are thought to contribute to the symptomatology and decline in functionality. These high

levels are caused by a dysfunction in glutamate transmission. In normal neurotransmission, glutamate plays an essential role in learning and memory by triggering NMDA receptors to allow a controlled amount of calcium to flow into a nerve cell. This creates the appropriate environment for information processing. In AD, there is a sustained release of glutamate, which results in a continuous influx of calcium into the nerve cells. This increased intracellular calcium concentration ultimately leads to disruption and death of the neurons. Memantine may protect cells against excess glutamate by partially blocking NMDA receptors. Memantine has been shown in clinical trials to be effective in improving cognitive function and the ability to perform ADLs in clients with moderate to severe AD. Although it does not stop or reverse the effects of the disease, it has been shown to slow down the progression of the decline in cognition and function (Salloway & Correia, 2009). Because memantine's action differs from that of the cholinesterase inhibitors, consideration is being given to possible co-administration of these medications. Ongoing research is revealing a greater improvement in cognitive function, ADLs, behavior, and clinical global status in clients who are administered a combination of memantine and a cholinesterase inhibitor than those administered either drug alone (Diamond, 2008).

Current drug trials are under way to test for a vaccine against AD. One recent study led by the Karolinska Institutet in Sweden reports positive use with CAD106, a vaccine designed to trigger the body's immune defense against beta-amyloid (Winblad et al., 2012). In a study funded by the U.S. Institutes of Health, three drugs are currently in clinical trials to be evaluated in the prevention of a rare and aggressive form of autosomal-dominant AD (Bateman et al., 2012). This study includes individuals who are mutation carriers, and are therefore genetically destined to develop AD at a young age, typically when they are in their 30s, 40s, or 50s. Because these individuals exhibit measurable biochemical and imaging changes up to 25 years before AD symptoms appear, the drugs will target these biomarkers to determine if the treatment can stop or slow the disease process.

Agitation, Aggression, Hallucinations, Thought Disturbances, and Wandering

Historically, physicians have prescribed antipsychotic medications to control agitation, aggression, hallucinations, thought disturbances, and wandering in clients with NCD. The atypical antipsychotic medications, such as risperidone, olanzapine, quetiapine, and ziprasidone, are often favored because of their lessened propensity to cause anticholinergic and extrapyramidal side effects. In 2005, however, following review of a number of studies, the FDA ordered black box warnings on drug labels of all the atypical antipsychotics noting that the drugs are associated with an increased risk of death in elderly patients with psychotic behaviors associated with NCD. Most of the deaths appeared to be cardiovascular related. In July 2008, based on the results of several studies, the FDA extended this warning to include all first-generation antipsychotics as well, such as haloperidol and perphenazine. This poses a clinical dilemma for physicians who have found these medications to be helpful to their clients, and some have chosen to continue to use them in clients without significant cerebrovascular disease, in which previous behavioral programs have failed, and with consent from relatives or guardians who are clearly aware of the risks and benefits.

Anticholinergic Effects

Many antipsychotic, antidepressant, and antihistaminic medications produce anticholinergic side effects, which include confusion, blurred vision, constipation, dry mouth, dizziness, and difficulty urinating. Older people, and especially those with NCD, are particularly sensitive to these effects because of decreased cholinergic reserves. Many elderly individuals are also at increased risk for developing an anticholinergic toxicity syndrome because of the additive anticholinergic effects of multiple medications (Hall, Hall, & Chapman, 2009).

Depression

It is estimated that up to 40 percent of people with AD also suffer from major depression (Alzheimer's Association, 2013b). Recognizing the symptoms of depression in these individuals is often a challenge. Depression—which affects thinking, memory, sleep, appetite, and interferes with daily life—is sometimes difficult to distinguish from NCD. Clearly, the existence of depression in the client with NCD complicates and worsens the individual's functioning.

Antidepressant medication is sometimes used in treatment of depression in NCD. The selective serotonin reuptake inhibitors (SSRIs) are considered by many to be the first-line drug treatment for depression in the elderly because of their favorable side effect profile. Although still used by some physicians, tricyclic antidepressants are often avoided because of cardiac and anticholinergic side effects. Trazodone may be a good choice, used at bedtime, for depression and insomnia. Dopaminergic agents (e.g., methylphenidate, amantadine, bromocriptine, and bupropion) may be helpful in the treatment of severe apathy (Rabins et al., 2006).

Not only is depression common in AD, but research has recently suggested that it may be a risk factor for the disease (Geerlings, den Heijer, Koudstaal, Hofman, & Breteler, 2008). This study found that individuals with a history of depression, particularly those with onset before age 60, had a 2.5 times greater risk of developing AD than people who had not suffered from depression. The authors suggest that further studies are required to understand the relationship between depression and AD. It is not completely understood whether depression contributes to the development of AD or whether another unknown factor is involved in the etiology of both. In another study, Caraci, Copani, Nicoletti, and Drago (2010) report that "molecular mechanisms and cascades that underlie the pathogenesis of major depression, such as chronic inflammation and hyperactivation of hypothalamic-pituitary-adrenal axis, are also involved in the pathogenesis of Alzheimer's disease" (p. 64).

Anxiety

The progressive loss of mental functioning is a significant source of anxiety in the early stages of NCD. It is important that clients be encouraged to verbalize their feelings and fears associated with this loss. These interventions may be useful in reducing the anxiety of clients with NCD.

Antianxiety medications may be helpful but should not be used routinely or for prolonged periods. The least toxic and most effective of the antianxiety medications are the benzodiazepines. Examples include diazepam (Valium), chlordiazepoxide (Librium), alprazolam (Xanax), lorazepam (Ativan), and oxazepam (Serax). The drugs with shorter half-lives (e.g., lorazepam and oxazepam) are preferred to those longer-acting medications (e.g., diazepam), which promote a higher risk of oversedation and falls. Barbiturates are not appropriate as antianxiety agents because they frequently induce confusion and paradoxical excitement in elderly individuals.

Sleep Disturbances

Sleep problems are common in clients with NCD and often intensify as the disease progresses. Wakefulness and nighttime wandering create much distress and anguish in family members who are charged with protection of their loved one. Indeed, sleep disturbances are among the problems that most frequently initiate the need for placement of the client in a long-term care facility.

Some physicians treat sleep problems with sedative-hypnotic medications. The benzodiazepines may be useful for some clients but are indicated for relatively brief periods only. Examples include flurazepam (Dalmane), temazepam (Restoril), and triazolam (Halcion). Daytime sedation and cognitive impairment, in addition to paradoxical agitation in elderly clients,

are of particular concern with these medications. The nonbenzodiazepine sedative-hypnotics zolpidem (Ambien), zaleplon (Sonata), eszopiclone (Lunesta), and ramelteon (Rozerem) and the antidepressants trazodone (Desyrel) and mirtazapine (Remeron) are also prescribed. Daytime sedation may also be a problem with these medications. As previously stated, barbiturates should not be used in elderly clients. Sleep problems are usually ongoing, and most clinicians prefer to use medications only to help an individual through a short-term stressful situation. Rising at the same time each morning; minimizing daytime sleep; participating in regular physical exercise (but no later than 4 hours before bedtime); getting proper nutrition; avoiding alcohol, caffeine, and nicotine; and retiring at the same time each night are behavioral approaches to sleep problems that may eliminate the need for sleep aids, particularly in the early stages of NCD. Because of the tremendous potential for adverse drug reactions in the elderly, many of whom are already taking multiple medications, pharmacological treatment of insomnia should be considered only after attempts at nonpharmacological strategies have failed.

CASE STUDY AND SAMPLE CARE PLAN

NURSING HISTORY AND ASSESSMENT

Carmen is an 81-year-old widow who has lived in the same small town, in the same house that she shared with her husband until his death 16 years ago. She and her husband reared two daughters, Joan and Nancy, who have been living with their husbands in a large city about 2 hours away from Carmen. They have always visited Carmen every 1 or 2 months. She has four grown grandchildren who live in distant states, and who see their grandmother on holidays.

About a year ago, Carmen's daughters began to receive reports from friends and other family members about incidents in which Carmen was becoming forgetful (e.g., forgetting to go to a cousin's birthday party, taking a wrong turn and getting lost on the way to a niece's house [where she had driven many times], returning to church to search for something she thought she "had forgotten" [although she could not explain what it was], sending birthday gifts to people when it was not their birthday). During routine visits, the elder daughter, Joan, found bills left unpaid, sometimes months overdue. Housekeepers and yard workers reported to Joan that Carmen would forget she had paid them, and try to pay them again . . . and sometimes a third time. She became very confused when she would attempt to fill her weekly pillboxes, a task she had completed in the past without difficulty. Hundreds of dollars would disappear from her wallet, and she could not tell Joan what happened to it.

Joan and her husband subsequently moved to the small town where Carmen lived. They bought a home, and Joan visited her mother every day, took care of finances, and ensured that Carmen took her daily medications, although Joan

worked in a job that required occasional out of town travel. As the months progressed, Carmen's cognitive abilities deteriorated. She burned food on the stove, left the house with the broiler-oven on, forgot to take her medication, got lost in her car, missed appointments, and forgot the names of her neighbors whom she had known for many years. She began to lose weight because she was forgetting to eat her meals.

Carmen was evaluated by a neurologist, who diagnosed her with neurocognitive disorder due to Alzheimer's disease. Because they believed that Carmen needed 24-hour care, Joan and Nancy made the painful decision to place Carmen in long-term care. In the nursing home, her condition has continued to deteriorate. Carmen wanders up and down the halls (day and night), and she has fallen twice, once while attempting to get out of bed. She requires assistance to shower and dress, and has become incontinent of urine. The nurses found her attempting to leave the building, saying, "I'm going across the street to visit my daughter." One morning at breakfast she appeared in her pajamas in the communal dining room, not realizing that she had not dressed. She is unable to form new memories, and sometimes uses confabulation to fill in the blanks. She asks the same questions repeatedly, sometimes struggling for the right word. She can no longer provide the correct names of items in her environment. She has no concept of time.

Joan visits Carmen daily, and Nancy visits weekly, each offering support to the other in person and by phone. Carmen always seems pleased to see them, but can no longer call either of them by name. They are unsure if she knows who they are.

CASE STUDY AND SAMPLE CARE PLAN—cont'd

NURSING DIAGNOSES/OUTCOME IDENTIFICATION

From the assessment data, the nurse develops the following nursing diagnoses for Carmen:

1. **Risk for trauma** related to impairments in cognitive and psychomotor functioning; wandering; falls
   a. **Outcome Criteria:** Carmen will remain injury free during her nursing home stay.
   b. **Short-Term Goals:**
      - Carmen will not fall while wandering the halls.
      - Carmen will not fall out of bed.
2. **Disturbed thought processes** related to cerebral degeneration evidenced by disorientation, confusion, and memory deficits
   a. **Outcome Criteria:** Carmen will maintain reality orientation to the best of her cognitive ability.
   b. **Short-Term Goals:**
      - Carmen will be able to find her room.
      - Carmen will be able to communicate her needs to staff.
3. **Self-care deficit** related to cognitive impairments, disorientation, confusion, and memory deficits
   a. **Outcome Criteria:** Carmen will accomplish ADLs to the best of her ability.
   b. **Short-Term Goals:**
      - Carmen will assist with dressing herself.
      - Carmen will cooperate with trips to the bathroom.
      - Carmen will wash herself in the shower, with help from the nurse.

PLANNING/IMPLEMENTATION

RISK FOR TRAUMA
The following nursing interventions may be implemented *in an effort to ensure client safety:*

1. Arrange the furniture in Carmen's room so that it will accommodate her moving around freely.
2. Store frequently used items within her easy reach.
3. Provide a "low bed," or possibly move her mattress from the bed to the floor, to prevent falls from bed.
4. Attach a bed alarm to alert the nurse's station when Carmen has alighted from her bed.
5. Keep a dim light on in her room at night.
6. During the day and evening, provide a well-lighted area where Carmen can safely wander.
7. Ensure that all outside doors are electronically controlled.
8. Play soft music and maintain a low level of stimuli in the environment.

DISTURBED THOUGHT PROCESSES
The following nursing interventions may be implemented *to help maintain orientation and aid in memory and recognition:*

1. Use clocks and calendars with large numbers that are easy to read.

2. Put a sign on Carmen's door with her name on it, and hang a personal item of hers on the door.
3. Ask Joan to bring some of Carmen's personal items for her room, even a favorite comfy chair, if possible. Ask also for some old photograph albums if they are available.
4. Keep staff and caregivers to a minimum to promote familiarity.
5. Speak slowly and clearly while looking into Carmen's face.
6. Use reminiscence therapy with Carmen. Ask her to share happy times from her life with you. This technique helps decrease depression and boost self-esteem.
7. Mention the date and time in casual conversation. Refer to "spring rain," "summer flowers," "fall leaves." Emphasize holidays.
8. Correct misperceptions gently and matter-of-factly, and focus on real events and real people if false ideas should occur. Validate her feelings associated with current and past life situations.
9. Monitor for medication side effects, because toxic effects from certain medications can intensify altered thought processes.

SELF-CARE DEFICIT
The following nursing interventions may be implemented *to ensure that all Carmen's needs are fulfilled:*

1. Assess what Carmen can do independently and with what she needs assistance.
2. Allow plenty of time for her to accomplish tasks that are within her ability. Clothing with easy removal or replacement, such as Velcro, facilitates independence.
3. Provide guidance and support for independent actions by talking her through tasks one step at a time.
4. Provide a structured schedule of activities that does not change from day to day.
5. Ensure that Carmen has snacks between meals.
6. Take Carmen to the bathroom regularly (according to her usual pattern, e.g., after meals, before bedtime, on arising).
7. To minimize nighttime wetness, offer fluid every 2 hours during the day and restrict fluid after 6 p.m.
8. To promote more restful nighttime sleep (and less wandering at night), reduce naps during late afternoon and encourage sitting exercises, walking, and ball toss. Carbohydrate snacks at bedtime may also be helpful.

EVALUATION

The outcome criteria identified for Carmen have been met. She has experienced no injury. She has not fallen out of bed. She continues to wander in a safe area. She can find her room by herself, but occasionally requires some assistance when she is anxious and more confused. She has some difficulty communicating her needs to the staff, but those who work with her on a consistent basis are able to anticipate her needs. All ADLs are being fulfilled, and Carmen assists with dressing and grooming, accomplishing about half on her own. Nighttime wandering has been minimized. Soft bedtime music helps to relax her.

Summary and Key Points

- Neurocognitive disorders (NCDs) constitute a large and growing public health concern.
- Delirium is a disturbance of awareness and a change in cognition that develop rapidly over a short period. Level of consciousness is often affected and psychomotor activity may fluctuate between agitated purposeless movements and a vegetative state resembling catatonic stupor.
- The symptoms of delirium usually begin quite abruptly and often are reversible and brief.
- Delirium may be caused by a general medical condition, substance intoxication or withdrawal, or ingestion of a medication or exposure to a toxin.
- NCD is a syndrome of acquired, persistent intellectual impairment with compromised function in multiple spheres of mental activity, such as memory, language, visuospatial skills, emotion or personality, and cognition.
- Symptoms of NCD are insidious and develop slowly over time. In most clients, the disorder runs a progressive, irreversible course.
- NCD may be caused by genetics, cardiovascular disease, infections, neurophysiological disorders, and other general medical conditions.

- Nursing care of the client with a NCD is presented around the six steps of the nursing process.
- Objectives of care for the client experiencing an acute syndrome are aimed at eliminating the etiology, promoting client safety, and returning to the highest possible level of functioning.
- Objectives of care for the client experiencing a chronic, progressive disorder are aimed at preserving the dignity of the individual, promoting deceleration of the symptoms, and maximizing functional capabilities.
- Nursing interventions are also directed toward helping the client's family or primary caregivers learn about a chronic, progressive neurocognitive disorder.
- Education is provided about the disease process, expectations of client behavioral changes, methods for facilitating care, and sources of assistance and support as they struggle, both physically and emotionally, with the demands brought on by a disease process that is slowly taking their loved one away from them.

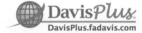

DavisPlus   Additional info available at
DavisPlus.fadavis.com   www.davisplus.com

Review Questions
Self-Examination/Learning Exercise

*Select the answer that is **most** appropriate for each of the following questions.*

1. An example of a treatable (reversible) form of neurocognitive disorder (NCD) is one that is caused by which of the following? (Select all that apply.)
   a. Multiple sclerosis
   b. Multiple small brain infarcts
   c. Electrolyte imbalances
   d. HIV disease
   e. Folate deficiency

2. Mrs. G has been diagnosed with NCD due to Alzheimer's disease. The cause of this disorder is which of the following?
   a. Multiple small brain infarcts
   b. Chronic alcohol abuse
   c. Cerebral abscess
   d. Unknown

3. Mrs. G has been diagnosed with NCD due to Alzheimer's disease. The *primary* nursing intervention in working with Mrs. G is which of the following?
   a. Ensuring that she receives food she likes, to prevent hunger
   b. Ensuring that the environment is safe, to prevent injury
   c. Ensuring that she meets the other patients, to prevent social isolation
   d. Ensuring that she takes care of her own ADLs, to prevent dependence

Continued

Review Questions—cont'd
Self-Examination/Learning Exercise

4. Which of the following medications have been indicated for improvement in cognitive functioning in mild to moderate Alzheimer's disease? (Select all that apply.)
   a. Donepezil (Aricept)
   b. Rivastigmine (Exelon)
   c. Risperidone (Risperdal)
   d. Sertraline (Zoloft)
   e. Galantamine (Razadyne)

5. Mrs. G, who has NCD due to Alzheimer's disease, says to the nurse, "I have a date tonight. I always have a date on Christmas." Which of the following is the most appropriate response?
   a. "Don't be silly. It's not Christmas, Mrs. G."
   b. "Today is Tuesday, Oct. 21, Mrs. G. We will have supper soon, and then your daughter will come to visit."
   c. "Who is your date with, Mrs. G?"
   d. "I think you need some more medication, Mrs. G. I'll bring it to you now."

6. In addition to disturbances in cognition and orientation, individuals with Alzheimer's disease may also show changes in which of the following? (Select all that apply.)
   a. Personality
   b. Vision
   c. Speech
   d. Hearing
   e. Mobility

7. Mrs. G, who has NCD due to Alzheimer's disease, has trouble sleeping and wanders around at night. Which of the following nursing actions would be *best* to promote sleep in Mrs. G?
   a. Ask the doctor to prescribe flurazepam (Dalmane).
   b. Ensure that Mrs. G gets an afternoon nap so she will not be overtired at bedtime.
   c. Make Mrs. G a cup of tea with honey before bedtime.
   d. Ensure that Mrs. G gets regular physical exercise during the day.

8. The night nurse finds Mrs. G, a client with Alzheimer's disease, wandering the hallway at 4 a.m. and trying to open the door to the side yard. Which statement by the nurse probably reflects the most accurate assessment of the situation?
   a. "That door leads out to the patio, Mrs. G. It's nighttime. You don't want to go outside now."
   b. "You look confused, Mrs. G. What is bothering you?"
   c. "This is the patio door, Mrs. G. Are you looking for the bathroom?"
   d. "Are you lonely? Perhaps you'd like to go back to your room and talk for a while."

9. A client says to the nurse: "I read an article about Alzheimer's and it said the disease is hereditary. My mother has Alzheimer's disease. Does that mean I'll get it when I'm old?" The nurse bases her response on the knowledge that which of the following factors is *not* associated with increased incidence of NCD due to Alzheimer's disease?
   a. Multiple small strokes
   b. Family history of Alzheimer's disease
   c. Head trauma
   d. Advanced age

10. Mr. Stone is a client in the hospital with a diagnosis of vascular NCD. In explaining this disorder to Mr. Stone's family, which of the following statements by the nurse is correct?
    a. "He will probably live longer than if his disorder was of the Alzheimer's type."
    b. "Vascular NCD shows step-wise progression. This is why he sometimes seems okay."
    c. "Vascular NCD is caused by plaques and tangles that form in the brain."
    d. "The cause of vascular NCD is unknown."

Review Questions—cont'd
Self-Examination/Learning Exercise

11. Which of the following interventions is most appropriate in helping a client with Alzheimer's disease with her ADLs? (Select all that apply.)
    a. Perform ADLs for her while she is in the hospital.
    b. Provide her with a written list of activities she is expected to perform.
    c. Assist her with step-by-step instructions.
    d. Tell her that if her morning care is not completed by 9 a.m. it will be performed for her by the nurse's aide so that she can attend group therapy.
    e. Encourage her and give her plenty of time to perform as many of her ADLs as possible independently.

IMPLICATIONS OF RESEARCH FOR EVIDENCE-BASED PRACTICE

Kovach, C.R., Noonan, P.E., Schlidt, A.M., & Wells, T. (2005). A model of consequences of need-driven, dementia-compromised behavior. *Journal of Nursing Scholarship, 37*(2), 134-140.

DESCRIPTION OF THE STUDY: Need-driven, dementia-compromised behavior (NDB) occurs because the caregiver is unable to comprehend needs, and the person with neurocognitive disorder (NCD) cannot make needs known. The behaviors are viewed as an attempt on the part of the person with the disorder to communicate a need and as a symptom that the need is not being met. The authors extend the primary need model to encompass secondary needs when primary needs go unresolved. From an extensive literature review, the authors proposed a framework for improving understanding of the person with a NCD and the consequences of behavioral symptoms and unmet needs.

RESULTS OF THE STUDY: The experiences of people with NCD who have unmet needs is described as having "cascading effects." In people with NCD, basic needs (e.g., thirst/need for fluid) result in primary NDB (e.g., restlessness/repetitive movements), which if left unmet may result in the negative outcome of constipation and abdominal discomfort. This need for relief may lead to the secondary NDB of aggression. The authors state, "Secondary NDBs are iatrogenic outcomes of these cascading effects and the response of a vulnerable person to the recurrent and unpredictable stress of treatment targeted inappropriately or care providers who dismiss the NDB communication." Common problematic behaviors that may be associated with unmet needs include resistance to care, verbal complaining, restlessness, facial grimacing, aggression, crying, moaning, calling out, exiting behavior, tense body parts, and rubbing or holding a body part. Unmet needs may also influence affective status (e.g., depression or anxiety), physical status (e.g., immune suppression), and acceleration in functional status.

IMPLICATIONS FOR NURSING PRACTICE: The authors of this study state, "The consequences of need-driven dementia-compromised behavior theory indicates that meeting needs of people with dementia will moderate the sequence of events that leads to negative outcomes." When caregivers cannot understand primary NDBs, they cannot provide anticipatory care. The anticipation and fulfillment of clients' needs is necessary to decrease the prevalence and severity of new unmet needs, thereby positively influencing comfort and quality of life for people with neurocognitive disorders.

IMPLICATIONS OF RESEARCH FOR EVIDENCE-BASED PRACTICE

Rusanen, M., Kivipelto, M., Quesenberry, C.P., Zhou, J., & Whitmer, R.A. (2011). Heavy smoking in midlife and long-term risk of Alzheimer disease and vascular dementia. *Archives of Internal Medicine, 171*(4), 333-339.

DESCRIPTION OF THE STUDY: The purpose of this study was to investigate the correlation between midlife smoking and long-term risk of all-cause neurocognitive disorders (NCDs) 2 to 3 decades later. The study began with 33,108 individuals enrolled in a medical health plan in Northern California. They participated in a voluntary health examination called the Multiphasic Health Checkup (MHC) during 1978 through 1985, when they were 50 to 60 years old. The MHC collected large amounts of data on health habits (including smoking), health status, and medical and family history, and was given as part of routine care. The study

IMPLICATIONS OF RESEARCH FOR EVIDENCE-BASED PRACTICE—cont'd

participants consisted of 21,123 people who were still alive and members of the health plan in 1994. Diagnoses of NCD were ascertained from electronic medical records between January 1, 1994, and July 31, 2008, and results were adjusted for age, sex, education, race, marital status, hypertension, hyperlipidemia, body mass index (BMI), diabetes, heart disease, stroke, and alcohol use. The average age in 1994 at the onset of the NCD follow-up was 71.6 years.

RESULTS OF THE STUDY: During a mean follow-up period of 23 years, about 25 percent of the group (5,367 people) were diagnosed as having a NCD, with 1,136 identified as Alzheimer disease and 416 as vascular NCD. The study revealed the following data:

- Those diagnosed with NCD were older, had fewer years of education, and were more likely to be female.
- Compared to whites, African Americans were more likely to have NCD, whereas Asians were less likely.
- A higher percentage of those with a NCD diagnosis were divorced, widowed, or separated.
- A higher percentage of those with a NCD diagnosis were "never drinkers" of alcohol.

- Those with a NCD diagnosis had a higher mean BMI and all associated comorbidities.
- Former smoking or smoking less than 0.5 pack per day at midlife was not associated with NCD in later life.
- Compared to nonsmokers, smoking less than 2 packs per day at midlife was associated with an increased risk of NCD, but study statistics were not significant.
- Those who smoked more than 2 packs per day in midlife had a greater than 100 percent risk of developing NCD.

IMPLICATIONS FOR NURSING PRACTICE: This study provides yet another reason for nurses to be involved in helping individuals to stop smoking, and for those who do not smoke, to emphasize the importance of not starting. Educational programs aimed at individuals of all ages that emphasize the health hazards associated with smoking are well within the scope of nursing practice. The authors of this study state, "The large detrimental impact that smoking already has on public health has the potential to become even greater as the population worldwide ages and dementia prevalence increases" (p. 338).

TEST YOUR CRITICAL THINKING SKILLS

Joe, a 62-year-old accountant, began having difficulty remembering details necessary to perform his job. He was also having trouble at home, failing to keep his finances straight, and forgetting to pay bills. It became increasingly difficult for him to function properly at work, and eventually he was forced to retire. Cognitive deterioration continued, and behavioral problems soon began. He became stubborn, verbally and physically abusive, and suspicious of most everyone in his environment. His wife and son convinced him to see a physician, who recommended hospitalization for testing.

At Joe's initial evaluation, he was fully alert and cooperative but obviously anxious and fidgety. He thought he was at his accounting office and he could not state what year it was. He could not say the names of his parents or siblings, nor did he know who was currently the president of the United States. He could not perform simple arithmetic calculations, write a proper sentence, or copy a drawing. He interpreted proverbs concretely and had difficulty stating similarities between related objects.

Laboratory serum studies revealed no abnormalities, but a CT scan showed marked cortical atrophy. The physician's diagnosis was neurocognitive disorder due to Alzheimer's disease.

Answer the following questions related to Joe:

1. Identify the pertinent assessment data from which nursing care will be devised.
2. What is the primary nursing diagnosis for Joe?
3. How would outcomes be identified?

Communication Exercises

1. Mrs. B is a patient on the Alzheimer's unit. The nurse hears her yelling, "Waitress! Waitress! Why can't I get some service around here?!"
   - How would the nurse respond appropriately to this statement by Mrs. B?
2. Mrs. B, who had breakfast an hour ago, says to the nurse, "I've been waiting and waiting for my breakfast. On the farm, we always had breakfast by 6 o'clock. Those were the good old days."
   - How would the nurse respond appropriately to this statement by Mrs. B?

References

Allen, J. (2000). Using validation therapy to manage difficult behaviors. *Prism Innovations. ElderCare Online.* Retrieved from http://www.ec-online.net/community/Activists/difficultbehaviors.htm

Alzheimer's Association (2013a). 2012 Alzheimer's disease facts and figures. *Alzheimer's & Dementia, 8*(2). Retrieved from http://www.alz.org/alzheimers_disease_facts_and_figures.asp

Alzheimer's Association (2013b). *Depression and Alzheimer's.* Retrieved from http://www.alz.org/care/alzheimers-dementia-depression.asp

Alzheimer's Disease Education & Referral (ADEAR). (2012). *Alzheimer's disease genetics.* National Institute on Aging.

Retrieved from http://www.nia.nih.gov/alzheimers/publication/alzheimers-disease-genetics-fact-sheet

American Psychiatric Association. (2000). *Diagnostic and statistical manual of mental disorders* (4th ed., text rev.). Washington, DC: Author.

American Psychiatric Association. (2013). *Diagnostic and statistical manual of mental disorders* (5th ed.). Washington, DC: Author.

Arvanitakis, Z. (2000). *Dementia and vascular disease.* Duval County Medical Society. Retrieved from http://www.dcmsonline.org/jax-medicine/2000journals/February2000/vascdement.htm

Bateman, R.J., Xiong, C., Benzinger, T.L.S., Fagan, A.M., Goate, A., Fox, N.C., Marcus, D.S., Caims, N.J., et al. (2012). Clinical and biomarker changes in dominantly inherited Alzheimer's disease. *New England Journal of Medicine, 367*(9), 795-804.

Black, D.W., & Andreasen, N.C. (2011). *Introductory textbook of psychiatry* (5th ed.). Washington, DC: American Psychiatric Publishing.

Blazer, D.G. (2008). Treatment of seniors. In R.E. Hales, S.C. Yudofsky, & G.O. Gabbard (Eds.), *Textbook of psychiatry* (5th ed., pp. 1449-1469). Washington, DC: American Psychiatric Publishing.

Bourgeois, J.A., Seaman, J.S., & Servis, M.E. (2008). Delirium, dementia, and amnestic disorders. In R.E. Hales, S.C. Yudofsky, & G.O. Gabbard (Eds.), *Textbook of clinical psychiatry* (5th ed., pp. 303-363). Washington, DC: American Psychiatric Publishing.

Caraci, F., Copani, A., Nicoletti, F., & Drago, F. (2010). Depression and Alzheimer's disease: Neurobiological links and common pharmacological targets. *European Journal of Pharmacology, 626*(1), 64-71.

Coelho Filho, J.M., & Birks, J. (2001). Physostigmine for dementia due to Alzheimer's disease (Cochrane Review). *The Cochrane Database of Systematic Reviews,* Issue 2. Art. No.: CD001499.

Cummings, J.L., & Mega, M.S. (2003). *Neuropsychiatry and behavioral neuroscience.* New York, NY: Oxford University Press.

Davis, C.P.(2012). Dementia: Treatable causes. Retrieved from http://www.emedicinehealth.com/script/main/art.asp?articlekey=59089&pf=38page3

Day, C.R. (2013). Validation therapy: A review of the literature. *The Validation Training Institute, Inc.* Retrieved from http://www.vfvalidation.org/web.php?request=article1

Diamond, J. (2008). *A report on Alzheimer's disease and current research.* Alzheimer Society of Canada. Retrieved from http://www.edu.gov.mb.ca/k12/dl/downloads/gr11_bio_alzheimer.pdf

Eisendrath, S.J., & Lichtmacher, J.E. (2012). Psychiatric disorders. In S.J. McPhee, M.A. Papadakis, & M.W. Rabow (Eds.), *Current medical diagnosis and treatment 2012* (pp. 1010-1064). New York, NY: McGraw-Hill.

Feil, N. (2013). It is never good to lie to a person who has dementia. *The Validation Training Institute, Inc.* Retrieved from http://www.vfvalidation.org//web.php?request=article5

Foroud, T., Gray, J., Ivashina, J., and Conneally, P.M. (1999). Differences in duration of Huntington's disease based on age at onset. *Journal of Neurology, Neurosurgery and Psychiatry, 66,* 52-56.

Geerlings, M.I., den Heijer, T., Koudstaal, P.J., Hofman, A., & Breteler, M.M.B. (2008). History of depression, depressive symptoms, and medial temporal lobe atrophy and the risk of Alzheimer disease. *Neurology, 70*(15), 1258-1264.

Hall, R., Hall, R., & Chapman, M.J. (2009). Anticholinergic syndrome: Presentations, etiological agents, differential diagnosis, and treatment. *Clinical Geriatrics, 17*(11), 22-28.

Institute of Medicine. (2003). *Health professions education: A bridge to quality.* Washington, DC: Author.

Langa, K.M., Foster, N.L., & Larson, E.B. (2004). Mixed dementia: Emerging concepts and therapeutic implications. *Journal of the American Medical Association, 292*(23), 2901-2908.

Mayo Clinic. (2011). *Frontotemporal dementia.* Retrieved from http://www.mayoclinic.com/health/frontotemporal-dementia/DS00874

McShane, R. (2000). *Hallucinations and delusions.* London: The Alzheimer's Society.

Munoz, D.G., & Feldman, H. (2000). Causes of Alzheimer's disease. *Canadian Medical Association Journal, 162*(1), 65-72.

NANDA International (NANDA-I). (2012). *Nursing diagnoses: Definitions & classification 2012-2014.* Hoboken, NJ: Wiley-Blackwell.

National Institute of Neurological Disorders and Stroke [NINDS]. (2012). *NINDS frontotemporal dementia information page.* National Institutes of Health. Retrieved from http://www.ninds.nih.gov/disorders/picks/picks.htm

National Institute on Aging [NIA]. (2011). *Alzheimer's disease: Unraveling the mystery.* NIH Publication No. 08-3782. Washington, DC: National Institutes of Health, U.S. Department of Health and Human Services.

National Institute on Aging [NIA]. (2013). About Alzheimer's disease: Symptoms. Retrieved from http://www.nia.nih.gov/alzheimers/topics/symptoms

Puri, B.K., & Treasaden, I.H. (2012). *Textbook of psychiatry* (3rd ed.). Philadelphia, PA: Churchill Livingstone Elsevier.

Rabins, P., Bland, W., Bright-Long, L., Cohen, E., Katz, I., Rovner, B., Schneider, L., & Blacker, D. (2006). Practice guideline for the treatment of patients with Alzheimer's disease and other dementias of late life. *American Psychiatric Association Practice Guidelines for the Treatment of Psychiatric Disorders, Compendium 2006.* Washington, DC: American Psychiatric Association.

Rentz, C. (2008). Nursing care of the person with sporadic Creutzfeldt-Jakob disease. *Journal of Hospice and Palliative Nursing, 10*(5), 272-282.

Rogaeva, E., Meng. Y., Lee, J.H., Gu, Y., Kawarai, T., Zou, F., Katayama, T., Baldwin, C.T., Cheng, R., et al. (2007). The neuronal sortilin-related receptor SOR1 is genetically associated with Alzheimer disease. *Nature Genetics, 39*(2), 168-177.

Sadock, B.J., & Sadock, V.A. (2007). *Synopsis of psychiatry: Behavioral sciences/clinical psychiatry* (10th ed.). Philadelphia, PA: Lippincott Williams & Wilkins.

Salloway, S., & Correia, S. (2009). Alzheimer disease: Time to improve its diagnosis and treatment. *Cleveland Clinic Journal of Medicine, 76*(1), 49-58.

Schatzberg, A.F., Cole, J.O., & DeBattista, C. (2010). *Manual of clinical psychopharmacology* (7th ed.). Washington, DC: American Psychiatric Publishing.

Small, G.W., Kepe, V., Ercoli, L.M., Siddarth, P., Bookheimer, S.Y., Miller, K.J., Lavretsky, H., et al. (2006). PET of brain amyloid and tau in mild cognitive impairment. *The New England Journal of Medicine, 355*(25), 2652-2663.

Smith, G. (2011). *Can a head injury cause or hasten Alzheimer's disease or other types of dementia?* The Mayo Clinic. Retrieved from http://www.mayoclinic.com/health/alzheimers-disease/AN01710

Spector, A., Davies, S., Woods, B., & Orrell, M. (2000). Reality orientation for dementia: A systematic review of the evidence of effectiveness from randomized controlled trials. *The Gerontologist, 40*(2), 206-212.

Srikanth, S., & Nagaraja, A.V. (2005). A prospective study of reversible dementias: Frequency, causes, clinical profile and results of treatment. *Neurology India, 53*(3), 291-294.

Stanley, M., Blair, K.A., & Beare, P.G. (2005). *Gerontological nursing: Promoting successful aging with older adults* (3rd ed.). Philadelphia, PA: F.A. Davis.

Steckl, C. (2008). *Alzheimer's disease and other cognitive disorders.* Retrieved from http://www.mentalhelp.net/poc/view_doc.php?type=doc &id=3237&cn=231

Winblad, B., Andreasen, N., Minthon, L., Floesser, A., Imbert, G., Dumortier, T., Maguire, R.P., Blennow, K., Lundmark, J., Staufenbiel, M., Orgogozo, J.M., & Graf, A. (2012). Safety, tolerability, and antibody response of active Aβ immunotherapy with CAD106 in patients with Alzheimer's disease: randomized, double-blind, placebo-controlled, first-in-human study. *The Lancet Neurology, 11*(7), 597-604.

@ INTERNET REFERENCES

• Additional information about Alzheimer's disease may be located at the following websites:
  • http://www.alz.org
  • http://www.nia.nih.gov/alzheimers
  • http://www.ninds.nih.gov/disorders/alzheimersdisease

• Information on caregiving can be located at the following website:
  • http://www.aarp.org

• Additional information about medications to treat Alzheimer's disease may be located at the following websites:
  • http://www.nlm.nih.gov/medlineplus/druginformation.html
  • http://www.nimh.nih.gov/health/publications/mental-health-medications/index.shtml
  • http://www.drugs.com

MOVIE CONNECTIONS

The Notebook (Alzheimer's disease) • *Away From Her* (Alzheimer's disease) • *Iris* (Alzheimer's disease)

Substance-Related and Addictive Disorders

23

CHAPTER OUTLINE

Objectives

Homework Assignment

Substance Use Disorder, Defined

Substance-Induced Disorder, Defined

Classes of Psychoactive Substances

Predisposing Factors to Substance-Related Disorders

The Dynamics of Substance-Related Disorders

Application of the Nursing Process

The Chemically-Impaired Nurse

Codependency

Treatment Modalities for Substance-Related Disorders

Non-Substance Addictions

Summary and Key Points

Review Questions

CORE CONCEPT

addiction

intoxication

withdrawal

KEY TERMS

Alcoholics Anonymous

amphetamines

ascites

cannabis

codependency

detoxification

disulfiram (Antabuse)

dual diagnosis

esophageal varices

Gamblers Anonymous

hepatic encephalopathy

Korsakoff's psychosis

opioids

peer assistance programs

phencyclidine

substitution therapy

Wernicke's encephalopathy

OBJECTIVES

After reading this chapter, the student will be able to:

1. Define *addiction, intoxication*, and *withdrawal*.
2. Discuss predisposing factors implicated in the etiology of substance-related and addictive disorders.
3. Identify symptomatology and use the information in assessment of clients with various substance-related and addictive disorders.
4. Identify nursing diagnoses common to clients with substance-related and addictive disorders, and select appropriate nursing interventions for each.
5. Identify topics for client and family teaching relevant to substance-related and addictive disorders.
6. Describe relevant outcome criteria for evaluating nursing care of clients with substance-related and addictive disorders.
7. Discuss the issue of substance-related and addictive disorders within the profession of nursing.
8. Define codependency and identify behavioral characteristics associated with the disorder.
9. Discuss treatment of codependency.
10. Describe various modalities relevant to treatment of individuals with substance-related and addictive disorders.

HOMEWORK ASSIGNMENT

Please read the chapter and answer the following questions:

1. What are the physical consequences of thiamine deficiency in chronic alcohol use?
2. Define *tolerance* as it relates to physical addiction to a substance.
3. Describe two types of toxic reactions that can occur with the use of hallucinogens.
4. What is substitution therapy?

Substance-related disorders are composed of two groups: the substance use disorders (addiction) and the substance-induced disorders (intoxication, withdrawal, delirium, neurocognitive disorder, psychosis, bipolar disorder, depressive disorder, obsessive-compulsive disorder, anxiety disorder, sexual dysfunction, and sleep disorders). This chapter discusses addiction, intoxication, and withdrawal. The remainder of the substance-induced disorders are included in the chapters with which they share symptomatology (e.g., substance-induced depressive disorder is included in Chapter 25; substance-induced anxiety disorder is included in Chapter 27). Also included in this chapter is a discussion of gambling disorder, a non-substance addiction disorder.

Drugs are a pervasive part of our society. Certain mood-altering substances are quite socially acceptable and are used moderately by many adult Americans. They include alcohol, caffeine, and nicotine. Society has even developed a relative indifference to an occasional abuse of these substances, despite documentation of their negative impact on health.

A wide variety of substances are produced for medicinal purposes. These include central nervous system (CNS) stimulants (e.g., **amphetamines**), CNS depressants (e.g., sedatives, tranquilizers), as well as numerous over-the-counter preparations designed to relieve nearly every kind of human ailment, real or imagined.

Some illegal substances have achieved a degree of social acceptance by various subcultural groups within our society. These drugs, such as marijuana and hashish, are by no means harmless, and the long-term effects are still being studied. On the other hand, the dangerous effects of other illegal substances (e.g., lysergic acid diethylamide [LSD], **phencyclidine**, cocaine, and heroin) have been well documented.

This chapter discusses the physical and behavioral manifestations and personal and social consequences related to the abuse of or addiction to alcohol, other CNS depressants, CNS stimulants, **opioids**, hallucinogens, cannabinoids, and the non-substance addiction to gambling. Wide cultural variations in attitudes exist regarding substance consumption and patterns of use. Substance abuse is especially prevalent among individuals between the ages of 18 and 24. Substance-related disorders are diagnosed more commonly in men than in women, but the gender ratios vary with the class of the substance.

Codependency is described in this chapter, as are aspects of treatment for the disorder. The issue of substance impairment within the profession of nursing is also explored. Nursing care for individuals with substance use and addictive disorders is presented in the context of the six steps of the nursing process. Various medical and other treatment modalities are also discussed.

Substance Use Disorder, Defined

> ### CORE CONCEPT
> **Addiction**
> A compulsive or chronic requirement. The need is so strong as to generate distress (either physical or psychological) if left unfulfilled.

Substance Addiction

The *Diagnostic and Statistical Manual of Mental Disorders, Fifth Edition (DSM-5)* (American Psychiatric Association [APA], 2013) lists diagnostic criteria for addiction to specific substances, including alcohol, cannabis, hallucinogens, inhalants, opioids, sedatives/hypnotics/anxiolytics, stimulants, and tobacco. Individuals are considered to have a substance use disorder when use of the substance interferes with their ability to fulfill role obligations, such as at work, school, or home. Often the individual would like to cut down or control use of the substance, but attempts fail, and use of the substance continues to increase. There is an intense craving for the substance, and an excessive amount of time is spent trying to procure more of the substance or recover from the effects of its use. Use of the substance causes problems with interpersonal relationships, and the individual may become socially isolated. Individuals with substance use disorders often participate in hazardous activities when they are impaired by the substance, and continue to use the substance despite knowing that its use is contributing to a physical or psychological problem. Addiction is evident when tolerance develops and the amount required to achieve the desired effect continues to increase. A syndrome of symptoms, characteristic of the specific substance, occurs when the individual with the addiction attempts to discontinue use of the substance.

Substance-Induced Disorder, Defined

> ### CORE CONCEPT
> **Intoxication**
> A physical and mental state of exhilaration and emotional frenzy or lethargy and stupor.

Substance Intoxication

Substance intoxication is defined as the development of a reversible syndrome of symptoms following excessive use of a substance. The symptoms are drug-specific, and occur during or shortly after the ingestion of the substance. There is a direct effect on the CNS, and a disruption in physical and psychological functioning occurs. Judgment is disturbed, resulting in inappropriate and maladaptive behavior, and social and occupational functioning are impaired.

CORE CONCEPT

Withdrawal
The physiological and mental readjustment that accompanies the discontinuation of an addictive substance.

Substance Withdrawal

Substance withdrawal occurs upon abrupt reduction or discontinuation of a substance that has been used regularly over a prolonged period of time. The substance-specific syndrome includes clinically significant physical signs and symptoms as well as psychological changes such as disturbances in thinking, feeling, and behavior.

Classes of Psychoactive Substances

The following classes of psychoactive substances are associated with substance use and substance-induced disorders:

1. Alcohol
2. Caffeine
3. Cannabis
4. Hallucinogens
5. Inhalants
6. Opioids
7. Sedatives/Hypnotics/Anxiolytics
8. Stimulants
9. Tobacco

Predisposing Factors to Substance-Related Disorders

A number of factors have been implicated in the predisposition to abuse of substances. At present, there is no single theory that can adequately explain the etiology of this problem. No doubt the interaction between various elements forms a complex collection of determinants that influence a person's susceptibility to abuse substances.

Biological Factors

Genetics

An apparent hereditary factor is involved in the development of substance use disorders. This is especially evident with alcoholism, but less so with other substances. Children of alcoholics are four times more likely than other children to become alcoholics (American Academy of Child and Adolescent Psychiatry, 2011). Studies with monozygotic and dizygotic twins have also supported the genetic hypothesis. Monozygotic (one egg, genetically identical) twins have a higher rate for concordance of alcoholism than dizygotic (two eggs, genetically nonidentical) twins (Black & Andreasen, 2011). Other studies have shown that biological offspring of alcoholic parents have a significantly greater incidence of alcoholism than offspring of nonalcoholic parents. This is true whether the child was reared by the biological parents or by nonalcoholic adoptive parents (Puri & Treasaden, 2011).

Biochemical

A second biological hypothesis relates to the possibility that alcohol may produce morphine-like substances in the brain that are responsible for alcohol addiction. These substances are formed by the reaction of biologically active amines (e.g., dopamine, serotonin) with products of alcohol metabolism, such as acetaldehyde (Jamal et al., 2003). Examples of these morphine-like substances include tetrahydropapaveroline and salsolinol. Some tests with animals have shown that injection of these compounds into the brain in small amounts results in patterns of alcohol addiction in animals who had previously avoided even the most dilute alcohol solutions (McCoy, Strawbridge, McMurtrey, Kane, & Ward, 2003).

Psychological Factors

Developmental Influences

The psychodynamic approach to the etiology of substance abuse focuses on a punitive superego and fixation at the oral stage of psychosexual development (Sadock & Sadock, 2007). Individuals with punitive superegos turn to alcohol to diminish unconscious anxiety and increase feelings of power and self-worth. Sadock and Sadock (2007) state, "As a form of self-medication, alcohol may be used to control panic, opioids to diminish anger, and amphetamines to alleviate depression" (p. 386).

Personality Factors

Certain personality traits have been associated with an increased tendency toward addictive behavior. Some clinicians believe a low self-esteem, frequent depression, passivity, the inability to relax or to defer gratification, and the inability to communicate effectively are common in individuals who abuse substances. These personality characteristics cannot be called *predictive* of addictive behavior, yet for reasons not completely understood, they have been found to accompany addiction in many instances.

Substance abuse has also been associated with antisocial personality and depressive response styles.

This may be explained by the inability of the individual with antisocial personality to anticipate the aversive consequences of his or her behavior. It is likely an effort on the part of the depressed person to treat the symptoms of discomfort associated with dysphoria. Achievement of relief then provides the positive reinforcement to continue abusing the substance.

Sociocultural Factors

Social Learning

The effects of modeling, imitation, and identification on behavior can be observed from early childhood onward. In relation to drug consumption, the family appears to be an important influence. Various studies have shown that children and adolescents are more likely to use substances if they have parents who provide a model for substance use. Peers often exert a great deal of influence in the life of the child or adolescent who is being encouraged to use substances for the first time. Modeling may continue to be a factor in the use of substances once the individual enters the workforce, particularly if the work setting provides plenty of leisure time with coworkers and drinking is valued as a way to express group cohesiveness.

Conditioning

Another important learning factor is the effect of the substance itself. Many substances create a pleasurable experience that encourages the user to repeat it. Thus, it is the intrinsically reinforcing properties of addictive drugs that "condition" the individual to seek out their use again and again. The environment in which the substance is taken also contributes to the reinforcement. If the environment is pleasurable, substance use is usually increased. Aversive stimuli within an environment are thought to be associated with a decrease in substance use within that environment.

Cultural and Ethnic Influences

Factors within an individual's culture help to establish patterns of substance use by molding attitudes, influencing patterns of consumption based on cultural acceptance, and determining the availability of the substance. For centuries, the French and Italians have considered wine an essential part of the family meal, even for the children. The incidence of alcohol addiction is low, and acute intoxication from alcohol is not common. However, the possibility of chronic physiological effects associated with lifelong alcohol consumption cannot be ignored.

Historically, a high incidence of alcohol addiction has existed within the Native American culture. Alcohol-related deaths among Native Americans are more than three times that of the U.S. general population (Indian Health Service, 2011). Veterans Administration records show that 45 percent of Native American veterans are addicted to alcohol, a rate two times that of non–Native American veterans. A number of reasons have been postulated for alcohol abuse among Native Americans: a possible physical cause (difficulty metabolizing alcohol), children modeling their parents' drinking habits, unemployment and poverty, and loss of the traditional Native American religion that some believe has led to the increased use of alcohol to fill the spiritual gap.

The incidence of alcohol addiction is higher among northern Europeans than southern Europeans. The Finns and the Irish use excessive alcohol consumption for the release of aggression, and the English and Irish "pubs" are known for their attraction as social meeting places (Ehrlander, 2007; Schim, 2013).

Incidence of alcohol addiction among Asians is relatively low. This may be a result of a possible genetic intolerance of the substance. Some Asians develop unpleasant symptoms, such as flushing, headaches, nausea, and palpitations, when they drink alcohol. Research indicates that this is because of an isoenzyme variant that quickly converts alcohol to acetaldehyde, as well as the absence of an isoenzyme that is needed to oxidize acetaldehyde. This results in a rapid accumulation of acetaldehyde, which produces the unpleasant symptoms (Hanley, 2013).

The Dynamics of Substance-Related Disorders

Alcohol Use Disorder

A Profile of the Substance

Alcohol is a natural substance formed by the reaction of fermenting sugar with yeast spores. Although there are many alcohols, the kind in alcoholic beverages is known scientifically as ethyl alcohol and chemically as C_2H_5OH. Its abbreviation, ETOH, is sometimes seen in medical records and in various other documents and publications.

By strict definition, alcohol is classified as a food because it contains calories; however, it has no nutritional value. Different alcoholic beverages are produced by using different sources of sugar for the fermentation process. For example, beer is made from malted barley, wine from grapes or berries, whiskey from malted grains, and rum from molasses. Distilled beverages (e.g., whiskey, scotch, gin, vodka, and other "hard" liquors) derive their name from further concentration of the alcohol through a process called distillation.

The alcohol content varies by type of beverage. For example, most American beers contain 3 to 6 percent alcohol, wines average 10 to 20 percent, and distilled beverages range from 40 to 50 percent alcohol. The average-sized drink, regardless of beverage, contains a similar amount of alcohol. That is, 12 ounces of beer, 3 to 5 ounces of wine, and a cocktail with 1 ounce of whiskey all contain approximately 0.5 ounce of alcohol. If consumed at the same rate, they all would have an equal effect on the body.

Alcohol exerts a depressant effect on the CNS, resulting in behavioral and mood changes. The effects of alcohol on the CNS are proportional to the alcoholic concentration in the blood. Most states consider that an individual is legally intoxicated with a blood alcohol level of 0.08 percent.

The body burns alcohol at the rate of about 0.5 ounce per hour, so behavioral changes would not be expected to occur in an individual who slowly consumed only one averaged-sized drink per hour. Other factors do influence these effects, however, such as individual size and whether or not the stomach contains food at the time the alcohol is consumed. Alcohol is also thought to have a more profound effect when an individual is emotionally stressed or fatigued.

Historical Aspects

The use of alcohol can be traced back to the Neolithic age. Beer and wine are known to have been used around 6400 BC. With the introduction of distillation by the Arabs in the Middle Ages, alchemists believed that alcohol was the answer to all of their ailments. The word *whiskey*, meaning "water of life," became widely known.

In America, Native Americans had been drinking beer and wine prior to the arrival of the first white immigrants. Refinement of the distillation process made beverages with high alcohol content readily available. By the early 1800s, one renowned physician of the time, Benjamin Rush, had begun to identify the widespread excessive, chronic alcohol consumption as a disease and an addiction. The strong religious mores on which this country was founded soon led to a driving force aimed at prohibiting the sale of alcoholic beverages. By the middle of the 19th century, 13 states had passed prohibition laws. The most notable prohibition of major proportions was that in effect in the United States from 1920 to 1933. The mandatory restrictions on national social habits resulted in the creation of profitable underground markets that led to flourishing criminal enterprises. Furthermore, millions of dollars in federal, state, and local revenues from taxes and import duties on alcohol were lost. It is difficult to measure the value of this dollar loss against the human devastation and social costs that occur as a result of alcohol abuse in the United States today.

Patterns of Use

About half of Americans aged 12 years and older report being current drinkers of alcohol (Substance Abuse and Mental Health Services Administration [SAMHSA], 2013). Of these, approximately 23 percent report participating in binge drinking, and 6.5 percent engage in heavy alcohol use.

Why do people drink? Drinking patterns in the United States show that people use alcoholic beverages to enhance the flavor of food with meals; at social gatherings to encourage relaxation and conviviality among the guests; and to promote a feeling of celebration at special occasions such as weddings, birthdays, and anniversaries. An alcoholic beverage (wine) is also used as part of the sacred ritual in some religious ceremonies. Therapeutically, alcohol is the major ingredient in many over-the-counter and prescription medicines that are prepared in concentrated form. Therefore, alcohol can be harmless and enjoyable—sometimes even beneficial—if it is used responsibly and in moderation. Like any other mind-altering drug, however, alcohol has the potential for abuse. Indeed, it is the most widely abused drug in the United States today. Alcoholism is the nation's number one health problem and the third leading lifestyle-related cause of death in the United States (National Council on Alcoholism and Drug Dependence, 2013). Thousands of Americans die each year as a result of alcohol use, and it is a factor in more than half of all homicides, suicides, and traffic accidents. Incidents of domestic violence are commonly alcohol-related. Heavy drinking contributes to illness in each of the top three causes of death: heart disease, cancer, and stroke. Fetal alcohol syndrome is the most common preventable cause of intellectual disability in the United States (Walton-Moss, Becker, Kub, & Woodruff, 2010).

Jellinek (1952) outlined four phases through which the alcoholic's pattern of drinking progresses. Some variability among individuals is to be expected within this model of progression.

Phase I: The Prealcoholic Phase

This phase is characterized by the use of alcohol to relieve the everyday stress and tensions of life. As a child, the individual may have observed parents or other adults drinking alcohol and enjoying the effects. The child learns that use of alcohol is an acceptable method of coping with stress. Tolerance develops, and the amount required to achieve the desired effect increases steadily.

Phase II: The Early Alcoholic Phase

This phase begins with blackouts—brief periods of amnesia that occur during or immediately following a period of drinking. Now the alcohol is no longer a source of pleasure or relief for the individual but rather a drug that is *required* by the individual. Common behaviors include sneaking drinks or secret drinking, preoccupation with drinking and maintaining the supply of alcohol, rapid gulping of drinks, and further blackouts. The individual feels enormous guilt and becomes very defensive about his or her drinking. Excessive use of denial and rationalization is evident.

Phase III: The Crucial Phase

In this phase, the individual has lost control, and physiological addiction is clearly evident. This loss of control has been described as the inability to choose whether or not to drink. Binge drinking, lasting from a few hours to several weeks, is common. These episodes are characterized by sickness, loss of consciousness, squalor, and degradation. In this phase, the individual is extremely ill. Anger and aggression are common manifestations. Drinking is the total focus, and he or she is willing to risk losing everything that was once important, in an effort to maintain the addiction. By this phase of the illness, it is not uncommon for the individual to have experienced the loss of job, marriage, family, friends, and most especially, self-respect.

Phase IV: The Chronic Phase

This phase is characterized by emotional and physical disintegration. The individual is usually intoxicated more than he or she is sober. Emotional disintegration is evidenced by profound helplessness and self-pity. Impairment in reality testing may result in psychosis. Life-threatening physical manifestations may be evident in virtually every system of the body. Abstention from alcohol results in a terrifying syndrome of symptoms that include hallucinations, tremors, convulsions, severe agitation, and panic. Depression and ideas of suicide are not uncommon.

Effects on the Body

Alcohol can induce a general, nonselective, reversible depression of the CNS. About 20 percent of a single dose of alcohol is absorbed directly and immediately into the bloodstream through the stomach wall. Unlike other "foods," it does not have to be digested. The blood carries it directly to the brain where the alcohol acts on the brain's central control areas, slowing down or depressing brain activity. The other 80 percent of the alcohol in one drink is processed only slightly slower through the upper intestinal tract and into the bloodstream. Only moments after alcohol is consumed, it can be found in all tissues, organs, and secretions of the body. Rapidity of absorption is influenced by various factors. For example, absorption is delayed when the drink is sipped, rather than gulped; when the stomach contains food, rather than being empty; and when the drink is wine or beer, rather than distilled beverages.

At low doses, alcohol produces relaxation, loss of inhibitions, lack of concentration, drowsiness, slurred speech, and sleep. Chronic abuse results in multisystem physiological impairments. These complications include (but are not limited to) those outlined in the following sections.

Peripheral Neuropathy

Peripheral neuropathy, characterized by peripheral nerve damage, results in pain, burning, tingling, or prickly sensations of the extremities. Researchers believe it is the direct result of deficiencies in the B vitamins, particularly thiamine. Nutritional deficiencies are common in chronic alcoholics because of insufficient intake of nutrients as well as the toxic effect of alcohol that results in malabsorption of nutrients. The process is reversible with abstinence from alcohol and restoration of nutritional deficiencies. Otherwise, permanent muscle wasting and paralysis can occur.

Alcoholic Myopathy

Alcoholic myopathy may occur as an acute or chronic condition. In the acute condition, the individual experiences a sudden onset of muscle pain, swelling, and weakness; a reddish tinge in the urine caused by myoglobin, a breakdown product of muscle excreted in the urine; and a rapid rise in muscle enzymes in the blood (Klopstock, Haller, & DiMauro, 2012). Muscle symptoms are usually generalized, but pain and swelling may selectively involve the calves or other muscle groups. Laboratory studies show elevations of the enzymes creatine phosphokinase (CPK), lactate dehydrogenase (LDH), aldolase, and aspartate aminotransferase (AST). The symptoms of chronic alcoholic myopathy include a gradual wasting and weakness in skeletal muscles. Neither the pain and tenderness nor the elevated muscle enzymes seen in acute myopathy are evident in the chronic condition.

Alcoholic myopathy is thought to be a result of the same B vitamin deficiency that contributes to peripheral neuropathy. Improvement is observed with abstinence from alcohol and the return to a nutritious diet with vitamin supplements.

Wernicke's Encephalopathy

Wernicke's encephalopathy represents the most serious form of thiamine deficiency in alcoholics. Symptoms include paralysis of the ocular muscles, diplopia, ataxia, somnolence, and stupor. If thiamine replacement therapy is not undertaken quickly, death will ensue.

Korsakoff's Psychosis

Korsakoff's psychosis is identified by a syndrome of confusion, loss of recent memory, and confabulation in alcoholics. It is frequently encountered in clients recovering from Wernicke's encephalopathy. In the

United States, the two disorders are usually considered together and are called *Wernicke-Korsakoff syndrome.* Treatment is with parenteral or oral thiamine replacement.

Alcoholic Cardiomyopathy

The effect of alcohol on the heart is an accumulation of lipids in the myocardial cells, resulting in enlargement and a weakened condition. The clinical findings of alcoholic cardiomyopathy generally relate to congestive heart failure or arrhythmia. Symptoms include decreased exercise tolerance, tachycardia, dyspnea, edema, palpitations, and nonproductive cough. Laboratory studies may show elevation of the enzymes CPK, AST, alanine aminotransferase (ALT), and LDH. Changes may be observed by electrocardiogram, and congestive heart failure may be evident on chest x-ray films (Bashore, Granger, Hranitzky, & Patel, 2012).

The treatment is total permanent abstinence from alcohol. Treatment of the congestive heart failure may include rest, oxygen, digitalization, sodium restriction, and diuretics. Prognosis is encouraging if treated in the early stages. The death rate is high for individuals with advanced symptomatology.

Esophagitis

Esophagitis—inflammation and pain in the esophagus—occurs because of the toxic effects of alcohol on the esophageal mucosa. It also occurs because of frequent vomiting associated with alcohol abuse.

Gastritis

The effects of alcohol on the stomach include inflammation of the stomach lining characterized by epigastric distress, nausea, vomiting, and distention. Alcohol breaks down the stomach's protective mucosal barrier, allowing hydrochloric acid to erode the stomach wall. Damage to blood vessels may result in hemorrhage.

Pancreatitis

Pancreatitis may be categorized as *acute* or *chronic.* Acute pancreatitis usually occurs 1 or 2 days after a binge of excessive alcohol consumption. Symptoms include constant, severe epigastric pain, nausea and vomiting, and abdominal distention. The chronic condition leads to pancreatic insufficiency resulting in steatorrhea, malnutrition, weight loss, and diabetes mellitus.

Alcoholic Hepatitis

Alcoholic hepatitis is inflammation of the liver caused by long-term heavy alcohol use. Clinical manifestations include an enlarged and tender liver, nausea and vomiting, lethargy, anorexia, elevated white blood cell count, fever, and jaundice. **Ascites** and weight loss may be evident in more severe cases. With treatment—which includes strict abstinence from

alcohol, proper nutrition, and rest—the individual can experience complete recovery. Severe cases can lead to cirrhosis or **hepatic encephalopathy**.

Cirrhosis of the Liver

Cirrhosis of the liver may be caused by anything that results in chronic injury to the liver. It is the end-stage of alcoholic liver disease and results from long-term chronic alcohol abuse. There is widespread destruction of liver cells, which are replaced by fibrous (scar) tissue. Clinical manifestations include nausea and vomiting, anorexia, weight loss, abdominal pain, jaundice, edema, anemia, and blood coagulation abnormalities. Treatment includes abstention from alcohol, correction of malnutrition, and supportive care to prevent complications of the disease. Complications of cirrhosis include the following:

- **Portal Hypertension.** Elevation of blood pressure through the portal circulation results from defective blood flow through the cirrhotic liver.
- **Ascites.** Ascites, a condition in which an excessive amount of serous fluid accumulates in the abdominal cavity, occurs in response to portal hypertension. The increased pressure results in the seepage of fluid from the surface of the liver into the abdominal cavity.
- **Esophageal Varices. Esophageal varices** are veins in the esophagus that become distended because of excessive pressure from defective blood flow through the cirrhotic liver. As this pressure increases, these varicosities can rupture, resulting in hemorrhage and sometimes death.
- **Hepatic Encephalopathy.** This serious complication occurs in response to the inability of the diseased liver to convert ammonia to urea for excretion. The continued rise in serum ammonia results in progressively impaired mental functioning, apathy, euphoria or depression, sleep disturbance, increasing confusion, and progression to coma and eventual death. Treatment requires complete abstention from alcohol, temporary elimination of protein from the diet, and reduction of intestinal ammonia using neomycin or lactulose (National Library of Medicine, 2011).

Leukopenia

The production, function, and movement of the white blood cells are impaired in chronic alcoholics. This condition, called leukopenia, places the individual at high risk for contracting infectious diseases as well as for complicated recovery.

Thrombocytopenia

Platelet production and survival is impaired as a result of the toxic effects of alcohol. This places the alcoholic at risk for hemorrhage. Abstinence from alcohol rapidly reverses this deficiency.

Sexual Dysfunction

Alcohol interferes with the normal production and maintenance of female and male hormones (Sadock & Sadock, 2007). For women, this can mean changes in the menstrual cycles and a decreased or loss of ability to become pregnant. For men, the decreased hormone levels result in a diminished libido, decreased sexual performance, and impaired fertility.

Use During Pregnancy

Fetal Alcohol Syndrome

Prenatal exposure to alcohol can result in a broad range of disorders to the fetus, known as fetal alcohol spectrum disorders (FASDs), the most common of which is fetal alcohol syndrome (FAS). Fetal alcohol syndrome includes physical, mental, behavioral, and/or learning disabilities with lifelong implications. There may be problems with learning, memory, attention span, communication, vision, hearing, or a combination of these (Centers for Disease Control and Prevention [CDC], 2011). Other FASDs include alcohol-related neurodevelopmental disorder (ARND) and alcohol-related birth defects (ARBD).

No amount of alcohol during pregnancy is considered safe, and alcohol can damage a fetus at any stage of pregnancy (Carmona, 2005). Therefore, drinking alcohol should be avoided by women who are pregnant or by women who could become pregnant. Estimates of the prevalence of FAS range from 0.2 to 1.5 per 1,000 live births (CDC, 2012a). The rate is higher among African Americans and Native Americans (possibly as high as 9 per 1,000 in the latter group) (Dannaway & Mulvihill, 2009). Maier and West (2013) stated:

> The number of women who engage in heavy alcohol consumption during pregnancy surpasses the total number of children diagnosed with either FAS or ARND, meaning that not every child whose mother drank alcohol during pregnancy develops FAS or ARND. Moreover, the degree to which people with FAS or ARND are impaired differs from person to person. Several factors may contribute to this variation in the consequences of maternal drinking. These factors include, but are not limited to, the following:
>
> ■ Maternal drinking pattern
> ■ Differences in maternal metabolism
> ■ Differences in genetic susceptibility
> ■ Timing of the alcohol consumption during pregnancy
> ■ Variation in the vulnerability of different brain regions

Children with FAS may have the following characteristics or exhibit the following behaviors (CDC, 2011):

■ Abnormal facial features (see Fig. 23-1)
■ Small head size
■ Shorter-than-average height
■ Low body weight
■ Poor coordination

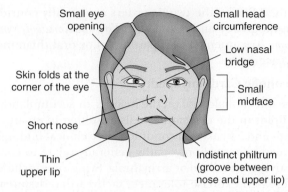

FIGURE 23-1 Facial features of FAS. (From the National Institute of Alcohol Abuse and Alcoholism of the National Institutes of Health, Washington, D.C.)

■ Hyperactive behavior
■ Difficulty paying attention
■ Poor memory
■ Difficulty in school
■ Learning disabilities
■ Speech and language delays
■ Intellectual disability or low IQ
■ Poor reasoning and judgment skills
■ Sleep and sucking problems as a baby
■ Vision or hearing problems
■ Problems with the heart, kidneys, or bones

Neuroimaging of children with FAS shows abnormalities in the size and shape of their brains. The frontal lobes and cerebellum are often smaller than normal, and the corpus callosum and basal ganglia are commonly affected (Dannaway & Mulvihill, 2009). Studies show that children with FAS are often at risk for psychiatric disorders, commonly attention-deficit/hyperactivity disorder, mood disorders, anxiety disorders, eating disorders, reactive attachment disorder, and conduct disorder (Coles, 2011; Hoffman, 2006).

Children with FAS require lifelong care and treatment. There is no cure for FAS, but it can be prevented. The Surgeon General's Advisory on Alcohol Use in Pregnancy states:

> Health professionals should inquire routinely about alcohol consumption by women of childbearing age, inform them of the risks of alcohol consumption during pregnancy, and advise them not to drink alcoholic beverages during pregnancy (Carmona, 2005, p. 1).

Alcohol Intoxication

Symptoms of alcohol intoxication include disinhibition of sexual or aggressive impulses, mood lability, impaired judgment, impaired social or occupational functioning, slurred speech, incoordination, unsteady gait, nystagmus, and flushed face. Intoxication usually occurs at blood alcohol levels between 100 and 200 mg/dL. Death has been reported at levels ranging from 400 to 700 mg/dL.

Alcohol Withdrawal

Within 4 to 12 hours of cessation of or reduction in heavy and prolonged (several days or longer) alcohol use, the following symptoms may appear: coarse tremor of hands, tongue, or eyelids; nausea or vomiting; malaise or weakness; tachycardia; sweating; elevated blood pressure; anxiety; depressed mood or irritability; transient hallucinations or illusions; headache; and insomnia. A complicated withdrawal syndrome may progress to *alcohol withdrawal delirium*. Onset of delirium is usually on the second or third day following cessation of or reduction in prolonged, heavy alcohol use. Symptoms include those described under the syndrome of delirium (Chapter 22).

Sedative, Hypnotic, or Anxiolytic Use Disorder

A Profile of the Substance

The sedative/hypnotic/anxiolytic compounds are drugs of diverse chemical structures that are all capable of inducing varying degrees of CNS depression, from tranquilizing relief of anxiety to anesthesia, coma, and even death. They are generally categorized as (1) barbiturates, (2) nonbarbiturate hypnotics, and (3) antianxiety agents. Effects produced by these substances depend on size of dose and potency of drug administered.

Table 23-1 presents a selected list of drugs included in these categories. Generic names are followed in parentheses by the trade names. Common street names for each category are also included.

Several principles have been identified that apply fairly uniformly to all CNS depressants:

1. **The effects of CNS depressants are additive with one another and with the behavioral state of the user.** For example, when these drugs are used in combination with each other or in combination with alcohol, the depressive effects are compounded. These intense depressive effects are often unpredictable and can even be fatal. Similarly, a person who is mentally depressed or physically fatigued may have an exaggerated response to a dose of the drug

TABLE 23–1 Sedative, Hypnotic, and Anxiolytic Drugs

CATEGORIES	GENERIC (TRADE) NAMES	COMMON STREET NAMES
Barbiturates	Amobarbital (Amytal) Pentobarbital (Nembutal) Secobarbital (Seconal) Butabarbital (Butisol) Phenobarbital	Blue birds; blue angels (amobarbital); Yellow jackets; yellow birds (pentobarbital); GBs; red birds; red devils (secobarbital)
Nonbarbiturate hypnotics	Chloral hydrate Estazolam Flurazepam Temazepam (Restoril) Triazolam (Halcion) Quazepam (Doral) Eszoplicone (Lunesta) Ramelteon (Rozerem) Zaleplon (Sonata) Zolpidem (Ambien)	Peter, Mickey (Chloral hydrate); Sleepers
Antianxiety agents	Alprazolam (Xanax) Chlordiazepoxide (Librium) Clonazepam (Klonopin) Clorazepate (Tranxene) Diazepam (Valium) Lorazepam (Ativan) Oxazepam (Serax) Meprobamate (Miltown)	Green and whites; roaches (Librium); Candy, downers (the benzodiazepines) Vs (Valium; color designates strength); Dolls; dollies (Meprobamate)
Club drugs	Flunitrazepam (Rohypnol) Gamma hydroxybutyric acid (gamma hydroxybutyrate; GHB)	Date rape drug; roofies, R-2, rope (Rohypnol); G, liquid X, grievous bodily harm, easy lay (GHB)

that would only slightly affect a person in a normal or excited state.

2. **CNS depressants are capable of producing physiological addiction.** If large doses of CNS depressants are repeatedly administered over a prolonged duration, a period of CNS hyperexcitability occurs on withdrawal of the drug. The response can be quite severe, even leading to convulsions and death.

3. **CNS depressants are capable of producing psychological addiction.** CNS depressants have the potential to generate within the individual a psychic drive for periodic or continuous administration of the drug to achieve a maximum level of functioning or feeling of well-being.

4. **Cross-tolerance and cross-dependence may exist between various CNS depressants.** Cross-tolerance is exhibited when one drug results in a lessened response to another drug. Cross-dependence is a condition in which one drug can prevent withdrawal symptoms associated with physical addiction to a different drug (Julien, 2008).

Historical Aspects

Anxiety and insomnia, two of the most common human afflictions, were treated during the 19th century with opiates, bromide salts, chloral hydrate, paraldehyde, and alcohol (Julien, 2008; Sateia, 2009). Because the opiates were known to produce physical addiction, the bromides carried the risk of chronic bromide poisoning, and chloral hydrate and paraldehyde had an objectionable taste and smell, alcohol became the prescribed depressant drug of choice. However, some people refused to use alcohol either because they did not like the taste or for moral reasons, and others tended to take more than was prescribed. Therefore, a search for a better sedative drug continued.

Although barbituric acid was first synthesized in 1864, it was not until 1912 that phenobarbital was introduced into medicine as a sedative drug, the first of the structurally classified group of drugs called barbiturates (Julien, 2008). Since that time, more than 2,500 barbiturate derivatives have been synthesized, but currently, fewer than a dozen remain in medical use. Illicit use of the drugs for recreational purposes grew throughout the 1930s and 1940s.

Efforts to create depressant medications that were not barbiturate derivatives accelerated. By the mid-1950s the market for depressants had been expanded by the appearance of the nonbarbiturates glutethimide, ethchlorvynol, methyprylon, and meprobamate. Introduction of the benzodiazepines occurred around 1960 with the marketing of chlordiazepoxide (Librium), followed shortly by its derivative diazepam (Valium). The use of these drugs, and others within their group, grew very rapidly, and they are prescribed widely in medical practice. Their margin of safety is greater than that of barbiturates and the other nonbarbiturates. However, prolonged use of even moderate doses is likely to result in physical and psychological addiction, with a characteristic syndrome of withdrawal that can be severe.

Patterns of Use

Sadock and Sadock (2007) reported that about 15 percent of all persons in the United States have had a benzodiazepine prescribed by a physician. Of all the drugs used in clinical practice, the sedative/hypnotic/anxiolytic drugs are among the most widely prescribed.

Two patterns of addiction are described. The first pattern is one of an individual whose physician originally prescribed the CNS depressant as treatment for anxiety or insomnia. Independently, the individual has increased the dosage or frequency from that which was prescribed. Use of the medication is justified on the basis of treating symptoms, but as tolerance grows, more and more of the medication is required to produce the desired effect. Substance-seeking behavior is evident as the individual seeks prescriptions from several physicians in order to maintain sufficient supplies.

The second pattern involves young people in their teens or early 20s who, in the company of their peers, use substances that were obtained illegally. The initial objective is to achieve a feeling of euphoria. The drug is usually used intermittently during recreational gatherings. This pattern of intermittent use leads to regular use and extreme levels of tolerance. Combining use with other substances is not uncommon. Physical and psychological addiction leads to intense substance-seeking behaviors, most often through illegal channels.

Effects on the Body

The sedative/hypnotic/anxiolytic compounds induce a general depressant effect; that is, they depress the activity of the brain, nerves, muscles, and heart tissue. They reduce the rate of metabolism in a variety of tissues throughout the body, and in general, they depress any system that uses energy (Julien, 2008). Large doses are required to produce these effects. In lower doses these drugs appear to be more selective in their depressant actions by exerting their action on the centers within the brain that are concerned with arousal (e.g., the ascending reticular activating system, in the reticular formation, and the diffuse thalamic projection system).

As stated previously, these drugs are capable of producing all levels of CNS depression—from mild sedation to death. The level is determined by dosage and potency of the drug used. In Figure 23-2, a continuum of the CNS depressant effects is presented

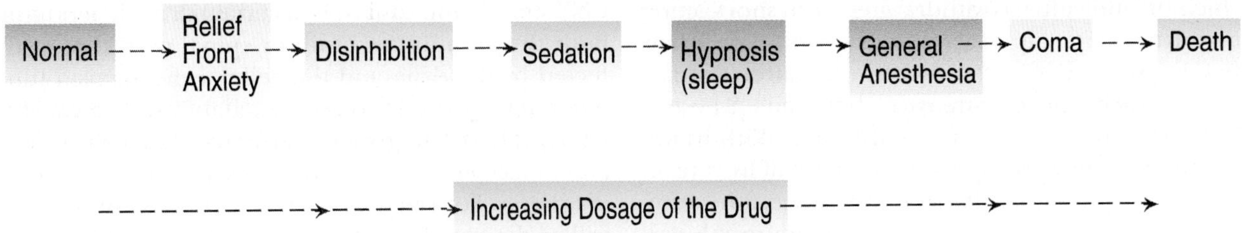

FIGURE 23-2 Continuum of behavioral depression with increasing doses of sedative-hypnotic drugs.

to demonstrate how increasing doses of sedative/hypnotic drugs affect behavioral depression.

The primary action of sedatives, hypnotics, and anxiolytics is on nervous tissue. However, large doses may have an effect on other organ systems. Following is a discussion of the physiological effects of these medications.

The Effects on Sleep and Dreaming

Barbiturate use decreases the amount of sleep time spent in dreaming. During drug withdrawal, dreaming becomes vivid and excessive. Rebound insomnia and increased dreaming (termed *REM rebound*) are not uncommon with abrupt withdrawal from long-term use of these drugs as sleeping aids (Julien, 2008).

Respiratory Depression

Barbiturates are capable of inhibiting the reticular activating system, resulting in respiratory depression (Sadock & Sadock, 2007). Additive effects can occur with the concurrent use of other CNS depressants, effecting a life-threatening situation.

Cardiovascular Effects

Hypotension may be a problem with large doses. Only a slight decrease in blood pressure is noted with normal oral dosage. High dosages of barbiturates may result in decreased cardiac output, decreased cerebral blood flow, and direct impairment of myocardial contractility (Lafferty & Abdel-Kariem, 2012).

Renal Function

In doses high enough to produce anesthesia, barbiturates may suppress urine function. At the usual sedative/hypnotic dosage, however, there is no evidence that they have any direct action on the kidneys.

Hepatic Effects

The barbiturates may produce jaundice with doses large enough to produce acute intoxication. Barbiturates stimulate the production of liver enzymes, resulting in a decrease in the plasma levels of both the barbiturates and other drugs metabolized in the liver. Preexisting liver disease may predispose an individual to additional liver damage with excessive barbiturate use.

Body Temperature

High doses of barbiturates can greatly decrease body temperature. It is not significantly altered with normal dosage levels.

Sexual Functioning

CNS depressants have a tendency to produce a biphasic response. There is an initial increase in libido, presumably from the primary disinhibitory effects of the drug. This initial response is then followed by a decrease in the ability to maintain an erection.

Sedative, Hypnotic, or Anxiolytic Intoxication

The *DSM-5* (APA, 2013) describes sedative, hypnotic, or anxiolytic intoxication as the presence of clinically significant maladaptive behavioral or psychological changes that develop during, or shortly after, use of one of these substances. These maladaptive changes may include inappropriate sexual or aggressive behavior, mood lability, impaired judgment, or impaired social or occupational functioning. Other symptoms that may develop with excessive use of CNS depressants include slurred speech, incoordination, unsteady gait, nystagmus, impairment in attention or memory, and stupor or coma.

"Club drugs" in this category include gamma hydroxybutyric acid (GHB) and flunitrazepam (Rohypnol). Like all of the depressants, they can produce a state of disinhibition, excitement, drunkenness, and amnesia. They have been widely implicated as "date rape" drugs, their presence being easily disguised in drinks. They produce anterograde amnesia, rendering the inability to remember events experienced while under their influence (Walton-Moss et al., 2010).

Sedative, Hypnotic, or Anxiolytic Withdrawal

Withdrawal from sedatives, hypnotics, or anxiolytics produces a characteristic syndrome of symptoms that develops after a marked decrease in or cessation of intake that has been heavy or prolonged (APA, 2013). Onset of the symptoms depends on the drug from which the individual is withdrawing. With short-acting anxiolytics (e.g., alprazolam, lorazepam), symptoms may begin between 12 and 24 hours after the last dose, reach peak intensity between 24 and 72 hours, and subside in 5 to 10 days. Withdrawal symptoms from substances with longer half-lives (e.g., diazepam, phenobarbital, chlordiazepoxide) may begin within 2 to 7 days, peak on the 5th to 8th day, and subside in 10 to 16 days (Gualtieri, 2004; Leamon, Wright, & Myrick, 2008).

Severe withdrawal is most likely to occur when a substance has been used at high dosages for prolonged periods. However, withdrawal symptoms also have been reported with moderate dosages taken over a relatively short duration. Withdrawal symptoms associated with sedatives, hypnotics, or anxiolytics include autonomic hyperactivity (e.g., sweating or pulse rate greater than 100), increased hand tremor, insomnia, nausea or vomiting, hallucinations, illusions, psychomotor agitation, anxiety, or grand mal seizures.

Stimulant Use Disorder

A Profile of the Substance

The CNS stimulants are identified by the behavioral stimulation and psychomotor agitation that they induce. They differ widely in their molecular structures and in their mechanisms of action. The amount of CNS stimulation caused by a certain drug depends on both the area in the brain or spinal cord that is affected by the drug and the cellular mechanism fundamental to the increased excitability. The *DSM-5* (APA, 2013) categorizes caffeine-related disorders and tobacco-related disorders as separate and distinct diagnoses. For purposes of this text, these substances will be discussed with the stimulant-related disorders.

Groups within this category are classified according to similarities in mechanism of action. The *psychomotor stimulants* induce stimulation by augmentation or potentiation of the neurotransmitters norepinephrine, epinephrine, or dopamine. The *general cellular stimulants* (caffeine and nicotine) exert their action directly on cellular activity. Caffeine inhibits the enzyme phosphodiesterase, allowing increased levels of 3', 5'-cyclic adenosine monophosphate (cAMP), a chemical substance that promotes increased rates of cellular metabolism. Nicotine stimulates ganglionic synapses. This results in increased acetylcholine, which stimulates nerve impulse transmission to the entire autonomic nervous system. A selected list of drugs included in these categories is presented in Table 23-2.

The two most prevalent and widely used stimulants are caffeine and nicotine. Caffeine is readily available in every supermarket and grocery store as a common ingredient in coffee, tea, colas, and chocolate. Nicotine

TABLE 23–2 CNS Stimulants

CATEGORIES	GENERIC (TRADE) NAMES	COMMON STREET NAMES
Amphetamines	Dextroamphetamine (Dexedrine) Methamphetamine (Desoxyn) 3,4-methylenedioxyamphetamine (MDMA)* Amphetamine + dextroamphetamine (Adderall)	Dexies, uppers, truck drivers Meth, speed, crystal, ice Adam, Ecstasy, EVE, XTC Beanies, pep pills, speed, uppers
Synthetic stimulants	3,4-methylenedioxypyrovalerone (MDPV)* 4-methylmethcathinone (mephedrone, 4-MMC)* Methylone*	Bath Salts (also called blue silk, cloud 9, ivory wave, vanilla sky, white knight, and others)
Nonamphetamine stimulants	Phendametrazine (Bontril) Benzphetamine (Didrex) Diethylpropion (Tenuate) Phentermine (Adipex-P; Ionamin) Sibutramine (Meridia)† Methylphenidate (Ritalin) Dexmethylphenidate (Focalin) Modafinil (Provigil)	Diet pills Speed, uppers
Cocaine	Cocaine hydrochloride	Coke, blow, toot, snow, lady, flake, crack
Caffeine	Coffee, tea, colas, chocolate	Java, mud, brew, cocoa
Nicotine	Cigarettes, cigars, pipe tobacco, snuff	Weeds, fags, butts, chaw, cancer sticks

*Cross-listed with the hallucinogens.
†No longer marketed in the United States.

is the primary psychoactive substance found in tobacco products. When used in moderation, these stimulants tend to relieve fatigue and increase alertness. They are a generally accepted part of our culture; however, with increased social awareness regarding the health risks associated with tobacco products, their use has become stigmatized in some circles.

The more potent stimulants, because of their potential for physiological addiction, are under regulation by the Controlled Substances Act. These controlled stimulants are available for therapeutic purposes by prescription only; however, they are also clandestinely manufactured and widely distributed on the illicit market. Most recently, the synthetic stimulants mephedrone, 3,4-methylenedioxypyrovalerone (MDPV), methylone, and others, have become available. Known as "bath salts," their street names include blue silk, cloud 9, ivory wave, vanilla sky, white knight, stardust, and purple wave. In October 2011, the United States Drug Enforcement Administration (DEA) issued emergency scheduling of these substances to make their possession and sales illegal (except as authorized by law). They are currently designated as Schedule I substances, the most restrictive category under the Controlled Substances Act. This action was taken in response to reports of episodes of violent behavior associated with use of the substances.

Historical Aspects

Cocaine is the most potent stimulant derived from nature. It is extracted from the leaves of the coca plant, which has been cultivated in the Andean highlands of South America since prehistoric times. Natives of the region chew the leaves of the plant for refreshment and relief from fatigue.

The coca leaves must be mixed with lime to release the cocaine alkaloid. The chemical formula for the pure form of the drug was developed in 1960. Physicians began using the drug as an anesthetic in eye, nose, and throat surgeries. It has also been used therapeutically in the United States in a morphine-cocaine elixir designed to relieve the suffering associated with terminal illness. These therapeutic uses are now obsolete.

Cocaine has achieved a degree of acceptability within some social circles. It is illicitly distributed as a white crystalline powder, often mixed with other ingredients to increase its volume and, therefore, create more profits. The drug is most commonly "snorted," and chronic users may manifest symptoms that resemble the congested nose of a common cold. The intensely pleasurable effects of the drug create the potential for extraordinary psychological addiction.

Another form of cocaine commonly used in the United States is made by processing powdered cocaine with ammonia or sodium bicarbonate and water, and heating it to remove the hydrochloride (*Street Drugs*, 2012). The term "crack," which is the street name for this form of the drug, refers to the crackling sound heard when the mixture is smoked. Because this type of cocaine can be easily vaporized and inhaled, its effects have an extremely rapid onset.

Amphetamine was first prepared in 1887. Various derivatives of the drug soon followed, and clinical use of the drug began in 1927. Amphetamines were used quite extensively for medical purposes through the 1960s, but recognition of their abuse potential has sharply decreased clinical use. Today, they are prescribed only to treat narcolepsy (a rare disorder resulting in an uncontrollable desire for sleep), to treat hyperactivity disorders in children, and in certain cases of obesity. Clandestine production of amphetamines for distribution on the illicit market has become a thriving business. U.S. government estimates report the economic cost to society of methamphetamine use at between $16.2 billion and $48.3 billion (Office of National Drug Control Policy [ONDCP], 2010). Most of these expenses are related to the costs "that addiction places on dependent users and their premature mortality and from crime and criminal justice costs" (ONDCP, p. 1). Methamphetamine can be smoked, snorted, injected, or taken orally. The effects include an intense rush from smoking or intravenous injection to a slower onset of euphoria as a result of snorting or oral ingestion. Another form of the drug, crystal methamphetamine, is produced by slowly recrystallizing powder methamphetamine from a solvent such as methanol, ethanol, isopropanol, or acetone (*Street Drugs*, 2012). It is a colorless, odorless, large-crystal form of *d*-methamphetamine, and is commonly called glass or ice because of its appearance. Crystal meth is usually smoked in a glass pipe like crack cocaine.

The earliest history of caffeine is unknown and is shrouded by legend and myth. Caffeine was first discovered in coffee in 1820 and in tea 7 years later. Both beverages have been widely accepted and enjoyed as a "pick-me-up" by many cultures.

Tobacco was used by the aborigines from remote times. Introduced in Europe in the mid-16th century, its use grew rapidly and soon became prevalent in the Orient. Tobacco came to America with the settlement of the earliest colonies. Today, it is grown in many countries of the world, and although smoking is decreasing in most industrialized nations, it continues to be a serious problem in developing areas.

Patterns of Use

Because of their pleasurable effects, CNS stimulants have a high abuse potential. In 2012, about 1.6 million Americans were current cocaine users (SAMHSA, 2013). Use was highest among Americans ages 18 to 34.

Many individuals who abuse or are addicted to CNS stimulants began using the substance for the appetite-suppressant effect in an attempt at weight control. Higher and higher doses are consumed in an effort to maintain the pleasurable effects. With continued use, the pleasurable effects diminish, and there is a corresponding increase in dysphoric effects. There is a persistent craving for the substance, however, even in the face of unpleasant adverse effects from the continued drug taking.

CNS stimulant use is usually characterized by either episodic or chronic daily, or almost daily, use. Individuals who use the substances on an episodic basis often "binge" on the drug with very high dosages followed by a day or two of recuperation. This recuperation period is characterized by extremely intense and unpleasant symptoms (called a "crash").

The daily user may take large or small doses and may use the drug several times a day or only at a specific time during the day. The amount consumed usually increases over time as tolerance develops. Chronic users tend to rely on CNS stimulants to feel more powerful, more confident, and more decisive. They often fall into a pattern of taking "uppers" in the morning and "downers," such as alcohol or sleeping pills, at night.

The average American consumes two cups of coffee (about 200 mg of caffeine) per day. Caffeine is consumed in various amounts by about 90 percent of the population. At a level of 500 to 600 mg of daily caffeine consumption, symptoms of anxiety, insomnia, and depression are not uncommon. It is also at this level that caffeine dependence and withdrawal can occur. Caffeine consumption is prevalent among children as well as adults. Table 23-3 lists some common sources of caffeine.

Next to caffeine, nicotine, an active ingredient in tobacco, is the most widely used psychoactive substance in U.S. society. Of the U.S. population aged 12 years or older, 26.7 percent reported current use of a tobacco product in 2012 (SAMHSA, 2013). Since 1964, when the results of the first public health report on smoking were issued, the percentage of total smokers has been on the decline. However, the percentage of women and teenage smokers has declined more slowly than that of adult men. The CDC (2012b) reports that an estimated 443,000 people die annually because of tobacco use or exposure to secondhand smoke, and more than $96 billion a year of the direct health-care costs in the United States go to treat tobacco-related illnesses.

Effects on the Body

The CNS stimulants are a group of pharmacological agents that are capable of exciting the entire nervous

TABLE 23-3 **Common Sources of Caffeine**	
SOURCE	CAFFEINE CONTENT (mg)
FOOD AND BEVERAGES	
5–6 oz. brewed coffee	90–125
5–6 oz. instant coffee	60–90
5–6 oz. decaffeinated coffee	3
5–6 oz. brewed tea	70
5–6 oz. instant tea	45
8 oz. green tea	15–30
8–12 oz. cola drinks	60
12 oz. Red Bull energy drink	115
2 oz. High Energy drinks	215–240
5–6 oz. cocoa	20
8 oz. chocolate milk	2–7
1 oz. chocolate bar	22
PRESCRIPTION MEDICATIONS	
APCs (aspirin, phenacetin, caffeine)	32
Cafergot	100
Fiorinal	40
Migralam	100
OVER-THE-COUNTER ANALGESICS	
Anacin, Empirin, Midol, Vanquish	32
Excedrin Migraine (aspirin, acetaminophen, caffeine)	65
OVER-THE-COUNTER STIMULANTS	
No Doz Tablets	100
Vivarin	200
Caffedrine	250

system. This is accomplished by increasing the activity or augmenting the capability of the neurotransmitter agents known to be directly involved in bodily activation and behavioral stimulation. Physiological responses vary markedly according to the potency and dosage of the drug.

Central Nervous System Effects

Stimulation of the CNS results in tremor, restlessness, anorexia, insomnia, agitation, and increased motor activity. Amphetamines, nonamphetamine stimulants, and cocaine produce increased alertness, decrease in fatigue, elation and euphoria, and subjective feelings of greater mental agility and muscular power. Chronic use of these drugs may result in compulsive behavior, paranoia, hallucinations, and aggressive behavior (*Street Drugs*, 2012).

Cardiovascular/Pulmonary Effects

Amphetamines can induce increased systolic and diastolic blood pressure, increased heart rate, and cardiac arrhythmias (*Street Drugs*, 2012). These drugs also relax bronchial smooth muscle.

Cocaine intoxication typically produces a rise in myocardial demand for oxygen and an increase in heart rate. Severe vasoconstriction may occur and can result in myocardial infarction, ventricular fibrillation, and sudden death. Inhaled cocaine can cause pulmonary hemorrhage, chronic bronchiolitis, and pneumonia. Nasal rhinitis is a result of chronic cocaine snorting.

Caffeine ingestion can result in increased heart rate, palpitations, extrasystoles, and cardiac arrhythmias. Caffeine induces dilation of pulmonary and general systemic blood vessels and constriction of cerebral blood vessels.

Nicotine stimulates the sympathetic nervous system, resulting in an increase in heart rate, blood pressure, and cardiac contractility, thereby increasing myocardial oxygen consumption and demand for blood flow. Contractions of gastric smooth muscle associated with hunger are inhibited, thereby producing a mild anorectic effect.

Gastrointestinal and Renal Effects

Gastrointestinal (GI) effects of amphetamines are somewhat unpredictable; however, a decrease in GI tract motility commonly results in constipation. Contraction of the bladder sphincter makes urination difficult. Caffeine exerts a diuretic effect on the kidneys. Nicotine stimulates the hypothalamus to release antidiuretic hormone, reducing the excretion of urine. Because nicotine increases the tone and activity of the bowel, it may occasionally cause diarrhea.

Most CNS stimulants induce a small rise in metabolic rate and various degrees of anorexia. Amphetamines and cocaine can cause a rise in body temperature.

Sexual Functioning

CNS stimulants appear to promote the coital urge in both men and women. Women, more than men, report that stimulants make them feel sexier and have more orgasms. In fact, some men may experience sexual dysfunction with the use of stimulants. For the majority of individuals, however, these drugs exert a powerful aphrodisiac effect.

Stimulant Intoxication

Stimulant intoxication produces maladaptive behavioral and psychological changes that develop during, or shortly after, use of these drugs. Amphetamine and cocaine intoxication typically produces euphoria or affective blunting; changes in sociability; hypervigilance; interpersonal sensitivity; anxiety, tension, or anger; stereotyped behaviors; or impaired judgment. Physical effects include tachycardia or bradycardia, pupillary dilation, elevated or lowered blood pressure, perspiration or chills, nausea or vomiting, weight loss, psychomotor agitation or retardation, muscular weakness, respiratory depression, chest pain, cardiac arrhythmias, confusion, seizures, dyskinesias, dystonias, or coma (APA, 2013).

Intoxication from caffeine usually occurs following consumption in excess of 250 mg. Symptoms include restlessness, nervousness, excitement, insomnia, flushed face, diuresis, GI disturbance, muscle twitching, rambling flow of thought and speech, tachycardia or cardiac arrhythmia, periods of inexhaustibility, and psychomotor agitation (APA, 2013).

Stimulant Withdrawal

Stimulant withdrawal is the presence of a characteristic withdrawal syndrome that develops within a few hours to several days after cessation of, or reduction in, heavy and prolonged use (APA, 2013). Black and Andreasen (2011) state:

> Cessation or reduction of amphetamine (or cocaine) use may lead to a withdrawal syndrome often referred to as a "crash." Symptoms include fatigue and depression, nightmares, headache, profuse sweating, muscle cramps, and hunger. Withdrawal symptoms usually peak in 2-4 days. Intense dysphoria can occur, peaking between 48 and 72 hours after the last dose of the stimulant. (p. 274)

The *DSM-5* (APA, 2013) states that a withdrawal syndrome can occur with abrupt cessation of caffeine intake after a prolonged daily use of the substance. The symptoms begin within 24 hours after last consumption and may include the following symptoms: headache, fatigue, drowsiness, dysphoric mood, irritability, difficulty concentrating, flu-like symptoms, nausea, vomiting, and/or muscle pain and stiffness.

Withdrawal from nicotine results in dysphoric or depressed mood; insomnia; irritability, frustration, or anger; anxiety; difficulty concentrating; restlessness; decreased heart rate; and increased appetite or weight gain (APA, 2013). A mild syndrome of nicotine withdrawal can appear when a smoker switches from regular cigarettes to low-nicotine cigarettes (Sadock & Sadock, 2007).

Inhalant Use Disorder

A Profile of the Substance

Inhalant disorders are induced by inhaling the aliphatic and aromatic hydrocarbons found in substances such as fuels, solvents, adhesives, aerosol propellants, and paint thinners.

Specific examples of these substances include gasoline, varnish remover, lighter fluid, airplane glue, rubber cement, cleaning fluid, spray paint, shoe conditioner, and typewriter correction fluid.

Patterns of Use

Inhalant substances are readily available, legal, and inexpensive. These three factors make inhalants the drug of choice among poor people and among children and young adults. Highest usage is by youths ages 12 to 17. By age 18, the usage drops dramatically. A national government survey of drug use indicated that 8.1 percent of people in the United States ages 12 years or older acknowledged having used inhalants (SAMHSA, 2013).

Methods of use include "huffing"—a procedure in which a rag soaked with the substance is applied to the mouth and nose and the vapors breathed in. Another common method is called "bagging," in which the substance is placed in a paper or plastic bag and inhaled from the bag by the user. The substance may also be inhaled directly from the container or sprayed in the mouth or nose.

Sadock and Sadock (2007) reported that:

> Inhalant use among adolescents may be most common in those whose parents or older siblings use illegal substances. Inhalant use among adolescents is also associated with an increased likelihood of conduct disorder or antisocial personality disorder. (p. 435)

Tolerance to inhalants has been reported with heavy use. A mild withdrawal syndrome has been documented but does not appear to be clinically significant. Among children with inhalant disorder, the products may be used several times a week, often on weekends and after school. Adults with inhalant addiction may use the substance at varying times during each day, or they may binge on the substance during a period of several days.

Effects on the Body

Inhalants are absorbed through the lungs and reach the CNS very rapidly. Inhalants generally act as CNS depressants (Black & Andreasen, 2011). The effects are relatively brief, lasting from several minutes to a few hours, depending on the specific substance and amount consumed.

Central Nervous System

Inhalants can cause both central and peripheral nervous system damage. Neurological damage, such as ataxia, peripheral and sensorimotor neuropathy, speech problems, and tremor, can occur (Leamon et al., 2008). Other CNS effects that have been reported with heavy inhalant use include ototoxicity, encephalopathy, parkinsonism, and damage to the protective sheath around certain nerve fibers in the brain and peripheral nervous system (Walton-Moss et al., 2010).

Respiratory Effects

Respiratory effects of inhalant use range from coughing and wheezing to dyspnea, emphysema, and pneumonia (Leamon et al., 2008). There is increased airway resistance due to inflammation of the passages. Walton-Moss and associates (2010) state, "Death can occur from suffocation, which may occur when inhaling from a paper or plastic bag in a closed area" (p. 208).

Gastrointestinal Effects

Abdominal pain, nausea, and vomiting may occur. A rash may be present around the individual's nose and mouth. Unusual breath odors are common. Long-term use has resulted in reports of liver toxicity (Leamon et al., 2008).

Renal System Effects

Acute and chronic renal failure and hepatorenal syndrome have occurred. Renal toxicity from toluene exposure has been reported, manifesting in renal tubular acidosis, hypokalemia, hypophosphatemia, hyperchloremia, azotemia, sterile pyuria, hematuria, and proteinuria (McKeown, 2011).

Inhalant Intoxication

The *DSM-5* defines inhalant intoxication as "clinically significant problematic behavioral or psychological changes that developed during or shortly after exposure to inhalants" (APA, 2013). Symptoms are similar to alcohol intoxication and may include the following (APA, 2013; Black & Andreasen, 2011):

- Dizziness; ataxia
- Euphoria; excitation; disinhibition
- Nystagmus; blurred vision; double vision
- Slurred speech
- Hypoactive reflexes
- Psychomotor retardation; lethargy
- Generalized muscle weakness
- Stupor or coma (at higher doses)

Opioid Use Disorder

A Profile of the Substance

The term *opioid* refers to a group of compounds that includes opium, opium derivatives, and synthetic substitutes. Opioids exert both a sedative and an analgesic effect, and their major medical uses are for the relief of pain, the treatment of diarrhea, and the relief of coughing. These drugs have addictive qualities; that is, they are capable of inducing tolerance and physiological and psychological addiction.

Opioids are popular drugs of abuse in that they desensitize an individual to both psychological and physiological pain and induce a sense of euphoria. Lethargy and indifference to the environment are common manifestations.

Opioid abusers usually spend much of their time nourishing their habit. Individuals who are addicted to opioids are seldom able to hold a steady job that will support their need. They must therefore secure funds from friends, relatives, or whomever they have not yet alienated with their addiction-related behavior. It is not uncommon for individuals who are addicted to opioids to resort to illegal means of obtaining funds, such as burglary, robbery, prostitution, or selling drugs.

Methods of administration of opioid drugs include oral, snorting, or smoking, and by subcutaneous, intramuscular, and intravenous injection. A selected list of opioid substances is presented in Table 23-4.

Under close supervision, opioids are indispensable in the practice of medicine. They are the most effective agents known for the relief of intense pain. However, they also induce a pleasurable effect on the CNS that promotes their abuse. The physiological and psychological addiction that occurs with opioids, as well as the development of profound tolerance, contribute to the addict's ongoing quest for more of the substance, regardless of the means.

Historical Aspects

In its crude form, opium is a brownish-black, gummy substance obtained from the ripened pods of the opium poppy. References to the use of opiates have been found in the Egyptian, Greek, and Arabian cultures as early as 3000 BC. The drug became widely used both medicinally and recreationally throughout Europe during the 16th and 17th centuries. Most of the opium supply came from China, where the drug was introduced by Arabic traders in the late 17th century. Morphine, the primary active ingredient of opium, was isolated in 1803 by the European chemist Frederich Serturner. Since that time, morphine, rather than crude opium, has been used throughout the world for the medical treatment of pain and diarrhea. This process was facilitated in 1853 by the development of the hypodermic syringe, which made it possible to deliver the undiluted morphine quickly into the body for rapid relief from pain.

This development also created a new variety of opiate user in the United States: one who was able to self-administer the drug by injection. During this time, there was also a large influx of Chinese immigrants into the United States, who introduced opium smoking to this country. By the early part of the 20th century, opium addiction was widespread.

In response to the concerns over widespread addiction, in 1914 the U.S. government passed the Harrison Narcotic Act, which created strict controls on the accessibility of opiates. Until that time, these substances had been freely available to the public without a prescription. The Harrison Act banned the use of opiates for other than medicinal purposes and drove the use of heroin underground. To this day, the beneficial uses of these substances are widely acclaimed within the medical profession, but the illicit trafficking of the drugs for recreational purposes continues to resist most efforts aimed at control.

Patterns of Use

The development of opioid addiction may follow one of two typical behavior patterns. The first occurs in

TABLE 23-4 **Opioids and Related Substances**		
CATEGORIES	GENERIC (TRADE) NAMES	COMMON STREET NAMES
Opioids of natural origin	Opium (ingredient in various antidiarrheal agents)	Black stuff, poppy, tar, big O
	Morphine (Astramorph)	M, white stuff, Miss Emma
	Codeine (ingredient in various analgesics and cough suppressants)	Terp, schoolboy, syrup, cody
Opioid derivatives	Heroin	H, horse, junk, brown sugar, smack, skag, TNT, Harry
	Hydromorphone (Dilaudid)	DLs, 4s, lords, little D
	Oxycodone (Percodan; OxyContin)	Perks, perkies, Oxy, O.C.
	Hydrocodone (Vicodin)	Vike
Synthetic opiate-like drugs	Meperidine (Demerol)	Doctors
	Methadone (Dolophine)	Dollies, done
	Pentazocine (Talwin)	Ts
	Fentanyl (Fentora)	Apache, China girl, China town, dance fever, goodfella, jackpot

the individual who has obtained the drug by prescription from a physician for the relief of a medical problem. Abuse and addiction occur when the individual increases the amount and frequency of use, justifying the behavior as symptom treatment. He or she becomes obsessed with obtaining more and more of the substance, seeking out several physicians in order to replenish and maintain supplies.

The second pattern of behavior associated with addiction to opioids occurs among individuals who use the drugs for recreational purposes and obtain them from illegal sources. Opioids may be used alone to induce the euphoric effects or in combination with stimulants or other drugs to enhance the euphoria or to counteract the depressant effects of the opioid. Tolerance develops and addiction occurs, leading the individual to procure the substance by whatever means is required to support the habit.

A recent government survey reported that there were 335,000 current heroin users aged 12 years and older in the United States in 2012 (SAMHSA, 2013). The same survey revealed an estimated 6.8 million persons in the same age group who used prescription psychotherapeutic drugs nonmedically. In the last 10 years, there has been a dramatic increase in the abuse of prescription pain medication, and it was the second most common type of illicit drug use in the United States in 2012 (SAMHSA, 2013).

Effects on the Body

Opiates are sometimes classified as *narcotic analgesics.* They exert their major effects primarily on the CNS, the eyes, and the GI tract. Chronic morphine use or acute morphine toxicity is manifested by a syndrome of sedation, chronic constipation, decreased respiratory rate, and pinpoint pupils. Intensity of symptoms is largely dose dependent. The following physiological effects are common with opioid use.

Central Nervous System

All opioids, opioid derivatives, and synthetic opioid-like drugs affect the CNS. Common manifestations include euphoria, mood changes, and mental clouding. Other common CNS effects include drowsiness and pain reduction. Pupillary constriction occurs in response to stimulation of the oculomotor nerve. CNS depression of the respiratory centers within the medulla results in respiratory depression. The antitussive response is due to suppression of the cough center within the medulla. The nausea and vomiting commonly associated with opiate ingestion is related to the stimulation of the centers within the medulla that trigger this response.

Gastrointestinal Effects

These drugs exert a profound effect on the GI tract. Both stomach and intestinal tone are increased, whereas peristaltic activity of the intestines is diminished. These effects lead to a marked decrease in the movement of food through the GI tract. This is a notable therapeutic effect in the treatment of severe diarrhea. In fact, no drugs have yet been developed that are more effective than the opioids for this purpose. However, constipation, and even fecal impaction, may be a serious problem for the chronic opioid user.

Cardiovascular Effects

In therapeutic doses, opioids have minimal effect on the action of the heart. Morphine is used extensively to relieve pulmonary edema and the pain of myocardial infarction in cardiac clients. At high doses, opioids induce hypotension, which may be caused by direct action on the heart or by opioid-induced histamine release.

Sexual Functioning

With opioid use, there is decreased sexual function and diminished libido (National Cancer Institute, 2012). Delayed ejaculation, impotence, and orgasm failure (in both men and women) may occur. Sexual side effects from opioids appear to be largely influenced by dosage.

Opioid Intoxication

Opioid intoxication constitutes clinically significant problematic behavioral or psychological changes that develop during, or shortly after, opioid use (APA, 2013). Symptoms include initial euphoria followed by apathy, dysphoria, psychomotor agitation or retardation, and impaired judgment. Physical symptoms include pupillary constriction (or dilation due to anoxia from severe overdose), drowsiness, slurred speech, and impairment in attention or memory (APA, 2013). Symptoms are consistent with the half-life of most opioid drugs, and usually last for several hours. Severe opioid intoxication can lead to respiratory depression, coma, and death.

Opioid Withdrawal

Opioid withdrawal produces a syndrome of symptoms that develops after cessation of, or reduction in, heavy and prolonged use of an opiate or related substance. Symptoms include dysphoric mood, nausea or vomiting, muscle aches, lacrimation or rhinorrhea, pupillary dilation, piloerection, sweating, diarrhea, yawning, fever, and insomnia (APA, 2013). With short-acting drugs such as heroin, withdrawal symptoms occur within 6 to 8 hours after the last dose, peak within 1 to 3 days, and gradually subside over a period of 5 to 10 days (Walton-Moss et al., 2010). With longer-acting drugs such as methadone, withdrawal symptoms begin within 1 to 3 days after the last dose, peak between days 4 and 6, and are complete in 14 to 21 days (Leamon et al., 2008). Withdrawal from the ultra-short-acting meperidine begins quickly, reaches a peak in 8 to 12 hours, and is complete in 4 to 5 days (Sadock & Sadock, 2007).

Hallucinogen Use Disorder

A Profile of the Substance

Hallucinogenic substances are capable of distorting an individual's perception of reality. They have the ability to alter sensory perception and induce hallucinations. For this reason they have sometimes been referred to as "mind expanding." Some of the manifestations have been likened to a psychotic break. The hallucinations experienced by an individual with schizophrenia, however, are most often auditory, whereas substance-induced hallucinations are usually visual (Mack, Franklin, & Frances, 2003). Perceptual distortions have been reported by some users as spiritual, as giving a sense of depersonalization (observing oneself having the experience), or as being at peace with self and the universe. Others, who describe their experiences as "bad trips," report feelings of panic and a fear of dying or going insane. A common danger reported with hallucinogenic drugs is that of "flashbacks," or a spontaneous reoccurrence of the hallucinogenic state without ingestion of the drug. These can occur months after the drug was last taken.

Recurrent use can produce tolerance, encouraging users to resort to higher and higher dosages. No evidence of physical addiction is detectable when the drug is withdrawn; however, recurrent use appears to induce a psychological addiction to the insight-inducing experiences that a user may associate with episodes of hallucinogen use (Sadock & Sadock,

2007). This psychological addiction varies according to the drug, the dose, and the individual user. Hallucinogens are highly unpredictable in the effects they may induce each time they are used.

Many of the hallucinogenic substances have structural similarities. Some are produced synthetically; others are natural products of plants and fungi. A selected list of hallucinogens is presented in Table 23-5.

Historical Aspects

Archeological data obtained with carbon-14 dating suggest that hallucinogens have been used as part of religious ceremonies and at social gatherings by Native Americans for as long as 7,000 years (Goldstein, 2002). Use of the peyote cactus as part of religious ceremonies in the southwestern part of the United States still occurs today, although this ritual use has greatly diminished.

LSD was first synthesized in 1943 by Dr. Albert Hoffman (Goldstein, 2002). It was used as a clinical research tool to investigate the biochemical etiology of schizophrenia. It soon reached the illicit market, however, and its abuse began to overshadow the research effort.

The abuse of hallucinogens reached a peak in the late 1960s, waned during the 1970s, and returned to favor in the 1980s with the so-called designer drugs (e.g., 3,4-methylene-dioxyamphetamine [MDMA] and methoxy-amphetamine [MDA]). One of the most commonly abused hallucinogens today is PCP, even

TABLE 23–5 **Hallucinogens**		
CATEGORIES	GENERIC (TRADE) NAMES	COMMON STREET NAMES
Naturally occurring hallucinogens	Mescaline (the primary active ingredient of the peyote cactus)	Cactus, mesc, mescal, half moon, big chief, bad seed, peyote
	Psilocybin and psilocin (active ingredients of *Psilocybe* mushrooms)	Magic mushroom, God's flesh, shrooms
	Ololiuqui (morning glory seeds)	Heavenly blue, pearly gates, flying saucers
Synthetic compounds	Lysergic acid diethylamide (LSD)—synthetically produced from a fungal substance found on rye or a chemical substance found in morning glory seeds	Acid, cube, big D, California sunshine, microdots, blue dots, sugar, orange wedges, peace tablets, purple haze, cupcakes
	Dimethyltryptamine (DMT) and diethyltryptamine (DET)—chemical analogues of tryptamine	Businessman's trip
	2,5-Dimethoxy-4-methylamphetamine (STP, DOM)	STP (serenity, tranquility, peace)
	Phencyclidine (PCP)	Angel dust, hog, peace pill, rocket fuel
	Ketamine (Ketalar)	Special K, vitamin K, kit kat
	3,4-Methylene-dioxyamphetamine (MDMA)*	XTC, ecstasy, Adam, Eve
	Methoxy-amphetamine (MDA)	Love drug
	3,4-methylenedioxypyrovalerone (MDPV)* 4-methylmethcathinone (mephedrone, 4-MMC)* Methylone*	Bath Salts (also called blue silk, cloud 9, ivory wave, vanilla sky, white knight, and others)

*Cross-listed with the CNS stimulants

though many of its effects are perceived as undesirable. A number of deaths have been directly attributed to the use of PCP, and numerous accidental deaths have occurred as a result of overdose and of the behavioral changes the drug precipitates. A derivative of PCP, ketamine, which is a preoperative anesthetic, also is abused for its psychedelic properties. It produces effects similar to, but somewhat less intense than, those of PCP.

Several therapeutic uses of LSD have been proposed, including the treatment of chronic alcoholism and the reduction of intractable pain such as occurs in malignant disease. A great deal more research is required regarding the therapeutic uses of LSD. At this time, there is no real evidence of the safety and efficacy of the drug in humans.

Patterns of Use

Use of hallucinogens is usually episodic. Because cognitive and perceptual abilities are so markedly affected by these substances, the user must set aside time from normal daily activities for indulging in the consequences. According to the SAMHSA (2013) report, hallucinogens were used in the previous 30-day period before the survey in 2012 by approximately 1.1 million persons (0.4 percent) aged 12 or older.

The use of LSD does not lead to the development of physical addiction or withdrawal symptoms (Sadock & Sadock, 2007). However, tolerance does develop quickly and to a high degree. In fact, an individual who uses LSD repeatedly for a period of 3 to 4 days may develop complete tolerance to the drug. Recovery from the tolerance also occurs very rapidly (in 4 to 7 days), so that the individual is able to achieve the desired effect from the drug repeatedly and often.

PCP is usually taken episodically, in binges that can last for several days. However, some chronic users take the substance daily. Physical addiction does not occur with PCP; however, psychological addiction characterized by craving for the drug has been reported in chronic users, as has the development of tolerance. Tolerance apparently develops quickly with frequent use.

Psilocybin is an ingredient of the *Psilocybe* mushroom indigenous to the United States and Mexico. Ingestion of these mushrooms produces an effect similar to that of LSD but of a shorter duration. This hallucinogenic chemical can now be produced synthetically.

Mescaline is the only hallucinogenic compound used legally for religious purposes today by members of the Native American Church of the United States. It is the primary active ingredient of the peyote cactus. Neither physical nor psychological addiction occurs with the use of mescaline, although, as with other hallucinogens, tolerance can develop quickly with frequent use.

Among the very potent hallucinogens of the current drug culture are those that are categorized as derivatives of amphetamines. These include 2,5-dimethoxy-4-methylamphetamine (DOM, STP), MDMA, and MDA. At lower doses, these drugs produce the "high" associated with CNS stimulants. At higher doses, hallucinogenic effects occur. These drugs have existed for many years but were *rediscovered* in the mid-1980s. Because of the rapid increase in recreational use, the DEA imposed an emergency classification of MDMA as a Schedule I drug in 1985. MDMA, or Ecstasy, is a synthetic drug with both stimulant and hallucinogenic qualities. It has a chemical structure similar to methamphetamine and mescaline, and it has become widely available throughout the world. Because of its growing popularity, the demand for this drug has led to tablets and capsules being sold as "Ecstasy," but which are not pure MDMA. Many contain drugs such as methamphetamine, PCP, amphetamine, ketamine, and *p*-methoxyamphetamine (PMA, a stimulant with hallucinogenic properties; more toxic than MDMA). This practice has increased the dangers associated with MDMA use.

Effects on the Body

The effects produced by the various hallucinogens are highly unpredictable. The variety of effects may be related to dosage, the mental state of the individual, and the environment in which the substance is used. Some common effects have been reported (APA, 2013; Julien, 2008; Sadock & Sadock, 2007):

Physiological Effects

■ Nausea and vomiting
■ Chills
■ Pupil dilation
■ Increased pulse, blood pressure, and temperature
■ Mild dizziness
■ Trembling
■ Loss of appetite
■ Insomnia
■ Sweating
■ A slowing of respirations
■ Elevation in blood sugar

Psychological Effects

■ Heightened response to color, texture, and sounds
■ Heightened body awareness
■ Distortion of vision
■ Sense of slowing of time
■ All feelings magnified: love, lust, hate, joy, anger, pain, terror, despair
■ Fear of losing control
■ Paranoia, panic
■ Euphoria, bliss
■ Projection of self into dreamlike images
■ Serenity, peace

■ Depersonalization
■ Derealization
■ Increased libido

The effects of hallucinogens are not always pleasurable for the user. Two types of toxic reactions are known to occur. The first is the *panic reaction*, or "bad trip." Symptoms include an intense level of anxiety, fear, and stimulation. The individual hallucinates and fears going insane. Paranoia and acute psychosis may be evident.

The second type of toxic reaction to hallucinogens is the *flashback*. This phenomenon refers to the transient, spontaneous repetition of a previous hallucinogen-induced experience that occurs in the absence of the substance. The *DSM-5* (APA, 2013) refers to this as *hallucinogen persisting perception disorder*. Various studies have reported that 15 to 80 percent of hallucinogen users report having experienced flashbacks (Sadock & Sadock, 2007).

Hallucinogen Intoxication

Symptoms of hallucinogen intoxication develop during, or shortly after hallucinogen use. Maladaptive behavioral or psychological changes include marked anxiety or depression, ideas of reference (a type of delusional thinking that all activity within one's environment is "referred to" [about] one's self), fear of losing one's mind, paranoid ideation, and impaired judgment (APA, 2013). Perceptual changes occur while the individual is fully awake and alert and include intensification of perceptions, depersonalization, derealization, illusions, hallucinations, and synesthesias (APA, 2013). Because hallucinogens are sympathomimetics, they can cause tachycardia, hypertension, sweating, blurred vision, pupillary dilation, and tremors (Black & Andreasen, 2011).

Symptoms of PCP intoxication are unpredictable. Specific symptoms are dose related and may be manifested by impulsiveness, impaired judgment, assaultiveness, and belligerence, or the individual may appear calm, stuporous, or comatose (Leamon et al., 2008; Walton-Moss et al., 2010). Physical symptoms include vertical or horizontal nystagmus, hypertension, tachycardia, ataxia, diminished pain sensation, muscle rigidity, and seizures (Leamon et al., 2008; Walton-Moss et al., 2010). Symptoms of ketamine intoxication appear similar to those of PCP.

General effects of MDMA (Ecstasy) include increased heart rate, blood pressure, and body temperature; dehydration; confusion; insomnia; and paranoia. Overdose can result in panic attacks, hallucinations, severe hyperthermia, dehydration, and seizures. Death can occur from kidney or cardiovascular failure.

Cannabis Use Disorder

A Profile of the Substance

Cannabis is second only to alcohol as the most widely abused drug in the United States. The major psychoactive ingredient of this class of substances is delta-9-tetrahydrocannabinol (THC). It occurs naturally in the plant *Cannabis sativa*, which grows readily in warm climates. Marijuana, the most prevalent type of cannabis preparation, is composed of the dried leaves, stems, and flowers of the plant. Hashish is a more potent concentrate of the resin derived from the flowering tops of the plant. Hash oil is a very concentrated form of THC made by boiling hashish in a solvent and filtering out the solid matter (*Street Drugs*, 2012). Cannabis products are usually smoked in the form of loosely rolled cigarettes. Cannabis can also be taken orally when it is prepared in food, but about two to three times the amount of cannabis must be ingested orally to equal the potency of that obtained by the inhalation of its smoke (Sadock & Sadock, 2007).

At moderate dosages, cannabis drugs produce effects resembling alcohol and other CNS depressants. By depressing higher brain centers, they release lower centers from inhibitory influences. There has been some controversy in the past over the classification of these substances. They are not narcotics, although they are legally classified as controlled substances. They are not hallucinogens, although in very high dosages they can induce hallucinations. They are not sedative-hypnotics, although they most closely resemble these substances. Like sedative-hypnotics, their action occurs in the ascending reticular activating system.

Psychological addiction has been shown to occur with cannabis, and tolerance can occur. Controversy has existed about whether physiological addiction occurs with cannabis. In the past, symptoms of cannabis withdrawal were considered less than clinically significant to include the diagnosis in the *DSM*. However, the *DSM-5* Substance-Related Work Group determined that subsequent research studies have provided significant data to support cannabis withdrawal as a valid and reliable syndrome that can negatively impact abstinence attempts of heavy cannabis users. The diagnosis of cannabis withdrawal is included in the *DSM-5*.

Common cannabis preparations are presented in Table 23-6.

TABLE 23–6 **Cannabinoids**		
CATEGORY	COMMON PREPARATIONS	STREET NAMES
Cannabis	Marijuana	Joint, weed, pot, grass, Mary Jane, Texas tea, locoweed, MJ, hay, stick
	Hashish	Hash, bhang, ganja, charas

Historical Aspects

Products of *Cannabis sativa* have been used therapeutically for nearly 5,000 years (Julien, 2008). Cannabis was first employed in China and India as an antiseptic and an analgesic. Its use later spread to the Middle East, Africa, and Eastern Europe.

In the United States, medical interest in the use of cannabis arose during the early part of the 19th century. Many articles were published espousing its use for many and varied reasons. The drug was almost as commonly used for medicinal purposes as aspirin is today and could be purchased without a prescription in any drug store. It was purported to have antibacterial and anticonvulsant capabilities, to decrease intraocular pressure, decrease pain, help in the treatment of asthma, increase appetite, and generally raise one's morale.

The drug went out of favor primarily because of the huge variation in potency within batches of medication caused by the variations in the THC content of different plants. Other medications were favored for their greater degree of solubility and faster onset of action than cannabis products. A federal law put an end to its legal use in 1937, after an association between marijuana and criminal activity became evident. In the 1960s, marijuana became the symbol of the "antiestablishment" generation, at which time it reached its peak as a drug of abuse.

Research continues in regard to the possible therapeutic uses of cannabis. It has been shown to be an effective agent for relieving the nausea and vomiting associated with cancer chemotherapy, when other antinausea medications fail. It has also been used in the treatment of chronic pain, glaucoma, multiple sclerosis, and acquired immune deficiency syndrome (Sadock & Sadock, 2007).

Advocates who praise the therapeutic usefulness and support the legalization of the cannabinoids persist within the United States today. Such groups as the Alliance for Cannabis Therapeutics (ACT) and the National Organization for the Reform of Marijuana Laws (NORML) have lobbied extensively to allow disease sufferers easier access to the drug. The medical use of marijuana has been legalized by a number of states. The U.S. Drug Enforcement Agency (USDEA, 2011) has stated:

> The DEA supports ongoing research into potential medicinal uses of marijuana's active ingredients. [Currently] there are 111 researchers registered with the DEA to perform studies with marijuana, marijuana extracts, and non-tetrahydrocannabinol marijuana derivatives that exist in the plant, such as cannabidiol and cannabinol. Studies include evaluation of abuse potential, physical/psychological effects, adverse effects, therapeutic potential, and detection. Fourteen of the researchers are approved to conduct research with smoked marijuana on human subjects. At present, however, the clear weight of the evidence is that smoked marijuana is harmful. No matter what medical condition has been studied, other drugs already approved by the FDA have been proven to be safer and more effective than smoked marijuana. (p. 5)

A great deal more research is required to determine the long-term effects of the drug. Until results indicate otherwise, it is safe to assume that the harmful effects of the drug outweigh the benefits.

Patterns of Use

In its 2012 National Survey on Drug Use and Health, SAMHSA (2013) reported that an estimated 23.8 million Americans aged 12 years or older were current illicit drug users, meaning they had used an illicit drug during the month before the survey interview. This estimate represents approximately 9.2 percent of the population aged 12 years old or older. Marijuana is the most commonly used illicit drug. In 2012, it was used by 79 percent of current illicit drug users. This constitutes about 18.8 million users of marijuana in the United States in the year 2012.

Many people incorrectly regard cannabis as a substance of low abuse potential. This lack of knowledge has promoted use of the substance by some individuals who believe it is harmless. Tolerance, although it tends to decline rapidly, does occur with chronic use. As tolerance develops, physical addiction also occurs, resulting in a withdrawal syndrome upon cessation of drug use.

One controversy that exists regarding marijuana is whether its use leads to the use of other illicit drugs. Leamon and associates (2008) stated, "A relationship has consistently been shown between early, regular cannabis use and subsequent abuse of other drugs" (p. 381).

Effects on the Body

Following is a summary of some of the effects that have been attributed to marijuana in recent years. Undoubtedly, as research continues, evidence of additional physiological and psychological effects will be made available.

Cardiovascular Effects

Cannabis ingestion induces tachycardia and orthostatic hypotension (National Institutes of Health [NIH], 2012). With the decrease in blood pressure, myocardial oxygen supply is decreased. Tachycardia in turn increases oxygen demand.

Respiratory Effects

Marijuana produces a greater amount of "tar" than its equivalent weight in tobacco. Because of the method by which marijuana is smoked—that is, the smoke is held in the lungs for as long as possible to achieve the desired effect—larger amounts of tar are deposited in the lungs, promoting deleterious effects to the lungs.

Although the initial reaction to the marijuana is bronchodilatation, thereby facilitating respiratory function, chronic use results in obstructive airway disorders (NIH, 2012). Frequent marijuana users often have laryngitis, bronchitis, cough, and hoarseness. Cannabis smoke contains more carcinogens than tobacco smoke; therefore, lung damage and cancer are real risks for heavy users (NIH, 2012).

Reproductive Effects

Some studies have shown that, with heavy marijuana use, men may have a decrease in sperm count, motility, and structure. In women, heavy marijuana use may result in a suppression of ovulation, disruption in menstrual cycles, and alteration of hormone levels.

Central Nervous System Effects

Acute CNS effects of marijuana are dose related. Many people report a feeling of being "high"—the equivalent of being "drunk" on alcohol. Symptoms include feelings of euphoria, relaxed inhibitions, disorientation, depersonalization, and relaxation. At higher doses, sensory alterations may occur, including impairment in judgment of time and distance, recent memory, and learning ability. Physiological symptoms may include tremors, muscle rigidity, and conjunctival redness. Toxic effects are generally characterized by panic reactions. Very heavy usage has been shown to precipitate an acute psychosis that is self-limited and short-lived once the drug is removed from the body (Julien, 2008).

Heavy long-term cannabis use is also associated with a condition called *amotivational syndrome*. When this syndrome occurs, the individual is totally preoccupied with using the substance. Symptoms include lethargy, apathy, social and personal deterioration, and lack of motivation. This syndrome appears to be more common in countries in which the most potent preparations are used and where the substance is more freely available than it is in the United States.

Sexual Functioning

Marijuana is reported to enhance the sexual experience in both men and women. The intensified sensory awareness and the subjective slowness of time perception are thought to increase sexual satisfaction. Marijuana also enhances the sexual functioning by releasing inhibitions for certain activities that would normally be restrained.

Cannabis Intoxication

Cannabis intoxication is evidenced by the presence of clinically significant problematic behavioral or psychological changes that develop during, or shortly after, cannabis use. Symptoms include impaired motor coordination, euphoria, anxiety, a sensation of slowed time, impaired judgment, and social withdrawal. Physical symptoms include conjunctival injection, increased appetite, dry mouth, and tachycardia (APA, 2013). The impairment of motor skills lasts for 8 to 12 hours and interferes with the operation of motor vehicles. These effects are additive to those of alcohol, which is commonly used in combination with cannabis (Sadock & Sadock, 2007).

Cannabis Withdrawal

The *DSM-5* describes a syndrome of symptoms that occur upon cessation of cannabis use that has been heavy and prolonged. Symptoms occur within a week following cessation of use and may include any of the following:

- Irritability, anger, or aggression
- Nervousness or anxiety
- Sleep difficulty (e.g., insomnia, disturbing dreams)
- Decreased appetite or weight loss
- Restlessness
- Depressed mood
- Physical symptoms, such as abdominal pain, tremors, sweating, fever, chills, or headache

Tables 23-7 and 23-8 include summaries of the psychoactive substances, including symptoms of intoxication, withdrawal, use, overdose, possible therapeutic uses, and trade and common names by which they may be referred. The dynamics of substance use disorders using the Transactional Model of Stress/Adaptation are presented in Figure 23-3.

Application of the Nursing Process

Assessment

In the pre-introductory phase of relationship development, the nurse must examine his or her feelings about working with a client who abuses substances. If these behaviors are viewed as morally wrong and the nurse has internalized these attitudes from very early in life, it may be very difficult to suppress judgmental feelings. The role that alcohol or other substances has played (or plays) in the life of the nurse most certainly will affect the way in which he or she interacts with a client who has a substance use disorder.

How are attitudes examined? Some individuals may have sufficient ability for introspection to be able to recognize on their own whether they have unresolved issues related to substance abuse. For others, it may be more helpful to discuss these issues in a group situation, where insight may be gained from feedback regarding the perceptions of others.

TABLE 23–7 Psychoactive Substances: A Profile Summary

CLASS OF DRUGS	SYMPTOMS OF USE	THERAPEUTIC USES	SYMPTOMS OF OVERDOSE	TRADE NAMES	COMMON NAMES
CNS DEPRESSANTS					
Alcohol	Relaxation, loss of inhibitions, lack of concentration, drowsiness, slurred speech, sleep	Antidote for methanol consumption; ingredient in many pharmacological concentrates	Nausea, vomiting; shallow respirations; cold, clammy skin; weak, rapid pulse; coma; possible death	Ethyl alcohol, beer, gin, rum, vodka, bourbon, whiskey, liqueurs, wine, brandy, sherry, champagne	Booze, alcohol, liquor, drinks, cocktails, highballs, nightcaps, moonshine, white lightning, firewater
Other (barbiturates and nonbarbiturates)	Same as alcohol	Relief from anxiety and insomnia; as anticonvulsants and anesthetics	Anxiety, fever, agitation, hallucinations, disorientation, tremors, delirium, convulsions, possible death	Seconal, Amytal, Nembutal Valium Librium Noctec Miltown	Red birds, yellow birds, blue birds Blues/yellows Green & whites Mickies Downers
CNS STIMULANTS					
Amphetamines and related drugs	Hyperactivity, agitation, euphoria, insomnia, loss of appetite	Management of narcolepsy, hyperkinesia, and weight control	Cardiac arrhythmias, headache, convulsions, hypertension, rapid heart rate, coma, possible death	Dexedrine, Didrex, Tenuate, Bontril, Ritalin, Focalin, Meridia, Provigil	Uppers, pep pills, wakeups, bennies, eye-openers, speed, black beauties, sweet As
Cocaine	Euphoria, hyperactivity, restlessness, talkativeness, increased pulse, dilated pupils, rhinitis		Hallucinations, convulsions, pulmonary edema, respiratory failure, coma, cardiac arrest, possible death	Cocaine hydrochloride	Coke, flake, snow, dust, happy dust, gold dust, girl, cecil, C, toot, blow, crack
Synthetic stimulants	Agitation, insomnia, irritability, dizziness, decreased ability to think clearly, increased heart rate, chest pains		Depression, paranoia, delusions, suicidal thoughts, seizures, panic attacks, nausea, vomiting, heart attack, stroke, hallucinations, aggresive behavior	Mephedrone, MDPV (3-4 methylene-dioxypyrovalerone)	Bath salts, bliss, vanilla sky, ivory wave, purple wave
OPIOIDS					
	Euphoria, lethargy, drowsiness, lack of motivation, constricted pupils	As analgesics; antidiarrheals, and antitussives; methadone in substitution therapy; heroin has no therapeutic use	Shallow breathing, slowed pulse, clammy skin, pulmonary edema, respiratory arrest, convulsions, coma, possible death	Heroin Morphine Codeine Dilaudid Demerol Dolophine Percodan Talwin Opium	Snow, stuff, H, harry, horse M, morph, Miss Emma Schoolboy Lords Doctors Dollies Perkies Ts Big O, black stuff

Categories	Symptoms	Therapeutic Uses	Symptoms of Overdose	Generic (Trade) Names	Common Street Names
HALLUCINOGENS	Visual hallucinations, disorientation, confusion, paranoid delusions, euphoria, anxiety, panic, increased pulse	LSD has been proposed in the treatment of chronic alcoholism, and in the reduction of intractable pain	Agitation, extreme hyperactivity, violence, hallucinations, psychosis, convulsions, possible death	LSD PCP Mescaline DMT STP, DOM MDMA Ketamine MDPV	Acid, cube, big D Angel dust, hog, peace pill Mesc Businessman's trip Serenity and peace Ecstasy, XTC Special K, vitamin K, kit kat Bath Salts
CANNABINOIDS	Relaxation, talkativeness, lowered inhibitions, euphoria, mood swings	Marijuana has been used for relief of nausea and vomiting associated with antineoplastic chemotherapy and to reduce eye pressure in glaucoma	Fatigue, paranoia, delusions, hallucinations, possible psychosis	Cannabis Hashish	Marijuana, pot, grass, joint, Mary Jane, MJ Hash, rope, Sweet Lucy

TABLE 23–8 **Summary of Symptoms Associated With the Syndromes of Intoxication and Withdrawal**

CLASS OF DRUGS	INTOXICATION	WITHDRAWAL	COMMENTS
Alcohol	Aggressiveness, impaired judgment, impaired attention, irritability, euphoria, depression, emotional lability, slurred speech, incoordination, unsteady gait, nystagmus, flushed face	Tremors, nausea/vomiting, malaise, weakness, tachycardia, sweating, elevated blood pressure, anxiety, depressed mood, irritability, hallucinations, headache, insomnia, seizures	Alcohol withdrawal begins within 4-12 hr after last drink. May progress to delirium tremens on 2nd or 3rd day. Use of Librium or Serax is common for substitution therapy.
Amphetamines and related substances	Fighting, grandiosity, hypervigilance, psychomotor agitation, impaired judgment, tachycardia, pupillary dilation, elevated blood pressure, perspiration or chills, nausea and vomiting	Anxiety, depressed mood, irritability, craving for the substance, fatigue, insomnia or hypersomnia, psychomotor agitation, paranoid and suicidal ideation	Withdrawal symptoms usually peak within 2–4 days, although depression and irritability may persist for months. Antidepressants may be used.
Caffeine	Restlessness, nervousness, excitement, insomnia, flushed face, diuresis, gastrointestinal complaints, muscle twitching, rambling flow of thought and speech, cardiac arrhythmia, periods of inexhaustibility, psychomotor agitation	Headache	Caffeine is contained in coffee, tea, colas, cocoa, chocolate, some over-the-counter analgesics, "cold" preparations, and stimulants.
Cannabis	Euphoria, anxiety, suspiciousness, sensation of slowed time, impaired judgment, social withdrawal, tachycardia, conjunctival redness, increased appetite, hallucinations	Restlessness, irritability, insomnia, loss of appetite, depressed mood, tremors, fever, chills, headache, abdominal pain	Intoxication occurs immediately and lasts about 3 hours. Oral ingestion is more slowly absorbed and has longer-lasting effects.
Cocaine	Euphoria, fighting, grandiosity, hypervigilance, psychomotor agitation, impaired judgment, tachycardia, elevated blood pressure, pupillary dilation, perspiration or chills, nausea/vomiting, hallucinations, delirium	Depression, anxiety, irritability, fatigue, insomnia or hypersomnia, psychomotor agitation, paranoid or suicidal ideation, apathy, social withdrawal	Large doses of the drug can result in convulsions or death from cardiac arrhythmias or respiratory paralysis.
Inhalants	Belligerence, assaultiveness, apathy, impaired judgment, dizziness, nystagmus, slurred speech, unsteady gait, lethargy, depressed reflexes, tremor, blurred vision, stupor or coma, euphoria, irritation around eyes, throat, and nose		Intoxication occurs within 5 minutes of inhalation. Symptoms last 60–90 minutes. Large doses can result in death from CNS depression or cardiac arrhythmia.
Nicotine		Craving for the drug, irritability, anger, frustration, anxiety, difficulty concentrating, restlessness, decreased heart rate, increased appetite, weight gain, tremor, headaches, insomnia	Symptoms of withdrawal begin within 24 hours of last drug use and decrease in intensity over days, weeks, or sometimes longer.
Opioids	Euphoria, lethargy, somnolence, apathy, dysphoria, impaired judgment, pupillary constriction, drowsiness, slurred speech, constipation, nausea, decreased respiratory rate and blood pressure	Craving for the drug, nausea/vomiting, muscle aches, lacrimation or rhinorrhea, pupillary dilation, piloerection or sweating, diarrhea, yawning, fever, insomnia	Withdrawal symptoms appear within 6–8 hours after last dose, reach a peak in the 2nd or 3rd day, and subside in 5–10 days. Times are shorter with meperidine and longer with methadone.

TABLE 23–8	**Summary of Symptoms Associated With the Syndromes of Intoxication and Withdrawal—cont'd**		
CLASS OF DRUGS	**INTOXICATION**	**WITHDRAWAL**	**COMMENTS**
Phencyclidine and related substances	Belligerence, assaultiveness, impulsiveness, psychomotor agitation, impaired judgment, nystagmus, increased heart rate and blood pressure, diminished pain response, ataxia, dysarthria, muscle rigidity, seizures, hyperacusis, delirium		Delirium can occur within 24 hours after use of phencyclidine, or may occur up to a week following recovery from an overdose of the drug.
Sedatives, hypnotics, and anxiolytics	Disinhibition of sexual or aggressive impulses, mood lability, impaired judgment, slurred speech, incoordination, unsteady gait, impairment in attention or memory disorientation, confusion	Nausea/vomiting, malaise, weakness, tachycardia, sweating, anxiety, irritability, orthostatic hypotension, tremor, insomnia, seizures	Withdrawal may progress to delirium, usually within 1 week of last use. Long-acting barbiturates or benzodiazepines may be used in withdrawal substitution therapy.

Whether alone or in a group, the nurse may gain a greater understanding about attitudes and feelings related to substance abuse by responding to the following types of questions. As written here, the questions are specific to alcohol, but they could be adapted for any substance.

■ What are my drinking patterns?
■ If I drink, why do I drink? When, where, and how much?
■ If I don't drink, why do I abstain?
■ Am I comfortable with my drinking patterns?
■ If I decided not to drink anymore, would that be a problem for me?
■ What did I learn from my parents about drinking?
■ Have my attitudes changed as an adult?
■ What are my feelings about people who become intoxicated?
■ Does it seem more acceptable for some individuals than for others?
■ Do I ever use terms like "sot," "drunk," or "boozer," to describe some individuals who overindulge, yet overlook it in others?
■ Do I ever overindulge myself?
■ Has the use of alcohol (by me or others) affected my life in any way?
■ Do I see alcohol/drug abuse as a sign of weakness? A moral problem? An illness?

Unless nurses fully understand and accept their own attitudes and feelings, they cannot be empathetic toward clients' problems. Clients in recovery need to know they are accepted for themselves, regardless of past behaviors. Nurses must be able to separate the client from the behavior and to accept that individual with unconditional positive regard.

Assessment Tools

Nurses are often the individuals who perform the admission interview. A variety of assessment tools are appropriate for use in chemical dependency units. A nursing history and assessment tool was presented in Chapter 9 of this text. With some adaptation, it is an appropriate instrument for creating a database on clients who abuse substances. Box 23-1 presents a drug history and assessment that could be used in conjunction with the general biopsychosocial assessment.

The Clinical Institute Withdrawal Assessment of Alcohol Scale, Revised (CIWA-Ar) is an excellent tool that is used by many hospitals to assess risk and severity of withdrawal from alcohol. It may be used for initial assessment as well as ongoing monitoring of alcohol withdrawal symptoms. A copy of the CIWA-Ar is presented in Box 23-2.

Other screening tools exist for determining whether an individual has a problem with substances. Two such tools developed by the American Psychiatric Association for the diagnosis of alcoholism include the Michigan Alcoholism Screening Test and the CAGE Questionnaire (Boxes 23-3 and 23-4). Some psychiatric units administer these surveys to all clients who are admitted to help determine if there is a secondary alcoholism problem in addition to the psychiatric problem for which the client is being admitted (sometimes called **dual diagnosis**). It would be possible to adapt these tools to use in diagnosing problems with other drugs as well.

Dual Diagnosis

If it is determined that the client has a coexisting substance disorder and mental illness, he or she may be

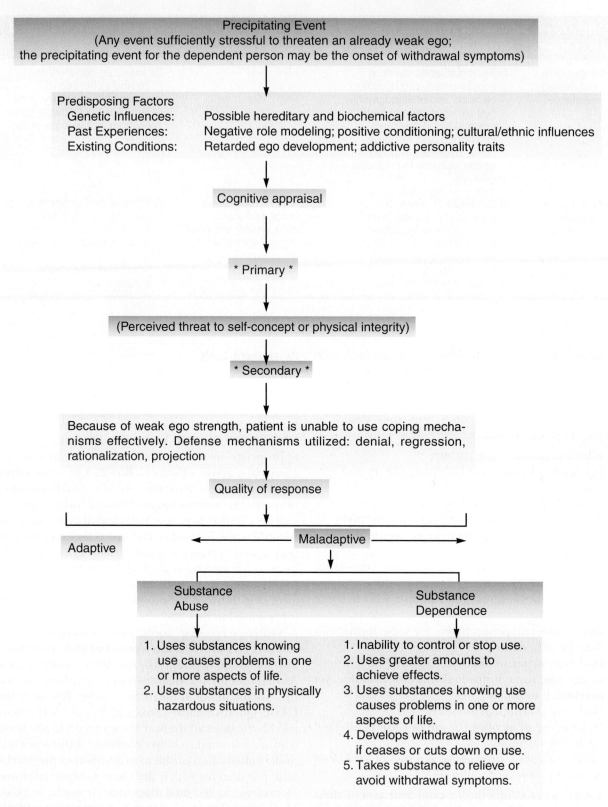

FIGURE 23–3 The dynamics of substance use disorders using the Transactional Model of Stress/Adaptation.

BOX 23-1 **Drug History and Assessment***

1. When you were growing up, did anyone in your family drink alcohol or take other kinds of drugs?
2. If so, how did the substance use affect the family situation?
3. When did you have your first drink/drugs?
4. How long have you been drinking/taking drugs on a regular basis?
5. What is your pattern of substance use?
    a. When do you use substances?
    b. What do you use?
    c. How much do you use?
    d. Where are you and with whom when you use substances?
6. When did you have your last drink/drug? What was it and how much did you consume?
7. Does using the substance(s) cause problems for you? Describe. Include family, friends, job, school, other.
8. Have you ever experienced injury as a result of substance use?
9. Have you ever been arrested or incarcerated for drinking/using drugs?
10. Have you ever tried to stop drinking/using drugs? If so, what was the result? Did you experience any physical symptoms, such as tremors, headache, insomnia, sweating, or seizures?
11. Have you ever experienced loss of memory for times when you have been drinking/using drugs?
12. Describe a typical day in your life.
13. Are there any changes you would like to make in your life? If so, what are they?
14. What plans or ideas do you have for seeing that these changes occur?

*To be used in conjunction with general biopsychosocial nursing history and assessment tool (Chapter 9).

BOX 23-2 **Clinical Institute Withdrawal Assessment of Alcohol Scale, Revised (CIWA-Ar)**

Patient: **Date:**   **Time:**

Pulse or heart rate, taken for one minute: **Blood pressure:**

Nausea and Vomiting—Ask "Do you feel sick to your stomach? Have you vomited?" Observation.

0 no nausea and no vomiting
1 mild nausea with no vomiting
2
3
4 intermittent nausea with dry heaves
5
6
7 constant nausea, frequent dry heaves and vomiting

Tremor—Arms extended and fingers spread apart. Observation.

0 no tremor
1 not visible, but can be felt fingertip to fingertip
2
3
4 moderate, with patient's arms extended
5
6
7 severe, even with arms not extended

Tactile Disturbances—Ask "Have you any itching, pins and needles sensations, any burning, any numbness, or do you feel bugs crawling on or under your skin?" Observation.

0 none
1 very mild itching, pins and needles, burning or numbness
2 mild itching, pins and needles, burning or numbness
3 moderate itching, pins and needles, burning or numbness
4 moderately severe hallucinations
5 severe hallucinations
6 extremely severe hallucinations
7 continuous hallucinations

Auditory Disturbances—Ask "Are you more aware of sounds around you? Are they harsh? Do they frighten you? Are you hearing anything that is disturbing to you? Are you hearing things you know are not there?" Observation.

0 not present
1 very mild harshness or ability to frighten
2 mild harshness or ability to frighten
3 moderate harshness or ability to frighten
4 moderately severe hallucinations
5 severe hallucinations
6 extremely severe hallucinations
7 continuous hallucinations

Continued

BOX 23-2 Clinical Institute Withdrawal Assessment of Alcohol Scale, Revised (CIWA-Ar)—cont'd

Paroxysmal Sweats—Observation.

0 no sweat visible
1 barely perceptible sweating, palms moist
2
3
4 beads of sweat obvious on forehead
5
6
7 drenching sweats

Anxiety—Ask "Do you feel nervous?" Observation.

0 no anxiety, at ease
1 mild anxious
2
3
4 moderately anxious, or guarded, so anxiety is inferred
5
6
7 equivalent to acute panic states as seen in severe delirium or acute schizophrenic reactions

AGITATION—Observation.

0 normal activity
1 somewhat more than normal activity
2
3
4 moderately fidgety and restless
5
6
7 paces back and forth during most of the interview, or constantly thrashes about

_____
_____

The CIWA-Ar is not copyrighted and may be reproduced freely. This assessment for monitoring withdrawal symptoms requires approximately 5 minutes to administer. The maximum score is 67 (see instrument). Patients scoring less than 10 do not usually need additional medication for withdrawal. _____
_____

Visual Disturbances—Ask "Does the light appear to be too bright? Is its color different? Does it hurt your eyes? Are you seeing anything that is disturbing to you? Are you seeing things you know are not there?" Observation.

0 not present
1 very mild sensitivity
2 mild sensitivity
3 moderate sensitivity
4 moderately severe hallucinations
5 severe hallucinations
6 extremely severe hallucinations
7 continuous hallucinations

Headache, Fullness In Head—Ask "Does your head feel different? Does it feel like there is a band around your head?" Do not rate for dizziness or lightheadedness. Otherwise, rate severity.

0 not present
1 very mild
2 mild
3 moderate
4 moderately severe
5 severe
6 very severe
7 extremely severe

Orientation And Clouding Of Sensorium—Ask "What day is this? Where are you? Who am I?"

0 oriented and can do serial additions
1 cannot do serial additions or is uncertain about date
2 disoriented for date by no more than 2 calendar days
3 disoriented for date by more than 2 calendar days
4 disoriented for place/or person

Total CIWA-Ar Score_____
Rater's Initials_____

From Sullivan, J.T., Sykora, K., Schneiderman, J., Naranjo, C.A., and Sellers, E.M. (1989). Assessment of alcohol withdrawal: The revised Clinical Institute Withdrawal Assessment for Alcohol scale (CIWA-Ar). British Journal of Addiction 84, 1353-1357.

assigned to a special program that targets both problems. Counseling for the mentally ill person who abuses substances takes a different approach than that which is directed at individuals who abuse substances but are not mentally ill. In the latter, many counselors use direct confrontation of the substance use behaviors. This approach is thought to be detrimental to the treatment of a person with mental illness (Mack et al., 2003). Most dual diagnosis programs take a more supportive and less confrontational approach.

BOX 23-3 Michigan Alcoholism Screening Test (MAST)

Answer the following questions by placing an X under yes or no.*	Yes	No
1. Do you enjoy a drink now and then?	0	0
2. Do you feel you are a normal drinker? (By normal we mean you drink less than or as much as most people.)		2
3. Have you ever awakened the morning after some drinking the night before and found that you could not remember a part of the evening?	2	
4. Does your wife, husband, parent, or other near relative ever worry or complain about your drinking?	1	
5. Can you stop drinking without a struggle after one or two drinks?		2
6. Do you ever feel guilty about your drinking?	1	
7. Do friends or relatives think you are a normal drinker?		2
8. Are you able to stop drinking when you want to?		2
9. Have you ever attended a meeting of Alcoholics Anonymous (AA)?	5	
10. Have you gotten into physical fights when drinking?	1	
11. Has your drinking ever created problems between you and your wife, husband, a parent, or other relative?	2	
12. Has your wife, husband, or another family member ever gone to anyone for help about your drinking?	2	
13. Have you ever lost friends because of your drinking?	2	
14. Have you ever gotten into trouble at work or school because of drinking?	2	
15. Have you ever lost a job because of drinking?	2	
16. Have you ever neglected your obligations, your family, or your work for 2 or more days in a row because you were drinking?	2	
17. Do you drink before noon fairly often?	1	
18. Have you ever been told you have liver trouble? Cirrhosis?	2	
19. After heavy drinking have you ever had delirium tremens (DTs) or severe shaking or heard voices or seen things that really were not there?	5	
20. Have you ever gone to anyone for help about your drinking?	5	
21. Have you ever been in a hospital because of drinking?	5	
22. Have you ever been a patient in a psychiatric hospital or on a psychiatric ward of a general hospital where drinking was part of the problem that resulted in hospitalization?	2	
23. Have you ever been seen at a psychiatric or mental health clinic or gone to any doctor, social worker, or clergyman for help with any emotional problem, where drinking was part of the problem?	2	
24. Have you ever been arrested for drunk driving, driving while intoxicated, or driving under the influence of alcoholic beverages? (If yes, how many times?_____)	2 ea	
25. Have you ever been arrested, or taken into custody, even for a few hours, because of other drunk behavior? (If yes, how many times?_____)	2 ea	

* Items are scored under the response that would indicate a problem with alcohol.
Method of scoring: 0–3 points = no problem with alcohol
        4 points = possible problem with alcohol
        5 or more = indicates problem with alcohol
From Selzer, M.L. (1971). The Michigan alcohol screening test: The quest for a new diagnostic instrument. American Journal of Psychiatry, 127, 1653-1658, with permission.

BOX 23-4 The CAGE Questionnaire

1. Have you ever felt you should **C**ut down on your drinking?
2. Have people **A**nnoyed you by criticizing your drinking?
3. Have you ever felt bad or **G**uilty about your drinking?
4. Have you ever had a drink first thing in the morning to steady your nerves or get rid of a hangover (**E**ye-opener)?

Scoring: 2 or 3 "yes" answers strongly suggest a problem with alcohol.
From Mayfield, D., McLeod, G., & Hall, P. (1974). The CAGE questionnaire: Validation of a new alcoholism screening instrument. American Journal of Psychiatry, 131, 1121-1123, with permission.

Peer support groups are an important part of the treatment program. Group members offer encouragement and practical advice to each other. Psychodynamic therapy can be useful for some individuals with dual diagnosis by delving into the personal history of how psychiatric disorders and substance abuse have reinforced one another and how the cycle can be broken (Harvard Medical School, 2003). Cognitive and behavioral therapies are helpful in training clients to monitor moods and thought patterns that lead to substance abuse. With these therapies, clients also learn to avoid substance use and to cope with cravings and the temptation to relapse (Harvard Medical School, 2003).

Individuals with dual diagnoses should be encouraged to attend 12-step recovery programs (e.g., Alcoholics Anonymous or Narcotics Anonymous). Dual diagnosis clients are sometimes resistant to attending 12-step programs, and they often do better in groups specifically designed for people with psychiatric disorders.

Substance-abuse groups are usually integrated into regular programming for the psychiatric client with a dual diagnosis. An individual in a psychiatric facility or day treatment program will attend a substance-abuse group periodically in lieu of another scheduled activity therapy. Topics are directed toward areas that are unique to clients with a mental illness, such as mixing medications with other substances, as well as topics that are common to primary substances abusers. Individuals are encouraged to discuss their personal problems. Mack and associates (2003) have stated:

> The dual diagnosis patient often falls through the cracks of the treatment system. Severe psychiatric disorders often preclude full treatment in substance abuse clinics or self-help groups. The addition of other [psychiatric] disorders to a substance use disorder greatly complicates diagnosis and makes treatment more difficult. (p. 359)

Continued attendance at 12-step group meetings is encouraged on discharge from treatment. Family involvement is enlisted, and preventive strategies are outlined. Individual case management is common, and success is often promoted by this close supervision.

Diagnosis/Outcome Identification

The next step in the nursing process is to identify appropriate nursing diagnoses by analyzing the data collected during the assessment phase. The individual who abuses or is dependent on substances undoubtedly has many unmet physical and emotional needs. Table 23-9 presents a list of client behaviors and the NANDA nursing diagnoses that correspond to those

---

TABLE 23–9 Assigning Nursing Diagnoses to Behaviors Commonly Associated With Substance Use Disorders

BEHAVIORS	NURSING DIAGNOSES
Makes statements such as, "I don't have a problem with (substance). I can quit any time I want to." Delays seeking assistance; does not perceive problems related to use of substances; minimizes use of substances; unable to admit impact of disease on life pattern	Ineffective denial
Abuse of chemical agents; destructive behavior toward others and self; inability to meet basic needs; inability to meet role expectations; risk taking	Ineffective coping
Loss of weight, pale conjunctiva and mucous membranes, decreased skin turgor, electrolyte imbalance, anemia, drinks alcohol instead of eating	Imbalanced nutrition: Less than body requirements/Deficient fluid volume
Risk factors: Malnutrition, altered immune condition, failing to avoid exposure to pathogens	Risk for infection
Criticizes self and others, self-destructive behavior (abuse of substances as a coping mechanism), dysfunctional family background	Chronic low self-esteem
Denies that substance is harmful; continues to use substance in light of obvious consequences	Deficient knowledge
FOR THE CLIENT WITHDRAWING FROM CNS DEPRESSANTS: Risk factors: CNS agitation (tremors, elevated blood pressure, nausea and vomiting, hallucinations, illusions, tachycardia, anxiety, seizures)	Risk for injury
FOR THE CLIENT WITHDRAWING FROM CNS STIMULANTS: Risk factors: Intense feelings of lassitude and depression; "crashing," suicidal ideation	Risk for suicide

behaviors, which may be used in planning care for the client with a substance use disorder.

Outcome Criteria

The following criteria may be used for measurement of outcomes in the care of the client with substance-related disorders.

The client:

- Has not experienced physical injury.
- Has not caused harm to self or others.
- Accepts responsibility for own behavior.
- Acknowledges association between personal problems and use of substance(s).
- Demonstrates more adaptive coping mechanisms that can be used in stressful situations (instead of taking substances).
- Shows no signs or symptoms of infection or malnutrition.
- Exhibits evidence of increased self-worth by attempting new projects without fear of failure and by demonstrating less defensive behavior toward others.
- Verbalizes importance of abstaining from use of substances in order to maintain optimal wellness.

Planning/Implementation

Implementation with clients who abuse substances is a long-term process, often beginning with **detoxification** and progressing to total abstinence. The following section presents a group of selected nursing diagnoses, with short- and long-term goals and nursing interventions for each.

Risk for Injury

Risk for injury is defined as "at risk for injury as a result of [internal or external] environmental conditions interacting with the individual's adaptive and defensive resources" (NANDA International [NANDA-I], 2012, p. 430).

Client Goals

Outcome criteria include short- and long-term goals. Timelines are individually determined.

Short-Term Goal

- Client's condition will stabilize within 72 hours.

Long-Term Goal

- Client will not experience physical injury.

Interventions

For the Client in Substance Withdrawal

- Assess the client's level of disorientation to determine specific requirements for safety.
- Obtain a drug history, if possible. It is important to determine the type of substance(s) used, the time and amount of last use, the length and frequency of use, and the amount used on a daily basis.
- Because subjective history is often not accurate, obtain a urine sample for laboratory analysis of substance content.
- It is important to keep the client in as quiet an environment as possible. Excessive stimuli may increase client agitation. A private room is ideal.
- Observe client behaviors frequently. If seriousness of the condition warrants, it may be necessary to assign a staff person on a one-to-one basis.
- Accompany and assist client when ambulating, and use a wheelchair for transporting the client long distances.
- Pad the headboard and side rails of the bed with thick towels to protect the client in case of a seizure.
- Suicide precautions may need to be instituted for the client withdrawing from CNS stimulants.
- Ensure that smoking materials and other potentially harmful objects are stored away from client's access.
- Frequently orient the client to reality and the surroundings.
- Monitor the client's vital signs every 15 minutes initially and less frequently as acute symptoms subside.
- Follow the medication regimen, as ordered by the physician. Common psychopharmacological intervention for substance intoxication and withdrawal is presented later in this chapter under the section titled "Treatment Modalities for Substance-Related Disorders."

Ineffective Denial

Ineffective denial is defined as "conscious or unconscious attempt to disavow the knowledge or meaning of an event to reduce anxiety/fear, but leading to the detriment of health" (NANDA-I, 2012, p. 358). Table 23-10 presents this nursing diagnosis in care plan format.

Client Goals

Outcome criteria include short- and long-term goals. Timelines are individually determined.

Short-Term Goal

- Client will divert attention away from external issues and focus on behavioral outcomes associated with substance use.

Long-Term Goal

- Client will verbalize acceptance of responsibility for own behavior and acknowledge association between substance use and personal problems.

Interventions

- Begin by working to develop a trusting nurse-client relationship. Be honest and keep all promises.
- Convey an attitude of acceptance to the client. Ensure that he or she understands "It is not *you* but

Table 23-10 | CARE PLAN FOR A CLIENT WITH A SUBSTANCE USE DISORDER

NURSING DIAGNOSIS: INEFFECTIVE DENIAL

RELATED TO: Weak, underdeveloped ego

EVIDENCED BY: Statements indicating no problem with substance use

OUTCOME CRITERIA	NURSING INTERVENTIONS	RATIONALE
Short-Term Goal • Client will divert attention away from external issues and focus on behavioral outcomes associated with substance use. **Long-Term Goal** • Client will verbalize acceptance of responsibility for own behavior and acknowledge association between substance use and personal problems.	1. Begin by working to develop a trusting nurse-client relationship. Be honest. Keep all promises. 2. Convey an attitude of acceptance to the client. Ensure that he or she understands "It is not *you* but your *behavior* that is unacceptable." 3. Provide information to correct misconceptions about substance abuse. Client may rationalize his or her behavior with statements such as, "I'm not an alcoholic. I can stop drinking any time I want. Besides, I only drink beer." Or "I only smoke pot to relax before class. So what? I know lots of people who do. Besides, you can't get hooked on pot." 4. Identify recent maladaptive behaviors or situations that have occurred in the client's life, and discuss how use of substances may have been a contributing factor. 5. 💬 Use confrontation with caring. Do not allow client to fantasize about his or her lifestyle (for example: "It is my understanding that the last time you drank alcohol, you . . ." or "The lab report shows that you were under the influence of alcohol when you had the accident that injured three people"). 6. Do not accept rationalization or projection as client attempts to make excuses for or blame his or her behavior on other people or situations. 7. Encourage participation in group activities.	1. Trust is the basis of a therapeutic relationship. 2. An attitude of acceptance promotes feelings of dignity and self-worth. 3. Many myths abound regarding use of specific substances. Factual information presented in a matter-of-fact, nonjudgmental way explaining what behaviors constitute substance-related disorders may help the client focus on his or her own behaviors as an illness that requires help. 4. The first step in decreasing use of denial is for client to see the relationship between substance use and personal problems. 5. Confrontation interferes with client's ability to use denial; a caring attitude preserves self-esteem and avoids putting the client on the defensive. 6. Rationalization and projection prolong denial that problems exist in the client's life because of substance use. 7. Peer feedback is often more accepted than feedback from authority figures. Peer pressure can be a strong factor as well as association with individuals who are experiencing or who have experienced similar problems.

Table 23-10	CARE PLAN FOR A CLIENT WITH A SUBSTANCE USE DISORDER–cont'd		
OUTCOME CRITERIA	**NURSING INTERVENTIONS**	**RATIONALE**
	8. Offer immediate positive recognition of client's expressions of insight gained regarding illness and acceptance of responsibility for own behavior.	8. Positive reinforcement enhances self-esteem and encourages repetition of desirable behaviors.

your *behavior* that is unacceptable." An attitude of acceptance helps to promote the client's feelings of dignity and self-worth.

■ Provide information to correct misconceptions about substance abuse. Client may rationalize his or her behavior with statements such as, "I'm not an alcoholic. I can stop drinking any time I want. Besides, I only drink beer." or "I only smoke pot to relax before class. So what? I know lots of people who do. Besides, you can't get hooked on pot." Many myths abound regarding use of specific substances. Factual information presented in a matter-of-fact, nonjudgmental way explaining what behaviors constitute substance use disorders may help the client focus on his or her own behaviors as an illness that requires help.

■ Identify recent maladaptive behaviors or situations that have occurred in the client's life, and discuss how use of substances may have been a contributing factor. The first step in decreasing use of denial is for client to see the relationship between substance use and personal problems.

■ Use confrontation with caring. Do not allow client to fantasize about his or her lifestyle. Confrontation interferes with client's ability to use denial; a caring attitude preserves self-esteem and avoids putting the client on the defensive.

CLINICAL PEARL 💬

It is important to speak objectively and nonjudgmentally to a person in denial. Examples: "It is my understanding that the last time you drank alcohol, you . . ." or "The lab report shows that your blood alcohol level was 250 when you were involved in that automobile accident."

■ Do not accept the use of rationalization or projection as client attempts to make excuses for or blame his or her behavior on other people or situations. Rationalization and projection prolong the stage of denial that problems exist in the client's life because of substance use.

■ Encourage participation in group activities. Peer feedback is often more accepted than feedback from authority figures. Peer pressure can be a strong factor as well as the association with individuals who are experiencing or who have experienced similar problems.

■ Offer immediate positive recognition of client's expressions of insight gained regarding illness and acceptance of responsibility for own behavior. Positive reinforcement enhances self-esteem and encourages repetition of desirable behaviors.

Ineffective Coping

Ineffective coping is defined as the "inability to form a valid appraisal of the stressors, inadequate choices of practiced responses, and/or inability to use available resources" (NANDA-I, 2012, p. 348).

Client Goals

Outcome criteria include short- and long-term goals. Timelines are individually determined.

Short-Term Goal

■ Client will express true feelings about using substances as a method of coping with stress.

Long-Term Goal

■ Client will be able to verbalize use of adaptive coping mechanisms, instead of substance abuse, in response to stress.

Interventions

■ Spend time with the client and establish a trusting relationship.

■ Set limits on manipulative behavior. Be sure that the client knows what is acceptable, what is not, and the consequences for violating the limits set. Ensure that all staff maintain consistency with this intervention. The client is unable to establish his or her own limits, so limits must be set for the client. Unless administration of consequences for violation of limits is consistent, manipulative behavior will not be eliminated.

■ Encourage the client to verbalize feelings, fears, and anxieties. Answer any questions he or she may have regarding the disorder. Verbalization of feelings in a nonthreatening environment may help the client come to terms with long-unresolved issues.

■ Explain the effects of substance abuse on the body. Emphasize that the prognosis is closely related to abstinence. Many clients lack knowledge regarding the deleterious effects of substance abuse on the body.

■ Explore with the client the options available to assist with stressful situations rather than resorting to substance use (e.g., contacting various members of Alcoholics Anonymous or Narcotics Anonymous; physical exercise; relaxation techniques; meditation). The client may have persistently resorted to chemical use and thus may possess little or no knowledge of adaptive responses to stress.

■ Provide positive reinforcement for evidence of gratification delayed appropriately. Encourage the client to be as independent as possible in performing his or her self-care. Provide positive feedback for independent decision-making and effective use of problem-solving skills.

Dysfunctional Family Processes

Dysfunctional family processes are defined as "psychosocial, spiritual, and physiological functions of the family unit are chronically disorganized, which leads to conflict, denial of problems, resistance to change, ineffective problem solving, and a series of self-perpetuating crises" (NANDA-I, 2012, p. 308).

Client Goals

Outcome criteria include short- and long-term goals. Timelines are individually determined.

Short-Term Goals

■ Family members will participate in individual family programs and support groups.
■ Family members will identify ineffective coping behaviors and consequences.
■ Family will initiate and plan for necessary lifestyle changes.

Long-Term Goal

■ Family members will take action to change self-destructive behaviors and alter behaviors that contribute to client's addiction.

Interventions

■ Review family history; explore roles of family members, circumstances involving alcohol use, strengths, and areas of growth. Explore how family members have coped with the client's addiction (e.g., denial, repression, rationalization, hurt, loneliness,

projection). Persons who enable also suffer from the same feelings as the client and use ineffective methods for dealing with the situation, necessitating help in learning new and effective coping skills.

■ Determine the family's understanding of the current situation and previous methods of coping with life's problems. Assess family members' current level of functioning.

■ Determine the extent of enabling behaviors being evidenced by family members; explore with each individual and client. Enabling is doing for the client what he or she needs to do for self (rescuing). People want to be helpful and do not want to feel powerless to help their loved one to stop substance use and change the behavior that is so destructive. However, the substance abuser often relies on others to cover up for his or her inability to cope with daily responsibilities.

■ Provide information about enabling behavior and addictive disease characteristics for both the user and nonuser. Achieving awareness and knowledge of behaviors (e.g., avoiding and shielding, taking over responsibilities, rationalizing, and subserving) provides an opportunity for individuals to begin the process of change.

■ Identify and discuss the possibility of sabotage behaviors by family members. Even though family member(s) may verbalize a desire for the individual to become substance-free, the reality of interactive dynamics is that they may unconsciously not want the individual to recover, as this would affect the family members' own role in the relationship. Additionally, they may receive sympathy or attention from others (secondary gain).

■ Assist the client's partner to understand that the client's abstinence and drug use are not the partner's responsibility, and that the client's use of substances may or may not change despite involvement in treatment. Partners must come to realize and accept that the only behavior they can control is their own.

■ Involve the family in plans for discharge from treatment. Alcohol abuse is a family illness. Because the family has been so involved in dealing with the substance use behavior, family members need help adjusting to the new behavior of sobriety/abstinence. Encourage involvement with self-help associations, such as Alcoholics Anonymous, Al-Anon, Alateen, and professional family therapy. This puts the client and family in direct contact with support systems necessary for continued sobriety and assists with problem resolution.

Concept Care Mapping

The concept map care plan is an innovative approach to planning and organizing nursing care (see Chapter 9). It is a diagrammatic teaching and learning strategy that allows visualization of interrelationships between medical diagnoses, nursing diagnoses, assessment data, and treatments. An example of a concept map care plan for a client with a substance use disorder is presented in Figure 23-4.

Client/Family Education

The role of client teacher is important in the psychiatric area, as it is in all areas of nursing. A list of topics for client/family education relevant to substance-related disorders is presented in Box 23-5. Sample client teaching guides can be found online at www.davisplus.com.

Evaluation

The final step of the nursing process involves reassessment to determine if the nursing interventions have been effective in achieving the intended goals of care.

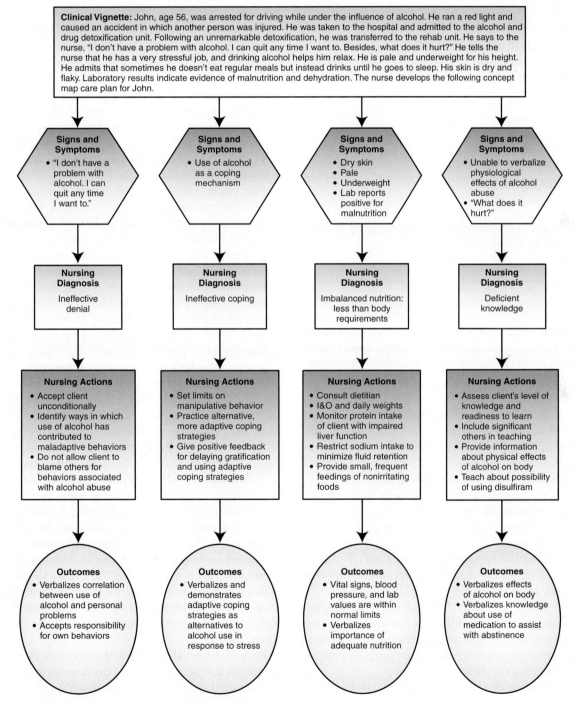

Clinical Vignette: John, age 56, was arrested for driving while under the influence of alcohol. He ran a red light and caused an accident in which another person was injured. He was taken to the hospital and admitted to the alcohol and drug detoxification unit. Following an unremarkable detoxification, he was transferred to the rehab unit. He says to the nurse, "I don't have a problem with alcohol. I can quit any time I want to. Besides, what does it hurt?" He tells the nurse that he has a very stressful job, and drinking alcohol helps him relax. He is pale and underweight for his height. He admits that sometimes he doesn't eat regular meals but instead drinks until he goes to sleep. His skin is dry and flaky. Laboratory results indicate evidence of malnutrition and dehydration. The nurse develops the following concept map care plan for John.

Signs and Symptoms
- "I don't have a problem with alcohol. I can quit any time I want to."

Signs and Symptoms
- Use of alcohol as a coping mechanism

Signs and Symptoms
- Dry skin
- Pale
- Underweight
- Lab reports positive for malnutrition

Signs and Symptoms
- Unable to verbalize physiological effects of alcohol abuse
- "What does it hurt?"

Nursing Diagnosis
Ineffective denial

Nursing Diagnosis
Ineffective coping

Nursing Diagnosis
Imbalanced nutrition: less than body requirements

Nursing Diagnosis
Deficient knowledge

Nursing Actions
- Accept client unconditionally
- Identify ways in which use of alcohol has contributed to maladaptive behaviors
- Do not allow client to blame others for behaviors associated with alcohol abuse

Nursing Actions
- Set limits on manipulative behavior
- Practice alternative, more adaptive coping strategies
- Give positive feedback for delaying gratification and using adaptive coping strategies

Nursing Actions
- Consult dietitian
- I&O and daily weights
- Monitor protein intake of client with impaired liver function
- Restrict sodium intake to minimize fluid retention
- Provide small, frequent feedings of nonirritating foods

Nursing Actions
- Assess client's level of knowledge and readiness to learn
- Include significant others in teaching
- Provide information about physical effects of alcohol on body
- Teach about possibility of using disulfiram

Outcomes
- Verbalizes correlation between use of alcohol and personal problems
- Accepts responsibility for own behaviors

Outcomes
- Verbalizes and demonstrates adaptive coping strategies as alternatives to alcohol use in response to stress

Outcomes
- Vital signs, blood pressure, and lab values are within normal limits
- Verbalizes importance of adequate nutrition

Outcomes
- Verbalizes effects of alcohol on body
- Verbalizes knowledge about use of medication to assist with abstinence

FIGURE 23-4 Concept map care plan for client with alcohol use disorder.

Evaluation of the client with a substance-related disorder may be accomplished by using information gathered from the following reassessment questions:

■ Has detoxification occurred without complications?
■ Is the client still in denial?
■ Does the client accept responsibility for his or her own behavior? Has he or she acknowledged a personal problem with substances?
■ Has a correlation been made between personal problems and the use of substances?
■ Does the client still make excuses or blame others for use of substances?
■ Has the client remained substance-free during hospitalization?
■ Does the client cooperate with treatment?
■ Does the client refrain from manipulative behavior and violation of limits?
■ Is the client able to verbalize alternative adaptive coping strategies to substitute for substance use? Has the use of these strategies been demonstrated? Does positive reinforcement encourage repetition of these adaptive behaviors?
■ Has nutritional status been restored? Does the client consume diet adequate for his or her size

and level of activity? Is the client able to discuss the importance of adequate nutrition?
■ Has the client remained free of infection during hospitalization?
■ Is the client able to verbalize the effects of substance abuse on the body?
■ Does the client verbalize that he or she wants to recover and lead a life free of substances?

The Chemically-Impaired Nurse

Substance abuse and addiction is a problem that has the potential for impairment in an individual's social, occupational, psychological, and physical functioning. This becomes an especially serious problem when the impaired person is responsible for the lives of others on a daily basis. Approximately 10 percent of the general population suffers from the disease of chemical addiction. It is estimated that 10 to 15 percent of nurses suffer from this disease (Thomas & Siela, 2011). Alcohol is the most widely abused drug, followed closely by narcotics.

For years, the impaired nurse was protected, promoted, transferred, ignored, or fired. These types of responses promoted the growth of the problem. Programs are needed that involve early reporting and treatment of chemical addiction as a disease, with a focus on public safety and rehabilitation of the nurse.

How does one identify the impaired nurse? It is still easiest to overlook what *might* be a problem. Denial, on the part of the impaired nurse as well as nurse colleagues, is still the strongest defense for dealing with substance-abuse problems. Some states have mandatory reporting laws that require observers to report substance-abusing nurses to the state board of nursing. They are difficult laws to enforce, and hospitals are not always compliant with mandatory reporting. Some hospitals may choose not to report to the state board of nursing if the impaired nurse is actively seeking treatment and is not placing clients in danger.

A number of clues for recognizing substance impairment in nurses have been identified (Ellis & Hartley, 2012; Thomas & Siela, 2011). They are not easy to detect and will vary according to the substance being used. There may be high absenteeism if the person's source is outside the work area, or the individual may rarely miss work if the substance source is at work. There may be an increase in "wasting" of drugs, higher incidences of incorrect narcotic counts, and a higher record of signing out drugs than for other nurses.

Poor concentration, difficulty meeting deadlines, inappropriate responses, and poor memory or recall are usually late in the disease process. The person may also have problems with relationships. Some other possible signs are irritability, mood swings, tendency to isolate, elaborate excuses for behavior, unkempt appearance, impaired motor coordination, slurred speech, flushed face, inconsistent job performance, and frequent use of the restroom. He or she may frequently medicate other nurses' patients, and there may be patient complaints of inadequate pain control. Discrepancies in documentation may occur.

If suspicious behavior occurs, it is important to keep careful, objective records. Confrontation with the impaired nurse will undoubtedly result in hostility and denial. Confrontation should occur in the presence of a supervisor or other nurse and should include the offer of assistance in seeking treatment. If a report is made to the state board of nursing, it should be a factual documentation of specific events and actions, not a diagnostic statement of impairment.

What will the state board do? Each case is generally decided on an individual basis. A state board may deny, suspend, or revoke a license based on a report of chemical abuse by a nurse. Several state boards of nursing have passed diversionary laws that allow impaired nurses to avoid disciplinary action by agreeing to seek treatment. Some of these state boards administer the treatment programs themselves, and others refer the nurse to community resources or state nurses' association assistance programs. This may require successful completion of inpatient, outpatient, group, or individual counseling treatment program(s); evidence of regular attendance at nurse support groups or 12-step program; random negative drug screens; and employment or volunteer activities during the suspension period. When a nurse is deemed safe to return to practice, he or she may be closely monitored for several years and required to undergo random drug screenings. The nurse also may be required to practice under specifically circumscribed conditions for a designated period of time.

In 1982, the American Nurses Association (ANA) House of Delegates adopted a national resolution to provide assistance to impaired nurses. Since that time, the majority of state nurses' associations have developed (or are developing) programs for nurses who are impaired by substances or psychiatric illness. The individuals who administer these efforts are nurse members of the state associations, as well as nurses who are in recovery themselves. For this reason, they are called **peer assistance programs**.

The peer assistance programs strive to intervene early, to reduce hazards to clients, and increase prospects for the nurse's recovery. Most states provide either a hotline number that the impaired nurse or intervening colleague may call or phone numbers of peer assistance committee members, which are made available for the same purpose. Typically, a contract is drawn up detailing the method of treatment, which may be obtained from various sources, such as employee assistance programs, Alcoholics Anonymous, Narcotics Anonymous, private counseling, or outpatient clinics. Guidelines for monitoring the course of treatment are established. Peer support is provided through regular contact with the impaired nurse, usually for a period of 2 years. Peer assistance programs serve to assist impaired nurses to recognize their impairment, to obtain necessary treatment, and to regain accountability within their profession.

Codependency

The concept of **codependency** arose out of a need to define the dysfunctional behaviors that are evident among members of the family of a chemically addicted person. The term has been expanded to include all individuals from families that harbor secrets of physical or emotional abuse, other cruelties, or pathological conditions. Living under these conditions results in unmet needs for autonomy and self-esteem and a profound sense of powerlessness. The codependent person is able to achieve a sense of control only through fulfilling the needs of others. Personal identity is relinquished and boundaries with the other person become blurred. The codependent person disowns his or her own needs and wants in order to respond to external demands and the demands of others. Codependence has been called "a dysfunctional relationship with oneself."

The traits associated with a codependent personality are varied. A codependent individual is confused about his or her own identity. In a relationship, the codependent person derives self-worth from that of the partner, whose feelings and behaviors determine how the codependent should feel and behave. In order for the codependent to feel good, his or her partner must be happy and behave in appropriate ways. If the partner is not happy, the codependent feels responsible for *making* him or her happy. The codependent's home life is fraught with stress. Ego boundaries are weak and behaviors are often enmeshed with those of the pathological partner. Denial that problems exist is common. Feelings are kept in control, and anxiety may be released in the form of stress-related illnesses or compulsive behaviors such as eating, spending, working, or use of substances.

Wesson (2013) describes the following behaviors characteristic of codependency. She stated that codependents:

■ Have a long history of focusing thoughts and behavior on other people.

■ Are "people pleasers" and will do almost anything to get the approval of others.

■ Outwardly appear very competent, but actually feel quite needy, helpless, or perhaps nothing at all.

■ Have experienced abuse or emotional neglect as a child.

■ Are outwardly focused towards others, and know very little about how to direct their own lives from their own sense of self.

The Codependent Nurse

Certain characteristics of codependence have been associated with the profession of nursing. A shortage of nurses combined with the increasing ranks of seriously ill clients may result in nurses providing care and fulfilling everyone's needs but their own. Many health-care workers who are reared in homes with a chemically addicted person or otherwise dysfunctional family are at risk for having any unresolved codependent tendencies activated. Nurses, who as children assumed the "fixer" role in their dysfunctional families of origin, may attempt to resume that role in their caregiving professions. They are attracted to a profession in which they are needed, but they nurture feelings of resentment for receiving so little in return. Their emotional needs go unmet; however, they continue to deny that these needs exist. Instead, these unmet emotional needs may be manifested through use of compulsive behaviors, such as work or spending excessively, or addictions, such as to food or substances.

Codependent nurses have a need to be in control. They often strive for an unrealistic level of achievement. Their self-worth comes from the feeling of being needed by others and of maintaining control over their environment. They nurture the dependence of others and accept the responsibility for the happiness and contentment of others. They rarely express their true feelings, and do what is necessary to preserve harmony and maintain control. They are at high risk for physical and emotional burnout.

Treating Codependency

Cermak (1986) identified four stages in the recovery process for individuals with codependent personality:

Stage I: The Survival Stage In this first stage, codependent persons must begin to let go of the denial that problems exist or that their personal capabilities are unlimited. This initiation of abstinence from blanket denial may be a very emotional and painful period.

Stage II: The Reidentification Stage Reidentification occurs when the individuals are able to glimpse their true selves through a break in the denial system. They accept the label of codependent and take responsibility for their own dysfunctional behavior. Codependents tend to enter reidentification only after being convinced that it is more painful not to. They accept their limitations and are ready to face the issues of codependence.

Stage III: The Core Issues Stage In this stage, the recovering codependent must face the fact that relationships cannot be managed by force of will. Each partner must be independent and autonomous. The goal of this stage is to detach from the struggles of life that exist because of prideful and willful efforts to control those things that are beyond the individual's power to control.

Stage IV: The Reintegration Stage This is a stage of self-acceptance and willingness to change when codependents relinquish the power *over others* that was not rightfully theirs but reclaim the *personal* power that they do possess. Integrity is achieved out of awareness, honesty, and being in touch with one's spiritual consciousness. Control is achieved through self-discipline and self-confidence.

Self-help groups have been found to be helpful in the treatment of codependency. Groups developed for families of chemically addicted people, such as Al-Anon, may be of assistance. Groups specific to the problem of codependency also exist. One of these groups, which bases its philosophy on the Twelve Steps of Alcoholics Anonymous (see the section that follows), is:

Co-Dependents Anonymous (CoDA)
P.O. Box 33577
Phoenix, AZ 85067-3577
888-444-2359
www.coda.org

Treatment Modalities for Substance-Related Disorders

Alcoholics Anonymous

Alcoholics Anonymous (AA) is a major self-help organization for the treatment of alcoholism. It was founded in 1935 by two alcoholics—a stockbroker, Bill Wilson, and a physician, Dr. Bob Smith—who discovered that they could remain sober through mutual support. This they accomplished not as professionals, but as peers who were able to share their common experiences. Soon they were working with other alcoholics, who in turn worked with others. The movement grew, and remarkably, individuals who had been treated unsuccessfully by professionals were able to maintain sobriety through helping one another.

Today AA chapters exist in virtually every community in the United States. The self-help groups are based on the concept of peer support—acceptance and understanding from others who have experienced the same problems in their lives. The only requirement for membership is a desire on the part of the alcoholic person to stop drinking. Each new member is assigned a support person from whom he or she may seek assistance when the temptation to drink occurs.

A survey by the General Service Office of Alcoholics Anonymous in 2011 (Alcoholics Anonymous [AA], 2012) revealed the following statistics: members ages 30 and younger comprised 13 percent of the membership and the average age of AA members was 49; women comprised 35 percent; 87 percent were white, 4 percent were African American, 5 percent were Hispanic, 2 percent were Native American, and 2 percent were Asian American and other minorities.

By occupation, the highest percentages included the following: 17 percent were retired; 10 percent were self-employed; 10 percent were unemployed; 9 percent were managers or administrators; and 8 percent were in professional or technical fields.

The sole purpose of AA is to help members stay sober. When sobriety has been achieved, they in turn are expected to help other alcoholic persons. The Twelve Steps that embody the philosophy of AA provide specific guidelines on how to attain and maintain sobriety (Box 23-6).

AA accepts alcoholism as an illness and promotes total abstinence as the only cure, emphasizing that the alcoholic person can never safely return to social

---

BOX 23-6 Alcoholics Anonymous

THE TWELVE STEPS

1. We admitted we were powerless over alcohol—that our lives have become unmanageable.
2. Came to believe that a Power greater than ourselves could restore us to sanity.
3. Made a decision to turn our will and our lives over to the care of God as we understood Him.
4. Made a searching and fearless moral inventory of ourselves.
5. Admitted to God, to ourselves, and to another human being the exact nature of our wrongs.
6. Were entirely ready to have God remove all these defects of character.
7. Humbly asked Him to remove our shortcomings.
8. Made a list of all persons we had harmed and became willing to make amends to them all.
9. Made direct amends to such people wherever possible except when to do so would injure them or others.
10. Continued to take personal inventory and when we were wrong promptly admitted it.
11. Sought through prayer and meditation to improve our conscious contact with God as we understood Him, praying only for knowledge of His will for us and the power to carry that out.
12. Having had a spiritual awakening as the result of these steps, we tried to carry this message to alcoholics and to practice these principles in all our affairs.

THE TWELVE TRADITIONS

1. Our common welfare should come first; personal recovery depends upon AA unity.
2. For our group purpose there is but one ultimate authority—a loving God as He may express Himself in our group conscience. Our leaders are but trusted servants; they do not govern.
3. The one requirement for AA membership is a desire to stop drinking.
4. Each group should be autonomous except in matters affecting other groups or AA as a whole.
5. Each group has but one primary purpose—to carry its message to the alcoholic who still suffers.
6. An AA group ought never endorse, finance, or lend the AA name to any related facility or outside enterprise, lest problems of money, property, and prestige divert us from our primary purpose.
7. Every AA group ought to be fully self-supporting, declining outside contributions.
8. Alcoholics Anonymous should remain forever nonprofessional, but our service centers may employ special workers.
9. Alcoholics Anonymous, as such, ought never be organized; but we may create service boards of committees directly responsible to those they serve.
10. Alcoholics Anonymous has no opinion on outside issues; hence, the Alcoholics Anonymous name ought never be drawn into public controversy.
11. Our public relations policy is based on attraction rather than promotion; we need always maintain personal anonymity at the level of press, radio, and films.
12. Anonymity is the spiritual foundation of all our traditions, ever reminding us to place principles before personalities.

drinking. They encourage the members to seek sobriety, taking one day at a time. The Twelve Traditions are the statements of principles that govern the organization (see Box 23-6).

AA has been the model for various other self-help groups associated with addiction problems. Some of these groups and the memberships for which they are organized are listed in Table 23-11. Nurses need to be fully and accurately informed about available self-help groups and their importance as a treatment resource on the health-care continuum so that they can use them as a referral source for clients with substance use disorders.

Pharmacotherapy

Disulfiram (Antabuse)

Disulfiram (Antabuse) is a drug that can be administered as a deterrent to drinking to individuals who abuse alcohol. Ingestion of alcohol while disulfiram is in the body results in a syndrome of symptoms that can produce a great deal of discomfort for the individual. It can even result in death if the blood alcohol level is high. The reaction varies according to the sensitivity of the individual and how much alcohol was ingested.

Disulfiram works by inhibiting the enzyme aldehyde dehydrogenase, thereby blocking the oxidation of alcohol at the stage when acetaldehyde is converted to acetate. This results in an accumulation of acetaldehyde in the blood, which is thought to produce the symptoms associated with the disulfiram-alcohol reaction. These symptoms persist as long as alcohol is being metabolized. The rate of alcohol elimination does not appear to be affected.

Symptoms of disulfiram-alcohol reaction can occur within 5 to 10 minutes of ingestion of alcohol. Mild reactions can occur at blood alcohol levels as low as 5 to 10 mg/dL. Symptoms are fully developed at approximately 50 mg/dL, and may include flushed skin, throbbing in the head and neck, respiratory difficulty, dizziness, nausea and vomiting, sweating, hyperventilation, tachycardia, hypotension, weakness, blurred vision, and confusion. With a blood alcohol level of approximately 125 to 150 mg/dL, severe reactions can occur, including respiratory depression, cardiovascular collapse, arrhythmias, myocardial infarction, acute congestive heart failure, unconsciousness, convulsions, and death.

Disulfiram should not be administered until it has been ascertained that the client has abstained from alcohol for at least 12 hours. If disulfiram is discontinued, it is important for the client to understand that the sensitivity to alcohol may last for as long as 2 weeks. Consuming alcohol or alcohol-containing

TABLE 23–11 **Addiction Self-Help Groups**	
GROUP	MEMBERSHIP
Adult Children of Alcoholics (ACOA)	Adults who grew up with an alcoholic in the home
Al-Anon	Families of alcoholics
Alateen	Adolescent children of alcoholics
Children Are People	School-age children with an alcoholic family member
Cocaine Anonymous	Cocaine addicts
Families Anonymous	Parents of children who abuse substances
Fresh Start	Nicotine addicts
Gamblers Anonymous	Gambling addicts
Narcotics Anonymous	Narcotics addicts
Nar-Anon	Families of narcotics addicts
Overeaters Anonymous	Food addicts
Pills Anonymous	Polysubstance addicts
Pot Smokers Anonymous	Marijuana smokers
Smokers Anonymous	Nicotine addicts
Women for Sobriety	Female alcoholics

substances during this 2-week period could result in the disulfiram-alcohol reaction.

The client receiving disulfiram therapy should be aware of the large number of alcohol-containing substances. These products, such as liquid cough and cold preparations, vanilla extract, aftershave lotions, colognes, mouthwash, nail polish removers, and isopropyl alcohol, if ingested or even rubbed on the skin, are capable of producing the symptoms described. The individual must read labels carefully and must inform any doctor, dentist, or other health-care professional from whom assistance is sought that he or she is taking disulfiram. In addition, it is important that the client carry a card explaining participation in disulfiram therapy, possible consequences of the therapy, and symptoms that may indicate an emergency situation.

The client must be assessed carefully before beginning disulfiram therapy. A thorough medical screening is performed before starting therapy, and written informed consent is usually required. The drug is contraindicated for clients who are at high risk for alcohol ingestion. It is also contraindicated for psychotic clients and clients with severe cardiac, renal, or hepatic disease.

Disulfiram therapy is not a cure for alcoholism. It provides a measure of control for the individual who desires to avoid impulse drinking. Clients receiving disulfiram therapy are encouraged to seek other assistance with their problem, such as AA or other support group, to aid in the recovery process.

Other Medications for Treatment of Alcoholism

The narcotic antagonist naltrexone (ReVia) was approved by the Food and Drug Administration (FDA) in 1994 for the treatment of alcohol addiction. Naltrexone, which was approved in 1984 for the treatment of heroin abuse, works on the same receptors in the brain that produce the feelings of pleasure when heroin or other opiates bind to them, but it does not produce the "narcotic high" and is not habit forming. Although alcohol does not bind to these same brain receptors, studies have shown that naltrexone works equally well against it (O'Malley et al., 1992; Volpicelli, Alterman, Hayashida, & O'Brien, 1992). In comparison to the placebo-treated clients, subjects on naltrexone therapy showed significantly lower overall relapse rates and fewer drinks per drinking day among those clients who did resume drinking. A study with an oral form of nalmefene (Revex) produced similar results (Mason et al., 1994).

Research on the efficacy of selective serotonin reuptake inhibitors (SSRIs) in decreasing alcohol craving among alcohol-dependent individuals has yielded mixed results (National Institute on Alcohol Abuse and Alcoholism [NIAAA], 2000). A greater degree of success was observed with moderate drinkers than with heavy drinkers.

In August 2004, the FDA approved acamprosate (Campral), which is indicated for the maintenance of abstinence from alcohol in patients with alcohol addiction who are abstinent at treatment initiation. The mechanism of action of acamprosate in maintenance of alcohol abstinence is not completely understood. It is hypothesized to restore the normal balance between neuronal excitation and inhibition by interacting with glutamate and gamma-aminobutyric acid (GABA) neurotransmitter systems. Acamprosate is ineffective in clients who have not undergone detoxification and not achieved alcohol abstinence prior to beginning treatment. It is recommended for concomitant use with psychosocial therapy.

Counseling

Counseling on a one-to-one basis is often used to help the client who abuses substances. The relationship is goal-directed, and the length of the counseling may vary from weeks to years. The focus is on current reality, development of a working treatment relationship, and strengthening ego assets. The counselor must be warm, kind, and nonjudgmental, yet able to set limits firmly. Research consistently demonstrates that personal characteristics of counselors are highly predictive of client outcome. In addition to technical counseling skills, many important therapeutic qualities affect the outcome of counseling, including insight, respect, genuineness, concreteness, and empathy (SAMHSA, 2009).

Counseling of the client who abuses substances passes through various phases, each of which is of indeterminate length. In the first phase, an assessment is conducted. Factual data are collected to determine whether the client does indeed have a problem with substances; that is, that substances are regularly impairing effective functioning in a significant life area.

Following the assessment, in the working phase of the relationship, the counselor assists the individual to work on acceptance of the fact that the use of substances causes problems in significant life areas and that he or she is not able to prevent it from occurring. The client states a desire to make changes. The strength of the denial system is determined by the duration and extent of substance-related adverse effects in the person's life. Thus, those individuals with rather minor substance-related problems of recent origin have less difficulty with this stage than those with long-term extensive impairment. The individual also works to gain self-control and abstain from substances.

Once the problem has been identified and sobriety is achieved, the client must have a concrete and workable plan for getting through the early weeks of abstinence. Anticipatory guidance through role-play helps the individual practice how he or she will respond when substances are readily obtainable and the impulse to partake is strong.

Counseling often includes the family or specific family members. In family counseling the therapist tries to help each member see how he or she has affected, and been affected by, the substance abuse behavior. Family strengths are mobilized, and family members are encouraged to move in a positive direction. Referrals are often made to self-help groups such as Al-Anon, Nar-Anon, Alateen, Families Anonymous, and Adult Children of Alcoholics.

Group Therapy

Group therapy with substance abusers has long been regarded as a powerful agent of change. In groups, individuals are able to share their experiences with others who are going through similar problems. They are able to "see themselves in others," and confront their defenses about giving up the substance. They may confront similar attitudes and defenses in others. Groups also give individuals the capacity for communicating needs and feelings directly.

Some groups may be task-oriented education groups in which the leader is charged with presenting material associated with substance abuse and its various effects on the person's life. Other educational groups that may be helpful with individuals who abuse substances include assertiveness techniques and relaxation training. Teaching groups differ from psychotherapy groups, whose focus is more on helping individuals understand and manage difficult feelings and situations, particularly as they relate to use of substances.

Therapy groups and self-help groups such as AA are complementary to each other. Whereas the self-help group focus is on achieving and maintaining sobriety, in the therapy group the individual may learn more adaptive ways of coping, how to deal with problems that may have arisen or were exacerbated by the former substance use, and ways to improve quality of life and to function more effectively without substances.

Psychopharmacology for Substance Intoxication and Substance Withdrawal

Various medications have been used to decrease the intensity of symptoms in an individual who is withdrawing from, or who is experiencing the effects of excessive use of, alcohol and other drugs. **Substitution therapy** may be required to reduce the life-threatening effects of intoxication or withdrawal from some substances. The severity of the withdrawal syndrome depends on the particular drug used, how long it has been used, the dose used, and the rate at which the drug is eliminated from the body.

Alcohol

Benzodiazepines are the most widely used group of drugs for substitution therapy in alcohol withdrawal. Chlordiazepoxide (Librium), oxazepam (Serax), lorazepam (Ativan), and diazepam (Valium) are the most commonly used agents. The approach to treatment with benzodiazepines for alcohol withdrawal is to start with relatively high doses and reduce the dosage by 20 to 25 percent each day until withdrawal is complete. Additional doses may be given for breakthrough signs or symptoms (Black & Andreasen, 2011). In clients with liver disease, accumulation of the longer-acting agents (chlordiazepoxide and diazepam) may be problematic, and use of the shorter-acting benzodiazepines (lorazepam or oxazepam) is more appropriate.

Some physicians may order anticonvulsant medication (e.g., carbamazepine, valproic acid, or gabapentin) for management of withdrawal seizures. These drugs are particularly useful in individuals who undergo repeated episodes of alcohol withdrawal. Repeated episodes of withdrawal appear to "kindle" even more serious withdrawal episodes, including the production of withdrawal seizures that can result in brain damage (Julien, 2008). These anticonvulsants have been used successfully in both acute withdrawal and longer-term craving situations.

Multivitamin therapy, in combination with daily injections or oral administration of thiamine, is common protocol. Thiamine is commonly deficient in chronic alcoholics. Replacement therapy is required to prevent neuropathy, confusion, and encephalopathy.

Opioids

Examples of drugs in the opioid classification include opium, morphine, codeine, heroin, hydromorphone, oxycodone, and hydrocodone. Synthetic opiate-like narcotic analgesics include meperidine, methadone, pentazocine, and fentanyl. With short-acting drugs such as heroin, withdrawal symptoms occur within 6 to 8 hours after the last dose, peak within 1 to 3 days, and gradually subside over a period of 5 to 7 days (Walton-Moss et al., 2010). With longer-acting drugs such as methadone, withdrawal symptoms begin within 1 to 3 days after the last dose, peak between days 4 and 6, and are complete in 14 to 21 days (Leamon et al., 2008). Withdrawal from the ultra-short-acting meperidine begins quickly, reaches a peak in 8 to 12 hours, and is complete in 4 to 5 days (Sadock & Sadock, 2007).

Opioid intoxication is treated with narcotic antagonists such as naloxone (Narcan), naltrexone (ReVia), or nalmefene (Revex). Withdrawal therapy includes rest, adequate nutritional support, and methadone substitution. Methadone is given on the first day in a dose sufficient to suppress withdrawal symptoms. The dose is then gradually tapered over a specified time. As the dose of methadone diminishes, renewed abstinence symptoms may be ameliorated by the addition of clonidine.

In October 2002, the FDA approved two forms of the drug buprenorphine for treating opiate addiction. Buprenorphine is less powerful than methadone but is considered to be somewhat safer and causes fewer side effects, making it especially attractive for clients who are mildly or moderately addicted. Individuals are able to access treatment with buprenorphine in office-based settings, providing an alternative to methadone clinics. Physicians are deemed qualified to prescribe buprenorphine if they hold an addiction certification from the American Society of Addiction Medicine, the American Academy of Addiction Psychiatry, the American Psychiatric Association, or other associations deemed appropriate. The number of patients to whom individual physicians may provide outpatient buprenorphine treatment is limited to 100 (Gordon, 2009). A sublingual formulation of a combination medication (buprenorphine and naloxone) is also available.

Clonidine (Catapres) also has been used to suppress opiate withdrawal symptoms. As monotherapy, it is not as effective as substitution with methadone, but it is nonaddicting and serves effectively as a bridge to enable the client to stay opiate free long enough to facilitate termination of methadone maintenance.

Depressants

Substitution therapy for CNS depressant withdrawal (particularly barbiturates) is most commonly with the long-acting barbiturate phenobarbital (Luminal). The dosage required to suppress withdrawal symptoms is administered. When stabilization has been achieved, the dose is gradually decreased by 30 mg/day until withdrawal is complete. Long-acting benzodiazepines are commonly used for substitution therapy when the abused substance is a nonbarbiturate CNS depressant (Ashton, 2002).

Stimulants

Treatment of stimulant intoxication usually begins with minor tranquilizers such as chlordiazepoxide and progresses to major tranquilizers such as haloperidol (Haldol). Antipsychotics should be administered with caution because of their propensity to lower seizure threshold (Mack et al., 2003). Repeated seizures are treated with intravenous diazepam.

Withdrawal from CNS stimulants is not the medical emergency observed with CNS depressants. Treatment is usually aimed at reducing drug craving and managing severe depression. The client is placed in

a quiet atmosphere and allowed to sleep and eat as much as is needed or desired. Suicide precautions may need to be instituted. Antidepressant therapy may be helpful in treating symptoms of depression. Desipramine has been especially successful with symptoms of cocaine withdrawal and abstinence (Mack et al., 2003).

Hallucinogens and Cannabinoids

Substitution therapy is not required with these drugs. When adverse reactions, such as anxiety or panic, occur, benzodiazepines (e.g., diazepam or chlordiazepoxide) may be prescribed to prevent harm to the client or others. Psychotic reactions may be treated with antipsychotic medications.

Non-Substance Addictions

Gambling Disorder

This disorder is defined by the *DSM-5* as persistent and recurrent problematic gambling behavior leading to clinically significant impairment or distress (APA, 2013). The preoccupation with and impulse to gamble often intensifies when the individual is under stress. Many impulsive gamblers describe a physical sensation of restlessness and anticipation that can only be relieved by placing a bet. Blume (2013) states:

> In some cases the initial change in gambling behavior leading to pathological gambling begins with a "big win," bringing a rapid development of preoccupation, tolerance, and loss of control. Winning brings feelings of special status, power, and omnipotence. The gambler increasingly depends on this activity to cope with disappointments, problems, and negative emotional states, pulling away from emotional attachment to family and friends.

As the need to gamble increases, the individual is forced to obtain money by any means available. This may include borrowing money from illegal sources or pawning personal items (or items that belong to others). As gambling debts accrue, or out of a need to continue gambling, the individual may desperately resort to forgery, theft, or even embezzlement. Family relationships are disrupted, and impairment in occupational functioning may occur because of absences from work in order to gamble.

Gambling behavior usually begins in adolescence; however, compulsive behaviors rarely occur before young adulthood. The disorder generally runs a chronic course, with periods of waxing and waning, largely dependent on periods of psychosocial stress. Prevalence estimates for pathological gambling range from 1.2 percent to 3.4 percent (Hollander, Berlin, & Stein, 2008). It is more common among men than women.

Various personality traits have been attributed to pathological gamblers. Unwin, Davis, and Leeuw (2000) stated:

Evidence points to the common existence of narcissistic personality characteristics and impulse control problems in pathologic gamblers. High rates of personality disorders (e.g., obsessive-compulsive, avoidant, schizotypal and paranoid) are noted in several studies. Personality profiles of persons who are alcoholics and pathologic gamblers are also similar in some studies. Some experts view pathologic gambling as an addictive disorder, citing as evidence the tolerance and withdrawal symptoms exhibited by pathologic gamblers because of debt escalation behaviors. However, no physical or biochemical markers exist to help physicians make the diagnosis. (p. 744)

The *DSM-5* suggests that gambling behavior can be episodic or chronic and vary by type and life circumstances. The following example is cited (APA, 2012):

An individual who wagers problematically only on football games may have Gambling Disorder during football season and not wager at all, or not wager problematically, throughout the remainder of the year. Gambling Disorder may also occur at one or more points in an individual's life, but be absent during other periods. Alternately, some individuals experience chronic Gambling Disorder throughout all or most of their lives.

The *DSM-5* diagnostic criteria for pathological gambling are presented in Box 23-7.

Predisposing Factors to Gambling Disorder

Biological Influences

Genetic Familial and twin studies show an increased prevalence of pathological gambling in family members of individuals diagnosed with the disorder. Hollander and associates (2008) report the results of research that indicates a common genetic vulnerability for pathological gambling and alcohol addiction in men.

Physiological Hodgins, Stea, and Grant (2011) suggest a correlation between pathological gambling and abnormalities in the serotonergic, noradrenergic, and dopaminergic neurotransmitter systems. They stated:

Dopamine is implicated in learning, motivation, and the salience of stimuli, including rewards. Alterations

---

BOX 23-7 **Diagnostic Criteria for Gambling Disorder**

A. Persistent and recurrent problematic gambling behavior leading to clinically significant impairment or distress, as indicated by the individual exhibiting four (or more) of the following in a 12-month period:
   1. Needs to gamble with increasing amounts of money in order to achieve the desired excitement.
   2. Is restless or irritable when attempting to cut down or stop gambling.
   3. Has made repeated unsuccessful efforts to control, cut back, or stop gambling.
   4. Is often preoccupied with gambling (e.g., persistent thoughts of reliving past gambling experiences, handicapping or planning the next venture, or thinking of ways to get money with which to gamble).
   5. Often gambles when feeling distressed (e.g., helpless, guilty, anxious, depressed).
   6. After losing money gambling, often returns another day to get even ("chasing" one's losses).
   7. Lies to conceal the extent of involvement with gambling.
   8. Has jeopardized or lost a significant relationship, job, or educational or career opportunity because of gambling.
   9. Relies on others to provide money to relieve desperate financial situations caused by gambling.
B. The gambling behavior is not better explained by a manic episode.

Specify if:

Episodic: meeting diagnostic criteria at more than one time point, with symptoms subsiding between periods of gambling disorder for at least several months.

Persistent: Experiencing continuous symptoms, to meet diagnostic criteria for multiple years.

Specify if:

In early remission: After full criteria for gambling disorder were previously met, none of the criteria for gambling disorder have been met for at least 3 months but for less than 12 months.

In sustained remission: After full criteria for gambling disorder were previously met, none of the criteria for gambling disorder have been met during a period of 12 months or longer.

Specify current severity:

Mild: 4–5 criteria met.

Moderate: 6–7 criteria met.

Severe: 8–9 criteria met.

Reprinted with permission from the Diagnostic and Statistical Manual of Mental Disorders, Fifth Edition *(Copyright 2013). American Psychiatric Association.*

in dopaminergic pathways might underlie the seeking of rewards (i.e., gambling) that trigger the release of dopamine and produce feelings of pleasure. (p. 1878)

Other studies have indicated alterations in the electroencephalographic patterns of pathologic gamblers (Regard, Knoch, Gutling, & Landis, 2003).

Psychosocial Influences

Sadock and Sadock (2007) report that the following may be predisposing factors to the development of pathological gambling: "loss of a parent by death, separation, divorce, or desertion before the child is 15 years of age; inappropriate parental discipline (absence, inconsistency, or harshness); exposure to and availability of gambling activities for the adolescent; a family emphasis on material and financial symbols; and a lack of family emphasis on saving, planning, and budgeting" (p. 779).

The early psychoanalytical view attempted to explain compulsive gambling in terms of psychosexual maturation. In this theory, the gambling is compared to masturbation; both of these activities derive motive force from a buildup of tension that is released through repetitive actions or the anticipation of them. Another view suggests a masochistic component to pathological gambling and the gambler's inherent need for punishment, which is then achieved through losing (Moreyra, Ibanez, Saiz-Ruiz, Nissenson, & Blanco, 2000).

Treatment Modalities for Gambling Disorder

Because most pathological gamblers deny that they have a problem, treatment is difficult. In fact, most gamblers only seek treatment due to legal difficulties, family pressures, or other psychiatric complaints. Behavior therapy, cognitive therapy, and psychoanalysis have been used with pathological gambling, with various degrees of success (Moreyra et al., 2000).

Some medications have been used with effective results in the treatment of pathological gambling. The SSRIs and clomipramine have been used successfully in the treatment of pathological gambling as a form of obsessive-compulsive disorder (Moreyra et al., 2000). Lithium, carbamazepine, and naltrexone have also been shown to be effective.

Possibly the most effective treatment of pathological gambling is participation by the individual in **Gamblers Anonymous** (GA). This organization of inspirational group therapy is modeled after Alcoholics Anonymous. The only requirement for GA membership is an expressed desire to stop gambling. Treatment is based on peer pressure, public confession, and the availability of other reformed gamblers to help individuals resist the urge to gamble. Gam-Anon (for family and spouses of compulsive gamblers) and Gam-a-Teen (for adolescent children of compulsive gamblers) are also important sources of treatment.

CASE STUDY AND SAMPLE CARE PLAN

NURSING HISTORY AND ASSESSMENT

The police bring Dan to the emergency department of the local hospital around 9 p.m. His wife, Carol, called 911 when Dan became violent and she began to fear for her safety. Dan was fired from his job as a foreman in a manufacturing plant for refusing to follow his supervisor's directions on a project. When cleaning up after his move, several partially used bottles of liquor were found in his work area.

Carol reports that Dan has been drinking since he came home shortly after noon today. He bloodied her nose and punched her in the stomach when she poured the contents of a bottle from which he was drinking down the kitchen sink. The police responded to her call and brought Dan to the hospital in handcuffs. By the time they arrive at the hospital, Dan has calmed down, and appears drugged and drowsy. His blood alcohol level measures 247 mg/dL. He is admitted to the detoxification unit of the hospital with a diagnosis of alcohol intoxication.

Carol tells the admitting nurse that she and Dan have been married for 12 years. He was a social drinker before they were married, but his drinking has increased over the years. He has been under a lot of stress at work, hates his job, his boss, and his coworkers, and is depressed a lot of the time. He never had a loving relationship with his parents, who

are now deceased. For the past few years, his pattern has been to come home, start drinking immediately, and drink until he passes out for the night. She states that she has tried to get him to go for help with his drinking, but he refuses, and says that he doesn't have a problem. Carol begins to cry and says to the nurse, "We can't go on like this. I don't know what to do!"

NURSING DIAGNOSES/OUTCOME IDENTIFICATION

From the assessment data, the nurse develops the following nursing diagnoses for Dan:

1. **Risk for injury** related to CNS agitation from alcohol withdrawal.
   a. **Short-Term Goal:** Dan's condition will stabilize within 72 hours.
   b. **Long-Term Goal:** Dan will not experience physical injury.
2. **Ineffective denial** related to low self-esteem, weak ego development, and underlying fears and anxieties.
   a. **Short-Term Goal:** Dan will focus immediate attention on behavioral changes required to achieve sobriety.
   b. **Long-Term Goal:** Dan will accept responsibility for his drinking behaviors, and acknowledge the association between his drinking and personal problems.

Continued

CASE STUDY AND SAMPLE CARE PLAN—cont'd

PLANNING/IMPLEMENTATION

RISK FOR INJURY

The following nursing interventions may be implemented *in an effort to ensure client safety:*

1. Assess his level of disorientation; frequently orient him to reality and his surroundings.
2. Obtain a drug history.
3. Obtain a urine sample for analysis.
4. Place Dan in a quiet room (private, if possible).
5. Ensure that smoking materials and other potentially harmful objects are stored away.
6. Observe Dan frequently. Take vital signs every 15 to 30 minutes.
7. Monitor for signs of withdrawal within a few hours after admission. Watch for signs of:
   - Increased heart rate
   - Tremors
   - Headache
   - Diaphoresis
   - Agitation; restlessness
   - Nausea
   - Fever
   - Convulsions
8. Follow medication regimen, as ordered by physician (commonly a benzodiazepine, thiamine, multivitamin).

INEFFECTIVE DENIAL

The following nursing interventions may be implemented *in an effort to help Dan accept responsibility for the behavioral consequences associated with his drinking:*

1. Develop Dan's trust by spending time with him, being honest, and keeping all promises.
2. Ensure that Dan understands that it is not *him*, but his *behavior*, that is unacceptable.
3. Provide Dan with accurate information about the effects of alcohol. Do this in a matter-of-fact, nonjudgmental way.

4. Point out recent negative events that have occurred in Dan's life, and associate the use of alcohol with these events. Help him to see the association.
5. Use confrontation with caring: "Yes, your wife called the police. You were physically abusive. She was afraid. And your blood alcohol level was 247 when you were brought in. You were obviously not in control of your behavior at the time."
6. Don't accept excuses for his drinking. Point out rationalization and projection behaviors. These behaviors prolong denial that he has a problem. He must directly accept responsibility for his drinking (not make excuses and blame it on the behavior of others). He must come to understand that only HE has control of his behavior.
7. Encourage Dan to attend group therapy during treatment, and Alcoholics Anonymous following treatment. Peer feedback is a strong factor in helping individuals recognize their problems and to ultimately remain sober.
8. Encourage Carol to attend Al-Anon meetings. She can benefit from the experiences of others who have experienced and are experiencing the same types of problems as she.
9. Help Dan to identify ways that he can cope besides using alcohol (e.g., exercise, sports, relaxation). He should choose what is most appropriate for him, and should be given positive feedback for efforts made toward change.

EVALUATION

The outcome criteria identified for Dan have been met. He experienced an uncomplicated withdrawal from alcohol and exhibits no evidence of physical injury. He verbalizes understanding of the relationship between his personal problems and his drinking, and accepts responsibility for his own behavior. He verbalizes understanding that alcohol addiction is an illness that requires ongoing support and treatment, and regularly attends AA meetings. Carol regularly attends Al-Anon meetings.

Summary and Key Points

- An individual is considered to be addicted to a substance when he or she is unable to control its use, even knowing that it interferes with normal functioning; when more and more of the substance is required to produce the desired effects; and when characteristic withdrawal symptoms develop upon cessation or drastic decrease in use of the substance.
- Substance intoxication is defined as the development of a reversible syndrome of maladaptive behavioral or psychological changes that are due to the direct physiological effects of a substance on the CNS and develop during or shortly after ingestion of (or exposure to) a substance.

- Substance withdrawal is the development of a substance-specific maladaptive behavioral change, with physiological and cognitive concomitants, that is due to the cessation of, or reduction in, heavy and prolonged substance use.
- The etiology of substance use disorders is unknown. Various contributing factors have been implicated, such as genetics, biochemical changes, developmental influences, personality factors, social learning, conditioning, and cultural and ethnic influences.
- Seven classes of substances are presented in this chapter in terms of a profile of the substance, historical aspects, patterns of use, and effects on the body. They include alcohol, other CNS depressants,

CNS stimulants, opioids, hallucinogens, inhalants, and cannabinoids.

■ The nurse uses the nursing process as the vehicle for delivery of care of the client with a substance-related disorder.

■ The nurse must first examine his or her own feelings regarding personal substance use and the substance use by others. Only the nurse who can be accepting and nonjudgmental of substance use behaviors will be effective in working with these clients.

■ Special care is given to clients with dual diagnoses of mental illness and substance use disorders.

■ Addiction to substances is a problem for many members of the nursing profession. Most state boards of nursing and state nurses' associations have established avenues for peer assistance to provide help to impaired members of the profession.

■ Individuals who are reared in families with chemically addicted persons learn patterns of dysfunctional behavior that carry over into adult life. These dysfunctional behavior patterns have been termed *codependence.* Codependent persons sacrifice their own needs for the fulfillment of others' in order to achieve a sense of control. Many nurses also have codependent traits.

■ Treatment modalities for substance-related disorders include self-help groups, deterrent therapy, individual counseling, and group therapy. Substitution pharmacotherapy is frequently implemented with clients experiencing substance intoxication or substance withdrawal. Treatment modalities are implemented on an inpatient basis or in outpatient settings, depending on the severity of the impairment.

■ Gambling disorder is defined by the *DSM-5* as persistent and recurrent problematic gambling behavior leading to clinically significant impairment or distress.

■ The preoccupation with and impulse to gamble intensifies when the individual is under stress. Many impulsive gamblers describe a physical sensation of restlessness and anticipation that can only be relieved by placing a bet.

■ Research indicates a possible genetic component in the etiology to gambling disorder. Abnormalities in the serotonergic, noradrenergic, and dopaminergic neurotransmitter systems have also been implicated.

■ A number of psychosocial influences have been implicated in the predisposition to gambling disorder, including dysfunctional family patterns.

■ Behavior therapy, cognitive therapy, and psychoanalysis have been used with gambling disorder, with various degrees of success. Various medications, such as the SSRIs, clomipramine, lithium, carbamazine, and naltrexone, have also been tried.

■ Gamblers Anonymous, an organization of inspirational group therapy modeled after Alcoholics Anonymous, has shown to be very effective in helping individuals who desire to stop gambling.

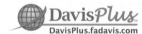 Additional info available at
DavisPlus.fadavis.com   www.davisplus.com

Review Questions
Self-Examination/Learning Exercise

Select the answer that is most appropriate for each of the following questions.

1. Mr. White is admitted to the hospital after an extended period of binge alcohol drinking. His wife reports that he has been a heavy drinker for a number of years. Lab reports reveal he has a blood alcohol level of 250 mg/dL. He is placed on the chemical addiction unit for detoxification. When would the first signs of alcohol withdrawal symptoms be expected to occur?
   a. Several hours after the last drink
   b. 2 to 3 days after the last drink
   c. 4 to 5 days after the last drink
   d. 6 to 7 days after the last drink

2. Symptoms of alcohol withdrawal include:
   a. Euphoria, hyperactivity, and insomnia
   b. Depression, suicidal ideation, and hypersomnia
   c. Diaphoresis, nausea and vomiting, and tremors
   d. Unsteady gait, nystagmus, and profound disorientation

Continued

Review Questions—cont'd
Self-Examination/Learning Exercise

3. Which of the following medications is the physician most likely to order for a client experiencing alcohol withdrawal syndrome?
   a. Haloperidol (Haldol)
   b. Chlordiazepoxide (Librium)
   c. Methadone (Dolophine)
   d. Phenytoin (Dilantin)

4. Dan, who has been admitted to the alcohol rehabilitation unit after being fired for drinking on the job, states to the nurse, "I don't have a problem with alcohol. I can handle my booze better than anyone I know. My boss is a jerk! I haven't missed any more days than my coworkers." The nurse's best response is:
   a. "Maybe your boss is mistaken, Dan."
   b. "You are here because your drinking was interfering with your work, Dan."
   c. "Get real, Dan! You're a boozer and you know it!"
   d. "Why do you think your boss sent you here, Dan?"

5. Dan, who has been admitted to the alcohol rehabilitation unit after being fired for drinking on the job, states to the nurse, "I don't have a problem with alcohol. I can handle my booze better than anyone I know. My boss is a jerk! I haven't missed any more days than my coworkers." The defense mechanism that Dan is using is:
   a. Denial
   b. Projection
   c. Displacement
   d. Rationalization

6. Dan has been admitted to the alcohol rehabilitation unit after being fired for drinking on the job. Dan's drinking buddies come for a visit, and when they leave, the nurse smells alcohol on Dan's breath. Which of the following would be the best intervention with Dan at this time?
   a. Search his room for evidence.
   b. Ask, "Have you been drinking alcohol, Dan?"
   c. Send a urine specimen from Dan to the lab for drug screening.
   d. Tell Dan, "These guys cannot come to the unit to visit you again."

7. Dan begins attendance at AA meetings. Which of the statements by Dan reflects the purpose of this organization?
   a. "They claim they will help me stay sober."
   b. "I'll dry out in AA, then I can have a social drink now and then."
   c. "AA is only for people who have reached the bottom."
   d. "If I lose my job, AA will help me find another."

8. From which of the following symptoms might the nurse identify a chronic cocaine user?
   a. Clear, constricted pupils
   b. Red, irritated nostrils
   c. Muscle aches
   d. Conjunctival redness

9. An individual who is addicted to heroin is likely to experience which of the following symptoms of withdrawal?
   a. Increased heart rate and blood pressure
   b. Tremors, insomnia, and seizures
   c. Incoordination and unsteady gait
   d. Nausea and vomiting, diarrhea, and diaphoresis

10. A polysubstance abuser makes the statement, "The green and whites do me good after speed." How might the nurse interpret the statement?
    a. The client abuses amphetamines and anxiolytics.
    b. The client abuses alcohol and cocaine.
    c. The client is psychotic.
    d. The client abuses narcotics and marijuana.

IMPLICATIONS OF RESEARCH FOR EVIDENCE-BASED PRACTICE

Stevenson, J.S., & Masters, J.A. (2005). Predictors of alcohol misuse and abuse in older women. *Journal of Nursing Scholarship, 37*(4), 329-335.

DESCRIPTION OF THE STUDY: The purpose of this study was to determine the predictive ability of self-report questions, physical measures, and biomarkers to detect alcohol misuse and abuse among older women. Older women are not routinely screened in health-care settings for alcohol use. Because they often have many other health concerns, health-care providers often fail to assess these older patients for an underlying alcohol problem. The sample included 135 healthy women aged 60 and older divided into two groups: drinkers (those who consumed 12 or more standard drinks [SD] in the past year) and nondrinkers (those who consumed no alcohol during the past year). A standard drink is identified by the National Institute on Alcohol Abuse and Alcoholism as 1.5 oz. of distilled liquor, 12 oz. of regular beer, or 5 oz. of wine. Data was gathered from an alcohol-enhanced assessment interview (the T-ACE), a physical examination, and biomarker-enhanced standard intake blood work. Biomarkers collected in this study were gamma glutamyltransferase (GGT), mean corpuscular volume (MCV), total cholesterol (TC), high-density lipoprotein (HDL), low-density lipoprotein (LDL), and the ratio of HDL to TC. Other physical data collected were systolic and diastolic blood pressures, body mass index (BMI), exercise habits, past experiences of trauma, hemoglobin (Hgb), and hematocrit (Hct).

RESULTS OF THE STUDY: The T-ACE questionnaire discriminated strongly between the two groups. This test is similar to the CAGE questionnaire, with one exception. The question related to "guilt" is replaced with a question related to "tolerance." ("How many drinks does it take to make you feel high?"). Analyses of the biomarkers showed significant differences in MCV, HDL, Hgb, Hct, and GGT, with drinkers showing higher levels. Drinkers also were found to consume more coffee and over-the-counter (OTC) drugs, and were more likely to be (or have been) smokers and to use alcohol to fall asleep. Nutrition, trauma, and blood pressure showed no significant differences between the groups.

IMPLICATIONS FOR NURSING PRACTICE: This study suggests a way in which to identify older women who may be at risk for problems related to alcohol abuse. Results reveal promising predictors of alcohol use and abuse that can be part of clinical data collection during intake assessments in primary care and acute care. Indications suggest that the best predictors of high-risk drinkers include the T-ACE tool (a score of 1 or higher), elevated MCV and Hgb levels, smoking or having been a smoker, drinking large amounts of coffee, using alcohol to sleep at night, and self-medicating with two or more OTC drugs on a routine basis. The authors suggest that biological markers are significant predictors because alcohol is documented to have a powerful physiological effect on women.

IMPLICATIONS OF RESEARCH FOR EVIDENCE-BASED PRACTICE

Gaffney, K.F. (2001). Infant exposure to environmental tobacco smoke. *Journal of Nursing Scholarship, 33*(4), 343-347.

DESCRIPTION OF THE STUDY: A review of 10 studies with a range of 100 to more than 1,000 participants was conducted. The studies took place in a variety of health-care settings in the United States, Australia, and Europe. The studies measured infant exposure to environmental tobacco smoke (ETS). Parents of the infants completed the self-reports that inquired about number of people in the household who smoked and the proximity of the infant to the smoking. The studies focused on children in the first year of life.

RESULTS OF THE STUDY: In one of the studies, questionnaire information was supported by hair analysis of the subjects. Median level of hair nicotine was over 1.5 times higher among infants in homes reported by means of questionnaires to have smokers than among those in homes reported to have no smokers. Eight of the 10 studies demonstrated increased risk for poor infant health outcomes associated with ETS exposure. Positive associations were found between infant ETS exposure and gastroesophageal reflux, colic, sudden infant death syndrome, lower respiratory tract infections, ear infections, and altered thyroid function.

IMPLICATIONS FOR NURSING PRACTICE: The author suggests that nurses may use these results to document the need for identifying mothers who smoke as an important target group for clinical intervention. She states, "This review shows the importance of identifying and assisting mothers who smoke so that this critical proximity with their infants may provide optimal health promotion. Nurses who care for infants as part of the regular health maintenance visits conducted during the first year of life are particularly well-prepared and logically situated to advise and assist these mothers as they initiate the long-term process of smoking cessation" (pp. 346-347).

TEST YOUR CRITICAL THINKING SKILLS

Kelly, age 23, is a first-year law student. She is engaged to a surgical resident at the local university hospital. She has been struggling to do well in law school because she wants to make her parents, two prominent local attorneys, proud of her. She had never aspired to do anything but go into law, and that is also what her parents expected her to do.

Kelly's mid-term grades were not as high as she had hoped, so she increased the number of hours of study time, staying awake all night several nights a week to study. She started drinking large amounts of coffee to stay awake, but still found herself falling asleep as she tried to study at the library and in her apartment. As final exams approached, she began to panic that she would not be able to continue the pace of studying she felt she needed in order to make the grades she hoped for.

One of Kelly's classmates told her that she needed some "speed" to give her that extra energy to study. Her classmate said, "All the kids do it. Hardly anyone I know gets through law school without it." She gave Kelly the name of a source.

Kelly contacted the source, who supplied her with enough amphetamines to see her through final exams. Kelly was excited, because she had so much energy, did not require sleep, and was able to study the additional hours she thought she needed for the exams. However, when the results were posted, Kelly had failed two courses and would have to repeat them in summer school if she was to continue with her class in the fall. She continued to replenish her supply of amphetamines from her "contact" until he told her he could not get her anymore. She became frantic and stole a prescription blank from her fiancé and forged his name for more pills.

She started taking more and more of the medication in order to achieve the "high" she wanted to feel. Her behavior became erratic. Yesterday, her fiancé received a call from a pharmacy to clarify an order for amphetamines that Kelly had written. He insisted that she admit herself to the chemical addiction unit for detoxification.

On the unit, she appears tired, depressed, moves very slowly, and wants to sleep all the time. She keeps saying to the nurse, "I'm a real failure. I'll never be an attorney like my parents. I'm too dumb. I just wish I could die."

Answer the following questions related to Kelly:

1. What is the primary nursing diagnosis for Kelly?
2. Describe important nursing interventions to be implemented with Kelly.
3. In addition to physical safety, what would be the primary short-term goal the nurses would strive to achieve with Kelly?

Communication Exercises

1. Tom is a patient on the Alcohol Treatment Unit. He says to the nurse, "My boss and my wife ganged up on me. They think I have a drinking problem. I don't have a drinking problem! I can quit any time I want to!"
   • How would the nurse respond appropriately to this statement by Tom?

2. Tom says to the nurse, "My head hurts. I didn't sleep very well last night. I'm getting shaky and it's hot in here! I could sure use a cup of coffee and a cigarette."
   • How would the nurse respond appropriately to this statement by Tom?

3. Tom says, "Sure, I missed a couple days of work. Everyone gets sick now and then. I don't think my wife cares about what happens to me. She and my boss got together and decided I needed to be here, or I lose my job!"
   • How would the nurse respond appropriately to this statement by Tom?

References

Alcoholics Anonymous [AA]. (2012). *Alcoholics Anonymous 2011 membership survey.* Retrieved from http://www.aa.org

American Academy of Child and Adolescent Psychiatry. (2011). *Children of alcoholics.* Retrieved from http://www.aacap.org/cs/root/facts_for_families/children_of_alcoholics

American Psychiatric Association. (2013). *Diagnostic and statistical manual of mental disorders* (5th ed.). Washington, DC: Author.

American Psychiatric Association. (2012). *Gambling disorder.* Retrieved from www.dsm5.org/ProposedRevision/Pages/proposedrevision.aspx?rid=210

Ashton, C.H. (2002). *Benzodiazepines: How they work and how to withdraw.* Newcastle upon Tyne, UK: University of Newcastle.

Bashore, T.M., Granger, C.B., Hranitzky, P., & Patel, M.R. (2012). Heart disease. In S.J. McPhee, M.A. Papadakis, and Rabow, M.W. (Eds.), *2012 Current medical diagnosis & treatment* (pp. 317-419). New York, NY: McGraw-Hill.

Black, D.W., & Andreasen, N.C. (2011). *Introductory textbook of psychiatry* (5th ed.). Washington, DC: American Psychiatric Publishing.

Blume, S.G. (2013). *Pathological gambling: Recognition and intervention.* Retrieved from http://education.iupui.edu/soe/programs/graduate/counselor/readings_n_docs/reading4.pdf

Carmona, R.H. (2005). *Surgeon General's advisory on alcohol use in pregnancy.* Washington, DC: U.S. Department of Health and Human Services.

Centers for Disease Control and Prevention (CDC). (2011). *Facts about FASDs.* Retrieved from http://www.cdc.gov/ncbddd/fasd/facts.html

Centers for Disease Control and Prevention (CDC). (2012a). *Fetal alcohol spectrum disorders: Data and statistics.* Retrieved from http://www.cdc.gov/ncbddd/fasd/data.html

Centers for Disease Control and Prevention (CDC). (2012b). *The burden of tobacco use.* Retrieved from http://www.cdc.gov/chronicdisease/resources/publications/aag/osh.htm

Coles, C.D. (2011). Discriminating the effects of prenatal alcohol exposure from other behavioral and learning disorders. *Alcohol Research & Health, 34*(1), 42-50.

Dannaway, D.C., & Mulvihill, J.J. (2009). Fetal alcohol spectrum disorder. *NeoReviews 10*(5), e230-e238.

Ehrlander, M. (2007). Alcohol cultures in Finland and Alaska: Explosive drinking patterns and their consequences. *Northern Review.* Number 27 (Fall 2007). Retrieved from http://www.highbeam.com/doc/1G1-185821604.html

Ellis, J.R., & Hartley, C.L. (2012). *Nursing in today's world: Trends, issues, and management* (10th ed.). Philadelphia, PA: Lippincott Williams & Wilkins.

Goldstein, A. (2002). Addiction: From biology to drug policy (2nd ed.). New York, NY: Oxford University Press.

Gordon, A.J. (2009). Buprenorphine resource guide—Version 9. *Buprenorphine initiative in the VA (BIV)*. Retrieved from http://www.mentalhealth.va.gov/providers/sud/docs/VA_Bup_Resource_Guidev9-1.pdf

Gualtieri, J. (2004). *Substance abuse: Sedative-hypnotics/alcohol withdrawal*. University of Minnesota, College of Pharmacy. Retrieved from http://www.courses.ahc.umn.edu/pharmacy/6124/handouts/sedatives.pdf

Hanley, C.E. (2013). Navajos. In J.N. Giger (Ed.), *Transcultural nursing: Assessment and intervention* (6th ed.). St. Louis, MO: Mosby.

Harvard Medical School. (2003, September). Dual diagnosis: Part II. *Harvard Mental Health Letter, 20*(3), 1-5.

Hoffman, M.T. (2006). ADHD related to fetal alcohol syndrome. *Medscape Psychiatry & Mental Health*. Retrieved from http://www.medscape.com/viewarticle/546475

Hodgins, D.C., Stea, J.N., & Grant, J.E. (2011). Gambling disorders. *The Lancet, 378*(9806), 1874-1888.

Hollander, E., Berlin, H.A., & Stein, D.J. (2008). Impulse-control disorders not elsewhere classified. In R.E. Hales, S.C. Yudofsky, & G.O. Gabbard (Eds.), *Textbook of psychiatry* (5th ed., pp. 777-820). Washington, DC: American Psychiatric Publishing.

Indian Health Service. (2011). *American Indian/Alaska Native behavioral health briefing book*. Retrieved from http://www.ihs.gov/medicalprograms/Behavioral/documents/AIANBHBriefingBook.pdf

Jamal, M., Ameno, K., Kubota, T., Ameno, S., Zhang, X., Kumihashi, M., & Ijiri, I. (2003). In vivo formation of salsolinol induced by high acetaldehyde concentration in rat striatum employing microdialysis. *Alcohol and Alcoholism, 38*(3), 197-201.

Julien, R.M. (2008). *A primer of drug action: A comprehensive guide to actions, uses and side effects of psychoactive drugs* (11th ed.). New York, NY: Worth Publishers.

Klopstock, T., Haller, R.G., & DiMauro, S. (2012). Alcoholic myopathy. *MedlinkNeurology*. Retrieved from http://www.medlink.com/CIP.ASP?UID=MLT000DF

Lafferty, K.A., & Abdel-Kariem, R. (2012). *Barbiturate toxicity*. Retrieved from http://emedicine.medscape.com/article/813155-overview

Leamon, M.H., Wright, T.M., & Myrick, H. (2008). Substance-related disorders. In R.E. Hales, S.C. Yudofsky, & G.O. Gabbard (Eds.), *Textbook of Psychiatry* (5th ed.). Washington, DC: American Psychiatric Publishing.

Mack, A.H., Franklin, J.E., & Frances, R.J. (2003). Substance use disorders. In R.E. Hales & S.C. Yudofsky (Eds.), *Textbook of clinical psychiatry* (4th ed.). Washington, DC: American Psychiatric Publishing.

Maier, S.E., & West, J.R. (2013). Drinking patterns and alcohol-related birth defects. *National Institute on Alcohol Abuse and Alcohol*. National Institutes of Health. Retrieved from http://pubs.niaaa.nih.gov/publications/arh25-3/168-174.htm

Mason, G.J., Ritvo, E.C., Morgan, R.O., Salvanto, F.R., Goldberg, G., Welch, B., & Mantero-Atienza, E. (1994). Double-blind, placebo-controlled pilot study to evaluate the efficacy and safety of oral nalmefene HCl for alcohol dependence. *Alcoholism, Clinical and Experimental Research, 18*(5), 1162-1167.

McCoy, J.G., Strawbridge, C., McMurtrey, K.D., Kane, V.B., & Ward, C.P. (2003). A re-evaluation of the role of tetrahydropapaveroline in ethanol consumption in rats. *Brain Research Bulletin, 60*(1-2), 59-65.

McKeown, N.J. (2011). Toluene toxicity. *Medscape Reference: Drugs, diseases, and procedures*. Retrieved from http://emedicine.medscape.com/article/818939-overview

Moreyra, P., Ibanez, A., Saiz-Ruiz, J., Nissenson, K., & Blanco, C. (2000). Review of the phenomenology, etiology and treatment of pathological gambling. *German Journal of Psychiatry, 3*, 37-52.

NANDA International (NANDA-I). (2012). *Nursing diagnoses: Definitions & classification 2012-2014*. Hoboken, NJ: Wiley-Blackwell.

National Cancer Institute. (2012). Pharmacological effects of supportive care medications on sexual function. Retrieved from http://www.cancer.gov/cancertopics/pdq/supportive-care/sexuality/HealthProfessional/page4

National Council on Alcoholism and Drug Dependence. (2013). *Facts about alcohol*. Retrieved from http://www.ncadd.org

National Institute on Alcohol Abuse and Alcoholism (NIAAA). (2000). *Tenth special report to the U.S. Congress on alcohol and health*. Bethesda, MD: The Institute.

National Institutes of Health (NIH). (2012). *Research Report Series—Marijuana Abuse*. NIH Publication Number 12-3859. Revised July 2012. Washington, DC: U.S. Department of Health and Human Services.

National Library of Medicine. (2011). *Hepatic encephalopathy*. Retrieved from http://www.nlm.nih.gov/medlineplus/ency/article/000302.htm

Office of National Drug Control Policy (ONDCP). (2010, May). *Methamphetamine trends in the United States*. Retrieved from http://www.whitehouse.gov/sites/default/files/ondcp/Fact_Sheets/pseudoephedrine_fact_sheet_7-16-10_0.pdf

O'Malley, S.S., Jaffe, A.J., Chang, G., Schottenfeld, R.S., Meyer, R.E., & Rounsaville, B. (1992). Naltrexone and coping skills therapy for alcohol dependence: A controlled study. *Archives of General Psychiatry, 49*(11), 881-887.

Puri, B.K., & Treasaden, I.H. (2011). *Textbook of psychiatry* (3rd ed.). Philadelphia, PA: Churchill Livingstone Elsevier.

Regard, M., Knoch, D., Gutling, E., & Landis, T. (2003). Brain damage and addictive behavior: A neuropsychological and electroencephalogram investigation with pathologic gamblers. *Cognitive and Behavioral Neurology, 16*(1), 47-53.

Sadock, B.J., & Sadock, V.A. (2007). *Synopsis of psychiatry: Behavioral sciences/clinical psychiatry* (10th ed.). Philadelphia, PA: Lippincott Williams & Wilkins.

Sateia, M.J. (2009). Description of insomnia. In C.A. Kushida (Ed.), *Handbook of sleep disorders* (2nd ed., pp. 3-13). New York, NY: Informa Healthcare.

Schim, S.M. (2013). People of Irish heritage. In L.D. Purnell (Ed.), *Transcultural health care: A culturally competent approach*. Philadelphia, PA: F.A. Davis.

Street Drugs. (2012). Long Lake, MN: The Publishers Group.

Substance Abuse and Mental Health Services Administration (SAMHSA). (2009). *Clinical supervision and professional development of the substance abuse counselor*. Treatment Improvement Protocol (TIP) Series 52, DHHS Publication No. SMA 09-4435. Rockville, MD: SAMHSA.

Substance Abuse and Mental Health Services Administration (SAMHSA). (2013). *Results from the 2012 national survey on drug use and health: Summary of national findings*. NSDUH Series H-46, HHS Publication No. (SMA) 13-4795. Rockville, MD: SAMHSA.

Sullivan, J.T., Sykora, K., Schneiderman, J., Naranjo, C.A. & Sellers, E.M. (1989). Assessment of alcohol withdrawal: The revised Clinical Institute Withdrawal Assessment for Alcohol scale (CIWA-Ar). *British Journal of Addiction, 84*, 1353-1357.

Thomas, C.M., & Siela, D. (2011). Would you know what to do if you suspected substance abuse? *American Nurse Today, 6*(8). Retrieved from http://www.americannursetoday.com/Article.aspx?id=8114&fid=8078#

U. S. Drug Enforcement Administration (USDEA). (2011). *The position on marijuana*. Retrieved from http://www.justice.gov/dea/docs/marijuana_position_2011.pdf

Unwin, B.K., Davis, M.K., & Leeuw, J.B. (2000). Pathologic gambling. *American Family Physician, 61*(3), 741-749.

Volpicelli, J.R., Alterman, A.I., Hayashida, M., & O'Brien, C.P. (1992). Naltrexone in the treatment of alcohol dependence. *Archives of General Psychiatry, 49*(11), 876-880.

Walton-Moss, B., Becker, K., Kub, J., & Woodruff, K. (2010). *Substance abuse: Commonly abused substances and the addiction process.* Brockton, MA: Western Schools.

Wesson, N. (2013). *Codependence: What is it? How do I know if I am codependent?* Retrieved from http://www.wespsych.com/codepend.html

Classical References

Cermak, T.L. (1986). *Diagnosing and treating co-dependence.* Center City, MN: Hazelton Publishing.

Jellinek, E.M. (1952). Phases of alcohol addiction. *Quarterly Journal of Studies on Alcohol, 13,* 673-684.

Mayfield, D., McLeod, G., & Hall, P. (1974). The CAGE questionnaire: Validation of a new alcoholism screening instrument. *American Journal of Psychiatry, 131,* 1121-1123.

Seltzer, M.L. (1971). The Michigan Alcoholism Screening Test: The quest for a new diagnostic instrument. *American Journal of Psychiatry, 127,* 1653-1658

@ INTERNET REFERENCES

- Additional information on addictions may be located at the following websites:
  - http://www.samhsa.gov/index.aspx
  - http://www.well.com/user/woa
  - http://www.addictions.org

- Additional information on self-help organizations may be located at the following websites:
  - http://www.ca.org (Cocaine Anonymous)
  - http://www.aa.org (Alcoholics Anonymous)
  - http://www.na.org (Narcotics Anonymous)
  - http://www.al-anon.org

- Additional information about medications for treatment of alcohol and drug addiction may be located at the following websites:
  - http://www.medicinenet.com/medications/article.htm
  - http://www.nlm.nih.gov/medlineplus
  - http://www.drugs.com/condition/alcoholism.html

MOVIE CONNECTIONS

Affliction (alcoholism) • *Days of Wine and Roses* (alcoholism) • *I'll Cry Tomorrow* (alcoholism) • *When a Man Loves a Woman* (alcoholism) • *Clean and Sober* (addiction-cocaine) • *28 Days* (alcoholism) • *Lady Sings the Blues* (addiction-heroin) • *I'm Dancing as Fast as I Can* (addiction-sedatives) • *The Rose* (polysubstance addiction) • *The Gambler* (gambling disorder)

Schizophrenia Spectrum and Other Psychotic Disorders

24

CORE CONCEPT

psychosis

KEY TERMS

agranulocytosis	echolalia	paranoia
akathisia	echopraxia	perseveration
akinesia	extrapyramidal symptoms	pseudoparkinsonism
amenorrhea	gynecomastia	religiosity
anhedonia	hallucinations	retrograde ejaculation
associative looseness	illusions	social skills training
catatonia	magical thinking	tangentiality
circumstantiality	neologisms	tardive dyskinesia
clang associations	neuroleptic malignant	waxy flexibility
delusions	syndrome	word salad
dystonia	oculogyric crisis	

OBJECTIVES
After reading this chapter, the student will be able to:

1. Discuss the concepts of schizophrenia and other psychotic disorders.
2. Identify predisposing factors in the development of these disorders.
3. Describe various types of schizophrenia and other psychotic disorders.
4. Identify symptomatology associated with these disorders and use this information in client assessment.
5. Formulate nursing diagnoses and outcomes of care for clients with schizophrenia and other psychotic disorders.
6. Identify topics for client and family teaching relevant to schizophrenia and other psychotic disorders.
7. Describe appropriate nursing interventions for behaviors associated with these disorders.
8. Describe relevant criteria for evaluating nursing care of clients with schizophrenia and other psychotic disorders.
9. Discuss various modalities relevant to treatment of schizophrenia and other psychotic disorders.

The term *schizophrenia* was coined in 1908 by the Swiss psychiatrist Eugen Bleuler. The word was derived from the Greek "skhizo" (split) and "phren" (mind).

Over the years, much debate has surrounded the concept of schizophrenia. Various definitions of the disorder have evolved, and numerous treatment strategies have been proposed, but none have proven to be uniformly effective or sufficient.

Although the controversy lingers, two general factors appear to be gaining acceptance among clinicians. The first is that schizophrenia is probably not a homogeneous disease entity with a single cause but results from a variable combination of genetic predisposition, biochemical dysfunction, physiological factors, and psychosocial stress. The second factor is that there is not now and probably never will be a single treatment that cures the disorder. Instead, effective treatment requires a comprehensive, multidisciplinary effort, including pharmacotherapy and various forms of psychosocial care, such as living skills and **social skills training**, rehabilitation and recovery, and family therapy.

Of all the mental illnesses that cause suffering in society, schizophrenia probably is responsible for lengthier hospitalizations, greater chaos in family life, more exorbitant costs to individuals and governments, and more fears than any other. Because it is such an enormous threat to life and happiness and because its causes are an unsolved puzzle, it has probably been studied more than any other mental disorder.

Potential for suicide is a major concern among patients with schizophrenia. About one-third of people with schizophrenia attempt suicide and about 1 in 10 die from the act (Black & Andreasen, 2011). Addington (2006) reports on studies that estimate the evidence of suicidal ideation in individuals with schizophrenia to be in the range of 40 to 55 percent and attempted suicide to be in the range of 20 to 50 percent.

Black and Andreasen (2011) stated:

> [Schizophrenia] is probably the most devastating illness that psychiatrists treat. [It] strikes people just when they are preparing to enter the phase of their lives in which they can achieve their highest growth and productivity—typically in the teens or early 20s—leaving most of them unable to return to normal young adult lives: to go to school, to find a job, or to marry and have children.

According to *The Global Burden of Disease,* a World Health Organization-sponsored study of the cost of medical illnesses worldwide, schizophrenia is among the 10 leading causes of disability in the world among people in the 15-44 age range. (p. 107)

This chapter explores various theories of predisposing factors that have been implicated in the development of schizophrenia. Symptomatology associated with different diagnostic categories of the disorder is discussed. Nursing care is presented in the context of the six steps of the nursing process. Various dimensions of medical treatment are explored.

Nature of the Disorder

CORE CONCEPT

Psychosis

A severe mental condition in which there is disorganization of the personality, deterioration in social functioning, and loss of contact with, or distortion of, reality. There may be evidence of hallucinations and delusional thinking. Psychosis can occur with or without the presence of organic impairment.

Perhaps no psychological disorder is more crippling than schizophrenia. Characteristically, disturbances in thought processes, perception, and affect invariably result in a severe deterioration of social and occupational functioning.

The lifetime prevalence of schizophrenia is about 1 percent in the general population (Puri & Treasaden, 2011). Symptoms generally appear in late adolescence or early adulthood, although they may occur in middle or late adult life. Symptoms that occur before age 17 suggest *early-onset schizophrenia* (EOS), and when symptoms occur before age 13, which is very rare, the condition is identified as *very early-onset schizophrenia* (VEOS) (Mattai, Hill, & Lenroot, 2010). Some studies have indicated that symptoms occur earlier in men than in women. The pattern of development of schizophrenia may be viewed in four phases: the premorbid phase, the prodromal phase, the active psychotic phase (schizophrenia), and the residual phase.

Phase I: The Premorbid Phase

The premorbid personality often indicates social maladjustment, social withdrawal, irritability, and antagonistic thoughts and behavior (Minzenberg, Yoon, & Carter, 2008). Premorbid personality and behavioral measurements that have been noted include being very shy and withdrawn, having poor peer relationships, doing poorly in school, and demonstrating antisocial behavior. Sadock and Sadock (2007) stated:

> In the typical, but not invariable, premorbid history of schizophrenia, patients had schizoid or schizotypal personalities characterized as quiet, passive, and introverted; as children, they had few friends. Preschizophrenic adolescents may have no close friends and no dates and may avoid team sports. They may enjoy [solitary activities] to the exclusion of social activities. (p. 481)

Phase II: The Prodromal Phase

The prodrome of an illness refers to certain signs and symptoms that precede the characteristic manifestations of the acute, fully developed illness. The prodromal phase of schizophrenia begins with a change from premorbid functioning and extends until the onset of frank psychotic symptoms. This phase can be as brief as a few weeks or months, but most studies indicate that the average length of the prodromal phase is between 2 and 5 years. Lehman and associates (2006) state:

> During the prodromal phase the person experiences substantial functional impairment and nonspecific symptoms such as a sleep disturbance, anxiety, irritability, depressed mood, poor concentration, fatigue, and behavioral deficits such as deterioration in role functioning and social withdrawal. Positive symptoms such as perceptual abnormalities, ideas of reference, and suspiciousness develop late in the prodromal phase and herald the imminent onset of psychosis. (pp. 625-626)

Recognition of the behaviors associated with the prodromal phase provides an opportunity for early intervention with a possibility for improvement in long-term outcomes. Current treatment guidelines suggest therapeutic interventions that offer support with identified problems, cognitive therapies to minimize functional impairment, family interventions to improve coping, and involvement with the schools to reduce the possibility of failure. Some controversy exists as to the benefit of using pharmaceutical therapy during the prodromal phase. Can providing interventions, including pharmacologic treatments, delay (or even prevent) the onset of psychosis? Minzenberg, Yoon, and Carter (2008) stated, "The use of [antipsychotic] medications to treat symptoms that are below the threshold of psychosis has to date been poorly studied" (p. 423).

Phase III: Schizophrenia

In the active phase of the disorder, psychotic symptoms are prominent. Following are the *Diagnostic and Statistical Manual of Mental Disorders, Fifth Edition (DSM-5)* (American Psychiatric Association [APA], 2013) diagnostic criteria for schizophrenia:*

A. Two (or more) of the following, each present for a significant portion of time during a 1-month period (or less if successfully treated). At least one of these must be (1), (2), or (3):
  1. **Delusions**
  2. **Hallucinations**
  3. Disorganized speech (e.g., frequent derailment or incoherence)
  4. Grossly disorganized or catatonic behavior
  5. Negative symptoms (i.e., diminished emotional expression or avolition)

B. For a significant portion of the time since the onset of the disturbance, level of functioning in one or more major areas, such as work, interpersonal relations, or self-care, is markedly below the level achieved prior to the onset (or when the onset is in childhood or adolescence, there is failure to achieve expected level of interpersonal, academic, or occupational functioning).

C. Continuous signs of the disturbance persist for at least 6 months. This 6-month period must include at least 1 month of symptoms (or less if successfully treated) that meet Criterion A (i.e., active-phase symptoms) and may include periods of prodromal or residual symptoms. During these prodromal or residual periods, the signs of the disturbance may be manifested by only negative symptoms or by two or more symptoms listed in Criterion A present in an attenuated form (e.g., odd beliefs, unusual perceptual experiences).

D. Schizoaffective disorder and depressive or bipolar disorder with psychotic features have been ruled out because either (1) no major depressive or manic episodes have occurred concurrently with the active-phase symptoms; or (2) if mood episodes have occurred during active-phase symptoms, they have been present for a minority of the total duration of the active and residual periods of the illness.

E. The disturbance is not attributable to the physiological effects of a substance (e.g., a drug of abuse, a medication) or another medical condition.

F. If there is a history of autism spectrum disorder or a communication disorder of childhood onset, the additional diagnosis of schizophrenia is made only if prominent delusions or hallucinations, in

---

*Reprinted with permission from the *Diagnostic and Statistical Manual of Mental Disorders, Fifth Edition* (Copyright 2013). American Psychiatric Association.

addition to the other required symptoms of schizophrenia, are also present for at least 1 month (or less if successfully treated).

Specify if: First episode, currently in acute, partial, or full remission; Multiple episodes, currently in acute, partial or full remission; Continuous; Unspecified.
Specify if: With **catatonia.**
Specify current severity.

Phase IV: Residual Phase

Schizophrenia is characterized by periods of remission and exacerbation. A residual phase usually follows an active phase of the illness (symptoms described in Phase III). During the residual phase, symptoms of the acute stage are either absent or no longer prominent. Negative symptoms may remain, and flat affect and impairment in role functioning are common. Residual impairment often increases between episodes of active psychosis.

Prognosis

Outcomes in schizophrenia are difficult to predict, but a complete return to full premorbid functioning is not common. However, several factors have been associated with a more positive outcome. These factors include good premorbid functioning, later age at onset, female gender, abrupt onset of symptoms with obvious precipitating factor (as opposed to gradual insidious onset of symptoms), associated mood disturbance, rapid resolution of active-phase symptoms, minimal residual symptoms, absence of structural brain abnormalities, normal neurological functioning, and no family history of schizophrenia (Black & Andreasen, 2011; Puri & Treasaden, 2011; Sadock & Sadock, 2007).

Predisposing Factors

The cause of schizophrenia is still uncertain. Most likely no single factor can be implicated in the etiology; rather, the disease probably results from a combination of influences including biological, psychological, and environmental factors.

Biological Factors

Refer to Chapter 4 for a more thorough review of the biological implications of psychiatric illness.

Genetics

The body of evidence for genetic vulnerability to schizophrenia is growing. Studies show that relatives of individuals with schizophrenia have a much higher probability of developing the disease than does the general population. Whereas the lifetime risk for developing schizophrenia is about 1 percent in most population studies, the siblings of an identified client have a 10 percent risk of developing schizophrenia, and offspring with one parent who has schizophrenia have a

5 to 6 percent chance of developing the disorder (Black & Andreasen, 2011).

How schizophrenia is inherited is uncertain. No definitive biological marker has as yet been found. Studies are ongoing to determine which genes are important in the vulnerability to schizophrenia, and whether one or many genes are implicated. Some individuals have a strong genetic link to the illness, whereas others may have only a weak genetic basis. This theory gives further credence to the notion of multiple causations.

Twin Studies

The rate of schizophrenia among monozygotic (identical) twins is four times that of dizygotic (fraternal) twins and approximately 50 times that of the general population (Sadock & Sadock, 2007). Identical twins reared apart have the same rate of development of the illness as do those reared together. Because in about half of the cases only one of a pair of monozygotic twins develops schizophrenia, some investigators believe environmental factors interact with genetic ones.

Adoption Studies

In studies conducted by both American and Danish investigators, adopted children born of schizophrenic mothers were compared with adopted children whose mothers had no psychiatric disorder. Children who were born to mothers with schizophrenia were more likely to develop the illness than the comparison control groups (Minzenberg et al., 2008). Studies also indicate that children born to nonschizophrenic parents, but reared by parents afflicted with the illness, do not seem to suffer more often from schizophrenia than general controls. These findings provide additional evidence for the genetic basis of schizophrenia.

Biochemical Factors

The oldest and most thoroughly explored biological theory in the explanation of schizophrenia attributes a pathogenic role to abnormal brain biochemistry. Notions of a "chemical disturbance" as an explanation for insanity were suggested by some theorists as early as the mid-19th century.

The Dopamine Hypothesis

This theory suggests that schizophrenia (or schizophrenia-like symptoms) may be caused by an excess of dopamine-dependent neuronal activity in the brain (Fig. 24-1). This excess activity may be related to increased production or release of the substance at nerve terminals, increased receptor sensitivity, too many dopamine receptors, or a combination of these mechanisms (Sadock & Sadock, 2007).

Pharmacological support for this hypothesis exists. Amphetamines, which increase levels of dopamine, induce psychotomimetic symptoms. The antipsychotics (e.g., chlorpromazine or haloperidol) lower brain

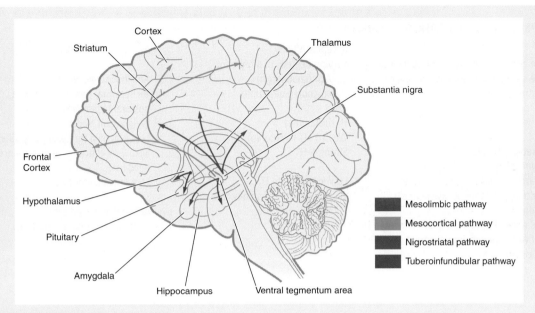

FIGURE 24–1 Neurobiology of schizophrenia.

NEUROTRANSMITTERS

A number of neurotransmitters have been implicated in the etiology of schizophrenia. These include dopamine, norepinephrine, serotonin, glutamate, and gamma-aminobutyric acid (GABA). The dopaminergic system has been most widely studied and closely linked to the symptoms associated with the disease.

AREAS OF THE BRAIN AFFECTED

Four major dopaminergic pathways have been identified:
- *Mesolimbic pathway:* originates in the ventral tegmentum area and projects to areas of the limbic system, including the nucleus accumbens, amygdala, and hippocampus. The mesolimbic pathway is associated with functions of memory, emotion, arousal, and pleasure. Excess activity in the mesolimbic tract has been implicated in the positive symptoms of schizophrenia (e.g., hallucinations, delusions).
- *Mesocortical pathway:* originates in the ventral tegmentum area and has projections into the cortex. The mesocortical pathway is concerned with cognition, social behavior, planning, problem solving, motivation, and reinforcement in learning. Negative symptoms of schizophrenia (e.g., flat affect, apathy, lack of motivation, and anhedonia) have been associated with diminished activity in the mesocortical tract.
- *Nigrostriatal pathway:* originates in the substantia nigra and terminates in the striatum of the basal ganglia. This pathway is associated with the function of motor control. Degeneration in this pathway is associated with Parkinson's disease and involuntary psychomotor symptoms of schizophrenia.
- *Tuberoinfundibular pathway:* originates in the hypothalamus and projects to the pituitary gland. It is associated with endocrine function, digestion, metabolism, hunger, thirst, temperature control, and sexual arousal. Implicated in certain endocrine abnormalities associated with schizophrenia.

Two major groups of dopamine receptors and their highest tissue locations include:
- The D_1 Family:
  D_1 receptors: basal ganglia, nucleus accumbens, and cerebral cortex
  D_5 receptors: hippocampus and hypothalamus, with lower concentrations in the cerebral cortex and basal ganglia
- The D_2 Family:
  D_2 receptors: basal ganglia, anterior pituitary, cerebral cortex, limbic structures
  D_3 receptors: limbic regions, with lower concentrations in basal ganglia
  D_4 receptors: frontal cortex, hippocampus, amygdala

ANTIPSYCHOTIC MEDICATIONS

Type	Receptor Affinity	Associated Side Effects
Conventional (typical) antipsychotics: Phenothiazines, haloperidol	Strong D_2 (dopamine)	EPS, hyperprolactinemia, neuroleptic malignant syndrome

Continued

ANTIPSYCHOTIC MEDICATIONS—cont'd

Type	Receptor Affinity	Associated Side Effects

Provide relief of psychosis, improvement in positive symptoms, worsening of negative symptoms.	Varying degrees of affinity for:
	    Ach (cholinergic)
	    α_1 (norepinephrine)
	
	H$_1$ (histamine)
	Weak 5-HT (serotonin)
		Anticholinergic effects
		Tachycardia, tremors, insomnia, postural hypotension
		Weight gain, sedation
		Low potential for ejaculatory difficulty

Novel (atypical) antipsychotics:
Clozapine, olanzepine, quetiapine, aripiprazole, risperdone, iloperidone, ziprasidone, paliperidone, asenapine, lurasidone
Provide relief of psychosis, improvement in positive symptoms, improvement in negative symptoms.
	Strong 5-HT
	
	Low to moderate D$_2$
	Varying degrees of affinity for:
	    Ach
	    α-adrenergic
	
	H$_1$
		Sexual dysfunction, GI disturbance, headache
		Low potential for EPS
		
		Anticholinergic effects
		Tachycardia, tremors, insomnia, postural hypotension
		Weight gain, sedation

levels of dopamine by blocking dopamine receptors, thus reducing the schizophrenic symptoms, including those induced by amphetamines.

Postmortem studies of brains of individuals who had schizophrenia have reported a significant increase in the average number of dopamine receptors in approximately two-thirds of the brains studied. This suggests that an increased dopamine response may not be important in *all* individuals with schizophrenia. Clients with acute manifestations (e.g., delusions and hallucinations) respond with greater efficacy to antipsychotic drugs than do clients with chronic manifestations (e.g., apathy, poverty of ideas, and loss of drive). The current position, in terms of the dopamine hypothesis, is that manifestations of acute schizophrenia may be related to increased numbers of dopamine receptors in the brain and respond to antipsychotic drugs that block these receptors. Manifestations of chronic schizophrenia are probably unrelated to numbers of dopamine receptors, and antipsychotic drugs are unlikely to be as effective in treating these chronic symptoms.

Other Biochemical Hypotheses

Various other biochemicals have been implicated in the predisposition to schizophrenia. Abnormalities in the neurotransmitters norepinephrine, serotonin, acetylcholine, and gamma-aminobutyric acid (GABA) and in the neuroregulators, such as prostaglandins and endorphins, have been suggested.

Recent research has implicated the neurotransmitter glutamate in the etiology of schizophrenia. The *N*-methyl-D-aspartate (NMDA) receptor is the receptor that is activated by the neurotransmitters glutamate and glycine. Psychopharmacological studies have shown that the drug class of glutamate antagonists (e.g., phencyclidine [PCP]; ketamine) can produce schizophrenic-like symptoms in individuals without the disorder (Hashimoto, 2006; Stahl, 2008). In one recent study, subjects who were experiencing ketamine-induced schizophrenia-like psychotic symptoms were treated with a drug trial of a glycine transporter-1 inhibitor (D'Souza et al., 2012). This medication was shown to reduce the effects induced by the NMDA receptor antagonism of the ketamine. The researchers suggest that "enhancing glutamate function by stimulating the glycine site of the NMDA receptor with glycine, D-serine, or with drugs that inhibit glycine reuptake may have therapeutic potential in schizophrenia" (p. 1036). Currently available conventional antipsychotic medications largely target the dopamine receptors in the brain. Newer novel antipsychotics have strong affinity for serotonergic receptors. The glutamate model of schizophrenia suggests possibilities for new therapeutic target options, including NMDA agonists, glycine transport inhibitors, and metabotropic glutamate receptor agonists (Citrome, 2011).

Physiological Factors

A number of physical factors of possible etiological significance have been identified in the medical literature. However, their specific mechanisms in the implication of schizophrenia are unclear.

Viral Infection

Sadock and Sadock (2007) report that epidemiological data indicate a high incidence of schizophrenia after prenatal exposure to influenza. They stated:

> Other data supporting a viral hypothesis are an increased number of physical anomalies at birth, an increased rate of pregnancy and birth complications, seasonality of birth consistent with viral infection, geographical clusters of adult cases, and seasonality of hospitalizations. (p. 469)

Another study found an association between viral infections of the central nervous system during childhood and adult onset schizophrenia (Rantakallio, Jones, Moring, & Von Wendt, 1997).

Anatomical Abnormalities

With the use of neuroimaging technologies, structural brain abnormalities have been observed in individuals with schizophrenia. Ventricular enlargement is the most consistent finding; however, sulci enlargement and cerebellar atrophy are also reported. Black and Andreasen (2011) have suggested that "ventricular enlargement is associated with poor premorbid functioning, negative symptoms, poor response to treatment, and cognitive impairment" (p. 122).

Magnetic resonance imaging (MRI) provides a greater ability to image in multiple planes. Studies with MRI have revealed a possible decrease in cerebral and intracranial size in clients with schizophrenia. Studies have also revealed a decrease in frontal lobe size, but this has been less consistently replicated. MRI has been used to explore possible abnormalities in specific subregions such as the amygdala, hippocampus, temporal lobes, and basal ganglia in the brains of people with schizophrenia.

Histological Changes

Cerebral changes in schizophrenia have also been studied at the microscopic level. A "disordering" or disarray of the pyramidal cells in the area of the hippocampus has been suggested (Jonsson, Luts, Guldberg-Kjaer, & Brun, 1997). This disarray of cells has been compared to the normal alignment of the cells in the brains of clients without the disorder. Some researchers have hypothesized that this alteration in hippocampal cells occurs during the second trimester of pregnancy and may be related to an influenza virus encountered by the mother during this period. Further research is required to determine the possible link between this birth defect and the development of schizophrenia.

Physical Conditions

Some studies have reported a link between schizophrenia and epilepsy (particularly temporal lobe), Huntington's disease, birth trauma, head injury in adulthood, alcohol abuse, cerebral tumor (particularly in the limbic system), cerebrovascular accidents, systemic lupus erythematosus, myxedema, parkinsonism, and Wilson's disease.

Psychological Factors

Early conceptualizations of schizophrenia focused on family relationship factors as major influences in the development of the illness, probably in light of the conspicuous absence of information related to a biological connection. These early theories implicated poor parent-child relationships and dysfunctional family systems as the cause of schizophrenia, but they no longer hold any credibility. Researchers now focus their studies in terms of schizophrenia as a brain disorder. Nevertheless, Sadock and Sadock (2007) have stated:

> Clinicians should consider both the psychosocial and biological factors affecting schizophrenia. The disorder affects individual patients, each of whom has a unique psychological makeup. Although many psychodynamic theories about the pathogenesis of schizophrenia seem outdated, perceptive clinical observations can help contemporary clinicians understand how the disease may affect a patient's psyche. (p. 474)

Environmental Influences

Sociocultural Factors

Many studies have been conducted that have attempted to link schizophrenia to social class. Indeed epidemiological statistics have shown that greater numbers of individuals from the lower socioeconomic classes experience symptoms associated with schizophrenia than do those from the higher socioeconomic groups (Puri & Treasaden, 2011). Explanations for this occurrence include the conditions associated with living in poverty, such as congested housing accommodations, inadequate nutrition, absence of prenatal care, few resources for dealing with stressful situations, and feelings of hopelessness for changing one's lifestyle of poverty.

An alternative view is that of the *downward drift hypothesis*, which suggests that, because of the characteristic symptoms of the disorder, individuals with schizophrenia have difficulty maintaining gainful employment and "drift down" to a lower socioeconomic level (or fail to rise out of a lower socioeconomic group). Proponents of this view consider poor social conditions to be a consequence rather than a cause of schizophrenia.

Stressful Life Events

Studies have been conducted in an effort to determine whether psychotic episodes may be precipitated by stressful life events. There is no scientific evidence to indicate that stress causes schizophrenia. It is very probable, however, that stress may contribute to the severity and course of the illness. It is known that extreme stress can precipitate psychotic episodes. Stress may indeed precipitate symptoms in an individual who possesses a genetic vulnerability to schizophrenia.

Stressful life events also may be associated with exacerbation of schizophrenic symptoms and increased rates of relapse.

The Transactional Model

The etiology of schizophrenia remains unclear. No single theory or hypothesis has been postulated that substantiates a clear-cut explanation for the disease. Indeed, it seems the more research that is conducted, the more evidence is compiled to support the concept of multiple causation in the development of schizophrenia. The most current theory seems to be that schizophrenia is a biologically based disease, the onset of which is influenced by factors within the environment (either internal or external). The dynamics of schizophrenia using the Transactional Model of Stress/Adaptation are presented in Figure 24-2.

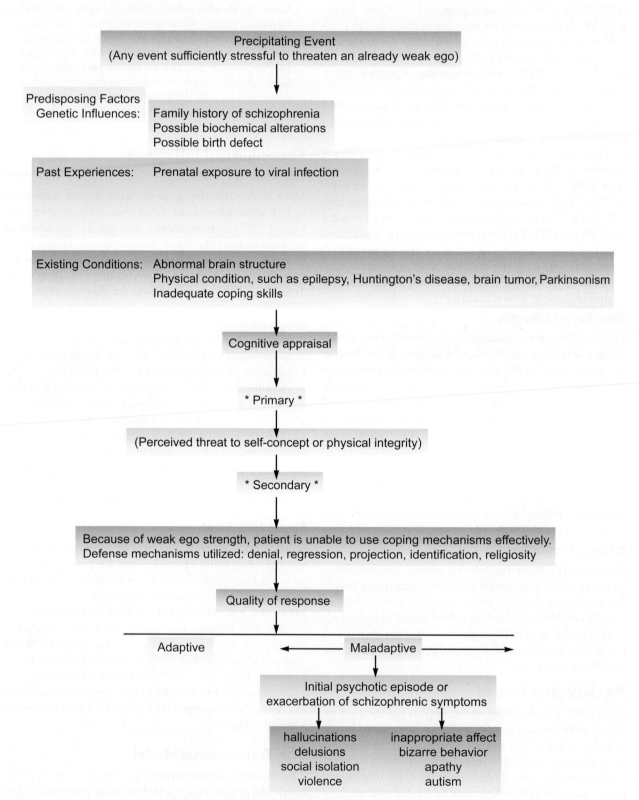

FIGURE 24–2 The dynamics of schizophrenia using the Transactional Model of Stress/Adaptation.

Types of Schizophrenia and Other Psychotic Disorders

The *DSM-5* (APA, 2013) identifies a spectrum of psychotic disorders that are organized to reflect a gradient of psychopathology from least to most severe. Degree of severity is determined by the level, number, and duration of psychotic signs and symptoms.

Several of the disorders may carry the additional specification of *with catatonic features*, the criteria for which are presented in Box 24-1. The disorders to which this specifier may be applied include brief psychotic disorder, schizophreniform disorder, schizophrenia, schizoaffective disorder, and substance-induced psychotic disorder. It may also be applied to neurodevelopmental disorders, major depressive disorder, and bipolar disorders I and II (APA, 2013).

The *DSM-5* initiates the spectrum of disorders with schizotypal personality disorder. For purposes of this textbook, this disorder is presented in Chapter 32, "Personality Disorders."

Delusional Disorder

Delusional disorder is characterized by the presence of delusions that have been experienced by the individual for at least 1 month (APA, 2013). If present at all, hallucinations are not prominent, and behavior is not bizarre. The subtype of delusional disorder is based on the predominant delusional theme. The *DSM-5* states that a specifier may be added to denote if the delusions are considered *bizarre* (i.e., if the thought is "clearly implausible, not understandable, and not derived from ordinary life experiences" [p. 91]). Subtypes of delusional disorder include the following:

Erotomanic Type

With this type of delusion, the individual believes that someone, usually of a higher status, is in love with him or her. Famous persons are often the subjects of erotomanic delusions. Sometimes the delusion is kept secret, but some individuals may follow, contact, or otherwise try to pursue the object of their delusion.

Grandiose Type

Individuals with grandiose delusions have irrational ideas regarding their own worth, talent, knowledge, or power. They may believe that they have a special relationship with a famous person, or even assume the identity of a famous person (believing that the actual person is an imposter). Grandiose delusions of a religious nature may lead to assumption of the identity of a deity or religious leader.

Jealous Type

The content of jealous delusions centers on the idea that the person's sexual partner is unfaithful. The idea is irrational and without cause, but the individual with the delusion searches for evidence to justify the belief. The sexual partner is confronted (and sometimes physically attacked) regarding the imagined infidelity. The imagined "lover" of the sexual partner may also be the object of the attack. Attempts to restrict the autonomy of the sexual partner in an effort to stop the imagined infidelity are common.

Persecutory Type

In persecutory delusions, which are the most common type, individuals believe they are being persecuted or malevolently treated in some way. Frequent themes include being plotted against, cheated or defrauded, followed and spied on, poisoned, or drugged. The individual may obsess about and exaggerate a slight rebuff (either real or imagined) until it becomes the focus of a delusional system. Repeated complaints may be directed at legal authorities, lack of satisfaction from which may result in violence toward the object of the delusion.

BOX 24-1 Diagnostic Criteria for Catatonia Specifier

The clinical picture is dominated by three (or more) of the following symptoms:

1. Stupor (i.e., no psychomotor activity; not actively related to environment)
2. Catalepsy (i.e., passive induction of a posture held against gravity)
3. Waxy flexibility (i.e., slight, even resistance to positioning by examiner)
4. Mutism (i.e., no, or very little, verbal response [exclude if known aphasia])
5. Negativism (i.e., opposition or no response to instructions or external stimuli)
6. Posturing (i.e., spontaneous and active maintenance of a posture against gravity)
7. Mannerism (i.e., odd, circumstantial caricature of normal actions)
8. Stereotypy (i.e., repetitive, abnormally frequent, non-goal-directed movements)
9. Agitation, not influenced by external stimuli
10. Grimacing
11. Echolalia (i.e., mimicking another's speech)
12. Echopraxia (i.e., mimicking another's movements)

Somatic Type

Individuals with somatic delusions believe they have some type of general medical condition.

Mixed Type

When the disorder is *mixed*, delusions are prominent, but no single theme is predominant.

Brief Psychotic Disorder

This disorder is identified by the sudden onset of psychotic symptoms that may or may not be preceded by a severe psychosocial stressor. These symptoms last at least 1 day but less than 1 month, and there is an eventual full return to the premorbid level of functioning (APA, 2013). The individual experiences emotional turmoil or overwhelming perplexity or confusion. Evidence of impaired reality testing may include incoherent speech, delusions, hallucinations, bizarre behavior, and disorientation. Individuals with preexisting personality disorders (most commonly histrionic, narcissistic, paranoid, schizotypal, and borderline personality disorders) appear to be susceptible to this disorder (Sadock & Sadock, 2007). Catatonic features may also be associated with this disorder (see Box 24-1).

Substance/Medication-Induced Psychotic Disorder

The prominent hallucinations and delusions associated with this disorder are found to be directly attributable to substance intoxication or withdrawal or to exposure to a medication or toxin. This diagnosis is made when the symptoms are more excessive and more severe than those usually associated with the intoxication or withdrawal syndrome (APA, 2013). The medical history, physical examination, or laboratory findings provide evidence that the appearance of the symptoms occurred in association with a substance intoxication or withdrawal or exposure to a medication or toxin. Substances that are believed to induce psychotic disorders are presented in Table 24-1. Catatonic features may also be associated with this disorder (see Box 24-1).

Psychotic Disorder Due to Another Medical Condition

The essential features of this disorder are prominent hallucinations and delusions that can be directly attributed to another medical condition (APA, 2013). The diagnosis is not made if the symptoms occur during the course of a delirium. A number of medical conditions that can cause psychotic symptoms are presented in Table 24-2.

TABLE 24–1	Substances That May Cause Psychotic Disorders
Drugs of abuse	Alcohol
	Amphetamines and related substances
	Cannabis
	Cocaine
	Hallucinogens
	Inhalants
	Opioids
	Phencyclidine and related substances
	Sedatives, hypnotics, and anxiolytics
Medications	Anesthetics and analgesics
	Anticholinergic agents
	Anticonvulsants
	Antidepressant medication
	Antihistamines
	Antihypertensive agents
	Cardiovascular medications
	Antimicrobial medications
	Antineoplastic medications
	Antiparkinsonian agents
	Corticosteroids
	Disulfiram
	Gastrointestinal medications
	Muscle relaxants
	Nonsteroidal anti-inflammatory agents
Toxins	Anticholinesterase
	Organophosphate insecticides
	Nerve gases
	Carbon dioxide
	Carbon monoxide
	Volatile substances (e.g., fuel, paint, gasoline, toluene)

SOURCES: APA (2013); Black & Andreasen (2011); Eisendrath & Lichtmacher (2012); Fohrman & Stein (2006); Freudenreich (2010).

Catatonic Disorder Due to Another Medical Condition

Catatonic disorder is identified by the symptoms described in Box 24-1. This diagnosis is made when the symptomatology is evidenced from medical history, physical examination, or laboratory findings to be directly attributable to the physiological consequences of another medical condition (APA, 2013). Types of medical conditions that have been associated with catatonic disorder include metabolic disorders (e.g., hepatic encephalopathy, hypo- and hyperthyroidism, hypo- and hyperadrenalism, and vitamin B_{12} deficiency) and neurological conditions (e.g., epilepsy, tumors, cerebrovascular disease, head trauma, and encephalitis) (Levenson, 2009).

TABLE 24-2	**General Medical Conditions That May Cause Psychotic Symptoms**

Acute intermittent porphyria
Cerebrovascular disease
CNS infections
CNS trauma
Deafness
Fluid or electrolyte imbalances
Hepatic disease
Herpes encephalitis
Huntington's disease
Hypoadrenocorticism
Hypo- or Hyperparathyroidism
Hypo- or Hyperthyroidism
Metabolic conditions (e.g., hypoxia, hypercarbia, hypoglycemia)
Migraine headache
Neoplasms
Neurosyphilis
Normal pressure hydrocephalus
Renal disease
Systemic lupus erythematosus
Temporal lobe epilepsy
Vitamin deficiency (e.g., B$_{12}$)
Wilson's disease

CNS, Central nervous system.
SOURCES: APA (2013); Black & Andreasen (2011); Freudenreich (2010); Sadock & Sadock (2007).

Schizophreniform Disorder

The essential features of schizophreniform disorder are identical to those of schizophrenia, with the exception that the duration, including prodromal, active, and residual phases, is at least 1 month but less than 6 months (APA, 2013). If the diagnosis is made while the individual is still symptomatic but has been so for less than 6 months, it is qualified as "provisional." The diagnosis is changed to schizophrenia if the clinical picture persists beyond 6 months. Schizophreniform disorder is thought to have a good prognosis if the individual's affect is not blunted or flat, if there is a rapid onset of psychotic symptoms from the time the unusual behavior is noticed, or if the premorbid social and occupational functioning was satisfactory (APA, 2013). Catatonic features may also be associated with this disorder (see Box 24-1).

Schizoaffective Disorder

This disorder is manifested by schizophrenic behaviors, with a strong element of symptomatology associated with the mood disorders (depression or mania). The client may appear depressed, with psychomotor retardation and suicidal ideation, or symptoms may include euphoria, grandiosity, and hyperactivity. The decisive factor in the diagnosis of schizoaffective disorder is the presence of hallucinations and/or delusions that occur for at least 2 weeks in the absence of a major mood episode (APA, 2013). However, prominent mood disorder symptoms must be evident for a majority of the time. The prognosis for schizoaffective disorder is generally better than that for other schizophrenic disorders but worse than that for mood disorders alone (Andreasen & Black, 2011). Catatonic features may also be associated with this disorder (see Box 24-1).

Application of the Nursing Process

Schizophrenia—Background Assessment Data

The diagnostic criteria for schizophrenia were presented earlier in this chapter. As previously stated, symptoms may present in phases, with schizophrenia representing the active phase of the disorder. Symptoms associated with the active phase are discussed in this section.

In the first step of the nursing process, the nurse gathers a database from which nursing diagnoses are derived and a plan of care is formulated. This first step of the nursing process is extremely important because without an accurate assessment, problem identification, objectives of care, and outcome criteria cannot be accurately determined.

Assessment of the client with schizophrenia may be a complex process, based on information gathered from a number of sources. Clients in an acute episode of their illness are seldom able to make a significant contribution to their history. Data may be obtained from family members, if possible; from old records, if available; or from other individuals who have been in a position to report on the progression of the client's behavior.

The nurse must be familiar with behaviors common to the disorder to be able to obtain an adequate assessment of the client with schizophrenia. Symptoms of schizophrenia are commonly described as positive or negative. Positive symptoms tend to reflect an alteration or distortion of normal mental functions, whereas negative symptoms reflect a diminution or loss of normal functions. Most clients exhibit a mixture of both types of symptoms.

Positive symptoms are associated with normal brain structures on computed tomography (CT) scan and relatively good responses to treatment. Regarding negative symptoms, Ho, Black, and Andreasen (2003) have stated, "Not only are [they] difficult to treat and respond less well to antipsychotics than positive symptoms, but they are also the most destructive because they render the patient inert and unmotivated" (p. 386).

The behavioral disturbances associated with schizophrenia are described in the following sections. They are categorized as positive or negative and considered in eight areas of functioning: content of thought, form of thought, perception, affect, sense of self, volition, interpersonal functioning and relationship to the external world, and psychomotor behavior. Additional impairments outside the limits of these eight areas are also presented. A summary of positive and negative symptoms is presented in Box 24-2.

Positive Symptoms

Content of Thought

Delusions Delusions are false personal beliefs that are inconsistent with the person's intelligence or cultural background. The individual continues to have the belief in spite of obvious proof that it is false or irrational. Delusions are subdivided according to their content. Some of the more common ones are listed here.

- **Delusion of Persecution.** The individual feels threatened and believes that others intend harm or persecution toward him or her in some way (e.g., "The FBI has 'bugged' my room and intends to kill me." "I can't take a shower in this bathroom;

the nurses have put a camera in there so that they can watch everything I do").

- **Delusion of Grandeur.** The individual has an exaggerated feeling of importance, power, knowledge, or identity (e.g., "I am Jesus Christ").
- **Delusion of Reference.** All events within the environment are referred by the psychotic person to him- or herself (e.g., "Someone is trying to get a message to me through the articles in this magazine [or newspaper or TV program]; I must break the code so that I can receive the message"). *Ideas* of reference are less rigid than delusions of reference. An example of an idea of reference is irrationally assuming that, when in the presence of others, one is the object of their discussion or ridicule.
- **Delusion of Control or Influence.** The individual believes certain objects or persons have control over his or her behavior (e.g., "The dentist put a filling in my tooth; I now receive transmissions through the filling that control what I think and do").
- **Somatic Delusion.** The individual has a false idea about the functioning of his or her body (e.g., "I'm 70 years old and I will be the oldest person ever to give birth. The doctor says I'm not pregnant, but I know I am.").

BOX 24-2 Positive and Negative Symptoms of Schizophrenia

POSITIVE SYMPTOMS

Content of Thought
Delusions
Religiosity
Paranoia
Magical thinking

Form of Thought
Associative looseness
Neologisms
Concrete thinking
Clang associations
Word salad
Circumstantiality
Tangentiality
Mutism
Perseveration

Perception
Hallucinations
Illusions

Sense of Self
Echolalia
Echopraxia
Identification and imitation
Depersonalization

NEGATIVE SYMPTOMS

Affect
Inappropriate affect
Bland or flat affect
Apathy

Volition
Inability to initiate goal-directed activity
Emotional ambivalence
Deteriorated appearance

Interpersonal Functioning and Relationship to the External World
Impaired social interaction
Social isolation

Psychomotor Behavior
Anergia
Waxy flexibility
Posturing
Pacing and rocking

Associated Features
Anhedonia
Regression

■ **Nihilistic Delusion.** The individual has a false idea that the self, a part of the self, others, or the world is nonexistent (e.g., "The world no longer exists." "I have no heart.").

Religiosity **Religiosity** is an excessive demonstration of or obsession with religious ideas and behavior. Because individuals vary greatly in their religious beliefs and level of spiritual commitment, religiosity is often difficult to assess. The individual with schizophrenia may use religious ideas in an attempt to provide rational meaning and structure to his or her behavior. Religious preoccupation in this vein may therefore be considered a manifestation of the illness. However, clients who derive comfort from their religious beliefs should not be discouraged from employing this means of support. An example of religiosity is the individual who believes the voice he or she hears is God and incessantly searches the Bible for interpretation.

Paranoia Individuals with **paranoia** have extreme suspiciousness of others and of their actions or perceived intentions (e.g., "I won't eat this food. I know it has been poisoned.").

Magical Thinking With **magical thinking,** the person believes that his or her thoughts or behaviors have control over specific situations or people (e.g., the mother who believed if she scolded her son in any way he would be taken away from her). Magical thinking is common in children (e.g., "It's raining; the sky is sad." "It snowed last night because I wished very, very hard that it would.").

Form of Thought

Associative Looseness Thinking is characterized by speech in which ideas shift from one unrelated subject to another. With **associative looseness,** the individual is unaware that the topics are unconnected. When the condition is severe, speech may be incoherent (e.g., "We wanted to take the bus, but the airport took all the traffic. Driving is the ticket when you want to get somewhere. No one needs a ticket to heaven. We have it all in our pockets.").

Neologisms The psychotic person invents new words, or **neologisms,** that are meaningless to others but have symbolic meaning to the psychotic person (e.g., "She wanted to give me a ride in her new *uniphorum.*").

Concrete Thinking Concreteness, or literal interpretations of the environment, represents a regression to an earlier level of cognitive development. Abstract thinking is very difficult. For example, the client with schizophrenia would have great difficulty describing the abstract meaning of sayings such as "I'm climbing the walls" or "It's raining cats and dogs."

Clang Associations Choice of words is governed by sounds. **Clang associations** often take the form of rhyming. For instance, "It is very cold. I am cold and bold. The gold has been sold."

Word Salad A **word salad** is a group of words that are put together randomly, without any logical connection (e.g., "Most forward action grows life double plays circle uniform.").

Circumstantiality With **circumstantiality**, the individual delays in reaching the point of a communication because of unnecessary and tedious details. The point or goal is usually met but only with numerous interruptions by the interviewer to keep the person on track of the topic being discussed.

Tangentiality **Tangentiality** differs from circumstantiality in that the person never really gets to the point of the communication. Unrelated topics are introduced, and the focus of the original discussion is lost.

Mutism Mutism is an individual's inability or refusal to speak.

Perseveration The individual who exhibits **perseveration** persistently repeats the same word or idea in response to different questions.

Perception

Hallucinations Hallucinations, or false sensory perceptions not associated with real external stimuli, may involve any of the five senses. Types of hallucinations include the following:

■ **Auditory.** Auditory hallucinations are false perceptions of sound. Most commonly they are of voices, but the individual may report clicks, rushing noises, music, and other noises. Command hallucinations may place the individual or others in a potentially dangerous situation. "Voices" that issue commands for violence to self or others may or may not be heeded by the psychotic person. Auditory hallucinations are the most common type in psychiatric disorders.
■ **Visual.** These are false visual perceptions. They may consist of formed images, such as of people, or of unformed images, such as flashes of light.
■ **Tactile.** Tactile hallucinations are false perceptions of the sense of touch, often of something on or under the skin. One specific tactile hallucination is formication, the sensation that something is crawling on or under the skin.
■ **Gustatory.** This type is a false perception of taste. Most commonly, gustatory hallucinations are described as unpleasant tastes.
■ **Olfactory.** Olfactory hallucinations are false perceptions of the sense of smell.

Illusions **Illusions** are misperceptions or misinterpretations of real external stimuli.

Sense of Self

Sense of self describes the uniqueness and individuality a person feels. Because of extremely weak ego boundaries, the individual with schizophrenia lacks this feeling of uniqueness and experiences a great deal of confusion regarding his or her identity.

Echolalia The client with schizophrenia may repeat words that he or she hears, which is called **echolalia**. This is an attempt to identify with the person speaking. (For instance, the nurse says, "John, it's time for lunch." The client may respond, "It's time for lunch, it's time for lunch" or sometimes, "Lunch, lunch, lunch, lunch").

Echopraxia The client who exhibits **echopraxia** may purposelessly imitate movements made by others.

Identification and Imitation Identification, which occurs on an unconscious level, and imitation, which occurs on a conscious level, are ego defense mechanisms used by individuals with schizophrenia and reflect their confusion regarding self-identity. Because they have difficulty knowing where their ego boundaries end and another person's begins, their behavior often takes on the form of that which they see in the other person.

Depersonalization The unstable self-identity of an individual with schizophrenia may lead to feelings of unreality (e.g., feeling that one's extremities have changed in size; or a sense of seeing oneself from a distance).

Negative Symptoms

Affect

Affect describes the behavior associated with an individual's feeling state or emotional tone.

Inappropriate Affect Affect is inappropriate when the individual's emotional tone is incongruent with the circumstances (e.g., a young woman who laughs when told of the death of her mother).

Bland or Flat Affect Affect is described as bland when the emotional tone is very weak. The individual with flat affect appears to be void of emotional tone (or overt expression of feelings).

Apathy The client with schizophrenia often demonstrates an indifference to or disinterest in the environment. The bland or flat affect is a manifestation of the emotional apathy.

Volition

Impaired volition has to do with the inability to initiate goal-directed activity. In the individual with schizophrenia, this may take the form of inadequate interest, motivation, or ability to choose a logical course of action in a given situation.

Emotional Ambivalence Ambivalence in the client with schizophrenia refers to the coexistence of opposite emotions toward the same object, person, or situation. These opposing emotions may interfere with the person's ability to make even a very simple decision (e.g., whether to have coffee or tea with lunch). Underlying the ambivalence is the difficulty the client with schizophrenia has in fulfilling a satisfying human relationship. This difficulty is based on the *need-fear dilemma*—the simultaneous need for and fear of intimacy.

Deteriorated Appearance Personal grooming and self-care activities may be neglected. The client with schizophrenia may appear disheveled and untidy and may need to be reminded of the need for personal hygiene.

Interpersonal Functioning and Relationship to the External World

Impairment in social functioning may be reflected in social isolation, emotional detachment, and lack of regard for social convention.

Impaired Social Interaction Some clients with acute schizophrenia cling to others and intrude on the personal space of others, exhibiting behaviors that are not socially and culturally acceptable.

Social Isolation Individuals with schizophrenia sometimes focus inward on themselves to the exclusion of the external environment.

Psychomotor Behavior

Anergia Anergia is a deficiency of energy. The individual with schizophrenia may lack sufficient energy to carry out activities of daily living or to interact with others.

Waxy Flexibility **Waxy flexibility** describes a condition in which the client with schizophrenia allows body parts to be placed in bizarre or uncomfortable positions. Once placed in position, the arm, leg, or head remains in that position for long periods, regardless of how uncomfortable it is for the client. For example, the nurse may position the client's arm in an outward position to take a blood pressure measurement. When the cuff is removed, the client may maintain the arm in the position in which it was placed to take the reading.

Posturing This symptom is manifested by the voluntary assumption of inappropriate or bizarre postures.

Pacing and Rocking Pacing back and forth and body rocking (a slow, rhythmic, backward-and-forward swaying of the trunk from the hips, usually while sitting) are common psychomotor behaviors of the client with schizophrenia.

Associated Features

Anhedonia **Anhedonia** is the inability to experience pleasure. This is a particularly distressing symptom that compels some clients to attempt suicide.

Regression Regression is the retreat to an earlier level of development. Regression, a primary defense mechanism of schizophrenia, is a dysfunctional attempt to reduce anxiety. It provides the basis for many of the behaviors associated with schizophrenia.

Diagnosis/Outcome Identification

Using information collected during the assessment, the nurse completes the client database, from which the selection of appropriate nursing diagnoses is determined. Table 24-3 presents a list of client behaviors and the NANDA International (NANDA-I) nursing

diagnoses that correspond to those behaviors, which may be used in planning care for clients with psychotic disorders.

Outcome Criteria

The following criteria may be used for measurement of outcomes in the care of the client with schizophrenia.

The client:

- Demonstrates an ability to relate satisfactorily with others
- Recognizes distortions of reality
- Has not harmed self or others
- Perceives self realistically
- Demonstrates the ability to perceive the environment correctly
- Maintains anxiety at a manageable level
- Relinquishes the need for delusions and hallucinations

TABLE 24–3 **Assigning Nursing Diagnoses to Behaviors Commonly Associated With Psychotic Disorders**	
BEHAVIORS	NURSING DIAGNOSES
Impaired communication (inappropriate responses), disordered thought sequencing, rapid mood swings, poor concentration, disorientation, stops talking in midsentence, tilts head to side as if to be listening	Disturbed sensory perception*
Delusional thinking; inability to concentrate; impaired volition; inability to problem solve, abstract, or conceptualize; extreme suspiciousness of others; inaccurate interpretation of the environment	Disturbed thought processes*
Withdrawal, sad dull affect, need-fear dilemma, preoccupation with own thoughts, expression of feelings of rejection or of aloneness imposed by others, uncommunicative, seeks to be alone	Social isolation
Risk factors: Aggressive body language (e.g., clenching fists and jaw, pacing, threatening stance), verbal aggression, catatonic excitement, command hallucinations, rage reactions, history of violence, overt and aggressive acts, goal-directed destruction of objects in the environment, self-destructive behavior, or active aggressive suicidal acts	Risk for violence: Self-directed or other-directed
Loose association of ideas, neologisms, word salad, clang associations, echolalia, verbalizations that reflect concrete thinking, poor eye contact, difficulty expressing thoughts verbally, inappropriate verbalization	Impaired verbal communication
Difficulty carrying out tasks associated with hygiene, dressing, grooming, eating, and toileting	Self-care deficit
Neglectful care of client in regard to basic human needs or illness treatment, extreme denial or prolonged overconcern regarding client's illness, depression, hostility and aggression	Disabled family coping
Inability to take responsibility for meeting basic health practices, history of lack of health-seeking behavior, lack of expressed interest in improving health behaviors, demonstrated lack of knowledge regarding basic health practices	Ineffective health maintenance
Unsafe, unclean, disorderly home environment; household members express difficulty in maintaining their home in a safe and comfortable condition	Impaired home maintenance

*These diagnoses have been retired from the NANDA-I taxonomy. They are used in this instance because they are most compatible with the identified behaviors.

■ Demonstrates the ability to trust others
■ Uses appropriate verbal communication in interactions with others
■ Performs self-care activities independently

Planning/Implementation

The following section presents a group of selected nursing diagnoses, with short- and long-term goals and nursing interventions for each.

Some institutions are using a case management model to coordinate care (see Chapter 9 for more detailed explanation). In case management models, the plan of care may take the form of a critical pathway.

Disturbed Sensory Perception: Auditory/Visual

Disturbed sensory perception has been retired from the NANDA-I taxonomy, but it is retained in this text because of its appropriateness in describing specific behaviors. In this instance, it is evidenced by behaviors that indicate the presence of auditory hallucinations. The diagnosis is defined as a "change in the amount or patterning of incoming stimuli accompanied by a diminished, exaggerated, distorted, or impaired response to such stimuli" (NANDA-I, 2012, p. 490). Table 24-4 presents this nursing diagnosis in care plan format.

Table 24-4 | CARE PLAN FOR THE CLIENT WITH SCHIZOPHRENIA

NURSING DIAGNOSIS: DISTURBED SENSORY PERCEPTION: AUDITORY/VISUAL

RELATED TO: Panic anxiety, extreme loneliness, and withdrawal into the self

EVIDENCED BY: Inappropriate responses, disordered thought sequencing, rapid mood swings, poor concentration, disorientation

OUTCOME CRITERIA	NURSING INTERVENTIONS	RATIONALE
Short-Term Goal • Client will discuss content of hallucinations with nurse or therapist within 1 week.	1. Observe client for signs of hallucinations (listening pose, laughing or talking to self, stopping in midsentence). Ask, "Are you hearing the voices again?"	1. Early intervention may prevent aggressive response to command hallucinations.
Long-Term Goal • Client will be able to define and test reality, reducing or eliminating the occurrence of hallucinations.	2. Avoid touching the client without warning him or her that you are about to do so.	2. Client may perceive touch as threatening and may respond in an aggressive manner.
This goal may not be realistic for the individual with severe and persistent illness who has experienced auditory hallucinations for many years. A more realistic goal may be: • Client will verbalize understanding that the voices are a result of his or her illness and demonstrate ways to interrupt the hallucination.	3. An attitude of acceptance will encourage the client to share the content of the hallucination with you. Ask, "What do you hear the voices saying to you?"	3. This is important to prevent possible injury to the client or others from command hallucinations.
	4. 💬 Do not reinforce the hallucination. Use "the voices" instead of words like "they" that imply validation. Let client know that you do not share the perception. Say, "Even though I realize the voices are real to you, I do not hear any voices speaking."	4. It is important for the nurse to be honest, and the client must accept the perception as unreal before hallucinations can be eliminated.
	5. Help the client understand the connection between increased anxiety and the presence of hallucinations.	5. If client can learn to interrupt escalating anxiety, hallucinations may be prevented.
	6. Try to distract the client from the hallucination.	6. Involvement in interpersonal activities and explanation of the actual situation will help bring the client back to reality.

Table 24-4 | CARE PLAN FOR THE CLIENT WITH SCHIZOPHRENIA—cont'd

OUTCOME CRITERIA	NURSING INTERVENTIONS	RATIONALE
	7. For some clients, auditory hallucinations persist after the acute psychotic episode has subsided. Listening to the radio or watching television helps distract some clients from attention to the voices. Others have benefited from an intervention called *voice dismissal.* With this technique, the client is taught to say loudly, "Go away!" or "Leave me alone!" in a conscious effort to dismiss the auditory perception.	7. These activities assist the client to exert some conscious control over the hallucination.

Client Goals

Outcome criteria include short- and long-term goals. Timelines are individually determined.

Short-Term Goal

■ Client will discuss content of hallucinations with nurse or therapist within 1 week.

Long-Term Goal

■ Client will be able to define and test reality, reducing or eliminating the occurrence of hallucinations.

This goal may not be realistic for the individual with severe and persistent illness who has experienced auditory hallucinations for many years. A more realistic goal may be:

■ Client will verbalize understanding that the voices are a result of his or her illness and demonstrate ways to interrupt the hallucination.

Interventions

■ Observe the client for signs of hallucinations (listening pose, laughing or talking to self, stopping in midsentence). Ask, "Are you hearing the voices again?" Early intervention may prevent aggressive responses to command hallucinations.

■ Avoid touching the client before warning him or her that you are about to do so. The client may perceive touch as threatening and respond in an aggressive or defensive manner.

■ An attitude of acceptance will encourage the client to share the content of the hallucination with you. Ask, "What do you hear the voices saying to you?" This is important in order to prevent possible injury to the client or others from command hallucinations.

> **CLINICAL PEARL**
>
> Do not reinforce the hallucination. Use "the voices" instead of words like "they" that imply validation. Let the client know that you do not share the perception. Say, "Even though I realize that the voices are real to you, I do not hear any voices speaking." It is important for the nurse to be honest, and the client must accept the perception as unreal before hallucinations can be eliminated.

■ Help the client to understand the connection between increased anxiety and the presence of hallucinations. If the client can learn to interrupt escalating anxiety, hallucinations may be prevented.

■ Try to distract the client from the hallucination. Involvement in interpersonal activities and explanation of the actual situation will help bring the client back to reality.

■ For some clients, auditory hallucinations persist after the acute psychotic episode has subsided. Listening to the radio or watching television helps distract some clients from attention to the voices. Others have benefited from an intervention called *voice dismissal.* With this technique, the client is taught to say loudly, "Go away!" or "Leave me alone!" thereby exerting some conscious control over the behavior.

Disturbed Thought Processes

Disturbed thought processes has been retired from the NANDA-I taxonomy, but it is retained in this text because of its appropriateness in describing specific behaviors. In this instance, it is evidenced by behaviors that indicate the presence of delusional thinking, suspiciousness, and inaccurate interpretation of the environment. The diagnosis is defined as a disruption in cognitive operations and activities.

Client Goals

Outcome criteria include short- and long-term goals. Timelines are individually determined.

Short-Term Goal

■ By the end of 2 weeks, client will recognize and verbalize that false ideas occur at times of increased anxiety.

Long-Term Goal

Depending on chronicity of the disease process, choose the most realistic long-term goal for the client:

■ By time of discharge from treatment, client's verbalizations will reflect reality-based thinking with no evidence of delusional ideation.
■ By time of discharge from treatment, the client will be able to differentiate between delusional thinking and reality.

Interventions

■ Convey acceptance of the client's need for the false belief, but indicate that you do not share the belief. The client must understand that you do not view the idea as real.
■ Do not argue or deny the belief. Arguing with the client or denying the belief serves no useful purpose, because delusional ideas are not eliminated by this approach, and the development of a trusting relationship may be impeded.

> **CLINICAL PEARL** 💬
>
> Use *reasonable doubt* as a therapeutic technique: "I understand that you believe this is true, but I personally find it hard to accept."

■ Reinforce and focus on reality. Discourage long ruminations about the irrational thinking. Talk about real events and real people. Discussions that focus on the false ideas are purposeless and useless, and may even aggravate the psychosis.
■ If the client is highly suspicious, the following interventions may be helpful:
   ■ To promote the development of trust, use the same staff as much as possible; be honest and keep all promises.
   ■ Avoid physical contact. Warn client before touching to perform a procedure, such as taking a blood pressure. Suspicious clients often perceive touch as threatening and may respond in an aggressive or defensive manner.
   ■ Avoid laughing, whispering, or talking quietly where the client can see but cannot hear what is being said.

■ Suspicious clients may believe they are being poisoned and refuse to eat food from an individually prepared tray. It may be necessary to provide canned food with a can opener or serve food family style.
■ They may believe they are being poisoned with their medication and attempt to discard the tablets or capsules. Mouth checks may be necessary following medication administration to verify whether client is actually swallowing the pills.
■ Competitive activities are very threatening to suspicious clients. Activities that encourage a one-to-one relationship with the nurse or therapist are best.
■ Maintain an assertive, matter-of-fact, yet genuine approach with suspicious clients. They do not have the capacity to relate to, and therefore often feel threatened by, a friendly or overly cheerful attitude.

Risk for Violence: Self-Directed or Other-Directed

Risk for self- or other-directed violence is defined as "at risk for behaviors in which an individual demonstrates that he or she can be physically, emotionally, and/or sexually harmful either to self or to others" (NANDA-I, 2012, pp. 447-448). **NOTE:** Please refer to Chapter 16 for additional concepts related to anger and aggression management.

Client Goals

Outcome criteria include short- and long-term goals. Timelines are individually determined.

Short-Term Goals

■ Within [a specified time], client will be able to recognize signs of increasing anxiety and agitation and report to staff (or other care provider) for assistance with intervention.
■ Client will not harm self or others.

Long-Term Goal

■ Client will not harm self or others.

Interventions

■ Maintain low level of stimuli in client's environment (low lighting, few people, simple decor, low noise level). Anxiety level rises in a stimulating environment. A suspicious, agitated client may perceive individuals as threatening.
■ Observe client's behavior frequently. Do this while carrying out routine activities so as to avoid creating suspiciousness in the individual. Close observation is necessary so that intervention can occur if required to ensure client (and others') safety.
■ Remove all dangerous objects from client's environment so that in his or her agitated, confused state client may not use them to harm self or others.

CLINICAL PEARL

Intervene at the first sign of increased anxiety, agitation, or verbal or behavioral aggression. Offer empathetic response to client's feelings: "You seem anxious (or frustrated, or angry) about this situation. How can I help?" Validation of the client's feelings conveys a caring attitude and offering assistance reinforces trust.

■ It is important to maintain a calm attitude toward the client. As the client's anxiety increases, offer some alternatives: to participate in a physical activity (e.g., punching bag, physical exercise), talking about the situation, taking some antianxiety medication. Offering alternatives to the client gives him or her a feeling of some control over the situation.

■ Have sufficient staff available to indicate a show of strength to client if it becomes necessary. This shows the client evidence of control over the situation and provides some physical security for staff.

■ If client is not calmed by "talking down" or by medication, use of mechanical restraints may be necessary. The avenue of the "least restrictive alternative" must be selected when planning interventions for a violent client. Restraints should be used only as a last resort, after all other interventions have been unsuccessful, and the client is clearly at risk of harm to self or others.

■ If restraint is deemed necessary, ensure that sufficient staff is available to assist. Follow protocol established by the institution. The Joint Commission (formerly the Joint Commission on Accreditation of Healthcare Organizations [JCAHO]) requires that an in-person evaluation by a physician or other licensed independent practitioner (LIP) be conducted within 1 hour of the initiation of the restraint or seclusion (The Joint Commission, 2010). The physician or LIP must reissue a new order for restraints every 4 hours for adults and every 1 to 2 hours for children and adolescents.

■ The Joint Commission requires that the client in restraints be observed at least every 15 minutes to ensure that circulation to extremities is not compromised (check temperature, color, pulses); to assist the client with needs related to nutrition, hydration, and elimination; and to position the client so that comfort is facilitated and aspiration is prevented. Some institutions may require continuous one-to-one monitoring of restrained clients, particularly those who are highly agitated, and for whom there is a high risk of self- or accidental injury.

■ As agitation decreases, assess the client's readiness for restraint removal or reduction. Remove one restraint at a time while assessing the client's response. This minimizes the risk of injury to client and staff.

Impaired Verbal Communication

Impaired verbal communication is defined as "decreased, delayed, or absent ability to receive, process, transmit, and/or use a system of symbols" (NANDA-I, 2012, p. 275).

Client Goals

Outcome criteria include short- and long-term goals. Timelines are individually determined.

Short-Term Goal

■ Client will demonstrate ability to remain on one topic, using appropriate, intermittent eye contact, for 5 minutes with the nurse or therapist.

Long-Term Goal

■ By time of discharge from treatment, the client will demonstrate ability to carry on a verbal communication in a socially acceptable manner with health-care providers and peers.

Interventions

■ Facilitate trust and understanding by maintaining staff assignments as consistently as possible. In a nonthreatening manner, explain to client how his or her behavior and verbalizations are viewed by and may alienate others.

CLINICAL PEARL

Attempt to decode incomprehensible communication patterns. Seek validation and clarification by stating, "Is it that you mean . . . ?" or "I don't understand what you mean by that. Would you please explain it to me?" These techniques reveal to the client how he or she is being perceived by others, and the responsibility for not understanding is accepted by the nurse.

■ Anticipate and fulfill the client's needs until functional communication has been established.

■ Orient the client to reality as required. Call the client by name. Validate those aspects of communication that help differentiate between what is real and not real. These techniques may facilitate restoration of functional communication patterns in the client.

CLINICAL PEARL

If the client is unable or unwilling to speak (mutism), using the technique of *verbalizing the implied* is therapeutic. (Example: "That must have been very difficult for you when your mother left. You must have felt very alone.") This approach conveys empathy, facilitates trust, and eventually may encourage the client to discuss painful issues.

■ Because concrete thinking prevails, abstract phrases and clichés must be avoided, as they are likely to be misinterpreted. Explanations must be provided at the client's level of comprehension.

CLINICAL PEARL

Speak plainly and clearly in words that cannot be misinterpreted. Example: "Pick up the spoon, scoop some mashed potatoes into it, and put it in your mouth."

Concept Care Mapping

The concept map care plan is an innovative approach to planning and organizing nursing care (see Chapter 9). It is a diagrammatic teaching and learning strategy that allows visualization of interrelationships between medical diagnoses, nursing diagnoses, assessment data, and treatments. An example of a concept map care plan for a client with schizophrenia is presented in Figure 24-3.

Client/Family Education

The role of client teacher is important in the psychiatric area, as it is in all areas of nursing. A list of topics for client/family education relevant to schizophrenia is presented in Box 24-3.

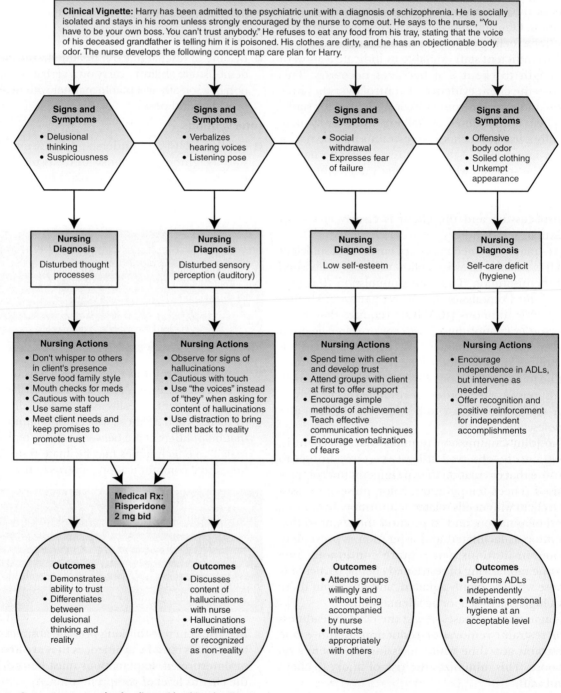

Clinical Vignette: Harry has been admitted to the psychiatric unit with a diagnosis of schizophrenia. He is socially isolated and stays in his room unless strongly encouraged by the nurse to come out. He says to the nurse, "You have to be your own boss. You can't trust anybody." He refuses to eat any food from his tray, stating that the voice of his deceased grandfather is telling him it is poisoned. His clothes are dirty, and he has an objectionable body odor. The nurse develops the following concept map care plan for Harry.

Signs and Symptoms
- Delusional thinking
- Suspiciousness

Signs and Symptoms
- Verbalizes hearing voices
- Listening pose

Signs and Symptoms
- Social withdrawal
- Expresses fear of failure

Signs and Symptoms
- Offensive body odor
- Soiled clothing
- Unkempt appearance

Nursing Diagnosis
Disturbed thought processes

Nursing Diagnosis
Disturbed sensory perception (auditory)

Nursing Diagnosis
Low self-esteem

Nursing Diagnosis
Self-care deficit (hygiene)

Nursing Actions
- Don't whisper to others in client's presence
- Serve food family style
- Mouth checks for meds
- Cautious with touch
- Use same staff
- Meet client needs and keep promises to promote trust

Nursing Actions
- Observe for signs of hallucinations
- Cautious with touch
- Use "the voices" instead of "they" when asking for content of hallucinations
- Use distraction to bring client back to reality

Nursing Actions
- Spend time with client and develop trust
- Attend groups with client at first to offer support
- Encourage simple methods of achievement
- Teach effective communication techniques
- Encourage verbalization of fears

Nursing Actions
- Encourage independence in ADLs, but intervene as needed
- Offer recognition and positive reinforcement for independent accomplishments

Medical Rx: Risperidone 2 mg bid

Outcomes
- Demonstrates ability to trust
- Differentiates between delusional thinking and reality

Outcomes
- Discusses content of hallucinations with nurse
- Hallucinations are eliminated or recognized as non-reality

Outcomes
- Attends groups willingly and without being accompanied by nurse
- Interacts appropriately with others

Outcomes
- Performs ADLs independently
- Maintains personal hygiene at an acceptable level

FIGURE 24–3 Concept map care plan for client with schizophrenia.

NATURE OF THE ILLNESS
1. What to expect as the illness progresses.
2. Symptoms associated with the illness.
3. Ways for family to respond to behaviors associated with the illness.

MANAGEMENT OF THE ILLNESS
1. Connection of exacerbation of symptoms to times of stress.
2. Appropriate medication management.
3. Side effects of medications.
4. Importance of not stopping medications.
5. When to contact health-care provider.
6. Relaxation techniques.
7. Social skills training.
8. Daily living skills training.

SUPPORT SERVICES
1. Financial assistance
2. Legal assistance
3. Caregiver support groups
4. Respite care
5. Home health care

Evaluation

In the final step of the nursing process, a reassessment is conducted in order to determine if the nursing actions have been successful in achieving the objectives of care. Evaluation of the nursing actions for the client with exacerbation of schizophrenic psychosis may be facilitated by gathering information utilizing the following types of questions:

■ Has the client established trust with at least one staff member?
■ Is the anxiety level maintained at a manageable level?
■ Is delusional thinking still prevalent?
■ Is hallucinogenic activity evident? Does the client share content of hallucinations, particularly if commands are heard?
■ Is the client able to interrupt escalating anxiety with adaptive coping mechanisms?
■ Is the client easily agitated?
■ Is the client able to interact with others appropriately?
■ Does the client voluntarily attend therapy activities?
■ Is verbal communication comprehensible?
■ Is the client compliant with medication? Does the client verbalize the importance of taking medication regularly and on a long-term basis? Does he or she verbalize understanding of possible side effects, and when to seek assistance from the physician?
■ Does the client spend time with others rather than isolating self?

■ Is the client able to carry out all activities of daily living independently?
■ Is the client able to verbalize resources from which he or she may seek assistance outside the hospital?
■ Does the family have information regarding support groups in which they may participate, and from which they may seek assistance in dealing with their family member who is ill?
■ If the client lives alone, does he or she have a source for assistance with home maintenance and health management?

Quality and Safety Education for Nurses (QSEN)

The Institute of Medicine (IOM), in its 2003 report, *Health Professions Education: A Bridge to Quality*, challenged faculties of medicine, nursing, and other health professions to ensure that their graduates have achieved a core set of competencies in order to meet the needs of the 21st-century health-care system. These competencies include *providing patient-centered care, working in interdisciplinary teams, employing evidence-based practice, applying quality improvement, ensuring safety,* and *utilizing informatics.* A QSEN teaching strategy is included in Box 24-4. The use of this type of activity is intended to arm the instructor and the student with guidelines for attaining the knowledge, skills, and attitudes necessary for achievement of quality and safety competencies in nursing.

Treatment Modalities for Schizophrenia and Other Psychotic Disorders

Psychological Treatments
Individual Psychotherapy

Ho and associates (2003) stated:

> Although intensive psychodynamic- and insight-oriented psychotherapy is generally not recommended, the form of individual psychotherapy that psychiatrists employ when providing pharmacological treatment typically involves a synthesis of various psychotherapeutic strategies and interventions. These include problem solving, reality testing, psychoeducation, and supportive and cognitive-behavioral techniques anchored on an empathetic therapeutic alliance with the patient. The goals of such individual psychotherapy are to improve medication compliance, enhance social and occupational functioning, and prevent relapse. (p. 419)

Reality-oriented individual therapy is the most suitable approach to individual psychotherapy for schizophrenia. The primary focus in all cases must reflect efforts to decrease anxiety and increase trust.

Establishing a relationship is often particularly difficult because the individual with schizophrenia is

BOX 24-4 QSEN TEACHING STRATEGY

Assignment: Using Evidence to Address Clinical Problems
Intervention With a Combative Client
Competency Domain: Evidence-Based Practice
Learning Objectives: Student will:
• Differentiate clinical opinion from research and evidence summaries.
• Explain the role of evidence in determining the best clinical practice for intervening with combative clients.
• Identify gaps between what is observed in the treatment setting to what has been identified as best practice.
• Discriminate between valid and invalid reasons for modifying evidence-based clinical practice based on clinical expertise or other reasons.
• Participate effectively in appropriate data collection and other research activities.
• Acknowledge own limitations in knowledge and clinical expertise before determining when to deviate from evidence-based best practices.

Strategy Overview:
1. Investigate the research related to intervening with a combative client.
2. Identify best practices described in the literature. How were these best practices determined?
3. Compare and contrast staff intervention with best practices described in the literature.
4. Investigate staff perceptions related to intervening with a combative client. How have they developed these perceptions?
5. Do staff members view any problems associated with their practice versus best practice described in the literature? If so, how would they like to see the problem addressed?
6. Describe ethical issues associated with intervening with a combative client.
7. What is your personal perception regarding the best evidence available to date related to intervening with a combative client? Are there situations that you can think of when you might deviate from the best practice model?
8. What questions do you have about intervening with a combative client that are not being addressed by current researchers?

Adapted from teaching strategy submitted by Pamela M. Ironside, Associate Professor, Indiana University School of Nursing, Indianapolis, Ind. © 2009 QSEN; http://qsen.org. With permission.

desperately lonely yet defends against closeness and trust. He or she is likely to respond to attempts at closeness with suspiciousness, anxiety, aggression, or regression. Successful intervention may be achieved with honesty, simple directness, and a manner that respects the client's privacy and human dignity. Exaggerated warmth and professions of friendship are likely to be met with confusion and suspicion.

Once a therapeutic interpersonal relationship has been established, reality orientation is maintained through exploration of the client's behavior within relationships. Education is provided to help the client identify sources of real or perceived danger and ways of reacting appropriately. Methods for improving interpersonal communication, emotional expression, and frustration tolerance are attempted.

Individual psychotherapy for clients with schizophrenia is seen as a long-term endeavor that requires patience on the part of the health-care provider, as well as the ability to accept that a great deal of change may not occur. Some cases report treatment durations of many years before clients regain some degree of independent functioning.

Group Therapy

Group therapy for individuals with schizophrenia has been shown to be effective, particularly with outpatients and when combined with drug treatment.

Sadock and Sadock (2007) stated:

Group therapy for persons with schizophrenia generally focuses on real-life plans, problems, and relationships. Some investigators doubt that dynamic interpretation and insight therapy are valuable for typical patients with schizophrenia. But group therapy is effective in reducing social isolation, increasing the sense of cohesiveness, and improving reality testing for patients with schizophrenia. (p. 492)

Group therapy in inpatient settings is less productive. Inpatient treatment usually occurs when symptomatology and social disorganization are at their most intense. At this time, the least amount of stimuli possible is most beneficial for the client. Because group therapy can be intensive and highly stimulating, it may be counterproductive early in treatment.

Group therapy for schizophrenia has been most useful over the long-term course of the illness. The social interaction, sense of cohesiveness, identification, and reality testing achieved within the group setting have proven to be highly therapeutic processes for these clients. Groups that offer a supportive environment appear to be more helpful to clients with schizophrenia than those that follow a more confrontational approach.

Behavior Therapy

Behavior modification has a history of qualified success in reducing the frequency of bizarre, disturbing, and deviant behaviors and increasing appropriate behaviors. Features that have led to the most positive results include:

- Clearly defining goals and how they will be measured.
- Attaching positive, negative, and aversive reinforcements to adaptive and maladaptive behavior.
- Using simple, concrete instructions and prompts to elicit the desired behavior.

Behavior therapy can be a powerful treatment tool for helping clients change undesirable behaviors. In the treatment setting, the health-care provider can use praise and other positive reinforcements to help the client with schizophrenia reduce the frequency of maladaptive or deviant behaviors. A limitation of this type of therapy is the inability of some individuals with schizophrenia to generalize what they have learned from the treatment setting to the community setting.

Social Skills Training

Social skills training has become one of the most widely used psychosocial interventions in the treatment of schizophrenia. Mueser, Bond, and Drake (2002) stated:

> The basic premise of social skills training is that complex interpersonal skills involve the smooth integration of a combination of simpler behaviors, including *nonverbal behaviors* (e.g., facial expression, eye contact); *paralinguistic features* (e.g., voice loudness and affect); *verbal content* (i.e., the appropriateness of what is said); and *interactive balance* (e.g., response latency, amount of time talking). These specific skills can be systematically taught, and, through the process of *shaping* (i.e., rewarding successive approximations toward the target behavior), complex behavioral repertoires can be acquired.

Social dysfunction is a hallmark of schizophrenia. Impairment in interpersonal relations is included as part of the defining diagnostic criteria for schizophrenia in the *DSM-5* (APA, 2013). Considerable attention is now being given to enhancement of social skills in these clients.

The educational procedure in social skills training focuses on role-play. A series of brief scenarios are selected. These should be typical of situations clients experience in their daily lives and be graduated in terms of level of difficulty. The health-care provider may serve as a role model for some behaviors. For example, "See how I sort of nod my head up and down and look at your face while you talk." This demonstration is followed by the client's role-playing. Immediate feedback is provided regarding the client's presentation. Only by countless repetitions does the response gradually become smooth and effortless.

Progress is geared toward the client's needs and limitations. The focus is on small units of behavior, and the training proceeds very gradually. Highly threatening issues are avoided, and emphasis is placed on functional skills that are relevant to activities of daily living.

Social Treatments

Milieu Therapy

Some clinicians believe that milieu therapy can be an appropriate treatment for the client with schizophrenia. Research suggests that psychotropic medication is more effective at all levels of care when used along with milieu therapy and that milieu therapy is more successful if used in conjunction with these medications.

Sadock and Sadock (2007) stated:

> Most milieu therapy programs emphasize group and social interaction; rules and expectations are mediated by peer pressure for normalization of adaptation. When patients are viewed as responsible human beings, the patient role becomes blurred. Milieu therapy stresses a patient's rights to goals and to have freedom of movement and informal relationship with staff; it also emphasizes interdisciplinary participation and goal-oriented, clear communication. (p. 970)

Individuals with schizophrenia who are treated with milieu therapy alone require longer hospital stays than do those treated with drugs and psychosocial therapy. Other economic considerations, such as the need for a high staff-to-client ratio, in addition to the longer admission, limit the use of milieu therapy in the treatment of schizophrenia. The milieu environment can be successfully employed in outpatient settings, however, such as day and partial hospitalization programs.

Family Therapy

Some health-care providers treat schizophrenia as an illness not of the client alone, but of the entire family. Even when families appear to cope well, there is a notable impact on the mental health status of relatives when a family member has the illness. Safier (1997) states:

> When a family member has a serious mental illness, the family must deal with a major upheaval in their lives, a terrible event that causes great pain and grief for the loss of a once-promising child or relationship. (p. 5)

The importance of the expanded role of family in the aftercare of relatives with schizophrenia has been recognized, thereby stimulating interest in family intervention programs designed to support the family system, prevent or delay relapse, and help to maintain the client in the community. These psychoeducational programs treat the family as a resource rather than a stressor, with the focus on concrete problem solving and specific helping behaviors for coping with stress. These programs recognize the biological basis for schizophrenia and the impact that stress has on the client's ability to function. By providing the family with information about the illness and suggestions for effective coping, psychoeducational programs reduce the likelihood of the client's relapse and the possible emergence of mental illness in previously nonaffected relatives.

Mueser and associates (2002) stated that although models of family intervention with schizophrenia differ in their characteristics and methods, effective treatment programs share a number of common features:

- All programs are long term (usually 9 months to 2 years or more).
- They all provide client and family with information about the illness and its management.
- They focus on improving adherence to prescribed medications.
- They strive to decrease stress in the family, and improve family functioning.

Asen (2002) suggested the following interventions with families of individuals with schizophrenia:

- Forming a close alliance with the caregivers
- Lowering the emotional intrafamily climate by reducing stress and burden on relatives
- Increasing the ability of relatives to anticipate and solve problems
- Reducing the expressions of anger and guilt by family members
- Maintaining reasonable expectations for how the ill family member should perform
- Encouraging relatives to set appropriate limits while maintaining some degree of separateness
- Promoting desirable changes in the relatives' behaviors and belief systems

Family therapy typically consists of a brief program of family education about schizophrenia, and a more extended program of family contact designed to reduce overt manifestations of conflict and to improve patterns of family communication and problem solving. The response to this type of therapy has been very dramatic. Studies have clearly revealed that a more positive outcome in the treatment of the client with schizophrenia can be achieved by including the family system in the program of care.

Program of Assertive Community Treatment (PACT)

The Program of Assertive Community Treatment (PACT) is a program of case management that takes a team approach in providing comprehensive, community-based psychiatric treatment, rehabilitation, and support to persons with serious and persistent mental illness such as schizophrenia. (The National Alliance on Mental Illness [NAMI] uses the terms PACT and Assertive Community Treatment [ACT] interchangeably. Some states use other terms for this type of treatment, such as Mobile Treatment Teams [MTTs] and Community Support Programs [CSPs].) Aggressive programs of treatment are individually tailored for each client and include the teaching of basic living skills, helping clients work with community agencies, and assisting clients in developing a social support network. There is emphasis on vocational expectations, and supported work settings (i.e., sheltered workshops) are an important part of the treatment program. Other services include substance abuse treatment, psychoeducational programs, family support and education, mobile crisis intervention, and attention to health-care needs.

Responsibilities are shared by multiple team members, including psychiatrists, nurses, social workers, vocational rehabilitation therapists, and substance abuse counselors. Services are provided in the person's home, within the neighborhood, in local restaurants, parks, stores, or wherever assistance by the client is required. These services are available to the client 24 hours a day, 365 days a year. NAMI (2013) lists the primary goals of ACT as follows:

- To meet basic needs and enhance quality of life
- To improve functioning in adult social and employment roles
- To enhance an individual's ability to live independently in his or her own community
- To lessen the family's burden of providing care
- To lessen or eliminate the debilitating symptoms of mental illness
- To minimize or prevent recurrent acute episodes of the illness

Individuals best served by PACT are identified by the Assertive Community Treatment Association (ACTA) (2013) as follows:

Clients served by ACT are individuals with serious and persistent mental illness or personality disorders, with severe functional impairments, who have avoided or not responded well to traditional outpatient mental health care and psychiatric rehabilitation services. Persons served by ACT often have co-existing problems such as homelessness, substance abuse problems, or involvement with the judicial system.

PACT has been shown to reduce the number of hospitalizations and decrease costs of care for these clients. Although it has been called "paternalistic" and "coercive" by its critics, PACT has provided a much-needed service and increased quality of life to many clients who are unable to manage in a less-structured environment.

The Recovery Model

Research provides support for recovery as an obtainable objective for individuals with schizophrenia (Lysaker, Roe, & Buck, 2010). Lysaker and associates (2010) state:

> Recovery from schizophrenia, in the sense of a state in which persons experience no difficulties associated with the illness, can occur but the modal outcome seems to be one in which difficulties linked to symptoms, social function, and work appear periodically but can be successfully confronted. (p. 40)

Conceptual models of recovery from mental illness are presented in Chapter 21. The recovery model has been used primarily in caring for individuals with serious mental illness, such as schizophrenia and bipolar disorder. However, concepts of the model are amenable to use with all individuals experiencing emotional conditions with which they require assistance and who have a desire to take control and manage their lives more independently.

Weiden (2010) identifies two types of recovery with schizophrenia: functional and process. Functional recovery focuses on the individual's level of functioning in such areas as relationships, work, independent living, and other kinds of life functioning. He or she may or may not be experiencing active symptoms of schizophrenia.

Weiden (2010) suggests that recovery can also be considered as a process. With process recovery, there is no defined endpoint, but recovery is viewed as a process that continues throughout the individual's life, and involves collaboration between client and clinician. The individual identifies goals based on personal values or what he or she defines as giving meaning and purpose to life. The clinician and client work together to develop a treatment plan that is in alignment with the goals set forth by the client. In the process recovery model, the individual may still be experiencing symptoms. Weiden (2010) states:

> Patients do not have to be in remission, nor does remission automatically have to be a desired (or likely) goal when embarking on a recovery-oriented treatment plan. As long as the patient (and family) understands that a process recovery treatment plan is not to be confused with a promise of "cure" or even "remission," then one does not overpromise.

The concept of recovery in schizophrenia remains controversial among clinicians, and many challenges lie ahead for continued study. Currently, there is a lack of consistency in what constitutes "recovery," and many concepts exist. Therefore, it is important to ensure that "recovery" is clearly defined anytime it is considered as the plan of care.

Organic Treatment

Psychopharmacology

Chlorpromazine (Thorazine) was first introduced in the United States in 1952. At that time, it was used in conjunction with barbiturates in surgical anesthesia. With increased use, the drug's psychic properties were recognized, and by 1954 it was marketed as an antipsychotic medication in the United States. The manufacture and sale of other antipsychotic drugs followed in rapid succession.

Antipsychotic medications are also called *neuroleptics* or major tranquilizers. They are effective in the treatment of acute and chronic manifestations of schizophrenia and in maintenance therapy to prevent exacerbation of schizophrenic symptoms. Without drug treatment, an estimated 72 percent of individuals who have experienced a psychotic episode relapse within a year. This relapse rate can be reduced to about 23 percent with continuous medication administration (Dixon, Lehman, & Levine, 2010).

The prognosis of schizophrenia has often been reported in a paradigm of thirds. One-third of the people achieve significant and lasting improvement. They may never experience another episode of psychosis following the initial occurrence. One-third may achieve some improvement with intermittent relapses and residual disability. Their occupational level may have decreased because of their illness, or they may be socially isolated. Finally, one-third experiences severe and permanent incapacity. They often do not respond to medication and remain severely ill for much of their lives. Men have poorer outcomes than women do; women respond better to treatment with antipsychotic medications.

As mentioned earlier, the efficacy of antipsychotic medications is enhanced by adjunct psychosocial therapy. Because the psychotic manifestations of the illness subside with use of the drugs, clients are generally more cooperative with the psychosocial therapies. However, it takes several weeks for the antipsychotics to effectively treat positive symptoms, a fact that often leads to discontinuation of the medication. Clients and families need to be educated about the importance of waiting, often for several weeks, to determine if the drug will be effective.

These medications are classified as either "typical" (first-generation, conventional antipsychotics) or "atypical" (the newer, novel antipsychotics). Examples of commonly used antipsychotic agents are presented in Table 24-5. A detailed description of these medications follows.

TABLE 24–5 **Antipsychotic Agents**			
CATEGORY	GENERIC (TRADE NAME)	PREGNANCY CATEGORIES/ HALF-LIFE (hr)	DAILY DOSAGE RANGE (mg)
Typical Antipsychotic Agents (First Generation; Conventional)	Chlorpromazine	C/ 24	40–400
	Fluphenazine	C/ HCl: 18 hr Decanoate: 6.8–9.6 days	2.5–10
	Haloperidol (Haldol)	C/ ~18 (oral); ~3 wk (IM decanoate)	1–100
	Loxapine	C/ 8	20–250
	Perphenazine	C/ 9–12	12–64
	Pimozide (Orap)	C/ ~55	1–10
	Prochlorperazine	C/ 3–5 (oral) 6.9 (IV)	15–150
	Thioridazine	C/ 24	150–800
	Thiothixene (Navane)	C/ 34	6–30
	Trifluoperazine	C/ 18	4–40
Atypical Antipsychotic Agents (Second Generation; Novel)	Aripiprazole (Abilify)	C/ 75–146	10–30
	Asenapine (Saphris)	C/ 24	10–20
	Clozapine (Clozaril)	B/ 8 (single dose); 12 (at steady state)	300–900
	Iloperidone (Fanapt)	C/ 18–33	12–24
	Lurasidone (Latuda)	B/ 18	40–80
	Olanzapine (Zyprexa)	C/ 21–54	5–20
	Paliperidone (Invega)	C/ 23	6–12
	Quetiapine (Seroquel)	C/ ~6	300–400
	Risperidone (Risperdal)	C/ 3–20	4–8
	Ziprasidone (Geodon)	C/ ~7 (oral); 2–5 (IM)	40–160

Indications

Antipsychotic medications are used in the treatment of schizophrenia and other psychotic disorders. Selected agents are used in the treatment of bipolar mania (olanzapine, aripiprazole, chlorpromazine, quetiapine, risperidone, asenapine, ziprasidone). Others are used as antiemetics (chlorpromazine, perphenazine, prochlorperazine), in the treatment of intractable hiccoughs (chlorpromazine), and for the control of tics and vocal utterances in Tourette's disorder (haloperidol, pimozide).

Action

Typical antipsychotics work by blocking postsynaptic dopamine receptors in the basal ganglia, hypothalamus, limbic system, brainstem, and medulla. They also demonstrate varying affinity for cholinergic, alpha$_1$-adrenergic, and histaminic receptors. Antipsychotic effects may also be related to inhibition of dopamine-mediated transmission of neural impulses at the synapses.

Atypical antipsychotics are weaker dopamine receptor antagonists than the conventional antipsychotics, but are more potent antagonists of the serotonin (5-hydroxytryptamine) type 2A (5HT$_{2A}$) receptors. They also exhibit antagonism for cholinergic, histaminic, and adrenergic receptors.

Contraindications/Precautions

Typical antipsychotics are contraindicated in clients with known hypersensitivity (cross-sensitivity may exist among phenothiazines). They should not be used in comatose states or when central nervous system (CNS) depression is evident; when blood dyscrasias exist; in clients with Parkinson's disease or narrow angle glaucoma; in those with liver, renal, or cardiac insufficiency; in individuals with poorly-controlled seizure disorders; or in elderly clients with psychosis related to neurocognitive disorder (NCD). Thioridazine, pimozide, and haloperidol have been shown to prolong the QT interval and are contraindicated if the client is taking other drugs that also produce this side effect.

Caution should be taken in administering these drugs to clients who are elderly, severely ill, or debilitated, and to diabetic clients or clients with respiratory insufficiency, prostatic hypertrophy, or intestinal obstruction. Antipsychotics may lower seizure threshold. Individuals should avoid exposure to extremes in temperature while taking antipsychotic medication. Safety in pregnancy and lactation has not been established.

Atypical antipsychotics are contraindicated in hypersensitivity, comatose or severely depressed patients, elderly patients with NCD-related psychosis, and lactation. Ziprasidone, resperidone, paliperidone, asenapine, and iloperidone are contraindicated in patients with a history of QT prolongation or cardiac arrhythmias, recent myocardial infarction (MI), uncompensated heart failure, and concurrent use with other drugs that prolong the QT interval. Clozapine is contraindicated in patients with myeloproliferative disorders, with a history of clozapine-induced agranulocytosis or severe granulocytopenia, and with uncontrolled epilepsy. Lurasidone is contraindicated in concomitant use with strong inhibitors of cytochrome P450 isozyme 3A4 (CYP3A4) (e.g., ketoconazole) and strong CYP3A4 inducers (e.g., rifampin).

Caution should be taken in administering these drugs to elderly or debilitated patients; patients with cardiac, hepatic, or renal insufficiency; to those with a history of seizures; to patients with diabetes or risk factors for diabetes; to clients exposed to temperature extremes; under conditions that cause hypotension (dehydration, hypovolemia, treatment with antihypertensive medication); and to pregnant clients or children (safety not established).

Interactions

Typical antipsychotics have additive hypotensive effects when taken with antihypertensive agents, additive CNS effects when taken with CNS depressants, and additive anticholinergic effects when taken with drugs that have anticholinergic properties. Phenothiazines may reduce the effectiveness of oral anticoagulants. Concurrent use of phenothiazines or haloperidol with epinephrine or dopamine may result in severe hypotension. Additive effects of QT prolongation occur when haloperidol, thioridazine, or pimozide are taken concurrently with other drugs that prolong the QT interval. Pimozide is contraindicated with CYP3A inhibitors, and thioridazine is contraindicated with cytochrome P450 isozyme 2D6 (CYP2D6) inhibitors. Concurrent use of haloperidol and carbamazepine results in decreased therapeutic effects of haloperidol and increased effects of carbamazepine.

Atypical antipsychotics have additive hypotensive effects when taken with antihypertensive agents and additive CNS effects with CNS depressants. There are additive anticholinergic effects when resperidone or paliperidone are taken with other drugs that have anticholinergic properties. Additive effects of QT prolongation occur when ziprasidone, risperidone, paliperidone, asenapine, and iloperidone are taken with other drugs that prolong the QT interval. Decreased effects of levodopa and dopamine agonists occur with concurrent use of ziprasidone, olanzapine, quetiapine, resperidone, or paliperidone. Increased effects of ziprasidone, clozapine, quetiapine, aripiprazole, lurasidone, and iloperidone occur with CYP3A4 inhibitors. Decreased effects of lurasidone occur with CYP3A4 inducers. Increased effects of iloperidone occur with CYP2D6 inhibitors. Decreased effects of ziprasidone, clozapine, olanzapine, risperidone, paliperidone, asenapine, and aripiprazole occur with cytochrome P450 isozyme 1A2 (CYP1A2) inducers, and increased effects occur with CYP1A2 inhibitors. Concurrent use of asenapine and paroxetine results in decreased therapeutic effects of asenapine and increased effects of paroxetine. Additive orthostatic hypotension occurs with resperidone, paliperidone, or iloperidone and other drugs that also cause this adverse reaction.

Side Effects

The effects of these medications are related to blockage of a number of receptors for which they exhibit various degrees of affinity. Blockage of the dopamine receptors is thought to be responsible for controlling positive symptoms of schizophrenia. Dopamine blockage also results in **extrapyramidal symptoms** (EPS) and prolactin elevation (galactorrhea; gynecomastia). Cholinergic blockade causes anticholinergic side effects (dry mouth, blurred vision, constipation, urinary retention, tachycardia). Blockage of the alpha$_1$-adrenergic receptors produces dizziness, orthostatic hypotension, tremors, and reflex tachycardia. Histamine blockade is associated with weight gain and sedation.

The plan of care should include monitoring for the following side effects from antipsychotic medications. Nursing implications related to each side effect are designated by an asterisk (*). A profile of side effects comparing various antipsychotic medications is presented in Table 24-6.

- Anticholinergic effects (see Table 24-6 for differences between typical and atypical antipsychotics)
  - Dry mouth
    *Provide the client with sugarless candy or gum, ice, and frequent sips of water.
    *Ensure that client practices strict oral hygiene.
  - Blurred vision
    *Explain that this symptom will most likely subside after a few weeks.
    *Advise client not to drive a car until vision clears.
    *Clear small items from pathway to prevent falls.
  - Constipation
    *Order foods high in fiber; encourage increase in physical activity and fluid intake if not contraindicated.
  - Urinary retention
    *Instruct client to report any difficulty urinating; monitor intake and output.
- Nausea; gastrointestinal (GI) upset (may occur with all classifications)
  *Tablets or capsules may be administered with food to minimize GI upset.

TABLE 24–6 Comparison of Side Effects Among Antipsychotic Agents

CLASS	GENERIC (TRADE) NAME	EPS†	SEDATION	ANTI-CHOLINERGIC	ORTHOSTATIC HYPOTENSION	WEIGHT GAIN
Typical Antipsychotic Agents	Chlorpromazine	3	4	3	4	*
	Fluphenazine	5	2	2	2	
	Haloperidol (Haldol)	5	2	2	2	
	Loxapine	3	2	2	2	*
	Perphenazine	4	2	2	2	*
	Pimozide (Orap)	4	2	3	2	*
	Prochlorperazine	3	2	2	2	*
	Thioridazine	2	4	4	4	*
	Thiothixene (Navane)	4	2	2	2	*
	Trifluoperazine	4	2	2	2	*
Atypicals	Aripiprazole (Abilify)	1	2	1	3	2
	Asenapine (Saphris)	1	3	1	3	4
	Clozapine (Clozaril)	1	5	5	4	5
	Iloperidone (Fanapt)	1	3	2	3	3
	Lurasidone (Latuda)	1	3	1	3	3
	Olanzapine (Zyprexa)	1	3	2	2	5
	Paliperidone (Invega)	1	2	1	3	2
	Quetiapine (Seroquel)	1	3	1	3	4
	Risperidone (Risperdal)	1	2	1	3	4
	Ziprasidone (Geodon)	1	3	1	2	2

Key: 1 = Very low; 2 = Low; 3 = Moderate; 4 = High; 5 = Very high

*Weight gain occurs, but incidence is unknown.

†EPS = Extrapyramidal symptoms.

SOURCE: Adapted from Black & Andreasen (2011); *Drug Facts and Comparisons* (2014); and Schatzberg, Cole, & DeBattista (2010).

*Concentrates may be diluted and administered with fruit juice or other liquid; they should be mixed immediately before administration.

■ Skin rash (may occur with all classifications)
*Report appearance of any rash on skin to physician.
*Avoid spilling any of the liquid concentrate on skin; contact dermatitis can occur with some medications.

■ Sedation (see Table 24-6 for differences between typical and atypical antipsychotics)
*Discuss with physician the possibility of administering the drug at bedtime.
*Discuss with physician a possible decrease in dosage or an order for a less sedating drug.
*Instruct client not to drive or operate dangerous equipment while experiencing sedation.

■ Orthostatic hypotension (see Table 26-6 for differences between typical and atypical antipsychotics)
*Instruct client to rise slowly from a lying or sitting position.
*Monitor blood pressure (lying and standing) each shift; document and report significant changes.

■ Photosensitivity (may occur with all classifications)
*Ensure that the client wears a sunblock lotion, protective clothing, and sunglasses while spending time outdoors.

■ Hormonal effects (may occur with all classifications, but more common with typical antipsychotics)
  ■ Decreased libido, **retrograde ejaculation** (the discharge of seminal fluid into the bladder rather than through the urethra), **gynecomastia** (men)
  *Provide explanation of the effects and reassurance of reversibility. If necessary, discuss with physician possibility of ordering alternate medication.
  ■ Amenorrhea (absence of menstruation) (women)
  *Offer reassurance of reversibility; instruct client to continue use of contraception, because **amenorrhea** does not indicate cessation of ovulation.
  ■ Weight gain (may occur with all classifications; has been problematic with the atypical antipsychotics)
  *Weigh client every other day; order calorie-controlled diet; provide opportunity for physical exercise; provide diet and exercise instruction.

■ Electrocardiogram (ECG) changes. ECG changes, including prolongation of the QT interval, are possible with most of the antipsychotics. This is particularly true with ziprasidone, thioridazine, pimozide, haloperidol, paliperidone, iloperidone, asenapine, and clozapine. Caution is advised in prescribing these medications to individuals with history of arrhythmias. Conditions that produce hypokalemia and/or hypomagnesemia, such as diuretic therapy or diarrhea, should be taken into consideration when prescribing. Routine ECG should be performed before initiation of therapy and periodically during therapy. Clozapine has also been associated with other cardiac events, such as ischemic changes, arrhythmias, congestive heart failure, myocarditis, and cardiomyopathy.

*Monitor vital signs every shift.

*Observe for symptoms of dizziness, palpitations, syncope, weakness, dyspnea, and peripheral edema.

■ Reduction of seizure threshold (more common with the typical than the atypical antipsychotics, with the exception of clozapine)

*Closely observe clients with history of seizures. *Note:* This is particularly important with clients taking clozapine (Clozaril), with which seizures have been frequently associated. Dose appears to be an important predictor, with a greater likelihood of seizures occurring at higher doses. Extreme caution is advised in prescribing clozapine for clients with a history of seizures.

■ Agranulocytosis (more common with the typical than the atypical antipsychotics, with the exception of clozapine)

*Agranulocytosis usually occurs within the first 3 months of treatment. Observe for symptoms of sore throat, fever, malaise. A complete blood count should be monitored if these symptoms appear.

*EXCEPTION: There is a significant risk of agranulocytosis with clozapine (Clozaril). Agranulocytosis is a potentially fatal blood disorder in which the client's white blood cell (WBC) count can drop to extremely low levels. A baseline WBC count and absolute neutrophil count (ANC) must be taken before initiation of treatment with clozapine and weekly for the first 6 months of treatment. Only a 1-week supply of medication is dispensed at a time. If the counts remain within the acceptable levels (i.e., WBC at least $3,500/mm^3$ and the ANC at least $2,000/mm^3$) during the 6-month period, blood counts may be monitored biweekly, and a 2-week supply of medication may then be dispensed. If the counts remain within the acceptable level for the biweekly period (6 months), counts may then be monitored every 4 weeks thereafter. When the medication is discontinued, weekly WBC counts are continued for an additional 4 weeks.

■ Hypersalivation (most common with clozapine)
*A significant number of clients receiving clozapine (Clozaril) therapy experience extreme salivation.

Offer support to the client because this may be an embarrassing situation. It may even be a safety issue (e.g., risk of aspiration) if the problem is very severe. Management has included the use of sugar-free gum to increase the swallowing rate, as well as the prescription of medications such as an anticholinergic (e.g., scopolamine patch) or alpha$_2$-adrenoceptor agonist (e.g., clonidine).

■ Extrapyramidal symptoms (see Table 24-6 for differences between typical and atypical antipsychotics)
*Observe for symptoms and report; administer antiparkinsonian drugs, as ordered (see Table 24-7).

  ■ **Pseudoparkinsonism** (tremor, shuffling gait, drooling, rigidity)
  *Symptoms may appear 1 to 5 days following initiation of antipsychotic medication; occurs most often in women, the elderly, and dehydrated clients.

  ■ **Akinesia** (muscular weakness)
  *Same as for pseudoparkinsonism.

  ■ **Akathisia** (continuous restlessness and fidgeting)
  *This occurs most frequently in women; symptoms may occur 50 to 60 days following initiation of therapy.

  ■ **Dystonia** (involuntary muscular movements [spasms] of face, arms, legs, and neck)
  *This occurs most often in men and in people younger than 25 years of age.

  ■ **Oculogyric crisis** (uncontrolled rolling back of the eyes)
  *This may appear as part of the syndrome described as dystonia. It may be mistaken for seizure activity. Dystonia and oculogyric crisis should be treated as an emergency situation. The physician should be contacted, and intravenous benztropine mesylate (Cogentin) is commonly administered. Stay with the client and offer reassurance and support during this frightening time.

■ **Tardive dyskinesia** (bizarre facial and tongue movements, stiff neck, and difficulty swallowing; may occur with all classifications, but more common with typical antipsychotics)
*All clients receiving long-term (months or years) antipsychotic therapy are at risk.
*The symptoms are potentially irreversible.
*The drug should be withdrawn at the first sign, which is usually vermiform movements of the tongue; prompt action may prevent irreversibility.
*The Abnormal Involuntary Movement Scale (AIMS) is a rating scale that was developed in the 1970s by the National Institute of Mental Health to measure involuntary movements associated with tardive dyskinesia. The AIMS aids in early

TABLE 24-7 Antiparkinsonian Agents Used to Treat Extrapyramidal Side Effects of Antipsychotic Drugs

Indication	Used to treat parkinsonism of various causes and drug-induced extrapyramidal reactions.
Action	Restores the natural balance of acetylcholine and dopamine in the CNS. The imbalance is a deficiency in dopamine that results in excessive cholinergic activity.
Contraindications/ Precautions	Antiparkinsonian agents are contraindicated in individuals with hypersensitivity.
	Anticholinergics should be avoided by individuals with angle-closure glaucoma; pyloric, duodenal, or bladder neck obstructions; prostatic hypertrophy; or myasthenia gravis.
	Caution should be used in administering these drugs to clients with hepatic, renal or cardiac insufficiency; elderly and debilitated clients; those with a tendency toward urinary retention; or those exposed to high environmental temperatures.
Common side effects	Anticholinergic effects (dry mouth, blurred vision, constipation, paralytic ileus, urinary retention, tachycardia, elevated temperature, decreased sweating), nausea/GI upset, sedation, dizziness, orthostatic hypotension, exacerbation of psychoses.

CHEMICAL CLASS	GENERIC (TRADE NAME)	PREGNANCY CATEGORIES/ HALF-LIFE (hr)	DAILY DOSAGE RANGE (mg)
Anticholinergics	Benztropine (Cogentin)	C/UKN	1–8
	Biperiden (Akineton)	C/18.4–24.3	2–6
	Trihexyphenidyl	C/5.6–10.2	1–15
Antihistamines	Diphenhydramine (Benadryl)	C/4–15	25–200
Dopaminergic Agonists	Amantadine	C/10–25	200–300

detection of movement disorders and provides a means for ongoing surveillance. The AIMS assessment tool, examination procedure, and interpretation of scoring are presented in Box 24-5.

■ **Neuroleptic malignant syndrome** (NMS) (more common with the typical than the atypical antipsychotics)

*This is a relatively rare, but potentially fatal, complication of treatment with antipsychotic drugs. Routine assessments should include temperature and observation for parkinsonian symptoms.

*Onset can occur within hours or even years after drug initiation, and progression is rapid over the following 24 to 72 hours.

BOX 24-5 Abnormal Involuntary Movement Scale (AIMS)

NAME _____ RATER NAME _____ DATE _____

INSTRUCTIONS: Complete the examination procedure before making ratings. For movement ratings, circle the highest severity observed. Rate movements that occur upon activation one *less* than those observed spontaneously. Circle movement as well as code number that applies.

Code: 0 = None
1 = Minimal, may be normal
2 = Mild
3 = Moderate
4 = Severe

Facial and Oral Movements

1. **Muscles of Facial Expression** 0 1 2 3 4
(e.g., movements of forehead, eyebrows, periorbital area, cheeks, including frowning, blinking, smiling, grimacing)

2. **Lips and Perioral Area** 0 1 2 3 4
(e.g., puckering, pouting, smacking)

3. **Jaw** 0 1 2 3 4
(e.g., biting, clenching, chewing, mouth opening, lateral movement)

4. **Tongue** 0 1 2 3 4
(Rate only increases in movement both in and out of mouth. NOT inability to sustain movement. Darting in and out of mouth.)

BOX 24-5 Abnormal Involuntary Movement Scale (AIMS)–cont'd

Extremity Movements	5. Upper (arms, wrists, hands, fingers) (Include choreic movements (i.e., rapid, objectively purposeless, irregular, spontaneous) and athetoid movements (i.e., slow, irregular, complex serpentine). *Do not include tremor* (i.e., repetitive, regular, rhythmic)	0 1 2 3 4
	6. Lower (legs, knees, ankles, toes) (e.g., lateral knee movement, foot tapping, heel dropping, foot squirming, inversion and eversion of foot)	0 1 2 3 4
Trunk Movements	7. Neck, shoulders, hips (e.g., rocking, twisting, squirming, pelvic gyrations)	0 1 2 3 4
Global Judgments	8. Severity of abnormal movements overall	0 1 2 3 4
	9. Incapacitation due to abnormal movements	0 1 2 3 4
	10. Patient's awareness of abnormal movements (Rate only the client's report)	
	No awareness	0
	Aware, no distress	1
	Aware, mild distress	2
	Aware, moderate distress	3
	Aware, severe distress	4
Dental Status	11. Current problems with teeth and/or dentures?	No Yes
	12. Are dentures usually worn?	No Yes
	13. Edentia?	No Yes
	14. Do movements disappear in sleep?	No Yes

AIMS EXAMINATION PROCEDURE

Either before or after completing the Examination Procedure, observe the client unobtrusively, at rest (e.g. in waiting room). The chair to be used in this examination should be a hard, firm one without arms.

1. Ask client to remove shoes and socks.
2. Ask client whether there is anything in his/her mouth (i.e., gum, candy, etc.), and if there is, to remove it.
3. Ask client about the current condition of his/her teeth. Ask client if he/she wears dentures. Do teeth or dentures bother client now?
4. Ask client whether he/she notices any movements in mouth, face, hands, or feet. If yes, ask to describe and to what extent they currently bother client or interfere with his/her activities.
5. Have client sit in chair with both hands on knees, legs slightly apart, and feet flat on floor. (Look at entire body for movements while in this position.)
6. Ask client to sit with hands hanging unsupported. If male, between legs, if female and wearing a dress, hanging over knees. (Observe hands and other body areas.)
7. Ask client to open mouth. (Observe tongue at rest within mouth.) Do this twice.
8. Ask client to protrude tongue. (Observe abnormalities of tongue movement.) Do this twice.
9. Ask client to tap thumb with each finger as rapidly as possible for 10 to 15 seconds; separately with right hand, then with left hand. (Observe facial and leg movements.)
10. Flex and extend client's left and right arms (one at a time). (Note any rigidity.)
11. Ask client to stand up. (Observe in profile. Observe all body areas again, hips included.)
12. Ask client to extend both arms outstretched in front with palms down. (Observe trunk, legs, and mouth.)
13. Have client walk a few paces, turn, and walk back to chair. (Observe hands and gait.) Do this twice.

INTERPRETATION OF AIMS SCORE

Add client scores and note areas of difficulty.
Score of:

- 0 to 1 = Low risk
- 2 in only ONE of the areas assessed = borderline/observe closely
- 2 in TWO or more of the areas assessed **or** 3 to 4 in ONLY ONE area = indicative of TD

From U.S. Department of Health and Human Services. Available for use in the public domain.

*Symptoms include severe parkinsonian muscle rigidity, very high fever, tachycardia, tachypnea, fluctuations in blood pressure, diaphoresis, and rapid deterioration of mental status to stupor and coma.

*Discontinue antipsychotic medication immediately.

*Monitor vital signs, degree of muscle rigidity, intake and output, level of consciousness.

*The physician may order bromocriptine (Parlodel) or dantrolene (Dantrium) to counteract the effects of neuroleptic malignant syndrome.

■ Hyperglycemia and diabetes (more common with atypical antipsychotics). Studies have suggested an increased risk of treatment-emergent hyperglycemia-related adverse events in clients using atypical antipsychotics (e.g., risperidone, clozepine, olanzapine, quetiapine, ziprasidone, paliperidone, iloperidone, asenapine, lurasidone, and aripiprazole). The U.S. Food and Drug Administration (FDA) recommends that clients with diabetes starting on atypical antipsychotic drugs be monitored regularly for worsening of glucose control. Clients with risk factors for diabetes should undergo fasting blood glucose testing at the beginning of treatment and periodically thereafter. All clients taking these medications should be monitored for symptoms of hyperglycemia (polydipsia, polyuria, polyphagia, and weakness). If these symptoms appear during treatment, the client should undergo fasting blood glucose testing.

■ Increased risk of mortality in elderly patients with psychosis related to neurocognitive disorder (NCD). Studies have indicated that elderly patients with NCD-related psychosis who are treated with antipsychotic drugs are at increased risk of death, compared with placebo. Causes of death are most commonly related to infections or cardiovascular problems. All antipsychotic drugs now carry black-box warnings to this effect. They are not approved for treatment of elderly patients with NCD-related psychosis.

Client/Family Education Related to Antipsychotics

The client should:

■ Use caution when driving or operating dangerous machinery. Drowsiness and dizziness can occur.

■ Not stop taking the drug abruptly after long-term use. To do so might produce withdrawal symptoms, such as nausea, vomiting, dizziness, gastritis, headache, tachycardia, insomnia, tremulousness.

■ Use sunblock lotion and wear protective clothing when spending time outdoors. Skin is more susceptible to sunburn, which can occur in as little as 30 minutes.

■ Report weekly (if receiving clozapine therapy) to have blood levels drawn and to obtain a weekly supply of the drug.

■ Report the occurrence of any of the following symptoms to the physician immediately: sore throat, fever, malaise, unusual bleeding, easy bruising, persistent nausea and vomiting, severe headache, rapid heart rate, difficulty urinating, muscle twitching, tremors, darkly colored urine, excessive urination, excessive thirst, excessive hunger, weakness, pale stools, yellow skin or eyes, muscular incoordination, or skin rash.

■ Rise slowly from a sitting or lying position to prevent a sudden drop in blood pressure.

■ Take frequent sips of water, chew sugarless gum, or suck on hard candy, if dry mouth is a problem. Good oral care (frequent brushing, flossing) is very important.

■ Consult the physician regarding smoking while on antipsychotic therapy. Smoking increases the metabolism of antipsychotics, requiring an adjustment in dosage to achieve a therapeutic effect.

■ Dress warmly in cold weather, and avoid extended exposure to very high or low temperatures. Body temperature is harder to maintain with this medication.

■ Avoid drinking alcohol while on antipsychotic therapy. These drugs potentiate each other's effects.

■ Avoid taking other medications (including over-the-counter products) without the physician's approval. Many medications contain substances that interact with antipsychotics in a way that may be harmful.

■ Be aware of possible risks of taking antipsychotics during pregnancy. Safe use during pregnancy has not been established. Antipsychotics are thought to readily cross the placental barrier; if so, a fetus could experience adverse effects of the drug. Inform the physician immediately if pregnancy occurs, is suspected, or is planned.

■ Be aware of side effects of antipsychotic drugs. Refer to written materials furnished by health-care providers for safe self-administration.

■ Continue to take the medication, even if feeling well and as though it is not needed. Symptoms may return if medication is discontinued.

■ Carry a card or other identification at all times describing medications being taken.

CASE STUDY AND SAMPLE CARE PLAN

NURSING HISTORY AND ASSESSMENT

Frank is 22 years old. He joined the Marines just out of high school at age 18 for a 3-year enlistment. His final year was spent in Afghanistan. When his 3-year enlistment was up, he returned to his hometown and married a young woman with whom he had been a high school classmate. Frank has always been quiet, somewhat withdrawn, and had very few friends. He was the only child of a single mom who never married, and he does not know his father. His mother was killed in an automobile accident the spring before he enlisted in the Marines.

During the past year, he has become more and more isolated and withdrawn. He is without regular employment, but finds work as a day laborer when he can. His wife, Suzanne, works as a secretary and is the primary wage earner. Lately he has become very suspicious of her, and sometimes follows her to work. He also drops in on her at work and accuses her of having affairs with some of the men in the office.

Last evening when Suzanne got home from work, Frank was hiding in the closet. She didn't know he was home. When she started to undress, he jumped out of the closet holding a large kitchen knife and threatened to kill her "for being unfaithful." Suzanne managed to flee their home and ran to the neighbor's house and called the police.

Frank told the police that he received a message over the radio from his Marine commanding officer telling him that he couldn't allow his wife to continue to commit adultery, and the only way he could stop it was to kill her. The police took Frank to the emergency department of the VA Hospital, where he was admitted to the psychiatric unit. Suzanne is helping with the admission history.

Suzanne tells the nurse that she has never been unfaithful to Frank and she doesn't know why he believes that she has. Frank tells the nurse that he has been "taking orders from my commanding officer through my car radio ever since I got back from Afghanistan." He survived a helicopter crash in Afghanistan in which all were killed except Frank and one other man. Frank says, "I have to follow my CO's orders. God saved me to annihilate the impure."

Following an evaluation, the psychiatrist diagnoses Frank with schizophrenia. He orders olanzapine 10 mg PO to be given daily and olanzapine 10 mg IM q6h prn for agitation.

NURSING DIAGNOSES/OUTCOME IDENTIFICATION

From the assessment data, the nurse develops the following nursing diagnoses for Frank:

1. **Risk for self-directed or other-directed violence** related to unresolved grief over loss of mother; survivor's guilt associated with helicopter crash; command hallucinations; and history of violence.
   a. **Short-Term Goals:**
      ■ Frank will seek out staff when anxiety and agitation start to increase.
      ■ Frank will not harm self or others.
   b. **Long-Term Goal:** Frank will not harm self or others.

2. **Disturbed sensory perception: Auditory** related to increased anxiety and agitation, withdrawal into self, and stress of sufficient intensity to threaten an already weak ego.
   a. **Short-Term Goals:**
      ■ Frank will discuss the content of the hallucinations with the nurse.
      ■ Frank will maintain anxiety at a manageable level.
   b. **Long-Term Goal:** Frank will be able to define and test reality, reducing or eliminating the occurrence of hallucinations.

PLANNING/IMPLEMENTATION

RISK FOR SELF-DIRECTED OR OTHER-DIRECTED VIOLENCE

1. Keep the stimuli as low as possible in Frank's environment.
2. Monitor Frank's behavior frequently, but in a manner of carrying out routine activities so as not to create suspiciousness on his part.
3. Watch for the following signs (considered the prodrome to aggressive behavior: increased motor activity, pounding, slamming, tense posture, defiant affect, clenched teeth and fists, arguing, demanding, and challenging or threatening staff).
4. If client should become aggressive, maintain a calm attitude. Try talking. Offer medication. Provide physical activities.
5. If these interventions fail, indicate a show of strength with a team of staff members.
6. Utilize restraints only as a last resort and if Frank is clearly at risk of harm to himself or others.
7. Help Frank recognize unresolved grief and fixation in denial or anger stage of grief process.
8. Encourage him to talk about the loss of his mother and fellow Marines in Afghanistan.
9. Encourage him to talk about guilt feelings associated with survival when others died.
10. Make a short-term contract with Frank that he will seek out staff if considering harming himself or others. When this contract expires, make another, etc.

DISTURBED SENSORY PERCEPTION: AUDITORY

1. Monitor Frank's behavior for signs that he is hearing voices: listening pose, talking and laughing to self, stopping in midsentence.
2. If these behaviors are observed, ask Frank, "Are you hearing the voices again?"
3. Encourage Frank to share the content of the hallucinations. This is important for early intervention in case the content contains commands to harm himself or others.
4. Say to Frank, "I understand that the voice is real to you, but I do not hear any voices speaking." It is important for him to learn the difference between what is real and what is not real.
5. Try to help Frank recognize that the voices often appear at times when he becomes anxious about something and his agitation increases.

Continued

CASE STUDY AND SAMPLE CARE PLAN—cont'd

6. Help him to recognize this increasing anxiety, and teach him methods to keep it from escalating.

7. Use distracting activities to bring him back to reality. Involvement with real people and real situations will help to distract him from the hallucination.

8. Teach him to use *voice dismissal.* When he hears the CO's (or others') voice, he should shout, "Go away!" or "Leave me alone!" These commands may help to diminish the sounds and give him a feeling of control over the situation.

EVALUATION

The outcome criteria identified for Frank have been met. When feeling especially anxious or becoming agitated, he seeks out staff for comfort and for assistance in maintaining his anxiety at a manageable level. He establishes short-term contracts with staff not to harm himself. He is experiencing fewer auditory hallucinations, and has learned to use voice dismissal to interrupt the behavior. He is beginning to recognize his position in the grief process, and working toward resolution at his own pace.

Summary and Key Points

■ Of all mental illness, schizophrenia undoubtedly results in the greatest amount of personal, emotional, and social costs. It presents an enormous threat to life and happiness, yet it remains an enigma to the medical community.

■ For many years there was little agreement as to a definition of the concept of schizophrenia. The *DSM-5* (APA, 2013) identifies specific criteria for diagnosis of the disorder.

■ The initial symptoms of schizophrenia most often occur in early adulthood. Development of the disorder can be viewed in four phases: (1) the premorbid phase, (2) the prodromal phase, (3) the active psychotic phase (schizophrenia), and (4) the residual phase.

■ The cause of schizophrenia remains unclear. Research continues, and most contemporary psychiatrists view schizophrenia as a brain disorder with little if any emphasis on psychosocial influences.

■ Schizophrenia most likely results from a combination of influences including genetics, biochemical dysfunction, and physiological and environmental factors.

■ A spectrum of schizophrenic and other psychotic disorders has been identified. These include (on a gradient of psychopathology from least to most severe): schizotypal personality disorder, delusional disorder, brief psychotic disorder, substance-induced psychotic disorder, psychotic disorder associated with another medical condition, catatonic disorder associated with another medical condition, schizophreniform disorder, schizoaffective disorder, and schizophrenia.

■ Nursing care of the client with schizophrenia is accomplished using the six steps of the nursing process.

■ Nursing assessment is based on knowledge of symptomatology related to thought content and form, perception, affect, sense of self, volition, interpersonal functioning and relationship to the external world, and psychomotor behavior.

■ These behaviors are categorized as *positive* (an excess or distortion of normal functions) or *negative* (a diminution or loss of normal functions).

■ Antipsychotic medications remain the mainstay of treatment for psychotic disorders. Atypical antipsychotics have become the first-line of therapy, and treat both positive and negative symptoms of schizophrenia. They have a more favorable side-effect profile than the conventional (typical) antipsychotics.

■ Individuals with schizophrenia require long-term integrated treatment with pharmacological and other interventions. Some of these include individual psychotherapy, group therapy, behavior therapy, social skills training, milieu therapy, family therapy, and assertive community treatment. For the majority of clients, the most effective treatment appears to be a combination of psychotropic medication and psychosocial therapy.

■ Some clinicians are choosing a course of therapy based on a model of recovery, somewhat like that which has been used for many years with problems of addiction. The basic premise of a recovery model is empowerment of the consumer. The recovery model is designed to allow consumers primary control over decisions about their own care, and to enable persons with mental health problems to live a meaningful life in a community of their choice while striving to achieve their full potential.

■ Families generally require support and education about psychotic illnesses. The focus is on coping with the diagnosis, understanding the illness and its course, teaching about medication, and learning ways to manage symptoms.

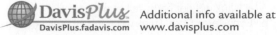

Review Questions
Self-Examination/Learning Exercise

Select the answer that is most appropriate for each of the following questions.

1. Tony, age 21, has been diagnosed with schizophrenia. He has been socially isolated and hearing voices telling him to kill his parents. He has been admitted to the psychiatric unit from the emergency department. The *initial* nursing intervention for Tony is to:
   a. Give him an injection of Thorazine.
   b. Ensure a safe environment for him and others.
   c. Place him in restraints.
   d. Order him a nutritious diet.

2. The primary goal in working with an actively psychotic, suspicious client would be to:
   a. Promote interaction with others.
   b. Decrease his anxiety and increase trust.
   c. Improve his relationship with his parents.
   d. Encourage participation in therapy activities.

3. The nurse is caring for a client with schizophrenia. Orders from the physician include 100 mg chlorpromazine IM STAT and then 50 mg PO bid; 2 mg benztropine PO bid prn. Why is chlorpromazine ordered?
   a. To reduce extrapyramidal symptoms
   b. To prevent neuroleptic malignant syndrome
   c. To decrease psychotic symptoms
   d. To induce sleep

4. The nurse is caring for a client with schizophrenia. Orders from the physician include 100 mg chlorpromazine IM STAT and then 50 mg PO bid; 2 mg benztropine PO bid prn. Because benztropine was ordered on a prn basis, which of the following assessments by the nurse would convey a need for this medication?
   a. The client's level of agitation increases.
   b. The client complains of a sore throat.
   c. The client's skin has a yellowish cast.
   d. The client develops tremors and a shuffling gait.

5. Clint, a client on the psychiatric unit, has been diagnosed with schizophrenia. He begins to tell the nurse about how the CIA is looking for him and will kill him if they find him. The most appropriate response by the nurse is:
   a. "That's ridiculous, Clint. No one is going to hurt you."
   b. "The CIA isn't interested in people like you, Clint."
   c. "Why do you think the CIA wants to kill you?"
   d. "I know you believe that, Clint, but it's really hard for me to believe."

6. Clint, a client on the psychiatric unit, has been diagnosed with schizophrenia. He begins to tell the nurse about how the CIA is looking for him and will kill him if they find him. Clint's belief is an example of a:
   a. Delusion of persecution
   b. Delusion of reference
   c. Delusion of control or influence
   d. Delusion of grandeur

7. The nurse is interviewing a client on the psychiatric unit. The client tilts his head to the side, stops talking in midsentence, and listens intently. The nurse recognizes from these signs that the client is likely experiencing:
   a. Somatic delusions
   b. Catatonic stupor
   c. Auditory hallucinations
   d. Pseudoparkinsonism

Continued

Review Questions—cont'd
Self-Examination/Learning Exercise

8. The nurse is interviewing a client on the psychiatric unit. The client tilts his head to the side, stops talking in midsentence, and listens intently. The nurse recognizes these behaviors as a symptom of the client's illness. The most appropriate nursing intervention for this symptom is to:
   a. Ask the client to describe his physical symptoms.
   b. Ask the client to describe what he is hearing.
   c. Administer a dose of benztropine.
   d. Call the physician for additional orders.

9. When a client suddenly becomes aggressive and violent on the unit, which of the following approaches would be best for the nurse to use *first?*
   a. Provide large motor activities to relieve the client's pent-up tension.
   b. Administer a dose of prn chlorpromazine to keep the client calm.
   c. Call for sufficient help to control the situation safely.
   d. Convey to the client that his behavior is unacceptable and will not be permitted.

10. The primary focus of family therapy for clients with schizophrenia and their families is:
   a. To discuss concrete problem solving and adaptive behaviors for coping with stress
   b. To introduce the family to others with the same problem
   c. To keep the client and family in touch with the health care system
   d. To promote family interaction and increase understanding of the illness

IMPLICATIONS OF RESEARCH FOR EVIDENCE-BASED PRACTICE

Trygstad, L., Buccheri, R., Dowling, G., Zin, R., White, K., Griffin, J.J., et al. (2002). Behavioral management of persistent auditory hallucinations in schizophrenia: Outcomes from a 10-week course. *Journal of the American Psychiatric Nurses Association, 8*(3), 84-91.

DESCRIPTION OF THE STUDY: The purpose of this study was to examine the effects of a 10-week course in which behavior management strategies were taught to participants with schizophrenia who experienced persistent auditory hallucinations. The primary aim was to examine the effects of the intervention on seven specific characteristics of auditory hallucinations: frequency, loudness, self-control, clarity, tone, distractibility, and distress. The secondary aim was to examine level of anxiety and depression. The sample consisted of 62 subjects who had been diagnosed with schizophrenia by a board-certified psychiatrist using *DSM-IV* diagnostic criteria. They all reported having persistent auditory hallucinations for at least 10 minutes a day for the past 3 months; reported a desire to learn new strategies to manage their auditory hallucinations; were taking stable doses of antipsychotic medication for at least 4 weeks before entry into the study; were able to read and write in English; and did not have a severe cognitive deficit. The 10-week course was taught in 9 different outpatient

settings by nurses who had experience caring for patients with schizophrenia and were knowledgeable in group facilitation skills. In each class, participants were taught and practiced one behavior strategy. The following strategies were taught in the course: self-monitoring, talking with someone, listening to music with or without earphones, watching television, saying "stop"/ignoring what the voices say to do, using ear plugs, learning relaxation techniques, keeping busy with an enjoyable activity and/or helping others, and practicing communication related to taking medication and not using drugs and alcohol. Measurement of the outcomes were based on subjects' scores on the Characteristics of Auditory Hallucinations Questionnaire (CAHQ), the Profile of Mood States (POMS) scale, and the Beck Depression Inventory, second edition (BDI-II).

RESULTS OF THE STUDY: The outcome of this study strongly supported the expectation that subjects who attended the behavior-management strategy classes for auditory hallucinations would experience improvement in the characteristics of their auditory hallucinations and have less anxiety and depression. Post-intervention scores on the POMS and BDI-II were significantly lower than pre-intervention scores, indicating an overall decrease in anxiety and depression. Post-intervention mean scores on the CAHQ were significantly

IMPLICATIONS OF RESEARCH FOR EVIDENCE-BASED PRACTICE—cont'd

lower than pre-intervention on all hallucination characteristics, with the exception of loudness, which did not change significantly. In a 5-point self-report rating helpfulness of the course, 25% of the participants reported that the course was *extremely helpful*, 42% reported that it was *helpful*, 23% *moderately helpful*, 8% *minimally helpful*, and 2% *not helpful*.

IMPLICATIONS FOR NURSING PRACTICE: This study shows that individuals can manage their auditory hallucinations by learning and using specific behavioral strategies. The group setting also proved to be beneficial, as clients were able to have their own experiences validated, to see that others had similar experiences, and to learn how others managed them. They gained encouragement and hope from learning that certain strategies were effective for others in the group. The authors stated, "This low cost, low-tech intervention could be incorporated into the practice of psychiatric nurses or other mental health professionals who have group training and experience facilitating groups with people who have schizophrenia. Teaching behavior management of persistent auditory hallucinations to clients who wish to learn has minimal risks and could be easily incorporated into existing outpatient programs" (p. 90).

IMPLICATIONS OF RESEARCH FOR EVIDENCE-BASED PRACTICE

Beebe, L.H., Smith, K., Crye, C., Addonizio, C., Strunk, D.J., Martin, W., & Poche, J. (2008). Telenursing intervention increases psychiatric medication adherence in schizophrenia outpatients. *Journal of the American Psychiatric Nurses Association, 14*(3), 217-224.

DESCRIPTION OF THE STUDY: The purpose of this study was to evaluate the impact of telephone intervention problem solving (TIPS), a problem-based telenursing intervention, on both psychiatric and nonpsychiatric medication adherence in outpatients with schizophrenia. The study sample included 25 outpatients (age range 25 to 69) receiving care at a Community Mental Health Center (CMHC) in the southeastern United States; 60% were male and 44% were African American. The majority lived alone and were unemployed. All had chart diagnoses of schizophrenia (any subtype) according to the criteria in the *DMS-IV-TR*. Thirteen study participants and 12 control subjects completed the research study. The intervention included weekly telephone calls throughout the 3-month study by registered nurses with graduate degrees who had received TIPS training from one of the authors. The calls were designed "to foster problem solving, offer coping alternatives, provide reminders so clients remember to use alternatives, and assess the effectiveness of coping efforts. Effective use of problem solving may assist patients to cope with common medication adherence barriers such as forgetfulness or lack of knowledge about prescribed medications. Nurses guide the participant through the problem-solving process for any difficulties identified, generating solutions, choosing a solution, and following up on the effectiveness of the solution at the next call" (p. 220). Medication adherence was measured by pill counts performed monthly in the participants' homes. Both psychiatric and nonpsychiatric medications were counted.

RESULTS OF THE STUDY: As had been expected, there was a statistically significant improvement in adherence to psychiatric medications in the experimental group compared to the control group. However, nonpsychiatric medication adherence was not significantly affected by the TIPS intervention. The authors suggest that this may have occurred "because participants were recruited at a CMHC, they associated TIPS providers with the CMHC and tended to generalize adherence suggestions to psychiatric medications for this reason" (p. 223).

IMPLICATIONS FOR NURSING PRACTICE: The telenursing intervention described in this study may provide nurses with a tool for assisting clients with schizophrenia to maintain greater medication adherence. Prior work by the primary author demonstrated fewer rehospitalizations in persons receiving TIPS, indicating that there is a strong association between lack of psychiatric medication adherence and symptom relapse and psychiatric readmission. TIPS may be considered as part of an outpatient or partial hospitalization program for clients with schizophrenia.

TEST YOUR CRITICAL THINKING SKILLS

Sara, a 23-year-old single woman, has just been admitted to the psychiatric unit by her parents. They explain that over the past few months she has become more and more withdrawn. She stays in her room alone, but lately has been heard talking and laughing to herself.

Sara left home for the first time at age 18 to attend college. She performed well during her first semester, but when she returned after Christmas, she began to accuse her roommate of stealing her possessions. She started writing to her parents that her roommate wanted to kill her and that her roommate was turning everyone against her. She said she feared for her life. She started missing classes and stayed in her bed most of the time. Sometimes she locked herself in her closet. Her parents took her home, and she was hospitalized and diagnosed with schizophrenia. She has since been maintained on antipsychotic medication while taking a few classes at the local community college.

Sara tells the admitting nurse that she quit taking her medication 4 weeks ago because the pharmacist who fills the prescriptions is plotting to have her killed. She believes he is trying to poison her. She says she got this information from a television message. As Sara speaks, the nurse notices that she sometimes stops in mid-sentence and listens; sometimes she cocks her head to the side and moves her lips as though she is talking.

Answer the following questions related to Sara:

1. From the assessment data, what would be the most immediate nursing concern in working with Sara?
2. What is the nursing diagnosis related to this concern?
3. What interventions must be accomplished before the nurse can be successful in working with Sara?

💬 Communication Exercises

1. Hal, a patient on the psychiatric unit, has a diagnosis of schizophrenia. He lives in a halfway house, where last evening he began yelling that "aliens were on the way to take over our bodies! The message is coming through loud and clear!" The residence supervisor became frightened and called 911. Hal tells the nurse, "I'm special! I get messages from a higher being! We are in for big trouble!"

   How would the nurse respond appropriately to this statement by Hal?

2. The nurse notices that Hal is sitting off to himself in a corner of the dayroom. He appears to be talking to himself and tilts his head to the side as if listening to something.

   How would the nurse intervene with Hal in this situation?

3. Hal says to the nurse, "We must choose to take a ride. All alone we slip and slide. Now it's time to take a bride."

   How would the nurse respond appropriately to this statement by Hal?

References

Addington, D.E. (2006). Reducing suicide risk in patients with schizophrenia. *Medscape Psychiatry & Mental Health.* Retrieved from http://www.medscape.com/viewprogram/5616

American Psychiatric Association (APA). (2013). *Diagnostic and statistical manual of mental disorders* (5th ed.) Washington, DC: American Psychiatric Publishing.

Asen, E. (2002). Outcome research in family therapy: Family intervention for psychosis. *Advances in Psychiatric Treatment, 8,* 230-238.

Assertive Community Treatment Association (ACTA). (2013). *ACT Model.* Retrieved from http://www.actassociation.org/actModel

Black, D.W., & Andreasen, N.C. (2011). *Introductory textbook of psychiatry* (5th ed.). Washington, DC: American Psychiatric Publishing.

Citrome, L. (2011). Neurochemical models of schizophrenia: Transcending dopamine. Supplement to *Current Psychiatry, 10*(9), S10-S14.

Dixon, L.B., Lehman, A.F., & Levine, J. (2010). *Conventional antipsychotic medications for schizophrenia.* Retrieved from http://www.mental-health-matters.com

Drug facts and comparisons. (2014). St. Louis, MO: Wolters Kluwer.

D'Souza, D.C., Singh, N., Elander, J., Carbuto, M., Pittman, B., Udo de Haes, J., Sjogren, M., Peeters, P., Ranganathan, M., & Schipper, J. (2012). Glycine transporter inhibitor attenuates the psychotomimetic effects of ketamine in healthy males: Preliminary evidence. *Neuropsychopharmacology, 37,* 1036-1046.

Eisendrath, S.J. & Lichtmacher, J.E. (2012). Psychiatric disorders. In S.J. McPhee, M.A. Papadakis, & M.W. Rabow (Eds.), *Current medical diagnosis and treatment 2012* (pp. 1010-1064). New York, NY: McGraw-Hill.

Fohrman, D.A., & Stein, M.T. (2006). Psychosis: Six steps rule out medical causes in kids. *The Journal of Family Practice Online, 5*(2). Retrieved from http://www.jfponline.com/pages.asp?aid=3887

Freudenreich, O. (2010). Differential diagnosis of psychotic symptoms: Medical "mimics." *Psychiatric Times, 27*(12), 52-61.

Hashimoto, K. (2006). Glycine transporter inhibitors as therapeutic agents for schizophrenia. *Recent Patents on CNS Drug Discovery, 1,* 43-53.

Ho, B.C., Black, D.W., & Andreasen, N.C. (2003). Schizophrenia and other psychotic disorders. In R.E. Hales & S.C. Yudofsky (Eds.), *Textbook of clinical psychiatry* (4th ed., pp. 379-438). Washington, DC: American Psychiatric Publishing.

Institute of Medicine. (2003). *Health professions education: A bridge to quality.* Washington, DC: Author.

Jonsson, S.A., Luts, A., Guldberg-Kjaer, N., & Brun, A. (1997). Hippocampal pyramidal cell disarray correlates negatively to cell number: Implications for the pathogenesis of schizophrenia. *European Archives of Psychiatry and Clinical Neuroscience, 247*(3), 120-127.

Lehman, A.F., Lieberman, J.A., Dixon, L.B., McGlashan, T.H., Miller, A.L., Perkins, D.O., & Kreyenbuhl, J. (2006). Practice guideline for the treatment of patients with schizophrenia, 2nd edition. *American Psychiatric Association practice guidelines for the treatment of psychiatric disorders, Compendium 2006.* Washington, DC: American Psychiatric Publishing.

Levenson, J.L. (2009). Medical aspects of catatonia. *Primary Psychiatry, 16*(3), 23-26.

Lysaker, P.H., Roe, D., & Buck, K.D. (2010). Recovery and wellness amidst schizophrenia: Definitions, evidence, and the implications for clinical practice. *Journal of the American Psychiatric Nurses Association, 16*(1), 36-42.

Mattai, A.K., Hill, J.L., & Lenroot, R.K. (2010). Treatment of early-onset schizophrenia. *Current Opinion in Psychiatry, 23*(4), 304-310.

Minzenberg, M.J., Yoon, J.H., & Carter, C.S. (2008). Schizophrenia. In R.E. Hales, S.C. Yudofsky, & G.O. Gabbard (Eds.), *Textbook of Psychiatry* (5th ed., pp. 407-456). Washington, DC: American Psychiatric Publishing.

Mueser, K.T., Bond, G.R., & Drake, R.E. (2002). Community-based treatment of schizophrenia and other severe mental disorders: Treatment outcomes. *Medscape Psychiatry & Mental Health eJournal.* Retrieved from http://www.medscape.com/viewarticle/430529

NANDA International (NANDA-I). (2012). *Nursing diagnoses: Definitions & classification 2012-2014.* Philadelphia, PA: NANDA-I.

National Alliance on Mental Illness (NAMI). (2013). *PACT: Program of assertive community treatment.* Retrieved from http://www.nami.org

Puri, B.K., & Treasaden, I.H. (2011). *Textbook of psychiatry* (3rd ed.). Philadelphia, PA: Churchill Livingstone Elsevier.

Rantakallio, P., Jones, P., Moring, J., & Von Wendt, L. (1997). Association between central nervous system infections during childhood and adult onset schizophrenia and other psychoses: A 28-year follow-up. *International Journal of Epidemiology, 26,* 837-843.

Sadock, B.J., & Sadock, V.A. (2007). *Synopsis of psychiatry: Behavioral sciences/clinical psychiatry* (10th ed.). Philadelphia, PA: Lippincott Williams & Wilkins.

Safier, E. (1997). Our families, the context of our lives. *Menninger Perspective, 28*(1), 4-9.

Schatzberg, A.F., Cole, J.O., & DeBattista, C. (2010). *Manual of clinical psychopharmacology* (7th ed.). Washington, DC: American Psychiatric Publishing.

Stahl, S.M. (2008). *Stahl's essential psychopharmacology: Neuroscientific basis and practical applications* (3rd ed.). New York, NY: Cambridge University Press.

The Joint Commission. (2010, January). *The comprehensive accreditation manual for hospitals: The official handbook.* Oakbrook Terrace, IL: Joint Commission Resources.

Weiden, P.J. (2010). Is recovery attainable in schizophrenia? *Medscape Psychiatry & Mental Health.* Retrieved from http://www.medscape.com/viewarticle/729750

@ INTERNET REFERENCES

- Additional information about schizophrenia may be located at the following websites:
  - http://www.schizophrenia.com
  - http://www.nimh.nih.gov
  - http://www.nami.org
  - http://mentalhealth.com
  - http://bbrfoundation.org

- Additional information about medications to treat schizophrenia may be located at the following websites:
  - http://www.medicinenet.com/medications/article.htm
  - http://www.nlm.nih.gov/medlineplus
  - http://www.drugs.com

MOVIE CONNECTIONS

I Never Promised You a Rose Garden (schizophrenia) • *A Beautiful Mind* (schizophrenia) • *The Fisher King* (schizophrenia) • *Bennie & Joon* (schizophrenia) • *Out of Darkness* (schizophrenia) • *Conspiracy Theory* (delusional disorder) • *The Fan* (delusional disorder)

25

Depressive Disorders

CHAPTER OUTLINE

KEY TERMS

OBJECTIVES

After reading this chapter, the student will be able to:

1. Recount historical perspectives of depression.
2. Discuss epidemiological statistics related to depression.
3. Describe various types of depressive disorders.
4. Identify predisposing factors in the development of depression.
5. Discuss implications of depression related to developmental stage.
6. Identify symptomatology associated with depression and use this information in client assessment.
7. Formulate nursing diagnoses and goals of care for clients with depression.
8. Identify topics for client and family teaching relevant to depression.
9. Describe appropriate nursing interventions for behaviors associated with depression.
10. Describe relevant criteria for evaluating nursing care of clients with depression.
11. Discuss various modalities relevant to treatment of depression.

HOMEWORK ASSIGNMENT

Please read the chapter and answer the following questions:

1. Alterations in which of the neurotransmitters are most closely associated with depression?
2. Depression in adolescence is very hard to differentiate from the normal stormy behavior associated with adolescence. What is the best clue for determining a problem with depression in adolescence?
3. Behaviors of depression often change with the diurnal variation in the level of neurotransmitters. Describe the difference in this phenomenon between moderate and severe depression.
4. All antidepressants carry a black box warning. What is it?

Depression is likely the oldest and still one of the most frequently diagnosed psychiatric illnesses. Symptoms of depression have been described almost as far back as there is evidence of written documentation.

An occasional bout with the "blues," a feeling of sadness or downheartedness, is common among healthy people and considered to be a normal response to everyday disappointments in life. These episodes are short-lived as the individual adapts to the loss, change, or failure (real or perceived) that has been experienced. Pathological depression occurs when adaptation is ineffective.

CORE CONCEPT

Mood

Also called *affect*. Mood is a pervasive and sustained emotion that may have a major influence on a person's perception of the world. Examples of mood include depression, joy, elation, anger, and anxiety. *Affect* is described as the emotional reaction associated with an experience.

This chapter focuses on the consequences of complicated grieving as it is manifested by depression. A historical perspective and epidemiological statistics related to depression are presented. Predisposing factors that have been implicated in the etiology of depression provide a framework for studying the dynamics of the disorder.

The implications of depression relevant to individuals of various developmental stages are discussed. An explanation of the symptomatology is presented as background knowledge for assessing the client with depression. Nursing care is described in the context of the six steps of the nursing process. Various medical treatment modalities are explored.

CORE CONCEPT

Depression

An alteration in mood that is expressed by feelings of sadness, despair, and pessimism. There is a loss of interest in usual activities, and somatic symptoms may be evident. Changes in appetite and sleep patterns are common.

Historical Perspective

Many ancient cultures (e.g., Babylonian, Egyptian, Hebrew) have believed in the supernatural or divine origin of mood disorders. The Old Testament states in the Book of Samuel that King Saul's depression was inflicted by an "evil spirit" sent from God to "torment" him.

A clearly nondivine point of view regarding depression was held by the Greek medical community from the 5th century BC through the 3rd century AD. This represented the thinking of Hippocrates, Celsus, and Galen, among others. They strongly rejected the idea of divine origin and considered the brain as the seat of all emotional states. Hippocrates believed that **melancholia** was caused by an excess of black bile, a heavily toxic substance produced in the spleen or intestine, which affected the brain. Melancholia is a severe form of depressive disorder in which symptoms are exaggerated and interest or pleasure in virtually all activities is lost.

During the Renaissance, several new theories evolved. Depression was viewed by some as being the result of obstruction of vital air circulation, excessive brooding, or helpless situations beyond the client's control. Depression was reflected in major literary works of the time, including Shakespeare's *King Lear*, *Macbeth*, and *Hamlet*.

Contemporary thinking has been shaped a great deal by the works of Sigmund Freud, Emil Kraepelin, and Adolf Meyer. Having evolved from these early 20th-century models, current thinking about mood disorders generally encompasses the intrapsychic, behavioral, and biological perspectives. These various perspectives support the notion of multiple causation in the development of mood disorders.

Epidemiology

Major depressive disorder (MDD) is one of the leading causes of disability in the United States. In 2012, 6.9 percent of persons aged 18 or older (16 million persons) had at least one major depressive episode in the past year (Substance Abuse and Mental Health Services Administration [SAMHSA], 2013). During their lifetime, about 21 percent of women and 13 percent of men will become clinically depressed. This preponderance has led to the consideration of depression by some researchers as "the common cold of psychiatric disorders" and this generation as an "age of melancholia."

Age and Gender

Research indicates that the incidence of depressive disorder is higher in women than it is in men by almost 2 to 1. Women experience more depression than men beginning at about age 10 and continuing through midlife (Kornstein, 2006). The gender difference is less pronounced between ages 44 and 65, but after the age of 65, women are again more likely to be depressed than men. This occurrence may be related to gender differences in social roles and economic and social opportunities and the shifts that occur with age. The construction of gender stereo-types, or *gender socialization*, promotes typical female characteristics, such as helplessness, passivity, and emotionality, which are associated with depression. In contrast, some studies have suggested that "mascu-line" characteristics are associated with higher self-esteem and less depression.

Social Class

Results of studies have indicated an inverse relation-ship between social class and report of depressive symptoms. However, there has yet to be a definitive causal structure in the socioeconomic status–mental illness relationship. Hudson (2005) stated:

> Do poor socioeconomic conditions predispose people to mental disability? Or do preexisting, bi-ologically based mental illnesses result in the drift of individuals into poor socioeconomic circum-stances? (p. 3)

Hudson (2005) reported that both depression and personality disorders have most commonly been found to be outcomes of low socioeconomic status.

Race and Culture

Studies have shown no consistent relationship be-tween race and affective disorder. One problem en-countered in reviewing racial comparisons has to do with the socioeconomic class of the race being inves-tigated. Sample populations of nonwhite clients are many times predominantly lower class and are often compared with white populations from middle and upper social classes.

Other studies suggest a second problematic factor in the study of racial comparisons. Clinicians tend to underdiagnose mood disorders and to overdiagnose schizophrenia in clients who have racial or cultural backgrounds different from their own (Sadock and Sadock, 2007). This misdiagnosis may result from lan-guage barriers between clients and physicians who are unfamiliar with cultural aspects of nonwhite clients' language and behavior.

Findings from the SAMHSA *National Survey on Drug Use and Health* (2013) reveal that depression is more prevalent in whites than it is in blacks. However, Williams and associates (2007) report that depression tends to be more severe, persistent, and disabling in blacks, and they are less likely to be treated. In their

---

▌IMPLICATIONS OF RESEARCH FOR EVIDENCE-BASED PRACTICE

Peden, A.R., Rayens, M.K., Hall, L.A., & Grant, E. (2004). Negative thinking and the mental health of low-income single mothers. *Journal of Nursing Scholarship, (36)*4, 337-344.

DESCRIPTION OF THE STUDY: The aims of this study were to: (1) examine the prevalence of a high level of depressive symptoms in low-income, single mothers with children 2 to 6 years of age; (2) evaluate the relationships of personal sociodemographic characteristics with self-esteem, chronic stressors, negative thinking, and depressive symptoms; and (3) determine whether negative thinking mediates the effects of self-esteem and chronic stressors on depressive symp-toms. Single mothers are a particularly high-risk group for clin-ical depression because of life circumstances such as poverty, low self-esteem, and few social resources. The average age of the mothers in the study was 27 years. The ethnicity of the sample was approximately half Caucasian and half African American. The majority had never been married; most were employed, but had annual incomes at or below $15,000. The Beck Depression Inventory was used to measure symptoms of depression, the Crandell Cognitions Inventory was used to measure negative thoughts, and the Rosenberg Self-Esteem Scale was used to measure self-worth and self-acceptance.

RESULTS OF THE STUDY: More than 75 percent of the mothers scored somewhere in the mild to high range for depression.

Negative thinking mediated the effect of self-esteem on de-pressive symptoms and partially mediated the effect of chronic stressors. Those subjects who were employed measured higher self-esteem, less negative thinking, fewer chronic stres-sors, and less depression. No differences in predictors of depression were found between Caucasian and African American mothers in this study.

IMPLICATIONS FOR NURSING PRACTICE: The results of this study suggest the importance of intervening to address negative thinking among low-income single mothers to help them lessen their stress and decrease their risk of depression. The authors state, "Depression may interfere with parenting and participation in educational and em-ployment opportunities, significantly undermining the quality of life in these families. A number of studies have indicated that mothers' depression may also negatively in-fluence their children's behavior." Psychiatric nurses may employ cognitive-behavioral strategies to help women minimize negative thinking. Strategies such as writing affirmations and use of positive self-talk have been sup-ported in nursing research. Targeting the symptom of neg-ative thinking, which can be modified, may serve to break the links of chronic stressors and low self-esteem to depressive symptoms, resulting in improved mental health for the mother and the subsequent well-being of her children.

study they found that, even among blacks whose symptoms were rated severe or very severe, only 48.5 percent of African Americans and 21.9 percent of Caribbean blacks received any treatment at all. The authors concluded that these findings highlight the importance of identifying high-risk subgroups in racial populations and the need for targeting cost-effective interventions to them.

Marital Status

A number of studies have suggested that marriage has a positive effect on the psychological well-being of an individual (as compared to those who are single or do not have a close relationship with another person). LaPierre (2004) suggested that marital status alone may lack validity, and that the effect of marital status on depression may be contingent on age. She found in her study that being single was a significant predictor of depression in the 37- to 49-year-old age group, but was not a significant predictor of depression in any of the other age groups (18 to 25; 26 to 36; 50+). She explained her findings in the following way:

> The realization that the normative ideal of marriage (and accompanying children) is becoming a remote possibility is likely to occur in the 37-49 year old age group, causing a decrease in mental health and corresponding increase in depressive symptomatology. This is particularly true for women who reach the end of their childbearing years in this age category, and feel they may have to forfeit the normative role of motherhood if they do not find a partner to have a child with. The subsequent decline in depressive symptomatology (observed in the 50+ age group) could occur because with time the never-married/childless individual comes to accept their non-normative behavior and find ways to adjust. (p. 14)

Other studies also have indicated that age may moderate the effect of marital status on depression. George (1992) found that marriage (versus separated/divorced) had a protective effect against major depression only in the oldest age category (65+). Her results also showed that being never married (versus separated/divorced) was associated with increased risk of major depression in the 40- to 64-year-old age group and the 65+ age group.

Seasonality

A number of studies have examined seasonal patterns associated with mood disorders. These studies have revealed two prevalent periods of seasonal involvement: one in the spring (March, April, and May) and one in the fall (September, October, and November). This pattern tends to parallel the seasonal pattern for suicide, which shows a large peak in the spring and a smaller one in October (Davidson, 2005). A number of etiologies

associated with this trend have been postulated (Hakko, 2000). Some of these include the following:

■ A meteorological factor, associating drastic temperature and barometric pressure changes to human mental instability
■ Sociodemographic variables, such as the seasonal increase in social intercourse (e.g., increased social activity with the commencement of an academic year)
■ Biochemical variables due to possible seasonal variations in peripheral and central aspects of serotonergic function involved in depression and suicide

Types of Depressive Disorders

Major Depressive Disorder

Major depressive disorder (MDD) is characterized by depressed mood or loss of interest or pleasure in usual activities. Evidence will show impaired social and occupational functioning that has existed for at least 2 weeks, no history of manic behavior, and symptoms that cannot be attributed to use of substances or a general medical condition. Additionally, the diagnosis of MDD is specified according to whether it is a *single episode* (the individual's first encounter with a major depressive episode) or *recurrent* (the individual has a history of previous major depressive episodes). The diagnosis will also identify the degree of severity of symptoms (mild, moderate, or severe) and whether there is evidence of psychotic, catatonic, or melancholic features. The presence of anxiety and severity of suicide risk may also be noted. The *Diagnostic and Statistical Manual of Mental Disorders, Fifth Edition (DSM-5)* (APA, 2013) diagnostic criteria for major depressive disorder are presented in Box 25-1.

Persistent Depressive Disorder (Dysthymia)

Characteristics of **dysthymia** are similar to, if somewhat milder than, those ascribed to MDD. Individuals with this mood disturbance describe their mood as sad or "down in the dumps." There is no evidence of psychotic symptoms. The essential feature is a chronically depressed mood (or possibly an irritable mood in children or adolescents) for most of the day, more days than not, for at least 2 years (1 year for children and adolescents). The diagnosis is identified as *early onset* (occurring before age 21 years) or *late onset* (occurring at age 21 years or older). The *DSM-5* diagnostic criteria for dysthymia are presented in Box 25-2.

Premenstrual Dysphoric Disorder

The essential features of **premenstrual dysphoric disorder** include markedly depressed mood, excessive anxiety, mood swings, and decreased interest in activities during the week prior to menses, improving

BOX 25-1 Diagnostic Criteria for Major Depressive Disorder

A. Five (or more) of the following symptoms have been present during the same 2-week period and represent a change from previous functioning; at least one of the symptoms is either (1) depressed mood, or (2) loss of interest or pleasure. *Note:* Do not include symptoms that are clearly due to another medical condition.

1. Depressed mood most of the day, nearly every day, as indicated by either subjective report (e.g., feels sad, empty, or hopeless) or observation made by others (e.g., appears tearful). *Note:* In children and adolescents, can be irritable mood.
2. Markedly diminished interest or pleasure in all, or almost all, activities most of the day, nearly every day (as indicated by either subjective account or observation).
3. Significant weight loss when not dieting or weight gain (e.g., a change of more than 5% of body weight in a month), or decrease or increase in appetite nearly every day. *Note:* In children, consider failure to make expected weight gain.
4. Insomnia or hypersomnia nearly every day.
5. Psychomotor agitation or retardation nearly every day (observable by others, not merely subjective feelings of restlessness or being slowed down).
6. Fatigue or loss of energy nearly every day.
7. Feelings of worthlessness or excessive or inappropriate guilt (which may be delusional) nearly every day (not merely self-reproach or guilt about being sick).
8. Diminished ability to think or concentrate, or indecisiveness, nearly every day (either by subjective account or as observed by others).
9. Recurrent thoughts of death (not just fear of dying), recurrent suicidal ideation without a specific plan, or a suicide attempt or a specific plan for committing suicide.

B. The symptoms cause clinically significant distress or impairment in social, occupational, or other important areas of functioning.

C. The episode is not attributable to the physiological effects of a substance or another medical condition.
   Note: Criteria A-C represent a major depressive episode.
   Note: Responses to a significant loss (e.g., bereavement, financial ruin, losses from a natural disaster, a serious medical illness or disability) may include the feelings of intense sadness, rumination about the loss, insomnia, poor appetite, and weight loss noted in Criterion A, which may resemble a depressive episode. Although such symptoms may be understandable or considered appropriate to the loss, the presence of a major depressive episode in addition to the normal response to a significant loss should also be carefully considered. This decision inevitably requires the exercise of clinical judgment based on the individual's history and the cultural norms for the expression of distress in the context of loss.

D. The occurrence of the major depressive episode is not better explained by schizoaffective disorder, schizophrenia, schizophreniform disorder, delusional disorder, or other specified and unspecified schizophrenia spectrum and other psychotic disorders.

E. There has never been a manic episode or a hypomanic episode.

Specify:
With anxious distress
With mixed features
With melancholic features
With atypical features
With mood-congruent psychotic features
With mood-incongruent psychotic features
With catatonia
With peripartum onset
With seasonal pattern

Reprinted with permission from the *Diagnostic and Statistical Manual of Mental Disorders, Fifth Edition* (Copyright 2013). American Psychiatric Association.

shortly after the onset of menstruation, and becoming minimal or absent in the week postmenses (APA, 2013). The *DSM-5* diagnostic criteria for premenstrual dysphoric disorder are presented in Box 25-3.

Substance/Medication-Induced Depressive Disorder

The symptoms associated with a substance/medication-induced depressive disorder are considered to be the direct result of physiological effects of a substance (e.g., a drug of abuse, a medication, or toxin exposure), and they cause clinically significant distress or impairment in social, occupational, or other important areas of functioning. The depressed mood is associated with *intoxication* or *withdrawal* from substances such as alcohol, amphetamines, cocaine, hallucinogens, opioids, phencyclidine-like substances, sedatives, hypnotics, or

anxiolytics. The symptoms meet the full criteria for a relevant depressive disorder (APA, 2013).

A number of medications have been known to evoke mood symptoms. Classifications include anesthetics, analgesics, anticholinergics, anticonvulsants, antihypertensives, antiparkinsonian agents, antiulcer agents, cardiac medications, oral contraceptives, psychotropic medications, muscle relaxants, steroids, and sulfonamides. Some specific examples are included in the discussion of predisposing factors to depressive disorders.

Depressive Disorder Due to Another Medical Condition

This disorder is characterized by symptoms associated with a major depressive episode that are the direct physiological consequence of another medical condition (APA, 2013). The depression causes clinically

BOX 25-2 **Diagnostic Criteria for Persistent Depressive Disorder (Dysthymia)**

A. Depressed mood for most of the day, for more days than not, as indicated by either subjective account or observation by others, for at least 2 years. *Note:* In children and adolescents, mood can be irritable and duration must be at least 1 year.

B. Presence, while depressed, of two (or more) of the following:
1. Poor appetite or overeating
2. Insomnia or hypersomnia
3. Low energy or fatigue
4. Low self-esteem
5. Poor concentration or difficulty making decisions
6. Feelings of hopelessness

C. During the 2-year period (1 year for children or adolescents) of the disturbance, the individual has never been without the symptoms in Criteria A and B for more than 2 months at a time.

D. Criteria for a major depressive disorder may be continuously present for 2 years.

E. There has never been a manic episode or a hypomanic episode, and criteria have never been met for cyclothymic disorder.

F. The disturbance is not better explained by a persistent schizoaffective disorder, schizophrenia, delusional disorder, or other specified or unspecified schizophrenia spectrum and other psychotic disorder.

G. The symptoms are not attributable to the physiological effects of a substance (e.g., a drug of abuse, a medication) or another medical condition (e.g., hypothyroidism).

H. The symptoms cause clinically significant distress or impairment in social, occupational, or other important areas of functioning.

Specify if:
With anxious distress
With mixed features
With melancholic features
With atypical features
With mood-congruent psychotic features
With mood-incongruent psychotic features
With peripartum onset

Specify if:
With pure dysthymic syndrome
With persistent major depressive episode
With intermittent major depressive episodes, with current episode
With intermittent major depressive episodes, without current episode

Specify if:
In partial remission
In full remission

Specify if:
Early onset (onset before age 21 years)
Late onset (onset at age 21 years or older)

Specify if:
Mild
Moderate
Severe

Reprinted with permission from the *Diagnostic and Statistical Manual of Mental Disorders, Fifth Edition* (Copyright 2013). American Psychiatric Association.

BOX 25-3 **Diagnostic Criteria for Premenstrual Dysphoric Disorder**

A. In the majority of menstrual cycles, at least five symptoms must be present in the final week before the onset of menses, start to *improve* within a few days after the onset of menses, and become *minimal* or absent in the week postmenses.

B. One (or more) of the following symptoms must be present:
1. Marked affective lability (e.g., mood swings; feeling suddenly sad or tearful or increased sensitivity to rejection).
2. Marked irritability or anger or increased interpersonal conflicts.
3. Marked depressed mood, feelings of hopelessness, or self-deprecating thoughts.
4. Marked anxiety, tension, feelings of being keyed up or on edge.

C. One (or more) of the following symptoms must additionally be present, to reach a total of *five* symptoms when combined with symptoms from Criterion B above.
1. Decreased interest in usual activities (e.g., work, school, friends, hobbies).
2. Subjective difficulty in concentration.
3. Lethargy, easy fatigability, or marked lack of energy.
4. Marked change in appetite; overeating; or specific food cravings.

5. Hypersomnia or insomnia
6. A sense of being overwhelmed or out of control.
7. Physical symptoms, such as breast tenderness or swelling, joint or muscle pain, a sensation of "bloating," weight gain.

Note: The symptoms in Criteria A-C must have been met for most menstrual cycles that occurred in the preceding year.

D. The symptoms are associated with clinically significant distress or interferences with work, school, usual social activities, or relationships with others (e.g., avoidance of social activities, decreased productivity, and efficiency at work, school or home).

E. The disturbance is not merely an exacerbation of the symptoms of another disorder, such as major depressive disorder, panic disorder, persistent depressive disorder (dysthymia), or a personality disorder (although it may co-occur with any of these disorders).

F. Criteria A should be confirmed by prospective daily ratings during at least two symptomatic cycles. (*Note:* The diagnosis may be made provisionally prior to this confirmation).

G. The symptoms are not attributable to the physiological effects of a substance (e.g., a drug of abuse, a medication, or other treatment) or another medical condition (e.g., hyperthyroidism).

Reprinted with permission from the *Diagnostic and Statistical Manual of Mental Disorders, Fifth Edition* (Copyright 2013). American Psychiatric Association.

significant distress or impairment in social, occupational, or other important areas of functioning. Types of physiological influences are included in the discussion on predisposing factors to depression.

Predisposing Factors

The etiology of depression is unclear. No single theory or hypothesis has been postulated that substantiates a clear-cut explanation for the disease. Evidence continues to mount in support of multiple causations, recognizing the combined effects of genetic, biochemical, and psychosocial influences on an individual's susceptibility to depression. A number of theoretical postulates are presented here.

Biological Theories

Genetics

Affective illness has been the subject of considerable research on the relevance of hereditary factors. A genetic link has been suggested in numerous studies; however, a definitive mode of genetic transmission has yet to be demonstrated.

Twin Studies

Twin studies suggest a strong genetic factor in the etiology of affective illness. Joska and Stein (2008) reported that studies of monozygotic twins indicate that heritability of recurrent major depression is approximately 37 percent. They stated:

> In individuals who share all or almost all of their genetic material, genes account for about 37 percent of the risk of developing major depression. The effect of the individual environment and the interaction between genes and the said environment probably account for a large portion of the remaining risk. (p. 474)

Family Studies

Most family studies have shown that major depression is more common among first-degree biological relatives of people with the disorder than among the general population (Black & Andreasen, 2011). Indeed, the evidence to support an increased risk of depressive disorder in individuals with positive family history is quite compelling. It is unlikely that random environmental factors could cause the concentration of illness that is seen within families.

Adoption Studies

Further support for heritability as an etiological influence in depression comes from studies of the adopted offspring of affectively ill biological parents. These studies have indicated that biological children of parents with mood disorders are at increased risk of developing a mood disorder, even when they are reared by adoptive parents who do not have the disorder (Puri & Treasaden, 2011).

Biochemical Influences

Biogenic Amines

It has been hypothesized that depressive illness may be related to a deficiency of the neurotransmitters norepinepherine, serotonin, and dopamine, at functionally important receptor sites in the brain. Historically, the biogenic amine hypothesis of mood disorders grew out of the observation that reserpine, which depletes the brain of amines, was associated with the development of a depressive syndrome (Slattery, Hudson, & Nutt, 2004). The catecholamine norepinephrine has been identified as a key component in the mobilization of the body to deal with stressful situations. Neurons that contain serotonin are critically involved in the regulation of many psychobiological functions, such as mood, anxiety, arousal, vigilance, irritability, thinking, cognition, appetite, aggression, and circadian rhythm (Dubovsky, Davies, & Dubovsky, 2003). Tryptophan, the amino acid precursor of serotonin, has been shown to enhance the efficacy of antidepressant medications and, on occasion, to be effective as an antidepressant itself. The level of dopamine in the mesolimbic system of the brain is thought to exert a strong influence over human mood and behavior. A diminished supply of these biogenic amines inhibits the transmission of impulses from one neuronal fiber to another, causing a failure of the cells to fire or become charged (see Figure 25-1).

More recently, the biogenic amine hypothesis has been expanded to include another neurotransmitter, acetylcholine. Because cholinergic agents do have profound effects on mood, electroencephalograms, sleep, and neuroendocrine function, it has been suggested that the problem in depression and mania may be an imbalance between the biogenic amines and acetylcholine. Cholinergic transmission is thought to be excessive in depression and inadequate in mania (Dubovsky et al., 2003).

The precise role that any of the neurotransmitters plays in the etiology of depression is unknown. As the body of research grows, there is no doubt that increased knowledge regarding the biogenic amines will contribute to a greater capacity for understanding and treating affective illness.

Neuroendocrine Disturbances

Neuroendocrine disturbances may play a role in the pathogenesis or persistence of depressive illness. This notion has arisen in view of the marked disturbances in mood observed with the administration of certain hormones or in the presence of spontaneously occurring endocrine disease.

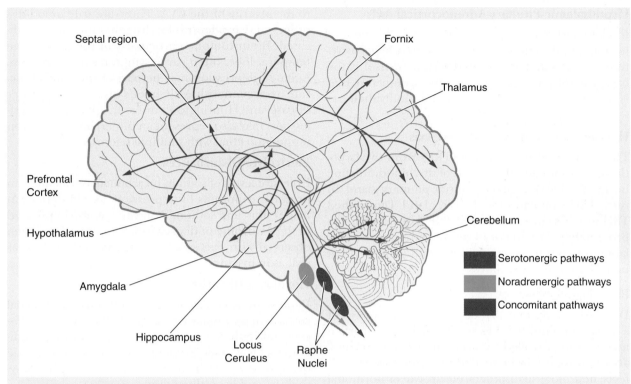

FIGURE 25-1 Neurobiology of depression.

NEUROTRANSMITTERS

Although other neurotransmitters have also been implicated in the pathophysiology of depression, disturbances in serotonin and norepinephrine have been the most extensively scrutinized.

Cell bodies of origin for the serotonin pathways lie within the raphe nuclei located in the brainstem. Those for norepinepherine originate in the locus ceruleus. Projections for both neurotransmitters extend throughout the forebrain, prefrontal cortex, cerebellum, and limbic system.

AREAS OF THE BRAIN AFFECTED

Areas of the brain affected by depression and the symptoms that they mediate include the following:
• Hippocampus: Memory impairments, feelings of worthlessness, hopelessness, and guilt
• Amygdala: Anhedonia, anxiety, reduced motivation
• Hypothalamus: Increased or decreased sleep and appetite; decreased energy and libido
• Other limbic structures: Emotional alterations
• Frontal cortex: Depressed mood; problems concentrating
• Cerebellum: Psychomotor retardation/agitation

MEDICATIONS AND THEIR EFFECTS IN THE BRAIN

All medications that increase serotonin, norepinephrine, or both can improve the emotional and vegetative symptoms of depression. Medications that produce these effects include those that block the presynaptic reuptake of the neurotransmitters or block receptors at nerve endings (tricyclics; SSRIs; SNRIs) and those that inhibit monoamine oxidase, an enzyme that is involved in the metabolism of the monoamines serotonin, norepinephrine, and dopamine (MAOIs).

Side effects of these medications relate to their specific neurotransmitter receptor-blocking action. Tricyclic and tetracyclic drugs (e.g., imipramine, amitriptyline, mirtazapine) block reuptake and/or receptors for serotonin, norepinephrine, acetylcholine, and histamine. SSRIs are selective serotonin reuptake inhibitors. Others, such as bupropion, venlafaxine, and duloxetine, block serotonin and norepinephrine reuptake and also are weak inhibitors of dopamine.

Blockade of norepinephrine reuptake results in side effects of tremors, cardiac arrhythmias, sexual dysfunction, and hypertension. Blockade of serotonin reuptake results in side effects of GI disturbances, increased agitation, and sexual dysfunction. Blockade of dopamine reuptake results in side effects of psychomotor activation. Blockade of acetylcholine reuptake results in dry mouth, blurred vision, constipation, and urinary retention. Blockade of histamine reuptake results in sedation, weight gain, and hypotension.

Hypothalamic-Pituitary-Adrenocortical Axis

In clients who are depressed, the normal system of hormonal inhibition fails, resulting in a hypersecretion of cortisol. This elevated serum cortisol is the basis for the dexamethasone suppression test that is sometimes used to determine if an individual has somatically treatable depression.

Hypothalamic-Pituitary-Thyroid Axis

Thyrotropin-releasing factor (TRF) from the hypothalamus stimulates the release of thyroid-stimulating hormone (TSH) from the anterior pituitary gland. In turn, TSH stimulates the thyroid gland. Diminished TSH response to administered TRF is observed in approximately 25 percent of depressed persons. This laboratory test has potential for identifying clients at high risk for affective illness.

Physiological Influences

Depressive symptoms that occur as a consequence of a non-mood disorder or as an adverse effect of certain medications are called a *secondary* depression. Secondary depression may be related to medication side effects, neurological disorders, electrolyte or hormonal disturbances, nutritional deficiencies, and other physiological or psychological conditions.

Medication Side Effects

A number of drugs, either alone or in combination with other medications, can produce a depressive syndrome. Most common among these drugs are those that have a direct effect on the central nervous system. Examples of these include the anxiolytics, antipsychotics, and sedative-hypnotics. Certain antihypertensive medications, such as propranolol and reserpine, have been known to produce depressive symptoms. One research study has found a statistically significant association between the acne medication isotretinoin (Accutane), and depression (Azoulay, Blais, Koren, LeLorier, & Berard, 2008). Depressed mood may also occur with any of the following medications, although the list is by no means all-inclusive (Sadock & Sadock, 2007):

■ Steroids: prednisone and cortisone
■ Hormones: estrogen and progesterone
■ Sedatives: barbiturates and benzodiazepines
■ Antibacterial and antifungal drugs: ampicillin, cycloserine, tetracycline, and sulfonamides
■ Antineoplastics: vincristine and zidovudine
■ Analgesics and anti-inflammatory drugs: opiates, ibuprofen, and phenylbutazone
■ Antiulcer: cimetidine

Neurological Disorders

An individual who has suffered a cardiovascular accident (CVA) may experience a despondency unrelated to the severity of the CVA. These are true mood disorders, and antidepressant drug therapy may be indicated. Brain tumors, particularly in the area of the temporal lobe, often cause symptoms of depression. Agitated depression may be part of the clinical picture associated with Alzheimer's disease, Parkinson's disease, and Huntington's disease. Agitation and restlessness may also represent an underlying depression in the individual with multiple sclerosis.

Electrolyte Disturbances

Excessive levels of sodium bicarbonate or calcium can produce symptoms of depression, as can deficits in magnesium and sodium. Potassium is also implicated in the syndrome of depression. Symptoms have been observed with excesses of potassium in the body, as well as in instances of potassium depletion.

Hormonal Disturbances

Depression is associated with dysfunction of the adrenal cortex and is commonly observed in both Addison's disease and Cushing's syndrome. Other endocrine conditions that may result in symptoms of depression include hypoparathyroidism, hyperparathyroidism, hypothyroidism, and hyperthyroidism.

An imbalance of the hormones estrogen and progesterone has been implicated in the predisposition to premenstrual dysphoric disorder. It is postulated that excess estrogen or a high estrogen-to-progesterone ratio during the luteal phase of the menstrual cycle is responsible for the symptoms associated with the disorder, although the exact etiology is unknown (Sadock & Sadock, 2007).

Nutritional Deficiencies

Deficiencies in vitamin B_1 (thiamine), vitamin B_6 (pyridoxine), vitamin B_{12}, niacin, vitamin C, iron, folic acid, zinc, calcium, and potassium may produce symptoms of depression (Schimelpfening, 2012).

A number of nutritional alterations have also been indicated in the etiology of premenstrual dysphoric disorder. They include deficiencies in the B vitamins, calcium, magnesium, manganese, vitamin E, and linolenic acid (Frackiewicz & Shiovitz, 2001). Glucose tolerance fluctuations, abnormal fatty acid metabolism, and sensitivity to caffeine and alcohol may also play a role in bringing about the symptoms associated with this disorder. No definitive evidence exists to support any specific nutritional alteration in the etiology of these symptoms.

Other Physiological Conditions

Other conditions that have been associated with secondary depression include collagen disorders, such as systemic lupus erythematosus (SLE) and polyarteritis nodosa; cardiovascular disease, such as cardiomyopathy, congestive heart failure, and myocardial infarction; infections, such as encephalitis, hepatitis, mononucleosis, pneumonia, and syphilis; and metabolic disorders, such as diabetes mellitus and porphyria.

Psychosocial Theories

Psychoanalytical Theory

Freud (1957) presented his classic paper "Mourning and Melancholia" in 1917. He defined the distinguishing features of melancholia as:

> . . . a profoundly painful dejection, cessation of interest in the outside world, loss of the capacity to love, inhibition of all activity, and a lowering of the self-regarding feelings to a degree that finds utterances in self-reproaches and self-revilings, and culminates in a delusional expectation of punishment.

He observed that melancholia occurs after the loss of a loved object, either actually by death or emotionally by rejection, or the loss of some other abstraction of value to the individual. Freud indicated that in melancholia, the depressed patient's rage is internally directed because of identification with the lost object (Sadock & Sadock, 2007).

Freud believed that the individual predisposed to melancholia experienced ambivalence in love relationships. He postulated, therefore, that once the loss had been incorporated into the self (ego), the hostile part of the ambivalence that had been felt for the lost object is then turned inward against the ego.

Learning Theory

The model of "learned helplessness" arises out of Seligman's (1973) experiments with dogs. The animals were exposed to electrical stimulation from which they could not escape. Later, when they were given the opportunity to avoid the traumatic experience, they reacted with helplessness and made no attempt to escape. A similar state of helplessness exists in humans who have experienced numerous failures (either real or perceived). The individual abandons any further attempt to succeed. Seligman theorized that learned helplessness predisposes individuals to depression by imposing a feeling of lack of control over their life situation. They become depressed because they feel helpless; they have learned that whatever they do is futile. This can be especially damaging very early in life, because the sense of mastery over one's environment is an important foundation for future emotional development.

Object Loss Theory

The theory of object loss suggests that depressive illness occurs as a result of having been abandoned by or otherwise separated from a significant other during the first 6 months of life. Because during this period the mother represents the child's main source of security, she is considered to be the "object." This absence of attachment, which may be either physical or emotional, leads to feelings of helplessness and despair that contribute to lifelong patterns of depression in response to loss.

The concept of "anaclitic depression" was introduced in 1946 by psychiatrist René Spitz to refer to children who became depressed after being separated from their mothers for an extended period of time during the first year of life (Cartwright, 2004). The condition included behaviors such as excessive crying, anorexia, withdrawal, **psychomotor retardation**, stupor, and a generalized impairment in the normal process of growth and development. Some researchers suggest that loss in adult life afflicts people much more severely in the form of depression if the subjects have suffered early childhood loss.

Cognitive Theory

Beck and colleagues (1979) proposed a theory suggesting that the primary disturbance in depression is cognitive rather than affective. The underlying cause of the depressive affect is seen as cognitive distortions that result in negative, defeated attitudes. Beck and colleagues identified three cognitive distortions that they believe serve as the basis for depression:

1. Negative expectations of the environment.
2. Negative expectations of the self.
3. Negative expectations of the future.

These cognitive distortions arise out of a defect in cognitive development, and the individual feels inadequate, worthless, and rejected by others. Outlook for the future is one of pessimism and hopelessness.

Cognitive theorists believe that depression is the product of negative thinking. This is in contrast to the other theorists, who suggest that negative thinking occurs when an individual is depressed. **Cognitive therapy** focuses on helping the individual to alter mood by changing the way he or she thinks. The individual is taught to control negative thought distortions that lead to pessimism, lethargy, procrastination, and low self-esteem (see Chapter 19).

The Transactional Model

As is clearly evident, no single theory or hypothesis exists to substantiate a clear-cut explanation for depressive disorder. Evidence continues to mount in support of multiple causation. The transactional model recognizes the combined effects of genetic, biochemical, and psychosocial influences on an individual's susceptibility to depression. The dynamics of depression using the Transactional Model of Stress/Adaptation are presented in Figure 25-2.

Developmental Implications

Childhood

Only in recent years has a consensus developed among investigators identifying major depressive

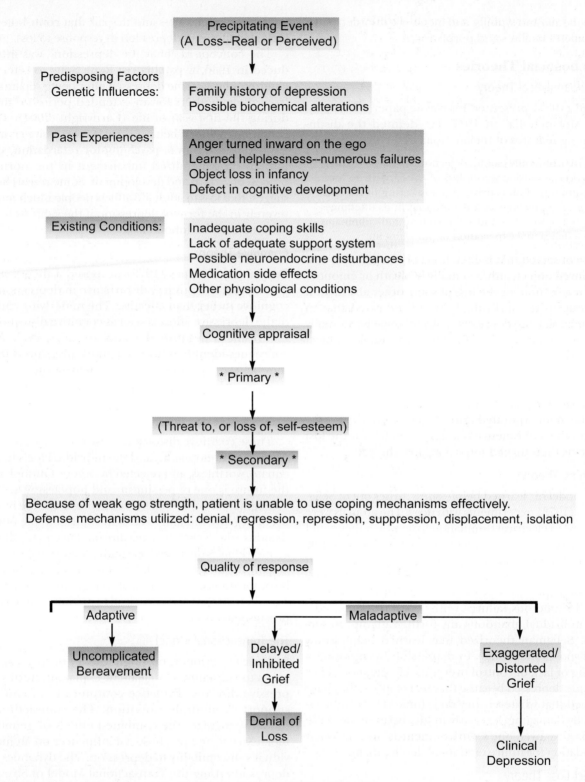

Precipitating Event
(A Loss--Real or Perceived)

Predisposing Factors
Genetic Influences:

Family history of depression
Possible biochemical alterations

Past Experiences:

Anger turned inward on the ego
Learned helplessness--numerous failures
Object loss in infancy
Defect in cognitive development

Existing Conditions:

Inadequate coping skills
Lack of adequate support system
Possible neuroendocrine disturbances
Medication side effects
Other physiological conditions

Cognitive appraisal

* Primary *

(Threat to, or loss of, self-esteem)

* Secondary *

Because of weak ego strength, patient is unable to use coping mechanisms effectively.
Defense mechanisms utilized: denial, regression, repression, suppression, displacement, isolation

Quality of response

Adaptive   Maladaptive

Uncomplicated   Delayed/   Exaggerated/
Bereavement   Inhibited   Distorted
                       Grief   Grief

                       Denial of
                       Loss
                                             Clinical
                                             Depression

FIGURE 25–2 The dynamics of depression using the Transactional Model of Stress/Adaptation.

disorder as an entity in children and adolescents that can be identified using criteria similar to those used for adults (Dubovsky et al., 2003). It is not uncommon, however, for the symptoms of depression to be manifested differently in childhood, and the picture changes with age (Dopheide, 2006; Joska & Stein, 2008; Tempfer, 2006):

1. **Up to age 3:** Signs may include feeding problems, tantrums, lack of playfulness and emotional expressiveness, failure to thrive, or delays in speech and gross motor development.
2. **From ages 3 to 5:** Common symptoms may include accident proneness, phobias, aggressiveness, and excessive self-reproach for minor infractions.
3. **From ages 6 to 8:** There may be vague physical complaints and aggressive behavior. They may cling to parents and avoid new people and challenges. They may lag behind their classmates in social skills and academic competence.
4. **From ages 9 to 12:** Common symptoms include morbid thoughts and excessive worrying. They may reason that they are depressed because they have disappointed their parents in some way. There may be lack of interest in playing with friends.

Other symptoms of childhood depression may include hyperactivity, delinquency, school problems, psychosomatic complaints, sleeping and eating disturbances, social isolation, delusional thinking, and suicidal thoughts or actions. The APA (2013) has included a new diagnostic category in the Depressive Disorders chapter of the *DSM-5*. This childhood disorder is called *disruptive mood dysregulation disorder*. The diagnostic criteria for disruptive mood dysregulation disorder are presented in Box 25-4.

Children may become depressed for various reasons. In many depressed children, there is a genetic predisposition toward the condition, which is then precipitated by a stressful situation. Common precipitating factors include physical or emotional detachment by the primary caregiver, parental separation or divorce, death of a loved one (person or pet), a move, academic failure, or physical illness. In any event, the common denominator is loss.

The focus of therapy with depressed children is to alleviate the child's symptoms and strengthen the child's coping and adaptive skills, with the hope of possibly preventing future psychological problems. Some studies have shown that untreated childhood depression may lead to subsequent problems in adolescence

BOX 25-4 Diagnostic Criteria for Disruptive Mood Dysregulation Disorder

A. Severe recurrent temper outbursts manifested verbally (e.g., verbal rages) and/or behaviorally (e.g., physical aggression toward people or property) that are grossly out of proportion in intensity or duration to the situation or provocation.
B. The temper outbursts are inconsistent with developmental level.
C. The temper outbursts occur, on average, three or more times per week.
D. The mood between temper outbursts is persistently irritable or angry most of the day, nearly every day, and is observable by others (e.g., parents, teachers, peers).
E. Criteria A-D have been present for 12 or more months. Throughout that time, the individual has not had a period lasting 3 or more consecutive months without all of the symptoms of Criteria A-D.
F. Criteria A and D are present in at least two of three settings (i.e., at home, at school, with peers) and are severe in at least one of these.
G. The diagnosis should not be made for the first time before age 6 or after age 18 years.
H. By history or observation, the age at onset of Criteria A-E is before 10 years.
I. There has never been a distinct period lasting more than 1 day during which the full symptom criteria, except

duration, for a manic or hypomanic episode have been met. *Note:* Developmentally appropriate mood elevation, such as occurs in the context of a highly positive event or its anticipation, should not be considered as a symptom of mania or hypomania.
J. The behaviors do not occur exclusively during an episode of major depressive disorder and are not better explained by another mental disorder (e.g., autism spectrum disorder, posttraumatic stress disorder, separation anxiety disorder, persistent depressive disorder [dysthymia]).
Note: This diagnosis cannot coexist with oppositional defiant disorder, intermittent explosive disorder, or bipolar disorder, though it can coexist with others, including major depressive disorder, attention-deficit/hyperactivity disorder, conduct disorder, and substance use disorders. Individuals whose symptoms meet criteria for both disruptive mood dysregulation disorder and oppositional defiant disorder should only be given the diagnosis of disruptive mood dysregulation disorder. If an individual has ever experienced a manic or hypomanic episode, the diagnosis of disruptive mood dysregulation disorder should not be assigned.
K. The symptoms are not attributable to the physiological effects of a substance or to another medical or neurological condition.

and adult life. Most children are treated on an outpatient basis. Hospitalization of the depressed child usually occurs only if he or she is actively suicidal, when the home environment precludes adherence to a treatment regimen, or if the child needs to be separated from the home because of psychosocial deprivation.

Parental and family therapy are commonly used to help the younger depressed child. Recovery is facilitated by emotional support and guidance to family members. Children older than age 8 years usually participate in family therapy. In some situations, individual treatment may be appropriate for older children. Medications, such as antidepressants, can be important in the treatment of children, especially for the more serious and recurrent forms of depression. The selective serotonin reuptake inhibitors (SSRIs) have been used with success, particularly in combination with psychosocial therapies. However, because there has been some concern that the use of antidepressant medications may cause suicidal behavior in young people, the U.S. Food and Drug Administration (FDA) has applied a "black box" label warning (described in the next section) to all antidepressant medications. The National Institute of Mental Health (2013) stated:

> Those who are prescribed an [antidepressant] medication should receive ongoing medical monitoring. Children already taking an [antidepressant] should remain on the medication if it has been helpful, but should be carefully monitored by a doctor for side effects. Parents should promptly seek medical advice and evaluation if their child or adolescent experiences suicidal thinking or behavior, nervousness, agitation, irritability, mood instability, or sleeplessness that either emerges or worsens during treatment with [antidepressant] medications.

Adolescence

Depression may be even harder to recognize in an adolescent than in a younger child. Feelings of sadness, loneliness, anxiety, and hopelessness associated with depression may be perceived as the normal emotional stresses of growing up. Therefore, many young people whose symptoms are attributed to the "normal adjustments" of adolescence do not get the help they need. Depression is a major cause of suicide among teens, and suicide is the second leading cause of death in the 15- to 24-year-old age group (National Center for Health Statistics [NCHS], 2012). The World Health Organization (WHO) recently reported that depression is the main cause of illness and disability in adolescents worldwide (WHO, 2014).

Common symptoms of depression in the adolescent are inappropriately expressed anger, aggressiveness, running away, delinquency, social withdrawal, sexual acting out, substance abuse, restlessness, and apathy.

Loss of self-esteem, sleeping and eating disturbances, and psychosomatic complaints are also common.

What, then, is the indicator that differentiates mood disorder from the typical stormy behavior of adolescence? A visible manifestation of *behavioral change that lasts for several weeks* is the best clue for a mood disorder. Examples include the normally outgoing and extroverted adolescent who has become withdrawn and antisocial, the good student who previously received consistently high marks but is now failing and skipping classes, and the usually self-confident teenager who is now inappropriately irritable and defensive with others.

Adolescents become depressed for all the same reasons that were discussed under childhood depression. In adolescence, however, depression is a common manifestation of the stress and independence conflicts associated with the normal maturation process. Depression may also be the response to death of a parent, other relative, or friend, or to a breakup with a boyfriend or girlfriend. This perception of abandonment by parents or closest peer relationship is thought to be the most frequent immediate precipitant to adolescent suicide.

Treatment of the depressed adolescent is often conducted on an outpatient basis. Hospitalization may be required in cases of severe depression or threat of imminent suicide, when a family situation is such that treatment cannot be carried out in the home, when the physical condition precludes self-care of biological needs, or when the adolescent has indicated possible harm to self or others in the family.

In addition to supportive psychosocial intervention, antidepressant therapy may be part of the treatment of adolescent mood disorders. However, as mentioned previously, the FDA has issued a public health advisory warning the public about the increased risk of suicidal thoughts and behavior in children and adolescents being treated with antidepressant medications. The black box warning label on all antidepressant medications describes this risk and emphasizes the need for close monitoring of clients started on these medications. The advisory language does not prohibit the use of antidepressants in children and adolescents. Rather, it warns of the risk of suicidality and encourages prescribers to balance this risk with clinical need.

Fluoxetine (Prozac) has been approved by the FDA to treat depression in children and adolescents, and escitalopram (Lexipro) was approved in 2009 for treatment of MDD in adolescents aged 12 to 17 years. The other SSRI medications, such as sertraline, citalopram, and paroxetine, and the SNRI antidepressants duloxetine, venlafaxine, and desvenlafaxine have not been approved for treatment of depression in children or adolescents, although they have been prescribed to children by physicians in "off-label use"—a use other than the

FDA-approved use. In June 2003, the FDA recommended that paroxetine not be used in children and adolescents for the treatment of major depressive disorder.

Senescence

Depression is the most common psychiatric disorder of the elderly, who make up 13.3 percent of the general population of the United States (Administration on Aging, 2013). This is not surprising considering the disproportionate value our society places on youth, vigor, and uninterrupted productivity. These societal attitudes continually nurture the feelings of low self-esteem, helplessness, and hopelessness that become more pervasive and intensive with advanced age. Further, the aging individual's adaptive coping strategies may be seriously challenged by major stressors, such as financial problems, physical illness, changes in bodily functioning, and an increasing awareness of approaching death. The problem is often intensified by the numerous losses individuals experience during this period in life, such as spouse, friends, children, home, and independence. A phenomenon called *bereavement overload* occurs when individuals experience so many losses in their lives that they are not able to resolve one grief response before another one begins. Bereavement overload predisposes elderly individuals to depressive illness.

Although they make up only slightly more than 13 percent of the population, the elderly account for approximately 16 percent of the suicides in the United States (NCHS, 2013). The highest number of suicides is among white men 85 years of age and older, at almost 4 times the national rate.

Symptoms of depression in the elderly are not very different from those in younger adults. However, depressive syndromes are often confused with other illnesses associated with the aging process. Symptoms of depression are often misdiagnosed as neurocognitive disorder (NCD), when in fact the memory loss, confused thinking, or apathy symptomatic of NCD actually may be the result of depression. The early awakening and reduced appetite typical of depression are common among many older people who are not depressed. Compounding this situation is the fact that many medical conditions, such as endocrinological, neurological, nutritional, and metabolic disorders, often present with classic symptoms of depression. Many medications commonly used by the elderly, such as antihypertensives, corticosteroids, and analgesics, can also produce a depressant effect.

Depression does accompany many of the illnesses that afflict older people, such as Parkinson's disease, cancer, arthritis, and the early stages of Alzheimer's disease. Treating depression in these situations can reduce unnecessary suffering and help afflicted individuals cope with their medical problems.

The most effective treatment of depression in the elderly individual is thought to be a combination of psychosocial and biological approaches. Antidepressant medications are administered with consideration for age-related physiological changes in absorption, distribution, elimination, and brain receptor sensitivity. Because of these changes, plasma concentrations of these medications can reach very high levels despite moderate oral doses.

Electroconvulsive therapy (ECT) remains one of the safest and most effective treatments for major depression in the elderly. The response to ECT appears to be slower with advancing age, and the therapeutic effects are of limited duration. However, it may be considered the treatment of choice for the elderly individual who is an acute suicidal risk or is unable to tolerate antidepressant medications.

Other therapeutic approaches include interpersonal, behavioral, cognitive, group, and family psychotherapies. Appropriate treatment of the depressed elderly individual can bring relief from suffering and offer a new lease on life with a feeling of renewed productivity.

Postpartum Depression

The severity of depression in the postpartum period varies from a feeling of the "blues," to moderate depression, to psychotic depression or melancholia. Of women who give birth, approximately 50 to 85 percent experience the "blues" following delivery (Mehta & Sheth, 2006). The incidence of moderate depression is 10 to 20 percent. Severe, or psychotic, depression occurs rarely, in about 1 or 2 out of 1000 postpartum women.

Symptoms of the "maternity blues" include tearfulness, despondency, anxiety, and subjectively impaired concentration appearing in the early puerperium. The symptoms usually begin within 48 hours of delivery, peak at about 3 to 5 days, and last approximately 2 weeks (Mehta & Sheth, 2006).

Symptoms of moderate **postpartum depression** have been described as depressed mood varying from day to day, with more bad days than good, tending to be worse toward evening and associated with fatigue, irritability, loss of appetite, sleep disturbances, and loss of libido. In addition, the new mother expresses a great deal of concern about her inability to care for her baby. These symptoms begin somewhat later than those described in the "maternity blues," and take from a few weeks to several months to abate.

Postpartum melancholia, or depressive psychosis, is characterized by depressed mood, agitation, indecision, lack of concentration, guilt, and an abnormal attitude toward bodily functions. There may be lack of interest in, or rejection of, the baby, or a morbid fear that the baby may be harmed. Risks of suicide and infanticide should not be overlooked. These symptoms usually develop during the first few days following birth, but may occur later (Mehta & Sheth, 2006).

The etiology of postpartum depression remains unclear. "Maternity blues" may be associated with hormonal changes, tryptophan metabolism, or alterations in membrane transport during the early postpartum period. Besides being exposed to these same somatic changes, the woman who experiences moderate to severe symptoms probably possesses a vulnerability to depression related to heredity, upbringing, early life experiences, personality, or social circumstances. A history of depression appears to be a risk factor for postpartum depression (Sword, Clark, Hegadoren, Brooks, & Kingston, 2012). The etiology of postpartum depression may very likely be a combination of hormonal, metabolic, and psychosocial influences.

Treatment of postpartum depression varies with the severity of the illness. Psychotic depression may be treated with antidepressant medication, along with supportive psychotherapy, group therapy, and possibly family therapy. Moderate depression may be relieved with supportive psychotherapy and continuing assistance with home management until the symptoms subside. "Maternity blues" usually needs no treatment beyond a word of reassurance from the physician or nurse that these feelings are common and will soon pass. Extra support and comfort from significant others also is important.

Application of the Nursing Process

Background Assessment Data

Symptomatology of depression can be viewed on a continuum according to severity of the illness. All individuals become depressed from time to time. These are the transient symptoms that accompany the everyday disappointments of life. Examples of the disappointments include failing an examination or breaking up with a boyfriend or girlfriend. Transient symptoms of depression subside relatively quickly as the individual advances toward other goals and achievements.

Mild depressive episodes occur when the grief process is triggered in response to the loss of a valued object. This can occur with the loss of a loved one, pet, friend, home, or significant other. As one is able to work through the stages of grief, the loss is accepted, symptoms subside, and activities of daily living are resumed within a few weeks. If this does not occur, grief is prolonged or exaggerated, and symptoms intensify.

Moderate depression occurs when grief is prolonged or exaggerated. The individual becomes fixed in the anger stage of the grief response, and the anger is turned inward on the self. All of the feelings associated with normal grieving are exaggerated out of proportion, and the individual is unable to function without assistance. Dysthymia is an example of moderate depression.

Severe depression is an intensification of the symptoms associated with the moderate level. The individual who is severely depressed may also demonstrate a loss of contact with reality. This level is associated with a complete lack of pleasure in all activities, and ruminations about suicide are common. Major depressive disorder is an example of severe depression. A continuum of depression is presented in Figure 25-3.

A number of assessment rating scales are available for measuring severity of depressive symptoms. Some are meant to be clinician administered, whereas others may be self-administered. Examples of self-rating scales include the Zung Self-Rating Depression Scale and the Beck Depression Inventory. One of the most widely used clinician-administered scales is the Hamilton Depression Rating Scale (HDRS). It has been reviewed and revised over the years, and exists today in several versions. The original version (see Box 25-5) contains 17 items and is designed to measure mood, guilty feelings, suicidal ideation, sleep disturbances, anxiety levels, and weight loss.

Symptoms of depression can be described as alterations in four spheres of human functioning: (1) affective, (2) behavioral, (3) cognitive, and (4) physiological. Alterations within these spheres differ according to degree of severity of symptomatology.

Transient Depression

Symptoms at this level of the continuum are not necessarily dysfunctional. Alterations include the following:

■ **Affective:** sadness, dejection, feeling downhearted, having the "blues."

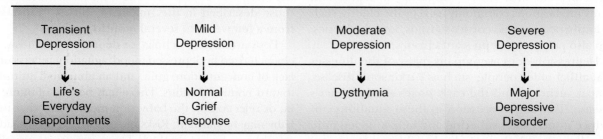

FIGURE 25–3 A continuum of depression.

BOX 25-5 **Hamilton Depression Rating Scale (HDRS)**

Instructions: For each item, circle the number to select the one "cue" that best characterizes the patient.

1. **Depressed Mood** (sadness, hopeless, helpless, worthless)
   0 = Absent.
   1 = These feeling states indicated only on questioning.
   2 = These feeling states spontaneously reported verbally.
   3 = Communicates feeling states nonverbally, i.e., through facial expression, posture, voice, tendency to weep.
   4 = Patient reports virtually only these feeling states in spontaneous verbal and nonverbal communication.

2. **Feelings of Guilt**
   0 = Absent.
   1 = Self reproach; feels he/she has let people down.
   2 = Ideas of guilt or rumination over past errors or sinful deeds.
   3 = Present illness is a punishment. Delusions of guilt.
   4 = Hears accusatory or denunciatory voices and/or experiences threatening visual hallucinations.

3. **Suicide**
   0 = Absent.
   1 = Feels life is not worth living.
   2 = Wishes he/she were dead or any thoughts of possible death to self.
   3 = Suicidal ideas or gesture.
   4 = Attempts at suicide (any serious attempt rates 4).

4. **Insomnia: Early in the Night**
   0 = No difficulty falling asleep.
   1 = Complains of occasional difficulty falling asleep, i.e., more than 1/2 hour.
   2 = Complains of nightly difficulty falling asleep.

5. **Insomnia: Middle of the Night**
   0 = No difficulty.
   1 = Complains of being restless and disturbed during the night.
   2 = Waking during the night—any getting out of bed rates 2 (except for purposes of voiding).

6. **Insomnia: Early Hours of the Morning**
   0 = No difficulty.
   1 = Waking in early hours of the morning, but goes back to sleep.
   2 = Unable to fall asleep again if he/she gets out of bed.

7. **Work and Activities**
   0 = No difficulty.
   1 = Thoughts and feelings of incapacity, fatigue, or weakness related to activities, work, or hobbies.
   2 = Loss of interest in activity, hobbies, or work—either directly reported by patient, or indirectly in listlessness, indecision, and vacillation (feels he/she has to push self to work or activities).

   3 = Decrease in actual time spent in activities or decrease in productivity. Rate 3 if patient does not spend at least 3 hours a day in activities (job or hobbies), excluding routine chores.
   4 = Stopped working because of present illness. Rate 4 if patient engages in no activities except routine chores, or if does not perform routine chores unassisted.

8. **Psychomotor Retardation** (slowness of thought and speech, impaired ability to concentrate, decreased motor activity)
   0 = Normal speech and thought.
   1 = Slight retardation during the interview.
   2 = Obvious retardation during the interview.
   3 = Interview difficult.
   4 = Complete stupor.

9. **Agitation**
   0 = None.
   1 = Fidgetiness.
   2 = Playing with hands, hair, etc.
   3 = Moving about, can't sit still.
   4 = Hand wringing, nail biting, hair pulling, biting of lips.

10. **Anxiety (Psychic)**
    0 = No difficulty.
    1 = Subjective tension and irritability.
    2 = Worrying about minor matters.
    3 = Apprehensive attitude apparent in face or speech.
    4 = Fears expressed without questioning.

11. **Anxiety (Somatic):** Physiological concomitants of anxiety (e.g., dry mouth, indigestion, diarrhea, cramps, belching, palpitations, headache, tremor, hyperventilation, sighing, urinary frequency, sweating, flushing)
    0 = Absent.   3 = Severe.
    1 = Mild.   4 = Incapacitating.
    2 = Moderate.

12. **Somatic Symptoms (Gastrointestinal)**
    0 = None.
    1 = Loss of appetite, but eating without encouragement. Heavy feelings in abdomen.
    2 = Difficulty eating without urging from others. Requests or requires medication for constipation or gastrointestinal symptoms.

13. **Somatic Symptoms (General)**
    0 = None.
    1 = Heaviness in limbs, back or head. Backaches, headache, muscle aches. Loss of energy and fatigability.
    2 = Any clear-cut symptom rates 2.

Continued

BOX 25-5 Hamilton Depression Rating Scale (HDRS)—cont'd

14. **Genital Symptoms** (e.g., loss of libido, impaired sexual performance, menstrual disturbances)
    0 = Absent.
    1 = Mild.
    2 = Severe.

15. **Hypochondriasis**
    0 = Not present.
    1 = Self-absorption (bodily).
    2 = Preoccupation with health.
    3 = Frequent complaints, requests for help, etc.
    4 = Hypochondriacal delusions.

16. **Loss of Weight (Rate *either* A *or* B)**
    A. **According to subjective patient history:**
       0 = No weight loss.
       1 = Probably weight loss associated with present illness.
       2 = Definite weight loss associated with present illness.

B. **According to objective weekly measurements:**
    0 = Less than 1 lb. weight loss in week.
    1 = Greater than 1 lb. weight loss in week.
    2 = Greater than 2 lb. weight loss in week.

17. **Insight**
    0 = Acknowledges being depressed and ill.
    1 = Acknowledges illness but attributes cause to bad food, climate, overwork, virus, need for rest, etc.
    2 = Denies being ill at all.

SCORING:
0–6 = No evidence of depressive illness
7–17 = Mild depression
18–24 = Moderate depression
> 24 = Severe depression

TOTAL SCORE_____

SOURCE: Hamilton, M. (1960). A rating scale for depression. *Journal of Neurology, Neurosurgery, & Psychiatry, 23,* 56-62. The HDRS is in the public domain.

- **Behavioral:** some crying possible.
- **Cognitive:** some difficulty getting mind off of one's disappointment.
- **Physiological:** feeling tired and listless.

Mild Depression

Symptoms at the mild level of depression are identified by those associated with uncomplicated grieving. Alterations at the mild level include the following:

- **Affective:** denial of feelings, anger, anxiety, guilt, helplessness, hopelessness, sadness, despondency.
- **Behavioral:** tearfulness, regression, restlessness, agitation, withdrawal.
- **Cognitive:** preoccupation with the loss, self-blame, ambivalence, blaming others.
- **Physiological:** anorexia or overeating, insomnia or hypersomnia, headache, backache, chest pain, or other symptoms associated with the loss of a significant other.

Moderate Depression

Dysthymia, which is an example of moderate depression, represents a more problematic disturbance. Symptoms associated with this disorder include the following:

- **Affective:** feelings of sadness, dejection, helplessness, powerlessness, hopelessness; gloomy and pessimistic outlook; low self-esteem; difficulty experiencing pleasure in activities.
- **Behavioral:** sluggish physical movements (i.e., psychomotor retardation); slumped posture; slowed speech; limited verbalizations, possibly consisting of ruminations about life's failures or regrets; social isolation with a focus on the self; increased use of substances possible; self-destructive behavior possible; decreased interest in personal hygiene and grooming.
- **Cognitive:** slowed thinking processes; difficulty concentrating and directing attention; obsessive and repetitive thoughts, generally portraying pessimism and negativism; verbalizations and behavior reflecting suicidal ideation.
- **Physiological:** anorexia or overeating; insomnia or hypersomnia; sleep disturbances; amenorrhea; decreased libido; headaches; backaches; chest pain; abdominal pain; low energy level; fatigue and listlessness; feeling best early in the morning and continually worse as the day progresses. This may be related to the diurnal variation in the level of neurotransmitters that affect mood and level of activity.

Severe Depression

Severe depression is characterized by an intensification of the symptoms described for moderate depression. Examples of severe depression include major depressive disorder and bipolar depression. Symptoms at the severe level of depression include the following:

- **Affective:** feelings of total despair, hopelessness, and worthlessness; flat (unchanging) affect, appearing devoid of emotional tone; prevalent feelings of nothingness and emptiness; apathy; loneliness; sadness; inability to feel pleasure.

- **Behavioral:** psychomotor retardation so severe that physical movement may literally come to a standstill, or psychomotor behavior manifested by rapid, agitated, purposeless movements; slumped posture; sitting in a curled-up position; walking slowly and rigidly; virtually nonexistent communication (when verbalizations do occur, they may reflect delusional thinking); no personal hygiene and grooming; social isolation is common, with virtually no inclination toward interaction with others.
- **Cognitive:** prevalent delusional thinking, with delusions of persecution and somatic delusions being most common; confusion, indecisiveness, and an inability to concentrate; hallucinations reflecting misinterpretations of the environment; excessive self-deprecation, self-blame, and thoughts of suicide.

NOTE: Because of the low energy level and slow thought processes, the individual may be unable to follow through on suicidal ideas. However, the desire is strong at this level.

- **Physiological:** a general slowdown of the entire body, reflected in sluggish digestion, constipation, and urinary retention; amenorrhea; impotence; diminished libido; anorexia; weight loss; difficulty falling asleep and awakening very early in the morning; feeling worse early in the morning and somewhat better as the day progresses. As with moderate depression, this may reflect the diurnal variation in the level of neurotransmitters that affect mood and activity.

Diagnosis/Outcome Identification

Using information collected during the assessment, the nurse completes the client database, from which the selection of appropriate nursing diagnoses is determined. Table 25-1 presents a list of client behaviors and the NANDA nursing diagnoses that correspond to those behaviors, which may be used in planning care for the depressed client.

Outcome Criteria

The following criteria may be used for measurement of outcomes in the care of the depressed client.

TABLE 25–1 **Assigning Nursing Diagnoses to Behaviors Commonly Associated With Depression**	
BEHAVIORS	NURSING DIAGNOSES
Depressed mood; feelings of hopelessness and worthlessness; anger turned inward on the self; misinterpretations of reality; suicidal ideation, plan, and available means	Risk for suicide
Depression, preoccupation with thoughts of loss, self-blame, grief avoidance, inappropriate expression of anger, decreased functioning in life roles	Complicated grieving
Expressions of helplessness, uselessness, guilt, and shame; hypersensitivity to slight or criticism; negative, pessimistic outlook; lack of eye contact; self-negating verbalizations	Low self-esteem
Apathy, verbal expressions of having no control, dependence on others to fulfill needs	Powerlessness
Expresses anger toward God, expresses lack of meaning in life, sudden changes in spiritual practices, refuses interactions with significant others or with spiritual leaders	Spiritual distress
Withdrawn, uncommunicative, seeks to be alone, dysfunctional interaction with others, discomfort in social situations	Social isolation/Impaired social interaction
Inappropriate thinking, confusion, difficulty concentrating, impaired problem-solving ability, inaccurate interpretation of environment, memory deficit	Disturbed thought processes*
Weight loss, poor muscle tone, pale conjunctiva and mucous membranes, poor skin turgor, weakness	Imbalanced nutrition: Less than body requirements
Difficulty falling asleep, difficulty staying asleep, lack of energy, difficulty concentrating, verbal reports of not feeling well rested	Insomnia
Uncombed hair, disheveled clothing, offensive body odor	Self-care deficit (hygiene, grooming)

*This diagnosis has been retired from the NANDA-I list of approved diagnoses. It is used in this instance because it is most compatible with the identified behaviors.

The client:

- Has experienced no physical harm to self.
- Discusses the loss with staff and family members.
- No longer idealizes or obsesses about the lost entity/concept.
- Sets realistic goals for self.
- Is no longer afraid to attempt new activities.
- Is able to identify aspects of self-control over life situation.
- Expresses personal satisfaction and support from spiritual practices.
- Interacts willingly and appropriately with others.
- Is able to maintain reality orientation.
- Is able to concentrate, reason, and solve problems.
- Eats a well-balanced diet with snacks, to prevent weight loss and maintain nutritional status.
- Sleeps 6 to 8 hours per night and reports feeling well rested.
- Bathes, washes and combs hair, and dresses in clean clothing without assistance.

Planning/Implementation

The following section presents a group of selected nursing diagnoses, with short- and long-term goals and nursing interventions for each.

Some institutions are using a case management model to coordinate care (see Chapter 9 for more detailed explanation). In case management models, the plan of care may take the form of a critical pathway.

Risk for Suicide

Risk for suicide is defined as "at risk for self-inflicted, life-threatening injury" (NANDA-International [NANDA-I], 2012, p. 452). For additional interventions and to view this nursing diagnosis in care plan format, see Chapter 17.

Client Goals

Outcome criteria include short- and long-term goals. Timelines are individually determined.

Short-Term Goals

- Client will seek out staff when feeling urge to harm self.
- Client will make short-term verbal (or written) contract with nurse not to harm self.
- Client will not harm self.

Long-Term Goal

- Client will not harm self.

Interventions

- Create a safe environment for the client. Remove all potentially harmful objects from client's access (sharp objects, straps, belts, ties, glass items, alcohol). Supervise closely during meals and medication administration. Perform room searches as deemed necessary.

> **CLINICAL PEARL**
> Ask the client directly, "Have you thought about killing yourself?" or "Have you thought about harming yourself in any way?" "If so, what do you plan to do? Do you have the means to carry out this plan?" The risk of suicide is greatly increased if the client has developed a plan and particularly if means exist for the client to execute the plan.

- Formulate a short-term verbal or written contract with the client that he or she will not harm self during a specific time period. When that contract expires, make another. Repeat this process for as long as required. Discussion of suicidal feelings with a trusted individual provides some relief to the client. A contract gets the subject out in the open and some of the responsibility for his or her safety is given to the client. An attitude of unconditional acceptance of the client as a worthwhile individual is conveyed. *Note:* Some clinicians believe that suicide prevention contracting is not helpful (Knoll, 2011). Obviously, the contract for safety comes with no guarantee, and it holds no legal credibility. It should never be used as a single intervention, but can be viewed as one among many that serve to ensure the client's safety.
- Secure a promise from the client that he or she will seek out a staff member or support person if thoughts of suicide emerge. Suicidal clients are often very ambivalent about their feelings. Discussion of feelings with a trusted individual may provide assistance before the client experiences a crisis situation.

> **CLINICAL PEARL** Be direct. Talk openly and matter-of-factly about suicide. Listen actively and encourage expression of feelings, including anger. Accept the client's feelings in a nonjudgmental manner.

- Maintain close observation of the client. Depending on level of suicide precaution, provide one-to-one contact, constant visual observation, or every-15-minute checks. Place in room close to the nurse's station; do not assign to a private room. Accompany to off-ward activities if attendance is indicated. May need to accompany to bathroom. Close observation is necessary to ensure that client does not harm self in any way. Being alert for suicidal and escape attempts facilitates being able to prevent or interrupt harmful behavior.
- Maintain special care in administration of medications. This prevents saving up to overdose or discarding and not taking.
- Make rounds at frequent, *irregular* intervals (especially at night, toward early morning, at change of

shift, or other predictably busy times for staff). This prevents staff surveillance from becoming predictable. To be aware of client's location is important, especially when staff is busy, unavailable, or less observable.

■ Encourage verbalizations of honest feelings. Through exploration and discussion, help the client to identify symbols of hope in his or her life.

■ Encourage the client to express angry feelings within appropriate limits. Provide a safe method of hostility release. Help the client to identify the true source of anger and to work on adaptive coping skills for use outside the treatment setting. Depression and suicidal behaviors may be viewed as anger turned inward on the self. If this anger can be verbalized in a nonthreatening environment, the client may be able to eventually resolve these feelings.

■ Identify community resources that the client may use as a support system and from whom he or she may request help if feeling suicidal. Having a concrete plan for seeking assistance during a crisis may discourage or prevent self-destructive behaviors.

■ Orient the client to reality, as required. Point out sensory misperceptions or misinterpretations of the environment. Take care not to belittle the client's fears or indicate disapproval of verbal expressions.

■ Most important, spend time with client. This provides a feeling of safety and security, while also conveying the message, "I want to spend time with you because I think you are a worthwhile person."

Complicated Grieving

Complicated grieving is defined as "a disorder that occurs after the death of a significant other [or any other loss of significance to the individual], in which the experience of distress accompanying bereavement fails to follow normative expectations and manifests in functional impairment" (NANDA-I, 2012, p. 365). Table 25-2 presents this nursing diagnosis in care plan format.

Client Goals

Outcome criteria include short- and long-term goals. Timelines are individually determined.

Short-Term Goals

■ Client will express anger about the loss.
■ Client will verbalize behaviors associated with normal grieving.

Table 25-2 | CARE PLAN FOR THE DEPRESSED CLIENT

NURSING DIAGNOSIS: COMPLICATED GRIEVING

RELATED TO: Real or perceived loss, bereavement overload

EVIDENCED BY: Denial of loss, inappropriate expression of anger, idealization of or obsession with lost object, inability to carry out activities of daily living

OUTCOME CRITERIA	NURSING INTERVENTIONS	RATIONALE
Short-Term Goals • Client will express anger about the loss. • Client will verbalize behaviors associated with normal grieving. **Long-Term Goal** • Client will be able to recognize his or her position in the grief process, while progressing at own pace toward resolution.	1. Determine the stage of grief in which the client is fixed. Identify behaviors associated with this stage. 2. Develop a trusting relationship with the client. Show empathy, concern, and unconditional positive regard. Be honest and keep all promises. 3. Convey an accepting attitude, and enable the client to express feelings openly. 4. Encourage the client to express anger. Do not become defensive if the initial expression of anger is displaced on the nurse or therapist. Help the client explore angry feelings so that they may be directed toward the actual intended person or situation.	1. Accurate baseline assessment data are necessary to effectively plan care for the grieving client 2. Trust is the basis for a therapeutic relationship. 3. An accepting attitude conveys to the client that you believe he or she is a worthwhile person. Trust is enhanced. 4. Verbalization of feelings in a nonthreatening environment may help the client come to terms with unresolved issues.

Continued

Table 25-2 | CARE PLAN FOR THE DEPRESSED CLIENT—cont'd

OUTCOME CRITERIA	NURSING INTERVENTIONS	RATIONALE
	5. Help the client to discharge pent-up anger through participation in large motor activities (e.g., brisk walks, jogging, physical exercises, volleyball, punching bag, exercise bike).	5. Physical exercise provides a safe and effective method for discharging pent-up tension.
	6. Teach the normal stages of grief and behaviors associated with each stage. Help the client to understand that feelings such as guilt and anger toward the lost concept are appropriate and acceptable during the grief process and should be expressed rather than held inside.	6. Knowledge of acceptability of the feelings associated with normal grieving may help to relieve some of the guilt that these responses generate.
	7. Encourage the client to review the relationship with the lost concept. With support and sensitivity, point out the reality of the situation in areas where misrepresentations are expressed.	7. The client must give up an idealized perception and be able to accept both positive and negative aspects about the lost concept before the grief process is complete.
	8. Communicate to the client that crying is acceptable. Use of touch may also be therapeutic.	8. Some cultures believe it is important to remain stoic and refrain from crying openly. Individuals from certain cultures are uncomfortable with touch. It is important to be aware of cultural influences before employing these interventions.
	9. Encourage the client to reach out for spiritual support during this time in whatever form is desirable to him or her. Assess spiritual needs of the client (see Chapter 6) and assist as necessary in the fulfillment of those needs.	9. Client may find comfort in religious rituals with which he or she is familiar.

Long-Term Goal

■ Client will be able to recognize his or her position in the grief process, while progressing at own pace toward resolution.

Interventions

■ Determine the stage of grief in which the client is fixed. Identify behaviors associated with this stage. It is important to obtain accurate baseline assessment data to effectively plan care for the grieving client.
■ Develop a trusting relationship with the client. Show empathy, concern, and unconditional positive regard. Be honest and keep all promises. Convey an accepting attitude, and encourage the client to express feelings openly.

■ Encourage the client to express anger. Do not become defensive if the initial expression of anger is displaced on the nurse or therapist. Help the client to explore angry feelings so that they may be directed toward the actual intended person or situation.
■ Help the client to discharge pent-up anger through participation in large motor activities (e.g., brisk walks, jogging, physical exercises, volleyball, punching bag, exercise bike). Physical exercise provides a safe and effective method for discharging pent-up tension.
■ Teach the normal stages of grief and behaviors associated with each stage. Help the client to understand that feelings such as guilt and anger toward the lost concept/entity are appropriate and

acceptable during the grief process, and should be expressed rather than held inside. Knowledge of acceptability of the feelings associated with normal grieving may help to relieve some of the guilt that these responses generate.

■ Encourage the client to review the relationship with the lost concept/entity. With support and sensitivity, point out the reality of the situation in areas where misrepresentations are expressed. The client must give up an idealized perception and be able to accept both positive and negative aspects about the lost concept/entity before the grief process is complete.

■ Communicate to the client that crying is acceptable. The use of touch is therapeutic and appropriate with most clients. Knowledge of cultural influences specific to the client is important before using this technique.

■ Assist the client in problem-solving as he or she attempts to determine methods for more adaptive coping with the experienced loss. Provide positive feedback for strategies identified and decisions made.

■ Encourage the client to reach out for spiritual support during this time in whatever form is desirable to him or her. Assess spiritual needs of the client (see Chapter 6) and assist as necessary in the fulfillment of those needs.

■ Encourage the client to attend a support group of individuals who are experiencing life situations similar to his or her own. Help the client to locate a group of this type.

Low Self-Esteem/Self-Care Deficit

Low self-esteem is defined as "negative self-evaluating/ feelings about self or self-capabilities [either long-standing or in response to a current situation]" (NANDA-I, 2012, pp. 287-288). *Self-care deficit* is defined as "impaired ability to perform or complete [activities of daily living (ADLs)] for self" (NANDA-I, 2012, pp. 250-253).

Client Goals

Short-Term Goals

■ Client will verbalize attributes he or she likes about self.

■ Client will participate in ADLs with assistance from health-care provider.

Long-Term Goals

■ By time of discharge from treatment, the client will exhibit increased feelings of self-worth as evidenced by verbal expression of positive aspects of self, past accomplishments, and future prospects.

■ By time of discharge from treatment, the client will exhibit increased feelings of self-worth by setting realistic goals and trying to reach them, thereby demonstrating a decrease in fear of failure.

■ By time of discharge from treatment, the client will satisfactorily accomplish ADLs independently.

Interventions

■ Be accepting of the client and spend time with him or her even though pessimism and negativism may seem objectionable. Focus on strengths and accomplishments and minimize failures.

■ Promote attendance in therapy groups that offer client simple methods of accomplishment. Encourage client to be as independent as possible.

■ Encourage the client to recognize areas of change and provide assistance toward this effort.

■ Teach assertiveness techniques: the ability to recognize the differences among passive, assertive, and aggressive behaviors, and the importance of respecting the human rights of others while protecting one's own basic human rights. Self-esteem is enhanced by the ability to interact with others in an assertive manner.

■ Teach effective communication techniques, such as the use of "I" messages. Emphasize ways to avoid making judgmental statements (see Chapter 14).

■ Encourage independence in the performance of ADLs, but intervene when client is unable to perform.

> **CLINICAL PEARL**
>
> Offer recognition and positive reinforcement for independent accomplishments. (Example: "Mrs. J., I see you have put on a clean dress and combed your hair.")

■ Show the client how to perform activities with which he or she is having difficulty. When a client is depressed, he or she may require simple, concrete demonstrations of activities that would be performed without difficulty under normal conditions.

■ Keep strict records of food and fluid intake. Offer nutritious snacks and fluids between meals. The client may be unable to tolerate large amounts of food at mealtimes and may therefore require additional nourishment at other times during the day to receive adequate nutrition.

■ Before bedtime, provide nursing measures that promote sleep, such as back rub; warm bath; warm, nonstimulating drinks; soft music; and relaxation exercises.

Powerlessness

Powerlessness is defined as "the lived experience of lack of control over a situation, including a perception that one's actions do not significantly affect an outcome" (NANDA-I, 2012, p. 370).

Client Goals

Short-Term Goal

■ Client will participate in decision-making regarding own care within 5 days.

Long-Term Goal

■ Client will be able to effectively problem-solve ways to take control of his or her life situation by time of discharge from treatment, thereby decreasing feelings of powerlessness.

Interventions

■ Encourage the client to take as much responsibility as possible for his or her own self-care practices. Providing the client with choices will increase feelings of control.

EXAMPLES

■ Include the client in setting the goals of care he or she wishes to achieve.
■ Allow the client to establish own schedule for self-care activities.
■ Provide the client with privacy as need is determined.
■ Provide positive feedback for decisions made. Respect the client's right to make those decisions independently, and refrain from attempting to influence him or her toward those that may seem more logical.

■ Help the client set realistic goals. Unrealistic goals set up the client for failure and reinforce feelings of powerlessness.
■ Help the client identify areas of his or her life situation that can be controlled. The client's emotional condition interferes with his or her ability to solve problems. Assistance is required to perceive the benefits and consequences of available alternatives accurately.
■ Discuss with the client areas of life that are not within his or her ability to control. Encourage verbalization of feelings related to this inability in an effort to deal with unresolved issues and accept what cannot be changed.

Concept Care Mapping

The concept map care plan is an innovative approach to planning and organizing nursing care (see Chapter 9). It is a diagrammatic teaching and learning strategy that allows visualization of interrelationships between medical diagnoses, nursing diagnoses, assessment data, and treatments. An example of a concept map care plan for a client with depression is presented in Figure 25-4.

Client/Family Education

The role of client teacher is important in the psychiatric area, as it is in all areas of nursing. A list of topics for client/family education relevant to depression is presented in Box 25-6. Sample client teaching guides may be found online at www.DavisPlus.com.

Evaluation of Care for the Depressed Client

In the final step of the nursing process, a reassessment is conducted to determine if the nursing actions have been successful in achieving the objectives of care. Evaluation of the nursing actions for the depressed client may be facilitated by gathering information using the following types of questions:

■ Has self-harm to the individual been avoided?
■ Have suicidal ideations subsided?
■ Does the individual know where to seek assistance outside the hospital when suicidal thoughts occur?
■ Has the client discussed the recent loss with staff and family members?
■ Is he or she able to verbalize feelings and behaviors associated with each stage of the grieving process and recognize own position in the process?
■ Have obsession with and idealization of the lost object subsided?
■ Is anger toward the lost object expressed appropriately?
■ Does the client set realistic goals for self?
■ Is he or she able to verbalize positive aspects about self, past accomplishments, and future prospects?
■ Can the client identify areas of life situation over which he or she has control?
■ Is the client able to participate in usual religious practices and feel satisfaction and support from them?
■ Is the client seeking out interaction with others in an appropriate manner?
■ Does the client maintain reality orientation with no evidence of delusional thinking?
■ Is he or she able to concentrate and make decisions concerning own self-care?
■ Is the client selecting and consuming foods sufficiently high in nutrients and calories to maintain weight and nutritional status?
■ Does the client sleep without difficulty and wake feeling rested?
■ Does the client show pride in appearance by attending to personal hygiene and grooming?
■ Have somatic complaints subsided?

Quality and Safety Education for Nurses (QSEN)

The 2003 report *Health Professions Education: A Bridge to Quality* (Greiner, Knebel, & Institute of Medicine, 2003) challenged faculties of medicine, nursing, and

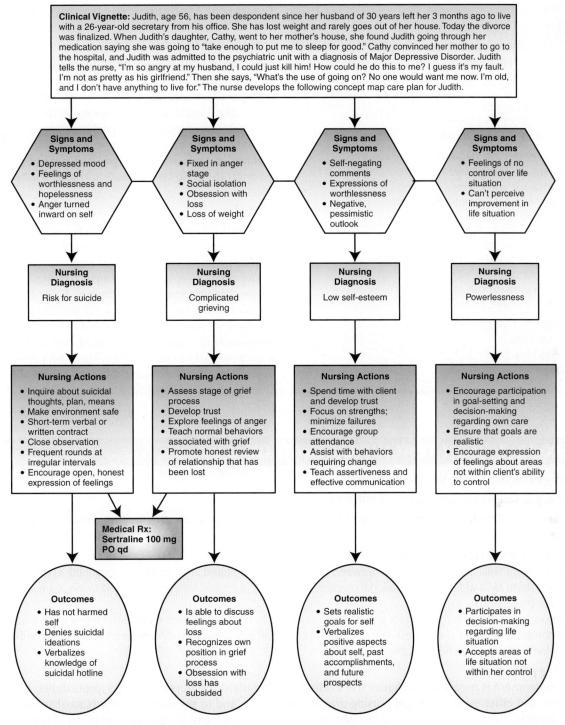

Clinical Vignette: Judith, age 56, has been despondent since her husband of 30 years left her 3 months ago to live with a 26-year-old secretary from his office. She has lost weight and rarely goes out of her house. Today the divorce was finalized. When Judith's daughter, Cathy, went to her mother's house, she found Judith going through her medication saying she was going to "take enough to put me to sleep for good." Cathy convinced her mother to go to the hospital, and Judith was admitted to the psychiatric unit with a diagnosis of Major Depressive Disorder. Judith tells the nurse, "I'm so angry at my husband, I could just kill him! How could he do this to me? I guess it's my fault. I'm not as pretty as his girlfriend." Then she says, "What's the use of going on? No one would want me now. I'm old, and I don't have anything to live for." The nurse develops the following concept map care plan for Judith.

Signs and Symptoms
- Depressed mood
- Feelings of worthlessness and hopelessness
- Anger turned inward on self

Signs and Symptoms
- Fixed in anger stage
- Social isolation
- Obsession with loss
- Loss of weight

Signs and Symptoms
- Self-negating comments
- Expressions of worthlessness
- Negative, pessimistic outlook

Signs and Symptoms
- Feelings of no control over life situation
- Can't perceive improvement in life situation

Nursing Diagnosis
Risk for suicide

Nursing Diagnosis
Complicated grieving

Nursing Diagnosis
Low self-esteem

Nursing Diagnosis
Powerlessness

Nursing Actions
- Inquire about suicidal thoughts, plan, means
- Make environment safe
- Short-term verbal or written contract
- Close observation
- Frequent rounds at irregular intervals
- Encourage open, honest expression of feelings

Nursing Actions
- Assess stage of grief process
- Develop trust
- Explore feelings of anger
- Teach normal behaviors associated with grief
- Promote honest review of relationship that has been lost

Nursing Actions
- Spend time with client and develop trust
- Focus on strengths; minimize failures
- Encourage group attendance
- Assist with behaviors requiring change
- Teach assertiveness and effective communication

Nursing Actions
- Encourage participation in goal-setting and decision-making regarding own care
- Ensure that goals are realistic
- Encourage expression of feelings about areas not within client's ability to control

Medical Rx:
Sertraline 100 mg PO qd

Outcomes
- Has not harmed self
- Denies suicidal ideations
- Verbalizes knowledge of suicidal hotline

Outcomes
- Is able to discuss feelings about loss
- Recognizes own position in grief process
- Obsession with loss has subsided

Outcomes
- Sets realistic goals for self
- Verbalizes positive aspects about self, past accomplishments, and future prospects

Outcomes
- Participates in decision-making regarding life situation
- Accepts areas of life situation not within her control

FIGURE 25–4 Concept map care plan for a client with depression.

other health professions to ensure that their graduates have achieved a core set of competencies in order to meet the needs of the 21st-century health-care system. These competencies include *providing patient-centered care, working in interdisciplinary teams, employing evidence-based practice, applying quality improvement,* *ensuring safety,* and *utilizing informatics.* A QSEN teaching strategy is included in Box 25-7. The use of this type of activity is intended to arm the instructor and the student with guidelines for attaining the knowledge, skills, and attitudes necessary for achievement of quality and safety competencies in nursing.

BOX 25-6 Topics for Client/Family Education Related to Depression

NATURE OF THE ILLNESS

1. Stages of grief and symptoms associated with each stage.
2. What is depression?
3. Why do people get depressed?
4. What are the symptoms of depression?

MANAGEMENT OF THE ILLNESS

1. Medication management
   a. Nuisance side effects
   b. Side effects to report to physician
   c. Importance of taking regularly
   d. Length of time to take effect
   e. Diet (related to MAO inhibitors)
2. Assertiveness techniques
3. Stress-management techniques
4. Ways to increase self-esteem
5. Electroconvulsive therapy

SUPPORT SERVICES

1. Suicide hotline
2. Support groups
3. Legal/financial assistance

Treatment Modalities for Depression

Individual Psychotherapy

Research has documented both the importance of close and satisfactory attachments in the prevention of depression and the role of disrupted attachments in the development of depression. With this concept in mind, interpersonal psychotherapy focuses on the client's current interpersonal relations. Interpersonal psychotherapy with the depressed person proceeds through the following phases and interventions.

Phase I

During the first phase, the client is assessed to determine the extent of the illness. Complete information is then given to the individual regarding the nature of depression, symptom pattern, frequency, clinical course, and alternative treatments. If the level of depression is severe, interpersonal psychotherapy has been shown to be more effective if conducted in combination with antidepressant medication. The client is encouraged to continue working and participating in regular activities during therapy. A mutually agreeable therapeutic contract is negotiated.

BOX 25-7 QSEN TEACHING STRATEGY

Assignment: Staff Work-Arounds
Placing a Client on Suicide Precautions

Competency Domains: Evidence-based Practice; Patient-centered Care; Quality Improvement; Safety; Teamwork and Collaboration

Learning Objectives: Student will:
- Demonstrate skills in identifying gaps between practice on the unit and what has been identified as best practice.
- Demonstrate skills at finding professional practice standards and research literature related to placing a client on suicide precautions.
- Demonstrate skills in accounting for patient preferences within the boundaries of safe and therapeutic practice.
- Demonstrate attitudes and behaviors that show that they value teamwork and want to contribute to maintaining standards of safe and effective care.

Strategy Overview:
This assignment is meant to familiarize the student with standardized nursing policies, procedures, standards of care, and other evidence-based nursing practice guidelines, and to encourage students to observe actual nursing practice on the units to note compliance with, deviations from, or "work arounds" by RNs when implementing nursing procedures. The following aspects of the assignment can guide students in preparation for clinical conference discussion, in writing a paper, or in putting together a poster presentation.

1. Identify a need to place a client on suicide precautions.
2. Find the current written nursing policy or procedure in place for your institution/unit and answer these questions:
   a. How easy/difficult was it to find the policy/procedure?
   b. Did the RNs know where to find the written policy/procedure?
   c. How was the policy/procedure originally disseminated to the staff?
   d. Is the policy/procedure evidence-based?
      (Review the current practice standards from professional organizations and/or oversight and accreditation groups [e.g.: The Joint Commission, CDC], and/or the research literature.)

BOX 25-7 QSEN TEACHING STRATEGY—cont'd

3. Observe RNs on the unit putting a client on suicide precautions and describe:
   a. What steps the RN took.
   b. In what ways the RN deviated from the written policy/procedure.
   c. What prompted the RN to make the deviations she/he did.
   d. As many details as you can recollect.
4. Discuss why RNs may or may not follow the institution's written policies and procedures. Reflect on the opportunities and challenges of evidence-based practice and the implementation into actual bedside nursing practice.
5. Discuss what the proper response should be when you as an RN discover unsafe practice that deviates from standards, policies, or procedures.

Adapted from teaching strategy submitted by Lisa Day, Assistant Clinical Professor, UCSF, School of Nursing, San Francisco, CA. © 2009 QSEN; http://qsen.org. With permission.

Phase II

Treatment at this phase focuses on helping the client resolve complicated grief reactions. This may include resolving the ambivalence with a lost relationship, serving as a temporary substitute for the lost relationship, and assistance with establishing new relationships. Other areas of treatment focus may include interpersonal disputes between the client and a significant other, difficult role transitions at various developmental life cycles, and correction of interpersonal deficits that may interfere with the client's ability to initiate or sustain interpersonal relationships.

Phase III

During the final phase of interpersonal psychotherapy, the therapeutic alliance is terminated. With emphasis on reassurance, clarification of emotional states, improvement of interpersonal communication, testing of perceptions, and performance in interpersonal settings, interpersonal psychotherapy has been successful in helping depressed persons recover enhanced social functioning.

Group Therapy

Group therapy forms an important dimension of multimodal treatment for the depressed client. Once an acute phase of the illness is passed, groups can provide an atmosphere in which individuals may discuss issues in their lives that cause, maintain, or arise out of having a serious affective disorder. The element of peer support provides a feeling of security, as troublesome or embarrassing issues are discussed and resolved. Some groups have other specific purposes, such as helping to monitor medication-related issues or serving as an avenue for promoting education related to the affective disorder and its treatment. Therapy groups help members gain a sense of perspective on their condition and tangibly encourage them to link up with others who have common problems. A sense of hope is conveyed when the individual is able to see that he or she is not alone or unique in experiencing affective illness.

Self-help groups offer another avenue of support for the depressed client. These groups are usually peer led and are not meant to substitute for, or compete with, professional therapy. They offer supplementary support that frequently enhances compliance with the medical regimen. Examples of self-help groups are the Depression and Bipolar Support Alliance (DBSA), Depressives Anonymous, Recovery International, and GriefShare (grief recovery support groups). Although self-help groups are not psychotherapy groups, they do provide important adjunctive support experiences, which often have therapeutic benefit for participants.

Family Therapy

The ultimate objectives in working with families of clients with mood disorders are to resolve the symptoms and initiate or restore adaptive family functioning. As with group therapy, the most effective approach appears to be with a combination of psychotherapeutic and pharmacotherapeutic treatments. Sadock and Sadock (2007) stated:

> Family therapy is indicated if the disorder jeopardizes the patient's marriage or family functioning or if the mood disorder is promoted or maintained by the family situation. Family therapy examines the role of the mood-disordered member in the overall psychological well-being of the whole family; it also examines the role of the entire family in the maintenance of the patient's symptoms. (p. 565)

Cognitive Therapy

In cognitive therapy, the individual is taught to control thought distortions that are considered to be a factor in the development and maintenance of mood disorders. In the cognitive model, depression is characterized by a triad of negative distortions related to expectations of the environment, self, and future. The environment and activities within it are viewed as unsatisfying, the self is unrealistically devalued, and the future is perceived as hopeless.

The general goals in cognitive therapy are to obtain symptom relief as quickly as possible, to assist the client in identifying dysfunctional patterns of thinking and behaving, and to guide the client to evidence and logic that effectively tests the validity of the dysfunctional thinking (see Chapter 19). Therapy focuses on changing "automatic thoughts" that occur spontaneously and contribute to the distorted affect. Examples of automatic thoughts in depression include:

- **Personalizing:** "I'm the only one who failed."
- **All or nothing:** "I'm a complete failure."
- **Mind reading:** "He thinks I'm foolish."
- **Discounting positives:** "The other questions were so easy. Any dummy could have gotten them right."

The client is asked to describe evidence that both supports and disputes the automatic thought. The logic underlying the inferences is then reviewed with the client. Another technique involves evaluating what would most likely happen if the client's automatic thoughts were true. Implications of the consequences are then discussed.

Clients should not become discouraged if one technique seems not to be working. No single technique works with all clients. He or she should be reassured that any of a number of techniques may be used, and both therapist and client may explore these possibilities.

Cognitive therapy has offered encouraging results in the treatment of depression. In fact, the results of several studies with depressed clients show that in some cases cognitive therapy may be equally or even more effective than antidepressant medication (Rupke, Blecke, & Renfrow, 2006).

Electroconvulsive Therapy

Electroconvulsive therapy (ECT) is the induction of a grand mal (generalized) seizure through the application of electrical current to the brain. ECT is effective with clients who are acutely suicidal and in the treatment of severe depression, particularly in those clients who are also experiencing psychotic symptoms and those with psychomotor retardation and neurovegetative changes, such as disturbances in sleep, appetite, and energy. It is often considered for treatment only after a trial of therapy with antidepressant medication has proved ineffective (see Chapter 20 for a detailed discussion of ECT).

Transcranial Magnetic Stimulation

Transcranial magnetic stimulation (TMS) is a procedure that is used to treat depression by targeting certain cells in the brain. TMS involves the use of very short pulses of magnetic energy to stimulate nerve cells in the brain, similar to the electrical activity observed with ECT. However, unlike ECT, the electrical waves generated by TMS do not result in generalized seizure activity (George, Taylor, & Short, 2013). The waves are passed through a coil placed on the scalp to areas of the brain involved in mood regulation. Some clinicians believe that TMS holds a great deal of promise in the treatment of depression, whereas others remain skeptical. In rare instances, seizures have been triggered with the use of TMS therapy (Lanocha, 2010). In a study at King's College in London, researchers compared the efficacy of TMS with ECT in the treatment of severe depression (Eranti et al., 2007). They concluded that ECT was substantially more effective for the short-term treatment of depression, and they indicated the need for further intense clinical evaluation of TMS.

George and associates (2013) stated:

> Since FDA approval, TMS has been generally safe and well tolerated with a low incidence of treatment discontinuation, and the therapeutic effects once obtained appear at least as durable as other antidepressant treatments. TMS also shows promise in several other psychiatric disorders, particularly treating acute and chronic pain. (p. 17)

Light Therapy

Between 15 and 25 percent of people with recurrent depressive disorder exhibit a seasonal pattern whereby symptoms are exacerbated during the winter months and subside during the spring and summer (Thase, 2007). The *DSM-5* identifies this disorder as Major Depressive Disorder, Recurrent, With Seasonal Pattern. It has commonly been known as seasonal affective disorder (SAD). Bright light therapy has been suggested as a first-line treatment for winter "blues" and as an adjunct in chronic major depressive disorder or dysthymia with seasonal exacerbations (Karasu, Gelenberg, Merriam, & Wang, 2006).

SAD is thought to be related to the presence of the hormone melatonin, which is produced by the pineal gland. Melatonin plays a role in the regulation of biological rhythms for sleep and activation. It is produced during the cycle of darkness and shuts off in the light of day. During the months of longer darkness hours, there is increased production of melatonin, which seems to trigger the symptoms of SAD in susceptible people.

Light therapy, or exposure to light, has been shown to be an effective treatment for SAD. The light therapy is administered by a 10,000-lux light box, which contains white fluorescent light tubes covered with a plastic screen that blocks ultraviolet rays. The individual sits in front of the box with the eyes open (although they should not look directly into the light). Therapy usually begins with 10- to 15-minute sessions, and gradually progresses to 30 to 45 minutes. Some people notice improvement rapidly, within a few days, whereas others may take several weeks to feel better. Side effects appear to be dosage related, and include headache, eyestrain, nausea, irritability, photophobia (eye sensitivity to light), insomnia (when light therapy is used late in the day), and (rarely) hypomania (Terman & Terman, 2005). Light therapy and antidepressants have shown comparable efficacy in studies of SAD treatment. One study compared the efficacy of light therapy for SAD to daily treatment with 20 mg of fluoxetine (Lam et al., 2006). The authors concluded that, "Light treatment showed earlier response onset and lower rate of some adverse events relative to fluoxetine, but there were no other significant differences in outcome between light therapy and antidepressant medication" (p. 805).

Psychopharmacology

Historical Aspects

Antidepressant medication had a serendipitous beginning. In the early 1950s, patients with tuberculosis were being treated with the monoamine oxidase inhibitor (MAOI) iproniazid. Although the drug proved ineffective for tuberculosis, it was found that patients exhibited a sustained elevation of mood while taking the medication (Schatzberg, Cole, & DeBattista, 2010). Following the initial enthusiasm about MAOIs, they fell into relative disuse for nearly two decades because of a perceived poor risk-to-benefit ratio.

The tricyclic antidepressants (TCAs) had a similar introduction. In the late 1950s, imipramine was being investigated as a treatment for schizophrenia, and although it did not relieve psychotic symptoms, it appeared to elevate mood. For almost 50 years, the TCAs have been widely used to treat depression. Since the initial discovery of their antidepressant properties, they have been subjected to hundreds of controlled trials, and their efficacy in treating depressive illness is now firmly established.

The success of these first two groups of antidepressants led the pharmaceutical industry to search for compounds with similar efficacy and fewer side effects than the MAOIs and the TCAs. Examples of commonly used antidepressant medications are presented in Table 25-3. A detailed description of these medications follows.

Indications

Antidepressant medications are used in the treatment of dysthymia; major depression with melancholia or psychotic symptoms; depression associated with organic disease, alcoholism, schizophrenia, or intellectual developmental disorder; depressive phase of bipolar disorder; and depression accompanied by anxiety. These drugs elevate mood and alleviate other symptoms associated with moderate to severe depression. Selected agents are also used to treat anxiety disorders, bulimia nervosa, and premenstrual dysphoric disorder.

Action

These drugs ultimately work to increase the concentration of norepinephrine, serotonin, and/or dopamine

TABLE 25–3	**Medications Used in the Treatment of Depression**			
CHEMICAL CLASS	GENERIC (TRADE) NAME*	PREGNANCY CATEGORIES/ HALF-LIFE (hr)	DAILY ADULT DOSAGE RANGE (mg)†	THERAPEUTIC PLASMA RANGES
Tricyclics	Amitriptyline	D/ 31–46	50–300	110–250 (including metabolite)
	Amoxapine	C/ 8	50–300	200–500
	Clomipramine (Anafranil)	C/ 19–37	25–250	80–100
	Desipramine (Norpramin)	C/ 12–24	25–300	125–300
	Doxepin	C/ 8–24	25-300	100–200 (including metabolite)
	Imipramine (Tofranil)	D/ 11–25	30–300	200–350 (including metabolite)
	Nortriptyline (Aventyl; Pamelor)	D/ 18–44	30–100	50–150
	Protriptyline (Vivactil)	C/ 67–89	15–60	100–200
	Trimipramine (Surmontil)	C/ 7–30	50–300	180 (including metabolite)

Continued

TABLE 25–3 Medications Used in the Treatment of Depression–cont'd

CHEMICAL CLASS	GENERIC (TRADE) NAME*	PREGNANCY CATEGORIES/ HALF-LIFE (hr)	DAILY ADULT DOSAGE RANGE (mg)†	THERAPEUTIC PLASMA RANGES
Selective Serotonin Reuptake Inhibitors (SSRIs)	Citalopram (Celexa)	C/ ~35	20–40	Not well established
	Escitalopram (Lexapro)	C/ 27–32	10–20	Not well established
	Fluoxetine (Prozac; Serafem)	C/ 1–16 days (including metabolite)	20–80	Not well established
	Fluvoxamine (Luvox)	C/ 13.6–15.6	50–300	Not well established
	Paroxetine (Paxil)	D/ 21 (CR: 15–20)	10–50 (CR: 12.5–75)	Not well established
	Sertraline (Zoloft)	C/ 26–104 (including metabolite)	25–200	Not well established
	Vilazodone (Viibryd) (also acts as a partial serotonergic agonist)	C/ 25	40	Not well established
	Vortioxetine (Brintellix)	C/ 66	5-20	Not well established
Monoamine Oxidase Inhibitors (MAOIs)	Isocarboxazid (Marplan)	C/ Not established	20–60	Not well established
	Phenelzine (Nardil)	C/ 11.6	45–90	Not well established
	Tranylcypromine (Parnate)	C/ 2.4–2.8	30–60	Not well established
	Selegiline Transdermal System (Emsam)	C/ 18–25 (including metabolites)	6/24 hr – 12/24 hr patch	Not well established
Heterocyclics	Bupropion (Wellbutrin)	C/ 8–24	200–450	Not well established
	Maprotiline	B/ 21–25	25–225	200–300 (incl. metabolite)
	Mirtazapine (Remeron)	C/ 20–40	15–45	Not well established
	Nefazodone‡	C/ 2–4	200–600	Not well established
	Trazodone	C/ 4-9	150–600	800–1600
Serotonin- Norepinephrine Reuptake Inhibitors (SNRIs)	Desvenlafaxine (Pristiq)	C/ 11	50–400	Not well established
	Levomilnacipran (Fetzima)	C/ 12	40-120	Not well established
	Duloxetine (Cymbalta)	C/ 8–17	40–60	Not well established
	Venlafaxine (Effexor)	C/ 5–11 (incl. metabolite)	75–375	Not well established
Psychotherapeutic Combinations	Olanzapine and fluoxetine (Symbyax)	C/ (see individual drugs)	6/25–12/50	Not well established
	Chlordiazepoxide and fluoxetine (Limbitrol)	D/ (see individual drugs)	20/50–40/100	Not well established
	Perphenazine and amitriptyline (Etrafon)	C–D/ (see individual drugs)	6/30–16/200	Not well established

*Drugs without trade names are available in generic form only.
†Dosage requires slow titration; onset of therapeutic response may be 1 to 4 weeks.
‡Bristol Myers Squibb voluntarily removed their brand of nefazodone (Serzone) from the market in 2004. The generic equivalent is currently available through various other manufacturers.

in the body. This is accomplished in the brain by blocking the reuptake of these neurotransmitters by the neurons (TCAs, heterocyclics, SSRIs, and SNRIs). It also occurs when an enzyme, monoamine oxidase, that is known to inactivate norepinephrine, serotonin, and dopamine, is inhibited at various sites in the nervous system (MAOIs).

Contraindications/Precautions

Antidepressant medications are contraindicated in individuals with hypersensitivity. TCAs are contraindicated in the acute recovery phase following myocardial infarction and in individuals with angle-closure glaucoma. TCAs, heterocyclics, SSRIs, and SNRIs are contraindicated with concomitant use of MAOIs.

Caution should be used in administering these medications to elderly or debilitated clients and those with hepatic, renal, or cardiac insufficiency. (The dosage usually must be decreased.) Caution is also required with psychotic clients, with clients who have benign prostatic hypertrophy, and with individuals who have a history of seizures (may decrease seizure threshold).

Interactions

Tricyclic Antidepressants

■ Increased effects of tricyclic antidepressants may occur with bupropion, cimetidine, haloperidol, SSRIs, and valproic acid.

■ Decreased effects of tricyclic antidepressants may occur with carbamazepine, barbiturates, and rifamycins.

■ Hyperpyretic crisis, convulsions, and death may occur with MAO inhibitors.

■ Coadministration with clonidine may produce hypertensive crisis.

■ Decreased effects of levodopa and guanethidine may occur with tricyclic antidepressants.

■ Potentiation of pressor response may occur with direct-acting sympathomimetics.

■ Increased anticoagulation effects may occur with dicumarol.

■ Increased serum levels of carbamazepine occur with concomitant use of tricyclics.

■ There is an increased risk of seizures with concomitant use of maprotiline and phenothiazines.

Monoamine Oxidase Inhibitors

■ Serious, potentially fatal adverse reactions may occur with concurrent use of all other antidepressants, carbamazepine, cyclobenzaprine, buspirone, sympathomimetics, tryptophan, dextromethorphan, anesthetic agents, CNS depressants, and amphetamines. Avoid using within 2 weeks of each other (5 weeks after therapy with fluoxetine).

■ Hypertensive crisis may occur with amphetamines, methyldopa, levodopa, dopamine, epinephrine, norepinephrine, guanethidine, guanadrel, reserpine, or vasoconstrictors.

■ Hypertension or hypotension, coma, convulsions, and death may occur with opioids (avoid use of meperidine within 14 to 21 days of MAOI therapy).

■ Excess CNS stimulation and hypertension may occur with methylphenidate.

■ Additive hypotension may occur with antihypertensives, thiazide diuretics, or spinal anesthesia.

■ Additive hypoglycemia may occur with insulins or oral hypoglycemic agents.

■ Doxapram may increase pressor response.

■ Serotonin syndrome may occur with concomitant use of St. John's wort.

■ Hypertensive crisis may occur with ingestion of foods or other products containing high concentrations of **tyramine** (Table 25-4).

■ Consumption of foods or beverages with high caffeine content increases the risk of hypertension and arrhythmias.

■ Bradycardia may occur with concurrent use of MAOIs and beta blockers.

■ There is a risk of toxicity from the 5-hydroxytryptamine (5-HT) receptor agonists with concurrent use of MAOIs.

Selective Serotonin Reuptake Inhibitors (SSRIs)

■ Toxic, sometimes fatal, reactions have occurred with concomitant use of MAOIs.

■ Increased effects of SSRIs may occur with cimetidine, L-tryptophan, lithium, linezolid, and St. John's wort.

■ Serotonin syndrome may occur with concomitant use of SSRIs and metoclopramide, sibutramine, tramadol, or 5-HT-receptor agonists (triptans), or any drug that increases levels of serotonin.

■ Concomitant use of SSRIs may increase effects of hydantoins, tricyclic antidepressants, cyclosporine, benzodiazepines, beta blockers, methadone, carbamazepine, clozapine, olanzapine, pimozide, haloperidol, mexiletine, phenothiazines, St. John's wort, trazodone, sumatriptan, sympathomimetics, theophylline, procyclidine, propafenone, risperidone, ropivacaine, warfarin, and zolpidem.

■ Concomitant use of SSRIs may decrease effects of buspirone and digoxin.

■ Lithium levels may be increased or decreased by concomitant use of SSRIs.

■ There may be decreased effects of SSRIs with concomitant use of carbamazepine and cyproheptadine.

■ Increased effects of vilazodone with strong inhibitors of CYP3A4 (e.g., ketoconazole).

■ Increased effects of vortioxetine with concomitant use of bupropion, fluoxetine, paroxetine, or quinidine.

■ Decreased effects of vortioxetine with concomitant use of CYP inducers (e.g., rifampicin, carbamazepine, phenytoin)

Others (Heterocyclics and SNRIs)

■ Concomitant use with MAOIs results in serious, sometimes fatal, effects resembling neuroleptic malignant syndrome. Coadministration is contraindicated.

■ Serotonin syndrome may occur when any of the following are used together: St. John's wort, sibutramine,

TABLE 25–4 **Diet and Drug Restrictions for Clients on MAOI Therapy**		
FOODS CONTAINING TYRAMINE		
HIGH TYRAMINE CONTENT *(AVOID WHILE ON MAOI THERAPY)*	**MODERATE TYRAMINE CONTENT** *(MAY EAT OCCASIONALLY WHILE ON MAOI THERAPY)*	**LOW TYRAMINE CONTENT** *(LIMITED QUANTITIES PERMISSIBLE WHILE ON MAOI THERAPY)*
Aged cheeses (cheddar, Swiss, Camembert, blue cheese, Parmesan, provolone, Romano, brie)	Gouda cheese, processed American cheese, mozzarella	Pasteurized cheeses (cream cheese, cottage cheese, ricotta)
Raisins, fava beans, flat Italian beans, Chinese pea pods	Yogurt, sour cream	Figs
Red wines (Chianti, burgundy, cabernet sauvignon)	Avocados, bananas	Distilled spirits (in moderation)
Smoked and processed meats (salami, bologna, pepperoni, summer sausage)	Beer, white wine, coffee, colas, tea, hot chocolate	
Caviar, pickled herring, corned beef, chicken or beef liver	Meat extracts, such as bouillon	
Soy sauce, brewer's yeast, meat tenderizer (MSG)	Chocolate	
DRUG RESTRICTIONS		

Ingestion of the following substances while on MAOI therapy could result in life-threatening hypertensive crisis. A 14-day interval is recommended between use of these drugs and an MAOI.
■ All other antidepressant medications (e.g., SSRIs, TCAs, SNRIs, heterocyclics)
■ Sympathomimetics: (epinephrine, dopamine, norepinephrine, ephedrine, pseudoephedrine, phenylephrine, phenyl-propanolamine, over-the-counter cough and cold preparations)
■ Stimulants (amphetamines, cocaine, diet drugs)
■ Antihypertensives (methyldopa, guanethidine, reserpine)
■ Meperidine and (possibly) other opioid narcotics (morphine, codeine)
■ Antiparkinsonian agents (levodopa)

SOURCES: Black & Andreasen (2010); Martinez, Marangell, & Martinez (2008); and Sadock & Sadock (2007).

trazodone, nefazodone, venlafaxine, desvenlafaxine, duloxetine, levomilnacipran, SSRIs, 5-HT-receptor agonists (triptans).
■ Increased effects of haloperidol, clozapine, and desipramine may occur when used concomitantly with venlafaxine.
■ Increased effects of venlafaxine may occur with cimetidine.
■ Increased effects of duloxetine may occur with cytochrome P450 (CYP) 1A2 inhibitors (e.g., fluvoxamine, quinolone antibiotics) and CYP2D6 inhibitors (e.g., fluoxetine, quinidine, paroxetine). Increased risk of liver injury occurs with concomitant use of alcohol and duloxteine.
■ Increased risk of toxicity or adverse effects from drugs extensively metabolized by CYP2D6 (e.g., flecainide, phenothiazines, propafenone, tricyclic antidepressants, thioridazine) when used concomitantly with duloxetine, desvenlafaxine, or bupropion.
■ Decreased effects of bupropion and trazodone may occur with carbamazepine.

■ Altered anticoagulant effect of warfarin may occur with bupropion, venlafaxine, desvenlafaxine, duloxetine, levomilnacipran, or trazodone.
■ Increased risk of seizures when bupropion is coadministered with drugs that lower the seizure threshold (e.g., antidepressants, antipsychotics, systemic steroids, theophylline, tramadol).
■ Decreased effects of midazolam with desvenlafaxine.
■ Increased effects of desvenlafaxine and levomilnacipran with concomitant use of potent CYP3A4 inhibitors (e.g., ketoconazole).

Side Effects

The plan of care should include monitoring for the following side effects from antidepressant medications. Nursing implications related to each side effect are designated by an asterisk (*).

May Occur With All Chemical Classes

■ Dry mouth
   *Offer the client sugarless candy, ice, frequent sips of water.
   *Strict oral hygiene is very important.

■ Sedation
*Request an order from the physician for the drug to be given at bedtime.
*Request that the physician decrease the dosage or perhaps order a less sedating drug.
*Instruct the client not to drive or use dangerous equipment while experiencing sedation.

■ Nausea
*Medication may be taken with food to minimize GI distress.

■ Discontinuation syndrome
*All classes of antidepressants have varying potentials to cause discontinuation syndromes. Abrupt withdrawal following long-term therapy with SSRIs, venlafaxine, desvenlafaxine, levomilnacipran, or duloxetine may result in dizziness, lethargy, headache, and nausea. Fluoxetine is less likely to result in withdrawal symptoms because of its long half-life. Abrupt withdrawal from tricyclics may produce hypomania, akathisia, cardiac arrhythmias, gastrointestinal upset, and panic attacks. The discontinuation syndrome associated with MAOIs includes flulike symptoms, confusion, hypomania, and worsening of depressive symptoms. All antidepressant medication should be tapered gradually to prevent withdrawal symptoms (Schatzberg et al., 2010).

Most Commonly Occur With Tricyclics and Heterocyclics

■ Blurred vision
*Offer reassurance that this symptom should subside after a few weeks.
*Instruct the client not to drive until vision is clear.
*Clear small items from routine pathway to prevent falls.

■ Constipation
*Order foods high in fiber; increase fluid intake if not contraindicated; and encourage the client to increase physical exercise, if possible.

■ Urinary retention
*Instruct the client to report hesitancy or inability to urinate.
*Monitor intake and output.
*Try various methods to stimulate urination, such as running water in the bathroom or pouring water over the perineal area.

■ Orthostatic hypotension
*Instruct the client to rise slowly from a lying or sitting position.
*Monitor blood pressure (lying and standing) frequently, and document and report significant changes.
*Avoid long hot showers or tub baths.

■ Reduction of seizure threshold
*Observe clients with history of seizures closely.

*Institute seizure precautions as specified in hospital procedure manual.
*Bupropion (Wellbutrin) should be administered in doses of no more than 150 mg and should be given at least 4 hours apart. Bupropion has been associated with a relatively high incidence of seizure activity in anorexic and cachectic clients.

■ Tachycardia; arrhythmias
*Carefully monitor blood pressure and pulse rate and rhythm, and report any significant change to the physician.

■ Photosensitivity
*Ensure that client wears sunblock lotion, protective clothing, and sunglasses while outdoors.

■ Weight gain
*Provide instructions for reduced-calorie diet.
*Encourage increased level of activity, if appropriate.

Most Commonly Occur With SSRIs and SNRIs

■ Insomnia; agitation
*Administer or instruct client to take dose early in the day.
*Instruct client to avoid caffeinated food and drinks.
*Teach relaxation techniques to use before bedtime.

■ Headache
*Administer analgesics, as prescribed.
*If relief is not achieved, physician may order another antidepressant.

■ Weight loss (may occur early in therapy)
*Ensure that client is provided with caloric intake sufficient to maintain desired weight.
*Caution should be taken in prescribing these drugs for anorectic clients.
*Weigh client daily or every other day, at the same time, and on the same scale, if possible.
*After prolonged use, some clients may gain weight on these drugs.

■ Sexual dysfunction
*Men may report abnormal ejaculation or impotence.
*Women may experience delay or loss of orgasm.
*If side effect becomes intolerable, a switch to another antidepressant may be necessary.

■ Serotonin syndrome (may occur when two drugs that potentiate serotonergic neurotransmission are used concurrently [see "Interactions"]).
*Most frequent symptoms include changes in mental status, restlessness, myoclonus, hyperreflexia, tachycardia, labile blood pressure, diaphoresis, shivering, and tremors.
*Discontinue the offending agent immediately.
*The physician may prescribe medications to block serotonin receptors, relieve hyperthermia and muscle rigidity, and prevent seizures. In severe cases, artificial ventilation may be required. The histamine-1 receptor antagonist cyproheptadine is

commonly used to treat the symptoms of serotonin syndrome.

*Supportive nursing measures include monitoring vital signs, providing safety measures to prevent injury when muscle rigidity and changes in mental status are present, cooling blankets and tepid baths to assist with temperature regulation, and monitoring intake and output (Cooper & Sejnowski, 2013).

*The condition will usually resolve on its own once the offending medication has been discontinued. However, if left untreated, the condition may progress to life-threatening complications such as seizures, coma, hypotension, ventricular arrhythmias, disseminated intravascular coagulation, rhabdomyolysis, metabolic acidosis, and renal failure (Cooper & Sejnowski, 2013).

Most Commonly Occur With MAOIs

■ Hypertensive crisis

*Hypertensive crisis occurs if the individual consumes foods containing tyramine while receiving MAOI therapy (see Table 25-4).

NOTE: Hypertensive crisis has not shown to be a problem with selegiline transdermal system at the 6 mg/24 hr dosage, and dietary restrictions at this dose are not recommended. Dietary modifications are recommended, however, at the 9 mg/24 hr and 12 mg/24 hr dosages.

*Symptoms of hypertensive crisis include severe occipital headache, palpitations, nausea/vomiting, nuchal rigidity, fever, sweating, marked increase in blood pressure, chest pain, and coma.

*Treatment of hypertensive crisis includes discontinuing the drug immediately; monitoring vital signs; administering short-acting antihypertensive medication, as ordered by the physician; and using external cooling measures to control hyperpyrexia.

■ Application site reactions (with selegiline transdermal system [Emsam])

*The most common reactions include rash, itching, erythema, irritation, swelling, or urticarial lesions. Most reactions resolve spontaneously, requiring no treatment. However, if reaction becomes problematic, it should be reported to the physician. Topical corticosteroids have been used in treatment.

Miscellaneous Side Effects

■ Priapism (with trazodone)

*Priapism is a rare side effect, but it has occurred in some men taking trazodone.

*If prolonged or inappropriate penile erection occurs, the medication should be withheld and the physician notified immediately.

*Priapism can become very problematic, requiring surgical intervention, and, if not treated successfully, can result in impotence.

■ Hepatic failure (with nefazodone)

*Cases of life-threatening hepatic failure have been reported in clients treated with nefazodone.

*Advise clients to be alert for signs or symptoms suggestive of liver dysfunction (e.g., jaundice, anorexia, GI complaints, or malaise) and to report them to the physician immediately.

Client/Family Education Related to Antidepressants

The client should:

■ Continue to take the medication even though the symptoms have not subsided. The therapeutic effect may not be seen for as long as 4 weeks. If after this length of time no improvement is noted, the physician may prescribe a different medication.

■ Use caution when driving or operating dangerous machinery. Drowsiness and dizziness can occur. If these side effects become persistent or interfere with activities of daily living, the client should report them to the physician. Dosage adjustment may be necessary.

■ Not discontinue use of the drug abruptly. To do so might produce withdrawal symptoms, such as nausea, vertigo, insomnia, headache, malaise, nightmares, and return of symptoms for which the medication was prescribed.

■ Use sunblock lotion and wear protective clothing when spending time outdoors. The skin may be sensitive to sunburn.

■ Report occurrence of any of the following symptoms to the physician immediately: sore throat, fever, malaise, yellowish skin, unusual bleeding, easy bruising, persistent nausea/vomiting, severe headache, rapid heart rate, difficulty urinating, anorexia/weight loss, seizure activity, stiff or sore neck, and chest pain.

■ Rise slowly from a sitting or lying position to prevent a sudden drop in blood pressure.

■ Take frequent sips of water, chew sugarless gum, or suck on hard candy if dry mouth is a problem. Good oral care (frequent brushing, flossing) is very important.

■ Not consume the following foods or medications while taking MAOIs: aged cheese, wine (especially Chianti), beer, chocolate, colas, coffee, tea, sour cream, smoked and processed meats, beef or chicken liver, canned figs, soy sauce, overripe and fermented foods, pickled herring, raisins, caviar, yogurt, yeast products, broad beans, cold remedies, diet pills. To do so could cause a life-threatening hypertensive crisis.

■ Avoid smoking while receiving tricyclic therapy. Smoking increases the metabolism of tricyclics, requiring an adjustment in dosage to achieve the therapeutic effect.

■ Avoid drinking alcohol while taking antidepressant therapy. These drugs potentiate the effects of each other.

■ Avoid use of other medications (including over-the-counter medications) without the physician's approval while receiving antidepressant therapy. Many medications contain substances that, in combination with antidepressant medication, could precipitate a life-threatening hypertensive crisis.

■ Notify physician immediately if inappropriate or prolonged penile erections occur while taking trazodone. If the erection persists longer than 1 hour, seek emergency department treatment. This condition is rare, but has occurred in some men who have taken trazodone. If measures are not instituted immediately, impotence can result.

■ Not "double up" on medication if a dose of bupropion (Wellbutrin) is missed, unless advised to do so by the physician. Taking bupropion in divided doses will decrease the risk of seizures and other adverse effects.

■ Follow the correct procedure for applying the selegiline transdermal patch:
  ■ Apply to dry, intact skin on upper torso, upper thigh, or outer surface of upper arm.
  ■ Apply approximately same time each day to new spot on skin, after removing and discarding old patch.
  ■ Wash hands thoroughly after applying the patch.
  ■ Avoid exposing application site to direct heat (e.g., heating pads, electric blankets, heat lamps, hot tub, or prolonged direct sunlight).
  ■ If patch falls off, apply new patch to a new site and resume previous schedule.

■ Be aware of possible risks of taking antidepressants during pregnancy. Safe use during pregnancy and lactation has not been fully established. These drugs are believed to readily cross the placental barrier; if so, the fetus could experience adverse effects of the drug. Inform the physician immediately if pregnancy occurs, is suspected, or is planned.

■ Be aware of the side effects of antidepressants. Refer to written materials furnished by health-care providers for safe self-administration.

■ Carry a card or other identification at all times describing the medications being taken.

CASE STUDY AND SAMPLE CARE PLAN

NURSING HISTORY AND ASSESSMENT

Sam is a 45-year-old white male admitted to the psychiatric unit of a general medical center by his family physician, Dr. Jones, who reported that Sam had become increasingly despondent over the past month. His wife reported that he had made statements such as, "Life is not worth living," and "I think I could just take all those pills Dr. Jones prescribed at one time; then it would all be over." Sam says he loves his wife and children and does not want to hurt them, but feels they no longer need him. He states, "They would probably be better off without me." His wife appears to be very concerned about his condition, although in his despondency, he seems oblivious to her feelings. His mother (a widow) lives in a neighboring state, and he sees her infrequently. His father was an alcoholic and physically abused Sam and his siblings. He admits that he is somewhat bitter toward his mother for allowing him and his siblings to "suffer from the physical and emotional brutality of their father." His siblings and their families live in distant states, and he sees them rarely, during holiday gatherings.

Sam earned a college degree working full-time at night to pay his way. He is employed in the administration department of a large corporation. Over the past 12 years, Sam has watched while a number of his peers were promoted to management positions. Sam has been considered for several of these positions but has never been selected. Last month a management position became available for which Sam felt he was qualified. He applied for this position, believing he had a good chance of being promoted. However, when the announcement was made, the position had been given to a younger man who had been with the company only 5 years. Sam seemed to accept the decision, but over the past few weeks he has become more and more withdrawn. He speaks to very few people at the office and is becoming more and more behind in his work. At home, he eats very little, talks to family members only when they ask a direct question, withdraws to his bedroom very early in the evening, and does not come out until time to leave for work the next morning. Today, he refused to get out of bed or to go to work. His wife convinced him to talk to their family doctor, who admitted him to the hospital. The referring psychiatrist diagnosed Sam with major depressive disorder.

NURSING DIAGNOSES/OUTCOME IDENTIFICATION

From the assessment data, the nurse develops the following nursing diagnoses for Sam:

1. **Risk for suicide** related to depressed mood and expressions of having nothing to live for.
   a. **Short-Term Goals:**
      ■ Sam will seek out staff when ideas of suicide occur.
      ■ Sam will maintain a short-term contract not to harm himself.

Continued

CASE STUDY AND SAMPLE CARE PLAN—cont'd

    b. Long-Term Goal:
- Sam will not harm himself during his hospitalization.

2. **Complicated grieving** related to unresolved losses (job promotion and unsatisfactory parent-child relationships) evidenced by anger turned inward on self and desire to end his life.

    a. Short-Term Goal:
- Sam will verbalize anger toward boss and parents within 1 week.

    b. Long-Term Goal:
- Sam will verbalize his position in the grief process and begin movement in the progression toward resolution by time of discharge from treatment.

PLANNING/IMPLEMENTATION

RISK FOR SUICIDE
The following nursing interventions have been identified for Sam:

1. Ask Sam directly, "Have you thought about killing yourself? If so, what do you plan to do? Do you have the means to carry out this plan?"
2. Create a safe environment. Remove all potentially harmful objects from immediate access (sharp objects, straps, belts, ties, glass items).
3. Formulate a short-term verbal contract with Sam that he will not harm himself during the next 24 hours. When that contract expires, make another. Continue with this intervention until Sam is discharged.
4. Secure a promise from Sam that he will seek out a staff member if thoughts of suicide emerge.
5. Encourage verbalizations of honest feelings. Through exploration and discussion, help him to identify symbols of hope in his life (participating in activities he finds satisfying outside of his job).
6. Allow Sam to express angry feelings within appropriate limits. Encourage use of the exercise room and punching bag each day. Help him to identify the true source of his anger, and work on adaptive coping skills for use outside the hospital (e.g., jogging, exercise club available to employees of his company).
7. Identify community resources that he may use as a support system and from whom he may request help if feeling suicidal (e.g., suicidal or crisis hotline; psychiatrist or social worker at community mental health center; hospital "HELP" line).
8. Introduce Sam to support and education groups for adult children of alcoholics (ACOA).
9. Spend time with Sam. This will help him to feel safe and secure while conveying the message that he is a worthwhile person.

COMPLICATED GRIEVING
The following nursing interventions have been identified for Sam:

1. Sam is fixed in the anger stage of the grieving process. Discuss with him behaviors associated with this stage, so that he may come to realize why he is feeling this way.
2. Develop a trusting relationship with Sam. Show empathy and caring. Be honest and keep all promises.
3. Convey an accepting attitude—one in which he is not afraid to express feelings openly.
4. Allow him to verbalize feelings of anger. The initial expression of anger may be displaced on to the healthcare provider. Do not become defensive if this should occur. Assist him to explore these angry feelings so that they may be directed toward the intended persons (boss, parents).
5. Have Sam write letters (not to be mailed) to his boss and to his parents stating his true feelings toward them. Discuss these feelings with him; then destroy the letters.
6. Assist Sam to discharge pent-up anger through participation in large motor activities (brisk walks, jogging, physical exercises, volleyball, punching bag, exercise bike, or other equipment).
7. Explain normal stages of grief, and the behaviors associated with each stage. Help Sam to understand that feelings such as guilt and anger toward his boss and parents are appropriate and acceptable during this stage of the grieving process. Help him also to understand that he must work through these feelings and move past this stage in order to eventually feel better. Knowledge of acceptability of the feelings associated with normal grieving may help to relieve some of the guilt that these responses generate. Knowing why he is experiencing these feelings may also help to resolve them.
8. Encourage Sam to review the relationship with his parents. With support and sensitivity, point out the reality of the situation in areas in which misrepresentations are expressed. Explain common roles and behaviors of members in an alcoholic family. Sam must give up the desire for an idealized family and accept the reality of his childhood situation and the effect it has had on his adult life, before the grief process can be completed.
9. Assist Sam in problem solving as he attempts to determine methods for more adaptive coping. Suggest alternatives to anger turned inward on the self when negative thinking sets in (e.g., thought-stopping techniques). Provide positive feedback for strategies identified and decisions made.
10. Encourage Sam to reach out for spiritual support during this time in whatever form is desirable to him. Assess spiritual needs (see Chapter 6), and assist as necessary in the fulfillment of those needs. Sam may find comfort in religious rituals with which he is familiar.

EVALUATION

The outcome criteria identified for Sam have been met. He sought out staff when feelings of suicide surfaced. He maintained an active no-suicide contract. He has not harmed himself in any way. He verbalizes no further thought of suicide and expresses hope for the future. He is able to

CASE STUDY AND SAMPLE CARE PLAN—cont'd

verbalize names of resources outside the hospital from whom he may request help if thoughts of suicide return. He is able to verbalize normal stages of the grief process and behaviors associated with each stage. He is able to identify his own position in the grief process and express honest feelings related to the loss of his job promotion and satisfactory parent-child relationships. He is no longer manifesting exaggerated emotions and behaviors related to complicated grieving, and is able to carry out self-care activities independently.

Summary and Key Points

■ Depression is one of the oldest recognized psychiatric illnesses that is still prevalent today. It is so common, in fact, that it has been referred to as the "common cold of psychiatric disorders."

■ The cause of depressive disorders is not entirely known. A number of factors, including genetics, biochemical influences, and psychosocial experiences, likely enter into the development of the disorder.

■ Secondary depression occurs in response to other physiological disorders.

■ Symptoms of depression occur along a continuum according to the degree of severity from transient to severe.

■ The disorder occurs in all developmental levels, including childhood, adolescence, senescence, and during the puerperium.

■ Treatment of depression includes individual therapy, group and family therapy, cognitive therapy, electroconvulsive therapy, light therapy, transcranial magnetic stimulation, and psychopharmacology.

■ Nursing care of the depressed client is provided using the six steps of the nursing process.

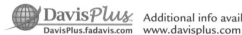 **DavisPlus** Additional info available at
DavisPlus.fadavis.com www.davisplus.com

Review Questions
Self-Examination/Learning Exercise

Select the answer that is most appropriate for each of the following questions.

1. Margaret, age 68, is a widow of 6 months. Since her husband died, her sister reports that Margaret has become socially withdrawn, has lost weight, and does little more each day than visit the cemetery where her husband was buried. She told her sister today that she "didn't have anything more to live for." She has been hospitalized with major depressive disorder. The *priority* nursing diagnosis for Margaret would be:
   a. Imbalanced nutrition: less than body requirements
   b. Complicated grieving
   c. Risk for suicide
   d. Social isolation

2. The physician orders sertraline (Zoloft) 50 mg PO bid for Margaret, a 68-year-old woman with major depressive disorder. After 3 days of taking the medication, Margaret says to the nurse, "I don't think this medicine is doing any good. I don't feel a bit better." What is the most appropriate response by the nurse?
   a. "Cheer up, Margaret. You have so much to be happy about."
   b. "Sometimes it takes a few weeks for the medicine to bring about an improvement in symptoms."
   c. "I'll report that to the physician, Margaret. Maybe he will order something different."
   d. "Try not to dwell on your symptoms, Margaret. Why don't you join the others down in the dayroom?"

3. The goal of cognitive therapy with depressed clients is to:
   a. Identify and change dysfunctional patterns of thinking.
   b. Resolve the symptoms and initiate or restore adaptive family functioning.
   c. Alter the neurotransmitters that are creating the depressed mood.
   d. Provide feedback from peers who are having similar experiences.

Continued

Review Questions—cont'd
Self-Examination/Learning Exercise

4. Education for the client who is taking MAOIs should include which of the following?
   a. Fluid and sodium replacement when appropriate, frequent drug blood levels, signs and symptoms of toxicity
   b. Lifetime of continuous use, possible tardive dyskinesia, advantages of an injection every 2 to 4 weeks
   c. Short-term use, possible tolerance to beneficial effects, careful tapering of the drug at end of treatment
   d. Tyramine-restricted diet, prohibitive concurrent use of over-the-counter medications without physician notification

5. In teaching a client about his antidepressant medication, fluoxetine, which of the following would the nurse include? (Select all that apply.)
   a. Don't eat chocolate while taking this medication.
   b. Keep taking this medication, even if you don't feel it is helping. It sometimes takes a while to take effect.
   c. Don't take this medication with the migraine drugs "triptans."
   d. Go to the lab each week to have your blood drawn for therapeutic level of this drug.
   e. This drug causes a high degree of sedation, so take it just before bedtime.

6. A client has just been admitted to the psychiatric unit with a diagnosis of major depressive disorder. Which of the following behavioral manifestations might the nurse expect to assess? (Select all that apply.)
   a. Slumped posture
   b. Delusional thinking
   c. Feelings of despair
   d. Feels best early in the morning and worse as the day progresses
   e. Anorexia

7. A client with depression has just been prescribed the antidepressant phenelzine (Nardil). She says to the nurse, "The doctor says I will need to watch my diet while I'm on this medication. What foods should I avoid?" Which of the following is the correct response by the nurse?
   a. Blue cheese, red wine, raisins
   b. Black beans, garlic, pears
   c. Pork, shellfish, egg yolks
   d. Milk, peanuts, tomatoes

8. A client whose husband died 6 months ago is diagnosed with major depressive disorder. She says to the nurse, "I start feeling angry that Harold died and left me all alone; he should have stopped smoking years ago! But then I start feeling guilty for feeling that way." What is an appropriate response by the nurse?
   a. "Yes, he should have stopped smoking. Then he probably wouldn't have gotten lung cancer."
   b. "I can understand how you must feel."
   c. "Those feelings are a normal part of the grief response."
   d. "Just think about the good times that you had while he was alive."

9. A newly admitted depressed client isolates herself in her room and just sits and stares into space. How best might the nurse begin an initial therapeutic relationship with this client?
   a. Say, "Come with me. I will go with you to group therapy."
   b. Make frequent short visits to her room and sit with her.
   c. Offer to introduce her to the other clients.
   d. Help her to identify stressors in her life that precipitate crises.

10. John is a client at the mental health clinic. He is depressed, has been expressing suicidal ideations, and has been seeing the psychiatric nurse every 3 days. He has been taking 100 mg of sertraline daily for about a month, receiving small amounts of the medication from his nurse at each visit. Today he comes to the clinic in a cheerful mood, much different than he seemed just 3 days ago. How might the nurse assess this behavioral change?
    a. The sertraline is finally taking effect.
    b. He is no longer in need of antidepressant medication.
    c. He has completed the grief response over loss of his wife.
    d. He may have decided to carry out his suicide plan.

IMPLICATIONS OF RESEARCH FOR EVIDENCE-BASED PRACTICE

Pessagno, R.A., & Hunker, D. (2012). Using short-term group psychotherapy as an evidence-based intervention for first-time mothers at risk for postpartum depression. *Perspectives in Psychiatric Care.* doi:10.1111/j.1744-6163.2012.00350.x

DESCRIPTION OF THE STUDY: The purpose of this study was to determine if an 8-week, short-term psychotherapy group decreased the risk of developing postpartum depression (PPD) among first-time mothers at risk for PPD. The sample consisted of 16 women between the ages of 20 and 38 (mean 28.5 yrs.). All were Caucasian, and the majority were Catholic. Thirteen were married, 2 were partnered, and one participant was single. Two psychotherapy groups with 8 women in each group met once a week for 8 weeks beginning 1 month after discharge from the hospital. Each session lasted 90 minutes, and both groups were led by the same advanced practice psychiatric nurse practitioner. All subjects had completed the Edinburgh Postnatal Depression Scale (EPDS) within 3 days of giving birth, and all had scored 11 or higher, which was targeted as a high-risk for PPD score by the participant hospital (a community hospital in New Jersey). The psychotherapy groups followed an unstructured format, with an interpersonal-focused theoretical model. The authors stated, "This focus was structured to provide optimal opportunity in developing skills relative to their new maternal roles as new mothers, coping with depression and stress, honing communication skills with their husbands and partners, and sharing their individual, weekly experiences. The EPDS was administered to all participants at the end of the 8 sessions.

RESULTS OF THE STUDY: The mean preintervention score on the EPDS for group 1 was 16.13, and for group 2, the mean score was 15.5, placing participants from both groups at high risk for PPD. Following the intervention, the mean score for group 1 participants was 6.38 and for group 2 was 6.63. The EPDS was administered at 6-months postintervention to determine the long-term effects. At that time, both groups demonstrated a significant decrease in scores on the EPDS, demonstrating a continued effect of the group intervention for participants. The authors stated, "This is suggestive that group psychotherapy can have long-term effects to reduce risk for PPD for first-time mothers."

IMPLICATIONS FOR NURSING PRACTICE: The results of this study indicate that, particularly in those states that mandate screening for PPD, implementing nonpharmacologic interventions such as short-term group psychotherapy provides a choice for women who decide against the use of medication. The authors stated, "In today's mental health services market, significant focus is paid on the importance of medication management skills of the psychiatric APN, yet the intervention in this project supports the need for continued education and training of advanced practice psychiatric nursing as psychotherapists with group psychotherapy skills."

TEST YOUR CRITICAL THINKING SKILLS

Carol is a 17-year-old high school senior. She will graduate in 1 month and has plans to attend the state university a few hours from her home. Carol has always made good grades in school, has participated in many activities, and has been a pep squad cheerleader. She had been dating the star quarterback, Alan, since last summer, and they had spoken a number of times about going to the senior prom together. About a month before the prom, Alan broke up with Carol and began dating Sally, whom he subsequently took to the prom. Since that time, Carol has become despondent. She doesn't go out with her friends; she dropped out of the pep squad; her grades have fallen; and she has lost 10 pounds. She attends classes most of the time, but evenings and weekends she spends in her room alone listening to her music, crying, and sleeping. Her parents have become very concerned and contacted the family physician, who has had Carol admitted to the psychiatric unit of the local hospital. The admitting psychiatrist has made the diagnosis of major depressive disorder. Carol tells the nurse, "Sometimes I drive around and try to find Alan and Sally. I don't know why he broke up with me. I hate myself! I just want to die!"

Answer the following questions related to Carol:

1. What is the primary nursing diagnosis that is identified for Carol?
2. To determine the seriousness of this problem, what are important nursing assessments that must be made?
3. What medication might the physician order for Carol?
4. What concern has the FDA identified that is associated with this medication?

Communication Exercises

- Carrie, age 75, is a patient on the psychiatric unit with a diagnosis of major depressive disorder. She says to the nurse, "I never knew my life would end up like this. I've lost my husband, all my friends, and my home."

  How would the nurse respond appropriately to this statement by Carrie?

- "I have spent my whole life taking care of others. Now someone else has to take care of me. I feel so useless."

  How would the nurse respond appropriately to this statement by Carrie?

- "I don't know why anyone would want to bother taking care of me. I really have nothing left to live for."

  How would the nurse respond appropriately to this statement by Carrie?

References

Abrams, R. (2002). *Electroconvulsive therapy* (4th ed). New York, NY: Oxford University Press.

Administration on Aging. (2013). *A profile of older Americans: 2012.* Washington, DC: U.S. Department of Health and Human Services.

American Psychiatric Association. (2013). *Diagnostic and statistical manual of mental disorders* (5th ed.). Washington, DC: American Psychiatric Publishing.

Azoulay, L., Blais, L., Koren, G., LeLorier, J. & Berard, A. (2008). Isotretinoin and the risk of depression in patients with acne vulgaris: A case-crossover study. *The Journal of Clinical Psychiatry, 69,* 526-532.

Black, D.W., & Andreasen, N.C. (2011). *Introductory textbook of psychiatry* (5th ed.). Washington, DC: American Psychiatric Publishing.

Cartwright, L. (2004). Emergencies of survival: Moral spectatorship and the new vision of the child in postwar child psychoanalysis. *Journal of Visual Culture, 3*(1), 35-49.

Cooper, B.E., & Sejnowski, C.A. (2013). Serotonin syndrome: Recognition and treatment. *AACN Advanced Critical Care, 24*(1), 15-20.

Davidson, L. (2005). *Suicide and season.* New York, NY: American Foundation for Suicide Prevention.

Dopheide, J.A. (2006). Recognizing and treating depression in children and adolescents. *American Journal of Health-System Pharmacy, 63*(3), 233-243.

Dubovsky, S.L., Davies, R., & Dubovsky, A.M. (2003). Mood disorders. In R.E. Hales & S.C. Yudofsky (Eds.). *Textbook of clinical psychiatry* (4th ed., pp. 439-542). Washington, DC: American Psychiatric Publishing.

Eranti, S., Mogg, A., Pluck, G., Landau, S., Purvis, R., Brown, R.G., Howard, R., Knapp, M., Philpot, M., Rabe-Hesketh, S., Romeo, R., Rothwell, J., Edwards, D., & McLoughlin, D.M. (2007). A randomized, controlled trial with 6-month follow-up of repetitive transcranial magnetic stimulation and electroconvulsive therapy for severe depression. *American Journal of Psychiatry, 164*(1), 73-81.

Frackiewicz, E.J., & Shiovitz, T.M. (2001). Evaluation and management of premenstrual syndrome. *Journal of the American Pharmaceutical Association, 41*(3), 437-447.

Frank, L.R. (2002). Electroshock: A crime against the spirit. *Ethical Human Sciences & Services, 4*(1), 63-71.

George, L.K. (1992). Social factors and depression. In K.W. Schaie, D. Blazer, & J.S. House (Eds.), *Aging, health behaviors, and health outcomes.* Hillsdale, NJ: Lawrence Erlbaum Associates.

George, M.S., Taylor, J.J., & Short, E.B. (2013). The expanding evidence base for rTMS treatment of depression. *Current Opinion in Psychiatry, 26*(1), 13-18.

Greiner, A., Knebel, E., & Institute of Medicine Board on Health Care Services and Committee on the Health Professions Education Summit. (2003). *Health professions education: A bridge to quality.* Washington, DC: National Academies Press.

Grover, S., Mattoo, S.K., & Gupta, N. (2005). Theories on mechanism of action of electroconvulsive therapy. *German Journal of Psychiatry, 8*(4), 70-84.

Hakko, H. (2000). *Seasonal variation of suicides and homicides in Finland.* Oulu, Finland: University of Oulu.

Hudson, C.G. (2005). Socioeconomic status and mental illness: Tests of the social causation and selection hypotheses. *American Journal of Orthopsychiatry, 75*(1), 3-18.

Joska, J.A., & Stein, D.J. (2008). Mood disorders. In R.E. Hales, S.C. Yudofsky, & G.O. Gabbard (Eds.), *Textbook of psychiatry* (5th ed., 457-503). Washington, DC: American Psychiatric Publishing.

Karasu, T.B., Gelenberg, A., Merriam, A., & Wang, P. (2006). Practice guideline for the treatment of patients with major depressive disorder (2nd ed.). *American Psychiatric Association Practice Guidelines for the Treatment of Psychiatric Disorders, Compendium 2006.* Washington, DC: American Psychiatric Publishing.

Knoll, J. (2011). The suicide prevention contract: Contracting for comfort. *Psychiatric Times.* Retrieved from http://www.psychiatrictimes.com/suicide/suicide-prevention-contract-contracting-comfort

Kornstein, S.G. (2006). Gender and depression. *MedscapeCME.* Retrieved from http://cme.medscape.com/viewarticle/527494

Lam, R.W., Levitt, A.J., Levitan, R.D., Enns, M.W., Morehouse, R., Michalak, E.E., & Tam, E.M. (2006). The Can-SAD Study: A randomized controlled trial of the effectiveness of light therapy and fluoxetine in patients with winter seasonal affective disorder. *The American Journal of Psychiatry, 163*(5), 805-812.

Lanocha, K. (2010). Presenting TMS to patients. *Current Psychiatry, 9*(12), S7-S8.

LaPierre, T.A. (2004). *An investigation of the role of age and life stage in the moderation and mediation of the effect of marital status on depression.* Paper presented at the annual meeting of the American Sociological Association, Hilton San Francisco & Renaissance Parc 55 Hotel, San Francisco, CA, August 14, 2004. Retrieved from http://www.allacademic.com/meta/p109917_index.html

Marangell, L.B., Silver, J.M., Goff, D.C., & Yudofsky, S.C. (2003). Psychopharmacology and electroconvulsive therapy. In R.E. Hales & S.C. Yudofsky (Eds.), *Textbook of clinical psychiatry* (4th ed., pp. 1047-1149). Washington, DC: American Psychiatric Publishing.

Martinez, M., Marangell, L.B., & Martinez, J.M. (2008). Psychopharmacology. In R.E. Hales, S.C. Yudofsky, & G.O. Gabbard (Eds.), *Textbook of Psychiatry* (5th ed., pp. 1053-1131). Washington, DC: American Psychiatric Publishing.

Mehta, A., & Sheth, S. (2006). Postpartum depression: How to recognize and treat this common condition. *Medscape Psychiatry & Mental Health, 11*(1). Retrieved from http://www.medscape.com/viewarticle/529390

NANDA International (NANDA-I). (2012). *Nursing diagnoses: Definitions and classification 2012-2014.* Hoboken, NJ: Wiley-Blackwell.

National Center for Health Statistics (NCHS). (2012). Deaths: Preliminary data for 2011. *National Vital Statistics Reports, 61*(6), October 10, 2012. Hyattsville, MD: NCHS.

National Center for Health Statistics (NCHS). (2013). Health, United States, 2012. DHS Publication No. 2013-1232. Hyattsville, MD: Author.

National Institute of Mental Health (NIMH). (2013). *Antidepressant medications for children and adolescents: Information for parents and caregivers.* Retrieved from http://www.nimh.nih.gov

Puri, B.K., & Treasaden, I.H. (2011). *Textbook of psychiatry* (3rd ed.). Philadelphia, PA: Churchill Livingstone Elsevier.

Rupke, S.J., Blecke, D., & Renfrow, M. (2006). Cognitive therapy for depression. *American Family Physician, 73*(1), 83-86.

Sadock, B.J., and Sadock, V.A. (2007). *Synopsis of psychiatry: Behavioral sciences/clinical psychiatry* (10th ed.). Philadelphia, PA: Lippincott Williams & Wilkins.

Schatzberg, A.F., Cole, J.O., & DeBattista, C. (2010). *Manual of clinical psychopharmacology* (7th ed.). Washington, DC: American Psychiatric Publishing.

Schimelpfening, N. (2012). *A good vitamin supplement could be just what the doctor ordered.* Retrieved from http://depression.about.com/cs/diet/a/vitamin.htm

Slattery, D.A., Hudson, A.L., & Nutt, D.J. (2004). Invited review: The evolution of antidepressant mechanisms. *Fundamental & Clinical Pharmacology, 18*(1): 1-21.

Substance Abuse and Mental Health Services Administration (SAMHSA). (2013). *Results from the 2012 National Survey on Drug Use and Health: Mental health findings.* NSDUH Series H- 47, HHS Publication No. (SMA) 13-4805. Rockville, MD: SAMHSA.

Sword, W., Clark, A.M., Hegadoren, K., Brooks, S., & Kingston, D. (2012). The complexity of postpartum mental health and illness: A critical realist study. *Nursing Inquiry, 19*(1), 51-62.

Tempfer, T.C. (2006). *Identifying childhood depression.* Highlights of the National Association of Pediatric Nurse Practitioners 27th Annual Conference. Retrieved from http://www.medscape.com/viewprogram/5458

Terman, M., & Terman, J.S. (2005). Light therapy for seasonal and nonseasonal depression: Efficacy, protocol, safety, and side effects. *CNS Spectrums, 10*(8), 647-663.

Thase, M.E. (2007). The new "blue light" intervention for seasonal affective disorder (SAD). *Medscape Psychiatry & Mental Health.* Retrieved from http://cme.medscape.com/viewarticle/550845

Williams, D.R., Gonzalez, H.M., Neighbors, H., Nesse, R., Abelson, J.M., Sweetman, J., and Jackson, J.S. (2007). Prevalence and distribution of major depressive disorder in African Americans, Caribbean Blacks, and Non-Hispanic Whites: Results from the National Survey of American Life. *Archives of General Psychiatry, 64*(3), 305-315.

World Health Organization (WHO). (2014). *Health for the world's adolescents: A second chance in the second decade.* Geneva, Switzerland: WHO.

Classical References

Beck, A.T., Rush, A.J., Shaw, B.F., & Emery, G. (1979). *Cognitive theory of depression.* New York, NY: Guilford Press.

Freud, S. (1957). *Mourning and melancholia* (Vol. 14; Standard ed.). London: Hogarth Press. (Original work published 1917.)

Seligman, M.E.P. (1973). Fall into helplessness. *Psychology Today, 7,* 43-48.

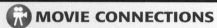

@ INTERNET REFERENCES

• Additional information about depression, including psychosocial and pharmacological treatment of these disorders, may be located at the following websites:
  • http://www.ndmda.org
  • http://www.mentalhealth.com
  • http://www.mental-health-matters.com
  • http://www.mentalhelp.net
  • http://www.nlm.nih.gov/medlineplus
  • http://nami.org
  • http://www.medicinenet.com/medications/article.htm
  • http://www.drugs.com

🎬 MOVIE CONNECTIONS

Prozac Nation (depression) • *The Butcher Boy* (depression) • *Night, Mother* (depression) • *The Prince of Tides* (depression/suicide)

26 Bipolar and Related Disorders

CORE CONCEPT

mania

KEY TERMS

bipolar disorder

cyclothymic disorder

delirious mania

hypomania

OBJECTIVES
After reading this chapter, the student will be able to:

1. Recount historical perspectives of bipolar disorder.
2. Discuss epidemiological statistics related to bipolar disorder.
3. Describe various types of bipolar disorders.
4. Identify predisposing factors in the development of bipolar disorder.
5. Discuss implications of bipolar disorder related to developmental stage.
6. Identify symptomatology associated with bipolar disorder and use this information in client assessment.

7. Formulate nursing diagnoses and goals of care for clients experiencing a manic episode.
8. Identify topics for client and family teaching relevant to bipolar disorder.
9. Describe appropriate nursing interventions for clients experiencing a manic episode.
10. Describe relevant criteria for evaluating nursing care of clients experiencing a manic episode.
11. Discuss various modalities relevant to the treatment of bipolar disorder.

HOMEWORK ASSIGNMENT
Please read the chapter and answer the following questions:

1. What is the most common medication that has been known to trigger manic episodes?
2. What is the speech pattern of a person experiencing a manic episode?
3. What is the difference between cyclothymic disorder and bipolar disorder?
4. Why should a person on lithium therapy have blood levels drawn regularly?

Mood was defined in the previous chapter as a pervasive and sustained emotion that may have a major influence on a person's perception of the world. Examples of mood include depression, joy, elation, anger, and anxiety. *Affect* is described as the emotional reaction associated with an experience.

The previous chapter focused on the consequences of complicated grieving as it is manifested by depressive disorders. This chapter addresses mood disorders as they are manifested by cycles of mania and depression—called **bipolar disorder**. A historical perspective and epidemiological statistics related to bipolar disorder are presented. Predisposing factors that have been implicated in the etiology of bipolar disorder provide a framework for studying the dynamics of the disorder.

The implications of bipolar disorder relevant to children and adolescents are discussed. An explanation of the symptomatology is presented as background knowledge for assessing the client with bipolar disorder. Nursing care is described in the context of the six steps of the nursing process. Various medical treatment modalities are explored.

CORE CONCEPT

Mania

An alteration in mood that is expressed by feelings of elation, inflated self-esteem, grandiosity, hyperactivity, agitation, and accelerated thinking and speaking. Mania can occur as a biological (organic) or psychological disorder, or as a response to substance use or a general medical condition.

Historical Perspective

Documentation of the symptoms associated with bipolar disorder dates back to about the second century in ancient Greece. Aretaeus of Cappadocia, a Greek physician, is credited with associating these extremes of mood as part of the same illness. It was not until much later, however, that his view gained some acceptance.

In early writings, mania was categorized with all forms of "severe madness." In 1025, the Persian physician Avicenna wrote *The Canon of Medicine*, in which he described mania as "bestial madness characterized by rapid onset and remission, with agitation and irritability." He considered rabies as a kind of mania. (Youssef, Youssef, & Dening, 1996, p. 57).

The modern concept of manic-depressive illness began to emerge in the 19th century. In 1854, Jules Baillarger presented information to the French Imperial Academy of Medicine in which he used the term *dual-form insanity* to describe the illness. In the same year, Jean-Pierre Falret described the same disorder, which he termed "circular insanity" (Nakate, 2011).

Contemporary thinking has been shaped a great deal by the works of Emil Kraepelin, who first coined the term manic-depressive in 1913. His approach became the most widely accepted theory of the early 1930s (Guadiz, 2011). In 1980, the American Psychiatric Association adopted the term *bipolar disorder* as the diagnostic category for manic-depressive illness in the third edition of the *Diagnostic and Statistical Manual of Mental Disorders (DSM-III)*.

Epidemiology

Bipolar disorder affects approximately 5.7 million American adults, or about 2.6 percent of the U.S. population age 18 and older in a given year (National Institute of Mental Health [NIMH], 2013). In terms of gender, the incidence of bipolar disorder is roughly equal, with a ratio of women to men of about 1.2 to 1. The average age of onset for bipolar disorder is the early 20s, and following the first manic episode, the disorder tends to be recurrent. As with depression, bipolar disorder appears to be more common in unmarried than in married persons (Joska & Stein, 2008). Unlike depressive disorders, bipolar disorder appears to occur more frequently among the higher socioeconomic classes (Sadock & Sadock, 2007). Bipolar disorder is the sixth leading cause of disability in the middle age group, and the loss of earnings and productivity attributable to mood disorders (depression and bipolar disorder) may amount to about $33 billion per year in the United States (Joska & Stein, 2008).

Types of Bipolar Disorders

A bipolar disorder is characterized by mood swings from profound depression to extreme euphoria (mania), with intervening periods of normalcy. Delusions or hallucinations may or may not be a part of the clinical picture, and onset of symptoms may reflect a seasonal pattern.

During a manic episode, the mood is elevated, expansive, or irritable. The disturbance is sufficiently severe to cause marked impairment in occupational functioning or in usual social activities or relationships with others or to require hospitalization to prevent harm to self or others. Motor activity is excessive and frenzied. Psychotic features may be present. The *Diagnostic and Statistical Manual of Mental Disorders, Fifth Edition (DSM-5)* (APA, 2013) diagnostic criteria for a manic episode are presented in Box 26-1.

A somewhat milder degree of this clinical symptom picture is called **hypomania**. Hypomania is not severe enough to cause marked impairment in social or occupational functioning or to require hospitalization, and it does not include psychotic features. The *DSM-5* diagnostic criteria for a hypomanic episode are presented in Box 26-2.

The diagnostic picture for depression associated with bipolar disorder is similar to that described for major depressive disorder, with one major distinction: the client must have a history of one or more manic episodes. When the symptom presentation includes rapidly alternating moods (sadness, irritability, euphoria) accompanied by symptoms associated with both

---

BOX 26-1 Diagnostic Criteria for Manic Episode

A. A distinct period of abnormally and persistently elevated, expansive, or irritable mood, and abnormally and persistently increased goal-directed activity or energy, lasting at least 1 week and present most of the day, nearly every day (or any duration if hospitalization is necessary).

B. During the period of mood disturbance and increased energy or activity, three (or more) of the following symptoms (four if the mood is only irritable) are present to a significant degree, and represent a noticeable change from usual behavior:
1. Inflated self-esteem or grandiosity.
2. Decreased need for sleep (e.g., feels rested after only 3 hours of sleep).
3. More talkative than usual or pressure to keep talking.
4. Flight of ideas or subjective experience that thoughts are racing.
5. Distractibility (i.e., attention too easily drawn to unimportant or irrelevant external stimuli), as reported or observed.
6. Increase in goal-directed activity (either socially, at work or school, or sexually) or psychomotor agitation (i.e., purposeless non-goal-directed activity).
7. Excessive involvement in activities that have a high potential for painful consequences (e.g., engaging in unrestrained buying sprees, sexual indiscretions, or foolish business investments).

C. The mood disturbance is sufficiently severe to cause marked impairment in social or occupational functioning or to necessitate hospitalization to prevent harm to self or others, or there are psychotic features.

D. The episode is not attributable to the physiological effects of a substance (e.g., a drug of abuse, a medication, or other treatment) or to another medical condition. *Note:* A full manic episode that emerges during antidepressant treatment (e.g., medication, electroconvulsive therapy), but persists at a fully syndromal level beyond the physiological effect of that treatment is sufficient evidence for a manic episode and, therefore, a bipolar I diagnosis.

Reprinted with permission from the *Diagnostic and Statistical Manual of Mental Disorders, Fifth Edition* (Copyright 2013). American Psychiatric Association.

BOX 26-2 Diagnostic Criteria for Hypomanic Episode

A. A distinct period of abnormally and persistently elevated, expansive, or irritable mood and abnormally and persistently increased activity or energy, lasting at least 4 consecutive days and present most of the day, nearly every day.

B. During the period of mood disturbance and increased energy and activity, three (or more) of the following symptoms (four if the mood is only irritable) have persisted, represent a noticeable change from usual behavior, and have been present to a significant degree:
1. Inflated self-esteem or grandiosity.
2. Decreased need for sleep (e.g., feels rested after only 3 hours of sleep).
3. More talkative than usual or pressure to keep talking.
4. Flight of ideas or subjective experience that thoughts are racing.
5. Distractibility (i.e., attention too easily drawn to unimportant or irrelevant external stimuli), as reported or observed.
6. Increase in goal-directed activity (either socially, at work or school, or sexually) or psychomotor agitation.
7. Excessive involvement in pleasurable activities that have a high potential for painful consequences (e.g., engaging in unrestrained buying sprees, sexual indiscretions, or foolish business investments).

C. The episode is associated with an unequivocal change in functioning that is uncharacteristic of the individual when not symptomatic.

D. The disturbance in mood and the change in functioning are observable by others.

E. The episode is not severe enough to cause marked impairment in social or occupational functioning or to necessitate hospitalization. If there are psychotic features, the episode is, by definition, manic.

F. The episode is not attributable to the physiological effects of a substance (e.g., a drug of abuse, a medication, or other treatment).

NOTE: A full hypomanic episode that emerges during antidepressant treatment (medication, electroconvulsive therapy) but persists at a fully syndromal level beyond the physiological effect of that treatment is sufficient evidence for a hypomanic episode diagnosis. However, caution is indicated so that one or two symptoms (particularly increased irritability, edginess or agitation following antidepressant use) are not taken as sufficient for diagnosis of a hypomanic episode, nor necessarily indicative of a bipolar diathesis.

Reprinted with permission from the *Diagnostic and Statistical Manual of Mental Disorders, Fifth Edition* (Copyright 2013). American Psychiatric Association.

depression and mania, the diagnosis is further specified as *with mixed features.*

Bipolar I Disorder

Bipolar I disorder is the diagnosis given to an individual who is experiencing a manic episode or has a history of one or more manic episodes. The client may also have experienced episodes of depression. This diagnosis is further specified by the current or most recent behavioral episode experienced. For example, the specifier might be *single manic episode* (to describe individuals having a first episode of mania) or the specifier may be identified as *current* (or most recent) *episode manic, hypomanic, mixed,* or *depressed* (to describe individuals who have had recurrent mood episodes). Psychotic or catatonic features may also be noted.

Bipolar II Disorder

The bipolar II disorder diagnostic category is characterized by recurrent bouts of major depression with episodic occurrence of hypomania. The individual who is assigned this diagnosis may present with symptoms (or history) of depression or hypomania. The client has never experienced a full manic episode. The diagnosis may specify whether the current or most recent episode is hypomanic, depressed, or with mixed features. If the current syndrome is a major depressive episode, psychotic or catatonic features may be noted.

Cyclothymic Disorder

The essential feature of **cyclothymic disorder** is a chronic mood disturbance of at least 2 years' duration, involving numerous periods of elevated mood that do not meet the criteria for a hypomanic episode and numerous periods of depressed mood of insufficient severity or duration to meet the criteria for major depressive episode. The individual is never without the symptoms for more than 2 months. The *DSM-5* criteria for cyclothymic disorder are presented in Box 26-3.

Substance/Medication-Induced Bipolar Disorder

The disturbance of mood associated with this disorder is considered to be the direct result of physiological effects of a substance (e.g., ingestion of or withdrawal from a drug of abuse or a medication). The mood disturbance may involve elevated, expansive, or irritable mood, with inflated self-esteem, decreased need for sleep, and distractibility. The disorder causes clinically significant distress or impairment in social, occupational, or other important areas of functioning.

Mood disturbances are associated with *intoxication* from substances such as alcohol, amphetamines, cocaine, hallucinogens, inhalants, opioids, phencyclidine, sedatives, hypnotics, and anxiolytics. Symptoms can occur with *withdrawal* from substances such as alcohol, amphetamines, cocaine, sedatives, hypnotics, and anxiolytics.

A number of medications have been known to evoke mood symptoms. Classifications include anesthetics, analgesics, anticholinergics, anticonvulsants, antihypertensives, antiparkinsonian agents, antiulcer agents, cardiac medications, oral contraceptives, psychotropic medications, muscle relaxants, steroids, and sulfonamides. Some specific examples are included in the discussion of predisposing factors associated with bipolar disorders.

BOX 26-3 Diagnostic Criteria for Cyclothymic Disorder

A. For at least 2 years (at least one year in children and adolescents) there have been numerous periods with hypomanic symptoms that do not meet criteria for hypomanic episode and numerous periods with depressive symptoms that do not meet the criteria for a major depressive episode.

B. During the above 2-year period (1 year in children and adolescents), the hypomanic and depressive periods have been present for at least half the time and the individual has not been without the symptoms for more than 2 months at a time.

C. Criteria for a major depressive, manic, or hypomanic episode have never been met.

D. The symptoms in Criterion A are not better explained by schizoaffective disorder, schizophrenia, schizophreniform disorder, delusional disorder, or other specified or unspecified schizophrenia spectrum and other psychotic disorder.

E. The symptoms are not attributable to the physiological effects of a substance (e.g., a drug of abuse, a medication) or another medical condition (e.g., hyperthyroidism).

F. The symptoms cause clinically significant distress or impairment in social, occupational, or other important areas of functioning.

Specify if:
With anxious distress

Bipolar Disorder Due to Another Medical Condition

This disorder is characterized by an abnormally and persistently elevated, expansive, or irritable mood and excessive activity or energy that is judged to be the result of direct physiological consequence of another medical condition (APA, 2013). The mood disturbance causes clinically significant distress or impairment in social, occupational, or other important areas of functioning. Types of physiological influences are included in the discussion of predisposing factors associated with bipolar disorders.

Predisposing Factors

The exact etiology of bipolar disorder has yet to be determined. Scientific evidence supports a chemical imbalance in the brain, although the cause of the imbalance remains unclear. Theories that consider a combination of hereditary factors and environmental triggers (stressful life events) appear to hold the most credibility.

Biological Theories

Genetics

Research suggests that bipolar disorder strongly reflects an underlying genetic vulnerability. Evidence from family, twin, and adoption studies exists to support this observation.

Twin Studies

Twin studies have indicated a concordance rate for bipolar disorder among monozygotic twins at 60 to 80 percent compared to 10 to 20 percent in dizygotic twins. Because monozygotic twins have identical genes and dizygotic twins share only approximately half their genes, this is strong evidence that genes play a major role in the etiology.

Family Studies

Family studies have shown that, if one parent has bipolar disorder, the risk that a child will have the disorder is around 28 percent (Dubovsky, Davies, & Dubovsky, 2003). If both parents have the disorder, the risk is 2 to 3 times as great. This has also been shown to be the case in studies of children born to parents with bipolar disorder who were adopted at birth and reared by adoptive parents without evidence of the disorder. These results strongly indicate that genes play a role separate from that of the environment.

Other Genetic Studies

Soreff and McInnes (2012) state:

> Studies from the first series of genome-wide association studies have given combined support for two particular genes, *ANK3* (ankyrin G) and *CACNA1C* (alpha

1C subunit of the L-type voltage-gated calcium channel) in a sample of 4,387 cases and 6,209 controls.

The *ANK3* protein is located on the first part of the axon and is involved in making the determination of whether a neuron will fire. Studies have shown that lithium carbonate, the most common medication used to prevent manic episodes, reduces expression of *ANK3* (NIMH, 2008). The *CACNA1C* protein regulates the influx and outflow of calcium from the cells, and is the site of action of the calcium channel blockers sometimes used in the treatment of bipolar disorder.

Biochemical Influences

Biogenic Amines

Early studies have associated symptoms of depression with a functional deficiency of norepinephrine and dopamine and mania with a functional excess of these amines. The neurotransmitter serotonin appears to remain low in both states. One study at the University of Michigan using a presynaptic marker and positron emission tomography revealed an increased density in the amine-releasing cells in the brains of people with bipolar disorder compared to control subjects (Zubieta et al., 2000). It was hypothesized that these excess cells result in the altered brain chemistry that is associated with the symptoms of bipolar disorder. Some support of this neurotransmitter hypothesis has been demonstrated by the effects of neuroleptic drugs that influence the levels of these biogenic amines to produce the desired effect.

More recently, the biogenic amine hypothesis has been expanded to include another neurotransmitter, acetylcholine. Because cholinergic agents do have profound effects on mood, electroencephalogram, sleep, and neuroendocrine function, it has been suggested that the problem in depression and mania may be an imbalance between the biogenic amines and acetylcholine. Cholinergic transmission is thought to be excessive in depression and inadequate in mania (Dubovsky et al., 2003).

Physiological Influences

Neuroanatomical Factors

Right-sided lesions in the limbic system, temporobasal areas, basal ganglia, and thalamus have been shown to induce secondary mania. Magnetic resonance imaging studies have revealed enlarged third ventricles and subcortical white matter and periventricular hyperintensities in clients with bipolar disorder (Dubovsky et al., 2003).

Medication Side Effects

Certain medications used to treat somatic illnesses have been known to trigger a manic response. The most common of these are the steroids frequently used to treat chronic illnesses such as multiple sclerosis and systemic lupus erythematosus (SLE). Some clients whose first episode of mania occurred during steroid therapy have reported spontaneous recurrence of manic symptoms years later. Amphetamines, antidepressants, and high doses of anticonvulsants and narcotics also have the potential for initiating a manic episode (Dubovsky et al., 2003).

Psychosocial Theories

The credibility of psychosocial theories has declined in recent years. Conditions such as schizophrenia and bipolar disorder are viewed as diseases of the brain with biological etiologies. The etiology of these illnesses remains unclear, however, and it is possible that both biological and psychosocial factors (such as environmental stressors) may be influential (Soreff & McInnes, 2012).

The Transactional Model

Bipolar disorder most likely results from interactions among genetic, biological, and psychosocial determinants. Soreff and McInnes (2012) state, "The cycle may be directly linked to external stresses or the external pressures may serve to exacerbate some underlying genetic or biochemical predisposition." The transactional model takes into consideration these various etiological influences, as well as those associated with past experiences, existing conditions, and the individual's perception of the event. Figure 26-1 depicts the dynamics of bipolar mania, using the Transactional Model of Stress/Adaptation.

Developmental Implications

Childhood and Adolescence

The lifetime prevalence of pediatric and adolescent bipolar disorders is estimated to be about 1 percent, but children and adolescents are often difficult to diagnose (Nandagopal & DelBello, 2008). The developmental courses and symptom profiles of psychiatric disorders in children are unique from those of adults; therefore, approaches to diagnosis and treatment cannot merely rely on strategies examined and implemented in a typical adult population.

A working group sponsored by the Child and Adolescent Bipolar Foundation (CABF) has developed consensus guidelines for the diagnosis and treatment of children with bipolar disorder. These guidelines were presented in the March 2005 issue of the *Journal of the American Academy of Child and Adolescent Psychiatry* and address diagnosis, comorbidity, acute treatment, and maintenance treatment (Kowatch et al., 2005).

Symptoms of bipolar disorder are often difficult to assess in children, and they may also present with comorbid conduct disorders or attention-deficit/hyperactivity disorder (ADHD). Because there is a genetic component and children of bipolar adults are at higher risk, family history may be particularly important (Nandagopal & DelBello, 2008). To differentiate between occasional spontaneous behaviors of childhood and behaviors associated with bipolar disorder, the Consensus Group recommends that clinicians use the FIND (frequency, intensity, number, and duration) strategy (Kowatch et al., 2005):

- **Frequency:** Symptoms occur most days in a week.
- **Intensity:** Symptoms are severe enough to cause extreme disturbance in one domain or moderate disturbance in two or more domains.
- **Number:** Symptoms occur three or four times a day.
- **Duration:** Symptoms occur 4 or more hours a day.

The symptoms associated with mania in children and adolescents are as follows. Regarding these symptoms, Kowatch and associates (2005) state:

> For any of these symptoms to be counted as a manic symptom, they must exceed the FIND threshold. Additionally, they must occur in concert with other manic symptoms because no one symptom is diagnostic of mania. (p. 215)

- **Euphoric/expansive mood.** Extremely happy, silly, or giddy.
- **Irritable mood.** Hostility and rage, often over trivial matters. The irritability may be accompanied by aggressive and/or self-injurious behavior.
- **Grandiosity.** Believing that his or her abilities are better than everyone else's.
- **Decreased need for sleep.** May sleep only 4 or 5 hours per night and wake up fresh and full of energy the next day. Or he or she may get up in the middle of the night and wander around the house looking for things to do.
- **Pressured speech.** Rapid speech that is loud, intrusive, and difficult to interrupt.
- **Racing thoughts.** Topics of conversation change rapidly, in a manner confusing to anyone listening.
- **Distractibility.** To consider distractibility a manic symptom, it needs to reflect a change from baseline functioning, needs to occur in conjunction with a "manic" mood shift, and cannot be accounted for exclusively by another disorder, particularly ADHD (Kowatch et al., 2005). Distractibility during a manic episode may be reflected in a child who is normally a B or C student and is unable to focus on any school lessons.
- **Increase in goal-directed activity/psychomotor agitation.** A child who is not usually highly productive, during a manic episode becomes very project

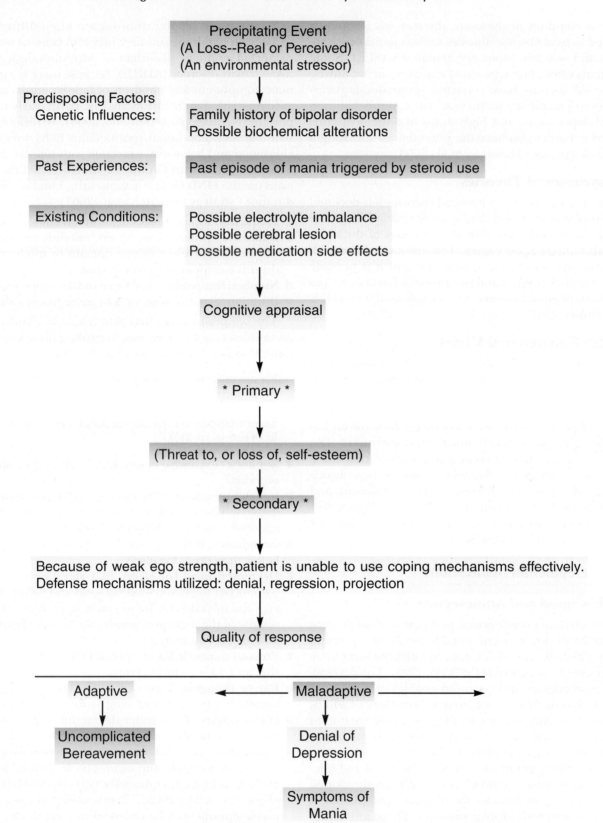

FIGURE 26–1   The dynamics of bipolar mania, using the Transactional Model of Stress/Adaptation.

oriented, increasing goal-directed activity to an obsessive level. Psychomotor agitation represents a distinct change from baseline behavior.

■ **Excessive involvement in pleasurable or risky activities.** Children with bipolar disorder are often hypersexual, exhibiting behavior that has an erotic, pleasure-seeking quality about it (Kowatch et al., 2005). Adolescents may seek out sexual activity multiple times in a day.

■ **Psychosis.** In addition to core symptoms of mania, psychotic symptoms, including hallucinations and delusions, are frequently present in children with bipolar disorder (Geller et al., 2002; Kafantaris, Dicker, Coletti, & Kane, 2001).

■ **Suicidality.** Although not a core symptom of mania, children with bipolar disorder are at risk of suicidal ideation, intent, plans, and attempts during a depressed or mixed episode or when psychotic (Geller et al., 2002).

Treatment Strategies

Psychopharmacology

Monotherapy with the traditional mood stabilizers (e.g., lithium, divalproex, carbamazepine) or atypical antipsychotics (e.g., olanzapine, quetiapine, risperidone, aripiprazole) was determined to be the first-line treatment (Kowatch et al., 2005). In the event of inadequate response to initial monotherapy, an alternate monotherapeutic agent is suggested. Augmentation with a second medication is indicated when monotherapy fails.

In a recent study to examine current research data, Hazell and Jairam (2012) reported "evidence favoring the use of second-generation antipsychotics (SGAs), limited evidence favoring the use of combinations of SGA with a mood stabilizer, and no evidence supporting the use of mood stabilizer monotherapy" (p. 264). From their study, they suggest that the first-line treatment for mania in children and adolescents is a SGA, with combination therapies offering no clear advantage.

ADHD has been identified as the most common comorbid condition in children and adolescents with bipolar disorder. Because stimulants can exacerbate mania, it is suggested that medication for ADHD be initiated only after bipolar symptoms have been controlled with a mood stabilizing agent (McClellan, Kowatch, & Findling, 2007). Nonstimulant medications indicated for ADHD (e.g., atomoxetine, bupropion, the tricyclic antidepressants) may also induce switches to mania or hypomania.

Bipolar disorder in children and adolescents appears to be a chronic condition with a high risk of relapse. Maintenance therapy incorporates the same medications used to treat acute symptoms, although few research studies exist that deal with long-term maintenance of bipolar disorder in children. The Consensus Group recommends that medication tapering or discontinuation be considered after remission has been achieved for a minimum of 12 to 24 consecutive months. It was acknowledged, however, that some clients may require long-term or even lifelong pharmacotherapy (McClellan et al., 2007).

Family Interventions

Although pharmacologic treatment is acknowledged as the primary method of stabilizing an acutely ill bipolar client, adjunctive psychotherapy has been recognized as playing an important role in preventing relapses and improving adjustment. Correll (2007) stresses the importance of psychoeducational therapy to familiarize both the patient and the family with the symptoms, course, and impact of the disorder and the available treatment options. Correll (2007) states, "Social and family function can be significantly disrupted by a child with bipolar disorder. Patients and their families may need counseling in ways to address these disruptions." Relapse prevention, including the importance of treatment adherence, must be emphasized.

Family dynamics and attitudes can play a crucial role in the outcome of a client's recovery. Interventions with family members must include education that promotes understanding that at least part of the client's negative behaviors are attributable to an illness that must be managed, as opposed to being willful and deliberate.

Studies show that family-focused psychoeducational treatment (FFT) is an effective method of reducing relapses and increasing medication adherence in bipolar clients (Miklowitz et al., 2003). FFT includes sessions that deal with psychoeducation about bipolar disorder (i.e., symptoms, early recognition, etiology, treatment, self-management), communication training, and problem-solving skills training. Allen (2003) states:

> There are several important goals of FFT, which include: improving communication within the family, teaching the family to recognize the early warning signs of a relapse, teaching the family how to respond to these warning signs, and educating them regarding the necessary treatments. This education helps families gain some control over the conflict that occurs in the post-episode phases.

There is evidence to suggest that the addition of psychosocial therapy enhances the effectiveness of psychopharmacological therapy in the maintenance of bipolar disorder in children and adolescents.

Application of the Nursing Process to Bipolar Disorder (Mania)

Background Assessment Data

Symptoms of manic states can be described according to three stages: hypomania, acute mania, and **delirious mania**. Symptoms of mood, cognition and perception, and activity and behavior are presented for each stage.

Stage I: Hypomania

At this stage the disturbance is not sufficiently severe to cause marked impairment in social or occupational functioning or to require hospitalization (APA, 2013).

Mood

The mood of a hypomanic person is cheerful and expansive. There is an underlying irritability that surfaces rapidly when the person's wishes and desires go unfulfilled, however. The nature of the hypomanic person is very volatile and fluctuating (see Box 26-2).

Cognition and Perception

Perceptions of the self are exalted—ideas of great worth and ability. Thinking is flighty, with a rapid flow of ideas. Perception of the environment is heightened, but the individual is so easily distracted by irrelevant stimuli that goal-directed activities are difficult.

Activity and Behavior

Hypomanic individuals exhibit increased motor activity. They are perceived as being very extroverted and sociable, and because of this they attract numerous acquaintances. However, they lack the depth of personality and warmth to formulate close friendships. They talk and laugh a great deal, usually very loudly and often inappropriately. Increased libido is common. Some individuals experience anorexia and weight loss. The exalted self-perception leads some hypomanic individuals to engage in inappropriate behaviors, such as phoning the President of the United States, or buying huge amounts on a credit card without having the resources to pay.

Stage II: Acute Mania

Symptoms of acute mania may be a progression in intensification of those experienced in hypomania, or they may be manifested directly. Most individuals experience marked impairment in functioning and require hospitalization (see Box 26-1).

Mood

Acute mania is characterized by euphoria and elation. The person appears to be on a continuous "high." However, the mood is always subject to frequent variation, easily changing to irritability and anger or even to sadness and crying.

Cognition and Perception

Cognition and perception become fragmented and often psychotic in acute mania. Rapid thinking proceeds to racing and disjointed thinking (flight of ideas) and may be manifested by a continuous flow of accelerated, pressured speech (loquaciousness), with abrupt changes from topic to topic. When flight of ideas is severe, speech may be disorganized and incoherent. Distractibility becomes all-pervasive. Attention can be diverted by even the smallest of stimuli. Hallucinations and delusions (usually paranoid and grandiose) are common.

Activity and Behavior

Psychomotor activity is excessive. Sexual interest is increased. There is poor impulse control, and the individual who is normally discreet may become socially and sexually uninhibited. Excessive spending is common. Individuals with acute mania have the ability to manipulate others to carry out their wishes, and if things go wrong, they can skillfully project responsibility for the failure onto others. Energy seems inexhaustible, and the need for sleep is diminished. They may go for many days without sleep and still not feel tired. Hygiene and grooming may be neglected. Dress may be disorganized, flamboyant, or bizarre, and the use of excessive makeup or jewelry is common.

Stage III: Delirious Mania

Delirious mania is a grave form of the disorder characterized by severe clouding of consciousness and an intensification of the symptoms associated with acute mania. This condition has become relatively rare since the availability of antipsychotic medication.

Mood

The mood of the delirious person is very labile. He or she may exhibit feelings of despair, quickly converting to unrestrained merriment and ecstasy or becoming irritable or totally indifferent to the environment. Panic anxiety may be evident.

Cognition and Perception

Cognition and perception are characterized by a clouding of consciousness, with accompanying confusion, disorientation, and sometimes stupor. Other common manifestations include religiosity, delusions of grandeur or persecution, and auditory or visual hallucinations. The individual is extremely distractible and incoherent.

Activity and Behavior

Psychomotor activity is frenzied and characterized by agitated, purposeless movements. The safety of these individuals is at stake unless this activity is curtailed. Exhaustion, injury to self or others, and eventually death could occur without intervention.

Diagnosis/Outcome Identification

Using information collected during the assessment, the nurse completes the client database, from which the selection of appropriate nursing diagnoses is determined. Table 26-1 presents a list of client behaviors and the NANDA nursing diagnoses that correspond

TABLE 26-1	Assigning Nursing Diagnoses to Behaviors Commonly Exhibited by Individuals Experiencing a Manic Episode
BEHAVIORS	**NURSING DIAGNOSES**
Extreme hyperactivity; increased agitation and lack of control over purposeless and potentially injurious movements	**Risk for injury**
Manic excitement, delusional thinking, hallucinations, impulsivity	**Risk for violence: Self-directed or other-directed**
Loss of weight, amenorrhea, refusal or inability to sit still long enough to eat	**Imbalanced nutrition: Less than body requirements**
Delusions of grandeur and persecution; inaccurate interpretation of the environment	**Disturbed thought processes***
Auditory and visual hallucinations; disorientation	**Disturbed sensory perception***
Inability to develop satisfying relationships, manipulation of others for own desires, use of unsuccessful social interaction behaviors	**Impaired social interaction**
Difficulty falling asleep, sleeping only short periods	**Insomnia**

*These diagnoses have been retired from the NANDA-I list of approved diagnoses. They are used in this instance because they are most compatible with the identified behaviors.

to those behaviors, which may be used in planning care for the client experiencing a manic episode.

Outcome Criteria

The following criteria may be used for measuring outcomes in the care of the client experiencing a manic episode.

The client:

■ Exhibits no evidence of physical injury
■ Has not harmed self or others
■ Is no longer exhibiting signs of physical agitation
■ Eats a well-balanced diet with snacks to prevent weight loss and maintain nutritional status
■ Verbalizes an accurate interpretation of the environment
■ Verbalizes that hallucinatory activity has ceased and demonstrates no outward behavior indicating hallucinations
■ Accepts responsibility for own behaviors
■ Does not manipulate others for gratification of own needs
■ Interacts appropriately with others
■ Is able to fall asleep within 30 minutes of retiring
■ Is able to sleep 6 to 8 hours per night without medication

Planning/Implementation

The following section presents a group of selected nursing diagnoses, with short- and long-term goals and nursing interventions for each.

Some institutions are using a case management model to coordinate care (see Chapter 9 for a more detailed explanation). In case management models, the plan of care may take the form of a critical pathway.

Risk for Violence: Self-Directed or Other-Directed

Risk for self- or other-directed violence is defined as "at risk for behaviors in which an individual demonstrates that he or she can be physically, emotionally, and/or sexually harmful to [self or to others]" (NANDA-I, 2012, pp. 447-448). **NOTE:** Please refer to Chapter 16 for additional concepts related to anger and aggression management.

Client Goals

Outcome criteria include short- and long-term goals. Timelines are individually determined.

Short-Term Goals

■ Within [a specified time], client will recognize signs of increasing anxiety and agitation and report to staff (or other care provider) for assistance with intervention.
■ Client will not harm self or others.

Long-Term Goal

■ Client will not harm self or others.

Interventions

■ Maintain a low level of stimuli in the client's environment (low lighting, few people, simple decor, low noise level). Anxiety level rises in a stimulating environment. A suspicious, agitated client may perceive individuals as threatening.
■ Observe the client's behavior frequently. Do this while carrying out routine activities so as to avoid

creating suspiciousness in the individual. Close observation is necessary so that intervention can occur if required to ensure client (and others') safety.

■ Remove all dangerous objects from the client's environment so that in his or her agitated, confused state the client may not use them to harm self or others.

■ 💬 Intervene at the first sign of increased anxiety, agitation, or verbal or behavioral aggression. Offer empathetic response to client's feelings: "You seem anxious (or frustrated, or angry) about this situation. How can I help?" Validation of the client's feelings conveys a caring attitude and offering assistance reinforces trust.

■ It is important to maintain a calm attitude toward the client. As the client's anxiety increases, offer some alternatives: participating in a physical activity (e.g., punching bag, physical exercise), talking about the situation, taking some antianxiety medication. Offering alternatives to the client gives him or her a feeling of some control over the situation.

■ Have sufficient staff available to indicate a show of strength to the client if it becomes necessary. This shows the client evidence of control over the situation and provides some physical security for staff.

■ If the client is not calmed by "talking down" or by medication, use of mechanical restraints may be necessary.

> **CLINICAL PEARL** The avenue of the "least restrictive alternative" must be selected when planning interventions for a violent client. Restraints should be used only as a last resort, after all other interventions have been unsuccessful, and the client is clearly at risk of harm to self or others.

■ If restraint is deemed necessary, ensure that sufficient staff is available to assist. Follow protocol established by the institution. The Joint Commission (formerly the Joint Commission on Accreditation of Healthcare Organizations [JCAHO]) requires that an in-person evaluation by a physician or other licensed independent practitioner (LIP) be conducted within 1 hour of the initiation of the restraint or seclusion (The Joint Commission, 2010). The physician or LIP must reissue a new order for restraints every 4 hours for adults and every 1 to 2 hours for children and adolescents.

■ The Joint Commission requires that the client in restraints be observed at least every 15 minutes to ensure that circulation to extremities is not compromised (check temperature, color, pulses); to assist the client with needs related to nutrition, hydration, and elimination; and to position the client so that comfort is facilitated and aspiration can be prevented. Some institutions may require

continuous one-to-one monitoring of restrained clients, particularly those who are highly agitated, and for whom there is a high risk of self- or accidental injury.

■ As agitation decreases, assess the client's readiness for restraint removal or reduction. Remove one restraint at a time while assessing the client's response. This minimizes the risk of injury to client and staff.

Impaired Social Interaction

Impaired social interaction is defined as "insufficient or excessive quantity or ineffective quality of social exchange" (NANDA-I, 2012, p. 320). Table 26-2 presents this nursing diagnosis in care plan format.

Client Goals

Outcome criteria include short- and long-term goals. Timelines are individually determined.

Short-Term Goal

■ Client will verbalize which of his or her interaction behaviors are appropriate and which are inappropriate within 1 week.

Long-Term Goal

■ Client will demonstrate use of appropriate interaction skills as evidenced by lack of, or marked decrease in, manipulation of others to fulfill own desires.

Interventions

■ Recognize the purpose these behaviors serve for the client: to reduce feelings of insecurity by increasing feelings of power and control. Understanding the motivation behind the manipulation may help to facilitate acceptance of the individual and his or her behavior.

■ Set limits on manipulative behaviors. Explain to the client what is expected and what the consequences are if the limits are violated. Terms of the limitations must be agreed on by all staff who will be working with the client. The client is unable to establish own limits, so this must be done for him or her. Unless administration of consequences for violation of limits is consistent, manipulative behavior will not be eliminated.

■ Do not argue, bargain, or try to reason with the client. Merely state the limits and expectations. Individuals with mania can be very charming in their efforts to fulfill their own desires. Confront the client as soon as possible when interactions with others are manipulative or exploitative. Follow through with established consequences for unacceptable behavior. Because of the strong id influence on the client's behavior, he or she should receive immediate feedback when behavior is unacceptable. Consistency in enforcing the consequences is essential if positive

Table 26-2 | CARE PLAN FOR THE CLIENT EXPERIENCING A MANIC EPISODE

NURSING DIAGNOSIS: IMPAIRED SOCIAL INTERACTION

RELATED TO: Delusional thought processes (grandeur and/or persecution); underdeveloped ego and low self-esteem

EVIDENCED BY: Inability to develop satisfying relationships and manipulation of others for own desires

OUTCOME CRITERIA	NURSING INTERVENTIONS	RATIONALE
Short-Term Goal • Client will verbalize which of his or her interaction behaviors are appropriate and which are inappropriate within 1 week. **Long-Term Goal** • Client will demonstrate use of appropriate interaction skills as evidenced by lack of, or marked decrease in, manipulation of others to fulfill own desires.	1. Recognize the purpose manipulative behaviors serve for the client: to reduce feelings of insecurity by increasing feelings of power and control. 2. Set limits on manipulative behaviors. Explain to the client what is expected and what the consequences are if the limits are violated. Terms of the limitations must be agreed on by all staff who will be working with the client. 3. Do not argue, bargain, or try to reason with the client. Merely state the limits and expectations. Confront the client as soon as possible when interactions with others are manipulative or exploitative. Follow through with established consequences for unacceptable behavior. 4. Provide positive reinforcement for nonmanipulative behaviors. Explore feelings and help the client seek more appropriate ways of dealing with them. 5. Help the client recognize that he or she must accept the consequences of own behaviors and refrain from attributing them to others. 6. Help the client identify positive aspects about self, recognize accomplishments, and feel good about them.	1. Understanding the motivation behind the manipulation may facilitate acceptance of the individual and his or her behavior. 2. The client is unable to establish own limits, so this must be done for him or her. Unless administration of consequences for violation of limits is consistent, manipulative behavior will not be eliminated. 3. Because of the strong id influence on client's behavior, he or she should receive immediate feedback when behavior is unacceptable. Consistency in enforcing the consequences is essential if positive outcomes are to be achieved. Inconsistency creates confusion and encourages testing of limits. 4. Positive reinforcement enhances self-esteem and promotes repetition of desirable behaviors. 5. The client must accept responsibility for own behaviors before adaptive change can occur. 6. As self-esteem is increased, client will feel less need to manipulate others for own gratification.

outcomes are to be achieved. Inconsistency creates confusion and encourages testing of limits.

■ Provide positive reinforcement for nonmanipulative behaviors. Explore feelings, and help the client seek more appropriate ways of dealing with them.

■ Help the client recognize that he or she must accept the consequences of own behaviors and refrain from attributing them to others. The client must accept responsibility for own behaviors before adaptive change can occur.

■ Help the client identify positive aspects about self, recognize accomplishments, and feel good about them. As self-esteem is increased, the client will feel less need to manipulate others for own gratification.

Imbalanced Nutrition: Less than Body Requirements/Insomnia

Imbalanced nutrition: Less than body requirements is defined as "intake of nutrients insufficient to meet metabolic needs" (NANDA-I, 2012, p. 174). *Insomnia* is defined as "a disruption in amount and quality of sleep that impairs functioning" (NANDA-I, 2012, p. 217).

Client Goals

Outcome criteria include short- and long-term goals. Timelines are individually determined.

Short-Term Goals

■ Client will consume sufficient finger foods and between-meal snacks to meet recommended daily allowances of nutrients.

■ Within 3 days, with the aid of a sleeping medication, client will sleep 4 to 6 hours without awakening.

Long-Term Goals

■ Client will exhibit no signs or symptoms of malnutrition.

■ By time of discharge from treatment, client will be able to acquire 6 to 8 hours of uninterrupted sleep without medication.

Interventions

■ In collaboration with the dietitian, determine the number of calories required to provide adequate nutrition for maintenance or realistic (according to body structure and height) weight gain. Determine client's likes and dislikes, and try to provide favorite foods, if possible. The client is more likely to eat foods that he or she particularly enjoys.

■ Provide the client with high-protein, high-calorie, nutritious finger foods and drinks that can be consumed "on the run." Because of the hyperactive state, the client has difficulty sitting still long enough to eat a meal. The likelihood is greater that he or she will consume food and drinks that can be carried around and eaten with little effort. Have juice and snacks available on the unit at all times. Nutritious intake is required on a regular basis to compensate for increased caloric requirements due to the hyperactivity.

■ Maintain an accurate record of intake, output, and calorie count. Weigh the client daily. Administer vitamin and mineral supplements, as ordered by the physician. Monitor laboratory values, and report significant changes to the physician. It is important to carefully monitor the data that provide an objective assessment of the client's nutritional status.

■ Assess the client's activity level. He or she may ignore or be unaware of feelings of fatigue. Observe for signs such as increasing restlessness; fine tremors; slurred speech; and puffy, dark circles under eyes.

The client could collapse from exhaustion if hyperactivity is uninterrupted and rest is not achieved.

■ Monitor sleep patterns. Provide a structured schedule of activities that includes established times for naps or rest. Accurate baseline data are important in planning care to help the client with this problem. A structured schedule, including time for short naps, will help the hyperactive client achieve much-needed rest.

■ Client should avoid intake of caffeinated drinks, such as tea, coffee, and colas. Caffeine is a CNS stimulant and may interfere with the client's achievement of rest and sleep.

■ Before bedtime, provide nursing measures that promote sleep, such as back rub; warm bath; warm, nonstimulating drinks; soft music; and relaxation exercises.

■ Administer sedative medications, as ordered, to assist client achieve sleep until normal sleep pattern is restored.

Concept Care Mapping

The concept map care plan is an innovative approach to planning and organizing nursing care (see Chapter 9). It is a diagrammatic teaching and learning strategy that allows visualization of interrelationships between medical diagnoses, nursing diagnoses, assessment data, and treatments. An example of a concept map care plan for a client experiencing a manic episode is presented in Figure 26-2.

Client/Family Education

The role of client teacher is important in the psychiatric area, as it is in all areas of nursing. A list of topics for client/family education relevant to bipolar disorder is presented in Box 26-4.

Evaluation of Care for the Client Experiencing a Manic Episode

In the final step of the nursing process, a reassessment is conducted to determine if the nursing actions have been successful in achieving the objectives of care. Evaluation of the nursing actions for the client experiencing a manic episode may be facilitated by gathering information using the following types of questions.

■ Has the individual avoided personal injury?

■ Has violence to client or others been prevented?

■ Has agitation subsided?

■ Have nutritional status and weight been stabilized? Is the client able to select foods to maintain adequate nutrition?

■ Have delusions and hallucinations ceased? Is the client able to interpret the environment correctly?

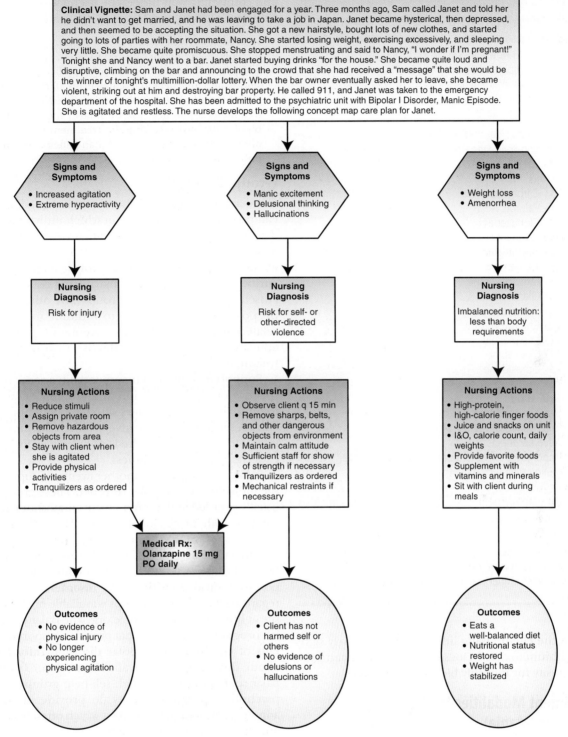

Clinical Vignette: Sam and Janet had been engaged for a year. Three months ago, Sam called Janet and told her he didn't want to get married, and he was leaving to take a job in Japan. Janet became hysterical, then depressed, and then seemed to be accepting the situation. She got a new hairstyle, bought lots of new clothes, and started going to lots of parties with her roommate, Nancy. She started losing weight, exercising excessively, and sleeping very little. She became quite promiscuous. She stopped menstruating and said to Nancy, "I wonder if I'm pregnant!" Tonight she and Nancy went to a bar. Janet started buying drinks "for the house." She became quite loud and disruptive, climbing on the bar and announcing to the crowd that she had received a "message" that she would be the winner of tonight's multimillion-dollar lottery. When the bar owner eventually asked her to leave, she became violent, striking out at him and destroying bar property. He called 911, and Janet was taken to the emergency department of the hospital. She has been admitted to the psychiatric unit with Bipolar I Disorder, Manic Episode. She is agitated and restless. The nurse develops the following concept map care plan for Janet.

Signs and Symptoms
- Increased agitation
- Extreme hyperactivity

Signs and Symptoms
- Manic excitement
- Delusional thinking
- Hallucinations

Signs and Symptoms
- Weight loss
- Amenorrhea

Nursing Diagnosis
Risk for injury

Nursing Diagnosis
Risk for self- or other-directed violence

Nursing Diagnosis
Imbalanced nutrition: less than body requirements

Nursing Actions
- Reduce stimuli
- Assign private room
- Remove hazardous objects from area
- Stay with client when she is agitated
- Provide physical activities
- Tranquilizers as ordered

Nursing Actions
- Observe client q 15 min
- Remove sharps, belts, and other dangerous objects from environment
- Maintain calm attitude
- Sufficient staff for show of strength if necessary
- Tranquilizers as ordered
- Mechanical restraints if necessary

Nursing Actions
- High-protein, high-calorie finger foods
- Juice and snacks on unit
- I&O, calorie count, daily weights
- Provide favorite foods
- Supplement with vitamins and minerals
- Sit with client during meals

Medical Rx: Olanzapine 15 mg PO daily

Outcomes
- No evidence of physical injury
- No longer experiencing physical agitation

Outcomes
- Client has not harmed self or others
- No evidence of delusions or hallucinations

Outcomes
- Eats a well-balanced diet
- Nutritional status restored
- Weight has stabilized

FIGURE 26–2 Concept map care plan for a client with bipolar mania.

- Is the client able to make decisions about own self-care? Has hygiene and grooming improved?
- Is behavior socially acceptable? Is client able to interact with others in a satisfactory manner? Has the client stopped manipulating others to fulfill own desires?

- Is the client able to sleep 6 to 8 hours per night and awaken feeling rested?
- Does the client understand the importance of maintenance medication therapy? Does he or she understand that symptoms may return if medication is discontinued?

BOX 26-4 Topics for Client/Family Education Related to Bipolar Disorder

NATURE OF THE ILLNESS
1. Causes of bipolar disorder
2. Cyclic nature of the illness
3. Symptoms of depression
4. Symptoms of mania

MANAGEMENT OF THE ILLNESS
1. Medication management
   a. Lithium
   b. Others
      1) Carbamazepine
      2) Valproic Acid
      3) Clonazepam
      4) Verapamil
      5) Lamotrigine
      6) Topiramate
      7) Oxcarbazepine
      8) Olanzapine
      9) Risperidone
      10) Chlorpromazine
      11) Aripiprazole
      12) Quetiapine
      13) Ziprasidone
      14) Asenapine
   c. Side effects
   d. Symptoms of lithium toxicity
   e. Importance of regular blood tests
   f. Adverse effects
   g. Importance of not stopping medication, even when feeling well
2. Assertive techniques
3. Anger management

SUPPORT SERVICES
1. Crisis hotline
2. Support groups
3. Individual psychotherapy
4. Legal and/or financial assistance

■ Can the client taking lithium verbalize early signs of lithium toxicity? Does he or she understand the necessity for monthly blood level checks?

Treatment Modalities for Bipolar Disorder (Mania)

Individual Psychotherapy

Historically, clients with mania have been difficult candidates for psychotherapy. They form a therapeutic relationship easily because they are eager to please and grateful for the therapist's interest. However, the relationship often tends to remain shallow and rigid. Some reports have indicated that psychotherapy (in conjunction with medication maintenance treatment)

and counseling may indeed be useful with these individuals. Goldberg and Hoop (2004) state:

> Interpersonal and social rhythm therapy is a form of interpersonal therapy tailored to bipolar patients. In addition to focusing on grief, role conflicts, role transitions, and interpersonal deficiencies, it includes psychoeducation about bipolar disorder and encourages treatment adherence. [Studies have] suggested that bipolar patients receiving the treatment were more often euthymic [stable mood] than patients receiving only clinical management.

Group Therapy

Once an acute phase of the illness is passed, groups can provide an atmosphere in which individuals may discuss issues in their lives that cause, maintain, or arise out of having a serious affective disorder. The element of peer support may provide a feeling of security, as troublesome or embarrassing issues are discussed and resolved. Some groups have other specific purposes, such as helping to monitor medication-related issues or serving as an avenue for promoting education related to the affective disorder and its treatment.

Support groups help members gain a sense of perspective on their condition and tangibly encourage them to link up with others who have common problems. A sense of hope is conveyed when the individual is able to see that he or she is not alone or unique in experiencing affective illness.

Self-help groups offer another avenue of support for the individual with bipolar disorder. These groups are usually peer led and are not meant to substitute for, or compete with, professional therapy. They offer supplementary support that frequently enhances compliance with the medical regimen. The Depression and Bipolar Support Alliance (DBSA) provides education and support for individuals with bipolar disorder. Information regarding local support groups is available on their website at http://www.dbsalliance.org. The Balanced Mind is a program of the DBSA that provides support for parents of children with bipolar disorder. Information about this program is available at http://www.thebalancedmind.org. Although self-help groups are not psychotherapy groups, they do provide important adjunctive support experiences, which often have therapeutic benefit for participants.

Family Therapy

The ultimate objectives in working with families of clients with mood disorders are to resolve the symptoms and initiate or restore adaptive family functioning. As with group therapy, the most effective approach appears to be with a combination of psychotherapeutic and pharmacotherapeutic treatments. Some studies with bipolar disorder have shown that behavioral family treatment combined with medication substantially reduces relapse rate compared with medication therapy alone.

Sadock and Sadock (2007) state:

> Family therapy is indicated if the disorder jeopardizes the patient's marriage or family functioning or if the mood disorder is promoted or maintained by the family situation. Family therapy examines the role of the mood-disordered member in the overall psychological well-being of the whole family; it also examines the role of the entire family in the maintenance of the patient's symptoms. (p. 555)

Cognitive Therapy

In cognitive therapy, the individual is taught to control thought distortions that are considered to be a factor in the development and maintenance of mood disorders. In the cognitive model, depression is characterized by a triad of negative distortions related to expectations of the environment, self, and future. The environment and activities within it are viewed as unsatisfying, the self is unrealistically devalued, and the future is perceived as hopeless. In the same model, mania is characterized by exaggeratedly positive cognitions and perceptions. The individual perceives the self as highly valued and powerful. Life is experienced with overstated self-assurance, and the future is viewed with unrealistic optimism.

The general goals in cognitive therapy are to obtain symptom relief as quickly as possible, to assist the client in identifying dysfunctional patterns of thinking and behaving, and to guide the client to evidence and logic that effectively tests the validity of the dysfunctional thinking (see Chapter 19). Therapy focuses on changing "automatic thoughts" that occur spontaneously and contribute to the distorted affect. Examples of automatic thoughts in bipolar mania include:

- **Personalizing:** "She's this happy only when she's with me."
- **All or nothing:** "Everything I do is great."
- **Mind reading:** "She thinks I'm wonderful."
- **Discounting negatives:** "None of those mistakes are really important."

The client is asked to describe evidence that both supports and disputes the automatic thought. The logic underlying the inferences is then reviewed with the client. Another technique involves evaluating what would most likely happen if the client's automatic thoughts were true. Implications of the consequences are then discussed.

Clients should not become discouraged if one technique seems not to be working. No single technique works with all clients. He or she should be reassured that any of a number of techniques may be used, and both therapist and client may explore these possibilities.

Finally, the use of cognitive therapy does not preclude the value of administering medication. Particularly in the treatment of bipolar mania, cognitive therapy should be considered a secondary treatment to pharmacological treatment.

The Recovery Model

Research provides support for recovery as an obtainable objective for individuals with bipolar disorder. Conceptual models of recovery from mental illness are presented in Chapter 21. The Recovery Model has been used primarily in caring for individuals with serious mental illness, such as schizophrenia and bipolar disorder. However, concepts of the model are amenable to use with all individuals experiencing emotional conditions with which they require assistance and who have a desire to take control and manage their lives more independently.

Davidson (2007) has stated:

> *Recovery from* refers to eradicating the symptoms and ameliorating the deficits caused by serious mental illnesses. *Recovery in* refers to learning how to live a safe, dignified, full, and self-determined life in the face of the enduring disability which may, at times, be associated with serious mental illness.

In bipolar disorder, recovery is a continuous process. The individual identifies goals based on personal values or what he or she defines as giving meaning and purpose to life. The clinician and client work together to develop a treatment plan that is in alignment with the goals set forth by the client. In the recovery process, the individual may still be experiencing symptoms. Weiden (2010) states:

> Patients do not have to be in remission, nor does remission automatically have to be a desired (or likely) goal when embarking on a recovery-oriented treatment plan. As long as the patient (and family) understands that a process recovery treatment plan is not to be confused with a promise of "cure" or even "remission," then one does not overpromise.

In the process of recovery, the client and clinician work on strategies to help the individual with bipolar disorder take control of and manage his or her illness. Some of these strategies include the following (National Alliance on Mental Illness [NAMI], 2008):

- Become an expert on the disorder
- Take medications regularly
- Become aware of earliest symptoms
- Develop a plan for emergencies
- Identify and reduce sources of stress: Know when to seek help
- Develop a personal support system

During the process of recovery, individuals actively work on the strategies they have identified to keep themselves well. The clinician serves as a support person to help the individual take the necessary steps to achieve the goals previously set forth by the client. Powell (2006) states:

> People with bipolar disorder have the power to create the lives they want for themselves. When they work on recovery and are able to look beyond their illness, the possibilities are limitless. (p. 7)

Although there is no cure for bipolar disorder, recovery is possible in the sense of learning to prevent and minimize symptoms, and to successfully cope with the effects of the illness on mood, career, and social life (Kiume, 2007).

Electroconvulsive Therapy

Episodes of acute mania are occasionally treated with electroconvulsive therapy (ECT), particularly when the client does not tolerate or fails to respond to lithium or other drug treatment, or when life is threatened by dangerous behavior or exhaustion (see Chapter 20 for a detailed discussion of ECT).

Psychopharmacology With Mood-Stabilizing Agents

For many years, the drug of choice for treatment and management of bipolar mania was lithium carbonate. However, in recent years, a number of investigators and clinicians in practice have achieved satisfactory results with several other medications, either alone or in combination with lithium. Table 26-3 provides information about the indication, action, and contraindications and precautions of various medications being used as mood stabilizers. Drug interactions associated with mood stabilizers are presented in Table 26-4.

Side Effects

The plan of care should include monitoring for side effects of therapy with mood stabilizing agents and intervening when required to prevent the occurrence of adverse events related to medication administration. Side effects and nursing implications for mood stabilizing agents are presented in Table 26-5.

Lithium Toxicity

The margin between the therapeutic and toxic levels of lithium carbonate is very narrow. The usual ranges of therapeutic serum concentrations are as follows (*Drug Facts and Comparisons*, 2014; Schatzberg, Cole, & DeBattista, 2010):

- For acute mania: 1.0 to 1.5 mEq/L
- For maintenance: 0.6 to 1.2 mEq/L

Serum lithium levels should be monitored once or twice a week after initial treatment until dosage and serum levels are stable, then monthly during maintenance therapy. Blood samples should be drawn 12 hours after the last dose.

Symptoms of lithium toxicity begin to appear at blood levels greater than 1.5 mEq/L and are dosage determinate. Symptoms include the following:

- **At serum levels of 1.5 to 2.0 mEq/L:** blurred vision, ataxia, tinnitus, persistent nausea and vomiting, severe diarrhea.
- **At serum levels of 2.0 to 3.5 mEq/L:** excessive output of dilute urine, increasing tremors, muscular irritability, psychomotor retardation, mental confusion, giddiness.
- **At serum levels above 3.5 mEq/L:** impaired consciousness, nystagmus, seizures, coma, oliguria/anuria, arrhythmias, myocardial infarction, cardiovascular collapse.

Lithium levels should be monitored prior to medication administration. The dosage should be withheld and the physician notified if the level reaches 1.5 mEq/L or at the earliest observation or report by the client of even the mildest symptom. If left untreated, lithium toxicity can be life threatening.

Lithium is similar in chemical structure to sodium, behaving in the body in much the same manner and competing at various sites in the body with sodium. If sodium intake is reduced or the body is depleted of its normal sodium (e.g., due to excessive sweating, fever, or diuresis), lithium is reabsorbed by the kidneys, increasing the possibility of toxicity. Therefore, the client must consume a diet adequate in sodium as well as 2,500 to 3,000 mL of fluid per day. Accurate records of intake, output, and client's weight should be kept on a daily basis.

Client/Family Education for Lithium

The client should:

- Take medication on a regular basis, even when feeling well. Discontinuation can result in return of symptoms.
- Not drive or operate dangerous machinery until lithium levels are stabilized. Drowsiness and dizziness can occur.
- Not skimp on dietary sodium intake. He or she should eat a variety of healthy foods and avoid "junk" foods. The client should drink 6 to 8 large glasses of water each day and avoid excessive use of beverages containing caffeine (coffee, tea, colas), which promote increased urine output.
- Notify the physician if vomiting or diarrhea occurs. These symptoms can result in sodium loss and an increased risk of lithium toxicity.
- Carry card or other identification noting that he or she is taking lithium.

TABLE 26–3 Mood Stabilizing Agents

CLASSIFICATION: GENERIC (TRADE)	PREGNANCY CATEGORY/ HALF-LIFE/INDICATIONS	MECHANISM OF ACTION	CONTRAINDICATIONS/ PRECAUTIONS	DAILY ADULT DOSAGE RANGE/ THERAPEUTIC PLASMA RANGE
Antimanic				
Lithium carbonate (Eskalith, Lithobid)	D/ 24 hr ■ Prevention and treatment of manic episodes of bipolar disorder *Unlabeled uses:* ■ Neutropenia ■ Cluster headaches (prophylaxis) ■ Alcohol dependence ■ Bulimia ■ Postpartum affective psychosis ■ Corticosteroid-induced psychosis	Not fully understood, but may modulate the effects of various neurotransmitters such as norepinephrine, serotonin, dopamine, glutamate, and GABA, that are thought to play a role in the symptomatology of bipolar disorder (may take 1-3 weeks for symptoms to subside).	Hypersensitivity Cardiac or renal disease, dehydration; sodium depletion; brain damage; pregnancy and lactation Caution with thyroid disorders, diabetes, urinary retention, history of seizures, and with the elderly	Acute mania: 1800-2400 mg Maintenance: 900-1200 mg/ Acute mania: 1.0-1.5 mEq/L Maintenance: 0.6-1.2 mEq/L
Anticonvulsants				
Carbamazepine (Tegretol)	D/ 25-65 hr (initial); 12-17 hr (repeated doses)/ ■ Epilepsy ■ Trigeminal neuralgia *Unlabeled uses:* ■ Bipolar disorder ■ Resistant schizophrenia ■ Management of alcohol withdrawal ■ Restless legs syndrome ■ Postherpetic neuralgia	Action in the treatment of bipolar disorder is unclear.	Hypersensitivity With MAOIs, lactation Caution with elderly, liver/renal/cardiac disease, pregnancy	200-1600 mg/ 4-12 mcg/mL
Clonazepam (Klonopin)	D/ 18-60 hr/ ■ Petit mal, akinetic, and myoclonic seizures ■ Panic disorder *Unlabeled uses:* ■ Acute manic episodes ■ Uncontrolled leg movements during sleep ■ Neuralgias	Action in the treatment of bipolar disorder is unclear.	Hypersensitivity, glaucoma, liver disease, lactation Caution in elderly, liver/renal disease, pregnancy	0.5-20 mg/ 20-80 ng/mL
Valproic acid (Depakene; Depakote)	D/ 5-20 hr/ ■ Epilepsy ■ Manic episodes ■ Migraine prophylaxis ■ Adjunct therapy in schizophrenia	Action in the treatment of bipolar disorder is unclear.	Hypersensitivity; liver disease Caution in elderly, renal/cardiac diseases, pregnancy and lactation	5 mg/kg to 60 mg/kg/ 50-150 mcg/mL

Continued

TABLE 26–3 Mood Stabilizing Agents—cont'd

CLASSIFICATION: GENERIC (TRADE)	PREGNANCY CATEGORY/ HALF-LIFE/INDICATIONS	MECHANISM OF ACTION	CONTRAINDICATIONS/ PRECAUTIONS	DAILY ADULT DOSAGE RANGE/ THERAPEUTIC PLASMA RANGE
Lamotrigine (Lamictal)	C/ ~33 hr/ ■ Epilepsy *Unlabeled use:* ■ Bipolar disorder	Action in the treatment of bipolar disorder is unclear.	Hypersensitivity Caution in renal and hepatic insufficiency, pregnancy, lactation, and children < 16 years old	100-200 mg/ Not established
Topiramate (Topamax)	C/ 21 hr/ ■ Epilepsy ■ Migraine prophylaxis *Unlabeled uses:* ■ Bipolar disorder ■ Cluster headaches ■ Bulimia ■ Binge eating disorder ■ Weight loss in obesity	Action in the treatment of bipolar disorder is unclear.	Hypersensitivity Caution in renal and hepatic impairment, pregnancy, lactation, children, and the elderly	50-400 mg/ Not established
Oxcarbazepine (Trileptal)	C/ 2-9 hr/ ■ Epilepsy *Unlabeled uses:* ■ Bipolar disorder ■ Diabetic neuropathy ■ Neuralgia	Action in the treatment of bipolar disorder is unclear.	Hypersensitivity Caution in renal and hepatic impairment, pregnancy, lactation, children, and the elderly	600-2400 mg/ Not established
Calcium Channel Blocker Verapamil (Calan; Isoptin)	C/ 3-7 hr (initially); 4.5-12 hr (repeated dosing) ■ Angina ■ Arrhythmias ■ Hypertension *Unlabeled uses:* ■ Bipolar mania ■ Migraine headache prophylaxis	Action in the treatment of bipolar disorder is unclear.	Hypersensitivity; severe left ventricular dysfunction, heart block, hypotension, cardiogenic shock, congestive heart failure Caution in liver or renal disease, cardiomyopathy, intracranial pressure, elderly patients, pregnancy and lactation	80-320 mg/ Not established
Antipsychotics Olanzapine (Zyprexa)	C/ 21-54 hr/ ■ Schizophrenia ■ Acute manic episodes ■ Management of bipolar disorder ■ Agitation associated with schizophrenia or mania *Unlabeled uses:* ■ Obsessive-compulsive disorder	**All antipsychotics:** Efficacy in schizophrenia is achieved through a combination of dopamine and serotonin type 2 ($5HT_2$) antagonism. Mechanism of action in the treatment of mania is unknown.	**All antipsychotics:** Contraindicated in hypersensitivity and during lactation. Caution with hepatic or cardiovascular disease, history of seizures, comatose or other CNS- depression, prostatic hypertrophy, narrow-angle glaucoma, diabetes or risk factors for diabetes, pregnancy, children, elderly, and debilitated patients	10-20 mg/ Not established

Drug	Pregnancy category/Half-life/Uses	Dose/Pediatric dose
Olanzapine and fluoxetine (Symbyax)	C/ (see individual drugs) / ■ For the treatment of depressive episodes associated with bipolar disorder	6/25-12/50 mg/ Not established
Aripiprazole (Abilify)	C/ 75-94/ ■ Bipolar mania ■ Schizophrenia	10-30 mg/ Not established
Chlorpromazine	C/ 24 hr/ ■ Bipolar mania ■ Schizophrenia ■ Emesis/hiccoughs ■ Acute intermittent porphyria ■ Preoperative apprehension *Unlabeled uses:* ■ Migraine headaches	75-400 mg/ Not established
Quetiapine (Seroquel)	C/ 6 hr/ ■ Schizophrenia ■ Acute manic episodes	100-800 mg/ Not established
Risperidone (Risperdal)	C/ 3-20 hr/ ■ Bipolar mania ■ Schizophrenia *Unlabeled uses:* ■ Severe behavioral problems in children ■ Behavioral problems associated with autism ■ Obsessive-compulsive disorder	1-6 mg/ Not established
Ziprasidone (Geodon)	C/ 7 hr (oral)/ ■ Bipolar mania ■ Schizophrenia ■ Acute agitation in schizophrenia	40-160 mg/ Not established
Asenapine (Saphris)	C/ 24 hr/ ■ Schizophrenia ■ Bipolar mania	10-20 mg/ Not established

TABLE 26–4 Interactions of Mood Stabilizing Agents

THE EFFECTS OF:	ARE INCREASED BY:	ARE DECREASED BY:	CONCURRENT USE MAY RESULT IN:
Antimanic: Lithium	Carbamazepine, fluoxetine, haloperidol, loop diuretics, methyldopa, NSAIDs, and thiazide diuretics	Acetazolamide, osmotic diuretics, theophylline, and urinary alkalinizers	Increased effects of neuromuscular blocking agents and tricyclic antidepressants; decreased pressor sensitivity of sympathomimetics; neurotoxicity may occur with phenothiazines or calcium channel blockers
Anticonvulsants: Clonazepam	CNS depressants, cimetidine, hormonal contraceptives, disulfiram fluoxetine, isoniazid, ketoconazole, metoprolol, propranolol, valproic acid, and probenecid	Rifampin, theophylline (↓ sedative effects), and phenytoin	Increased phenytoin levels; decreased efficacy of levodopa
Carbamazepine	Verapamil, diltiazem, erythromycin, clarithromycin, SSRIs, tricyclic antidepressants, cimetidine, isoniazid, danazol, lamotrigine, niacin, acetazolamide, dalfopristin, valproate, and nefazodone	Cisplatin, doxorubicin, felbamate, rifampin, barbiturates, hydantoins, primidone, and theophylline	Decreased levels of corticosteroids, doxycycline, quinidine, warfarin, estrogen-containing contraceptives, cyclosporine, benzodiazepines, theophylline, lamotrigine, valproic acid, bupropion, haloperidol, olanzapine, tiagabine, topiramate, voriconazole, ziprasidone, felbamate, levothyroxine, or antidepressants; increased levels of lithium; life-threatening hypertensive reaction with MAOIs
Valproic acid	Chlorpromazine, cimetidine, erythromycin, felbamate, and salicylates	Rifampin, carbamazepine, cholestyramine, lamotrigine, phenobarbital, ethosuximide, and hydantoins	Increased effects of tricyclic antidepressants, carbamazepine, CNS depressants, ethosuximide, lamotrigine, phenobarbital, warfarin, zidovudine, and hydantoins
Lamotragine	Valproic acid	Primidone, phenobarbital, phenytoin, rifamycin, succinimides, oral contraceptives, oxcarbazepine, carbamazepine, and acetaminophen	Decreased levels of valproic acid; increased levels of carbamazepine and topiramate
Topiramate	Metformin and hydrochlorothiazide	Phenytoin, carbamazepine, valproic acid, and lamotrigine	Increased risk of CNS depression with alcohol or other CNS depressants; increased risk of kidney stones with carbonic anhydrase inhibitors; increased effects of phenytoin, metformin, amitriptyline; decreased effects of oral contraceptives, digoxin, lithium, riseridone, and valproic acid
Oxcarbazepine		Carbamazepine, phenobarbital, phenytoin, valproic acid, and verapamil	Increased concentrations of phenobarbital and phenytoin; decreased effects of oral contraceptives, felodipine, and lamotrigine

TABLE 26–4 Interactions of Mood Stabilizing Agents—cont'd

THE EFFECTS OF:	ARE INCREASED BY:	ARE DECREASED BY:	CONCURRENT USE MAY RESULT IN:
Calcium Channel Blocker: Verapamil	Amiodarone, beta blockers, cimetidine, ranitidine, and grapefruit juice	Barbiturates, calcium salts, hydantoins, rifampin, and antineoplastics	Increased effects of beta blockers, disopyramide, flecainide, doxorubicin, benzodiazepines, buspirone, carbamazepine, digoxin, dofetilide, ethanol, imipramine, nondepolarizing muscle relaxants, prazosin, quinidine, sirolimus, tacrolimus, and theophylline; altered lithium levels
Antipsychotics: Olanzapine	Fluvoxamine and other CYP1A2 inhibitors, and fluoxetine	Carbamazepine and other CYP1A2 inducers, omeprazole, and rifampin	Decreased effects of levodopa and dopamine agonists; increased hypotension with antihypertensives; increased CNS depression with alcohol or other CNS depressants
Aripiprazole	Ketoconazole and other CYP3A4 inhibitors; quinidine, fluoxetine, paroxetine, or other potential CYP2D6 inhibitors	Carbamazepine, famotidine, and valproate	Increased CNS depression with alcohol or other CNS depressants; increased hypotension with antihypertensives
Chlorpromazine	Beta-blockers and paroxetine	Centrally acting anticholinergics	Increased effects of beta blockers; excessive sedation and hypotension with meperidine; decreased hypotensive effect of guanethidine; decreased effect of oral anticoagulants; decreased or increased phenytoin levels; increased orthostatic hypotension with thiazide diuretics; increased CNS depression with alcohol or other CNS depressants; increased hypotension with antihypertensives; increased anticholinergic effects with anticholinergic agents
Quetiapine	Cimetidine; ketoconazole, itraconazole, fluconazole, erythromycin, or other CYP3A4 inhibitors	Phenytoin, thioridazine	Decreased effects of levodopa and dopamine agonists; increased CNS depression with alcohol or other CNS depressants; increased hypotension with antihypertensives
Risperidone	Clozapine, fluoxetine, paroxetine, or ritonavir	Carbamazepine	Decreased effects of levodopa and dopamine agonists; increased effects of clozapine and valproate; increased CNS depression with alcohol or other CNS depressants; increased hypotension with antihypertensives
Ziprasidone	Ketoconazole and other CYP3A4 inhibitors	Carbamazepine	Life-threatening prolongation of QT interval with quinidine, dofetilide, other class Ia and III antiarrhythmics, pimozide, sotalol, thioridazine, chlorpromazine, pentamadine, arsenic trioxide, mefloquine, dolasetron, tacrolimus, droperidol, gatifloxacin, or moxifloxacin; decreased effects of levodopa and dopamine agonists; increased CNS depression with alcohol or other CNS depressants; increased hypotension with antihypertensives

Continued

TABLE 26–4 Interactions of Mood Stabilizing Agents—cont'd

THE EFFECTS OF:	ARE INCREASED BY:	ARE DECREASED BY:	CONCURRENT USE MAY RESULT IN:
Asenapine	Fluvoxamine, imipramine, and valproate	Carbamazepine, cimetidine, and paroxetine	Increased effects of paroxetine and dextromathorphan; increased CNS depression with alcohol or other CNS depressants; increased hypotension with antihypertensives; additive effects of QT interval prolongation with quinidine, dofetilide, other class Ia and III antiarrhythmics, pimozide, sotalol, thioridazine, chlorpromazine, pentamadine, arsenic trioxide, mefloquine, dolasetron, tacrolimus, droperidol, gatifloxacin, or moxifloxacin

TABLE 26–5 Side Effects and Nursing Implications of Mood Stabilizing Agents

MEDICATION	SIDE EFFECTS	NURSING IMPLICATIONS
Antimanic: Lithium carbonate (Eskalith, Lithane, Lithobid)	1. Drowsiness, dizziness, headache 2. Dry mouth; thirst 3. GI upset; nausea/vomiting 4. Fine hand tremors 5. Hypotension; arrhythmias; pulse irregularities 6. Polyuria; dehydration 7. Weight gain	1. Ensure that client does not participate in activities that require alertness, or operate dangerous machinery. 2. Provide sugarless candy, ice, frequent sips of water. Ensure that strict oral hygiene is maintained. 3. Administer medications with meals to minimize GI upset. 4. Report to physician, who may decrease dosage. Some physicians prescribe a small dose of beta-blocker propranolol to counteract this effect. 5. Monitor vital signs two or three times a day. Physician may decrease dose of medication. 6. May subside after initial week or two. Monitor daily intake and output and weight. Monitor skin turgor daily. 7. Provide instructions for reduced-calorie diet. Emphasize importance of maintaining adequate intake of sodium.
Anticonvulsants: Clonazepam (Klonopin) Carbamazepine (Tegretol) Valproic acid (Depakote; Depakene) Lamotrigine (Lamictal) Topiramate (Topamax) Oxcarbazepine (Trileptal)	1. Nausea/vomiting 2. Drowsiness; dizziness 3. Blood dyscrasias 4. Prolonged bleeding time (with valproic acid) 5. Risk of severe rash (with lamotrigine) 6. Decreased efficacy with oral contraceptives (with topiramate) 7. Risk of suicide with all antiepileptic drugs (warning by FDA, December 2008)	1. May give with food or milk to minimize GI upset. 2. Ensure that client does not operate dangerous machinery or participate in activities that require alertness 3. Ensure that client understands the importance of regular blood tests while receiving anticonvulsant therapy. 4. Ensure that platelet counts and bleeding time are determined before initiation of therapy with valproic acid. Monitor for spontaneous bleeding or bruising. 5. Ensure that client is informed that he or she must report evidence of skin rash to physician immediately. 6. Ensure that client is aware of decreased efficacy of oral contraceptives with concomitant use. 7. Monitor for worsening of depression, suicidal thoughts or behavior, or any unusual changes in mood or behavior.
Calcium Channel Blocker: Verapamil (Calan; Isoptin)	1. Drowsiness, dizziness 2. Hypotension; bradycardia 3. Nausea 4. Constipation	1. Ensure that client does not operate dangerous machinery or participate in activities that require alertness. 2. Take vital signs just before initiation of therapy and before daily administration of the medication. Physician will provide acceptable parameters for administration. Report marked changes immediately. 3. May give with food to minimize GI upset 4. Encourage increased fluid (if not contraindicated) and fiber in the diet.

TABLE 26–5	**Side Effects and Nursing Implications of Mood Stabilizing Agents—cont'd**	
MEDICATION	SIDE EFFECTS	NURSING IMPLICATIONS
Antipsychotics: Aripiprazole (Abilify) Asenapine (Saphris) Chlorpromazine Olanzapine (Zyprexa) Quetiapine (Seroquel) Risperidone (Risperdal) Ziprasidone (Geodon)	1. Drowsiness, dizziness 2. Dry mouth, constipation 3. Increased appetite, weight gain 4. ECG changes 5. Extrapyramidal symptoms 6. Hyperglycemia and diabetes	1. Ensure that client does not operate dangerous machinery or participate in activities that require alertness. 2. Provide sugarless candy or gum, ice, and frequent sips of water. Provide foods high in fiber. Encourage physical activity and fluid if not contraindicated. 3. Provide calorie-controlled diet; provide opportunity for physical exercise; provide diet and exercise instruction. 4. Monitor vital signs. Observe for symptoms of dizziness, palpitations, syncope, or weakness. 5. Monitor for symptoms. Administer prn medications at first sign. 6. Monitor blood glucose regularly. Observe for the appearance of symptoms of polydipsia, polyuria, polyphagia, and weakness at any time during therapy.

■ Be aware of appropriate diet should weight gain become a problem. Include adequate sodium and other nutrients while decreasing number of calories.

■ Be aware of risks of becoming pregnant while receiving lithium therapy. Use information furnished by health-care providers regarding methods of contraception. Notify the physician as soon as possible if pregnancy is suspected or planned.

■ Be aware of side effects and symptoms associated with toxicity. Notify the physician if any of the following symptoms occur: persistent nausea and vomiting, severe diarrhea, ataxia, blurred vision, tinnitus, excessive output of urine, increasing tremors, or mental confusion.

■ Refer to written materials furnished by health-care providers while receiving self-administered maintenance therapy. Keep appointments for outpatient follow-up; have serum lithium level checked every 1 to 2 months, or as advised by physician.

Client/Family Education for Anticonvulsants

The client should:

■ Refrain from discontinuing the drug abruptly. Physician will administer orders for tapering the drug when therapy is to be discontinued.

■ Report the following symptoms to the physician immediately: skin rash, unusual bleeding, spontaneous bruising, sore throat, fever, malaise, dark urine, and yellow skin or eyes.

■ Not drive or operate dangerous machinery until reaction to the medication has been established.

■ Avoid consuming alcoholic beverages and nonprescription medications without approval from physician.

■ Carry card at all times identifying the name of medications being taken.

CLINICAL PEARL The U.S. Food and Drug Administration requires that all antiepileptic (anticonvulsant) drugs carry a warning label indicating that use of the drugs increases risk for suicidal thoughts and behaviors. Patients being treated with these medications should be monitored for the emergence or worsening of depression, suicidal thoughts or behavior, or any unusual changes in mood or behavior.

Client/Family Education for Calcium Channel Blocker

The client should:

■ Take medication with meals if gastrointestinal (GI) upset occurs.

■ Use caution when driving or when operating dangerous machinery. Dizziness, drowsiness, and blurred vision can occur.

■ Refrain from discontinuing the drug abruptly. To do so may precipitate cardiovascular problems. Physician will administer orders for tapering the drug when therapy is to be discontinued.

■ Report occurrence of any of the following symptoms to physician immediately: irregular heartbeat, shortness of breath, swelling of the hands and feet, pronounced dizziness, chest pain, profound mood swings, severe and persistent headache.

■ Rise slowly from a sitting or lying position to prevent a sudden drop in blood pressure.

■ Avoid taking other medications (including over-the-counter medications) without physician's approval.

■ Carry card at all times describing medications being taken.

Client/Family Education for Antipsychotics

The client should:

■ Use caution when driving or operating dangerous machinery. Drowsiness and dizziness can occur.

■ Refrain from discontinuing the drug abruptly after long-term use. To do so might produce withdrawal symptoms, such as nausea, vomiting, dizziness, gastritis, headache, tachycardia, insomnia, tremulousness. Physician will administer orders for tapering the drug when therapy is to be discontinued.

■ Use sunblock lotion and wear protective clothing when spending time outdoors. Skin is more susceptible to sunburn, which can occur in as little as 30 minutes.

■ Report the occurrence of any of the following symptoms to the physician immediately: sore throat, fever, malaise, unusual bleeding, easy bruising, persistent nausea and vomiting, severe headache, rapid heart rate, difficulty urinating, muscle twitching, tremors, darkly colored urine, excessive urination, excessive thirst, excessive hunger, weakness, pale stools, yellow skin or eyes, muscular incoordination, or skin rash.

■ Rise slowly from a sitting or lying position to prevent a sudden drop in blood pressure.

■ Take frequent sips of water, chew sugarless gum, or suck on hard candy, if dry mouth is a problem. Good oral care (frequent brushing, flossing) is very important.

■ Consult the physician regarding smoking while on antipsychotic therapy. Smoking increases the metabolism of these drugs, requiring an adjustment in dosage to achieve a therapeutic effect.

■ Dress warmly in cold weather, and avoid extended exposure to very high or low temperatures. Body temperature is harder to maintain with this medication.

■ Avoid drinking alcohol while on antipsychotic therapy. These drugs potentiate each other's effects.

■ Avoid taking other medications (including over-the-counter products) without the physician's approval. Many medications contain substances that interact with antipsychotic medications in a way that may be harmful.

■ Be aware of possible risks of taking antipsychotics during pregnancy. Safe use during pregnancy has not been established. Antipsychotics are thought to readily cross the placental barrier; if so, a fetus could experience adverse effects of the drug. Inform the physician immediately if pregnancy occurs, is suspected, or is planned.

■ Be aware of side effects of antipsychotic medications. Refer to written materials furnished by health-care providers for safe self-administration.

■ Continue to take the medication, even if feeling well and as though it is not needed. Symptoms may return if medication is discontinued.

■ Carry a card or other identification at all times describing medications being taken.

CASE STUDY AND SAMPLE CARE PLAN

NURSING HISTORY AND ASSESSMENT

Candace, age 32, recently moved to New York City from Omaha, Nebraska, where she had been working as a television reporter. She felt that Omaha had become "too boring" and wanted to experience the big city life. Candace has a history of Bipolar I Disorder, and has been maintained on lithium since she was 23 years old. Since she arrived in New York City, she has run out of her medication and has not found a doctor to have her prescription renewed. She has been staying in an inexpensive apartment, using her savings to live on. She has been seeking employment in her chosen line of work, but it has been 2 months now, and she has been unable to find a job. She is becoming anxious, because her savings are becoming depleted. She has lost weight and has trouble sleeping.

Today, after two failed interviews, Candace went to a bar and began drinking. She ordered several rounds of drinks for everyone in the bar, and told the bartender to "put it on my tab." The bartender called the police when Candace refused to pay her tab and became loud and belligerent. He said she began shouting that she knew the mayor, and he was going to help her find a job, and if they didn't leave her alone, she would tell the mayor how they were treating her. She took out her cell phone and said she was calling the mayor. When others in the room began laughing at her, she began cursing and saying that "they would be sorry one day that they laughed at her." When the police arrived, Candace was resistant and had to be physically restrained. The police took Candace to the emergency department of the community hospital, where she was admitted with a diagnosis of Bipolar I Disorder, current episode manic. The psychiatrist ordered olanzapine 10 mg IM STAT, olanzapine 10 mg PO qd, lithium carbonate 600 mg PO bid, and vitamin supplement daily. He ordered lithium level to be drawn prior to first dose of lithium.

NURSING DIAGNOSES/OUTCOME IDENTIFICATION

From the assessment data, the admitting nurse develops the following nursing diagnoses for Candace:

1. **Risk for self- or other-directed violence** related to manic hyperactivity, delusional thinking, impulsivity
   a. **Short-Term Goal:**
      ■ Agitation and hyperactivity will be maintained at manageable level with the administration of tranquilizing medication.

CASE STUDY AND SAMPLE CARE PLAN—cont'd

b. Long-Term Goal:
- Candace will not harm self or others during hospitalization.

2. Imbalanced nutrition: Less than body requirements
related to lack of appetite and excessive physical agitation, evidenced by loss of weight.
a. Short-Term Goal:
- Candace will consume sufficient finger foods and between-meal snacks to meet recommended daily allowances of nutrients.
b. Long-Term Goal:
- Candace will begin to regain weight and exhibit no signs or symptoms of malnutrition.

PLANNING/IMPLEMENTATION

RISK FOR SELF- OR OTHER-DIRECTED VIOLENCE
The following nursing interventions have been identified for Candace:

1. Place Candace in a private room near the nurse's station. Observe her behavior frequently.
2. Remove all dangerous objects from her environment.
3. Plan some physical activities for Candace (e.g., treadmill, punching bag) and regular rest periods during the day.
4. Administer tranquilizing medication as ordered by physician.
5. Monitor lithium levels 3 times during first week of therapy. Monitor for signs and symptoms of toxicity (e.g., ataxia, blurred vision, severe diarrhea, persistent nausea and vomiting, tinnitus).
6. Ensure that sufficient staff is available to intervene should Candace become agitated and aggressive.

IMBALANCED NUTRITION: LESS THAN BODY REQUIREMENTS
The following nursing interventions have been identified for Candace:

1. Consult dietitian to determine appropriate diet for Candace to restore nutrition and gain weight. Ensure that her diet includes foods that she particularly likes.
2. Ensure that Candace has access to "finger foods" and between meal snacks if she cannot or will not sit still to eat off a meal tray.
3. Maintain an accurate record of intake, output, and calorie count.
4. Obtain daily weights.
5. Administer vitamin supplement, as ordered by physician.
6. Sit with Candace during mealtime.

EVALUATION

The outcome criteria identified for Candace have been met. She has not harmed herself or others in any way. She is able to verbalize names of resources outside the hospital from whom she may request help if needed. With help from the social worker, she has applied for unemployment assistance, and will begin receiving help within 2 weeks. She has gained 3 pounds in the hospital, and verbalizes understanding of the importance of maintaining good nutrition. She is taking her medication regularly, and has a follow-up appointment with the psychiatric nurse practitioner who will see Candace biweekly and ensure that Candace is compliant with medication and lab requirements. Candace verbalizes understanding of the importance of taking her medication on a continuous basis. She has a hopeful, but realistic, attitude about finding work in New York City, and states that she will give herself a deadline, after which she plans to return to her home in Omaha, where she may be near family and friends.

Summary and Key Points

- Bipolar disorder is manifested by mood swings from profound depression to extreme elation and euphoria.
- Genetic influences have been strongly implicated in the development of bipolar disorder. Various other physiological factors, such as biochemical and electrolyte alterations, as well as cerebral structural changes, have been implicated. Side effects of certain medications may also induce symptoms of mania. No single theory can explain the etiology of bipolar disorder, and it is likely that the illness is caused by a combination of factors.
- Symptoms of mania may be observed on a continuum of three phases, each identified by the degree of severity: phase I, hypomania; phase II, acute mania; and phase III, delirious mania.
- The symptoms of bipolar disorder may occur in children and adolescents, as well as adults.
- Treatment of bipolar disorders includes individual therapy, group and family therapy, cognitive therapy, electroconvulsive therapy, and psychopharmacology. For the majority of clients, the most effective treatment appears to be a combination of psychotropic medication and psychosocial therapy.
- Some clinicians are choosing a course of therapy based on a model of recovery, somewhat like that which has been used for many years with problems of addiction. The basic premise of a recovery model is empowerment of the individual. The recovery model is designed to allow individuals primary control over decisions about their own care, and to enable a person with a mental health problem to live a meaningful life in a community of choice while striving to achieve his or her full potential.

■ For many years, the pharmacological treatment of choice for bipolar mania was lithium carbonate. A number of other medications are now being used with satisfactory results, including anticonvulsants and antipsychotics.

■ There is a narrow margin between the therapeutic and toxic levels of lithium. Serum lithium levels

must be monitored regularly while on maintenance therapy.

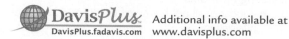 Additional info available at
DavisPlus.fadavis.com   www.davisplus.com

Review Questions
Self-Examination/Learning Exercise

*Select the answer that is **most** appropriate for each of the following questions.*

1. Margaret, a 68-year-old widow, is brought to the emergency department by her sister-in-law. Margaret has a history of bipolar disorder and has been maintained on medication for many years. Her sister-in-law reports that Margaret quit taking her medication a few months ago, thinking she didn't need it anymore. She is agitated, pacing, demanding, and speaking very loudly. Her sister-in-law reports that Margaret eats very little, is losing weight, and almost never sleeps. "I'm afraid she's going to just collapse!" Margaret is admitted to the psychiatric unit. The *priority* nursing diagnosis for Margaret is:
   a. Imbalanced nutrition: less than body requirements related to not eating
   b. Risk for injury related to hyperactivity
   c. Disturbed sleep pattern related to agitation
   d. Ineffective coping related to denial of depression

2. Margaret, age 68, is diagnosed with bipolar I disorder, current episode manic. She is extremely hyperactive and has lost weight. One way to promote adequate nutritional intake for Margaret is to:
   a. Sit with her during meals to ensure that she eats everything on her tray.
   b. Have her sister-in-law bring all her food from home because she knows Margaret's likes and dislikes.
   c. Provide high-calorie, nutritious finger foods and snacks that Margaret can eat "on the run."
   d. Tell Margaret that she will be on room restriction until she starts gaining weight.

3. The physician orders lithium carbonate 600 mg tid for a newly diagnosed client with Bipolar I Disorder. There is a narrow margin between the therapeutic and toxic levels of lithium. Therapeutic range for acute mania is:
   a. 1.0 to 1.5 mEq/L
   b. 10 to 15 mEq/L
   c. 0.5 to 1.0 mEq/L
   d. 5 to 10 mEq/L

4. Although historically lithium has been the medication of choice for mania, several others have been used with good results. Which of the following are used in the treatment of bipolar disorder? (Select all that apply.)
   a. Olanzepine (Zyprexa)
   b. Paroxetine (Paxil)
   c. Carbamazepine (Tegretol)
   d. Lamotrigine (Lamictal)
   e. Tranylcypromine (Parnate)

5. Margaret, a 68-year-old widow experiencing a manic episode, is admitted to the psychiatric unit after being brought to the emergency department by her sister-in-law. Margaret yells, "My sister-in-law is just jealous of me! She's trying to make it look like I'm insane!" This behavior is an example of:
   a. A delusion of grandeur
   b. A delusion of persecution
   c. A delusion of reference
   d. A delusion of control or influence

Review Questions—cont'd
Self-Examination/Learning Exercise

6. The most common comorbid condition in children with bipolar disorder is:
   a. Schizophrenia
   b. Substance disorders
   c. Oppositional defiant disorder
   d. Attention-deficit/hyperactivity disorder

7. A nurse is educating a client about his lithium therapy. She is explaining signs and symptoms of lithium toxicity. Which of the following would she instruct the client to be on the alert for?
   a. Fever, sore throat, malaise
   b. Tinnitus, severe diarrhea, ataxia
   c. Occipital headache, palpitations, chest pain
   d. Skin rash, marked rise in blood pressure, bradycardia

8. A client experiencing a manic episode enters the milieu area dressed in a provocative and physically revealing outfit. Which of the following is the most appropriate intervention by the nurse?
   a. Tell the client she cannot wear this outfit while she is in the hospital.
   b. Do nothing and allow her to learn from the responses of her peers.
   c. Quietly walk with her back to her room and help her change into something more appropriate.
   d. Explain to her that if she wears this outfit she must remain in her room.

9. The nurse is prioritizing nursing diagnoses in the plan of care for a client experiencing a manic episode. Number the diagnoses in order of the appropriate priority.
   _____a. Disturbed sleep pattern evidenced by sleeping only 4-5 hours per night
   _____b. Risk for injury related to manic hyperactivity
   _____c. Impaired social interaction evidenced by manipulation of others
   _____d. Imbalanced nutrition: Less than body requirements evidenced by loss of weight and poor skin turgor

10. A child with bipolar disorder also has attention-deficit/hyperactivity disorder (ADHD). How would these co-morbid conditions most likely be treated?
    a. No medication would be given for either condition.
    b. Medication would be given for both conditions simultaneously.
    c. The bipolar condition would be stabilized first before medication for the ADHD would be given.
    d. The ADHD would be treated before consideration of the bipolar disorder.

IMPLICATIONS OF RESEARCH FOR EVIDENCE-BASED PRACTICE

Zauszniewski, J.A., Bekhet, A.K., & Suresky, M.J. (2008). Factors associated with perceived burden, resourcefulness, and quality of life in female family members of adults with serious mental illness. *Journal of the American Psychiatric Association*, 14(2), 125-135.

DESCRIPTION OF THE STUDY: About 10 to 17.5 million persons experience serious mental illness (SMI) each year. Most of their caregivers are female family members. The authors state, "Caregiver burden is affected by disruptive behaviors of the mentally ill person, changes in household routines, strained social relationships, lack of social support, deteriorating finances, diminished opportunity for leisure, exhaustion, and the stigma associated with mental illness, termed *stigma by association*" (p. 125). Depression is not uncommon among caregivers, who are largely female. The purpose of this study was to examine the associations between characteristics of female family members, adults with SMI, and the family situation and caregivers' burden, stigma, depressive cognitions, resourcefulness, and quality of life. The sample consisted of 60 female family members of adults with SMI (i.e., schizophrenia, bipolar disorder, major depressive disorder, and anxiety disorders). Thirty were Caucasian and 30 were African American. Age range was

Continued

IMPLICATIONS OF RESEARCH FOR EVIDENCE-BASED PRACTICE—cont'd

18 to 65. The majority of the women lived in the same household and provided care for their family members with mental illness. Most had some college education.

RESULTS OF THE STUDY: Age and level of education were not associated with burden, stigma, depressive cognitions, resourcefulness, or quality of life. However, Caucasian women reported greater burden than did African American women. Perceived burden was inversely associated with length of caregiving time, suggesting that women adapt over time to having a family member with mental illness. A greater burden and stigma by association was expressed by caregivers of adults with bipolar disorder than those with schizophrenia. Mothers of adults with SMI expressed greater feelings of burden and stigma than other female family members (e.g., sisters, daughters, wives). The authors suggest that this may be related to mothers' feelings of being in some way responsible for the mental illness in their offspring. In-home caregivers expressed greater burden than out-of-home caregivers. The characteristics that related to lowest personal resourcefulness of caregivers included Caucasian race, relationship of mother, younger age of the individual with mental illness, and diagnosis of bipolar disorder.

IMPLICATIONS FOR NURSING PRACTICE: These findings have direct implications for psychiatric nursing of female caregivers of family members with SMI. The authors suggest that teaching personal resourcefulness skills in a systematic way to women with newly diagnosed family members may be beneficial in maintaining their optimal quality of life. The population at highest risk was suggested by this study to be Caucasian mothers of younger aged offspring with bipolar disorder. The authors state, "These women may benefit from programs that teach the cognitive-behavioral, self-help skills that constitute personal resourcefulness, because such skills have been associated with optimal quality of life" (p. 133)

TEST YOUR CRITICAL THINKING SKILLS

Alice, age 29, had been working in the typing pool of a large corporation for 6 years. Her immediate supervisor recently retired and Alice was promoted to supervisor, in charge of 20 people in the department. Alice was flattered by the promotion but anxious about the additional responsibility of the position. Shortly after the promotion, she overheard two of her former coworkers saying, "Why in the world did they choose her? She's not the best one for the job. I know *I* certainly won't be able to respect her as a boss!" Hearing these comments added to Alice's anxiety and self-doubt.

Shortly after Alice began her new duties, her friends and coworkers noticed a change. She had a great deal of energy and worked long hours on her job. She began to speak very loudly and rapidly. Her roommate noticed that Alice slept very little, yet seldom appeared tired. Every night she would go out to bars and dances. Sometimes she brought men she had just met home to the apartment, something she had never done before. She bought lots of clothes and makeup and had her hair restyled in a more youthful look. She failed to pay her share of the rent and bills but came home with a brand new convertible. She lost her temper and screamed at her roommate to "Mind your own business!" when asked to pay her share.

She became irritable at work, and several of her subordinates reported her behavior to the corporate manager. When the manager confronted Alice about her behavior, she lost control, shouting, cursing, and striking out at anyone and anything that happened to be within her reach. The security officers restrained her and took her to the emergency department of the hospital, where she was admitted to the psychiatric unit. She had no previous history of psychiatric illness.

The psychiatrist assigned a diagnosis of Bipolar I Disorder, and wrote orders for olanzapine (Zyprexa) 10 mg IM STAT, olanzapine 15 mg PO daily, and lithium carbonate 600 mg qid.

Answer the following questions related to Alice:

1. What are the most important considerations with which the nurse who is taking care of Alice should be concerned?
2. Why was Alice given the diagnosis of Bipolar I Disorder?
3. The doctor should order a lithium level drawn after 4 to 6 days. For what symptoms should the nurse be on the alert?
4. Why did the physician order olanzapine in addition to the lithium carbonate?

References

Allen, M.H. (2003). Approaches to the treatment of mania. *Medscape Psychiatry.* Retrieved from http://www.medscape.com/viewprogram/2639

American Psychiatric Association. (2013). *Diagnostic and statistical manual of mental disorders* (5th ed.). Washington, DC: American Psychiatric Publishing.

Correll, C.U. (2007). Current understanding in the development of bipolar disorder in pediatric patients. *Medscape Psychiatry.* Retrieved from http://www.medscape.com/viewarticle/566531

Davidson, L. (2007). *Recovery and serious mental illness: What it is and how to promote it.* Presentation at the Medical College of Georgia Psychiatry Grand Rounds (January 11, 2007).

Drug facts and comparisons. (2014). St. Louis, MO: Wolters Kluwer.

Dubovsky, S.L., Davies, R., & Dubovsky, A.M. (2003). Mood disorders. In R.E. Hales & S.C. Yudofsky (Eds.), *Textbook of clinical psychiatry* (4th ed., pp. 439-542). Washington, DC: American Psychiatric Publishing.

Geller, B., Zimerman, B., Williams, M., Delbello, M.P., Frazier, J., & Beringer, L. (2002). Phenomenology of prepubertal and early adolescent bipolar disorder: Examples of elated mood, grandiose behaviors, decreased need for sleep, racing thoughts, and hypersexuality. *Journal of Child and Adolescent Psychopharmacology, 12,* 3-9.

Goldberg, J.F., & Hoop, J. (2004). Bipolar depression: Long-term challenges for the clinician. *Medscape Psychiatry*. Retrieved from http://cme.medscape.com/viewprogram/3350

Guadiz, B. (2011). *History of bipolar disorder: Bipolar disorder already existed centuries ago*. Retrieved from http://doctorhelps.com/articles/57/fghaeffghahfcdfeefdfe

Hazell, P., & Jairam, R. (2012). Acute treatment of mania in children and adolescents. *Current Opinion in Psychiatry, 25*(4), 264-270.

Joska, J.A., & Stein, D.J. (2008). Mood disorders. In R.E. Hales, S.C. Yudofsky, & G.O. Gabbard (Eds.), *Textbook of Psychiatry* (5th ed., pp. 457-503). Washington, DC: American Psychiatric Publishing.

Kafantaris, V., Dicker, R., Coletti, D.J., & Kane, J.M. (2001). Adjunctive antipsychotic treatment is necessary for adolescents with psychotic mania. *Journal of Child and Adolescent Psychopharmacology, 11*(4), 409-413.

Kiume, S. (2007). Bipolar recovery guides. *Psych Central*. Retrieved from http://psychcentral.com/blog/archives/2007/03/05/bipolar-recovery-guides

Kowatch, R.A., Fristad, M., Birmaher, B., Wagner, K.D., Findling, R.L., & Hellander, M. (2005). Treatment guidelines for children and adolescents with bipolar disorder. *Journal of the American Academy of Child and Adolescent Psychiatry, 44*(3), 213-235.

McClellan, J., Kowatch, R., & Findling, R.L. (2007). Practice parameter for the assessment and treatment of children and adolescents with bipolar disorder. *Journal of the American Academy of Child and Adolescent Psychiatry, 46*(1), 107-125.

Miklowitz, D.J., George, E.L., Richards, J.A., Simoneau, T.L. & Suddath, R.L. (2003). A randomized study of family-focused psychoeducation and pharmacotherapy in the outpatient management of bipolar disorder. *Archives of General Psychiatry, 60*(9), 904-912.

Nakate, S. (2011). *History of bipolar disorder (manic depression)*. Retrieved from http://www.buzzle.com/articles/history-of-bipolar-disorder-manic-depression.html

NANDA International (NANDA-I). (2012). *Nursing diagnoses: Definitions and classification 2012-2014*. Hoboken, NJ: Wiley-Blackwell.

Nandagopal, J.J., & DelBello, M.P. (2008). Diagnosis and treatment of pediatric bipolar disorder. *Medscape Psychiatry*. Retrieved from http://www.medscape.com/viewprogram/15741

National Alliance on Mental Illness (NAMI). (2008). *Understanding bipolar disorder and recovery*. Retrieved from http://www.nami.org

National Institute of Mental Health (NIMH). (2008). Bipolar disorder and gene abnormalities: Sodium, calcium imbalances linked to manic depressive episodes. *ScienceDaily*. Retrieved from http://www.sciencedaily.com/releases/2008/08/080817223548.htm

National Institute of Mental Health (NIMH). (2013). *Mental disorders in America: The numbers count*. Bethesda, MD: National Institutes of Health.

Powell, I. (2006). *Family and friends' guide to recovery from depression and bipolar disorder*. The Empowerment Project of the Depression and Bipolar Support Alliance. Retrieved from http://www.dbsalliance.org/pdfs/FamilyBookFinal.pdf

Sadock, B.J., and Sadock, V.A. (2003). *Synopsis of psychiatry: Behavioral sciences/clinical psychiatry* (9th ed.). Philadelphia, PA: Lippincott Williams & Wilkins.

Schatzberg, A.F., Cole, J.O., & DeBattista, C. (2010). *Manual of clinical psychopharmacology* (7th ed.). Washington, DC: American Psychiatric Publishing.

Soreff, S., & McInnes, L.A. (2012). Bipolar affective disorder. *E-medicine: Psychiatry*. Retrieved from http://emedicine.medscape.com/article/286342-overview

The Joint Commission. (2010, January). *The comprehensive accreditation manual for hospitals: The official handbook*. Oakbrook Terrace, IL: Joint Commission Resources.

Weiden, P.J. (2010). Is recovery attainable in schizophrenia? *Medscape Psychiatry & Mental Health*. Retrieved from http://www.medscape.com/viewarticle/729750

Youssef, H.A., Youssef, F.A., & Dening, T.R. (1996). Evidence for the existence of schizophrenia in medieval Islamic society. *History of Psychiatry, 7*(25), 55-62.

Zubieta, J.K., Huguelet, P., Koeppe, R.A., Kilbourn, M.R., Carr, J.M., Giordani, B.J., & Frey, K.A. (2000). High vesicular monoamine transporter binding in asymptomatic bipolar I disorder: Sex differences and cognitive correlates. *American Journal of Psychiatry, 157*, 1619-1628.

@ INTERNET REFERENCES

- Additional information about bipolar disorders, including psychosocial and pharmacological treatment of these disorders, may be located at the following websites:
  - www.ndmda.org
  - www.mentalhealth.com
  - www.nami.org
  - www.mental-health-matters.com
  - www.mentalhelp.net
  - www.nlm.nih.gov/medlineplus
  - www.drugs.com

🎬 MOVIE CONNECTIONS

Lust for Life (bipolar disorder) • *Call Me Anna* (bipolar disorder) • *Blue Sky* (bipolar disorder) • *A Woman Under the Influence* (bipolar disorder)

27

Anxiety, Obsessive-Compulsive, and Related Disorders

CORE CONCEPTS

anxiety

compulsions

obsessions

panic

phobia

KEY TERMS

agoraphobia

body dysmorphic disorder

flooding

generalized anxiety disorder

habit-reversal therapy

hoarding disorder

implosion therapy

obsessive-compulsive
   disorder

panic disorder

social anxiety disorder

specific phobia

systematic desensitization

trichotillomania

OBJECTIVES
After reading this chapter, the student will be able to:

1. Differentiate among the terms *stress, anxiety,* and *fear.*
2. Discuss historical aspects and epidemiological statistics related to anxiety, obsessive-compulsive, and related disorders.
3. Differentiate between normal anxiety and psychoneurotic anxiety.
4. Describe various types of anxiety, obsessive-compulsive, and related disorders and identify symptomatology associated with each. Use this information in client assessment.
5. Identify predisposing factors in the development of anxiety, obsessive-compulsive, and related disorders.

6. Formulate nursing diagnoses and outcome criteria for clients with anxiety, obsessive-compulsive, and related disorders.
7. Describe appropriate nursing interventions for behaviors associated with anxiety, obsessive-compulsive, and related disorders.
8. Identify topics for client and family teaching relevant to anxiety, obsessive-compulsive, and related disorders.
9. Evaluate nursing care of clients with anxiety, obsessive-compulsive, and related disorders.
10. Discuss various modalities relevant to treatment of anxiety, obsessive-compulsive, and related disorders.

HOMEWORK ASSIGNMENT
Please read the chapter and answer the following questions:

1. What are the symptoms of a person with agoraphobia?
2. What neurotransmitter has been implicated in the development of obsessive-compulsive disorder?

3. What are some predisposing factors that have been associated with hair-pulling disorder?
4. What is the primary nursing intervention for a person in panic anxiety?

The following is an account by singer-songwriter Michael Johnson (1994) relating his experience with performance anxiety:

> You've got your Jolly Roger clothes on, you've got the microphone, the lights are on you, the owner has just told the crowd to shut up, and you are getting that kind of "show and tell" sickness that you used to get at grade school pageants or college recitals. Suddenly your mouth is so dry that your lips are sticking to your teeth and you find yourself gesturing oddly with your shoulder and wondering if they think that maybe something unfortunate happened to you. And they're trying to cope with the whole thing. It is now, of course, it hits you that you started with the second verse, you're doing a live rewrite, and you have no idea how this song is going to end. Your vocal range has shrunk and your heartbeat is interfering with your vibrato. Your palms are wet and your mouth is dry—a great combination!

CORE CONCEPT

Anxiety

Apprehension, tension, or uneasiness from anticipation of danger, the source of which is largely unknown or unrecognized. Anxiety may be regarded as pathological when it interferes with social and occupational functioning, achievement of desired goals, or emotional comfort (Black & Andreasen, 2011, pp. 590-591)

Individuals face anxiety on a daily basis. Anxiety, which provides the motivation for achievement, is a necessary force for survival. The term *anxiety* is often used interchangeably with the word *stress*; however, they are not the same. Stress, or more properly, a *stressor*, is an external pressure that is brought to bear on the individual. Anxiety is the subjective emotional response to that stressor. (See Chapter 2 for an overview of anxiety as a psychological response to stress.)

Anxiety may be distinguished from *fear* in that the former is an emotional process, whereas fear is a cognitive one. Fear involves the intellectual appraisal of a threatening stimulus; anxiety involves the emotional response to that appraisal.

This chapter focuses on disorders that are characterized by exaggerated and often disabling anxiety reactions. Historical aspects and epidemiological statistics are presented. Predisposing factors that have been implicated in the etiology of the disorders provide a framework for studying the dynamics of phobias, obsessive-compulsive disorders, generalized anxiety disorder, panic disorder, and other anxiety disorders. Various theories of causation are presented, although it is most likely that a combination of factors contribute to the etiology of these disorders. The neurobiology of anxiety disorders is presented in Figure 27-1.

An explanation of the symptomatology is presented as background knowledge for assessing the client with an anxiety or obsessive-compulsive disorder. Nursing care is described in the context of the nursing process. Various treatment modalities are explored.

Historical Aspects

Individuals have experienced anxiety throughout the ages. Yet anxiety, like fear, was not clearly defined or isolated as a separate entity by psychiatrists or psychologists until the 19th and 20th centuries. In fact, what we now know as anxiety was once solely identified by its physiological symptoms, focusing largely on the cardiovascular system. Clinicians used a myriad of diagnostic terms in attempting to identify these symptoms. For example, cardiac neurosis, DaCosta's syndrome, irritable heart, nervous tachycardia, neurocirculatory asthenia, soldier's heart, vasomotor neurosis, and vasoregulatory asthenia are just a few of the names under which anxiety has been concealed over the years (Sadock & Sadock, 2007).

Freud first introduced the term *anxiety neurosis* in 1895. Freud wrote, "I call this syndrome 'anxiety neurosis' because all its components can be grouped round the chief symptom of anxiety" (Freud, 1959). This notion attempted to negate the previous concept of the problem as strictly physical, although it was some time before physicians of internal medicine were ready to accept the psychological implications for the symptoms. In fact, it was not until the years during World War II that the psychological dimensions of these various functional heart conditions were recognized.

For many years, anxiety disorders were viewed as purely psychological or purely biological in nature. Researchers have begun to focus on the interrelatedness of mind and body, and anxiety disorders provide an excellent example of this complex relationship. It is likely that various factors, including genetic, developmental, environmental, and psychological, play a role in the etiology of anxiety disorders.

Epidemiological Statistics

Anxiety disorders are the most common of all psychiatric illnesses and result in considerable functional impairment and distress (Hollander & Simeon, 2008). Statistics vary widely, but most agree that anxiety disorders are more common in women than in men by at least 2 to 1. Prevalence rates for anxiety disorders within the general population have been given at 3 to 5 percent for generalized anxiety disorder and panic disorder, 13 percent for social anxiety disorder, and 25 percent for phobias. Obsessive-compulsive

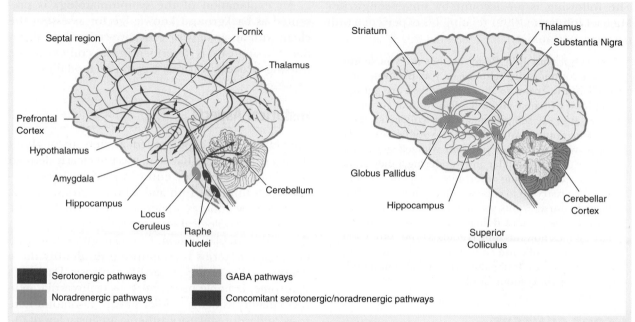

FIGURE 27-1 Neurobiology of anxiety disorders.

NEUROTRANSMITTERS

Although other neurotransmitters have also been implicated in the pathophysiology of anxiety disorders, disturbances in serotonin, norepinephrine, and gamma-aminobutyric acid (GABA) appear to be most significant.

Cell bodies of origin for the serotonin pathways lie within the raphe nuclei located in the brain stem. Serotonin is thought to be decreased in anxiety disorders. Cell bodies for norepinephrine originate in the locus ceruleus. Norepinephrine is thought to be increased in anxiety disorders. GABA is the major inhibitory neurotransmitter in the brain. It is involved in the reduction and slowing of cellular activity. It is synthesized from glutamic acid, with vitamin B_6 as a cofactor. It is found in almost every region of the brain. GABA is thought to be decreased in anxiety disorders (allowing for increased cellular excitability).

AREAS OF THE BRAIN AFFECTED

Areas of the brain affected by anxiety disorders and the symptoms that they mediate include the following:
- Amygdala: Fear; particularly important in panic and phobic disorders
- Hippocampus: Associated with memory related to fear responses
- Locus ceruleus: Arousal
- Brainstem: Respiratory activation; heart rate
- Hypothalamus: Activation of stress response
- Frontal cortex: Cognitive interpretations
- Thalamus: Integration of sensory stimuli
- Basal ganglia: Tremor

Anxiolytic Agents	Action	Side Effects
Benzodiazepines	Increases the affinity of the $GABA_A$ receptor for GABA	Sedation, dizziness, weakness, ataxia, decreased motor performance, dependence, withdrawal
SSRIs	Block reuptake of serotonin into the presynaptic nerve terminal, increasing synaptic concentration of serotonin	Nausea, diarrhea, headache, insomnia, somnolence, sexual dysfunction
SNRIs	Inhibit reuptake of neuronal serotonin and norepinephrine; mild reuptake of dopamine	Headache, dry mouth, nausea, somnolence, dizziness, insomnia, asthenia, constipation, diarrhea
Noradrenergic agents (e.g., propranolol, clonidine)	Propranolol: blocks beta adrenergic receptor activity	Propranolol: bradycardia, hypotension, weakness, fatigue, impotence, GI upset, bronchospasm
	Clonidine: stimulates alpha-adrenergic receptors	Clonidine: dry mouth, sedation, fatigue, hypotension
Barbiturates	CNS depression. Also produces effects in the hepatic and cardiovascular systems	Somnolence, agitation, confusion, ataxia, dizziness, bradycardia, hypotension, constipation
Buspirone	Partial agonist of $5-HT_{1A}$ receptor	Dizziness, drowsiness, dry mouth, headache, nervousness, nausea, insomnia

disorders account for 2 to 3 percent (Rowney, Hermida, & Malone, 2010). A review of the literature revealed a wide range of reports regarding the prevalence of anxiety disorders in children (2 percent to 43 percent). Epidemiological studies suggest that the symptoms are more prevalent among girls than boys, and that minority children and children from low socioeconomic environments may be at greater risk for all emotional illness (National Mental Health Association [NMHA], 2005). Studies of familial patterns suggest that a familial predisposition to anxiety disorders probably exists.

How Much Is Too Much?

Anxiety is usually considered a normal reaction to a realistic danger or threat to biological integrity or self-concept. Normal anxiety dissipates when the danger or threat is no longer present.

It is difficult to draw a precise line between normal and abnormal anxiety. Normality is determined by societal standards; what is considered normal in Chicago, Illinois, may not be considered so in Cairo, Egypt. There may even be regional differences within a country or cultural differences within a region. So what criteria can be used to determine if an individual's anxious response is normal? Anxiety can be considered abnormal or pathological if:

1. *It is out of proportion to the situation that is creating it.*

EXAMPLE

Mrs. K. witnessed a serious automobile accident 4 weeks ago when she was out driving in her car, and since that time refuses to drive even to the grocery store a few miles from her house. When he is available, her husband must take her wherever she needs to go.

2. *The anxiety interferes with social, occupational, or other important areas of functioning.*

EXAMPLE

Because of the anxiety associated with driving her car, Mrs. K. has been forced to quit her job in a downtown bank for lack of transportation.

Application of the Nursing Process– Assessment

CORE CONCEPT

Panic

A sudden overwhelming feeling of terror or impending doom. This most severe form of emotional anxiety is usually accompanied by behavioral, cognitive, and physiological signs and symptoms considered to be outside the expected range of normalcy.

Panic Disorder

Background Assessment Data

Panic disorder is characterized by recurrent panic attacks, the onset of which is unpredictable, and manifested by intense apprehension, fear, or terror, often associated with feelings of impending doom and accompanied by intense physical discomfort. The symptoms

IMPLICATIONS OF RESEARCH FOR EVIDENCE-BASED PRACTICE

Johnson, J.G., Cohen, P., Pine, D.S., Klein, D.F., Kasen, S., & Brook, J.S. (2000, November 8). Association between cigarette smoking and anxiety disorders during adolescence and early adulthood. *Journal of the American Medical Association, 284*(18), 2348-2351.

DESCRIPTION OF THE STUDY: The main objective of this study was to investigate the longitudinal association between cigarette smoking and anxiety disorders among adolescents and young adults. The study sample included 688 teenagers (51 percent female and 49 percent male) from upstate New York. The youths were interviewed at a mean age of 16 years, during the years 1985 to 1986, and again at a mean age of 22 years, during the years 1991 to 1993. At age 16, 6 percent of the participants smoked 20 or more cigarettes a day. The number increased to 15 percent by age 22.

RESULTS OF THE STUDY: Of the participants who smoked 20 cigarettes or more a day during adolescence, a significant number developed an anxiety disorder during young adulthood: 20.5 percent developed generalized anxiety disorder, 10.3 percent developed agoraphobia, and 7.7 percent developed panic disorder. According to the researchers, cigarette smoking does not appear to increase the risk of developing OCD or social anxiety disorder.

IMPLICATIONS FOR NURSING PRACTICE: The results of this study present just one more reason why adolescents should be encouraged not to smoke or not to begin smoking. The implications for nursing practice are serious. Nurses can initiate and become involved in educational programs to discourage cigarette smoking. Many negative health concerns are related to smoking, and this study provides additional information to include in educational programs designed specifically for adolescents.

come on unexpectedly; that is, they do not occur immediately before or on exposure to a situation that usually causes anxiety (as in specific phobia). They are not triggered by situations in which the person is the focus of others' attention (as in social anxiety disorder). The role of organic factors in the etiology has been ruled out.

The *Diagnostic and Statistical Manual of Mental Disorders, Fifth Edition (DSM-5)* (American Psychiatric Association [APA], 2013) states that at least four of the following symptoms must be present to identify the presence of a panic attack.

■ Palpitations, pounding heart, or accelerated heart rate
■ Sweating
■ Trembling or shaking
■ Sensations of shortness of breath or smothering
■ Feelings of choking
■ Chest pain or discomfort
■ Nausea or abdominal distress
■ Feeling dizzy, unsteady, light-headed, or faint
■ Chills or heat sensations
■ Paresthesias (numbness or tingling sensations)
■ Derealization (feelings of unreality) or depersonalization (feelings of being detached from oneself)
■ Fear of losing control or going crazy
■ Fear of dying

The attacks usually last minutes, or more rarely, hours. The individual often experiences varying degrees of nervousness and apprehension between attacks. Symptoms of depression are common.

The average age of onset of panic disorder is the late 20s. Frequency and severity of the panic attacks vary widely. Some individuals may have attacks of moderate severity weekly; others may have less severe or limited-symptom attacks several times a week. Still others may experience panic attacks that are separated by weeks or months. The disorder may last for a few weeks or months or for a number of years. Sometimes the individual experiences periods of remission and exacerbation. In times of remission, the person may have recurrent limited-symptom attacks. Panic disorder may or may not be accompanied by **agoraphobia** (discussed later in the chapter).

Generalized Anxiety Disorder

Background Assessment Data

Generalized anxiety disorder (GAD) is characterized by persistent, unrealistic, and excessive anxiety and worry, which have occurred more days than not for at least 6 months, and cannot be attributed to specific organic factors, such as caffeine intoxication or hyperthyroidism. The symptoms cause clinically significant distress or impairment in social, occupational, or other important areas of functioning. The anxiety and worry are associated with muscle tension, restlessness,

or feeling keyed up or on edge (APA, 2013). The individual often avoids activities or events that may result in negative outcomes, or spends considerable time and effort preparing for such activities. Anxiety and worry often result in procrastination in behavior or decision-making, and the individual repeatedly seeks reassurance from others.

The disorder may begin in childhood or adolescence, but onset is not uncommon after age 20. Depressive symptoms are common, and numerous somatic complaints may also be a part of the clinical picture. GAD tends to be chronic, with frequent stress-related exacerbations and fluctuations in the course of the illness.

Predisposing Factors to Panic and Generalized Anxiety Disorders

Psychodynamic Theory

The psychodynamic view focuses on the inability of the ego to intervene when conflict occurs between the id and the superego, producing anxiety. For various reasons (unsatisfactory parent-child relationship; conditional love or provisional gratification), ego development is delayed. When developmental defects in ego functions compromise the capacity to modulate anxiety, the individual resorts to unconscious mechanisms to resolve the conflict. Overuse or ineffective use of ego defense mechanisms results in maladaptive responses to anxiety.

Cognitive Theory

The main thesis of the cognitive view is that faulty, distorted, or counterproductive thinking patterns accompany or precede maladaptive behaviors and emotional disorders (Sadock & Sadock, 2007). When there is a disturbance in this central mechanism of cognition, there is a consequent disturbance in feeling and behavior. Because of distorted thinking, anxiety is maintained by erroneous or dysfunctional appraisal of a situation. There is a loss of ability to reason regarding the problem, whether it is physical or interpersonal. The individual feels vulnerable in a given situation, and the distorted thinking results in an irrational appraisal, fostering a negative outcome.

Biological Aspects

Research investigations into the psychobiological correlation of panic and generalized anxiety disorders have implicated a number of possibilities.

Genetics Panic disorder has a strong genetic element (Harvard Medical School, 2006). The concordance rate for identical twins is 30 percent, and the risk for the disorder in a close relative is 10 to 20 percent. Hollander and Simeon (2008) report on research findings of an association between panic disorder and a variant of the gene that controls the manufacture of the protein cholecystokinin, which has been known to induce panic attacks when it is injected.

Neuroanatomical Modern theory on the physiology of emotional states places the key in the lower brain centers, including the limbic system, the diencephalon (thalamus and hypothalamus), and the reticular formation. Structural brain imaging studies in patients with panic disorder have implicated pathological involvement in the temporal lobes, particularly the hippocampus (Sadock & Sadock, 2007).

Biochemical Abnormal elevations of blood lactate have been noted in clients with panic disorder. Likewise, infusion of sodium lactate into clients with anxiety neuroses produced symptoms of panic disorder. Although several laboratories have replicated these findings of increased lactate sensitivity in panic-prone individuals, no specific mechanism that triggers the panic symptoms can be explained (Hollander & Simeon, 2008).

Neurochemical Stronger evidence exists for the involvement of the neurotransmitter norepinephrine in the etiology of panic disorder. Norepinephrine is known to mediate arousal, and it causes hyperarousal and anxiety. This fact has been demonstrated by a notable increase in anxiety following the administration of drugs that increase the synaptic availability of norepinephrine, such as yohimbine. The neurotransmitters serotonin and gamma aminobutyric acid (GABA)

are thought to be decreased in anxiety disorders (Harvard Medical School, 2006).

CORE CONCEPT
Phobia

Fear cued by the presence or anticipation of a specific object or situation, exposure to which almost invariably provokes an immediate *anxiety* response or *panic attack* even though the subject recognizes that the fear is excessive or unreasonable. The phobic stimulus is avoided or endured with marked distress (Shahrokh & Hales, 2003).

Phobias
Agoraphobia
Background Assessment Data

The literal Greek translation of the word *agoraphobia* is "fear of the marketplace." This defines the fear that some patients have of being in open shops and markets, although "their true fear is being separated from a source of security" (Black & Andreasen, 2011, p. 171). The individual experiences fear of being in places or situations from which escape might be difficult or in which help might not be available in the event that panic symptoms should occur. It is possible that the individual may have experienced the symptom(s) in the past and is preoccupied with fears of their recurrence. The *DSM-5* diagnostic criteria for agoraphobia are presented in Box 27-1.

BOX 27-1 Diagnostic Criteria for Agoraphobia

A. Marked fear or anxiety about two (or more) of the following five situations:
   1. Using public transportation (e.g., automobiles, buses, trains, ships, planes)
   2. Being in open spaces (e.g., parking lots, marketplaces, bridges)
   3. Being in enclosed places (e.g., shops, theaters, cinemas)
   4. Standing in line or being in a crowd
   5. Being outside of the home alone
B. The individual fears these situations because of thoughts that escape might be difficult or help might not be available in the event of panic-like symptoms or other incapacitating or embarrassing symptoms (e.g., fear of falling in the elderly, fear of incontinence).
C. The agoraphobic situations almost always provoke fear or anxiety.
D. The agoraphobic situations are actively avoided, require the presence of a companion, or are endured with intense fear or anxiety.
E. The fear or anxiety is out of proportion to the actual danger posed by the agoraphobic situations and to the sociocultural context.

F. The fear, anxiety, or avoidance is persistent, typically lasting 6 months or more.
G. The fear, anxiety, or avoidance causes clinically significant distress or impairment in social, occupational, or other important areas of functioning.
H. If another medical condition (e.g., inflammatory bowel disease, Parkinson's disease) is present, the fear, anxiety, or avoidance is clearly excessive.
I. The fear, anxiety, or avoidance is not better explained by the symptoms of another mental disorder—for example, the symptoms are not confined to specific phobia, situational type; do not involve only social situations (as in social anxiety disorder); and are not related exclusively to obsessions (as in obsessive-compulsive disorder), perceived defects or flaws in physical appearance (as in body dysmorphic disorder), reminders of traumatic events (as in posttraumatic stress disorder), or fear of separation (as in separation anxiety disorder).

Reprinted with permission from the Diagnostic and Statistical Manual of Mental Disorders, Fifth Edition *(Copyright 2013). American Psychiatric Association.*

Onset of symptoms most commonly occurs in the 20s and 30s and persists for many years. It is diagnosed more commonly in women than in men. Impairment can be severe. In extreme cases the individual is unable to leave his or her home without being accompanied by a friend or relative. If this is not possible the person may become totally confined to his or her home.

Social Anxiety Disorder (Social Phobia)

Background Assessment Data

Social anxiety disorder is an excessive fear of situations in which a person might do something embarrassing or be evaluated negatively by others. The individual has extreme concerns about being exposed to possible scrutiny by others and fears social or performance situations in which embarrassment may occur (APA, 2013). In some instances, the fear may be quite defined, such as the fear of speaking or eating in a public place, fear of using a public restroom, or fear of writing in the presence of others. In other cases, the social phobia may involve general social situations, such as saying things or answering questions in a manner that would provoke laughter on the part of others. Exposure to the phobic situation usually results in feelings of panic anxiety, with sweating, tachycardia, and dyspnea.

Onset of symptoms of this disorder often begins in late childhood or early adolescence and runs a chronic, sometimes lifelong, course. It appears to be more common in women than in men (Puri & Treasaden, 2011). Impairment interferes with social or occupational functioning, or causes marked distress. The *DSM-5* diagnostic criteria for social anxiety disorder are presented in Box 27-2.

Specific Phobia

Background Assessment Data

Specific phobia is identified by fear of specific objects or situations that could conceivably cause harm (e.g., snakes, heights), but the person's reaction to them is excessive, unreasonable, and inappropriate.

Specific phobias are often identified when other anxiety disorders have become a focus of clinical attention. Treatment is generally aimed at the primary diagnosis because it usually produces the greatest distress and interferes with functioning more so than does a specific phobia. A diagnosis of specific phobia is made only when the irrational fear restricts the individual's activities and interferes with his or her daily living.

The phobic person may be no more (or less) anxious than anyone else until exposed to the phobic object or situation. Exposure to the phobic stimulus produces overwhelming symptoms of panic, including palpitations, sweating, dizziness, and difficulty breathing. In fact, these symptoms may occur in response to the individual's merely *thinking* about the

---

BOX 27-2 Diagnostic Criteria for Social Anxiety Disorder (Social Phobia)

A. Marked fear or anxiety about one or more social situations in which the individual is exposed to possible scrutiny by others. Examples include social interactions (e.g., having a conversation, meeting unfamiliar people), being observed (e.g., eating or drinking), and performing in front of others (e.g., giving a speech). *Note:* In children, the anxiety must occur in peer settings and not just during interactions with adults.

B. The individual fears that he or she will act in a way or show anxiety symptoms that will be negatively evaluated (i.e., will be humiliating or embarrassing; will lead to rejection or offend others).

C. The social situations almost always provoke fear or anxiety. *Note:* In children, the fear or anxiety may be expressed by crying, tantrums, freezing, clinging, shrinking, or failing to speak in social situations.

D. The social situations are avoided or endured with intense fear or anxiety.

E. The fear or anxiety is out of proportion to the actual threat posed by the social situation and to the sociocultural context.

F. The fear, anxiety, or avoidance is persistent, typically lasting 6 months or more.

G. The fear, anxiety, or avoidance causes clinically significant distress or impairment in social, occupation, or other important areas of functioning.

H. The fear, anxiety, or avoidance is not attributable to the physiological effects of a substance (e.g., a drug of abuse, a medication) or another medical condition.

I. The fear, anxiety, or avoidance is not better explained by the symptoms of another mental disorder, such as panic disorder, body dysmorphic disorder, or autism spectrum disorder.

J. If another medical condition (e.g., Parkinson's disease, obesity, disfigurement from burns or injury) is present, the fear, anxiety, or avoidance is clearly unrelated or is excessive.

Specify if:
Performance only: If the fear is restricted to speaking or performing in public

---

Reprinted with permission from the Diagnostic and Statistical Manual of Mental Disorders, Fifth Edition *(Copyright 2013). American Psychiatric Association.*

phobic stimulus. Invariably the person recognizes that his or her fear is excessive or unreasonable, but is powerless to change, even though the individual may occasionally endure the phobic stimulus when experiencing intense anxiety.

Phobias may begin at almost any age. Those that begin in childhood often disappear without treatment, but those that begin or persist into adulthood usually require assistance with therapy. The disorder is diagnosed more often in women than in men.

Even though the disorder is relatively common among the general population, people seldom seek treatment unless the phobia interferes with ability to function. Obviously the individual who has a fear of snakes, but who lives on the 23rd floor of an urban, high-rise apartment building, is not likely to be bothered by the phobia unless he or she decides to move to an area where snakes are prevalent. On the other hand, a fear of elevators may very well interfere with this individual's daily functioning.

Specific phobias have been classified according to the phobic stimulus. A list of some of the more common ones appears in Table 27-1. This list is by no means all-inclusive. People can become phobic about almost any object or situation, and anyone with a little knowledge of Greek or Latin can produce a phobia classification, thereby making possibilities for the list almost infinite.

Predisposing Factors to Phobias

The cause of phobias is unknown. However, various theories exist that may offer insight into the etiology.

Psychoanalytic Theory

Freud believed that phobias developed when a child experiences normal incestuous feelings toward the opposite-gender parent (Oedipal/Electra complex) and fears aggression from the same-gender parent (castration anxiety). To protect themselves, these children *repress* this fear of hostility from the same-gender parent, and *displace* it onto something safer and more neutral, which becomes the phobic stimulus. The phobic stimulus becomes the symbol for the parent, but the child does not realize this.

Modern-day psychoanalysts believe in the same concept of phobic development, but believe that castration anxiety is not the sole source of phobias. They believe that other unconscious fears may also be expressed in a symbolic manner as phobias. For example, a female child who was sexually abused by an adult male family friend when he was taking her for a ride in his boat grew up with an intense, irrational fear of all water vessels. Psychoanalytic theory postulates that fear of the man was repressed and displaced onto boats. Boats became an unconscious symbol for the feared person, but one that the young girl viewed

TABLE 27–1 **Classifications of Specific Phobias**	
CLASSIFICATION	FEAR
Acrophobia	Height
Ailurophobia	Cats
Algophobia	Pain
Anthophobia	Flowers
Anthropophobia	People
Aquaphobia	Water
Arachnophobia	Spiders
Astraphobia	Lightning
Belonephobia	Needles
Brontophobia	Thunder
Claustrophobia	Closed spaces
Cynophobia	Dogs
Dementophobia	Insanity
Equinophobia	Horses
Gamophobia	Marriage
Herpetophobia	Lizards, reptiles
Homophobia	Homosexuality
Murophobia	Mice
Mysophobia	Dirt, germs, contamination
Numerophobia	Numbers
Nyctophobia	Darkness
Ochophobia	Riding in a car
Ophidiophobia	Snakes
Pyrophobia	Fire
Scoleciphobia	Worms
Siderodromophobia	Railroads or train travel
Taphophobia	Being buried alive
Thanatophobia	Death
Trichophobia	Hair
Triskaidekaphobia	The number 13
Xenophobia	Strangers
Zoophobia	Animals

as safer since her fear of boats prevented her from having to confront the real fear.

Learning Theory

Classic conditioning in the case of phobias may be explained as follows: a stressful stimulus produces an "unconditioned" response of fear. When the stressful stimulus is repeatedly paired with a harmless object, eventually the harmless object alone produces a "conditioned" response: fear. This becomes a phobia when the individual consciously avoids the harmless object to escape fear.

Some learning theorists hold that fears are conditioned responses and, thus, they are learned by imposing rewards for certain behaviors. In the instance of phobias, when the individual avoids the phobic object, he or she escapes fear, which is indeed a powerful reward.

Phobias also may be acquired by direct learning or imitation (modeling) (e.g., a mother who exhibits fear toward an object will provide a model for the child, who may also develop a phobia of the same object).

Cognitive Theory

Cognitive theorists espouse that anxiety is the product of faulty cognitions or anxiety-inducing self-instructions. Two types of faulty thinking have been investigated: negative self-statements and irrational beliefs. Cognitive theorists believe that some individuals engage in negative and irrational thinking that produces anxiety reactions. The individual begins to seek out avoidance behaviors to prevent the anxiety reactions, and phobias result.

Somewhat related to the cognitive theory is the involvement of locus of control. Johnson and Sarason (1978) suggested that individuals with internal locus of control and those with external locus of control might respond differently to life change. These researchers proposed that locus of control orientation may be an important variable in the development of phobias. Individuals with an external control orientation experiencing anxiety attacks in a stressful period are likely to mislabel the anxiety and attribute it to external sources (e.g., crowded areas) or to a disease (e.g., heart attack). They may perceive the experienced anxiety as being outside of their control. Figure 27-2 depicts a graphic model of the relationship between locus of control and the development of phobias.

Biological Aspects

Temperament Children experience fears as a part of normal development. Most infants are afraid of loud noises. Common fears of toddlers and preschoolers include strangers, animals, darkness, and fears of being separated from parents or attachment figures. During the school-age years, there is fear of death and anxiety

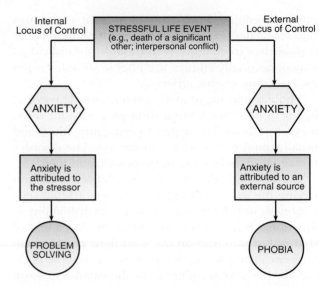

FIGURE 27-2 Locus of control as a variable in the etiology of phobias.

about school achievement. Fears of social rejection and sexual anxieties are common among adolescents.

Innate fears represent a part of the overall characteristics or tendencies with which one is born that influence how he or she responds throughout life to specific situations. Innate fears usually do not reach phobic intensity but may have the capacity for such development if reinforced by events in later life. For example, a 4-year-old girl is afraid of dogs. By age 5, however, she has overcome her fear and plays with her own dog and the neighbors' dogs without fear. Then, when she is 19, she is bitten by a stray dog and develops a phobia of dogs.

Life Experiences

Certain early experiences may set the stage for phobic reactions later in life. Some researchers believe that phobias, particularly specific phobias, are symbolic of original anxiety-producing objects or situations that have been repressed. Examples include:

■ A child who is punished by being locked in a closet develops a phobia for elevators or other closed places.

■ A child who falls down a flight of stairs develops a phobia for high places.

■ A young woman who, as a child, survived a plane crash in which both her parents were killed has a phobia of airplanes.

Anxiety Disorder Due to Another Medical Condition and Substance/Medication-Induced Anxiety Disorder

Background Assessment Data

The symptoms associated with these disorders are judged to be the direct physiological consequence of another medical condition or due to the direct physiological effects of substance intoxication or withdrawal or exposure to a medication. A number of medical conditions have been associated with the development of anxiety symptoms. Some of these include cardiac conditions, such as myocardial infarction, congestive heart failure, and mitral valve prolapse; endocrine conditions, such as hypoglycemia, hypo- or hyperthyroidism, and pheochromocytoma; respiratory conditions, such as chronic obstructive pulmonary disease and hyperventilation; and neurological conditions, such as complex partial seizures, neoplasms, and encephalitis.

Nursing care of clients with this disorder must take into consideration the underlying cause of the anxiety. Holistic nursing care is essential to ensure that the client's physiological and psychosocial needs are met. Nursing actions appropriate for the specific medical condition must be considered.

The diagnosis of substance-induced anxiety disorder is made only if the anxiety symptoms are in excess of those usually associated with the intoxication or withdrawal syndrome and warrant independent clinical attention. Evidence of intoxication or withdrawal must be available from history, physical examination, or laboratory findings to substantiate the diagnosis. Substance-induced anxiety disorder may be associated with use of the following substances: alcohol, amphetamines, cocaine, hallucinogen, sedatives, hypnotics, anxiolytics, caffeine, cannabis, or other substances (APA, 2013). Nursing care of the client with substance-induced anxiety disorder must take into consideration the nature of the substance and the context in which the symptoms occur—that is, intoxication or withdrawal.

CORE CONCEPT
Obsessions
Recurrent and persistent thoughts, impulses, or images experienced as intrusive and stressful. Recognized as being excessive and unreasonable even though they are a product of one's mind. The thought, impulse, or image cannot be expunged by logic or reasoning (Black & Andreasen, 2011, p. 611).

CORE CONCEPT
Compulsions
Repetitive ritualistic behavior or thoughts, the purpose of which is to prevent or reduce distress or to prevent some dreaded event or situation. The person feels driven to perform such actions in response to an obsession or according to rules that must be applied rigidly, even though the behaviors or thoughts are recognized to be excessive or unreasonable (Black & Andreasen, 2011, p. 596).

Obsessive-Compulsive Disorder
Background Assessment Data

The manifestations of **obsessive-compulsive disorder** (OCD) include the presence of obsessions, compulsions, or both, the severity of which is significant enough to cause distress or impairment in social, occupational, or other important areas of functioning (APA, 2013). The individual recognizes that the behavior is excessive or unreasonable but, because of the feeling of relief from discomfort that it promotes, is compelled to continue the act. Common compulsions include hand washing, ordering, checking, praying, counting, and repeating words silently (APA, 2013).

The disorder is equally common among men and women. It may begin in childhood, but more often begins in adolescence or early adulthood. The course is usually chronic, and may be complicated by depression or substance abuse. Single people are affected by OCD more often than are married people (Sadock & Sadock, 2007). The *DSM-5* diagnostic criteria for OCD are presented in Box 27-3.

Body Dysmorphic Disorder
Background Assessment Data

Body dysmorphic disorder is characterized by the exaggerated belief that the body is deformed or defective in some specific way. The most common complaints involve imagined or slight flaws of the face or head, such as wrinkles or scars, the shape of the nose, excessive facial hair, and facial asymmetry (Puri & Treasaden, 2011). Other complaints may have to do with some aspect of the ears, eyes, mouth, lips, or teeth. Some clients may present with complaints involving other parts of the body, and in some instances a true defect is present. The significance of the defect is unrealistically exaggerated, however, and the person's concern is grossly excessive.

Symptoms of depression and characteristics associated with obsessive-compulsive personality are common in individuals with body dysmorphic disorder. Social and occupational impairment may occur because of the excessive anxiety experienced by the individual in relation to the imagined defect. The person's medical history may reflect numerous visits to plastic surgeons and dermatologists in an unrelenting drive to correct the imagined defect. He or she may undergo unnecessary surgical procedures toward this effort.

This disorder has been closely associated with delusional thinking, and the condition must be differentiated from delusional disorder, somatic type. Black and Andreasen (2011) state:

[In Delusional Disorder, Somatic Type] a patient has a delusional belief that a body part is grossly

BOX 27-3 **Diagnostic Criteria for Obsessive-Compulsive Disorder**

A. Presence of obsessions, compulsions, or both:

Obsessions are defined by (1) and (2):

1. Recurrent and persistent thoughts, urges, or images that are experienced, at some time during the disturbance, as intrusive and unwanted, and that in most individuals cause marked anxiety or distress.
2. The individual attempts to ignore or suppress such thoughts, urges, or images, or to neutralize them with some other thought or action (i.e., by performing a compulsion).

Compulsions are defined by (1) and (2):

1. Repetitive behaviors (e.g., hand washing, ordering, checking) or mental acts (e.g., praying, counting, repeating words silently) that the person feels driven to perform in response to an obsession or according to rules that must be applied rigidly.
2. The behaviors or mental acts are aimed at preventing or reducing anxiety or distress, or preventing some dreaded event or situation; however, these behaviors or mental acts either are not connected in a realistic way with what they are designed to neutralize or prevent, or are clearly excessive. *Note:* Young children may not be able to articulate the aims of these behaviors or mental acts.

B. The obsessions or compulsions are time-consuming (e.g., take more than 1 hour a day) or cause clinically significant distress or impairment in social, occupational, or other important areas of functioning.

C. The obsessive-compulsive symptoms are not attributable to the direct physiological effects of a substance (e.g., a drug of abuse, a medication) or another medical condition.

D. The disturbance is not better explained by the symptoms of another mental disorder (e.g., excessive worries, as in generalized anxiety disorder; preoccupation with appearance, as in body dysmorphic disorder; difficulty discarding or parting with possessions, as in hoarding disorder; hair pulling, as in trichotillomania [hair-pulling disorder]; skin picking, as in excoriation [skin-picking] disorder; stereotypies, as in stereotypic movement disorder; ritualized eating behavior, as in eating disorders; preoccupation with substances or gambling, as in substance-related and addictive disorders; preoccupation with having an illness, as in illness anxiety disorder; sexual urges or fantasies, as in paraphilic disorders; impulses, as in disruptive, impulse-control, and conduct disorders; guilty ruminations, as in major depressive disorder; thought insertion or delusional preoccupations, as in schizophrenia spectrum and other psychotic disorders; or repetitive patterns of behavior, as in autism spectrum disorder).

Specify if:
   With good or fair insight
   With poor insight
   With absent insight/delusional beliefs
Specify if:
   Tic-related

Reprinted with permission from the Diagnostic and Statistical Manual of Mental Disorders, Fifth Edition *(Copyright 2013). American Psychiatric Association.*

deformed and distorted. In Body Dysmorphic Disorder, the patient is not delusional and is able to acknowledge that his or her concerns are exaggerated. (p. 221)

Traits associated with schizoid, obsessive-compulsive, and narcissistic personality disorders are not uncommon (Sadock & Sadock, 2007). The *DSM-5* diagnostic criteria for body dysmorphic disorder are presented in Box 27-4.

Trichotillomania (Hair-Pulling Disorder)

Background Assessment Data

The *DSM-5* defines **trichotillomania** as the recurrent pulling out of one's hair that results in hair loss (APA, 2013). The impulse is preceded by an increasing sense of tension and results in a sense of release or gratification from pulling out the hair. The most common sites for hair pulling are the scalp, eyebrows, and eyelashes but may occur in any area of the body on which hair grows. These areas of hair loss are often found on the opposite side of the body from the dominant hand.

Pain is seldom reported to accompany the hair pulling, although tingling and pruritus in the area are not uncommon.

Comorbid psychiatric disorders are common with hair-pulling disorder. Some of these include mood disorders, eating disorders, anxiety disorders, substance abuse disorders, and personality disorders—most commonly histrionic, borderline, and obsessive-compulsive (Hollander & Simeon, 2008).

The disorder usually begins in childhood and may be accompanied by nail biting, head banging, scratching, biting, or other acts of self-mutilation. This relatively rare phenomenon occurs more often in women than in men. Studies indicate that it affects 1 to 4 percent of adolescents and college students (Black & Andreasen, 2011).

Hoarding Disorder

Background Assessment Data

The *DSM-5* defines the essential feature of **hoarding disorder** as "persistent difficulties discarding or parting

---

BOX 27-4 **Diagnostic Criteria for Body Dysmorphic Disorder**

A. Preoccupation with one or more perceived defects or flaws in physical appearance that are not observable or appear slight to others.

B. At some point during the course of the disorder, the individual has performed repetitive behaviors (e.g., mirror checking, excessive grooming, skin picking, reassurance seeking) or mental acts (e.g., comparing his or her appearance with that of others) in response to the appearance concerns.

C. The preoccupation causes clinically significant distress or impairment in social, occupational, or other important areas of functioning.

D. The appearance preoccupation is not better explained by concerns with body fat or weight in an individual whose symptoms meet diagnostic criteria for an eating disorder.

Specify if:
   With muscle dysmorphia
Specify if:
   With good or fair insight
   With poor insight
   With absent insight/delusional beliefs

Reprinted with permission from the Diagnostic and Statistical Manual of Mental Disorders, Fifth Edition *(Copyright 2013). American Psychiatric Association.*

---

with possessions, regardless of their actual value" (APA, 2013, p. 248). Additionally, the diagnosis may be specified as "with excessive acquisition," which identifies the excessive need for continual acquiring of items (either by buying them or by other means). In previous editions of the *DSM*, hoarding was considered a symptom of OCD. However, in the *DSM-5*, it has been reclassified as a diagnostic disorder.

Individuals with this disorder collect items until virtually all surfaces within the home are covered. There may be only narrow pathways, winding through stacks of clutter, in which to walk. Some individuals also hoard food and animals, keeping dozens or hundreds of pets, often in unsanitary conditions (The Mayo Clinic, 2011).

Hoarding disorder affects an estimated 700,000 to 1.4 million Americans, but few receive adequate treatment (Symonds & Janney, 2013). More men than women are diagnosed with the disorder, and it is almost three times more prevalent in older adults (ages 55 to 94) compared with younger adults (ages 34 to 44) (APA, 2013). The severity of the symptoms, regardless of when they begin, appears to become more severe with each decade of life. Associated symptoms include perfectionism, indecisiveness, anxiety, depression, distractibility, and difficulty planning and organizing tasks (APA, 2013; Symonds & Janney, 2013).

Treatment of hoarding disorder has been met with mixed results. It is often difficult to convince individuals with the disorder that they are actually ill. Change is slow, and the relapse rate is high, with patients and family members showing various levels of understanding about their hoarding behaviors (Valente, 2009). Psychoeducation about the disorder is almost always the initial intervention, and treatment is most commonly a combination of cognitive behavioral therapy and psychopharmacology with the selective serotonin reuptake inhibitors (SSRIs).

Predisposing Factors to Obsessive-Compulsive and Related Disorders

Psychoanalytic Theory

Psychoanalytic theorists propose that individuals with OCD have weak, underdeveloped egos (for any of a variety of reasons: unsatisfactory parent-child relationship, conditional love, or provisional gratification). The psychoanalytical concept views clients with OCD as having regressed to earlier developmental stages of the infantile superego—the harsh, exacting, punitive characteristics that now reappear as part of the psychopathology. Regression to the pre-Oedipal anal-sadistic phase, combined with use of specific ego defense mechanisms (isolation, undoing, displacement, reaction formation), produces the clinical symptoms of obsessions and compulsions (Sadock & Sadock, 2007). Aggressive impulses (common during the anal-sadistic developmental phase) are channeled into thoughts and behaviors that prevent the feelings of aggression from surfacing and producing intense anxiety fraught with guilt (generated by the punitive superego).

Learning Theory

Learning theorists explain obsessive-compulsive behavior as a conditioned response to a traumatic event. The traumatic event produces anxiety and discomfort, and the individual learns to prevent the anxiety and discomfort by avoiding the situation with which they are associated. This type of learning is called *passive avoidance* (staying away from the source). When passive avoidance is not possible, the individual learns to engage in behaviors that provide relief from the anxiety and discomfort associated with the traumatic situation. This type of learning is called *active avoidance* and describes the behavior pattern of the individual with OCD (Sadock & Sadock, 2007).

According to this classic conditioning interpretation, a traumatic event should mark the beginning of the obsessive-compulsive behaviors. However, in a significant number of cases, the onset of the behavior is gradual and the clients relate the onset of their problems to life stress in general rather than to one or more traumatic events.

Psychosocial Influences

The onset of trichotillomania can be related to stressful situations in more than one-quarter of cases. Additional factors that have been implicated include disturbances in mother-child relationship, fear of abandonment, and recent object loss. Studies also have shown a possible correlation between trichotillomania and body dysmorphic disorder and a history of childhood abuse (e.g., physical, emotional, or sexual) or emotional neglect (Lochner et al., 2002; Phillips, 2009).

Biological Aspects

Genetics Trichotillomania has commonly been associated with obsessive-compulsive disorders among first-degree relatives, leading researchers to conclude that the disorder has a possible hereditary or familial predisposition. Structural abnormalities in various areas of the brain, as well as alterations in the serotonin and endogenous opioid systems, have also been noted.

Genetics also may play a role in the development of hoarding disorder. Family and twin studies indicate that approximately 50 percent of individuals who hoard report having a relative who also hoards (APA, 2013).

Neuroanatomy Recent findings suggest that neurobiological disturbances may play a role in the pathogenesis and maintenance of OCD. Abnormalities in various regions of the brain have been implicated in the neurobiology of OCD. Functional neuroimaging techniques have shown abnormal metabolic rates in the basal ganglia and orbitofrontal cortex of individuals with the disorder (Hollander & Simeon, 2008). In individuals with hoarding disorder, neuroimaging studies have indicated less activity in the cingulate cortex, the area of the brain that connects the emotional part of the brain with the parts that control higher-level thinking (Saxena, 2013).

Physiology Electrophysiological studies, sleep electroencephalogram studies, and neuroendocrine studies have suggested that there are commonalities between depressive disorders and OCD (Sadock & Sadock, 2007). Neuroendocrine commonalities were suggested in studies in which about one-third of OCD clients show nonsuppression on the dexamethasone-suppression test and decreased growth hormone secretion with clonidine infusions.

Biochemical Factors A number of studies have implicated the neurotransmitter serotonin as influential in the etiology of obsessive-compulsive behaviors. Drugs that have been used successfully in alleviating the symptoms of OCD are clomipramine and the SSRIs, all of which are believed to block the neuronal reuptake of serotonin, thereby potentiating serotoninergic activity in the central nervous system (see Figure 27-1). The serotonergic system may also be a factor in the etiology of body dysmorphic disorder. This can be reflected in a high incidence of comorbidity with major mood disorder and anxiety disorder and the positive responsiveness of the condition to the serotonin-specific drugs.

Transactional Model of Stress/Adaptation

Anxiety, obsessive-compulsive, and related disorders are most likely caused by multiple factors. In Figure 27-3, a graphic depiction of this theory of multiple causation is presented in the Transactional Model of Stress/Adaptation.

Assessment Scales

A number of assessment rating scales are available for measuring severity of anxiety symptoms. Some are meant to be clinician administered, whereas others may be self-administered. Examples of self-rating scales include the Beck Anxiety Inventory and the Zung Self-Rated Anxiety Scale. One of the most widely used clinician-administered scales is the Hamilton Anxiety Rating Scale (HAM-A), which is used in both clinical and research settings. The scale consists of 14 items and measures both psychic and somatic anxiety symptoms (psychological distress and physical complaints associated with anxiety). A copy of the HAM-A is presented in Box 27-5.

Diagnosis/Outcome Identification

Nursing diagnoses are formulated from the data gathered during the assessment phase and with background knowledge regarding predisposing factors to the disorder. Table 27-2 presents a list of client behaviors and the NANDA International (NANDA-I) nursing diagnoses that correspond to those behaviors, which may be used in planning care for clients with anxiety, obsessive-compulsive, and related disorders.

Outcome Criteria

The following criteria may be used for measurement of outcomes in the care of the client with anxiety disorders.

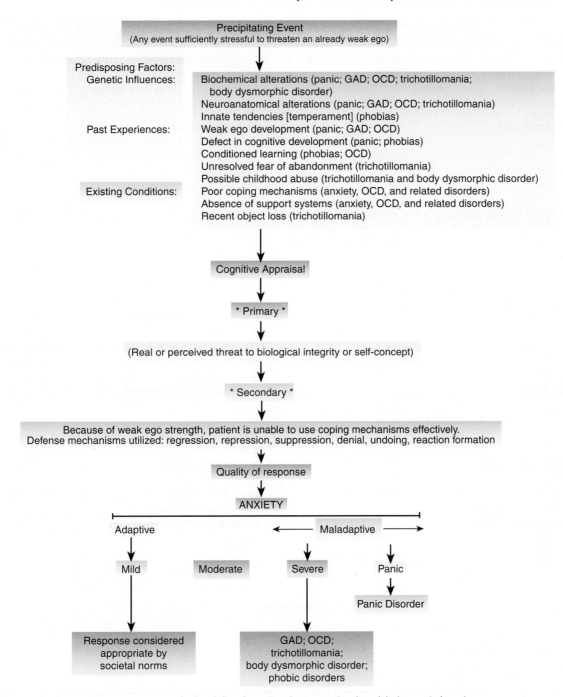

FIGURE 27–3 The dynamics of anxiety, OCD, and related disorders using the Transactional Model of Stress/Adaptation.

The client:

■ Is able to recognize signs of escalating anxiety and intervene before reaching panic level (*panic and generalized anxiety disorders*)

■ Is able to maintain anxiety at manageable level and make independent decisions about life situation (*panic and generalized anxiety disorders*)

■ Functions adaptively in the presence of the phobic object or situation without experiencing panic anxiety (*phobic disorder*)

■ Verbalizes a future plan of action for responding in the presence of the phobic object or situation without developing panic anxiety (*phobic disorder*)

■ Is able to maintain anxiety at a manageable level without resorting to the use of ritualistic behavior (*OCD*)

■ Demonstrates more adaptive coping strategies for dealing with anxiety than ritualistic behaviors (*OCD*)

■ Verbalizes a realistic perception of his or her appearance and expresses feelings that reflect a positive body image (*body dysmorphic disorder*)

BOX 27-5 Hamilton Anxiety Rating Scale (HAM-A)

Below are descriptions of symptoms commonly associated with anxiety. Assign the client the rating between 0 and 4 (for each of the 14 items) that best describes the extent to which he/she has these symptoms.

0 = Not present   1 = Mild   2 = Moderate   3 = Severe   4 = Very severe

Rating

1. **Anxious mood**

   _____

   Worries, anticipation of the worst, fearful anticipation, irritability

2. **Tension**

   _____

   Feelings of tension, fatigability, startle response, moved to tears easily, trembling, feelings of restlessness, inability to relax

3. **Fears**

   _____

   Of dark, of strangers, of being left alone, of animals, of traffic, of crowds

4. **Insomnia**

   _____

   Difficulty in falling asleep, broken sleep, unsatisfying sleep and fatigue on waking, dreams, nightmares, night terrors

5. **Intellectual**

   _____

   Difficulty in concentration, poor memory

6. **Depressed mood**

   _____

   Loss of interest, lack of pleasure in hobbies, depression, early waking, diurnal swing

7. **Somatic (muscular)**

   _____

   Pains and aches, twitching, stiffness, myoclonic jerks, grinding of teeth, unsteady voice, increased muscular tone

Rating

8. **Somatic (sensory)**

   _____

   Tinnitus, blurred vision, hot/cold flushes, feelings of weakness, tingling sensation

9. **Cardiovascular symptoms**

   _____

   Tachycardia, palpitations, pain in chest, throbbing of vessels, feeling faint

10. **Respiratory symptoms**

    _____

    Pressure or constriction in chest, choking feelings, sighing, dyspnea

11. **Gastrointestinal symptoms**

    _____

    Difficulty swallowing, flatulence, abdominal pain and full-ness, burning sensations, nausea/vomiting, borborygmi, diarrhea, constipation, weight loss

12. **Genitourinary symptoms**

    _____

    Urinary frequency, urinary urgency, amenorrhea, menorrhagia, loss of libido, premature ejaculation, impotence

13. **Autonomic symptoms**

    _____

    Dry mouth, flushing, pallor, tendency to sweat, giddi-ness, tension headache

14. **Behavior at interview**

    _____

    Fidgeting, restlessness or pacing, tremor of hands, fur-rowed brow, strained face, sighing or rapid respiration, facial pallor, swallowing, clearing throat

Client's Total Score _____

SCORING:
14 – 17 = Mild Anxiety
18 – 24 = Moderate Anxiety
25 – 30 = Severe Anxiety

SOURCE: Hamilton, M. (1959). The assessment of anxiety states by rating. British Journal of Medical Psychology, 32, 50-55. The HAM-A is in the public domain.

TABLE 27–2 Assigning Nursing Diagnoses to Behaviors Commonly Associated with Anxiety, Obsessive-Compulsive, and Related Disorders

BEHAVIORS	NURSING DIAGNOSES
Palpitations, trembling, sweating, chest pain, shortness of breath, fear of going crazy, fear of dying (*panic disorder*). Excessive worry, difficulty concentrating, sleep disturbance (*generalized anxiety disorder*).	**Anxiety (severe/panic)**
Verbal expressions of having no control over life situation; nonparticipation in decision making related to own care or life situation; expressions of doubt regarding role performance (*panic and generalized anxiety disorders*).	**Powerlessness**

TABLE 27–2	**Assigning Nursing Diagnoses to Behaviors Commonly Associated with Anxiety, Obsessive-Compulsive, and Related Disorders—cont'd**
BEHAVIORS	**NURSING DIAGNOSES**
Behavior directed toward avoidance of a feared object or situation (*phobic disorder*).	Fear
Stays at home alone, afraid to venture out alone (*agoraphobia*).	Social isolation
Ritualistic behavior; obsessive thoughts, inability to meet basic needs; severe level of anxiety (*OCD*).	Ineffective coping
Inability to fulfill usual patterns of responsibility because of need to perform rituals (*OCD*).	Ineffective role performance
Preoccupation with imagined defect; verbalizations that are out of proportion to any actual physical abnormality that may exist; numerous visits to plastic surgeons or dermatologists seeking relief (*body dysmorphic disorder*).	Disturbed body image
Repetitive and impulsive pulling out of one's hair (*trichotillomania*).	Ineffective impulse control

■ Verbalizes and demonstrates more adaptive strategies for coping with stressful situations (*trichotillomania*)

Planning/Implementation

Care Plan for the Client with Anxiety, OCD, and Related Disorders

The following section presents a group of selected nursing diagnoses, with short- and long-term goals and nursing interventions for each.

Some institutions are using a case management model to coordinate care (see Chapter 9 for more detailed explanation). In case management models, the plan of care may take the form of a critical pathway.

Anxiety (Panic)

Anxiety is defined as a "vague uneasy feeling of discomfort or dread accompanied by an autonomic response (the source often nonspecific or unknown to the individual); a feeling of apprehension caused by anticipation of danger. It is an alerting signal that warns of impending danger and enables the individual to take measures to deal with threat" (NANDA International [NANDA-I], 2012, p. 344). Table 27-3 presents this nursing diagnosis in care plan format.

Table 27-3 | CARE PLAN FOR THE CLIENT WITH ANXIETY, OBSESSIVE-COMPULSIVE, AND RELATED DISORDERS

NURSING DIAGNOSIS: PANIC ANXIETY

RELATED TO: Real or perceived threat to biological integrity or self-concept

EVIDENCED BY: Any or all of the physical symptoms identified by the *DSM-5*

OUTCOME CRITERIA	NURSING INTERVENTIONS	RATIONALE
Short-Term Goal • The client will verbalize ways to intervene in escalating anxiety within 1 week.	1. Stay with the client and offer reassurance of safety and security. Do not leave the client in panic anxiety alone.	1. The client may fear for his or her life. Presence of a trusted individual provides a feeling of security and assurance of personal safety.
	2. Maintain a calm, nonthreatening, matter-of-fact approach.	2. Anxiety is contagious and may be transferred from staff to client or vice versa. Client develops a feeling of security in the presence of a calm staff person.

Continued

Table 27-3 | CARE PLAN FOR THE CLIENT WITH ANXIETY, OBSESSIVE-COMPULSIVE, AND RELATED DISORDERS—cont'd

OUTCOME CRITERIA	NURSING INTERVENTIONS	RATIONALE
Long-Term Goal • By time of discharge from treatment, the client will be able to recognize symptoms of onset of anxiety and intervene before reaching panic level.	3. Use simple words and brief messages, spoken calmly and clearly, to explain hospital experiences.	3. In an intensely anxious situation, the client is unable to comprehend anything but the most elemental communication.
	4. Hyperventilation may occur during periods of extreme anxiety. Hyperventilation causes the amount of carbon dioxide (CO_2) in the blood to decrease, possibly resulting in lightheadedness, rapid heart rate, shortness of breath, numbness or tingling in the hands or feet, and syncope. If hyperventilation occurs, assist the client to breathe into a small paper bag held over the mouth and nose. Six to 12 natural breaths should be taken, alternating with short periods of diaphragmatic breathing.	4. Hyperventilation may result in injury to the patient, and patient safety is a nursing priority. The technique here should not be used with clients who have coronary or respiratory disorders, such as coronary artery disease, asthma, or chronic obstructive pulmonary disease.
	5. Keep immediate surroundings low in stimuli (dim lighting, few people, simple decor).	5. A stimulating environment may increase level of anxiety.
	6. Administer tranquilizing medication, as ordered by physician. Assess for effectiveness and for side effects.	6. Antianxiety medication provides relief from the immobilizing effects of anxiety.
	7. When level of anxiety has been reduced, explore possible reasons for occurrence.	7. Recognition of precipitating factor(s) is the first step in teaching client to interrupt escalation of anxiety.
	8. Teach signs and symptoms of escalating anxiety, and ways to interrupt its progression (relaxation techniques, such as deep-breathing exercises and meditation, or physical exercise, such as brisk walks and jogging).	8. Relaxation techniques result in a physiological response opposite that of the anxiety response. Physical activities discharge excess energy in a healthful manner.

Client Goals

Outcome criteria include short- and long-term goals. Timelines are individually determined.

Short-Term Goal

■ The client will verbalize ways to intervene in escalating anxiety within 1 week.

Long-Term Goal

■ By time of discharge from treatment, client will be able to recognize symptoms of onset of anxiety and intervene before reaching panic stage.

Interventions

■ Do not leave a client who is experiencing panic anxiety alone. Stay with him or her and offer reassurance of safety and security. At this level of anxiety, clients often express a fear of dying or of "going crazy." They need the presence and assurance of their safety from a trusted individual.

■ Maintain a calm, nonthreatening, matter-of-fact approach. Anxiety is contagious and can be transferred from staff to client or vice versa. The presence of a calm person provides a feeling of security to an anxious client.

■ Use simple words and brief messages, spoken calmly and clearly, to explain hospital experiences to the client. In an intensely anxious situation, the client is unable to comprehend anything but the most elementary communication.

■ Hyperventilation may occur during periods of extreme anxiety. Hyperventilation causes the amount of carbon dioxide (CO_2) in the blood to decrease, possibly resulting in light-headedness, rapid heart rate, shortness of breath, numbness or tingling in the hands or feet, and syncope. If hyperventilation occurs, assist the client to breathe into a small paper bag held over the mouth and nose. Six to 12 natural breaths should be taken, alternating with short periods of diaphragmatic breathing. This technique should not be used with clients who have coronary or respiratory disorders, such as coronary artery disease, asthma, or chronic obstructive pulmonary disease.

■ Keep the immediate surroundings low in stimuli (dim lighting, few people, simple decor). A stimulating environment may increase the level of anxiety.

■ Administer tranquilizing medication, as ordered by the physician. Assess the medication for effectiveness and for adverse side effects.

■ When the level of anxiety has been reduced, explore with the client possible reasons for its occurrence. If the client is going to learn to interrupt escalating anxiety, he or she must first learn to recognize the factors that precipitate its onset.

■ Teach the client the signs and symptoms of escalating anxiety. Discuss ways to interrupt its progression, such as relaxation techniques, deep-breathing exercises, physical exercises, brisk walks, jogging, and meditation. The client will determine which method is most appropriate for him or her. Relaxation techniques result in a physiological response opposite that of the anxiety response, and physical activities discharge excess energy in a healthful manner.

Fear

Fear is defined as the "response to perceived threat that is consciously recognized as a danger" (NANDA-I, 2012, p. 361).

Client Goals

Outcome criteria include short- and long-term goals. Timelines are individually determined.

Short-Term Goal

■ Client will discuss the phobic object or situation with the health-care provider within (time specified).

Long-Term Goal

■ By time of discharge from treatment, client will be able to function in the presence of the phobic object or situation without experiencing panic anxiety.

Interventions

■ Explore the client's perception of threat to physical integrity or threat to self-concept. Reassure the client of his or her safety and security. It is important to understand the client's perception of the phobic object or situation in order to assist with the desensitization process.

■ Discuss the reality of the situation with the client in order to recognize aspects that can be changed and those that cannot. The client must accept the reality of the situation (aspects that cannot change) before the work of reducing the fear can progress. For example, a man who has a fear of flying and whose employment position requires long-distance air travel must accept that he needs to conquer the fear of flying if he is going to stay in this particular job.

■ Include the client in making decisions related to the selection of alternative coping strategies. For example, the client may choose either to avoid the phobic stimulus or attempt to eliminate the fear associated with it. Encouraging the client to make choices promotes feelings of empowerment and serves to increase feelings of self-worth.

■ If the client elects to work on elimination of the fear, the techniques of systematic desensitization or implosion therapy may be employed. (See the explanation of these techniques under "Treatment Modalities" at the end of this chapter.) Systematic desensitization is a plan of behavior modification, designed to expose the individual gradually to the situation or object (either in reality or through fantasizing) until the fear is no longer experienced. With implosion therapy the individual is "flooded" with stimuli related to the phobic situation or object (rather than in gradual steps) until anxiety associated with the object or situation is no longer experienced. Fear is decreased as the physical and psychological sensations diminish in response to repeated exposure to the phobic stimulus under nonthreatening conditions.

■ Encourage the client to explore underlying feelings that may be contributing to irrational fears, and to face them rather than suppress them. Exploring underlying feelings may help the client to confront unresolved conflicts and develop more adaptive coping abilities.

Ineffective Coping

Ineffective coping is defined as the "inability to form a valid appraisal of the stressors, inadequate choices of practiced responses, and/or inability to use available resources" (NANDA-I, 2012, p. 348).

Client Goals

Outcome criteria include short- and long-term goals. Timelines are individually determined.

Short-Term Goal

■ Within 1 week, the client will decrease participation in ritualistic behavior by half.

Long-Term Goal

■ By the time of discharge from treatment, the client will demonstrate the ability to cope effectively without resorting to obsessive-compulsive behaviors or increased dependency.

Interventions

■ Work with the client to determine the types of situations that increase anxiety and result in ritualistic behaviors. If the client is going to learn to interrupt escalating anxiety, he or she must first learn to recognize the factors that precipitate its onset.

■ Initially meet the client's dependency needs as required. To suddenly and completely eliminate all avenues for dependency would create intense anxiety on the part of the client. Encourage independence and give positive reinforcement for independent behaviors. Positive reinforcement enhances self-esteem and may encourage repetition of the desired behaviors.

■ In the beginning of treatment, allow plenty of time for rituals. Do not be judgmental or verbalize disapproval of the behavior. To deny the client this activity may precipitate panic level of anxiety.

■ Support the client's efforts to explore the meaning and purpose of the behavior. He or she is most likely unaware of the relationship between emotional problems and compulsive behaviors. Knowledge and recognition of this fact is important before change can occur.

■ Provide a structured schedule of activities for the client, including adequate time for the completion of rituals. The anxious individual needs a great deal of structure in his or her life. Assistance is needed with decision making, and structure provides a sense of security and comfort to deal with activities of daily living.

■ Gradually begin to limit the amount of time allotted for ritualistic behavior as the client becomes more involved in other activities. Anxiety is minimized when the client is able to replace ritualistic behaviors with more adaptive ones. Give positive reinforcement for nonritualistic behaviors.

■ Help the client learn ways of interrupting obsessive thoughts and ritualistic behavior with techniques such as thought stopping (see Chapter 14), relaxation techniques (see Relaxation Therapy chapter online at www.DavisPlus.com), physical exercise, or other constructive activity with which client feels comfortable. Knowledge and practice of coping techniques that are more adaptive will help the client change and let go of maladaptive responses to anxiety.

Disturbed Body Image

Disturbed body image is defined as the "confusion in mental picture of one's physical self" (NANDA-I, 2012, p. 291).

Client Goals

Outcome criteria include short- and long-term goals. Timelines are individually determined.

Short-Term Goal

■ Client will verbalize understanding that perceptions of changes in bodily structure or function are exaggerated out of proportion to the change that actually exists. (Time frame for this goal must be determined according to individual client's situation.)

Long-Term Goal

■ Client will verbalize perception of own body that is realistic to actual structure or function by time of discharge from treatment.

Interventions

■ Assess client's perception of his or her body image. Keep in mind that this image is real to the client. Assessment information is necessary in developing an accurate plan of care. Denial of the client's feelings impedes the development of a trusting, therapeutic relationship.

■ Help client to see that his or her body image is distorted or that it is out of proportion in relation to the significance of an actual physical anomaly. Recognition that a misperception exists is necessary before the client can accept reality and reduce the significance of the imagined defect.

■ Encourage verbalization of fears and anxieties associated with identified stressful life situations. Discuss alternative adaptive coping strategies. Verbalization of feelings with a trusted individual may help the client come to terms with unresolved issues. Knowledge of alternative coping strategies may help the client respond to stress more adaptively in the future.

■ Involve client in activities that reinforce a positive sense of self not based on appearance. When the client is able to develop self-satisfaction based on accomplishments and unconditional acceptance, significance of the imagined defect or minor physical anomaly will diminish.

■ Make referrals to support groups of individuals with similar histories (e.g., Adult Children of Alcoholics [ACOA], Victims of Incest, Survivors of Suicide [SOS], Adults Abused as Children).

Ineffective Impulse Control

Ineffective impulse control is defined as "a pattern of performing rapid, unplanned reactions to internal or external stimuli without regard for the negative consequences of these reactions to the impulsive individual or to others" (NANDA-I, 2012, p. 269).

Client Goals

Outcome criteria include short- and long-term goals. Timelines are individually determined.

Short-Term Goal

■ Client will verbalize adaptive ways to cope with stress by means other than pulling out own hair (time dimension to be individually determined).

Long-Term Goal

■ Client will be able to demonstrate adaptive coping strategies in response to stress and a discontinuation of pulling out own hair (time dimension to be individually determined).

Interventions

■ Support client in his or her effort to stop hair pulling. Help client understand that it is possible to discontinue the behavior. Client realizes that the behavior is maladaptive, but feels helpless to stop. Support from the nurse builds trust.

■ Ensure that a nonjudgmental attitude is conveyed, and criticism of the behavior is avoided. An attitude of acceptance promotes feelings of dignity and self-worth.

■ Assist the client with **habit-reversal therapy** (HRT), which has been shown to be an effective tool in treatment of hair-pulling disorder. Components of HRT include the following:

  ■ **Awareness training.** Help the client become aware of times when the hair pulling most often occurs (e.g., client learns to recognize urges, thoughts, or sensations that precede the behavior; the therapist points out to the client each time the behavior occurs). This helps the client identify situations in which the behavior occurs, or is most likely to occur. Awareness gives the client a feeling of increased self-control.

  ■ **Competing response training.** In this step, the client learns to substitute another response to the urge to pull his or her hair. For example, when a client experiences a hair-pulling urge, suggest that the individual ball up his or her hands into fists, tightening arm muscles, and "locking" his or her arms so as to make hair pulling impossible at that moment (Golomb et al., 2011). Substituting an incompatible behavior may help to extinguish the undesirable behavior.

  ■ **Social support.** Encourage family members to participate in the therapy process and to offer positive feedback for attempts at habit reversal. Positive feedback enhances self-esteem and increases the client's desire to continue with the therapy. It also provides cues for family members to use in their attempts to help the client in treatment.

■ Once the client has become aware of hair-pulling times, suggest that the client hold something (a ball, paperweight, or other item) in his or her hand at times when hair pulling is anticipated. This would help to prevent behaviors occurring without the client being aware that they are happening.

■ Practice stress management techniques: deep breathing, meditation, stretching, physical exercise, listening to soft music. Hair pulling is thought to occur at times of increased anxiety.

■ Offer support and encouragement when setbacks occur. Help the client to understand the importance of not quitting when it seems that change is not happening as quickly as he or she would like. Although some people see a decrease in the behavior within a few days, most will take several months to notice the greatest change.

Concept Care Mapping

The concept map care plan is an innovative approach to planning and organizing nursing care (see Chapter 9). It is a diagrammatic teaching and learning strategy that allows visualization of interrelationships between medical diagnoses, nursing diagnoses, assessment data, and treatments. An example of a concept map care plan for the client with an anxiety disorder is presented in Figure 27–4.

Client/Family Education

The role of client teacher is important in the psychiatric area, as it is in all areas of nursing. A list of topics for client/family education relevant to anxiety disorders is presented in Box 27–6.

Evaluation

In the final step of the nursing process, a reassessment is conducted to determine if the nursing actions have been successful in achieving the objectives of care. Evaluation of the nursing actions for the client with an anxiety, obsessive-compulsive, or related disorder may be facilitated by gathering information utilizing the following types of questions:

■ Can the client recognize signs and symptoms of escalating anxiety?

■ Can the client use skills learned to interrupt the escalating anxiety before it reaches the panic level?

■ Can the client demonstrate the activities most appropriate for him or her that can be used to

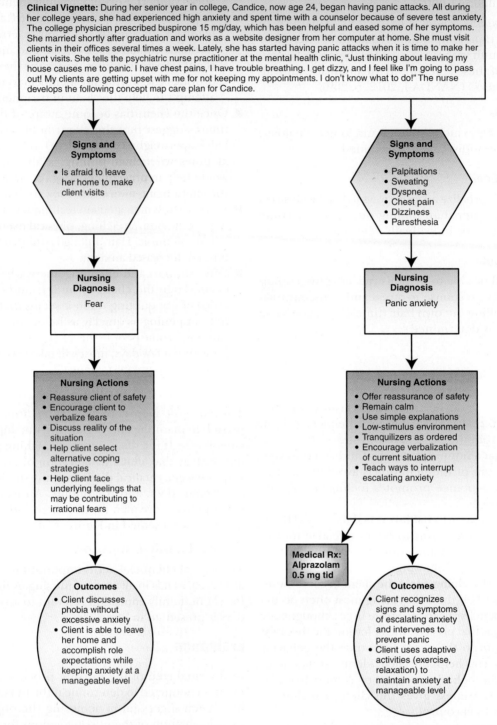

Clinical Vignette: During her senior year in college, Candice, now age 24, began having panic attacks. All during her college years, she had experienced high anxiety and spent time with a counselor because of severe test anxiety. The college physician prescribed buspirone 15 mg/day, which has been helpful and eased some of her symptoms. She married shortly after graduation and works as a website designer from her computer at home. She must visit clients in their offices several times a week. Lately, she has started having panic attacks when it is time to make her client visits. She tells the psychiatric nurse practitioner at the mental health clinic, "Just thinking about leaving my house causes me to panic. I have chest pains, I have trouble breathing. I get dizzy, and I feel like I'm going to pass out! My clients are getting upset with me for not keeping my appointments. I don't know what to do!" The nurse develops the following concept map care plan for Candice.

Signs and Symptoms

- Is afraid to leave her home to make client visits

Signs and Symptoms

- Palpitations
- Sweating
- Dyspnea
- Chest pain
- Dizziness
- Paresthesia

Nursing Diagnosis

Fear

Nursing Diagnosis

Panic anxiety

Nursing Actions

- Reassure client of safety
- Encourage client to verbalize fears
- Discuss reality of the situation
- Help client select alternative coping strategies
- Help client face underlying feelings that may be contributing to irrational fears

Nursing Actions

- Offer reassurance of safety
- Remain calm
- Use simple explanations
- Low-stimulus environment
- Tranquilizers as ordered
- Encourage verbalization of current situation
- Teach ways to interrupt escalating anxiety

Medical Rx: Alprazolam 0.5 mg tid

Outcomes

- Client discusses phobia without excessive anxiety
- Client is able to leave her home and accomplish role expectations while keeping anxiety at a manageable level

Outcomes

- Client recognizes signs and symptoms of escalating anxiety and intervenes to prevent panic
- Client uses adaptive activities (exercise, relaxation) to maintain anxiety at manageable level

FIGURE 27–4 Concept map care plan for a client with agoraphobia.

maintain anxiety at a manageable level (e.g., relaxation techniques; physical exercise)?

■ Can the client maintain anxiety at a manageable level without medication?

■ Can the client verbalize a long-term plan for preventing panic anxiety in the face of a stressful situation?

■ Can the client discuss the phobic object or situation without becoming anxious?

■ Can the client function in the presence of the phobic object or situation without experiencing panic anxiety?

■ Can the OCD client refrain from performing rituals when anxiety level rises?

■ Can the OCD client demonstrate substitute behaviors to maintain anxiety at a manageable level?
■ Does the OCD client recognize the relationship between escalating anxiety and the dependence on ritualistic behaviors for relief?
■ Can the client with trichotillomania refrain from hair pulling?
■ Can the client with trichotillomania successfully substitute a more adaptive behavior when urges to pull hair occur?
■ Does the client with body dysmorphic disorder verbalize a realistic perception and satisfactory acceptance of personal appearance?

Treatment Modalities

Individual Psychotherapy

Most clients experience a marked lessening of anxiety when given the opportunity to discuss their difficulties with a concerned and sympathetic therapist. Sadock & Sadock (2007) state:

> [Insight-oriented psychotherapy] focuses on helping patients understand the hypothesized unconscious meaning of the anxiety, the symbolism of the avoided situation, the need to repress impulses, and the secondary gains of the symptoms. (p. 596)
>
> With continuous and regular contact with an interested, sympathetic, and encouraging professional person, patients may be able to function by virtue of this help, without which their symptoms would incapacitate them. (p. 612)

The psychotherapist also can use logical and rational explanations to increase the client's understanding about various situations that create anxiety in his or her life. Psychoeducational information may also be presented in individual psychotherapy.

Cognitive Therapy

The cognitive model relates how individuals respond in stressful situations to their subjective cognitive appraisal of the event. Anxiety is experienced when the cognitive appraisal is one of danger with which the individual perceives that he or she is unable to cope. Impaired cognition can contribute to anxiety and related disorders when the individual's appraisals are chronically negative. Automatic negative appraisals provoke self-doubts, negative evaluations, and negative predictions. Anxiety is maintained by this dysfunctional appraisal of a situation.

Cognitive therapy strives to assist the individual to reduce anxiety responses by altering cognitive distortions. Anxiety is described as being the result of exaggerated, *automatic* thinking.

Cognitive therapy for anxiety is brief and time limited, usually lasting from 5 to 20 sessions. Brief therapy discourages the client's dependency on the therapist, which is prevalent in anxiety disorders, and encourages the client's self-sufficiency.

A sound therapeutic relationship is a necessary condition for effective cognitive therapy. For the therapeutic process to occur, the client must be able to talk openly about fears and feelings. A major part of treatment consists of encouraging the client to face frightening situations to be able to view them realistically, and talking about them is one way of achieving this. Treatment is a collaborative effort between client and therapist.

Rather than offering suggestions and explanations, the therapist uses questions to encourage the client to correct his or her anxiety-producing thoughts. The client is encouraged to become aware of the thoughts, examine them for cognitive distortions, substitute more balanced thoughts, and eventually develop new patterns of thinking.

Cognitive therapy is very structured and orderly, which is important for the client with an anxiety or related disorder who is often confused and lacks self-assurance. The focus is on solving current problems. Together, the client and therapist work to identify and correct maladaptive thoughts and behaviors that maintain a problem and block its solution.

Cognitive therapy is based on education. The premise is that one develops anxiety because he or she has learned inappropriate ways of handling life experiences. The belief is that with practice, individuals can learn more effective ways of responding to these experiences. Homework assignments, a central feature of cognitive therapy, provide an experimental, problem-solving approach to overcoming long-held anxieties. Through fulfillment of these personal "experiments," the effectiveness of specific strategies and techniques is determined.

Behavior Therapy

Behavior modification has been used to treat trichotillomania. Various techniques have been tried, including covert desensitization and HRT (habit-reversal therapy). These may include a system of positive and negative reinforcements in an effort to modify the hair-pulling behaviors. With HRT, in an attempt to extinguish the unwanted behavior, the individual learns to become more aware of the hair pulling, identify times of occurrence, and substitute a more adaptive coping strategy. (See interventions listed under the nursing diagnosis section "Ineffective Impulse Control.")

Other forms of behavior therapy include **systematic desensitization** and **implosion therapy** (**flooding**). They are commonly used to treat clients with phobic disorders and to modify the stereotyped behavior of clients with OCD. They have also been shown to be effective in a variety of other anxiety-producing situations.

Systematic Desensitization

In systematic desensitization, the client is gradually exposed to the phobic stimulus, either in a real or imagined situation. The concept was introduced by Joseph Wolpe in 1958, and is based on behavioral conditioning principles. Emphasis is placed on reciprocal inhibition or counterconditioning.

Reciprocal inhibition is described as the restriction of anxiety prior to the effort of reducing avoidance behavior. The rationale behind this concept is that because relaxation is antagonistic to anxiety, individuals cannot be anxious and relaxed at the same time.

Systematic desensitization with reciprocal inhibition involves two main elements:

1. Training in relaxation techniques.
2. Progressive exposure to a hierarchy of fear stimuli while in the relaxed state.

The individual is instructed in the art of relaxation using techniques most effective for him or her (e.g., progressive relaxation, mental imagery, tense and relax, meditation). When the individual has mastered the relaxation technique, exposure to the phobic stimulus is initiated. He or she is asked to present a hierarchal arrangement of situations pertaining to the phobic stimulus in order from most disturbing to least disturbing. While in a state of maximum relaxation, the client may be asked to imagine the phobic stimulus. Initial exposure is focused on a concept of the phobic stimulus that produces the least amount of fear or anxiety. In subsequent sessions, the individual is gradually exposed to stimuli that are more fearful. Sessions may be executed in fantasy, in real-life (*in vivo*) situations, or sometimes in a combination of both. Following is a case study describing systematic desensitization.

CASE STUDY: SYSTEMATIC DESENSITIZATION

John was afraid to ride on elevators. He had been known to climb 24 flights of stairs in an office building to avoid riding the elevator. John's own insurance office had plans for moving the company to a high-rise building soon, with offices on the 32nd floor. John sought assistance from a therapist for help to treat this fear. He was taught to achieve a sense of calmness and well-being by using a combination of mental imagery and progressive relaxation techniques. In the relaxed state, John was initially instructed to imagine the entry level of his office building, with a clear image of the

CASE STUDY: SYSTEMATIC DESENSITIZATION—cont'd

bank of elevators. In subsequent sessions, and always in the relaxed state, John progressed to images of walking onto an elevator, having the elevator door close after he had entered, riding the elevator to the 32nd floor, and emerging from the elevator once the doors were opened. The progression included being accompanied in the activities by the therapist and eventually accomplishing them alone.

Therapy for John also included *in vivo* sessions in which he was exposed to the phobic stimulus in real-life situations (always after achieving a state of relaxation). This technique, combining imagined and *in vivo* procedures, proved successful for John, and his employment in the high-rise complex was no longer in jeopardy because of his fear of elevators.

Implosion Therapy (Flooding)

Implosion therapy, or *flooding*, is a therapeutic process in which the client must imagine situations or participate in real-life situations that he or she finds extremely frightening, for a prolonged period of time. Relaxation training is not a part of this technique. Plenty of time must be allowed for these sessions because brief periods may be ineffective or even harmful. A session is terminated when the client responds with considerably less anxiety than at the beginning of the session.

In implosion therapy, the therapist "floods" the client with information concerning situations that trigger anxiety in him or her. The therapist describes anxiety-provoking situations in vivid detail and is guided by the client's response; the more anxiety provoked, the more expedient is the therapeutic endeavor. The same theme is continued as long as it arouses anxiety. The therapy is continued until a topic

no longer elicits inappropriate anxiety on the part of the client. Sadock and Sadock (2007) state:

> Many patients refuse flooding because of the psychological discomfort involved. It is also contraindicated when intense anxiety would be hazardous to a patient (e.g., those with heart disease or fragile psychological adaptation). The technique works best with specific phobias. (p. 955)

Psychopharmacology

Antianxiety Agents

Antianxiety drugs are also called *anxiolytics* and *minor tranquilizers*. Examples of commonly used antianxiety agents are presented in Table 27-4.

Indications

Antianxiety agents are used in the treatment of anxiety disorders, anxiety symptoms, acute alcohol withdrawal,

TABLE 27–4 Antianxiety Agents

CHEMICAL CLASS	GENERIC NAME (TRADE)	CONTROLLED CATEGORIES	PREGNANCY CATEGORIES (HALF-LIFE) (hr)	DAILY ADULT DOSAGE RANGE (mg)	COMMON SIDE EFFECTS OF ALL ANTIANXIETY AGENTS
Antihistamines	Hydroxyzine (Vistaril)		C (3)	100–400	■ Drowsiness, confusion, lethargy
Benzodiazepines	Alprazolam (Xanax)	C-IV	D (6.3–26.9)	0.75–4	■ Tolerance; physical and psychological dependence (does not apply to buspirone). Client should be tapered off long-term use.
	Chlordiazepoxide (Librium)	C-IV	D (5–30)	15–100	
	Clonazepam (Klonopin)	C-IV	D (18–50)	1.5–20	
	Clorazepate (Tranxene)	C-IV	D (40-50)	15–60	■ Potentiates the effects of other CNS depressants. Client should not take alcohol or other CNS depressants with the medication.
	Diazepam (Valium)	C-IV	D (20-80)	4–40	
	Lorazepam (Ativan)	C-IV	D (10–20)	2–6	
	Oxazepam	C-IV	D (5–20)	30–120	
Carbamate derivative	Meprobamate	C-IV	D (6–17)	400–1600	■ May aggravate symptoms of depression.

Continued

TABLE 27–4 Antianxiety Agents—cont'd

CHEMICAL CLASS	GENERIC NAME (TRADE)	CONTROLLED CATEGORIES	PREGNANCY CATEGORIES (HALF-LIFE) (hr)	DAILY ADULT DOSAGE RANGE (mg)	COMMON SIDE EFFECTS OF ALL ANTIANXIETY AGENTS
Azaspirodecanedione	Buspirone		B (2–3)	15–60	■ Orthostatic hypotension. Client should rise slowly from lying or sitting position. ■ Paradoxical excitement. If symptoms opposite of desired effect occur, notify physician immediately. ■ Dry mouth. ■ Nausea and vomiting. May be taken with food or milk. ■ Blood dyscrasias. Symptoms of sore throat, fever, malaise, easy bruising, or unusual bleeding should be reported to the physician immediately. ■ Delayed onset (with Buspirone). Lag time of 10 to 14 days for anxiety symptoms to diminish with buspirone. Buspirone is not recommended for prn administration.

skeletal muscle spasms, convulsive disorders, status epilepticus, and preoperative sedation. Their use and efficacy for periods greater than 4 months have not been evaluated.

Action

Antianxiety drugs depress subcortical levels of the CNS, particularly the limbic system and reticular formation. They may potentiate the effects of the powerful inhibitory neurotransmitter gamma-aminobutyric acid (GABA) in the brain, thereby producing a calmative effect. All levels of CNS depression can be affected, from mild sedation to hypnosis to coma. *Note:* Buspirone does not depress the CNS. Although its action is unknown, the drug is believed to produce the desired effects through interactions with serotonin, dopamine, and other neurotransmitter receptors.

Contraindications/Precautions

Antianxiety drugs are contraindicated in individuals with known hypersensitivity to any of the drugs within the classification (e.g., benzodiazepines). They should not be taken in combination with other CNS depressants and are contraindicated in pregnancy and lactation, narrow-angle glaucoma, shock, and coma.

Caution should be taken in administering these drugs to elderly or debilitated clients and clients with hepatic or renal dysfunction. (The dosage usually has to be decreased.) Caution is also required with individuals who have a history of drug abuse or addiction and with those who are depressed or suicidal. In depressed clients, CNS depressants can exacerbate symptoms.

Interactions

Increased effects of antianxiety agents can occur when taken concomitantly with alcohol, barbiturates, narcotics, antipsychotics, antidepressants, antihistamines, neuromuscular blocking agents, cimetidine, or disulfiram. Increased effects can also occur with herbal depressants (e.g., kava, valerian). Decreased effects can be noted with cigarette smoking and caffeine consumption.

Medications for Specific Disorders

For Panic and Generalized Anxiety Disorders

Anxiolytics The benzodiazepines have been used with success in the treatment of generalized anxiety disorder. They can be prescribed on an as-needed basis when the client is feeling particularly anxious. Alprazolam, lorazepam, and clonazepam have been particularly effective in the treatment of panic disorder. The major risks with benzodiazepine therapy are physical dependence and tolerance, which may encourage abuse. Because withdrawal symptoms can be life threatening, clients must be warned against abrupt discontinuation of the drug and should be tapered off the medication at the end of therapy. Because of this addiction potential, the benzodiazepines have been surpassed as first-line choice of treatment by the selective serotonin reuptake inhibitors (SSRIs), the serotonin and norepinephrine reuptake inhibitors (SNRIs), and buspirone.

The antianxiety agent buspirone is effective in about 60 to 80 percent of clients with generalized anxiety disorder (Sadock & Sadock, 2007). One disadvantage of buspirone is its 10- to 14-day delay in alleviating symptoms. However, the benefit of lack of physical dependence and tolerance with buspirone may make it the drug of choice in the treatment of generalized anxiety disorder.

Antidepressants Several antidepressants are effective as major antianxiety agents. The tricyclics clomipramine and imipramine have been used with success in clients experiencing panic disorder. However, since the advent of SSRIs, the tricyclics are less widely used because of their tendency to produce severe side effects at the high doses required to relieve symptoms of panic disorder.

The SSRIs have been effective in the treatment of panic disorder. Paroxetine, fluoxetine, and sertraline have been approved by the U.S. Food and Drug Administration (FDA) for this purpose. The dosage of these drugs must be titrated slowly because clients with panic disorder appear to be sensitive to the over-stimulation caused by SSRIs.

The use of antidepressants in the treatment of generalized anxiety disorder is still being investigated. Some success has been reported with the tricyclic imipramine and with the SSRIs. The FDA has approved paroxetine, escitalopram, duloxetine, and extended-release venlafaxine in the treatment of generalized anxiety disorder. Complete information about antidepressants is presented in Chapter 25.

Antihypertensive Agents Several studies have called attention to the effectiveness of beta blockers (e.g., propranolol) and alpha$_2$-receptor agonists (e.g., clonidine) in the amelioration of anxiety symptoms (Hollander & Simeon, 2008). Propranolol has potent effects on the somatic manifestations of anxiety (e.g., palpitations, tremors), with less dramatic effects on the psychic component of anxiety. It appears to be most effective in the treatment of acute situational anxiety (e.g., performance anxiety, test anxiety), but it is not the first-line drug of choice in the treatment of panic disorder and generalized anxiety disorder.

Clonidine is effective in blocking the acute anxiety effects in conditions such as opioid and nicotine withdrawal. However, it has had limited usefulness in the long-term treatment of panic and generalized anxiety disorders, particularly because of the development of tolerance to its antianxiety effects.

For Phobic Disorders

Anxiolytics The benzodiazepines have been successful in the treatment of social anxiety disorder (social phobia) (Hollander & Simeon, 2008). Controlled studies have shown the efficacy of alprazolam and clonazepam in reducing symptoms of social anxiety. Both are well tolerated and have a rapid onset of action. However, because of their potential for abuse and dependence, they are not considered first-line choice of treatment for social anxiety disorder.

Antidepressants The tricyclic imipramine and the monoamine oxidase inhibitor (MAOI) phenelzine have been effective in diminishing symptoms of agoraphobia and social anxiety disorder. In recent years, the SSRIs have become the first-line treatment of choice for social anxiety disorder, and paroxetine and sertraline have been approved for this purpose. Additional clinical trials have also indicated efficacy with other antidepressants, including nefazodone, venlafaxine, and bupropion. Specific phobias are generally not treated with medication unless panic attacks accompany the phobia.

Antihypertensive Agents The beta blockers propranolol and atenolol have been tried with success in clients experiencing anticipatory performance anxiety or "stage fright" (Hollander & Simeon, 2008). This type of phobic response produces symptoms such as sweaty palms, racing pulse, trembling hands, dry mouth, labored breathing, nausea, and memory loss. The beta blockers appear to be quite effective in reducing these symptoms in some individuals.

For Obsessive-Compulsive Disorder

Antidepressants The SSRIs fluoxetine, paroxetine, sertraline, and fluvoxamine have been approved by the FDA for the treatment of OCD. Doses in excess of what is effective for treating depression may be required for OCD. Common side effects include sleep disturbances, headache, and restlessness. These effects are often transient, and are less troublesome than those of the tricyclics.

The tricyclic antidepressant clomipramine was the first drug approved by the FDA in the treatment of OCD. Clomipramine is more selective for serotonin reuptake than any of the other tricyclics. Its efficacy in the treatment of OCD is well established, although the adverse effects, such as those associated with all the tricyclics, may make it less desirable than the SSRIs.

For Body Dysmorphic Disorder

Antidepressants The most positive results of pharmacological therapy with body dysmorphic disorder have been with clomipramine (Anafranil) and fluoxetine (Prozac). These medications have been shown to reduce symptoms in more than 50 percent of clients with the disorder (Sadock & Sadock, 2007).

For Trichotillomania (Hair-Pulling Disorder)

Various psychopharmacological agents, including chlorpromazine, amitriptyline, and lithium carbonate, have been tried in the treatment of trichotillomania, with moderate results. Recent success with SSRIs augmented with pimozide has been reported. One recent study showed olanzapine to be a safe and effective treatment for trichotillomania (Van Ameringen, Mancini, Patterson, Bennett, & Oakman, 2010).

CASE STUDY AND SAMPLE CARE PLAN

NURSING HISTORY AND ASSESSMENT

Karen is a 34-year-old mother of a 7-year-old girl named April. Karen's husband, Jake, brought Karen to the emergency department when she began complaining of chest pain and shortness of breath. Diagnostic testing ruled out cardiac problems, and Karen was referred for psychiatric evaluation. Jake is present at the admission interview. He explained to the nurse that Karen has become increasingly "nervous and high-strung" over the past few years. Four years ago, April, then 3 years old, was attending nursery school 2 days a week. April came down with a very severe case of influenza that developed into pneumonia. She was hospitalized and her prognosis was questionable for a short while, although she eventually made a complete recovery. Since that time, however, Karen has been extremely anxious about her family's health. She is fastidious about housekeeping, and scrubs her floors three times a week. She launders the bedclothes daily, and uses bleach on all the countertops and door handles several times a day. She washes the woodwork twice a week. She washes her hands incessantly, and they are red and noticeably chapped. Jake explained that Karen becomes very upset if she is not able to perform all of her cleaning "chores" according to her self-assigned schedule. This afternoon, April came home from school with a note from the teacher saying that a child in April's class had been diagnosed with a case of meningitis. Jake told the nurse, "Karen just lost it. She got all upset and started crying and had trouble breathing. Then she got those pains in her chest. That's when I brought her to the hospital." Karen is admitted to the psychiatric unit with a diagnosis of obsessive-compulsive disorder. The physician orders alprazolam 0.5 mg tid and paroxetine 20 mg every morning.

The night nurse finds her up at 2 a.m. scrubbing the shower with a hand towel. She refuses to sleep in the bed, stating that it must certainly be contaminated. When the day nurse makes morning rounds, she finds Karen in the bathroom washing her hands.

NURSING DIAGNOSES/OUTCOME IDENTIFICATION

From the assessment data, the nurse develops the following nursing diagnoses for Karen:

1. **Panic anxiety** related to perceived threat to biological integrity evidenced by chest pain and shortness of breath.
   a. **Short-Term Goal:** Client will be able to relax with effects of medication.
   b. **Long-Term Goal:** Client will be able to maintain anxiety at manageable level.
2. **Ineffective coping** related to panic anxiety and weak ego strength evidenced by compulsive cleaning and washing hands.
   a. **Short-Term Goal:** Client will reduce amount of time performing rituals within 3 days.
   b. **Long-Term Goal:** Client will demonstrate ability to cope effectively without resorting to ritualistic behavior.

PLANNING/IMPLEMENTATION

PANIC ANXIETY
The following nursing interventions have been identified for Karen:

1. Stay with Karen and reassure her that she is safe and that she is not going to die.
2. Maintain a calm, nonthreatening manner with Karen.
3. Speak very clearly, calmly, and use simple words and messages to communicate with Karen.
4. Keep the lights low, the noise level down as much as possible, and as few people in her environment as is necessary.
5. Administer the alprazolam and paroxetine as ordered by the physician. Monitor for effectiveness and side effects.
6. After several days, when the anxiety has subsided, discuss with her the reasons that precipitated this attack.
7. Teach her the signs that indicate her anxiety level is rising.

CASE STUDY AND SAMPLE CARE PLAN—cont'd

8. Teach strategies that she may employ to interrupt the escalation of the anxiety. She could choose which is best for her: relaxation exercises, physical exercise, meditation.

INEFFECTIVE COPING

The following nursing interventions have been identified for Karen:

1. Initially, allow Karen all the time she needs to wash her hands, straighten up her room, change her own sheets, etc. To deny her these rituals would result in panic anxiety.
2. Initiate discussions with Karen about her behavior. She ultimately must come to understand that these rituals are her way of keeping her anxiety under control.
3. Within a couple of days, begin to limit the amount of time Karen may spend on her rituals. Assign her to groups and activities that take up her time and distract her from her obsessions.
4. Explore with Karen the types of situations that cause her anxiety to rise. Help her to correlate these times of increased anxiety to initiation of the ritualistic behavior.
5. Help her with problem-solving and with making decisions about more adaptive ways to respond to situations that cause her anxiety to rise.
6. Explore her fears surrounding the health of her daughter. Help her to recognize which fears are legitimate and which are irrational.

7. Discuss possible activities in which she may participate that may distract from obsessions about contamination. Make suggestions, and encourage her to follow through. Examples may include enrollment in classes at the local community college, volunteer work at the local hospital, or part-time employment.
8. Explain to her that she will likely be discharged from the hospital with a prescription for paroxetine. Teach her about the medication, how it should be taken, possible side effects, and what to report to the physician.
9. Suggest that she may benefit from attendance in an anxiety disorder support group. If she is interested, help locate one that would be convenient and appropriate for her.

EVALUATION

The outcome criteria for Karen have been met. She has remained calm during her hospital stay with the use of the medication. The use of ritualistic behavior in the hospital setting diminished rapidly. She has discussed situations that she knows cause her anxiety to rise. She has learned relaxation exercises and practices them daily. She plans to start jogging and has the phone number for an anxiety support group that she plans to call. She says that she hopes the support group will help her maintain rationality about her daughter's health. She knows about paroxetine and plans to take it every morning.

Summary and Key Points

- Anxiety is a necessary force for survival and has been experienced by humanity throughout the ages.
- Anxiety was first described as a physiological disorder and identified by its physical symptoms, particularly the cardiac symptoms. The psychological implications for the symptoms were not recognized until the early 1900s.
- Anxiety is considered a normal reaction to a realistic danger or threat to biological integrity or self-concept.
- Normality of the anxiety experienced in response to a stressor is defined by societal and cultural standards.
- Anxiety disorders are more common in women than in men by at least two to one.
- Studies of familial patterns suggest that a familial predisposition to anxiety disorders probably exists.
- The *DSM-5* identifies several broad categories of anxiety and related disorders. They include panic and generalized anxiety disorders, phobic disorders, and OCD and related disorders, such as body dysmorphic disorder, trichotillomania, and hoarding disorder. Anxiety disorders may also be the result of other medical conditions and intoxication or withdrawal from substances.
- Panic disorder is characterized by recurrent panic attacks, the onset of which are unpredictable and

manifested by intense apprehension, fear, and physical discomfort.
- Generalized anxiety disorder is characterized by chronic, unrealistic, and excessive anxiety and worry.
- Social anxiety disorder is an excessive fear of situations in which a person might do something embarrassing or be evaluated negatively by others.
- Specific phobia is a marked, persistent, and excessive or unreasonable fear when in the presence of, or when anticipating an encounter with, a specific object or situation.
- Agoraphobia is a fear of being in places or situations from which escape might be difficult or in which help might not be available in the event that the person becomes anxious.
- OCD involves recurrent obsessions or compulsions that are severe enough to interfere with social and occupational functioning.
- Body dysmorphic disorder is an exaggerated belief that the body is deformed or defective in some specific way.
- Trichotillomania (also known as hair-pulling disorder) is a disorder of impulse control characterized by the recurrent pulling out of one's own hair that results in noticeable hair loss.
- Hoarding disorder is defined by the persistent difficulty of discarding or parting with possessions, regardless of their actual value.

■ A number of elements, including psychosocial factors, biological influences, and learning experiences most likely contribute to the development of these disorders.

■ Treatment of anxiety and related disorders includes individual psychotherapy, cognitive therapy, behavior therapy (including implosion therapy, systematic desensitization, and habit-reversal therapy), and psychopharmacology.

■ Nurses can help clients with anxiety and related disorders gain insight and increase self-awareness in relation to their illness.

■ Intervention focuses on assisting clients to learn techniques with which they may interrupt the escalation of anxiety before it reaches unmanageable proportions, and to replace maladaptive behavior patterns with new, more adaptive, coping skills.

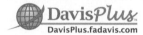 Additional info available at
DavisPlus.fadavis.com www.davisplus.com

Review Questions
Self-Examination/Learning Exercise

*Select the answer that is **most** appropriate for each of the following questions.*

1. Ms. T. has been diagnosed with agoraphobia. Which behavior would be most characteristic of this disorder?
   a. Ms. T. experiences panic anxiety when she encounters snakes.
   b. Ms. T. refuses to fly in an airplane.
   c. Ms. T. will not eat in a public place.
   d. Ms. T. stays in her home for fear of being in a place from which she cannot escape.

2. Which of the following is the most appropriate therapy for a client with agoraphobia?
   a. 10 mg Valium qid
   b. Group therapy with other agoraphobics
   c. Facing her fear in gradual step progression
   d. Hypnosis

3. With implosion therapy, a client with phobic anxiety would be:
   a. Taught relaxation exercises
   b. Subjected to graded intensities of the fear
   c. Instructed to stop the therapeutic session as soon as anxiety is experienced
   d. Presented with massive exposure to a variety of stimuli associated with the phobic object/situation

4. A client with OCD spends many hours each day washing her hands. The most likely reason she washes her hands so much is that it:
   a. Relieves her anxiety
   b. Reduces the probability of infection
   c. Gives her a feeling of control over her life
   d. Increases her self-concept

5. The *initial* care plan for a client with OCD who washes her hands obsessively would include which of the following nursing interventions?
   a. Keep the client's bathroom locked so she cannot wash her hands all the time.
   b. Structure the client's schedule so that she has plenty of time for washing her hands.
   c. Place the client in isolation until she promises to stop washing her hands so much.
   d. Explain the client's behavior to her, since she is probably unaware that it is maladaptive.

6. A client with OCD says to the nurse, "I've been here 4 days now, and I'm feeling better. I feel comfortable on this unit, and I'm not ill-at-ease with the staff or other patients anymore." In light of this change, which nursing intervention is most appropriate?
   a. Give attention to the ritualistic behaviors each time they occur and point out their inappropriateness.
   b. Ignore the ritualistic behaviors, and they will be eliminated for lack of reinforcement.
   c. Set limits on the amount of time Sandy may engage in the ritualistic behavior.
   d. Continue to allow Sandy all the time she wants to carry out the ritualistic behavior.

Review Questions—cont'd
Self-Examination/Learning Exercise

7. Annie has trichotillomania. She is receiving treatment at the mental health clinic with habit-reversal therapy. Which of the following elements would be included in this therapy? (Select all that apply.)
   a. Awareness training
   b. Competing response training
   c. Social support
   d. Hypnotherapy
   e. Aversive therapy

8. Joanie is a new patient at the mental health clinic. She has been diagnosed with body dysmorphic disorder. Which of the following medications is the psychiatric nurse practitioner most likely to prescribe for Joanie?
   a. Alprazolam (Xanax)
   b. Diazepam (Valium)
   c. Fluoxetine (Prozac)
   d. Olanzapine (Zyprexa)

9. A client who is experiencing a panic attack has just arrived at the emergency department. Which is the *priority* nursing intervention for this client?
   a. Stay with the client and reassure of safety.
   b. Administer a dose of diazepam.
   c. Leave the client alone in a quiet room so that she can calm down.
   d. Encourage the client to talk about what triggered the attack.

10. Janet has a diagnosis of generalized anxiety disorder. Her physician has prescribed buspirone 15 mg daily. Janet says to the nurse, "Why do I have to take this every day? My friend's doctor ordered Xanax for her, and she only takes it when she is feeling anxious." Which of the following would be an appropriate response by the nurse?
    a. "Xanax is not effective for generalized anxiety disorder."
    b. "Buspirone must be taken daily in order to be effective."
    c. "I will ask the doctor if he will change your dose of buspirone to prn so that you don't have to take it every day."
    d. "Your friend really should be taking the Xanax every day."

TEST YOUR CRITICAL THINKING SKILLS

Sarah, age 25, was taken to the emergency department by her friends. They were at a dinner party when Sarah suddenly clasped her chest and started having difficulty breathing. She complained of nausea and was perspiring profusely. She had calmed down some by the time they reached the hospital. She denied any pain, and electrocardiogram and laboratory results were unremarkable.

Sarah told the admitting nurse that she had a history of these "attacks." She began having them in her sophomore year of college. She knew her parents had expectations that she should follow in their footsteps and become an attorney. They also expected her to earn grades that would promote acceptance by a top Ivy League university. Sarah experienced her first attack when she made a "B" in English during her third semester of college. Since that time, she

has experienced these symptoms sporadically, often in conjunction with her perception of the need to excel. She graduated with top honors from Harvard.

Last week Sarah was promoted within her law firm. She was assigned her first solo case of representing a couple whose baby had died at birth and who were suing the physician for malpractice. She has experienced these panic symptoms daily for the past week, stating, "I feel like I'm going crazy!"

Sarah is transferred to the psychiatric unit. The psychiatrist diagnoses panic disorder.

Answer the following questions related to Sarah:

1. What would be the priority nursing diagnosis for Sarah?
2. What is the priority nursing intervention with Sarah?
3. What medical treatment might you expect the physician to prescribe?

References

American Psychiatric Association. (2013). *Diagnostic and statistical manual of mental disorders* (5th ed.) Washington, DC: American Psychiatric Publishing.

Black, D.W., & Andreasen, N.C. (2011). *Introductory textbook of psychiatry* (5th ed.).Washington, DC: American Psychiatric Publishing.

Golomb, R., Franklin, M., Grant, J.E., Keuthen, N.J., Mansueto, C.S., Mouton-Odum, S., Novak, C., & Woods, D. (2011). *Expert consensus: Treatment guidelines for trichotillomania, skin picking, and other body-focused repetitive behaviors.* Santa Cruz, CA: Trichotillomania Learning Center.

Harvard Medical School. (2006). *Coping with anxiety and phobias.* Boston, MA: Harvard Health Publications.

Hollander, E., & Simeon, D. (2008). Anxiety disorders. In R.E. Hales, S.C. Yudofsky, & G.O. Gabbard (Eds.), *Textbook of psychiatry* (5th ed., pp. 507-607). Washington, DC: American Psychiatric Publishing.

Johnson, M. (1994, May/June). Stage fright. From *Performing Songwriter 1*(6). Retrieved from http://www.mjblue.com/pfright.html

Lochner, C., duToit, P.L., Zungu-Dirwayi, N., Marais, A., vanKradenburg, J., Curr, B., Seedat, S., Niehaus, D.J.H., & Stein, D.J. (2002). Childhood trauma in obsessive-compulsive disorder, trichotillomania, and controls. *Depression and Anxiety, 15*(2), 66-68.

NANDA International (NANDA-I). (2012). *Nursing diagnoses: Definitions and classification 2012-2014.* Hoboken, NJ: Wiley-Blackwell.

National Mental Health Association (NMHA). (2005). *Children with emotional disorders in the juvenile justice system.* Alexandria, VA: NMHA.

Phillips, K.A. (2009). *Understanding body dysmorphic disorder.* New York, NY: Oxford University Press.

Puri, B.K., & Treasaden, I.H. (2011). *Textbook of psychiatry* (3rd ed.). Philadelphia, PA: Churchill Livingstone Elsevier.

Rowney, J., Hermida, T., & Malone, D. (2010). Anxiety disorders. In W.D. Carey (Ed.), *Current clinical medicine* (2nd ed.). Philadelphia, PA: Saunders Elsevier.

Sadock, B.J., & Sadock, V.A. (2007). *Synopsis of psychiatry: Behavioral sciences/clinical psychiatry* (10th ed.). Philadelphia, PA: Lippincott Williams & Wilkins.

Saxena, S. (2013). *Medicines for the treatment of hoarding.* International OCD Foundation. Retrieved from http://www.ocfoundation.org/hoarding/medication.aspx

Shahrokh, N.C., & Hales, R.E. (2003). *American psychiatric glossary.* Washington, DC: American Psychiatric Publishing.

Symonds, A., & Janney, R. (2013). Shining a light on hoarding disorder. *Nursing2013, 43*(10), 22-28.

The Mayo Clinic. (2011). *Hoarding.* Retrieved from http://www.mayoclinic.com/health/hoarding/DS00966

Valente, S.M. (2009). The hoarding syndrome: Screening and treatment. *Home Healthcare Nurse, 27*(7), 432-440.

Van Ameringen, M., Mancini, C., Patterson, B., Bennett, M., & Oakman, J. (2010). A randomized, double-blind, placebo-controlled trial of olanzapine in the treatment of trichotillomania. *Journal of Clinical Psychiatry, 71*(10), 1336-1343.

Classical References

Freud, S. (1959). On the grounds for detaching a particular syndrome from neurasthenia under the description 'anxiety neurosis.' In *The standard edition of the complete psychological works of Sigmund Freud* (Vol. 3). London: Hogarth Press.

Johnson, J.H., & Sarason, I.B. (1978). Life stress, depression and anxiety: Internal-external control as moderator variable. *Journal of Psychosomatic Research, 22*(3), 205-208.

@ INTERNET REFERENCES

- Additional information about anxiety disorders and medications to treat these disorders may be located at the following websites:
  - http://www.adaa.org
  - http://www.mentalhealth.com
  - http://www.nami.org
  - http://www.mental-health-matters.com/disorders
  - http://www.drugs.com
  - http://www.nimh.nih.gov/health/publications/mental-health-medications/index.shtml

---

 MOVIE CONNECTIONS

As Good As It Gets (OCD) • *The Aviator* (OCD) • *What About Bob?* (phobias) • *Copycat* (agoraphobia) • *Analyze This* (panic disorder) • *Vertigo* (specific phobia)

Trauma- and Stressor-Related Disorders

28

CORE CONCEPTS

stress

trauma

KEY TERMS

acute stress disorder

adjustment disorder

posttraumatic stress disorder

OBJECTIVES
After reading this chapter, the student will be able to:

1. Discuss historical aspects and epidemiological statistics related to trauma- and stressor-related disorders.
2. Describe various types of trauma- and stressor-related disorders and identify symptomatology associated with each; use this information in client assessment.
3. Identify predisposing factors in the development of trauma- and stressor-related disorders.

4. Formulate nursing diagnoses and goals of care for clients with trauma- and stressor-related disorders.
5. Describe appropriate nursing interventions for behaviors associated with trauma- and stressor-related disorders.
6. Evaluate the nursing care of clients with trauma- and stressor-related disorders.
7. Discuss various modalities relevant to treatment of trauma- and stressor-related disorders.

HOMEWORK ASSIGNMENT
Please read the chapter and answer the following questions:

1. What two variables are considered to be the best predictors of posttraumatic stress disorder (PTSD) according to the psychosocial theory?
2. What is associated with the onset of an adjustment disorder?

3. What are the elements that determine one's response (and subsequent adjustment) to a stressful situation?
4. What agents are considered first-line psychopharmacological treatment for PTSD?

The *Diagnostic and Statistical Manual of Mental Disorders, Fourth Edition, Text Revision (DSM-IV-TR)* (American Psychiatric Association [APA], 2000) classified **posttraumatic stress disorder** (PTSD) and **acute stress disorder** with the anxiety disorders. **Adjustment disorder** carried its own classification, and was identified as "a psychological response to an identifiable stressor or stressors" (APA, 2000, p. 679). In the *DSM-5* (APA,

2013), these disorders have been combined into a single chapter titled "Trauma- and Stressor-Related Disorders." The movement of these disorders in this manner "reflects increased recognition of trauma as a precipitant, emphasizing common etiology over common phenomenology" (Friedman et al., 2011, p. 737).

This chapter focuses on disorders that occur following exposure to an identifiable stressor or to an extreme traumatic event. Epidemiological statistics are presented, and predisposing factors associated with the etiology of these disorders are discussed. An explanation of the symptomatology is presented as background knowledge for assessing clients with trauma- and stressor-related disorders. Nursing care is described in the context of the nursing process. Various treatment modalities are explored.

Historical and Epidemiological Data

The concept of a post-trauma response is not new. It has been known throughout the centuries by terms such as shell shock, battle fatigue, accident neurosis, and posttraumatic neurosis. Reports of symptoms and syndromes with PTSD-like features have existed in writing throughout the centuries. In the early part of the 20th century, traumatic neurosis was viewed as the ego's inability to master the degree of disorganization brought about by a traumatic experience. Very little was written about posttraumatic neurosis during the years between 1950 and 1970. This absence was followed in the 1970s and 1980s with an explosion in the amount of research and writing on the subject. Many of the papers written during this time were about Vietnam veterans. Clearly, the renewed interest in PTSD was linked to the psychological casualties of the Vietnam War.

The diagnostic category of PTSD did not appear until the third edition of the *Diagnostic and Statistical Manual of Mental Disorders* (*DSM-III*) in 1980, after a need was indicated by increasing numbers of problems with Vietnam veterans and victims of multiple disasters. The *DSM-IV-TR* (2000) described the trauma that precedes PTSD as an event that is outside the range of usual human experience, such as rape, war, physical attack, torture, or natural or man-made disaster.

About 60 percent of men and 50 percent of women are exposed to a traumatic event in their lifetime (Department of Veterans Affairs, 2012). Women are more likely to experience sexual assault and childhood sexual abuse, whereas men are more likely to experience accidents, physical assaults, combat, or to witness death or injury. Although the exposure to trauma is high, less than 10 percent of trauma victims develop PTSD (Breslau, 2009). The disorder appears to be more common in women than in men.

Historically, as previously stated, individuals who experienced stress reactions that followed exposure to an extreme traumatic event were given the diagnosis of PTSD. Accordingly, stress reactions from "normal" daily events (e.g., divorce, failure, rejection) were characterized as adjustment disorders, rather than PTSD (Friedman, 1996).

A number of studies have indicated that adjustment disorders are probably quite common. Sadock and Sadock (2007) report:

> Adjustment disorders are one of the most common psychiatric diagnoses for disorders of patients hospitalized for medical and surgical problems. In one study, 5 percent of people admitted to a hospital over a 3-year period were classified as having an adjustment disorder. (p. 786)

Adjustment disorders are more common in women, unmarried persons, and younger people (Black & Andreasen, 2011). It can occur at any age, from childhood to senescence.

Application of the Nursing Process—Trauma-Related Disorders

> ### CORE CONCEPT
> **Trauma**
> An extremely distressing experience that causes severe emotional shock and may have long-lasting psychological effects.

Posttraumatic Stress Disorder and Acute Stress Disorder

Background Assessment Data

Puri and Treasaden (2011) describe PTSD as "a reaction to an extreme trauma, which is likely to cause pervasive distress to almost anyone, such as natural or man-made disasters, combat, serious accidents, witnessing the violent death of others, being the victim of torture, terrorism, rape, or other crimes" (p. 197). PTSD symptoms are not related to common experiences such as uncomplicated bereavement, marital conflict, or chronic illness, but are associated with events that would be markedly distressing to almost anyone. The individual may experience the trauma alone or in the presence of others.

Characteristic symptoms include reexperiencing the traumatic event, a sustained high level of anxiety or arousal, or a general numbing of responsiveness. Intrusive recollections or nightmares of the event are common. Some individuals may be unable to remember certain aspects of the trauma.

Symptoms of depression are common with this disorder and may be severe enough to warrant a diagnosis of a depressive disorder. In the case of a life-threatening trauma shared with others, survivors often describe painful guilt feelings about surviving when others did not or about the things they had to do to survive. Substance abuse, anger and aggressive behavior, and relationship problems are common.

The full symptom picture must be present for more than 1 month and cause significant interference with social, occupational, and other areas of functioning. The disorder can occur at any age. Symptoms may begin within the first 3 months after the trauma, or there may be a delay of several months or even years. The *DSM-5* diagnostic criteria for PTSD are presented in Box 28-1.

The *DSM-5* describes another disorder that is similar to PTSD called acute stress disorder (ASD). There are similarities between the two disorders in terms of precipitating traumatic events and symptomatology, but in ASD, the symptoms are time limited, up to 1 month following the trauma. By definition, if the symptoms last longer than 1 month, the diagnosis would be PTSD. The *DSM-5* diagnostic criteria for ASD are presented in Box 28-2.

Predisposing Factors to Trauma-Related Disorders

Psychosocial Theory

One psychosocial model that has become widely accepted seeks to explain why certain persons exposed

---

BOX 28-1 Diagnostic Criteria for Posttraumatic Stress Disorder

Note: The following criteria apply to adults, adolescents, and children older than 6 years.

A. Exposure to actual or threatened death, serious injury, or sexual violence, in one (or more) of the following ways:
1. Directly experiencing the traumatic event(s).
2. Witnessing, in person, the event(s) as it occurred to others.
3. Learning that the traumatic event(s) occurred to a close family member or close friend. In cases of actual or threatened death of a family member or friend, the event(s) must have been violent or accidental.
4. Experiencing repeated or extreme exposure to aversive details of the traumatic event(s) (e.g., first responders collecting human remains; police officers repeatedly exposed to details of child abuse). *Note:* Criterion A4 does not apply to exposure through electronic media, television, movies, or pictures, unless this exposure is work-related.

B. Presence of one (or more) of the following intrusion symptoms associated with the traumatic event(s), beginning after the traumatic event(s) occurred:
1. Recurrent, involuntary, and intrusive distressing memories of the traumatic event(s). *Note:* In children older than 6 years, repetitive play may occur in which themes or aspects of the traumatic event(s) are expressed.
2. Recurrent distressing dreams in which the content and/or affect of the dream is related to the traumatic event(s). *Note:* In children, there may be frightening dreams without recognizable content.
3. Dissociative reactions (e.g., flashbacks) in which the individual feels or acts as if the traumatic event(s) were recurring. (Such reactions may occur on a continuum, with the most extreme expression being a complete loss of awareness of present surroundings.) *Note:* In children, trauma-specific reenactment may occur in play.
4. Intense or prolonged psychological distress at exposure to internal or external cues that symbolize or resemble an aspect of the traumatic event(s).
5. Marked physiological reactions to internal or external cues that symbolize or resemble an aspect of the traumatic event(s).

C. Persistent avoidance of stimuli associated with the traumatic event(s) beginning after the traumatic event(s) occurred, as evidenced by one or both of the following:
1. Avoidance of or efforts to avoid distressing memories, thoughts, or feelings about or closely associated with the traumatic event(s).
2. Avoidance of or efforts to avoid external reminders (people, places, conversations, activities, objects, situations) that arouse distressing memories, thoughts, or feelings about or closely associated with the traumatic event(s).

D. Negative alterations in cognitions and mood associated with the traumatic event(s), beginning or worsening after the traumatic event(s) occurred, as evidenced by two or more of the following:
1. Inability to remember an important aspect of the traumatic event(s) (typically due to dissociative amnesia and not to other factors such as head injury, alcohol, or drugs).
2. Persistent and exaggerated negative beliefs or expectations about oneself, others, or the world (e.g., "I am bad," "No one can be trusted," "The world is completely dangerous," "My whole nervous system is permanently ruined").
3. Persistent, distorted cognitions about the cause or consequences of the traumatic event(s) that lead the individual to blame himself/herself or others.
4. Persistent negative emotional state (e.g., fear, horror, anger, guilt, or shame).
5. Markedly diminished interest or participation in significant activities.
6. Feelings of detachment or estrangement from others.
7. Persistent inability to experience positive emotions (e.g., inability to experience happiness, satisfaction, or loving feelings).

E. Marked alterations in arousal and reactivity associated with the traumatic event(s), beginning or worsening after the traumatic event(s) occurred, as evidenced by two or more of the following:
1. Irritable behavior and angry outbursts (with little or no provocation) typically expressed as verbal or physical aggression toward people or objects.
2. Reckless or self-destructive behavior.

Continued

BOX 28-1 **Diagnostic Criteria for Posttraumatic Stress Disorder—cont'd**

3. Hypervigilance.
4. Exaggerated startle response.
5. Problems with concentration.
6. Sleep disturbance (e.g., difficulty falling or staying asleep or restless sleep).

F. Duration of the disturbance (Criteria B, C, D, and E) is more than 1 month.

G. The disturbance causes clinically significant distress or impairment in social, occupational, or other important areas of functioning.

H. The disturbance is not attributable to the physiological effects of a substance (e.g., medication, alcohol) or another medical condition.

Specify whether:

With dissociative symptoms (depersonalization or derealization)

With delayed expression (full diagnostic criteria not met until at least 6 months after the event)

Reprinted with permission from the Diagnostic and Statistical Manual of Mental Disorders, Fifth Edition *(Copyright 2013). American Psychiatric Association.*

BOX 28-2 **Diagnostic Criteria for Acute Stress Disorder**

A. Exposure to actual or threatened death, serious injury, or sexual violation, in one (or more) of the following ways:
   1. Directly experiencing the traumatic event(s).
   2. Witnessing, in person, the event(s) as it occurred to others.
   3. Learning that the event(s) occurred to a close family member or close friend. *Note:* In cases of actual or threatened death of a family member or friend, the event(s) must have been violent or accidental.
   4. Experiencing repeated or extreme exposure to aversive details of the traumatic event(s) (e.g., first responders collecting human remains, police officers repeatedly exposed to details of child abuse). *Note:* This does not apply to exposure through electronic media, television, movies, or pictures, unless this exposure is work related.

B. Presence of nine (or more) of the following symptoms from any of the five categories of intrusion, negative mood, dissociation, avoidance, and arousal, beginning or worsening after the traumatic event(s) occurred:

Intrusion Symptoms
   1. Recurrent, involuntary, and intrusive distressing memories of the traumatic event(s). *Note:* In children, repetitive play may occur in which themes or aspects of the traumatic event(s) are expressed.
   2. Recurrent distressing dreams in which the content and/or affect of the dream are related to the event(s). *Note:* In children, there may be frightening dreams without recognizable content.
   3. Dissociative reactions (e.g., flashbacks) in which the individual feels or acts as if the traumatic event(s) were recurring. (Such reactions may occur on a continuum, with the most extreme expression being a complete loss of awareness of present surroundings.) *Note:* In children, trauma-specific reenactment may occur in play.
   4. Intense or prolonged psychological distress or marked physiological reactions in response to internal or external cues that symbolize or resemble an aspect of the traumatic event(s).

Negative Mood
   5. Persistent inability to experience positive emotions (e.g., inability to experience happiness, satisfaction, or loving feelings).

Dissociative Symptoms
   6. An altered sense of the reality of one's surroundings or oneself (e.g., seeing oneself from another's perspective, being in a daze, time slowing).
   7. Inability to remember an important aspect of the traumatic event(s) (typically due to dissociative amnesia and not to other factors such as head injury, alcohol, or drugs).

Avoidance Symptoms
   8. Efforts to avoid distressing memories, thoughts, or feelings about or closely associated with the traumatic event(s).
   9. Efforts to avoid external reminders (people, places, conversations, activities, objects, situations) that arouse distressing memories, thoughts, or feelings about or closely associated with the traumatic event(s).

Arousal Symptoms
   10. Sleep disturbance (e.g., difficulty falling or staying asleep, or restless sleep).
   11. Irritable behavior and angry outbursts (with little or no provocation), typically expressed as verbal or physical aggression toward people or objects.
   12. Hypervigilance.
   13. Problems with concentration.
   14. Exaggerated startle response.

C. Duration of the disturbance (symptoms in Criteria B) is 3 days to 1 month after trauma exposure. *Note:* Symptoms typically begin immediately after the trauma, but persistence for at least 3 days and up to a month is needed to meet disorder criteria.

D. The disturbance causes clinically significant distress or impairment in social, occupational, or other important areas of functioning.

E. The disturbance is not attributable to the direct physiological effects of a substance (e.g., medication or alcohol) or another medical condition (e.g., mild traumatic brain injury), and is not better explained by brief psychotic disorder.

Reprinted with permission from the Diagnostic and Statistical Manual of Mental Disorders, Fifth Edition *(Copyright 2013). American Psychiatric Association.*

to massive trauma develop trauma-related disorders and others do not. Variables include characteristics that relate to (1) the traumatic experience, (2) the individual, and (3) the recovery environment.

The Traumatic Experience

Specific characteristics relating to the trauma have been identified as crucial elements in the determination of an individual's long-term response to stress. They include:

■ Severity and duration of the stressor
■ Extent of anticipatory preparation for the event
■ Exposure to death
■ Numbers affected by life threat
■ Amount of control over recurrence
■ Location where the trauma was experienced (e.g., familiar surroundings, at home, in a foreign country)

The Individual

Variables that are considered important in determining an individual's response to trauma include:

■ Degree of ego-strength
■ Effectiveness of coping resources
■ Presence of preexisting psychopathology
■ Outcomes of previous experiences with stress/trauma
■ Behavioral tendencies (temperament)
■ Current psychosocial developmental stage
■ Demographic factors (e.g., age, socioeconomic status, education)

The Recovery Environment

It has been suggested that the quality of the environment in which the individual attempts to work through the traumatic experience is correlated with the outcome. Environmental variables include:

■ Availability of social supports
■ The cohesiveness and protectiveness of family and friends
■ The attitudes of society regarding the experience
■ Cultural and subcultural influences

In research with Vietnam veterans, it was shown that the best predictors of PTSD were the severity of the stressor and the degree of psychosocial isolation in the recovery environment.

Learning Theory

Learning theorists view negative reinforcement as behavior that leads to a reduction in an aversive experience, thereby reinforcing and resulting in repetition of the behavior. The avoidance behaviors and psychic numbing in response to a trauma are mediated by negative reinforcement (behaviors that decrease the emotional pain of the trauma). Behavioral disturbances, such as anger and aggression and drug and alcohol abuse, are the behavioral patterns that are reinforced by their capacity to reduce objectionable feelings.

Cognitive Theory

These models take into consideration the cognitive appraisal of an event and focus on assumptions that an individual makes about the world. Epstein (1991) outlines three fundamental beliefs that most people construct within a personal theory of reality:

■ The world is benevolent and a source of joy.
■ The world is meaningful and controllable.
■ The self is worthy (e.g., lovable, good, and competent).

As life situations occur, some disequilibrium is expected to occur until accommodation for the change has been made and it has become assimilated into one's personal theory of reality. An individual is vulnerable to trauma-related disorders when the fundamental beliefs are invalidated by a trauma that cannot be comprehended and a sense of helplessness and hopelessness prevails. One's appraisal of the environment can be drastically altered.

Biological Aspects

It has been suggested that an individual who has experienced previous trauma is more likely to develop symptoms after a stressful life event (Hollander & Simeon, 2008). These individuals with previous traumatic experiences may be more likely to become exposed to future traumas, as they can be inclined to reactivate the behaviors associated with the original trauma.

Hollander and Simeon also report on studies that suggest an endogenous opioid peptide response may assist in the maintenance of chronic PTSD. The hypothesis supports a type of "addiction to the trauma," which is explained in the following manner.

Opioids, including endogenous opioid peptides, have the following psychoactive properties:

■ Tranquilizing action
■ Reduction of rage/aggression
■ Reduction of paranoia
■ Reduction of feelings of inadequacy
■ Antidepressant action

These studies suggest that physiological arousal initiated by reexposure to trauma-like situations enhances production of endogenous opioid peptides and results in increased feelings of comfort and control. When the stressor terminates, the individual may experience opioid withdrawal, the symptoms of which bear strong resemblance to those of PTSD.

Other biological systems have also been implicated in the symptomatology of PTSD. Hageman and associates (2001) state:

It is reasonable to suggest that any disorder such as PTSD that can persist for decades (e.g., Holocaust survivors and Vietnam veterans) is associated with measurable biological features. Evidence suggests that biological dysregulation of the opioid, glutamatergic, noradrenergic, serotonergic, and neuroendocrine pathways are involved in the pathophysiology of PTSD. (p. 412)

Diagnosis/Outcome Identification

Nursing diagnoses are formulated from the data gathered during the assessment phase and with background knowledge regarding predisposing factors to the disorder. Some common nursing diagnoses for clients with trauma-related disorders include:

■ Post-trauma syndrome related to distressing event considered to be outside the range of usual human experience evidenced by flashbacks, intrusive recollections, nightmares, psychological numbness related to the event, dissociation, or amnesia.

■ Complicated grieving related to loss of self as perceived before the trauma or other actual or perceived losses incurred during or after the event evidenced by irritability and explosiveness, self-destructiveness, substance abuse, verbalization of survival guilt, or guilt about behavior required for survival.

The following criteria may be used for measurement of outcomes in the care of the client with a trauma-related disorder.

The client:

■ Can acknowledge the traumatic event and the impact it has had on his or her life

■ Is experiencing fewer flashbacks, intrusive recollections, and nightmares than he or she was on admission (or at the beginning of therapy)

■ Can demonstrate adaptive coping strategies (e.g., relaxation techniques, mental imagery, music, art)

■ Can concentrate and has made realistic goals for the future

■ Includes significant others in the recovery process and willingly accepts their support

■ Verbalizes no ideas or intent of self-harm

■ Has worked through feelings of survivor's guilt

■ Gets enough sleep to avoid risk of injury

■ Verbalizes community resources from which he or she may seek assistance in times of stress

■ Attends support group of individuals who have recovered or are recovering from similar traumatic experiences

■ Verbalizes desire to put the trauma in the past and progress with his or her life

Planning/Implementation

The following section presents a group of selected nursing diagnoses, with short- and long-term goals and nursing interventions for each.

Post-trauma Syndrome

Post-trauma syndrome is defined as "a sustained maladaptive response to a traumatic, overwhelming event" (NANDA-International [NANDA-I], 2012, p. 335). Table 28-1 presents this nursing diagnosis in care plan format.

Client Goals

Outcome criteria include short- and long-term goals. Timelines are individually determined.

Table 28-1 | CARE PLAN FOR THE CLIENT WITH A TRAUMA-RELATED DISORDER

NURSING DIAGNOSIS: POST-TRAUMA SYNDROME

RELATED TO: Distressing event considered to be outside the range of usual human experience

EVIDENCED BY: Flashbacks, intrusive recollections, nightmares, psychological numbness related to the event, dissociation, or amnesia

OUTCOME CRITERIA	NURSING INTERVENTIONS	RATIONALE
Short-Term Goals • Client will begin a healthy grief resolution, initiating the process of psychological healing (within time frame specific to individual). • Client will demonstrate ability to deal with emotional reactions in an individually appropriate manner.	1. a. Assign the same staff as often as possible. b. Use a nonthreatening, matter-of-fact, but friendly approach. c. Respect client's wishes regarding interaction with individuals of the opposite gender at this time (especially important if the trauma was rape). d. Be consistent; keep all promises; convey acceptance; spend time with client.	1. A post-trauma client may be suspicious of others in his or her environment. All of these interventions serve to facilitate a trusting relationship.

Table 28-1 | CARE PLAN FOR THE CLIENT WITH A TRAUMA-RELATED DISORDER–cont'd

Long-Term Goal

• The client will integrate the traumatic experience into his or her persona, renew significant relationships, and establish meaningful goals for the future.

2. Stay with client during periods of flashbacks and nightmares. Offer reassurance of safety and security and that these symptoms are not uncommon following a trauma of the magnitude he or she has experienced.

3. Obtain accurate history from significant others about the trauma and the client's specific response.

4. Encourage the client to talk about the trauma at his or her own pace. Provide a nonthreatening, private environment, and include a significant other if the client wishes. Acknowledge and validate client's feelings as they are expressed.

5. Discuss coping strategies used in response to the trauma, as well as those used during stressful situations in the past. Determine those that have been most helpful, and discuss alternative strategies for the future. Include available support systems, including religious and cultural influences. Identify maladaptive coping strategies (e.g., substance use, psychosomatic responses) and practice more adaptive coping strategies for possible future post-trauma responses.

6. Assist the individual to try to comprehend the trauma if possible. Discuss feelings of vulnerability and the individual's "place" in the world following the trauma.

2. Presence of a trusted individual may calm fears for personal safety and reassure client that he or she is not "going crazy."

3. Various types of traumas elicit different responses in clients (e.g., human-engendered traumas often generate a greater degree of humiliation and guilt in victims than trauma associated with natural disasters).

4. This debriefing process is the first step in the progression toward resolution.

5. Resolution of the post-trauma response is largely dependent on the effectiveness of the coping strategies employed.

6. Post-trauma response is largely a function of the shattering of basic beliefs the victim holds about self and world. Assimilation of the event into one's persona requires that some degree of meaning associated with the event be incorporated into the basic beliefs, which will affect how the individual eventually comes to reappraise self and world (Epstein, 1991).

Short-Term Goals

■ The client will begin a healthy grief resolution, initiating the process of psychological healing (within time frame specific to individual).

■ The client will demonstrate ability to deal with emotional reactions in an individually appropriate manner.

Long-Term Goal

■ The client will integrate the traumatic experience into his or her persona, renew significant relationships, and establish meaningful goals for the future.

Interventions

■ A post-trauma client may be suspicious of others in his or her environment. Establishing a trusting relationship with this individual is essential before care can be given. To do this, assign the same staff as often as possible. Use a nonthreatening, matter-of-fact but friendly approach. Respect the client's wishes regarding interaction with individuals of the opposite gender at this time (especially important if the trauma was rape). Be consistent and keep all promises, and convey an attitude of unconditional acceptance.

■ Stay with the client during periods of flashbacks and nightmares. Offer reassurance of safety and security and that these symptoms are not uncommon following a trauma of the magnitude he or she has experienced. The presence of a trusted individual may help to calm fears for personal safety and reassure the anxious client that he or she is not "going crazy."

■ Obtain an accurate history from significant others about the trauma and the client's specific response. Various types of traumas elicit different responses in clients. For example, human-engendered traumas often generate a greater degree of humiliation and guilt in victims than trauma associated with natural disasters.

■ Encourage the client to talk about the trauma at his or her own pace. Provide a nonthreatening, private environment, and include a significant other if the client wishes. Acknowledge and validate the client's feelings as they are expressed. This debriefing process is the first step in the progression toward resolution.

■ Discuss coping strategies used in response to the trauma, as well as those used during stressful situations in the past. Determine those that have been most helpful, and discuss alternative strategies for the future. Include available support systems, including religious and cultural influences. Identify maladaptive coping strategies, such as substance use or psychosomatic responses, and practice more adaptive coping strategies for possible future post-trauma responses. Resolution of the posttrauma response is largely dependent on the effectiveness of the coping strategies employed.

■ Assist the individual to try to comprehend the trauma if possible. Discuss feelings of vulnerability and the individual's "place" in the world following the trauma. Post-trauma response is largely a function of the shattering of basic beliefs the survivor holds about self and world. Assimilation of the event into one's persona requires that some degree of meaning associated with the event be incorporated into the basic beliefs, which will affect how the individual eventually comes to reappraise self and world (Epstein, 1991).

Complicated Grieving

Complicated grieving is defined as "a disorder that occurs after the death of a significant other [or any other loss of significance to the individual], in which the experience of distress accompanying bereavement fails to follow normative expectations and manifests in functional impairment" (NANDA-I, 2012, p. 365).

Client Goals

Outcome criteria include short- and long-term goals. Timelines are individually determined.

Short-Term Goal

■ Client will verbalize feelings (guilt, anger, self-blame, hopelessness) associated with the trauma.

Long-Term Goal

■ Client will demonstrate progress in dealing with stages of grief and will verbalize a sense of optimism and hope for the future.

Interventions

■ Acknowledge feelings of guilt or self-blame that client may express. Guilt at having survived a trauma in which others died is common. The client needs to discuss these feelings and recognize that he or she is not responsible for what happened but must take responsibility for own recovery.

■ Assess stage of grief in which the client is fixed. Discuss normalcy of feelings and behaviors related to stages of grief. Knowledge of grief stage is necessary for accurate intervention. Guilt may be generated if client believes it is unacceptable to have these feelings. Knowing they are normal can provide a sense of relief.

■ Assess impact of the trauma on client's ability to resume regular activities of daily living. Consider employment, marital relationship, and sleep patterns. Following a trauma, individuals are at high risk for physical injury because of disruption in ability to concentrate and problem-solve and because of lack of sufficient sleep. Isolation and avoidance behaviors may interfere with interpersonal relatedness.

■ Assess for self-destructive ideas and behavior. The trauma may result in feelings of hopelessness and worthlessness, leading to high risk for suicide.

■ Assess for maladaptive coping strategies, such as substance abuse. These behaviors interfere with and delay the recovery process.

■ Identify available community resources from which the individual may seek assistance if problems with complicated grieving persist. Support groups for victims of various types of traumas exist within most communities. The presence of support systems in the recovery environment has been identified as a major predictor in the successful recovery from trauma.

Concept Care Mapping

The concept map care plan is an innovative approach to planning and organizing nursing care (see Chapter 9). It is a diagrammatic teaching and learning strategy that allows visualization of interrelationships between medical diagnoses, nursing diagnoses, assessment data, and treatments. An example of a concept map care plan for a client with a trauma-related disorder is presented in Figure 28-1.

Evaluation

Reassessment is conducted in order to determine if the nursing actions have been successful in achieving the objectives of care. Evaluation of the nursing actions for the client with a trauma-related disorder may be facilitated by gathering information using the following types of questions:

■ Can the client discuss the traumatic event without experiencing panic anxiety?

■ Does the client voluntarily discuss the traumatic event?

■ Can the client discuss changes that have occurred in his or her life because of the traumatic event?

■ Does the client have "flashbacks?"

■ Can the client sleep without medication?

■ Does the client have nightmares?

■ Has the client learned new, adaptive coping strategies for assistance with recovery?

■ Can the client demonstrate successful use of these new coping strategies in times of stress?

■ Can the client verbalize stages of grief and the normal behaviors associated with each?

■ Can the client recognize his or her own position in the grieving process?

■ Is guilt being alleviated?

■ Has the client maintained or regained satisfactory relationships with significant others?

■ Can the client look to the future with optimism?

■ Does the client attend a regular support group for victims of similar traumatic experiences?

■ Does the client have a plan of action for dealing with symptoms, if they return?

Application of the Nursing Process—Stressor-Related Disorders

Adjustment Disorders—Background Assessment Data

> ## CORE CONCEPT
> **Stress**
> Mental, emotional, or physical strain experienced by an individual in response to stimuli from the external or internal environment.

An adjustment disorder is characterized by a maladaptive reaction to an identifiable stressor or stressors that results in the development of clinically significant emotional or behavioral symptoms (APA, 2013). The response occurs within 3 months after onset of the stressor and has persisted for no longer than 6 months after the stressor or its consequences have ended.

The individual shows impairment in social and occupational functioning or exhibits symptoms that are in excess of an expected reaction to the stressor. The symptoms are expected to remit soon after the stressor is relieved, or if the stressor persists, when a new level of adaptation is achieved. The *DSM-5* diagnostic criteria for adjustment disorders are presented in Box 28-3.

The stressor itself can be almost anything, but an individual's response to any particular stressor cannot be predicted. If an individual is highly predisposed or vulnerable to maladaptive response, a severe form of the disorder may follow what most people would consider only a mild or moderate stressor. On the other hand, a less vulnerable individual may develop only a mild form of the disorder in response to what others might consider a severe stressor.

A number of clinical presentations are associated with adjustment disorders. The following categories, identified by the *DSM-5* (APA, 2013), are distinguished by the predominant features of the maladaptive response.

Adjustment Disorder With Depressed Mood

This category is the most commonly diagnosed adjustment disorder. The clinical presentation is one of predominant mood disturbance, although less pronounced than that of major depressive disorder (MDD). The symptoms, such as depressed mood, tearfulness, and feelings of hopelessness, exceed what is an expected or normative response to an identified stressor.

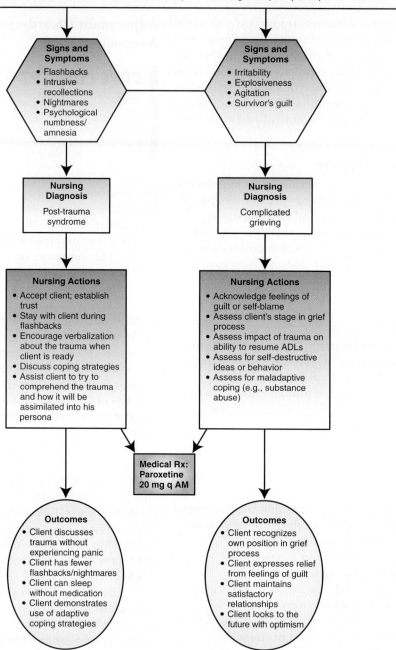

Clinical Vignette: Charles is a 29-year-old veteran of two deployments to Afghanistan. He was honorably discharged from the army 2 years ago and has resumed his position as an assemblyman with a large automobile manufacturing company. His wife reports that he has begun having nightmares, seems angry and bitter, and feels guilty that he survived while many of his friends had not. Recently, while working in their backyard, he threw himself on the ground at the sound of a helicopter flying overhead. Lately, at work, he becomes very agitated and irritable at the sounds of loud noises in the factory, a behavior that is interfering with his productivity. Charles has been diagnosed with Posttraumatic Stress Disorder. The mental health nurse develops the following concept map care plan for Charles.

Signs and Symptoms
- Flashbacks
- Intrusive recollections
- Nightmares
- Psychological numbness/ amnesia

Signs and Symptoms
- Irritability
- Explosiveness
- Agitation
- Survivor's guilt

Nursing Diagnosis
Post-trauma syndrome

Nursing Diagnosis
Complicated grieving

Nursing Actions
- Accept client; establish trust
- Stay with client during flashbacks
- Encourage verbalization about the trauma when client is ready
- Discuss coping strategies
- Assist client to try to comprehend the trauma and how it will be assimilated into his persona

Nursing Actions
- Acknowledge feelings of guilt or self-blame
- Assess client's stage in grief process
- Assess impact of trauma on ability to resume ADLs
- Assess for self-destructive ideas or behavior
- Assess for maladaptive coping (e.g., substance abuse)

Medical Rx: Paroxetine 20 mg q AM

Outcomes
- Client discusses trauma without experiencing panic
- Client has fewer flashbacks/nightmares
- Client can sleep without medication
- Client demonstrates use of adaptive coping strategies

Outcomes
- Client recognizes own position in grief process
- Client expresses relief from feelings of guilt
- Client maintains satisfactory relationships
- Client looks to the future with optimism

FIGURE 28–1 Concept map care plan for a client with posttraumatic stress disorder.

Adjustment Disorder With Anxiety

This category denotes a maladaptive response to a stressor in which the predominant manifestation is anxiety. For example, the symptoms may reveal nervousness, worry, and jitteriness. The clinician must differentiate this diagnosis from those of anxiety disorders.

Adjustment Disorder With Mixed Anxiety and Depressed Mood

The predominant features of this category include disturbances in mood (depression, feelings of hopelessness and sadness) and manifestations of anxiety (nervousness, worry, jitteriness) that are more intense

BOX 28-3 **Diagnostic Criteria for Adjustment Disorders**

A. The development of emotional or behavioral symptoms in response to an identifiable stressor(s) occurring within three months of the onset of the stressor(s).

B. These symptoms or behaviors are clinically significant, as evidenced by one or both of the following:
1. Marked distress that is out of proportion to the severity or intensity of the stressor, taking into account the external context and the cultural factors that might influence symptom severity and presentation.
2. Significant impairment in social, occupational, or other important areas of functioning.

C. The stress-related disturbance does not meet the criteria for another mental disorder and is not merely an exacerbation of a preexisting mental disorder.

D. The symptoms do not represent normal bereavement.

E. Once the stressor or its consequences have terminated, the symptoms do not persist for more than an additional 6 months.

Specify whether:

With depressed mood: Low mood, tearfulness, or feelings of hopelessness are predominant.

With anxiety: Nervousness, worry, jitteriness, or separation anxiety is predominant.

With mixed anxiety and depressed mood: A combination of depression and anxiety is predominant.

With disturbance of conduct: Disturbance of conduct is predominant.

With mixed disturbance of emotions and conduct: Both emotional symptoms (e.g., depression, anxiety) and a disturbance of conduct are predominant.

Unspecified: For maladaptive reactions that are not classifiable as one of the specific subtypes of adjustment disorder.

Reprinted with permission from the Diagnostic and Statistical Manual of Mental Disorders, Fifth Edition *(Copyright 2013). American Psychiatric Association.*

than what would be expected or considered to be a normative response to an identified stressor.

Adjustment Disorder With Disturbance of Conduct

This category is characterized by conduct in which there is violation of the rights of others or of major age-appropriate societal norms and rules. Examples include truancy, vandalism, reckless driving, fighting, and defaulting on legal responsibilities. Differential diagnosis must be made from conduct disorder or antisocial personality disorder.

Adjustment Disorder With Mixed Disturbance of Emotions and Conduct

The predominant features of this category include emotional disturbances (e.g., anxiety or depression) as well as disturbances of conduct in which there is violation of the rights of others or of major age-appropriate societal norms and rules (e.g., truancy, vandalism, fighting).

Adjustment Disorder Unspecified

This subtype is used when the maladaptive reaction is not consistent with any of the other categories. The individual may have physical complaints, withdraw from relationships, or exhibit impaired work or academic performance, but without significant disturbance in emotions or conduct.

Predisposing Factors to Adjustment Disorders

Biological Theory

Chronic disorders, such as neurocognitive disorder or intellectual disability, are thought to impair the ability of an individual to adapt to stress, causing increased vulnerability to adjustment disorder. Sadock and Sadock (2007) suggest that genetic factors also may influence individual risks for maladaptive response to stress.

Psychosocial Theories

Some proponents of psychoanalytic theory view adjustment disorder as a maladaptive response to stress that is caused by early childhood trauma, increased dependency, and retarded ego development. Other psychoanalysts put considerable weight on the constitutional factor, or birth characteristics that contribute to the manner in which individuals respond to stress. In many instances, adjustment disorder is precipitated by a specific meaningful stressor having found a point of vulnerability in an individual of otherwise adequate ego strength.

Some studies relate a predisposition to adjustment disorder to factors such as developmental stage, timing of the stressor, and available support systems. When a stressor occurs, and the individual does not have the developmental maturity, available support systems, or adequate coping strategies to adapt, normal functioning is disrupted, resulting in psychological or somatic symptoms. The disorder also may be related to a dysfunctional grieving process. The individual may remain in the denial or anger stage, with inadequate defense mechanisms to complete the grieving process.

Transactional Model of Stress/Adaptation

Why are some individuals able to confront stressful situations adaptively and even gain strength from the experience, whereas others not only fail to cope adaptively, but may even encounter psychopathological dysfunction? The Transactional Model of Stress/Adaptation takes into consideration the interaction between the individual and the environment.

The type of stressor that one experiences may influence one's adaptation. Sudden-shock stressors occur without warning, and continuous stressors are those that an individual is exposed to over an extended period. Although many studies have been directed to individuals' responses to sudden-shock stressors, it has been found that continuous stressors were more commonly cited than sudden-shock stressors as precipitants to maladaptive functioning.

Both situational and intrapersonal factors most likely contribute to an individual's stress response. Situational factors include personal and general economic conditions; occupational and recreational opportunities; and the availability of social supports such as family, friends, neighbors, and cultural or religious support groups.

Intrapersonal factors such as constitutional vulnerability have also been implicated in the predisposition to adjustment disorder. Some studies have indicated that a child with a difficult temperament (defined as one who cries loudly and often; adapts to changes slowly; and has irregular patterns of hunger, sleep, and elimination) is at greater risk of developing a behavior disorder. Freud (1964) theorized that traumatic childhood experiences created points of fixation to which the individual, during times of stress, would be likely to regress. This might also apply to other unresolved conflicts or developmental issues. Other intrapersonal factors that might influence one's ability to adjust to a painful life change include social skills, coping strategies, the presence of psychiatric illness, degree of flexibility, and level of intelligence.

Diagnosis/Outcome Identification

Nursing diagnoses are formulated from the data gathered during the assessment phase and with background knowledge regarding predisposing factors to the disorder. Nursing diagnoses that may be used for the client with an adjustment disorder include:

■ Complicated grieving related to real or perceived loss of any concept of value to the individual, evidenced by interference with life functioning, developmental regression, or somatic complaints.

■ Risk-prone health behavior related to change in health status requiring modification in lifestyle (e.g., chronic illness, physical disability), evidenced by inability to problem-solve or set realistic goals for the future. **NOTE:** This diagnosis would be appropriate for the person with adjustment disorder if the precipitating stressor was a change in health status.

■ Anxiety (moderate to severe) related to situational and/or maturational crisis evidenced by restlessness, increased helplessness, and diminished productivity.

Outcome Criteria

The following criteria may be used for measurement of outcomes in the care of the client with an adjustment disorder.

The client:

■ Verbalizes acceptable behaviors associated with each stage of the grief process
■ Demonstrates a reinvestment in the environment
■ Accomplishes activities of daily living independently
■ Demonstrates ability for adequate occupational and social functioning
■ Verbalizes awareness of change in health status and the effect it will have on lifestyle
■ Solves problems and sets realistic goals for the future
■ Demonstrates ability to cope effectively with change in lifestyle

Planning/Implementation

The following section presents a group of selected nursing diagnoses, with short- and long-term goals and nursing interventions for each.

Complicated Grieving

Complicated grieving is defined as "a disorder that occurs after the death of a significant other [or any other loss of significance to the individual], in which the experience of distress accompanying bereavement fails to follow normative expectations and manifests in functional impairment" (NANDA International [NANDA-I], 2012, p. 365).

Client Goals

Outcome criteria include short- and long-term goals. Timelines are individually determined.

Short-Term Goal

■ By end of 1 week, client will express anger toward lost entity.

Long-Term Goal

■ The client will be able to verbalize behaviors associated with the normal stages of grief and identify own position in grief process, while progressing at own pace toward resolution.

Interventions

■ Determine the stage of grief in which client is fixed. Identify behaviors associated with this stage. Accurate baseline assessment data are necessary to plan effective care for the grieving client.

■ Develop a trusting relationship with the client. Show empathy and caring. Be honest and keep all promises. Trust is the basis for a therapeutic relationship.

■ Convey an accepting attitude so that the client is not afraid to express feelings openly. An accepting attitude conveys to the client that you believe he or she is a worthwhile person. Trust is enhanced.

■ Allow the client to express anger. Do not become defensive if the initial expression of anger is displaced on the nurse or therapist. Help the client explore angry feelings so that they may be directed toward the intended object or person. Verbalization of feelings in a nonthreatening environment may help the client come to terms with unresolved issues.

■ Assist the client to discharge pent-up anger through participation in large motor activities (e.g., brisk walks, jogging, physical exercises, volleyball, punching bag, exercise bike). Physical exercise provides a safe and effective method for discharging pent-up tension.

■ Explain to the client the normal stages of grief and the behaviors associated with each stage. Help the client to understand that feelings such as guilt and anger toward the lost entity/concept are natural and acceptable during the grief process. Knowledge of the acceptability of the feelings associated with normal grieving may help to relieve some of the guilt that these responses generate.

■ Encourage the client to review his or her perception of the loss or change. With support and sensitivity, point out the reality of the situation in areas where misrepresentations are expressed. The client must give up an idealized perception and be able to accept both positive and negative aspects about the painful life change before the grief process is complete.

■ Communicate to the client that crying is acceptable. The use of touch is therapeutic and appropriate with most clients. Knowledge of cultural influences specific to the client is important before employing this technique. Touch is considered inappropriate in some cultures.

■ Help the client to solve problems as he or she attempts to determine methods for more adaptive coping with the stressor. Provide positive feedback for strategies identified and decisions made. Positive reinforcement enhances self-esteem and encourages repetition of desirable behaviors.

■ Encourage the client to reach out for spiritual support during this time in whatever form is desirable. Assess client's spiritual needs, and assist as necessary in the fulfillment of those needs. For some individuals, spiritual support can enhance successful adaptation to painful life experiences.

Risk-Prone Health Behavior

Risk-prone health behavior is defined as "impaired ability to modify lifestyle/behaviors in a manner that improves health status" (NANDA-I, 2012, p. 155).

Client Goals

Short-Term Goals

■ The client and primary nurse will discuss the kinds of lifestyle changes that will occur because of the change in health status.

■ With the help of the primary nurse, the client will formulate a plan of action for incorporating those changes into his or her lifestyle.

■ The client will demonstrate movement toward independence, considering the change in health status.

Long-Term Goal

■ The client will demonstrate competence to function independently to his or her optimal ability, considering the change in health status, by the time of discharge from treatment.

Interventions

■ Encourage the client to talk about his or her lifestyle prior to the change in health status. Discuss coping mechanisms that were used at stressful times in the past. It is important to identify the client's strengths so that they may be used to facilitate adaptation to the change or loss that has occurred.

■ Encourage the client to discuss the change or loss and particularly to express anger associated with it. Anger is a normal stage in the grieving process and if not released in an appropriate manner, may be turned inward on the self, leading to pathological depression.

■ Encourage the client to express fears associated with the change or loss or alteration in lifestyle that it has created. Change often creates a feeling of disequilibrium and the individual may respond with fears that are irrational or unfounded. The client may benefit from feedback that corrects misperceptions about how life will be with the change in health status.

■ Provide assistance with activities of daily living as required, but encourage independence to the limit that client's ability will allow. Give positive feedback for activities accomplished independently. Independent accomplishments and positive feedback enhance self-esteem and encourage repetition of desired behaviors. Successes also provide hope that adaptive functioning is possible and decrease feelings of powerlessness.

■ Help the client with decision making regarding incorporation of the change or loss into his or her lifestyle. Identify problems the change or loss is likely to create. Discuss alternative solutions, weighing potential benefits and consequences of each alternative. Support the client's decision in the selection of an alternative. The great amount of anxiety that usually accompanies a major lifestyle change often interferes with an individual's ability to solve problems and to make appropriate decisions. Client may need assistance with this process in an effort to progress toward successful adaptation.

■ Use role-play to practice stressful situations that might occur in relation to the health status change. Role-playing decreases anxiety and provides a feeling of security by providing the client with a plan of action for responding in an appropriate manner when a stressful situation occurs.

■ Ensure that the client and family are fully knowledgeable regarding the physiology of the change in health status and understand the necessity of such knowledge for optimal wellness. Encourage them to ask questions, and provide printed material explaining the change to which they may refer. Having knowledge about the health status and knowing what to expect regarding the change or loss decreases anxiety and enhances the capacity for wellness.

■ Ensure that the client can identify resources within the community from which he or she may seek assistance in adapting to the change in health status. Examples include self-help or support groups and public health nurse, counselor, or social worker. Encourage the client to keep follow-up appointments with his or her physician, or to call the physician's office prior to the follow-up date if problems or concerns arise. Support services provide a feeling of security that one is not alone and provide a means to prevent decompensation when stress becomes intolerable.

Concept Care Mapping

An example of a concept map care plan for a client with an adjustment disorder is presented in Figure 28-2.

Evaluation

Reassessment is conducted to determine if the nursing actions have been successful in achieving the objectives of care. Evaluation of the nursing actions for the client with an adjustment disorder may be facilitated by gathering information using the following types of questions:

■ Does the client verbalize understanding of the grief process and his or her position in the process?

■ Does the client recognize his or her adaptive and maladaptive behaviors associated with the grief response?

■ Does the client demonstrate evidence of progression along the grief response?

■ Can the client accomplish activities of daily living independently?

■ Does the client demonstrate the ability to perform occupational and social activities adequately?

■ Does the client discuss the change in health status and modification of lifestyle it will affect?

■ Does the client demonstrate acceptance of the modification?

■ Can the client participate in decision making and problem-solving for his or her future?

■ Does the client set realistic goals for the future?

■ Does the client demonstrate new adaptive coping strategies for dealing with the change in lifestyle?

■ Can the client verbalize available resources to whom he or she may go for support or assistance should it be necessary?

Treatment Modalities

Trauma-Related Disorders
Cognitive Therapy

Cognitive therapy for PTSD and ASD strives to help the individual recognize and modify trauma-related thoughts and beliefs. The individual learns to modify the relationships between thoughts and feelings, and to identify and challenge inaccurate or extreme automatic negative thoughts. The goal is to replace these negative thoughts with more accurate and less distressing thoughts, and to cope more effectively with feelings such as anger, guilt, and fear. The individual is assisted to modify the appraisal of self and the world as it has been affected by the trauma, and to regain hope and optimism about safety, trust, power and control, esteem, and intimacy.

Prolonged Exposure Therapy

Prolonged exposure therapy (PE) is a type of behavioral therapy somewhat similar to implosion therapy or flooding (see Chapter 27). It can be conducted in an imagined or real (in vivo) situation. In the imagined situation, the individual is exposed to repeated and prolonged mental recounting of the traumatic experience. In vivo exposure involves systematic confrontation, within safe limits, of trauma-related situations that are feared and avoided. This intense emotional processing of the traumatic event serves to neutralize the memories so that they no longer result in anxious arousal or escape and avoidance behaviors. PE has four main parts: (1) education about the treatment, (2) breathing retraining for relaxation, (3) imagined exposure through repeated discussion about the

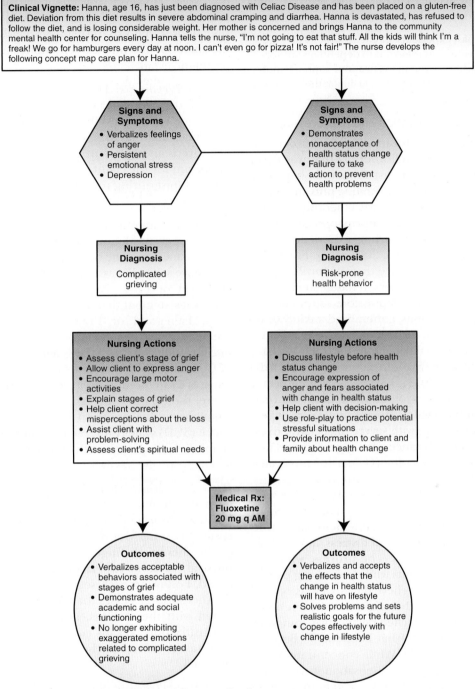

Clinical Vignette: Hanna, age 16, has just been diagnosed with Celiac Disease and has been placed on a gluten-free diet. Deviation from this diet results in severe abdominal cramping and diarrhea. Hanna is devastated, has refused to follow the diet, and is losing considerable weight. Her mother is concerned and brings Hanna to the community mental health center for counseling. Hanna tells the nurse, "I'm not going to eat that stuff. All the kids will think I'm a freak! We go for hamburgers every day at noon. I can't even go for pizza! It's not fair!" The nurse develops the following concept map care plan for Hanna.

Signs and Symptoms
• Verbalizes feelings of anger
• Persistent emotional stress
• Depression

Signs and Symptoms
• Demonstrates nonacceptance of health status change
• Failure to take action to prevent health problems

Nursing Diagnosis
Complicated grieving

Nursing Diagnosis
Risk-prone health behavior

Nursing Actions
• Assess client's stage of grief
• Allow client to express anger
• Encourage large motor activities
• Explain stages of grief
• Help client correct misperceptions about the loss
• Assist client with problem-solving
• Assess client's spiritual needs

Nursing Actions
• Discuss lifestyle before health status change
• Encourage expression of anger and fears associated with change in health status
• Help client with decision-making
• Use role-play to practice potential stressful situations
• Provide information to client and family about health change

Medical Rx:
Fluoxetine
20 mg q AM

Outcomes
• Verbalizes acceptable behaviors associated with stages of grief
• Demonstrates adequate academic and social functioning
• No longer exhibiting exaggerated emotions related to complicated grieving

Outcomes
• Verbalizes and accepts the effects that the change in health status will have on lifestyle
• Solves problems and sets realistic goals for the future
• Copes effectively with change in lifestyle

FIGURE 28–2 Concept map care plan for a client with an adjustment disorder.

trauma with a therapist, and (4) exposure to real-world situations related to the trauma.

Group/Family Therapy

Group therapy has been strongly advocated for clients with PTSD. It has proved especially effective with military veterans (Sadock & Sadock, 2007). The importance of being able to share their experiences with empathetic fellow veterans, to talk about problems in social adaptation, and to discuss options for managing their aggression toward others has been emphasized. Some PTSD groups are informal and leaderless, such as self-help or support groups, and some are led by experienced group therapists who may have had some firsthand experience with the trauma. Some groups involve family members, thereby recognizing that the symptoms of PTSD may also severely affect them. Hollander and Simeon (2008) state:

> Because of past experiences, [clients with PTSD] are often mistrustful and reluctant to depend on authority figures, whereas the identification, support, and hopefulness of peer settings can facilitate therapeutic change. (p. 579)

Eye Movement Desensitization and Reprocessing

Eye movement desensitization and reprocessing (EMDR) is a type of psychotherapy that was developed in 1989 by psychologist Francine Shapiro. It "has evolved from a simple technique into an integrative psychotherapy approach with a theoretical model that emphasizes the brain's information processing system and memories of disturbing experiences as the basis of pathology" (Shapiro, 2007, p. 3). EMDR has been shown to be an effective therapy for PTSD and other trauma-related disorders. It has been used with other disorders, including depression, adjustment disorder, phobias, addictions, generalized anxiety disorder, and panic disorder. However, at present, EMDR has been empirically validated only for trauma-related disorders such as PTSD and acute stress disorder (Aetna Healthcare, 2013). EMDR is contraindicated in clients who have neurological impairments (e.g., seizure disorders), clients who are suicidal or experiencing psychosis, those with severe dissociative disorders or unstable substance abuse, and those with detached retina or glaucoma (Center for Integrative Medicine, 2013).

The exact biological mechanisms by which EMDR achieves its therapeutic effects are unknown. Some studies have indicated that eye movements cause a decrease in imagery vividness and distress, as well as an increase in memory access. The process, which involves rapid eye movements while processing painful emotions, is thought to "relieve the anxiety associated with the trauma so that the original event can be examined from a more detached perspective, somewhat like watching a movie of what happened" (Bartson, Smith, & Corcoran, 2011). While concentrating on a particular emotion or physical sensation surrounding the traumatic event, the client is asked to focus his or her eye movements on the therapist's fingers as the therapist moves them from left to right and back again. Although some individuals report rapid results with this therapy, research has indicated that from 5 to 12 sessions are required to achieve lasting treatment effects. The EMDR treatment encompasses the following eight-phase process.

Phase 1: History and treatment planning In the first phase, the therapist takes a thorough history and develops a treatment plan. The problem for which the client is seeking treatment and current symptoms are discussed. However, the client is not required to discuss the traumatic event in detail, unless he or she chooses to do so. Instead, emphasis is placed on the emotions and physical sensations surrounding the traumatic event.

Phase 2: Preparation During this phase, the therapist teaches the client certain self-care techniques (e.g., relaxation techniques) for dealing with emotional disturbances that may arise during or between sessions. Self-care is an important component of EMDR. It is important for the client to develop a sense of trust in the therapist during this phase.

Phase 3: Assessment During this phase, the therapist asks the client to identify a specific scene or picture from the target event identified in phase 1 that best represents the memory. The client is then directed to express a negative self-belief associated with the memory (e.g., "I am bad" or "I'm in danger"). The next step is to identify a self-statement that he or she would *rather* believe (e.g., "I am good" or "I'm safe now"). When the self-statements have been identified, the client is asked to rate the validity of each of the statements on the Validity of Cognition (VOC) scale from "completely false" (a score of 1) to "completely true" (a score of 7). In this phase, the client is also asked to rank the disturbing emotions on the zero to 10 Subjective Units of Disturbance (SUD) scale (with zero meaning the disturbance is not disturbing at all and 10 meaning it is the worst feeling he or she has ever had).

Phase 4: Desensitization During this phase, the client gives attention to the negative beliefs and disturbing emotions associated with the traumatic event while focusing his or her vision on the back-and-forth motion of the therapist's finger. All personal feelings and physical reactions experienced during this time are noted. Following each set of rapid eye movements, the therapist reassesses the level of disturbance associated with the feelings, images, and beliefs. This desensitization process continues until the distress level (as measured by the SUD scale) is reduced to zero or 1.

Phase 5: Installation In phase 5, the client gives attention to the positive belief that he or she has identified to replace the negative belief associated with the trauma. This is accomplished while simultaneously visually tracking the therapist's finger. Following each set of rapid eye movements, the client is asked to rate the positive belief on the VOC scale. The goal is to strengthen the positive belief or self-statement until it is accepted as completely true (a score of 7 on the VOC scale).

Phase 6: Body scan When the positive cognition has been strengthened, the therapist asks the client to concentrate on any lingering physical sensations.

While focusing on the traumatic event, the client is asked to identify any areas of the body where residual tension is experienced. Because positive self-beliefs must be believed on more than just an intellectual level, phase 6 is not complete until the client is able to think about or discuss the traumatic event (or the feelings associated with it) without experiencing bodily tension.

Phase 7: Closure Closure ensures that the client leaves each session feeling better than he or she felt at the beginning. If the processing that took place during the session is not complete, the therapist will direct the client through a variety of self-calming relaxation techniques to help him or her regain emotional equilibrium. The client is briefed about what to expect between sessions. Until processing of the trauma is complete, disturbing images, thoughts, and emotions may arise between therapy sessions. The therapist instructs the client to record these experiences in a journal so that they may be used as targets for processing in future therapy sessions.

Phase 8: Reevaluation Reevaluation begins each new therapy session. The therapist assesses whether the positive changes have been maintained, determines if previous target areas need reprocessing, and identifies any new target areas that need attention.

Clients often feel relief quite rapidly with EMDR. However, to achieve lasting results, it is important that each of the eight phases be completed. Treatment is not complete until "EMDR therapy has focused on the past memories that are contributing to the problem, the present situations that are disturbing, and what skills the client may need for the future" (EMDR Network, 2013).

Psychopharmacology

Antidepressants The selective serotonin reuptake inhibitors (SSRIs) are now considered first-line treatment of choice for PTSD because of their efficacy, tolerability, and safety ratings (Sadock & Sadock, 2007). Paroxetine and sertraline have been approved by the Food and Drug Administration (FDA) for this purpose. The tricyclic antidepressants (e.g., amitriptyline and imipramine), the MAO inhibitors (e.g., phenelzine), and trazodone have also been effective in the treatment of PTSD.

Anxiolytics Alprazolam has been prescribed for PTSD clients for its antidepressant and antipanic effects. Other benzodiazepines have also been used, despite the absence of controlled studies demonstrating their efficacy in PTSD. Their addictive properties make them less desirable than some of the other medications in the treatment of post-trauma patients. Buspirone, which has serotonergic properties similar to

the SSRIs, may also be useful. Further controlled trials with this drug are needed to validate its efficacy in treating PTSD.

Antihypertensives The beta blocker propranolol and alpha$_2$-receptor agonist clonidine have been successful in alleviating some of the symptoms associated with PTSD. In clinical trials, marked reductions in nightmares, intrusive recollections, hypervigilance, insomnia, startle responses, and angry outbursts were reported with the use of these drugs (Hollander & Simeon, 2008).

Other Medications Carbamazepine, valproic acid, and lithium carbonate have been reported to alleviate symptoms of intrusive recollections, flashbacks, nightmares, impulsivity, irritability, and violent behavior in PTSD clients. Sadock and Sadock (2007) report that little positive evidence exists concerning the use of antipsychotics in PTSD. They suggest that these drugs "should be reserved for the short-term control of severe aggression and agitation" (p. 621).

Adjustment Disorders

Various treatments are used for clients with adjustment disorder. Strain, Klipstein, and Newcorn (2008) cite the following as major goals of therapy for these individuals:

1. To relieve symptoms associated with a stressor.
2. To enhance coping with stressors that cannot be reduced or removed.
3. To establish support systems that maximize adaptation.

Individual Psychotherapy

Individual psychotherapy is the most common treatment for adjustment disorder. Individual psychotherapy allows the client to examine the stressor that is causing the problem, possibly assign personal meaning to the stressor, and confront unresolved issues that may be exacerbating this crisis. Treatment works to remove these blocks to adaptation so that normal developmental progression can resume. Techniques are used to clarify links between the current stressor and past experiences, and to assist with the development of more adaptive coping strategies.

Family Therapy

The focus of treatment is shifted from the individual to the system of relationships in which the individual is involved. The maladaptive response of the identified client is viewed as symptomatic of a dysfunctional family system. All family members are included in the therapy, and treatment serves to improve the functioning within the family network. Emphasis is placed on communication, family rules, and interaction patterns among the family members.

Behavior Therapy

The goal of behavior therapy is to replace ineffective response patterns with more adaptive ones. The situations that promote ineffective responses are identified, and carefully designed reinforcement schedules, along with role-playing and coaching, are used to alter the maladaptive response patterns. This type of treatment is very effective when implemented in an inpatient setting where the client's behavior and its consequences may be more readily controlled.

Self-Help Groups

Group experiences, with or without a professional facilitator, provide an arena in which members may consider and compare their responses to individuals with similar life experiences. Members benefit from learning that they are not alone in their painful experiences. Hope is derived from knowing that others have survived and even grown from similar experiences. Members of the group exchange advice, share coping strategies, and provide support and encouragement for each other.

Crisis Intervention

In crisis intervention the therapist, or other intervener, becomes a part of the individual's life situation. Because of increased anxiety, the individual with adjustment disorder is unable to problem-solve, so he or she requires guidance and support from another to help mobilize the resources needed to resolve the crisis. Crisis intervention is short-term, and relies heavily on orderly problem-solving techniques and structured activities that are focused on change. The ultimate goal of crisis intervention in the treatment of adjustment disorder is to resolve the immediate crisis, restore adaptive functioning, and promote personal growth.

Psychopharmacology

Adjustment disorder is not commonly treated with medications, for the following reasons: (1) their effect may be temporary and only mask the real problem, interfering with the possibility of finding a more permanent solution, and (2) psychoactive drugs carry the potential for physiological and psychological dependence.

When the client with adjustment disorder has symptoms of anxiety or depression, the physician may prescribe antianxiety or antidepressant medication. These medications are considered only adjuncts to psychotherapy and should not be given as the primary therapy. In these instances they are given to alleviate symptoms so that the individual may more effectively cope while attempting to adapt to the stressful situation.

CASE STUDY AND SAMPLE CARE PLAN

NURSING HISTORY AND ASSESSMENT

Linda, age 22, was born in a small town in Oklahoma. She lived there her whole life, even living at home while she attended a nearby college to earn a baccalaureate degree in education. She is an only child, and her parents were in their 40s when she was born. She was engaged throughout her college years to her high school sweetheart, Tony, who graduated 6 months ago from the state university with a degree in aeronautical engineering. Upon his graduation, he accepted a position with NASA at Kennedy Space Center in Florida. Linda and Tony were married 5 months ago and moved to a small apartment in Cape Canaveral, where Tony began his work with NASA. The plan was for Linda to seek employment upon their arrival, but she has been unable to move ahead with those plans. She stays in the apartment most days, talking on the phone to her parents, and crying about how much she misses them and her home in Oklahoma. She has met very few people, and has no desire to do so. She sleeps a lot and has lost weight. She has been having severe headaches. Her husband has become very concerned about her, and made an appointment for her with a private physician. Following a complete and unremarkable physical examination, the physician referred Linda to the mental health clinic where she was admitted to the Day Treatment Center with a diagnosis of adjustment disorder with depressed mood.

NURSING DIAGNOSES/OUTCOME IDENTIFICATION

From the assessment data, the nurse develops the following nursing diagnoses for Linda:

1. **Complicated grieving** related to feelings of loss associated with leaving her parents and her lifetime home.
   a. **Short-Term Goal:** Within 1 week, Linda will express anger about the loss associated with her move.
   b. **Long-Term Goal:** Linda will be able to verbalize behaviors associated with the normal stages of grief and identify her own position in the grief process, while progressing at her own pace toward resolution.
2. **Relocation stress syndrome** related to move away from parents and familiar environment in which she had spent her whole life.
   a. **Short-Term Goal:** Within 1 week, Linda will verbalize at least one positive aspect regarding relocation to her new environment.
   b. **Long-Term Goal:** Within 1 month, Linda will demonstrate positive adaptation to her new environment as evidenced by involvement in activities, expression of satisfaction with new acquaintances, and elimination of previously evident physical and psychological symptoms associated with the relocation.

CASE STUDY AND SAMPLE CARE PLAN—cont'd

PLANNING/IMPLEMENTATION

COMPLICATED GRIEVING

The following nursing interventions have been identified for Linda:

1. Determine the stage of grief in which Linda is fixed. Identify behaviors associated with this stage.
2. Develop a trusting relationship with Linda. Show empathy and caring. Be honest and keep all promises.
3. Convey an accepting attitude so that Linda is not afraid to express her feelings openly.
4. Allow Linda to express her anger. Do not become defensive if the initial expression of anger is displaced on nurse or therapist. Help Linda explore angry feelings so that they may be directed toward the intended object or situation.
5. Help Linda discharge pent-up anger through participation in large motor activities (e.g., brisk walks, jogging, physical exercises, or activity of her choice).
6. Explain to Linda the normal stages of grief and the behaviors associated with each stage. Help her to understand that these feelings are normal and acceptable during a grief process.
7. Encourage Linda to review her personal perception of the move. With support and sensitivity, point out the reality of the situation in areas where misrepresentations are expressed.
8. Help Linda solve problems as she attempts to determine methods for more adaptive coping with the life change. Provide positive feedback for strategies identified and decisions made.
9. Encourage Linda to reach out for spiritual support during this time in whatever form is desirable to her. Assess her spiritual needs and assist as necessary in the fulfillment of those needs.

RELOCATION STRESS SYNDROME

The following nursing interventions have been identified for Linda:

1. Encourage Linda to discuss feelings (concerns, fears, anger) regarding this relocation.
2. Encourage Linda to discuss how the change will affect her life. Ensure that Linda is involved in decision making and problem-solving regarding the move.
3. Help Linda identify positive aspects about the move.
4. Help Linda identify resources within the new community from which assistance with various types of services may be obtained.
5. Identify groups within the community that specialize in helping individuals adapt to relocation. Examples include Newcomers' Club, Welcome Wagon International, and school and church organizations.
6. Refer Linda to a support group (e.g., Depression and Bipolar Support Alliance [DBSA]).

EVALUATION

The outcome criteria for Linda have been met. She is no longer having headaches, and she has regained some of her weight. She has joined a chapter of DBSA, and has made some new acquaintances. She has applied to become a substitute teacher in the local school district, and she and Tony have joined the local Methodist church, where they have started to socialize with several couples their age. They have also adopted Molly, a 2-year-old mutt from the local shelter, who showers Linda with love and keeps her company when no one else is around. They take daily walks together. Linda still talks to her parents on the phone daily, but no longer has feelings of despair about living so far away from them. Her parents provide encouragement and give her positive feedback for achieving a satisfactory adaptation to her new environment. They are planning a visit to see Linda and Tony in the near future.

Summary and Key Points

■ Posttraumatic stress disorder (PTSD) is the development of characteristic symptoms following exposure to an extreme traumatic stressor involving a personal threat to physical integrity or to the integrity of others. Symptoms may begin within the first 3 months after the trauma, or there may be a delay of several months or even years.

■ The symptoms of PTSD are associated with events that would be markedly distressing to almost anyone, and include reexperiencing the trauma, a sustained high level of anxiety or arousal, or a general numbing of responsiveness.

■ A disorder that is similar in terms of precipitating traumatic events and symptomatology to PTSD is called acute stress disorder (ASD). In ASD, the symptoms are time limited, up to 1 month following the trauma. If the symptoms last longer than 1 month, the diagnosis would be PTSD.

■ Predisposing factors to trauma-related disorders include psychosocial, learning, cognitive, and biological influences.

■ Adjustment disorders are relatively common. In fact, some studies indicate they are the most commonly ascribed psychiatric diagnoses.

■ Clinical symptoms associated with adjustment disorders include inability to function socially or occupationally in response to an identifiable stressor.

■ Adjustment disorder is distinguished by the predominant features of the maladaptive response. These include depression, anxiety, mixed anxiety and depression, disturbance of conduct, and mixed disturbance of emotions and conduct.

■ Of the two types of stressors discussed (i.e., sudden-shock and continuous), more individuals respond with maladaptive behaviors to long-term continuous stressors.

■ Treatment modalities for PTSD include cognitive therapy, prolonged exposure therapy, group/family therapy, eye movement desensitization and reprocessing (EMDR), and psychopharmacology.

■ Treatment modalities for adjustment disorders include individual psychotherapy, family therapy,

behavior therapy, self-help groups, crisis intervention, and medications to treat anxiety or depression.

■ Nursing care of individuals with trauma- and stressor-related disorders is accomplished using the steps of the nursing process.

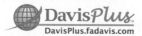 Additional info available at
DavisPlus.fadavis.com   www.davisplus.com

Review Questions
Self-Examination/Learning Exercise

Select the answer that is most appropriate for each of the following questions.

1. John, a veteran of the war in Iraq, is diagnosed with PTSD. He says to the nurse, "I can't figure out why God took my buddy instead of me." From this statement, the nurse assesses which of the following in John?
   a. Repressed anger
   b. Survivor's guilt
   c. Intrusive thoughts
   d. Spiritual distress

2. John, a veteran of the war in Iraq, is diagnosed with PTSD. He experiences a nightmare during his first night in the hospital. He explains to the nurse that he was dreaming about gunfire all around and people being killed. The nurse's most appropriate *initial* intervention is to:
   a. Administer alprazolam as ordered prn for anxiety.
   b. Call the physician and report the incident.
   c. Stay with John and reassure him of his safety.
   d. Have John listen to a tape of relaxation exercises.

3. John, a veteran of the war in Iraq, is diagnosed with PTSD. Which of the following therapy regimens would most appropriately be ordered for John?
   a. Paroxetine and group therapy
   b. Diazepam and implosion therapy
   c. Alprazolam and behavior therapy
   d. Carbamazepine and cognitive therapy

4. Which of the following may be influential in the predisposition to PTSD?
   a. Unsatisfactory parent/child relationship
   b. Excess of the neurotransmitter serotonin
   c. Distorted, negative cognitions
   d. Severity of the stressor and availability of support systems

5. Nina recently left her husband of 10 years. She was very dependent on her husband and is having difficulty adjusting to an independent lifestyle. She has been hospitalized with a diagnosis of adjustment disorder with depressed mood. The *priority* nursing diagnosis for Nina would be:
   a. Risk-prone health behavior related to loss of dependency
   b. Complicated grieving related to breakup of marriage
   c. Ineffective coping related to problems with dependency
   d. Social isolation related to depressed mood

6. Nina, who is depressed following the breakup of a very stormy marriage, says to the nurse, "I feel so bad. I thought I would feel better once I left, but I feel worse!" Which is the *best* response by the nurse?
   a. "Cheer up, Nina. You have a lot to be happy about."
   b. "You are grieving for the marriage you did not have. It's natural for you to feel bad."
   c. "Try not to dwell on how you feel. If you don't think about it, you'll feel better."
   d. "You did the right thing, Nina. Knowing that should make you feel better."

Review Questions—cont'd
Self-Examination/Learning Exercise

7. Nina has been hospitalized with adjustment disorder with depressed mood following the breakup of her marriage. Which of the following is true regarding the diagnosis of adjustment disorder?
   a. Nina will require long-term psychotherapy to achieve relief.
   b. Nina likely inherited a genetic tendency for the disorder.
   c. Nina's symptoms will likely remit once she has accepted the change in her life.
   d. Nina probably would not have experienced adjustment disorder if she had a higher level of intelligence.

8. The physician orders sertraline (Zoloft) for a client who is hospitalized with adjustment disorder with depressed mood. This medication is intended to:
   a. Increase energy and elevate mood.
   b. Stimulate the central nervous system.
   c. Prevent psychotic symptoms.
   d. Produce a calming effect.

9. The category of adjustment disorder with disturbance of conduct identifies the individual who:
   a. Violates the rights of others to feel better
   b. Expresses symptoms that reveal a high level of anxiety
   c. Exhibits severe social isolation and withdrawal
   d. Is experiencing a complicated grieving process

10. Carol, age 16, has recently been diagnosed with diabetes mellitus. She must watch her diet and take an oral hypoglycemic medication daily. She has become very depressed and her mother reports that Carol refuses to change her diet and often skips her medication. Carol has been hospitalized for stabilization of her blood sugar. The psychiatric nurse practitioner has been called in as a consult. Which of the following nursing diagnoses by the psychiatric nurse would be a priority for Carol at this time?
    a. Anxiety related to hospitalization evidenced by noncompliance
    b. Low self-esteem related to feeling different from her peers evidenced by social isolation
    c. Risk for suicide related to new diagnosis of diabetes mellitus
    d. Risk-prone health behavior related to denial of seriousness of her illness evidenced by refusal to follow diet and take medication

TEST YOUR CRITICAL THINKING SKILLS

Alice, age 48, underwent a mastectomy of the right breast after her mammogram revealed a lump that proved to be malignant when biopsied. Since her surgery 6 weeks ago, Alice has refused to see any of her friends. She stays in her bedroom, speaks to her husband only when he speaks first, is having difficulty sleeping, and eats very little. She refuses to look at the mastectomy scar and has refused to see the Reach to Recovery representative who has tried several times to help fit her with a prosthesis. Her husband has become very worried about her and spoke to the family doctor, who recommended a psychiatrist. She has been admitted to the psychiatric unit with a diagnosis of adjustment disorder with depressed mood.

Answer the following questions about Alice:

1. What would be the primary nursing diagnosis for Alice?
2. Describe a short-term goal and a long-term goal for Alice.
3. Discuss a priority nursing intervention in working with Alice.

References

Aetna Healthcare. (2013). *Clinical policy bulletin: Eye movement desensitization and Reprocessing (EMDR) therapy.* Retrieved from www.aetna.com/cpb/medical/data/500_599/0583.html

American Psychiatric Association (APA). (2000) *Diagnostic and statistical manual of mental disorders* (4th ed., text rev.) Washington, DC: Author.

American Psychiatric Association (APA). (2013) *Diagnostic and statistical manual of mental Disorders* (5th ed.). Washington, DC: Author.

Bartson, S., Smith, M., & Corcoran, C. (2011). *EMDR therapy: A guide to making an informed choice.* Retrieved from www.anapsys.co.uk/emdr.pdf

Black, D.W., & Andreasen, N.C. (2011). *Introductory textbook of psychiatry.* Washington, DC: American Psychiatric Publishing.

Breslau, N. (2009, July). The epidemiology of trauma, PTSD, and other post-trauma disorders. *Trauma, Violence, & Abuse, 10*(3), 198-210.

Center for Integrative Medicine. (2013). *Eye movement desensitization and reprocessing.* Retrieved from www.upmc.com/Services/integrative-medicine/outpatient-services/Pages/eye-movement.aspx

Department of Veterans Affairs. (2012). *How common is PTSD?* Retrieved from www.ptsd.va.gov/public/pages/how-common-is-ptsd.asp

EMDR Network. (2013). *A brief description of EMDR therapy: Eight phases of treatment.* Retrieved from www.emdrnetwork.org/description.html

Epstein, S. (1991). Beliefs and symptoms in maladaptive resolutions of the traumatic neurosis. In D. Ozer, J.M. Healy, Jr., & A. J. Stewart (Eds.), *Perspectives on personality* (Vol. 3). London: Jessica Kingsley.

Friedman, M.J. (1996). PTSD Diagnosis and treatment for mental health clinicians. *Community Mental Health Journal, 32*(2), 173-189.

Friedman, M.J., Resick, P.A., Bryant, R.A., Strain, J., Horowitz, M., & Spiegel, D. (2011). Classification of trauma and stressor-related disorders in DSM-5. *Depression and Anxiety, 28*(9), 737-749.

Hageman, I., Anderson, H.S., & Jergensen, M.B. (2001). Post-traumatic stress disorder: A review of psychobiology and pharmacotherapy. *ACTA Psychiatrica Scandinavica, 104,* 411-422.

Hollander, E., & Simeon, D. (2008). Anxiety disorders. In R.E. Hales, S.C. Yudofsky, & G.O. Gabbard (Eds.), *Textbook of psychiatry* (5th ed., 505-607). Washington, DC: American Psychiatric Publishing.

NANDA International (NANDA-I). (2012). *Nursing diagnoses: Definitions and classification 2012-2014.* Hoboken, NJ: Wiley-Blackwell.

Puri, B.K., & Treasaden, I.H. (2011). *Textbook of psychiatry.* Philadelphia, PA: Churchill Livingstone Elsevier.

Sadock, B.J., & Sadock, V.A. (2007). *Synopsis of psychiatry: Behavioral sciences/clinical psychiatry* (10th ed.). Philadelphia, PA: Lippincott Williams & Wilkins.

Shapiro, F. (2007). EMDR and case conceptualization from an adaptive information processing perspective. In F. Shapiro, F.W. Kaslow, & L. Maxfield (Eds.), *Handbook of EMDR and family therapy processes* (pp. 3-34). Hoboken, NJ: John Wiley & Sons.

Strain, J.J., Klipstein, K.G., & Newcorn, J.H. (2008). Adjustment disorders. In R.E. Hales, S.C. Yudofsky, & G.O. Gabbard (Eds.), *Textbook of psychiatry* (5th ed., pp. 755-775). Washington, DC: American Psychiatric Publishing.

Classical References

Freud, S. (1964). New introductory lectures on psychoanalysis and other works. In *The standard edition of the complete psychological works of Sigmund Freud* (Vol. 22). London: Hogarth Press.

@ INTERNET REFERENCES

- Additional information about trauma- and stressor-related disorders may be located at the following websites:
  - http://www.mentalhealth.com/rx/p23-aj01.html
  - http://www.psyweb.com/Mdisord/jsp/adjd.jsp
  - http://emedicine.medscape.com/article/2192631-overview
  - http://www.athealth.com/Consumer/disorders/Adjustment.html
  - http://www.nlm.nih.gov/medlineplus/ency/article/000932.htm
  - http://www.mayoclinic.com/health/adjustment-disorders/DS00584
  - http://www.ptsd.va.gov/
  - http://www.nimh.nih.gov/health/topics/post-traumatic-stress-disorder-ptsd/index.shtml
  - http://www.ptsd.va.gov/professional/treatment/early/acute-stress-disorder.asp

Somatic Symptom and Dissociative Disorders

29

CORE CONCEPTS

amnesia

dissociation

hysteria

KEY TERMS

abreaction

anosmia

aphonia

depersonalization

derealization

factitious disorder

fugue

integration

Munchausen syndrome

primary gain

pseudocyesis

secondary gain

tertiary gain

OBJECTIVES
After reading this chapter, the student will be able to:

1. Discuss historical aspects and epidemiological statistics related to somatic symptom and dissociative disorders.
2. Describe various types of somatic symptom and dissociative disorders and identify symptomatology associated with each; use this information in client assessment.
3. Identify predisposing factors in the development of somatic symptom and dissociative disorders.
4. Formulate nursing diagnoses and goals of care for clients with somatic symptom and dissociative disorders.

5. Describe appropriate nursing interventions for behaviors associated with somatic symptom and dissociative disorders.
6. Evaluate the nursing care of clients with somatic symptom and dissociative disorders.
7. Discuss various modalities relevant to treatment of somatic symptom and dissociative disorders.

HOMEWORK ASSIGNMENT
Please read the chapter and answer the following questions:

1. Past experience with serious or life-threatening physical illness, either personal or that of a close family member, can predispose an individual to what somatic symptom disorder?
2. In an individual with dissociative identity disorder, what most commonly precipitates transition from one personality to another?

3. Conversion symptoms most commonly occur in an individual for what reason?
4. Somatic symptom and dissociative disorders are the physical/behavioral responses to what unconscious phenomenon?

Somatic symptom disorders are characterized by physical symptoms suggesting medical disease, but without demonstrable organic pathology or known pathophysiological mechanism to account for them. They are classified as mental disorders because pathophysiological processes are not demonstrable or understandable by existing laboratory procedures, and there is either evidence or strong presumption that psychological factors are the major cause of the symptoms. It is now well documented that a large proportion of clients in general medical outpatient clinics and private medical offices do not have organic disease requiring medical treatment. It is likely that many of these clients have somatic symptom disorders, but they do not perceive themselves as having a psychiatric problem and thus do not seek treatment from psychiatrists.

Dissociative disorders are defined by a disturbance of or alteration in the usually integrated functions of consciousness, memory, and identity (Black & Andreasen, 2011). Dissociative responses occur when anxiety becomes overwhelming and the personality becomes disorganized. Defense mechanisms that normally govern consciousness, identity, and memory break down, and behavior occurs with little or no participation on the part of the conscious personality. Types of dissociative disorders described by the *Diagnostic and Statistical Manual of Mental Disorders (DSM-5)*:

- Depersonalization-derealization disorder
- Dissociative amnesia
- Dissociative identity disorder
- Other specified dissociative disorder
- Unspecified dissociative disorder

This chapter focuses on disorders characterized by severe anxiety that has been repressed and is being expressed in the form of physiological symptoms and dissociative behaviors. Historical and epidemiological statistics are presented. Predisposing factors that have been implicated in the etiology of these responses provide a framework for studying the dynamics of somatic symptom and dissociative disorders. An explanation of the symptomatology of these disorders is presented as background knowledge for assessing the client, and nursing care is described in the context of the nursing process. Additional treatment modalities are explored.

Historical Aspects

CORE CONCEPT

Hysteria

A polysymptomatic disorder that usually begins in adolescence (rarely after the 20s), chiefly affects women, and is characterized by recurrent multiple somatic complaints that are unexplained by organic pathology. It is thought to be associated with repressed anxiety.

Historically, somatic symptom disorders were identified as *hysterical neuroses*. The concept of hysteria is at least 4,000 years old and probably originated in Egypt. The name has been in use since the time of Hippocrates.

Over the years, symptoms of hysterical neuroses have been associated with witchcraft, demonology, and sorcery; dysfunction of the nervous system; and unexpressed emotion. Somatic symptom disorders are thought to occur in response to repressed severe anxiety. Freud observed that, under hypnosis, clients with hysterical neurosis could recall past memories and emotional experiences that would relieve their symptoms. This led to his proposal that unexpressed emotion can be "converted" into physical symptoms.

CORE CONCEPT

Dissociation

The splitting off of clusters of mental contents from conscious awareness, a mechanism central to hysterical conversion and dissociative disorder (Shahrokh & Hales, 2003).

Freud (1962) viewed dissociation as a type of repression, an active defense mechanism used to remove threatening or unacceptable mental contents from conscious awareness. He also described the defense of splitting of the ego in the management of incompatible mental contents. Despite the fact that the study of dissociative processes dates back to the 19th century, scientists still know remarkably little about the phenomena. Questions still remain unanswered: Are dissociative disorders psychopathological processes or ego-protective devices? Are dissociative processes under voluntary control, or are they a totally unconscious effort? Maldonado and Spiegel (2008) state:

> [These disorders] have much to teach us about the way humans adapt to traumatic stress, and about information processing in the brain. (p. 665)

The syndrome of fabricating symptoms for emotional gain was first described by Richard Asher in 1951 in an article in *The Lancet*. He described a pattern of behavior in which individuals fabricated or embellished their histories and signs and symptoms of illness. He termed this condition **Munchausen syndrome** after Baron Friedrich Hieronymus Freiherr von Munchhausen, a German cavalry officer and nobleman, who was known for his fabricated stories and fanciful exaggerations about himself (Asher, 1951).

Epidemiological Statistics

The prevalence of somatic symptom disorder is thought to be about 5 to 7 percent in the general population (APA, 2013). It is more common in women than in men, in rural areas, and in less educated persons (Black & Andreasen, 2011).

Lifetime prevalence rates of conversion disorder vary widely. Statistics within the general population have ranged from 5 to 30 percent. The disorder occurs more frequently in women than in men and more frequently in adolescents and young adults than in other age groups. A higher prevalence exists in lower socioeconomic groups, rural populations, and among those with less education (Black & Andreasen, 2011; Sadock & Sadock, 2007).

The disorder previously known as hypochondriasis (fear of having a serious disease) affects 1 to 5 percent of the general population. The disorder is equally common among men and women, and onset most commonly occurs in early adulthood. This disorder, which appeared in the *DSM-IV-TR* (APA, 2000), no longer appears as such in the *DSM-5*. Rationale for the change was that about 75 percent of individuals with hypochondriasis fall into a subgroup in which somatic symptoms are the primary complaint. The other 25 percent fall into a subgroup in which there are minimal or no somatic complaints, but who present with intense anxiety and suspiciousness of the presence of an undiagnosed, serious medical illness (APA, 2013). Therefore, the 75 percent of individuals with somatic symptoms are considered to have somatic symptom disorder, and those with minimal or no somatic symptoms would be diagnosed with illness anxiety disorder, a diagnosis new to the *DSM-5*. The diagnosis previously known as pain disorder has also been subsumed under the diagnosis of somatic symptom disorder. Body dysmorphic disorder is now a category under the Obsessive-Compulsive and Related Disorders classification.

Data on the prevalence of **factitious disorder** (discussed later in the chapter) is limited and frequency of the disorder is unknown. Estimates suggest that individuals with factitious disorder may comprise about 0.8 to 1.0 percent of psychiatric consultation clients (Sadock & Sadock, 2007).

Dissociative syndromes are statistically quite rare, but when they do occur they may present very dramatic clinical pictures of severe disturbances in normal personality functioning. Dissociative amnesia is relatively rare, occurring most frequently under conditions of war or during natural disasters. However, in recent years, there has been an increase in the number of reported cases, possibly attributed to increased awareness of the phenomenon, and identification of cases that were previously undiagnosed. It appears to be equally common in men and women. Dissociative amnesia can occur at any age but is difficult to diagnose in children because it is easily confused with inattention or oppositional behavior.

Estimates of the prevalence of dissociative identity disorder (DID) vary widely. Historically, it was thought to be quite rare; however, the number of reported cases has grown rapidly in the past few decades. The disorder occurs from five to nine times more frequently in women than in men (Sadock & Sadock, 2007). Onset likely occurs in childhood, although manifestations of the disorder may not be recognized until much later. Clinical symptoms usually are not recognized until late adolescence or early adulthood, although they have probably existed for a number of years prior to diagnosis. There appears to be some evidence that the disorder is more common in first-degree biological relatives of people with the disorder than in the general population.

The prevalence of severe episodes of depersonalization-derealization disorder is unknown. It is thought that single brief episodes may occur at some time in as many as half of all adults, particularly when under severe psychosocial stress, when sleep deprived, during travel to unfamiliar places, or when intoxicated with hallucinogens, marijuana, or alcohol (Black & Andreasen, 2011). Symptoms usually begin in adolescence or early adulthood. The disorder is chronic, with periods of remission and exacerbation. The incidence of depersonalization-derealization disorder is high under conditions of sustained traumatization, such as in military combat or prisoner-of-war camps. It has also been reported in many individuals who endure near-death experiences.

Application of the Nursing Process

Background Assessment Data: Types of Somatic Symptom Disorders

Somatic Symptom Disorder

Somatic symptom disorder is a syndrome of multiple somatic symptoms that cannot be explained medically and are associated with psychosocial distress and long-term seeking of assistance from health-care professionals. Symptoms may be vague, dramatized, or exaggerated in their presentation, and an excessive amount of time and energy is devoted to worry and concern about the symptoms. Individuals with somatic symptom disorder are so totally convinced that their symptoms are related to organic pathology that they adamantly reject, and are often irritated by, any implication that stress or psychosocial factors play any role in their condition. The disorder is chronic, with symptoms beginning before age 30. Anxiety and depression are frequently manifested, and suicidal threats and attempts are not uncommon.

The disorder usually runs a fluctuating course, with periods of remission and exacerbation. Clients often receive medical care from several physicians, sometimes concurrently, leading to the possibility of dangerous combinations of treatments. They have a tendency to seek relief through overmedicating with prescribed analgesics or antianxiety agents. Drug abuse and dependence are common complications of somatic symptom disorder. When suicide results, it is usually in association with substance abuse (Sadock & Sadock, 2007).

It has been suggested that, in somatic symptom disorder, there may be some overlapping of personality characteristics and features associated with histrionic personality disorder. These symptoms include heightened emotionality, impressionistic thought and speech, seductiveness, strong dependency needs, and a preoccupation with symptoms and oneself.

The *DSM-5* diagnostic criteria for somatic symptom disorder are presented in Box 29-1.

Illness Anxiety Disorder

Illness anxiety disorder may be defined as an unrealistic or inaccurate interpretation of physical symptoms or sensations, leading to preoccupation and fear of having a serious disease. The fear becomes disabling and persists despite appropriate reassurance that no organic pathology can be detected. Symptoms may be minimal or absent, but the individual is highly anxious about and suspicious of the presence of an undiagnosed, serious medical illness (APA, 2013).

Individuals with illness anxiety disorder are extremely conscious of bodily sensations and changes, and may become convinced that a rapid heart rate indicates they have heart disease or that a small sore is skin cancer. They are profoundly preoccupied with their bodies and are totally aware of even the slightest change in feeling or sensation. Their response to these small changes, however, is usually unrealistic and exaggerated.

Some individuals with illness anxiety disorder have a long history of "doctor shopping" and are convinced that they are not receiving the proper care. Others avoid seeking medical assistance because to do so would increase their anxiety to intolerable levels. Depression is common, and obsessive-compulsive traits frequently accompany the disorder. Preoccupation with the fear of serious disease may interfere with social or occupational functioning. Some individuals are able to function appropriately on the job, however, while limiting their physical complaints to non-work time.

Individuals with illness anxiety disorder are so apprehensive and fearful that they become alarmed at the slightest intimation of serious illness. Even reading about a disease or hearing that someone they know has been diagnosed with an illness precipitates alarm on their part.

The *DSM-5* diagnostic criteria for illness anxiety disorder are presented in Box 29-2.

Conversion Disorder (Functional Neurological Symptom Disorder)

Conversion disorder is a loss of or change in body function that cannot be explained by any known medical disorder or pathophysiological mechanism. There is most likely a psychological component involved in the initiation, exacerbation, or perpetuation of the symptom, although it may or may not be obvious or identifiable.

BOX 29-1 Diagnostic Criteria for Somatic Symptom Disorder

A. One or more somatic symptoms that are distressing or result in significant disruption in daily life.
B. Excessive thoughts, feelings, or behaviors related to the somatic symptoms or associated health concerns as manifested by at least one of the following:
   1. Disproportionate and persistent thoughts about the seriousness of one's symptoms.
   2. Persistently high level of anxiety about health or symptoms.
   3. Excessive time and energy devoted to these symptoms or health concerns.
C. Although any one symptom may not be continuously present, the state of being symptomatic is persistent (typically more than 6 months).

Specify if:
   With predominant pain (the somatic symptoms predominantly involve pain)
   Persistent (a persistent course is characterized by severe symptoms, marked impairment, and long duration [more than 6 months])
Specify current severity:
   Mild (only one of the symptoms specified in Criterion B is fulfilled)
   Moderate (two or more of the symptoms specified in Criterion B are fulfilled)
   Severe (two or more of the symptoms specified in Criterion B are fulfilled, plus there are multiple somatic complaints [or one very severe somatic symptom])

Conversion symptoms affect voluntary motor or sensory functioning suggestive of neurological disease. Examples include paralysis, **aphonia** (inability to produce voice), seizures, coordination disturbance, difficulty swallowing, urinary retention, akinesia, blindness, deafness, double vision, **anosmia** (inability to perceive smell), loss of pain sensation, and hallucinations. **Pseudocyesis** (false pregnancy) is a conversion symptom and may represent a strong desire to be pregnant.

Previous criteria in the *DSM-IV-TR* (APA, 2000) stated that the precipitation of conversion symptoms must be explained by psychological factors. This criterion has been removed in the *DSM-5*, which states, "The potential etiological relevance of stress or trauma may be suggested by a close temporal relationship. However, while assessment for stress and trauma is important, the diagnosis should not be withheld if none is found" (APA, 2013, pp. 319-320). It is likely that multiple causes play a role in the etiology.

Most symptoms of conversion disorder resolve within a few weeks. About 20 percent of individuals with the diagnosis have a relapse within 1 year. Black and Andreasen (2011) state, "A favorable outcome is generally associated with acute onset, a precipitating stressful event, good premorbid adjustment, and the absence of medical or neurological comorbidity" (p. 216).

The *DSM-5* diagnostic criteria for conversion disorder are presented in Box 29-3.

Psychological Factors Affecting Other Medical Conditions

Psychological factors may play a role in virtually any medical condition. In this disorder, it is evident that psychological or behavioral factors have been implicated in the development, exacerbation, or delayed recovery from a medical condition. Historically, mind and body have been viewed as two distinct entities, each subject to different laws of causality. Indeed, in many instances—particularly in highly specialized areas of medicine—the biological and psychological components of disease remain separate. However, medical research shows that a change is occurring. Research associated with biological functioning is being expanded to include the psychological and social determinants of health and disease. This psychobiological approach to illness reflects a more holistic perspective and one that promotes concern for helping clients achieve optimal functioning.

With this diagnosis, there is objective evidence of a general medical condition that has been precipitated by or is being perpetuated by psychological or behavioral circumstances. The *DSM-5* diagnostic criteria for psychological factors affecting other medical conditions are presented in Box 29-4.

Factitious Disorder

Factitious disorder involves conscious, intentional feigning of physical or psychological symptoms (Black & Andreasen, 2011). Individuals with factitious disorder pretend to be ill in order to receive emotional care and support commonly associated with the role of "patient." Even though the behaviors are deliberate and intentional, there may be an associated compulsive element that diminishes personal control. Individuals may aggravate existing symptoms, induce new ones, or even inflict painful injuries on themselves (Sadock & Sadock, 2007). The disorder may also be identified as *Munchausen syndrome*, and symptoms may be psychological, physical, or a combination of both.

BOX 29-3 Diagnostic Criteria for Conversion Disorder (Functional Neurological Symptom Disorder)

A. One or more symptoms of altered voluntary motor or sensory function.
B. Clinical findings provide evidence of incompatibility between the symptom and recognized neurological or medical conditions.
C. The symptom or deficit is not better explained by another medical or mental disorder.
D. The symptom or deficit causes clinically significant distress or impairment in social, occupational, or other important areas of functioning or warrants medical evaluation.

Specify symptom type:
　　With weakness or paralysis
　　With abnormal movement
　　With swallowing symptoms
　　With speech symptom
　　With attacks or seizures
　　With anesthesia or sensory loss
　　With special sensory symptom
　　With mixed symptoms
Specify if:
　　Acute episode
　　Persistent
Specify if:
　　With psychological stressor
　　Without psychological stressor

Reprinted with permission from the *Diagnostic and Statistical Manual of Mental Disorders, Fifth Edition* (Copyright 2013). American Psychiatric Association.

BOX 29-4 Diagnostic Criteria for Psychological Factors Affecting Other Medical Conditions

A. A medical symptom or condition (other than a mental disorder) is present.
B. Psychological or behavioral factors adversely affect the general medical condition in one of the following ways:
　1. The factors have influenced the course of the medical condition as shown by a close temporal association between the psychological factors and the development or exacerbation of, or delayed recovery from, the medical condition.
　2. The factors interfere with the treatment of the medical condition (e.g., poor adherence).
　3. The factors constitute additional well-established health risks for the individual.
　4. The factors influence the underlying pathophysiology, precipitating or exacerbating symptoms or necessitating medical attention.
C. The psychological and behavioral factors in Criterion B are not better explained by another mental disorder (e.g., panic disorder, major depressive disorder, posttraumatic stress disorder).

Specify current severity:
　　Mild: Increases medical risk
　　Moderate: Aggravates underlying medical condition
　　Severe: Results in medical hospitalization or emergency room visit
　　Extreme: Results in severe, life-threatening risk

Reprinted with permission from the *Diagnostic and Statistical Manual of Mental Disorders, Fifth Edition* (Copyright 2013). American Psychiatric Association.

The disorder may be imposed on oneself, or on another person (previously called *factitious disorder by proxy*). In the latter case, physical symptoms are intentionally imposed on a person under the care of the perpetrator. Diagnosis of factitious disorder can be very difficult, as individuals become very inventive in their quest to produce symptoms. Examples include self-inflicted wounds, injection or insertion of contaminated substances, manipulating a thermometer to feign a fever, urinary tract manipulation, and surreptitious use of medications (Black & Andreasen, 2011, p. 236).

The *DSM-5* diagnostic criteria for factitious disorder are presented in Box 29-5.

Predisposing Factors Associated With Somatic Symptom Disorders

Genetic

Studies have shown an increased incidence of somatic symptom disorder, conversion disorder, and illness anxiety disorder in first-degree relatives, implying a possible inheritable predisposition (Sadock

---

BOX 29-5 Diagnostic Criteria for Factitious Disorder

Factitious Disorder Imposed on Self

A. Falsification of physical or psychological signs or symptoms, or induction of injury or disease, associated with identified deception.
B. The individual presents himself or herself to others as ill, impaired, or injured.
C. The deceptive behavior is evident even in the absence of obvious external rewards.
D. The behavior is not better explained by another mental disorder, such as delusional disorder or other psychotic disorder.

Specify:
   Single episode
   Recurrent episodes

Factitious Disorder Imposed on Another (Previously Factitious Disorder by Proxy)

A. Falsification of physical or psychological signs or symptoms, or induction of injury or disease in another, associated with identified deception.
B. The individual presents another individual (victim) to others as ill, impaired, or injured.
C. The deceptive behavior is evident even in the absence of obvious external rewards.
D. The behavior is not better explained by another mental disorder, such as delusional disorder or other psychotic disorder.
   Note: The perpetrator, not the victim, receives this diagnosis.

Specify:
   Single episode
   Recurrent episodes

Reprinted with permission from the *Diagnostic and Statistical Manual of Mental Disorders, Fifth Edition* (Copyright 2013). American Psychiatric Association.

& Sadock, 2007; Soares & Grossman, 2012; Yutzy & Parish, 2008).

Biochemical

Decreased levels of serotonin and endorphins may play a role in the etiology of somatic symptom disorder, predominantly pain. Serotonin is probably the main neurotransmitter involved in inhibiting the firing of afferent pain fibers (Parcell, 2008). The deficiency of endorphins seems to correlate with an increase of incoming sensory (pain) stimuli (Wootton, 2008).

Neuroanatomical

Brain dysfunction has been proposed by some researchers as a factor in factitious disorders (Sadock & Sadock, 2007). The hypothesis is that impairment in information processing contributes to the aberrant behaviors associated with the disorder. However, no genetic patterns have been identified, nor have specific electroencephalographic (EEG) abnormalities been noted in clients with factitious disorder.

Psychodynamic

Some psychodynamicists view illness anxiety disorder as an ego defense mechanism. Physical complaints are the expression of low self-esteem and feelings of worthlessness, because it is easier to feel something is wrong with the body than to feel something is wrong with the self. Another psychodynamic view of illness anxiety disorder (as well as somatic symptom disorder, predominantly pain) is related to a defense against guilt. The individual views the self as "bad," based on real or imagined past misconduct, and views physical suffering as the deserved punishment required for atonement. This view has also been related to individuals with factitious disorders.

The psychodynamic theory of conversion disorder proposes that emotions associated with a traumatic event that the individual cannot express because of moral or ethical unacceptability are "converted" into physical symptoms. The unacceptable emotions are repressed and converted to a somatic hysterical symptom that is symbolic in some way of the original emotional trauma.

Some reports suggest that individuals with factitious disorders were victims of child abuse or neglect. Frequent childhood hospitalizations provided a reprieve from the traumatic home situation and a loving and caring environment that was absent in the child's family. This theory proposes that the individual with factitious disorder is attempting to recapture the only positive support he or she may have known by seeking out the environment in which it was received as a child. Regarding factitious disorder imposed on another, Sadock and Sadock (2007) have stated, "One apparent purpose of the behavior is for the caretaker to indirectly assume the sick role; another is to be relieved of the caretaking role by having the child hospitalized" (p. 661).

Family Dynamics

Some families have difficulty expressing emotions openly and resolving conflicts verbally. When this occurs, the child may become ill, and a shift in focus is made from the open conflict to the child's illness, leaving unresolved the underlying issues that the family cannot confront openly. Thus, somatization in the child brings some stability to the family, as harmony replaces discord and the child's welfare becomes the common concern. The child in turn receives positive reinforcement for the illness. This shift in focus from family discord to concern for the child is sometimes called **tertiary gain** (see following section).

Learning Theory

Somatic complaints are often reinforced when the sick role relieves the individual from the need to deal with a stressful situation, whether it be within society or within the family. The sick person learns that he or she may avoid stressful obligations, may postpone unwelcome challenges, and is excused from troublesome duties (**primary gain**); becomes the prominent focus of attention because of the illness (**secondary gain**); or relieves conflict within the family as concern is shifted to the ill person and away from the real issue (tertiary gain). These types of positive reinforcements virtually guarantee repetition of the response.

Past experience with serious or life-threatening physical illness, either personal or that of close family members, can predispose an individual to illness anxiety disorder. Once an individual has experienced a threat to biological integrity, he or she may develop a fear of recurrence. The fear of recurring illness generates an exaggerated response to minor physical changes, leading to excessive anxiety and health concerns.

Transactional Model of Stress/Adaptation

The etiology of somatic symptom disorders is most likely influenced by multiple factors. In Figure 29-1, a graphic depiction of this theory of multiple causation is presented in the Transactional Model of Stress/Adaptation.

Background Assessment Data: Types of Dissociative Disorders

Dissociative Amnesia

> ### ▌ CORE CONCEPT
>
> **Amnesia**
>
> Pathologic loss of memory; a phenomenon in which an area of experience becomes inaccessible to conscious recall. The loss in memory may be organic, emotional, dissociative, or of mixed origin, and may be permanent or limited to a sharply circumscribed period of time. (Shahrokh & Hales, 2003)

Dissociative amnesia is an inability to recall important personal information, usually of a traumatic or stressful nature, that is too extensive to be explained by ordinary forgetfulness, and is not due to the direct effects of substance use or a neurological or other medical condition (APA, 2013). The *DSM-5* states that the most common types of dissociative amnesia are localized, selective, and generalized. Localized and selective amnesia are related to a specific stressful event that has occurred. For example, the individual with *localized amnesia* is unable to recall all incidents associated with a stressful event. It may be broader than just a single event, however, such as being unable to remember months or years of child abuse (APA, 2013). In *selective amnesia*, the individual can recall only certain incidents associated with a stressful event for a specific period after the event. In the *generalized* type, the individual has amnesia for his or her identity and total life history.

The individual with amnesia usually appears alert and may give no indication to observers that anything is wrong, although some clients may present with alterations in consciousness, with conversion symptoms, or in trance states. Clients suffering from amnesia are often brought to general hospital emergency departments by police who have found them wandering confusedly around the streets.

Onset of an amnestic episode usually follows severe psychosocial stress. Termination is typically abrupt and followed by complete recovery. Recurrences are unusual. A specific subtype of dissociative amnesia is *with dissociative fugue*. Dissociative **fugue** is characterized by a sudden, unexpected travel away from customary place of daily activities, or by bewildered wandering, with the inability to recall some or all of one's past. An individual in a fugue state may not be able to recall personal identity and sometimes assumes a new identity (Black & Andreasen, 2011).

The *DSM-5* diagnostic criteria for dissociative amnesia are presented in Box 29-6.

Dissociative Identity Disorder

Dissociative identity disorder (DID) was formerly called multiple personality disorder. This disorder is characterized by the existence of two or more personalities in a single individual. Only one of the personalities is evident at any given moment, and one of them is dominant most of the time over the course of the disorder. Each personality is unique and composed of a complex set of memories, behavior patterns, and social relationships that surface during the dominant interval. Transition from one personality to another may be sudden or gradual, and is sometimes quite dramatic. Black and Andreasen (2011) state, "Switches have been observed with stressful situations, disputes among the alters, and psychological conflicts" (p. 230). A switch may occur with a sudden disruption in the individual's train of thought. There

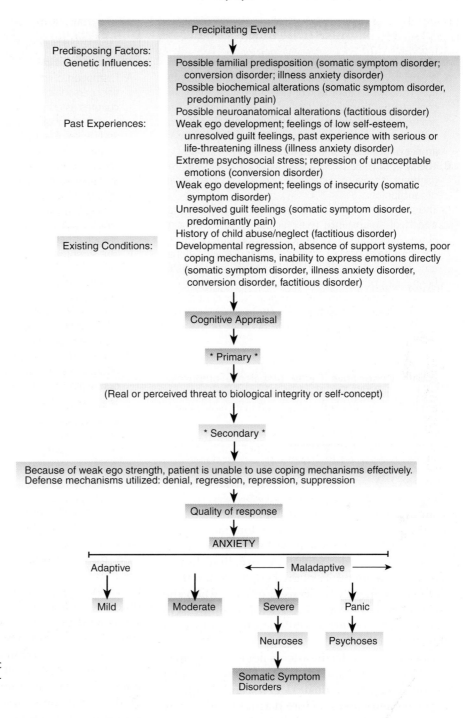

FIGURE 29–1 The dynamics of somatic symptom disorders using the Transactional Model of Stress/Adaptation.

may be rapid eye blinking and changes in voice or facial expression.

Before therapy, the original personality usually has no knowledge of the other personalities, but when there are two or more subpersonalities, they are usually aware of each other's existence. Most often, the various subpersonalities have different names, but they may be unnamed and may be of a different gender, race, and age. The various personalities are almost always quite disparate and may even appear to be the exact opposite of the original

personality. For example, a normally shy, socially withdrawn, faithful husband may become a gregarious womanizer and heavy drinker with the emergence of another personality.

Generally, there is amnesia for the events that took place when another personality was in the dominant position, and clients report "gaps" in autobiographical histories. Sometimes, however, one personality does not experience such amnesia and retains complete awareness of the existence, qualities, and activities of the other personalities. Subpersonalities that

BOX 29-6 Diagnostic Criteria for Dissociative Amnesia

A. An inability to recall important autobiographical information, usually of a traumatic or stressful nature, that is inconsistent with ordinary forgetting. *Note:* Dissociative amnesia most often consists of localized or selective amnesia for a specific event or events; or generalized amnesia for identity and life history.

B. The symptoms cause clinically significant distress or impairment in social, occupational, or other important areas of functioning.

C. The disturbance is not attributable to the physiological effects of a substance (e.g., alcohol or other drug of abuse, a medication) or a neurological or other medical condition (e.g., partial complex seizures, transient global amnesia, sequelae of a closed head injury/traumatic brain injury, other neurological condition).

D. The disturbance is not better explained by dissociative identity disorder, posttraumatic stress disorder, acute stress disorder, somatic symptom disorder, or major or mild neurocognitive disorder.

Specify if:

With Dissociative Fugue (Apparently purposeful travel or bewildered wandering that is associated with amnesia for identity or for other important autobiographical information.)

Reprinted with permission from the *Diagnostic and Statistical Manual of Mental Disorders, Fifth Edition* (Copyright 2013). American Psychiatric Association.

BOX 29-7 Diagnostic Criteria for Dissociative Identity Disorder

A. Disruption of identity characterized by two or more distinct personality states, which may be described in some cultures as an experience of possession. The disruption in identity involves marked discontinuity in sense of self and sense of agency, accompanied by related alterations in affect, behavior, consciousness, memory, perception, cognition, and/or sensory-motor functioning. These signs and symptoms may be observed by others or reported by the individual.

B. Recurrent gaps in the recall of everyday events, important personal information, and/or traumatic events that are inconsistent with ordinary forgetting.

C. The symptoms cause clinically significant distress or impairment in social, occupational, or other important areas of functioning.

D. The disturbance is not a normal part of a broadly accepted cultural or religious practice. *Note:* In children, the symptoms are not better explained by imaginary playmates or other fantasy play.

E. The symptoms are not attributable to the physiological effects of a substance (e.g., blackouts or chaotic behavior during alcohol intoxication) or another medical condition (e.g., complex partial seizures).

Reprinted with permission from the *Diagnostic and Statistical Manual of Mental Disorders, Fifth Edition* (Copyright 2013). American Psychiatric Association.

are amnestic for the other subpersonalities experience the periods when others are dominant as "lost time" or blackouts. They may "wake up" in unfamiliar situations with no idea where they are, how they got there, or of the identities of the people around them. They may frequently be accused of lying when they deny remembering or being responsible for events or actions that occurred while another personality controlled the body.

Dissociative identity disorder is not always incapacitating. Some individuals with DID maintain responsible positions, complete graduate degrees, and are successful spouses and parents before diagnosis and while in treatment. Before they are diagnosed with DID, many individuals are misdiagnosed with depression, borderline and antisocial personality disorders, schizophrenia, epilepsy, or bipolar disorder.

The *DSM-5* diagnostic criteria for DID are presented in Box 29-7.

Depersonalization-Derealization Disorder

Depersonalization-derealization disorder is characterized by a temporary change in the quality of self-awareness, which often takes the form of feelings of unreality, changes in body image, feelings of detachment from the environment, or a sense of observing oneself from outside the body. **Depersonalization** (a disturbance in the perception of oneself) is differentiated from **derealization**, which describes an alteration in the perception of the external environment. Both of these phenomena also occur in a variety of psychiatric illnesses such as schizophrenia, depression, anxiety states, and neurocognitive disorders. As previously stated, the symptoms of depersonalization and derealization are very common. It is estimated that approximately half of all adults have experienced transient episodes of the symptoms. Diagnosis of the disorder is made only if the symptoms cause significant distress or impairment in functioning.

The *DSM-5* describes this disorder as the persistence or recurrence of episodes of depersonalization, derealization, or both (APA, 2013). There may be a mechanical or dreamlike feeling or a belief that the body's physical characteristics have changed. If derealization is present, objects in the environment are perceived as altered in size or shape. Other people in the environment may seem automated or mechanical.

These distorted perceptions are experienced as disturbing, and are often accompanied by anxiety, depression, fear of going insane, obsessive thoughts, somatic complaints, and an alteration in the subjective sense of time. The disorder occurs more often in women than it does in men and is a disorder of younger people, rarely occurring in individuals older than 40 years of age (Black & Andreasen, 2011).

The *DSM-5* diagnostic criteria for depersonalization-derealization disorder are presented in Box 29-8.

Predisposing Factors Associated With Dissociative Disorders

Genetics

Regarding DID, Maldonado and Spiegel (2008) report on twin studies with monozygotic and dizygotic pairs in which the results suggested "common genetic factors underlying pathological and nonpathological dissociative capacity" (p. 685). Further research is required to determine if there is a true genetic influence associated with the etiology of DID.

Neurobiological

Some clinicians have suggested a possible correlation between neurological alterations and dissociative disorders. Although available information is inadequate, it is possible that dissociative amnesia may be related to neurophysiological dysfunction. Areas of the brain that have been associated with memory include the hippocampus, amygdala, fornix, mammillary bodies, thalamus, and frontal cortex. Brunet, Holowka, and Laurence (2003) state:

> Given the intimate relationship between dissociation, memory, and trauma, researchers have begun to investigate the brain structures and neurochemical systems that mediate functions. Several substances such as sodium-lactate, yohimbine, and metachlorophenylpiperazine have been shown to elicit dissociative symptoms in patients with PTSD or panic disorder, but not in normal controls. Such findings suggest a role for the locus coeruleus/noradrenergic system, which is implicated in fear and arousal regulation and influence a number of cortical structures such as the prefrontal, sensory and parietal cortex, the hippocampus, the hypothalamus, the amygdala, and the spinal cord. Still the relationship between trauma exposure, cortisol, hippocampus damage, memory, and dissociation is tentative at best, and remains to be thoroughly investigated. (p. 26)

Some studies have suggested a possible link between DID and certain neurological conditions, such as temporal lobe epilepsy and severe migraine headaches. Electroencephalographic abnormalities have been observed in some clients with DID.

Psychodynamic Theory

Freud (1962) believed that dissociative behaviors occurred when individuals repressed distressing mental contents from conscious awareness. He believed that the unconscious was a dynamic entity in which repressed mental contents were stored and unavailable to conscious recall. Current psychodynamic explanations of dissociation are based on Freud's concepts. The repression of mental contents is perceived as a coping mechanism for protecting the client from emotional pain that has arisen from either disturbing external circumstances or anxiety-provoking internal urges and feelings (Maldonado & Spiegel, 2008). In the case of depersonalization and derealization, the pain and anxiety are expressed as feelings of unreality or detachment from the environment of the painful situation.

Psychological Trauma

A growing body of evidence points to the etiology of DID as a set of traumatic experiences that overwhelms the individual's capacity to cope by any means other than dissociation. These experiences usually take the form of severe physical, sexual, or psychological abuse

---

BOX 29-8 **Diagnostic Criteria for Depersonalization-Derealization Disorder**

A. The presence of persistent or recurrent depersonalization, derealization, or both:
1. **Depersonalization:** Experiences of unreality, detachment, or being an outside observer with respect to one's thoughts, feelings, sensations, body, or actions (e.g., perceptual alterations, distorted sense of time, unreal or absent self, emotional and/or physical numbing).
2. **Derealization:** Experiences of unreality or detachment with respect to surroundings (e.g., individuals or objects are experienced as unreal, dreamlike, foggy, lifeless, or visually distorted).

B. During the depersonalization or derealization experiences, reality testing remains intact.

C. The symptoms cause clinically significant distress or impairment in social, occupational, or other important areas of functioning.

D. The disturbance is not attributable to the physiological effects of a substance (e.g., a drug of abuse, medication) or another medical condition (e.g., seizures).

E. The disturbance is not better explained by another mental disorder, such as schizophrenia, panic disorder, major depressive disorder, acute stress disorder, posttraumatic stress disorder, or another dissociative disorder.

IMPLICATIONS OF RESEARCH FOR EVIDENCE-BASED PRACTICE

Brunner, R., Parzer, P., Schuld, V., & Resch, F. (2000, February). Dissociative symptomatology and traumatogenic factors in adolescent psychiatric patients. *The Journal of Nervous and Mental Disease, 188*(2), 71-77.

DESCRIPTION OF THE STUDY: This study describes the relationship between different types of childhood trauma to the degree of dissociative experiences. Subjects were 198 consecutively admitted adolescent psychiatric patients, 11 to 19 years old (89 inpatients and 109 outpatients). All patients completed the Adolescent Dissociative Experiences Scale (ADES), a self-administered questionnaire with 30 items that quantifies the frequency of dissociative experiences on an 11-point scale ranging from 0 (never) to 10 (always). The instrument has been shown to discriminate patients with dissociative disorders from patients in several other diagnostic categories, as well as from adolescents in the general population. Subjects' therapists were asked to complete the Checklist of Traumatic Childhood Events, based on assessments, client self-reports, and reports by caregivers and custodial and social services. The checklist covered four main areas of traumatic experiences: sexual abuse, physical abuse, neglect, and stressful life events. Each area was further categorized by experiences considered from minor to severe. Examples of these abuse extremes included:

- Sexual: From sexualized communication to fondling to masturbation to penetration
- Physical: From being hit with a hand to punching, kicking, lacerations, burns, fractures

- Neglect: From physical and educational neglect to social/environmental neglect to emotional and psychological involvement (rejection; hostility)
- Stressful life events: From loss related to family members to physical/mental illness of family members to "others" (e.g., personal physical illness, witnessing an accident or violence, institutional placement)

RESULTS OF THE STUDY: All mean scores by traumatized adolescents were elevated in comparison to those of the control (nontraumatized) group. Increased dissociative symptomatology was unrelated to the degree of severity of sexual abuse experiences. Interestingly, the study found an increased amount of dissociative symptomatology associated with minor forms of physical abuse, as compared to the severe forms. Only severe forms of stressful life events contributed significantly to a higher degree of dissociative experiences. The study revealed that emotional neglect appears to be the best predictor of dissociative symptoms.

IMPLICATIONS FOR NURSING PRACTICE: The authors state: "In contrast to the current psychopathogenic model of dissociation which maintains that particularly severe traumatic events lead to dissociative symptomatology, moderate but chronic emotional stress may be equal or even more important in the development of dissociation." This is important information for the nursing database. Nurses should be aware that even less severe forms of abuse and neglect may have a significant impact on the development of dissociative psychopathology in adolescents.

---

by a parent or significant other in the child's life. The most widely accepted explanation for DID is that it begins as a survival strategy that serves to help children cope with the horrifying sexual, physical, or psychological abuse. In this traumatic environment, the child uses dissociation to become a passive victim of the cruel and unwanted experience. He or she creates a new being who is able to endure the overwhelming pain of the cruel reality, while the primary self can then escape awareness of the pain. Each new personality has as its nucleus a means of responding without anxiety and distress to various painful or dangerous stimuli.

Transactional Model of Stress/Adaptation

The etiology of dissociative disorders is most likely influenced by multiple factors. In Figure 29-2, a graphic depiction of this theory of multiple causation is presented in the Transactional Model of Stress/Adaptation.

Diagnosis/Outcome Identification

Nursing diagnoses are formulated from the data gathered during the assessment phase and with background

knowledge regarding predisposing factors to the disorder. Table 29-1 presents a list of client behaviors and the NANDA nursing diagnoses that correspond to those behaviors, which may be used in planning care for clients with somatic symptom and dissociative disorders.

Outcome Criteria

The following criteria may be used for measurement of outcomes in the care of the client with somatic symptom and dissociative disorders.

The client:

■ Effectively uses adaptive coping strategies during stressful situations without resorting to physical symptoms (*somatic symptom disorder*)

■ Verbalizes relief from pain and demonstrates adaptive coping strategies during stressful situations to prevent the onset of pain (*somatic symptom disorder*)

■ Interprets bodily sensations rationally; verbalizes understanding of the significance the irrational fear held for him or her; and has decreased the

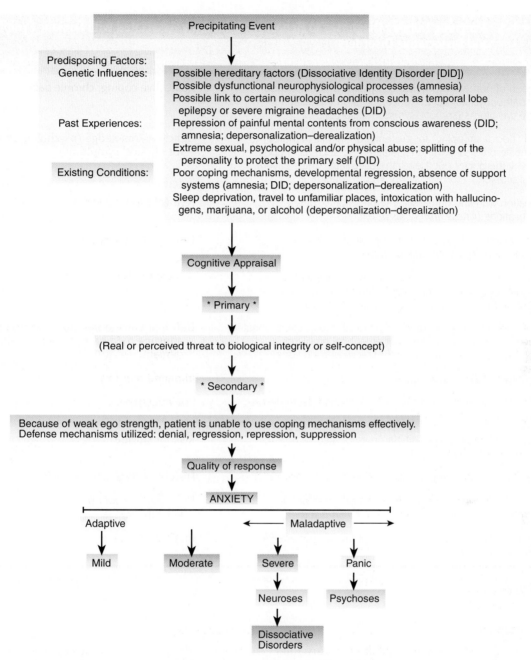

FIGURE 29–2 The dynamics of dissociative disorders using the Transactional Model of Stress/Adaptation.

number and frequency of physical complaints (*illness anxiety disorder*)

■ Is free of physical disability and is able to verbalize understanding of the possible correlation between the loss of or alteration in function and extreme emotional stress (*conversion disorder*)

■ Can recall events associated with a traumatic or stressful situation (*dissociative amnesia*)

■ Has recovered lost memories for events of past life (*dissociative amnesia*)

■ Can verbalize the extreme anxiety that precipitated the dissociation (*depersonalization-derealization disorder*)

■ Can demonstrate more adaptive coping strategies to avert dissociative behaviors in the face of severe anxiety (*depersonalization-derealization disorder*)

■ Verbalizes understanding of the existence of multiple personalities and the purposes they serve (*dissociative identity disorder*)

■ Is able to maintain a sense of reality during stressful situations (*depersonalization-derealization disorder*)

Planning/Implementation

The following section presents a group of selected nursing diagnoses, with short- and long-term goals and nursing interventions for each.

TABLE 29–1 Assigning Nursing Diagnoses to Behaviors Commonly Associated with Somatic Symptom and Dissociative Disorders

BEHAVIORS	NURSING DIAGNOSES
Verbalization of numerous physical complaints in the absence of any pathophysiological evidence; focus on the self and physical symptoms (*somatic symptom disorder*)	Ineffective coping; chronic pain
History of "doctor shopping" for evidence of organic pathology to substantiate physical symptoms; statements such as, "I don't know why the doctor put me on the psychiatric unit. I have a physical problem." (*somatic symptom disorder*)	Deficient knowledge (psychological causes for physical symptoms)
Preoccupation with and unrealistic interpretation of bodily signs and sensations (*illness anxiety disorder*)	Fear (of having a serious disease)
Loss or alteration in physical functioning without evidence of organic pathology (*conversion disorder*)	Disturbed sensory perception*
Need for assistance to carry out self-care activities such as eating, dressing, maintaining hygiene, and toileting due to alteration in physical functioning (*conversion disorder*)	Self-care deficit
History of numerous exacerbations of physical illness; inappropriate or exaggerated behaviors; denial of emotional problems (*psychological factors affecting other medical conditions*)	Deficient knowledge (psychological factors affecting medical condition); Ineffective denial
Loss of memory (*dissociative amnesia*)	Impaired memory
Verbalizations of frustration over lack of control and dependence on others (*dissociative amnesia*)	Powerlessness
Unresolved grief; depression; self-blame associated with childhood abuse (*DID*)	Risk for suicide
Presence of more than one personality within the individual (*DID*)	Disturbed personality identity
Alteration in the perception or experience of the self or the environment (*depersonalization-derealization disorder*)	Disturbed sensory perception (visual/kinesthetic)*
Feigning of physical or psychological symptoms to gain attention (*factitious disorder*)	Ineffective coping

*This diagnosis has been retired from the NANDA-I list of approved diagnoses. It is used in this instance because it is most compatible with the identified behaviors.

Ineffective coping

Ineffective coping is defined as the "inability to form a valid appraisal of the stressors, inadequate choices of practiced responses, and/or inability to use available resources" (NANDA International [NANDA-I], 2012, p. 348).

Client Goals

Outcome criteria include short- and long-term goals. Timelines are individually determined.

Short-Term Goal

■ Within (specified time), client will verbalize understanding of correlation between physical symptoms and psychological problems.

Long-Term Goal

■ By time of discharge from treatment, client will demonstrate ability to cope with stress by means other than preoccupation with physical symptoms.

Interventions

■ Monitor the physician's ongoing assessments, laboratory reports, and other data to maintain assurance that the possibility of organic pathology is clearly ruled out. Review findings with the client. Accurate medical assessment is vital for the provision of adequate and appropriate care. Honest explanation may help the client understand the psychological implications.

■ Recognize and accept that the physical complaint is real to the client, even though no organic etiology can be identified. Denial of the client's feelings is nontherapeutic and interferes with establishment of a trusting relationship.

■ Provide pain medication as prescribed by physician. Client comfort and safety are nursing priorities.

■ Identify gains that the physical symptoms are providing for the client: increased dependency, attention, and distraction from other problems. Identification of underlying motivation is important in assisting the client with problem resolution.

■ Initially, fulfill the client's most urgent dependency needs, but gradually withdraw attention to physical symptoms. Minimize time given in response to physical complaints. Anxiety and maladaptive behaviors will increase if dependency needs are ignored initially. Gradual withdrawal of positive reinforcement will discourage repetition of maladaptive behaviors.

■ Explain to the client that any new physical complaints will be referred to the physician and give no further attention to them. Follow up on the physician's assessment of the complaint. The possibility of organic pathology must always be considered. Failure to do so could jeopardize client safety.

■ Encourage the client to verbalize fears and anxieties. Explain that attention will be withdrawn if rumination about physical complaints begins. Follow through. Without consistency of limit setting, change will not occur.

■ Help the client recognize that physical symptoms often occur because of, or are exacerbated by, specific stressors. Discuss alternative coping strategies that client may use in response to stress (e.g., relaxation exercises, physical activities, assertiveness skills). The client may need help with problem-solving. Give positive reinforcement for adaptive coping strategies.

■ Have the client keep a diary of appearance, duration, and intensity of physical symptoms. A separate record of situations that the client finds especially stressful should also be kept. Comparison of these records may provide objective data from which to observe the relationship between physical symptoms and stress.

■ Help the client identify ways to achieve recognition from others without resorting to physical symptoms. Positive recognition from others enhances self-esteem and minimizes the need for attention through maladaptive behaviors.

■ Discuss how interpersonal relationships are affected by the client's narcissistic behavior. Explain how this behavior alienates others. The client may not realize how he or she is perceived by others.

■ Provide instruction in relaxation techniques and assertiveness skills. These approaches decrease anxiety and increase self-esteem, which facilitate adaptive responses to stressful situations.

Fear (of Having a Serious Disease)

Fear is defined as the "response to perceived threat that is consciously recognized as a danger" (NANDA-I, 2012, p. 361).

Client Goals

Outcome criteria include short- and long-term goals. Timelines are individually determined.

Short-Term Goal

■ Client will verbalize that fears associated with bodily sensations are irrational (within time limit deemed appropriate for specific individual).

Long-Term Goal

■ Client interprets bodily sensations correctly.

Interventions

■ Monitor the physician's ongoing assessments and laboratory reports. Organic pathology must be clearly ruled out.

■ Refer all new physical complaints to the physician. To ignore all physical complaints could place the client's safety in jeopardy.

■ Assess what function the client's illness is fulfilling for him or her (e.g., unfulfilled needs for dependency, nurturing, caring, attention, or control). This information may provide insight into reasons for maladaptive behavior and provide direction for planning client care.

■ Identify times during which the preoccupation with physical symptoms is worse. Determine the extent of correlation of physical complaints with times of increased anxiety. The client may be unaware of the psychosocial implications of the physical complaints. Knowledge of the relationship is the first step in the process for creating change.

■ Convey empathy. Let the client know that you understand how a specific symptom may conjure up fears of previous life-threatening illness. Unconditional acceptance and empathy promote a therapeutic nurse-client relationship.

■ Initially allow the client a limited amount of time (e.g., 10 minutes each hour) to discuss physical symptoms. Because this has been his or her primary method of coping for so long, complete prohibition of this activity would likely raise the client's anxiety level significantly, further exacerbating the behavior.

■ Help the client determine what techniques may be most useful for him or her to implement when fear and anxiety are exacerbated (e.g., relaxation techniques, mental imagery, thought-stopping techniques, physical exercise). All of these techniques are effective in reducing anxiety and may assist the client in the transition from focusing on fear of physical illness to the discussion of honest feelings.

■ Gradually increase the limit on amount of time spent each hour in discussing physical symptoms. If the client violates the limits, withdraw attention. Lack of positive reinforcement may help to extinguish the maladaptive behavior.

■ Encourage the client to discuss feelings associated with fear of serious illness. Verbalization of feelings in a nonthreatening environment facilitates expression and resolution of disturbing emotional issues. When the client can express feelings directly, there is less need to express them through physical symptoms.

■ Role-play the client's plan for dealing with the fear the next time it assumes control and before anxiety becomes disabling. Anxiety and fears are minimized when the client has achieved a degree of comfort through practicing a plan for dealing with stressful situations in the future.

Disturbed Sensory Perception

Disturbed sensory perception is defined as a "change in the amount or patterning of incoming stimuli accompanied by a diminished, exaggerated, distorted, or impaired response to such stimuli" (NANDA-I, 2012, p. 490). Table 29-2 presents this nursing diagnosis in care plan format.

Client Goals

Outcome criteria include short- and long-term goals. Timelines are individually determined.

Short-Term Goal

■ The client will verbalize understanding of emotional problems as a contributing factor to the alteration in physical functioning (within time limit appropriate for specific individual).

Long-Term Goal

■ The client will demonstrate recovery of lost or altered function.

Interventions

■ Monitor the physician's ongoing assessments, laboratory reports, and other data to ensure that the

---

Table 29-2 | CARE PLAN FOR THE CLIENT WITH CONVERSION DISORDER

NURSING DIAGNOSIS: DISTURBED SENSORY PERCEPTION

RELATED TO: Repressed severe anxiety

EVIDENCED BY: Loss or alteration in physical functioning, without evidence of organic pathology

OUTCOME CRITERIA	NURSING INTERVENTIONS	RATIONALE
Short-Term Goal • Client will verbalize understanding of emotional problems as a contributing factor to the alteration in physical functioning (within time limit appropriate for specific individual). **Long-Term Goal** • Client will demonstrate recovery of lost or altered function.	1. Monitor physician's ongoing assessments, laboratory reports, and other data to ensure that possibility of organic pathology is clearly ruled out. 2. Identify primary or secondary gains that the physical symptom may be providing for the client (e.g., increased dependency, attention, protection from experiencing a stressful event). 3. Do not focus on the disability, and encourage client to be as independent as possible. Intervene only when client requires assistance. 4. Maintain nonjudgmental attitude when providing assistance to the client. The physical symptom is not within the client's conscious control and is very real to him or her. 5. Do not allow the client to use the disability as a manipulative tool to avoid participation in therapeutic activities. Withdraw attention if client continues to focus on physical limitation.	1. Failure to do so may jeopardize client safety. 2. Primary and secondary gains are often etiological factors and may be used to assist in problem resolution. 3. Positive reinforcement would encourage continual use of the maladaptive response for secondary gains, such as dependency. 4. A judgmental attitude interferes with the nurse's ability to provide therapeutic care for the client. 5. Lack of reinforcement may help to extinguish the maladaptive response.

Table 29-2 | CARE PLAN FOR THE CLIENT WITH CONVERSION DISORDER—cont'd

OUTCOME CRITERIA	NURSING INTERVENTIONS	RATIONALE
	6. Encourage the client to verbalize fears and anxieties. Help identify physical symptoms as a coping mechanism that is used in times of extreme stress.	6. Clients with conversion disorder are usually unaware of the psychological implications of their illness.
	7. Help client identify coping mechanisms that he or she could use when faced with stressful situations, rather than retreating from reality with a physical disability.	7. Client needs assistance with problem solving at this severe level of anxiety.
	8. Give positive reinforcement for identification or demonstration of alternative, more adaptive coping strategies.	8. Positive reinforcement enhances self-esteem and encourages repetition of desirable behaviors.

possibility of organic pathology is clearly ruled out. Failure to do so may jeopardize the client's safety.

■ Identify primary or secondary gains that the physical symptom is providing for the client (e.g., increased dependency, attention, protection from experiencing a stressful event). These are considered to be etiological factors and may be used to assist in problem resolution.

■ Do not focus on the disability, and encourage the client to be as independent as possible. Intervene only when the client requires assistance. Positive reinforcement would encourage continued use of the maladaptive response for secondary gains, such as dependency.

■ Maintain a nonjudgmental attitude when providing assistance with self-care activities to the client. The physical symptom is not within the client's conscious control and is very real to him or her.

■ Do not allow the client to use the disability as a manipulative tool to avoid participating in therapeutic activities. Withdraw attention if the client continues to focus on the physical limitation. Lack of reinforcement may help to extinguish the maladaptive response.

■ Encourage the client to verbalize fears and anxieties. Help identify physical symptoms as a coping mechanism that is used in times of extreme stress. Clients with conversion disorder are usually unaware of the psychological implications of their illness.

■ Help the client identify coping mechanisms that he or she could use when faced with stressful situations, rather than retreating from reality with a physical disability. The client needs assistance with problem solving at this severe level of anxiety.

■ Give positive reinforcement for identification or demonstration of alternative, more adaptive coping strategies.

Deficient Knowledge (Psychological Factors Affecting Medical Condition)

Deficient knowledge is defined as "absence or deficiency of cognitive information related to a specific topic" (NANDA-I, 2012, p. 271).

Client Goals

Outcome criteria include short- and long-term goals. Timelines are individually determined.

Short-Term Goal

■ Client will cooperate with plan for teaching provided by primary nurse.

Long-Term Goal

■ By time of discharge from treatment, client will be able to verbalize psychological factors affecting his or her physical condition.

Interventions

■ Assess client's level of knowledge regarding effects of psychological problems on the body. An adequate database is necessary for the development of an effective teaching plan.

■ Assess client's level of anxiety and readiness to learn. Learning does not occur beyond the moderate level of anxiety.

■ Discuss physical examinations and laboratory tests that have been conducted. Explain purpose and results of each. Fear of the unknown may contribute to elevated level of anxiety. Client has the right to know about and accept or refuse any medical treatment.

■ Explore client's feelings and fears. Go slowly. These feelings may have been suppressed or repressed for so long that their disclosure may be a very painful experience. Be supportive. Expression of feelings in the presence of a trusted individual and in a nonthreatening environment may encourage the individual to confront unresolved issues.

■ Have client keep a diary of appearance, duration, and intensity of physical symptoms. A separate record of situations that the client finds especially stressful should also be kept. Comparison of these records may provide objective data from which to observe the relationship between physical symptoms and stress.

■ Help client identify needs that are being met through the sick role. Together, formulate more adaptive means for fulfilling these needs. Practice by role-playing. Repetition through practice serves to reduce discomfort in the actual situation.

■ Provide instruction in assertiveness techniques, especially the ability to recognize the differences among passive, assertive, and aggressive behaviors and the importance of respecting the rights of others while protecting one's own basic rights. These skills will preserve the client's self-esteem while also improving his or her ability to form satisfactory interpersonal relationships.

■ Discuss adaptive methods of stress management, such as relaxation techniques, physical exercise, meditation, breathing exercises, and autogenics. Use of these adaptive techniques may decrease appearance of physical symptoms in response to stress.

Impaired Memory

Impaired memory is defined as an "inability to remember or recall bits of information or behavioral skills" (NANDA-I, 2012, p. 273).

Client Goals

Outcome criteria include short- and long-term goals. Timelines are individually determined.

Short-Term Goal

■ The client will verbalize understanding that the loss of memory is related to a stressful situation and begin discussing the stressful situation with nurse or therapist.

Long-Term Goal

■ The client will recover deficits in memory and develop more adaptive coping mechanisms to deal with stressful situations.

Interventions

■ Obtain as much information as possible about the client from family and significant others if possible.

Consider likes, dislikes, important people, activities, music, and pets. A comprehensive baseline assessment is necessary for the development of an effective plan of care.

■ Do not flood the client with data regarding his or her past life. Individuals who are exposed to painful information from which the amnesia is providing protection may decompensate even further into a psychotic state.

■ Instead, expose the client to stimuli that represent pleasant experiences from the past, such as smells associated with enjoyable activities, beloved pets, and music known to have been pleasurable to the client. As memory begins to return, engage the client in activities that may provide additional stimulation. Recall often occurs during activities such as these that simulate life experiences.

■ Encourage the client to discuss situations that have been especially stressful and to explore the feelings associated with those times. Verbalization of feelings in a nonthreatening environment may help the client come to terms with unresolved issues that may be contributing to the dissociative process.

■ Identify specific conflicts that remain unresolved and help the client identify possible solutions. Provide instruction regarding more adaptive ways to respond to anxiety. Unless these underlying conflicts are resolved, any improvement in coping behaviors must be viewed as only temporary.

■ Provide positive feedback for decisions made. Respect the client's right to make those decisions independently, and refrain from attempting to influence him or her toward those that may seem more logical. Independent choice provides a feeling of control, decreases feelings of powerlessness, and increases self-esteem.

Disturbed Personal Identity

Disturbed personal identity is defined as the "inability to maintain an integrated and complete perception of self" (NANDA-I, 2012, p. 282).

Client Goals

Outcome criteria include short- and long-term goals. Timelines are individually determined.

Short-Term Goals

■ The client will verbalize understanding about the existence of multiple personalities within the self.
■ The client will be able to recognize stressful situations that precipitate transition from one personality to another.

Long-Term Goals

■ The client will verbalize understanding of the reason for existence of each personality and the role each plays for the individual.

■ The client will enter into and cooperate with long-term therapy, with the ultimate goal being integration into one personality.

Interventions

■ The nurse must develop a trusting relationship with the original personality and with each of the subpersonalities. Trust is the basis of a therapeutic relationship. Each of the personalities views itself as a separate entity and initially must be treated as such.

■ Help the client understand the existence of the subpersonalities and the need each serves in the personal identity of the individual. The client may initially be unaware of the dissociative response. Knowledge of the needs each personality fulfills is the first step in the integration process and the client's ability to face unresolved issues without dissociation.

■ Help the client identify stressful situations that precipitate transition from one personality to another. Carefully observe and record these transitions. Identification of stressors is required to assist the client in responding more adaptively and to eliminate the need for transition to another personality.

■ Use nursing interventions necessary to deal with maladaptive behaviors associated with individual subpersonalities. For example, if one personality is suicidal, precautions must be taken to guard against the client's self-harm. If another personality has a tendency toward physical hostility, precautions must be taken to protect others.

> **CLINICAL PEARL** It may be possible to seek assistance from one of the personalities. For example, a strong-willed personality may help to control the behaviors of a "suicidal" personality.

■ Help subpersonalities understand that their "being" will not be destroyed, but rather integrated into a unified identity within the individual. Because the subpersonalities function as separate entities, the idea of total elimination generates fear and defensiveness.

■ Provide support during disclosure of painful experiences and reassurance when the client becomes discouraged with lengthy treatment.

Disturbed Sensory Perception (Visual/Kinesthetic)

Disturbed sensory perception is defined as a "change in the amount or patterning of incoming stimuli accompanied by a diminished, exaggerated, distorted, or impaired response to such stimuli" (NANDA-I, 2012, p. 490).

Client Goals

Outcome criteria include short- and long-term goals. Timelines are individually determined.

Short-Term Goal

■ Client will verbalize adaptive ways of coping with stress.

Long-Term Goal

■ Client will demonstrate the ability to perceive stimuli correctly and maintain a sense of reality during stressful situations.

Interventions

■ Provide support and encouragement during times of depersonalization. Clients manifesting these symptoms may express fear and anxiety. They do not understand the response and may express a fear of going insane. Support and encouragement from a trusted individual provide a feeling of security when fears and anxieties are manifested.

■ Explain the depersonalization behaviors and the purpose they usually serve for the client. This knowledge may help to minimize fears and anxieties associated with their occurrence.

■ Explain the relationship between severe anxiety and depersonalization behaviors. Help relate these behaviors to times of severe psychological stress that client has experienced. The client may be unaware that the occurrence of depersonalization behaviors is related to severe anxiety. Knowledge of this relationship is the first step in the process of behavioral change.

■ Explore past experiences and possibly repressed painful situations such as trauma or abuse. Traumatic experiences may predispose individuals to dissociative disorders.

■ Discuss these painful experiences with client, and encourage him or her to deal with the feelings associated with these situations. Work to resolve the conflicts these repressed feelings have nurtured. Conflict resolution will serve to decrease the need for the dissociative response to anxiety.

■ Discuss ways the client may more adaptively respond to stress, and use role-play to practice using these new methods. Having practiced through role-play helps to prepare client to face stressful situations by using these new behaviors when they occur in real life.

Concept Care Mapping

The concept map care plan is an innovative approach to planning and organizing nursing care (see Chapter 9). It is a diagrammatic teaching and learning strategy that allows visualization of interrelationships between medical diagnoses, nursing diagnoses, assessment data, and treatments. Examples of concept map care plans for clients with somatic symptom and dissociative disorders are presented in Figures 29-3 and 29-4.

Evaluation

Reassessment is conducted to determine if the nursing actions have been successful in achieving the objectives of care. Evaluation of the nursing actions for the client with a somatic symptom disorder may be facilitated by

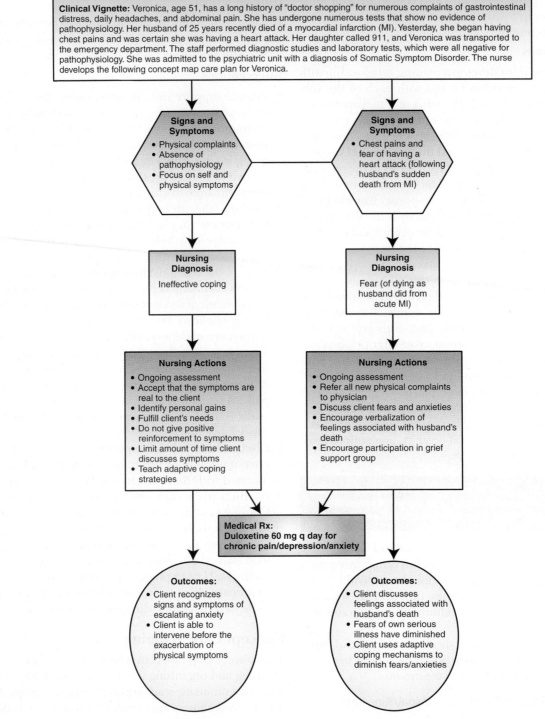

Clinical Vignette: Veronica, age 51, has a long history of "doctor shopping" for numerous complaints of gastrointestinal distress, daily headaches, and abdominal pain. She has undergone numerous tests that show no evidence of pathophysiology. Her husband of 25 years recently died of a myocardial infarction (MI). Yesterday, she began having chest pains and was certain she was having a heart attack. Her daughter called 911, and Veronica was transported to the emergency department. The staff performed diagnostic studies and laboratory tests, which were all negative for pathophysiology. She was admitted to the psychiatric unit with a diagnosis of Somatic Symptom Disorder. The nurse develops the following concept map care plan for Veronica.

Signs and Symptoms
• Physical complaints
• Absence of pathophysiology
• Focus on self and physical symptoms

Signs and Symptoms
• Chest pains and fear of having a heart attack (following husband's sudden death from MI)

Nursing Diagnosis
Ineffective coping

Nursing Diagnosis
Fear (of dying as husband did from acute MI)

Nursing Actions
• Ongoing assessment
• Accept that the symptoms are real to the client
• Identify personal gains
• Fulfill client's needs
• Do not give positive reinforcement to symptoms
• Limit amount of time client discusses symptoms
• Teach adaptive coping strategies

Nursing Actions
• Ongoing assessment
• Refer all new physical complaints to physician
• Discuss client fears and anxieties
• Encourage verbalization of feelings associated with husband's death
• Encourage participation in grief support group

Medical Rx:
Duloxetine 60 mg q day for chronic pain/depression/anxiety

Outcomes:
• Client recognizes signs and symptoms of escalating anxiety
• Client is able to intervene before the exacerbation of physical symptoms

Outcomes:
• Client discusses feelings associated with husband's death
• Fears of own serious illness have diminished
• Client uses adaptive coping mechanisms to diminish fears/anxieties

FIGURE 29-3 Concept map care plan for a client with somatic symptom disorder.

gathering information using the following types of questions:

■ Can the client recognize signs and symptoms of escalating anxiety?
■ Can the client intervene with adaptive coping strategies to interrupt the escalating anxiety before physical symptoms are exacerbated?

■ Can the client verbalize an understanding of the correlation between physical symptoms and times of escalating anxiety?
■ Does the client have a plan for dealing with increased stress to prevent exacerbation of physical symptoms?
■ Does the client demonstrate a decrease in ruminations about physical symptoms?

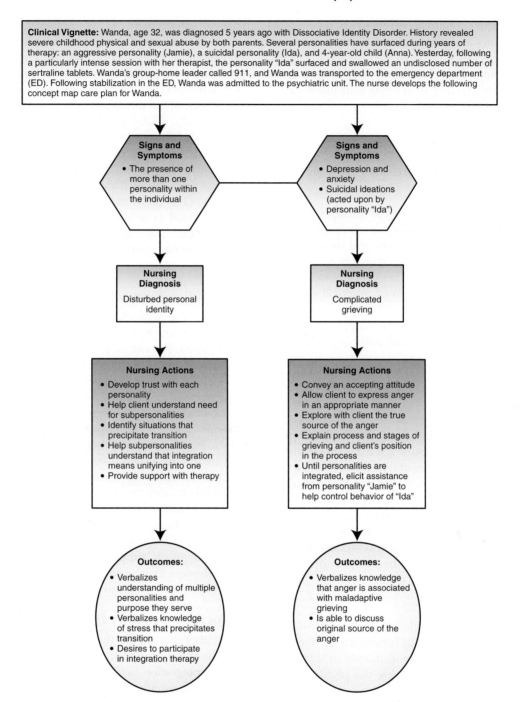

Clinical Vignette: Wanda, age 32, was diagnosed 5 years ago with Dissociative Identity Disorder. History revealed severe childhood physical and sexual abuse by both parents. Several personalities have surfaced during years of therapy: an aggressive personality (Jamie), a suicidal personality (Ida), and 4-year-old child (Anna). Yesterday, following a particularly intense session with her therapist, the personality "Ida" surfaced and swallowed an undisclosed number of sertraline tablets. Wanda's group-home leader called 911, and Wanda was transported to the emergency department (ED). Following stabilization in the ED, Wanda was admitted to the psychiatric unit. The nurse develops the following concept map care plan for Wanda.

Signs and Symptoms
• The presence of more than one personality within the individual

Signs and Symptoms
• Depression and anxiety
• Suicidal ideations (acted upon by personality "Ida")

Nursing Diagnosis
Disturbed personal identity

Nursing Diagnosis
Complicated grieving

Nursing Actions
• Develop trust with each personality
• Help client understand need for subpersonalities
• Identify situations that precipitate transition
• Help subpersonalities understand that integration means unifying into one
• Provide support with therapy

Nursing Actions
• Convey an accepting attitude
• Allow client to express anger in an appropriate manner
• Explore with client the true source of the anger
• Explain process and stages of grieving and client's position in the process
• Until personalities are integrated, elicit assistance from personality "Jamie" to help control behavior of "Ida"

Outcomes:
• Verbalizes understanding of multiple personalities and purpose they serve
• Verbalizes knowledge of stress that precipitates transition
• Desires to participate in integration therapy

Outcomes:
• Verbalizes knowledge that anger is associated with maladaptive grieving
• Is able to discuss original source of the anger

FIGURE 29–4 Concept map care plan for a client with dissociative identity disorder.

■ Have fears of serious illness diminished?
■ Does the client demonstrate full recovery from previous loss or alteration of physical functioning?

Evaluation of the nursing actions for the client with a dissociative disorder may be facilitated by gathering information using the following types of questions:

■ Has the client's memory been restored?
■ Can the client connect occurrence of psychological stress to loss of memory?

■ Does the client discuss fears and anxieties with members of the staff in an effort toward resolution?
■ Can the client discuss the presence of various personalities within the self?
■ Can he or she verbalize why these personalities exist?
■ Can the client verbalize situations that precipitate transition from one personality to another?
■ Can the client maintain a sense of reality during stressful situations?

■ Can the client verbalize a correlation between stressful situations and the onset of depersonalization behaviors?

■ Can the client demonstrate more adaptive coping strategies for dealing with stress without resorting to dissociation?

Treatment Modalities

Somatic Symptom Disorders

Individual Psychotherapy

The goal of psychotherapy is to help clients develop healthy and adaptive behaviors, encourage them to move beyond their somatization, and manage their lives more effectively. The focus is on personal and social difficulties that the client is experiencing in daily life as well as the achievement of practical solutions for these difficulties.

Treatment is initiated with a complete physical examination to rule out organic pathology. Once this has been ensured, the physician turns his or her attention to the client's social and personal problems and away from the somatic complaints.

Group Psychotherapy

Group therapy may be helpful for somatic symptom disorders because it provides a setting where clients can share their experiences of illness, can learn to verbalize thoughts and feelings, and can be confronted by group members and leaders when they reject responsibility for maladaptive behaviors. It has been reported to be the treatment of choice for both somatic symptom disorder and illness anxiety disorder, in part because it provides the social support and social interaction that these clients need.

Behavior Therapy

Behavior therapy is more likely to be successful in instances when secondary gain is prominent. This may involve working with the client's family or significant others who may be perpetuating the physical symptoms by rewarding passivity and dependency and by being overly solicitous and helpful. Behavioral therapy focuses on teaching these individuals to reward the client's autonomy, self-sufficiency, and independence. This process becomes more difficult when the client is very regressed and the sick role well established.

Psychopharmacology

Antidepressants are often used with somatic symptom disorder when the predominant symptom is pain. They have been shown to be effective in relieving pain, independent of influences on mood. The tricyclic antidepressants (TCAs) have been used extensively, and their efficacy in relieving pain has been demonstrated.

Adverse effects with TCAs, however, make their use problematic with some individuals. Leo (2008) reported that "the serotonin and norepinephrine reuptake inhibitors (SNRIs) venlafaxine and duloxetine have demonstrated utility as analgesic agents and bypass several of the untoward effects commonly associated with the TCAs" (p. 1038). Selective serotonin reuptake inhibitors (SSRIs) have not exhibited the consistent analgesic efficacy demonstrated by the TCAs and SNRIs (Leo, 2008).

Anticonvulsants such as phenytoin (Dilantin), carbamazepine (Tegregol), and clonazepam (Klonopin) have been reported to be effective in treating neuropathic and neuralgic pain, at least for short periods. Their efficacy in other somatic symptom (pain) disorders is less clear.

Dissociative Amnesia

Many cases of dissociative amnesia resolve spontaneously when the individual is removed from the stressful situation. For other, more refractory conditions, intravenous administration of amobarbital is useful in the retrieval of lost memories. Most clinicians recommend supportive psychotherapy as well to reinforce adjustment to the psychological impact of the retrieved memories and the emotions associated with them.

In some instances, psychotherapy is used as the primary treatment. Techniques of persuasion and free or directed association are used to help the client remember. In other cases, hypnosis may be required to mobilize the memories. Hypnosis is sometimes facilitated by the use of pharmacological agents, such as sodium amobarbital. Once the memories have been obtained through hypnosis, supportive psychotherapy or group psychotherapy may be employed to help the client integrate the memories into his or her conscious state.

Dissociative Identity Disorder

The goal of therapy for the client with DID is to optimize the client's function and potential. The achievement of **integration** (a blending of all the personalities into one) is usually considered desirable, but some clients choose not to pursue this lengthy therapeutic regimen. In these cases resolution, or a smooth collaboration among the subpersonalities, may be all that is realistic.

Intensive, long-term psychotherapy with the DID client is directed toward uncovering the underlying psychological conflicts, helping him or her gain insight into these conflicts, and striving to synthesize the various identities into one integrated personality. Clients are assisted to recall past traumas in detail. They must mentally reexperience the abuse that caused their illness. This process, called **abreaction**, or "remembering with feeling," is so painful that clients may actually cry, scream, and feel the pain that they felt at the time of the abuse.

During therapy, each personality is actively explored and encouraged to become aware of the others across previously amnestic barriers. Traumatic memories associated with the different personality manifestations, especially those related to childhood abuse, are examined. The course of treatment is often difficult and anxiety provoking to client and therapist alike, especially when aggressive or suicidal personalities are in the dominant role. In these instances, brief periods of hospitalization may be necessary as an interim supportive measure.

When integration is achieved, the individual becomes a total of all the feelings, experiences, memories, skills, and talents that were previously in the command of the various personalities. He or she learns how to function effectively without the necessity for creating new personalities to cope with life. This is possible only after years of intense psychotherapy, and even then, recovery is often incomplete.

Depersonalization-Derealization Disorder

Information about the treatment of depersonalization-derealization disorder is sparse and inconclusive. Various psychiatric medications have been tried, both singly and in combination: antidepressants, mood stabilizers, anticonvulsants, and antipsychotics. Results have been sporadic at best. If other psychiatric disorders, such as schizophrenia, are evident, they too may be treated pharmacologically. A study by Simeon, Stein, and Hollander (1998) found the antidepressant clomipramine (Anafranil) to be a promising pharmacological treatment for primary depersonalization-derealization disorder. For clients with evident intrapsychic conflict, analytically oriented insight psychotherapy may be useful. Some clients with depersonalization-derealization disorder have benefited from hypnotherapy or cognitive-behavioral therapy (CBT). With CBT, these clients "learn to confront their distorted thoughts and challenge their feelings of unreality" (Black & Andreasen, 2011, p. 234).

CASE STUDY AND SAMPLE CARE PLAN

NURSING HISTORY AND ASSESSMENT

Jake is a 54-year-old client of the psychiatric outpatient department of the VA Medical Center. At age 42, Jake was diagnosed with colon cancer and underwent a colon resection. Since that time, he has had regular follow-up exams, with no recurrence of the cancer and no residual effects. He did not require follow-up chemotherapy or radiation therapy. For 10 years, Jake has had yearly physical and laboratory examinations. He regularly complains to his family physician of mild abdominal pain, sensations of "fullness," "bowel rumblings," and what he calls a "firm mass," which he says he can sometimes feel in his lower left quadrant. The physician has performed x-rays of the entire gastrointestinal (GI) tract, an esophagoscopy, gastroscopy, and colonoscopy. All results were negative for organic pathology. Rather than being relieved, Jake appears to be resentful and disappointed that the physician has not been able to reveal a pathological problem. Jake's job is in jeopardy because of excessive use of sick leave. The family physician has referred Jake for psychiatric evaluation. Jake was admitted as an outpatient with the diagnosis of illness anxiety disorder. He has been assigned to Lisa, a psychiatric nurse practitioner.

In her assessment, Lisa learns that Jake has pretty much lived his adult life in isolation. He was never close to his parents, who worked and seldom had time for Jake or his sister. Jake told Lisa that, "My parents really didn't care about me. They were too busy taking care of the farm. Dad wanted me to take over the farm, but I was never interested. I liked working on cars, and went to vocational

school to learn how to be a mechanic. I thought they would be proud of me, but they never cared. I think they only had kids so they would have some help on the farm. When I left home, they really didn't care if they ever saw me again." He has never been married nor had a really serious relationship. "Women don't like me much. I spend most of my time alone. I guess I don't really like people, and they don't really like me."

NURSING DIAGNOSES/OUTCOME IDENTIFICATION

From the assessment data, the nurse develops the following nursing diagnoses for Jake:

1. **Fear** (of cancer recurrence) related to history of colon cancer evidenced by numerous complaints of the GI tract and insistence that something is wrong despite objective tests that rule out pathophysiology.
   a. **Short-Term Goal:** Client will verbalize that fears associated with bodily sensations are irrational.
   b. **Long-Term Goal:** Client interprets bodily sensations correctly.
2. **Chronic low self-esteem** related to unfulfilled childhood needs for nurturing and caring evidenced by transformation of internalized anger into physical complaints and hostility toward others.
   a. **Short-Term Goal:** Within 2 weeks, client will verbalize aspects about self that he likes.
   b. **Long-Term Goal:** By discharge from treatment, client will demonstrate acceptance of self as a person of worth, as evidenced by setting realistic goals, limiting

Continued

CASE STUDY AND SAMPLE CARE PLAN—cont'd

physical complaints and hostility toward others, and verbalizing positive prospects for the future.

PLANNING/IMPLEMENTATION

FEAR (OF CANCER RECURRENCE)
The following nursing interventions have been identified for Jake:

1. Monitor the physician's ongoing assessments and laboratory reports to ensure that pathology is clearly ruled out.
2. Refer any new physical complaints to the physician.
3. Assess what function these physical complaints are fulfilling for Jake. Is it a way for him to get attention that he can't get in any other way?
4. Show empathy for his feelings. Let him know that you understand how GI symptoms may bring about fears of the colon cancer.
5. Encourage Jake to talk about his fears of cancer recurrence. What feelings did he have when it was first diagnosed? How did he deal with those feelings? What are his fears at this time?
6. Have Jake keep a diary of the appearance of the symptoms. In a separate diary, have Jake keep a record of situations that create stress for him. Compare these two records. Correlate whether symptoms appear at times of increased anxiety.
7. Help Jake determine what techniques may be useful for him to implement when fear and anxiety are exacerbated (e.g., relaxation techniques, mental imagery, thought-stopping techniques, physical exercise).
8. Offer positive feedback when Jake responds to stressful situations with coping strategies other than physical complaints.

CHRONIC LOW SELF-ESTEEM
The following nursing interventions have been identified for Jake:

1. Convey acceptance, unconditional positive regard, and remain nonjudgmental at all times.
2. Encourage Jake to participate in decision-making regarding his care, as well as in life situations.

3. Help Jake to recognize and focus on strengths and accomplishments. Minimize attention given to past (real or perceived) failures.
4. Encourage Jake to talk about feelings related to his unsatisfactory relationship with his parents.
5. Discuss things in his life that Jake would like to change. Help him determine what *can* be changed and what changes are not realistic.
6. Encourage participation in group activities and in therapy groups that offer simple methods of achievement. Give recognition and positive feedback for actual accomplishments.
7. Teach assertiveness techniques and effective communication techniques.
8. Offer positive feedback for appropriate social interactions with others. Role-play with Jake situations that he finds particularly stressful. Help him to understand that ruminations about himself and his health may cause others to reject him socially.
9. Help Jake to set realistic goals for his future.

EVALUATION

Some of the outcome criteria for Jake have been met, and some are ongoing. He has come to realize that the fears about his "symptoms" are not rational. He understands that the physician has performed adequate diagnostic procedures to rule out illness. He still has fears of cancer occurrence, and discusses these fears with the nurse practitioner on a weekly basis. He has kept his symptoms/stressful situations diary, and has correlated the appearance of some of the symptoms to times of increased anxiety. He has started running, and tries to use this as a strategy to keep the anxiety from escalating out of proportion and bringing on new physical symptoms. He continues to discuss feelings associated with his childhood, and the nurse has helped him see that he has had numerous accomplishments in his life, even though they were not recognized by his parents or others. He has joined a support group for depressed persons, and states that he "has made a few friends." He has made a long-term goal of joining a church with the hope of meeting new people. He is missing fewer workdays because of illness, and his job is no longer in jeopardy.

Summary and Key Points

■ Somatic symptom disorders and dissociative disorders are associated with anxiety that occurs at the severe level. The anxiety is repressed and manifested in the form of symptoms and behaviors associated with these disorders.

■ Somatic symptom disorders, known historically as hysteria, affect about 5 to 7 percent of the general population. Types of somatic symptom disorders include somatic symptom disorder, illness anxiety

disorder, conversion disorder, psychological factors affecting other medical conditions, factitious disorder, and other specified or unspecified somatic symptom disorders.

■ Somatic symptom disorder is manifested by physical symptoms that may be vague, dramatized, or exaggerated in their presentation. No evidence of organic pathology can be identified.

■ Illness anxiety disorder is an unrealistic preoccupation with fear of having a serious illness. This disorder may follow a personal experience, or the experience of a close family member, with serious or life-threatening illness.

■ The individual with conversion disorder experiences a loss of or alteration in bodily functioning, unsubstantiated by medical or pathophysiological explanation. Psychological factors may be evident by the primary or secondary gains the individual achieves from experiencing the physiological manifestation.

■ With the diagnosis of psychological factors affecting other medical conditions, psychological or behavioral factors have been implicated in the development, exacerbation, or delayed recovery from a medical condition.

■ In factitious disorder, the individual falsifies physical or psychological signs or symptoms, or induces injury, on the self or another person in order to receive attention from medical personnel.

■ A dissociative response has been described as a defense mechanism to protect the ego in the face of overwhelming anxiety.

■ Dissociative responses result in an alteration in the normally integrative functions of identity, memory, or consciousness.

■ Classification of dissociative disorders includes dissociative amnesia, dissociative identity disorder (DID), depersonalization-derealization disorder, and other specified or unspecified dissociative disorders.

■ The individual with dissociative amnesia is unable to recall important personal information that is too extensive to be explained by ordinary forgetfulness.

■ The prominent feature of DID is the existence of two or more personalities within a single individual. An individual may have many personalities, each of which serves a purpose for that individual of enduring painful stimuli that the original personality is too weak to face.

■ Depersonalization-derealization disorder is characterized by an alteration in the perception of oneself and/or the environment. Depersonalization is described as a feeling of unreality or detachment from one's body. Derealization is an experience of unreality or detachment with respect to one's surroundings.

■ Individuals with somatic symptom and dissociative disorders often receive health care initially in areas other than psychiatry.

■ Nurses can assist clients with these disorders by helping them to understand their problem and identify and establish new, more adaptive behavior patterns.

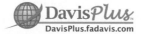
DavisPlus   Additional info available at
DavisPlus.fadavis.com   www.davisplus.com

Review Questions
Self-Examination/Learning Exercise

*Select the answer that is **most** appropriate for each of the following questions.*

1. Lorraine has been diagnosed with somatic symptom disorder. Which of the following symptom profiles would you expect when assessing Lorraine?
   a. Multiple somatic symptoms in several body systems
   b. Fear of having a serious disease
   c. Loss or alteration in sensorimotor functioning
   d. Belief that her body is deformed or defective in some way

2. Which of the following ego defense mechanisms describes the underlying psychodynamics of somatic symptom disorder?
   a. Denial of depression
   b. Repression of anxiety
   c. Suppression of grief
   d. Displacement of anger

3. Nursing care for a client with somatic symptom disorder would focus on helping her to:
   a. Eliminate the stress in her life.
   b. Discontinue her numerous physical complaints.
   c. Take her medication only as prescribed.
   d. Learn more adaptive coping strategies.

Continued

Review Questions—cont'd
Self-Examination/Learning Exercise

4. Lorraine, a client diagnosed with somatic symptom disorder, states, "My doctor thinks I should see a psychiatrist. I can't imagine why he would make such a suggestion." What is the basis for Lorraine's statement?
   a. She thinks her doctor wants to get rid of her as a client.
   b. She does not understand the correlation of symptoms and stress.
   c. She thinks psychiatrists are only for "crazy" people.
   d. She thinks her doctor has made an error in diagnosis.

5. Lorraine, a client diagnosed with somatic symptom disorder, tells the nurse about a pain in her side. She says she has not experienced it before. Which is the most appropriate response by the nurse?
   a. "I don't want to hear about another physical complaint. You know they are all in your head. It's time for group therapy now."
   b. "Let's sit down here together and you can tell me about this new pain you are experiencing. You'll just have to miss group therapy today."
   c. "I will report this pain to your physician. In the meantime, group therapy starts in 5 minutes. You must leave now to be on time."
   d. "I will call your physician and see if he will order a new pain medication for your side. The one you have now doesn't seem to provide relief. Why don't you get some rest for now?"

6. Ellen has a history of childhood physical and sexual abuse. She was diagnosed with dissociative identity disorder (DID) 6 years ago. She has been admitted to the psychiatric unit following a suicide attempt. The primary nursing diagnosis for Ellen would be:
   a. Disturbed personal identity related to childhood abuse
   b. Disturbed sensory perception related to repressed anxiety
   c. Impaired memory related to disturbed thought processes
   d. Risk for suicide related to unresolved grief

7. In establishing trust with Ellen, a client with the diagnosis of DID, the nurse must:
   a. Try to relate to Ellen as though she did not have multiple personalities.
   b. Establish a relationship with each of the personalities separately.
   c. Ignore behaviors that Ellen attributes to other subpersonalities.
   d. Explain to Ellen that he or she will work with her only if she maintains the status of the primary personality.

8. The ultimate goal of therapy for a client with DID is:
   a. Integration of the personalities into one
   b. For the client to have the ability to switch from one personality to another voluntarily
   c. For the client to select which personality he or she wants to be the dominant self
   d. For the client to recognize that the various personalities exist

9. The ultimate goal of therapy for a client with DID is most likely achieved through:
   a. Crisis intervention and directed association
   b. Psychotherapy and hypnosis
   c. Psychoanalysis and free association
   d. Insight psychotherapy and dextroamphetamines

10. Lucille has a diagnosis of somatic symptom disorder, predominantly pain. Which of the following medications would the psychiatric nurse practitioner most likely prescribe for Lucille?
    a. Chlorpromazine (Thorazine)
    b. Diazepam (Valium)
    c. Carbamazepine (Tegretol)
    d. Duloxetine (Cymbalta)

TEST YOUR CRITICAL THINKING SKILLS

Tom was admitted to the psychiatric unit from the emergency department of a general hospital in the Midwest. The owner of a local bar called the police when Tom suddenly seemed to "lose control. He just went ballistic." The police reported that Tom did not know where he was or how he got there. He kept saying, "My name is John Brown, and I live in Philadelphia." When the police ran an identity check on Tom, they found that he was indeed John Brown from Philadelphia and his wife had reported him missing a month ago. Mrs. Brown explained that about 12 months before his disappearance, her husband, who was a shop foreman at a large manufacturing plant, had been having considerable difficulty at work. He had been passed over for a promotion, and his supervisor had been very critical of his work. Several of his staff had left the company for other jobs, and without enough help, Tom had been unable to meet shop deadlines. Work stress made him very difficult to live with at home. Previously an easygoing, extroverted individual, he became withdrawn and extremely critical of his wife and children. Immediately preceding his disappearance, he had had a violent argument with his 18-year-old son, who called Tom a "loser" and stormed out of the house to stay with some friends. It was the day after this argument that Tom disappeared. The psychiatrist assigns a diagnosis of dissociative amnesia, with dissociative fugue.

Answer the following questions related to Tom:

1. Describe the *priority* nursing intervention with Tom as he is admitted to the psychiatric unit.
2. What approach should be taken to help Tom with his problem?
3. What is the long-term goal of therapy for Tom?

References

American Psychiatric Association. (2000). *Diagnostic and statistical manual of mental disorders* (4th ed., text rev.). Washington, DC: Author.

American Psychiatric Association. (2013). *Diagnostic and statistical manual of mental disorders* (5th ed.). Washington, DC: Author.

Black, D.W., & Andreasen, N.C. (2011). *Introductory textbook of psychiatry* (5th ed.). Washington, DC: American Psychiatric Publishing.

Brunet, A., Holowka, D.W., & Laurence, J.R. (2003). Dissociation. In M.J. Aminoff & R.B. Daroff (Eds.), *Encyclopedia of the neurological sciences* (Vol. 2). New York, NY: Elsevier.

Leo, R.J. (2008). Pain disorders. In R.E. Hales, S.C. Yudofsky, & G.O. Gabbard (Eds.), *Textbook of psychiatry* (5th ed., pp. 1025-1050). Washington, DC: American Psychiatric Publishing.

Maldonado, J.R., & Spiegel, D. (2008). Dissociative disorders. In R.E. Hales, S.C. Yudofsky, & G.O. Gabbard (Eds.), *Textbook of psychiatry* (5th ed., pp. 665-710). Washington, DC: American Psychiatric Publishing.

NANDA International (NANDA-I). (2012). *Nursing diagnoses: Definitions and classification 2012-2014*. Hoboken, NJ: Wiley-Blackwell.

Parcell, S. (2008). Biochemical and nutritional influences on pain. In J.F. Audette & A. Bailey (Eds.), *Integrative pain medicine*. New York, NY: Springer-Vertag.

Sadock, B.J., & Sadock, V.A. (2007). *Synopsis of psychiatry: Behavioral sciences/clinical psychiatry* (10th ed.). Philadelphia, PA: Lippincott Williams & Wilkins.

Shahrokh, N.C., & Hales, R.E. (2003). *American Psychiatric glossary* (8th ed.). Washington, DC: American Psychiatric Publishing.

Simeon, D., Stein, D.J., & Hollander, E. (1998). Treatment of depersonalization disorder with clomipramine. *Biological Psychiatry, 44*(4), 302-303.

Soares, N., and Grossman, L. (2012, November 29). Conversion disorder. *Emedicine Pediatrics*. Retrieved from http://emedicine.medscape.com/article/917864-overview

Wootton, J. (2008). Meditation and chronic pain. In J.F. Audette & A. Bailey (Eds.), *Integrative pain medicine*. New York, NY: Springer-Vertag.

Yutzy, S.H., & Parish, B.S. (2008). Somatoform disorders. In R.E. Hales, S.C. Yudofsky, & G.O. Gabbard (Eds.), *Textbook of psychiatry* (5th ed., pp, 609-664). Washington, DC: American Psychiatric Publishing.

Classical References

Asher, R. (1951). Munchausen's syndrome. *The Lancet, 257*(6650), 339-341.

Freud, S. (1962). The neuro-psychoses of defense. In J. Strachey (Ed.), *Standard edition of the complete psychological works of Sigmund Freud* (Vol. 3). London: Hogarth Press. (Original work published 1894).

@ INTERNET REFERENCES

- Additional information about somatic symptom disorders may be located at the following websites:
  - http://www.psyweb.com/Mdisord/somatd.html
  - http://my.clevelandclinic.org/disorders/hypochondriasis/hic_hypochondriasis.aspx
  - http://emedicine.medscape.com/article/805361-overview
  - http://emedicine.medscape.com/article/291304-overview

- Additional information about dissociative disorders may be located at the following websites:
  - http://www.nami.org/helpline/dissoc.htm
  - http://www.isst-d.org
  - http://www.mental-health-matters.com/disorders
  - http://emedicine.medscape.com/article/294508-overview

🎥 MOVIE CONNECTIONS

Bandits (illness anxiety disorder) • *Hanna and Her Sisters* (illness anxiety disorder) • Send Me No Flowers (illness anxiety disorder) • *Dead Again* (amnesia) • *Mirage* (amnesia) • *Suddenly Last Summer* (amnesia) • *Sybil* (DID) • *The Three Faces of Eve* (DID) • *Identity* (DID)

30 Issues Related to Human Sexuality and Gender Dysphoria

CHAPTER OUTLINE

KEY TERMS

anorgasmia

delayed ejaculation

premature (early) ejaculation

exhibitionistic disorder

fetishistic disorder

frotteuristic disorder

homosexuality

lesbianism

orgasm

pedophilic disorder

sensate focus

sexual masochism disorder

sexual sadism disorder

transvestic disorder

voyeuristic disorder

OBJECTIVES
After reading this chapter, the student will be able to:

1. Describe developmental processes associated with human sexuality.
2. Discuss historical and epidemiological aspects of paraphilic and sexual dysfunction disorders.
3. Identify various types of paraphilic and sexual dysfunction disorders and gender dysphoria.
4. Discuss predisposing factors associated with the etiology of paraphilic and sexual dysfunction disorders and gender dysphoria.
5. Describe the physiology of the human sexual response.
6. Conduct a sexual history.
7. Formulate nursing diagnoses and goals of care for clients with sexual dysfunctions and gender dysphoria in children.
8. Identify appropriate nursing interventions for clients with sexual dysfunctions and gender dysphoria in children.
9. Identify topics for client/family education relevant to sexual disorders.
10. Evaluate care of clients with sexual dysfunctions and gender dysphoria in children.
11. Describe various treatment modalities for clients with sexual disorders.
12. Discuss variations in sexual orientation.
13. Identify various types of sexually transmitted diseases and discuss the consequences of each.

HOMEWORK ASSIGNMENT
Please read the chapter and answer the following questions:

1. At about what age do children become aware of their own gender?
2. What types of psychosocial factors may predispose individuals to sexual desire disorders?
3. What medications have been implicated in the etiology of erectile disorder?
4. To disturbances in what physiological mechanism are sexual dysfunctions related?

Humans are sexual beings. Sexuality is a basic human need and an innate part of the total personality. It influences our thoughts, actions, and interactions, and is involved in aspects of physical and mental health.

Society's attitude toward sexuality is changing. Clients are more open to seeking assistance in matters that pertain to sexuality. Although not all nurses need to be educated as sex therapists, they can readily integrate information on sexuality into the care they give by focusing on preventive, therapeutic, and educational interventions to assist individuals to attain, regain, or maintain sexual wellness.

This chapter focuses on disorders associated with sexual functioning and gender dysphoria. Primary consideration is given to the categories of paraphilic disorders and sexual dysfunctions as classified in the *Diagnostic and Statistical Manual of Mental Disorders, Fifth Edition (DSM-5)* (American Psychiatric Association [APA], 2013). An overview of human sexual development throughout the life span is presented. Historical and epidemiological information associated with sexual disorders is included. Predisposing factors that have been implicated in the etiology of sexual disorders and gender dysphoria provide a framework for studying the dynamics of these conditions. Various medical treatment modalities are explored. A discussion of variations in sexual orientation is included. Various types of sexually transmitted diseases (STDs) are described, and an explanation of the consequences of each is presented.

Symptomatology is presented as background knowledge for assessing clients with sexual disorders and gender dysphoria. A tool for acquiring a sexual history is included. Nursing care is described in the context of the nursing process.

CORE CONCEPT

Sexuality

Sexuality is the constitution and life of an individual relative to characteristics regarding intimacy. It reflects the totality of the person and does not relate exclusively to the sex organs or sexual behavior.

Development of Human Sexuality

Birth Through Age 12

Although the sexual identity of an infant is determined before birth by chromosomal factors and physical appearance of the genitals, postnatal factors can greatly influence the way developing children perceive themselves sexually. Masculinity and femininity, as well as gender roles, are for the most part culturally defined. For example, differentiation of roles may be initiated at birth by painting a child's room pink or blue and by clothing the child in frilly, delicate dresses or tough, sturdy rompers.

It is not uncommon for infants to touch and explore their genitals. In fact, research on infantile sexuality indicates that both male and female infants are capable of sexual arousal and **orgasm** (Berman & Berman, 2005).

By age 2 or 2½ years, children know what gender they are. They know that they are like the parent of the same gender and different from the parent of the opposite gender and from other children of the opposite gender. They become acutely aware of anatomical gender differences during this time.

By age 4 or 5, children engage in heterosexual play. "Playing doctor" can be a popular game at this age. Through heterosexual play, children form a concept of marriage to a member of the opposite gender.

Children increasingly gain experience with masturbation during childhood, although certainly not all children masturbate during this period. Most children begin self-exploration and genital self-stimulation as soon as they are able to gain sufficient control over their physical movements (King, 2011).

Late childhood and preadolescence may be characterized by heterosexual or homosexual play. Generally the activity involves no more than touching the other's genitals, but may include a wide range of sexual behaviors (Masters, Johnson, & Kolodny, 1995). Girls at this age become interested in menstruation, and both genders are interested in learning about fertility, pregnancy, and birth. Interest in the opposite gender increases. Children of this age become self-conscious about their bodies and are concerned with physical attractiveness.

Children ages 10 to 12 are preoccupied with pubertal changes and the beginnings of romantic sexual attraction. Prepubescent boys may engage in group sexual activities such as genital exhibition or group masturbation. Homosexual sex play is not uncommon. Prepubescent girls may engage in some genital exhibition but they are usually not as preoccupied with the genitalia as are boys of this age.

Adolescence

Adolescence represents an acceleration in terms of biological changes and psychosocial and sexual development. This time of turmoil is nurtured by awakening endocrine forces and a new set of psychosocial tasks to undertake. Included in these tasks are issues relating to sexuality, such as how to deal with new or more powerful sexual feelings, whether to participate in various types of sexual behavior, how to recognize love, how to prevent unwanted pregnancy, and how to define age-appropriate gender roles.

Biologically, puberty begins for the female adolescent with breast enlargement, widening of the hips, and growth of pubic and ancillary hair. The onset of menstruation usually occurs between the ages of 11 and 13 years. In the male adolescent, growth of pubic hair and enlargement of the testicles begin at 12 to 16 years of age. Penile growth and the ability to ejaculate usually occur from the ages of 13 to 17. There is a marked growth of the body between ages 11 and 17, accompanied by the growth of body and facial hair, increased muscle mass, and a deeper voice.

Sexuality is slower to develop in the female than in the male adolescent. Women show steady increases in sexual responsiveness that peak in their middle 20s or early 30s. Sexual maturity for men is usually reached in the late teens, but their sexual drive remains high through young adulthood (Murray, Zentner, & Yakimo, 2009). Masturbation is a common sexual activity among male and female adolescents.

Many individuals have their first experience with sexual intercourse during the adolescent years. Although studies indicate a variety of statistics related to incidence of adolescent coitus, three notable trends have become evident:

1. More adolescents are engaging in premarital intercourse.
2. The incidence of premarital intercourse for girls has increased.
3. The average age of first intercourse has decreased.

The most recent data collected on this topic by the Centers for Disease Control and Prevention (CDC) indicated that there is a trend toward safer sex among adolescents. The survey revealed that, among those who reported being sexually active, condom use has increased since 2001 (CDC, 2012b).

The American culture has ambivalent feelings about adolescent sexuality. Psychosexual development is desired, but most parents want to avoid anything that may encourage teenage sex. The rise in number of cases of STDs, some of which are life-threatening, also contributes to fears associated with unprotected sexual activity in all age groups.

In June 2006, the U.S. Food and Drug Administration (FDA) licensed Gardasil, the first vaccine developed to prevent cervical cancer and other diseases caused by certain strains of human papillomavirus (HPV). A second vaccine, Cervarix, was approved by the FDA in October 2009. If administered prior to exposure to the sexually transmitted virus, these vaccines can protect women from ultimately developing cervical cancer caused by these specific strains. The CDC recommends routine administration of the vaccine to all girls ages 11 or 12 years with 3 doses of either vaccine (CDC, 2012a). The vaccine is also recommended for girls and women ages 13 through 26 years who have not already received the vaccine or have not completed all booster shots. In October 2011, the CDC's Advisory Committee on Immunization Practices (ACIP) recommended routine use of the quadrivalent vaccine, Gardasil, in males aged 11 or 12 years (CDC, 2011). The ACIP also recommended vaccination for males aged 13 through 21 years who have not been vaccinated previously or who have not completed the 3-dose series; males aged 22 through 26 years may also be vaccinated. Some state legislatures have proposed making administration of the HPV vaccine mandatory for girls ages 9 to 12 years. However, some parents believe these types of laws circumvent their rights, and may send the message that these young women are protected and therefore promote promiscuity. One recent study regarding this issue indicates that this concern is unfounded (Bednarczyk, Davis, Ault, Orenstein, & Omer, 2012). These researchers found that HPV vaccination in the recommended age group was not associated with increased sexual-activity-related outcome rates. Currently the controversy is ongoing, with supporters of a mandate saying that states have a rare opportunity to fight a cancer that kills 3,700 American women every year, and it must be given before a woman has been infected with the virus to be effective. But opponents say states—and parents—should be trying to prevent premarital sex instead of requiring a vaccination with the assumption that it is going to happen.

Adulthood

This period of the life cycle begins at approximately 20 years of age and continues to age 65. Sexuality associated with ages 65 and older is discussed in Chapter 34.

Marital Sex

Choosing a marital partner or developing a sexual relationship with another individual is one of the major tasks in the early years of this life-cycle stage. Current cultural perspective reflects that the institution of marriage has survived. About 80 to 90 percent of all people in the United States marry, and of those who divorce, a high percentage remarries. Intimacy in marriage is one of the most common forms of sexual expression for adults. The average American couple has coitus about two or three times per week when they are in their 20s, with the frequency gradually declining to about once weekly for those 45 years of age and over. Many adults continue to masturbate even though they are married and have ready access to heterosexual sex. This behavior is perfectly normal, although it often evokes feelings of guilt and may be kept secret.

Extramarital Sex

A number of studies present various results for surveys of extramarital sex. The estimates are that about one-third of married men and one-fourth of married women have engaged in extramarital sex at some time during their marriages (King, 2011). Although the incidence of extramarital sex for men seems to be holding constant, some evidence exists to suggest that the incidence for women may be increasing.

Although attitudes toward premarital sex have changed substantially during the last several decades, attitudes toward extramarital sex have remained relatively stable. Most women and men say they believe sexual exclusivity should be a goal in marriage, although they were less certain about what would happen if their partner did not live up to that ideal. Some estimates place the incidence of divorce caused by infidelity or adultery at around 20 percent of all divorce cases.

Sex and the Single Person

Attitudes about sexual intimacy among singles—never married, divorced, or widowed—vary from individual to individual. Some single people will settle for any kind of relationship, casual or committed, that they believe will enrich their lives. Others deny any desire for marriage or sexual intimacy, cherishing instead the independence they retain by being "unattached." Still others may search desperately for a spouse, with the desperation increasing as the years wear on.

Most divorced men and women return to having an active sex life following separation from their spouse. More widowed men than widowed women return to an active sex life after the loss of their partner. This may have in part to do with the fact that men choose women partners younger than themselves, and because widows outnumber widowers by more than 3 to 1 (Administration on Aging, 2014).

The "Middle" Years—40 to 65

With the advent of the middle years, a decrease in hormonal production initiates a number of changes in the sex organs, as well as the rest of the body. The average age of onset of menopause for the woman is around 50, although changes can be noted from about 40 to 60 years of age. Approximately 1 percent of women experience symptoms as early as age 35 (Murray et al., 2009). The decrease in the amount of estrogen can result in loss of vaginal lubrication, making intercourse painful. Other symptoms may include insomnia, "hot flashes," headaches, heart palpitations, and depression. Hormonal supplements may alleviate some of these symptoms, although controversy currently exists within the medical community regarding the safety of hormone replacement therapy.

With the decrease of androgen production during these years, men also experience sexual changes. The amount of ejaculate may decrease, and ejaculation may be less forceful. The testes decrease in size, and erections may be less frequent and less rigid. By age 50, the refractory period increases, and men may require 8 to 24 hours after orgasm before another erection can be achieved.

Biological drives decrease, and interest in sexual activity may decrease during these "middle" years. Although men need longer stimulation to reach orgasm and intensity of pleasure may decrease, women stabilize at the same level of sexual activity as at the previous stage in the life cycle and often have a greater capacity for orgasm in middle adulthood than in young adulthood (Sadock & Sadock, 2007). Murray and associates (2009) state:

> The enjoyment of sexual relations in younger years, rather than the frequency, is a key factor for maintenance of desire and activity in females, whereas frequency of relations and enjoyment are important factors for males. (p. 561)

Sexual Disorders

Paraphilic Disorders

The term *paraphilia* is used to identify repetitive or preferred sexual fantasies or behaviors that involve (1) nonhuman objects, (2) suffering or humiliation of oneself or one's partner, or (3) nonconsenting persons (Black & Andreasen, 2011).

In a paraphilic *disorder*, these sexual fantasies or behaviors are recurrent over a period of at least 6 months and cause the individual clinically significant distress or impairment in social, occupational, or other important areas of functioning (APA, 2013).

Historical Aspects

Historically, some restrictions on human sexual expression have always existed. Under the code of Orthodox Judaism, masturbation was punishable by death. In ancient Catholicism it was considered a carnal sin. In the late 19th century, masturbation was viewed as a major cause of insanity.

The sexual exploitation of children was condemned in ancient cultures, as it continues to be today. Incest remains the one taboo that crosses cultural barriers. It was punishable by death in Babylonia, Judea, and ancient China, and offenders were given the death penalty as late as 1650 in England.

Oral-genital, anal, homosexual, and animal sexual contacts were viewed by the early Christian church as unnatural and, in fact, were considered greater transgressions than extramarital sexual activity because they did not lead to biological reproduction.

Epidemiological Statistics

Relatively limited data exist on the prevalence or course of paraphilic disorders. Most available information has been obtained from studies of incarcerated sex offenders. Another source of information has been from outpatient psychiatric services for individuals with paraphilic disorders outside the criminal justice system.

Because few individuals with paraphilic disorders experience personal distress from their behavior, most come for treatment because of pressure from their partners or the authorities (Becker & Johnson, 2008). Data suggest that most people with paraphilic disorders who seek outpatient treatment do so for pedophilic disorder (45 percent), exhibitionistic disorder (25 percent), or voyeuristic disorder (12 percent).

Most individuals with paraphilic disorders are men, and the behavior is generally established in adolescence (Black & Andreasen, 2011). The behavior peaks between ages 15 and 25 and gradually declines so that, by age 50, the occurrence of paraphilic acts is very low, except for those behaviors that occur in isolation or with a cooperative partner. Some individuals experience multiple paraphilic disorders.

Types of Paraphilic Disorders

The following types of paraphilic disorders are identified by the *DSM-5:*

Exhibitionistic Disorder

Exhibitionistic disorder is characterized by recurrent and intense sexual arousal (manifested by fantasies, urges, or behaviors of at least 6 months' duration) from the exposure of one's genitals to an unsuspecting individual (APA, 2013). Masturbation may occur during the exhibitionism. In most cases of exhibitionism, the perpetrators are men and the victims are women (King, 2011).

The urges for genital exposure intensify when the exhibitionist has excessive free time or is under significant stress. Most people who engage in exhibitionism have rewarding sexual relationships with adult partners but concomitantly expose themselves to others.

Fetishistic Disorder

Fetishistic disorder involves recurrent and intense sexual arousal (manifested by fantasies, urges, or behaviors of at least 6 months' duration) from the use of either non-living objects or specific non-genital body part(s) (APA, 2013). A common sexual focus is on objects intimately associated with the human body (e.g., shoes, gloves, stockings). The fetish object is usually used during masturbation or incorporated into sexual activity with another person in order to produce sexual excitation.

Requirement of the fetish object for sexual arousal may become so intense in some individuals that to be without it may result in impotence. Onset of the disorder usually occurs during adolescence.

The disorder is chronic, and the complication arises when the individual becomes progressively more intensely aroused by sexual behaviors that exclude a sexual partner. The person with the fetish and his partner may become so distant that the partner eventually terminates the relationship.

Frotteuristic Disorder

Frotteuristic disorder is the recurrent and intense sexual arousal (manifested by urges, behaviors, or fantasies of at least 6 months' duration) involving touching or rubbing against a nonconsenting person (APA, 2013). Sexual excitement is derived from the actual touching or rubbing, not from the coercive nature of the act. Almost without exception, the gender of the frotteur is male.

The individual usually chooses to commit the act in crowded places, such as on buses or subways during rush hour. In this way, he can provide rationalization for his behavior, should someone complain, and can more easily escape arrest. The frotteur waits in a crowd until he identifies a victim, then he follows her and allows the rush of the crowd to push him against her. He fantasizes a relationship with his victim while rubbing his genitals against her thighs and buttocks or touching her genitalia or breasts with his hands. He often escapes detection because of the victim's initial shock and denial that such an act has been committed in this public place.

Pedophilic Disorder

The essential feature of **pedophilic disorder** is sexual arousal from prepubescent or early pubescent children equal to or greater than that derived from physically mature persons. *DSM-5* criteria specify that the behavior has lasted at least 6 months and is manifested by fantasies or sexual urges on which the individual has acted, or which cause significant distress or impairment in social, occupational, or other important areas of functioning (APA, 2013). The age of the molester is at least 16 years, and he or she is at least 5 years older than the child. This category of paraphilic disorder is the most common of sexual assaults.

Most child molestations involve genital fondling or oral sex. Vaginal or anal penetration of the child is most common in cases of incest. Sexual abuse of a child may include a wide range of behaviors, including speaking to the child in a sexual manner, indecent exposure and masturbation in the presence of the child, and inappropriate touching or acts of penetration (oral, vaginal, and anal) (King, 2011). Onset usually occurs during adolescence, and the disorder often runs a chronic course.

Sexual Masochism Disorder

The identifying feature of **sexual masochism disorder** is recurrent and intense sexual arousal (manifested by urges, behaviors, or fantasies of at least 6 months' duration) from the act of being humiliated, beaten, bound, or otherwise made to suffer (APA, 2013). These masochistic activities may be fantasized (e.g., being raped) and may be performed alone (e.g., self-inflicted pain) or with a partner (e.g., being restrained, spanked, or beaten by the partner). Some masochistic activities have resulted in death, in particular those that involve sexual arousal by oxygen deprivation. The disorder is usually chronic and can progress to the point at which the individual cannot achieve sexual satisfaction without masochistic fantasies or activities.

Sexual Sadism Disorder

The *DSM-5* identifies the essential feature of **sexual sadism disorder** as recurrent and intense sexual arousal (manifested by urges, behaviors, or fantasies of at least 6 months' duration) from the physical or psychological suffering of another individual (APA, 2013). The sadistic activities may be fantasized or acted on with a consenting or nonconsenting partner. In all instances, sexual excitation occurs in response to the suffering of the victim. Examples of sadistic acts include restraint, beating, burning, rape, cutting, torture, and even killing.

The course of the disorder is usually chronic, with the severity of the sadistic acts often increasing over time. Activities with nonconsenting partners are usually terminated by legal apprehension.

Transvestic Disorder

Transvestic disorder involves recurrent and intense sexual arousal (as manifested by fantasies, urges, or behaviors of at least 6 months' duration) from dressing in the clothes of the opposite gender. The individual is commonly a heterosexual man who keeps a collection of women's clothing that he intermittently uses to dress in when alone. The sexual arousal may be produced by an accompanying fantasy of the individual as a woman with female genitalia, or merely by the view of himself fully clothed as a woman without attention to the genitalia. The disorder causes marked distress to the individual, or interferes with social, occupational, or other important areas of functioning.

Voyeuristic Disorder

Voyeuristic disorder is identified by recurrent and intense sexual arousal (manifested by urges, behaviors, or fantasies of at least at least 6 months' duration) involving the act of observing an unsuspecting individual who is naked, in the process of disrobing, or engaging in sexual activity (APA, 2013). Sexual excitement is achieved through the act of looking, and no contact with the person is attempted. Masturbation usually accompanies the "window peeping" but may occur later as the individual fantasizes about the voyeuristic act.

Onset of voyeuristic behavior commonly occurs during adolescence, but the minimum age for a diagnosis of voyeuristic disorder is 18 years (APA, 2013). Many individuals who engage in this behavior enjoy satisfying sexual relationships with an adult partner. Few apprehensions occur because most targets of voyeurism are unaware that they are being observed.

Predisposing Factors to Paraphilic Disorders

Biological Factors

Various studies have implicated several organic factors in the etiology of paraphilic disorder. Destruction of parts of the limbic system in animals has been shown to cause hypersexual behavior (Becker & Johnson, 2008). Temporal lobe diseases, such as psychomotor seizures or temporal lobe tumors, have been implicated in some individuals with paraphilic disorder. Abnormal levels of androgens also may contribute to inappropriate sexual arousal. The majority of studies have involved violent sex offenders, and the results cannot accurately be generalized.

Psychoanalytic Theory

The psychoanalytic approach defines an individual with paraphilic disorder as one who has failed the normal developmental process toward heterosexual adjustment (Sadock & Sadock, 2007). This occurs when the individual fails to resolve the Oedipal crisis and either identifies with the parent of the opposite gender or selects an inappropriate object for libido cathexis. Becker and Johnson (2008) offered the following explanation:

> Severe castration anxiety during the Oedipal phase of development leads to the substitution of a symbolic object (inanimate or an anatomic part) for the mother, as in fetishism and transvestitism. Similarly, anxiety over arousal to the mother can lead to the choice of "safe," inappropriate sexual partners, as in pedophilia and zoophilia, or safe sexual behaviors in which there is no sexual contact, as in exhibitionism and voyeurism. (p. 740)

Behavioral Theory

The behavioral model hypothesizes that whether or not an individual engages in paraphilic behavior depends on the type of reinforcement he or she receives following the behavior. The initial act may be committed for various reasons. Some examples include recalling memories of experiences from an individual's early life (especially the first shared sexual experience), modeling behavior of others who have carried out paraphilic acts, mimicking sexual behavior depicted in the media, and recalling past trauma such as one's own molestation (Sadock & Sadock, 2007).

Once the initial act has been committed, the individual with paraphilic disorder consciously evaluates the behavior and decides whether to repeat it. A fear of punishment or perceived harm or injury to the victim, or a lack of pleasure derived from the experience, may extinguish the behavior. However, when negative consequences do not occur, when the act itself is highly pleasurable, or when the person with the paraphilic disorder immediately escapes and thereby avoids seeing any negative consequences experienced by the victim, the activity is more likely to be repeated.

Transactional Model of Stress/Adaptation

One model alone is probably not sufficient to explain the etiology of paraphilic disorders. It is most likely that the integration of learning experiences, sociocultural factors, and biological processes must occur to account for these deviant sexual behaviors. A combination of biological, psychosocial, and cultural factors, along with aspects of the learning paradigm previously described, probably provides the most comprehensive etiological explanation for paraphilic disorders to date. In Figure 30-1, a graphic depiction of the theory of multiple causation is presented in the Transactional Model of Stress/Adaptation.

Treatment Modalities for Paraphilic Disorders

Biological Treatment

Biological treatment of individuals with paraphilic disorders has focused on blocking or decreasing the level of circulating androgens. The most extensively used of the antiandrogenic medications are the progestin derivatives that block testosterone synthesis or block androgen receptors. They do not influence the direction of sexual drive toward appropriate adult partners. Instead they act to decrease libido, and thus break the individual's pattern of compulsive deviant sexual behavior (Becker & Johnson, 2008). They are not meant to be the sole source of treatment and work best when given in conjunction with participation in individual or group psychotherapy.

Psychoanalytic Therapy

Psychoanalytic approaches have been tried in the treatment of paraphilic disorders. In this type of therapy, the therapist helps the client to identify unresolved conflicts and traumas from early childhood. The therapy focuses on helping the individual resolve these early conflicts, thus relieving the anxiety that prevents him or her from forming appropriate sexual relationships. In turn the individual has no further need for paraphilic fantasies.

Behavior Therapy

Aversion techniques have been used to modify undesirable behavior. Aversion therapy methods in the treatment of paraphilic disorders involve pairing noxious stimuli, such as electric shocks and bad odors, with the impulse, which then diminishes. Behavioral therapy also includes skills training and cognitive restructuring in an effort to change the individual's maladaptive beliefs.

Other behavioral approaches to decreasing inappropriate sexual arousal have included covert sensitization and satiation. With covert sensitization, the individual combines inappropriate sexual fantasies with aversive, anxiety-provoking scenes under the guidance of the therapist (Becker & Johnson, 2008). Satiation is a technique in which the postorgasmic individual repeatedly fantasizes deviant behaviors to the point of saturation with the deviant stimuli, consequently making the fantasies and behavior unexciting.

Role of the Nurse

Treatment of the person with a paraphilic disorder is often very frustrating for both the client and the therapist. Most individuals with paraphilic disorders deny that they have a problem and seek psychiatric care only after their inappropriate behavior comes to the attention of others. In secondary prevention, the focus is to diagnose and treat the problem as early as possible to minimize difficulties. These individuals should be referred to specialists who are accustomed to working with this special population.

Nursing may best become involved in the primary prevention process. The focus of primary prevention in sexual disorders is to intervene in home life or other facets of childhood in an effort to prevent problems from developing. An additional concern of primary prevention is to assist in the development of adaptive coping strategies to deal with stressful life situations.

Three major components of sexual development have been identified: (1) gender identity (one's sense of maleness or femaleness), (2) sexual responsiveness (arousal to appropriate stimuli), and (3) the ability to establish relationships with others. A disturbance in one or more of these components may lead to a variety of sexual deviations.

Different developmental components seem to be disturbed in the various sexual deviations. For example, gender identity may be disturbed in transvestic disorder. The second component, sexual responsiveness to appropriate stimuli, may be disturbed in the case of the individual with fetishistic disorder. In the case of individuals with exhibitionistic or the frotteuristic disorders, the ability to form relationships may be disturbed.

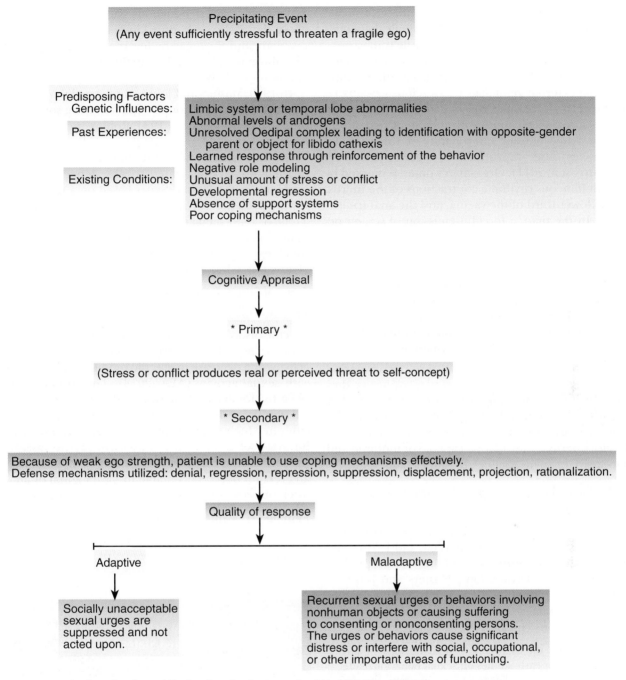

FIGURE 30-1 The dynamics of paraphilic disorder using the Transactional Model of Stress/Adaptation.

Nurses can participate in the regular evaluation of these developmental components to ensure that as children mature, their development in each of these three components is healthy, thereby preventing deviant sexual behaviors. Nurses who work in pediatrics, psychiatry, public health, ambulatory clinics, schools, and any other facility requiring contact with children must be knowledgeable about human sexual development. Accurate assessment and early intervention by these nurses can contribute a great deal toward primary prevention of sexual disorders.

Sexual Dysfunctions

The Sexual Response Cycle

Because sexual dysfunctions occur as disturbances in any of the phases of the sexual response cycle, an understanding of anatomy and physiology is a prerequisite to considerations of pathology and treatment.

■ **Phase I—Desire:** During this phase, the desire to have sexual activity occurs in response to verbal, physical, or visual stimulation. Sexual fantasies can also bring about this desire.

■ **Phase II—Excitement:** This is the phase of sexual arousal and erotic pleasure. Physiological changes occur. The male responds with penile tumescence and erection. Female changes include vasocongestion in the pelvis, vaginal lubrication, and swelling of the external genitalia.

■ **Phase III—Orgasm:** Orgasm is identified as a peaking of sexual pleasure, with release of sexual tension and rhythmic contraction of the perineal muscles and reproductive organs (Black & Andreasen, 2011). Orgasm in women is marked by simultaneous rhythmic contractions of the uterus, the lower third of the vagina, and the anal sphincter. In the man, a forceful emission of semen occurs in response to rhythmic spasms of the prostate, seminal vesicles, vas, and urethra.

■ **Phase IV—Resolution:** If orgasm has occurred, this phase is characterized by disgorgement of blood from the genitalia, creating a sense of general relaxation and well-being. If orgasm is not achieved, resolution may take several hours, producing pelvic discomfort and a feeling of irritability.

After orgasm, men experience a refractory period that may last from a few minutes to many hours, during which time they cannot be stimulated to further orgasm. Commonly, the length of the refractory period increases with age. Because women have no refractory period, they may be capable of multiple and successive orgasms (Sadock & Sadock, 2007).

Historical and Epidemiological Aspects Related to Sexual Dysfunction

Concurrent with the cultural changes occurring during the sexual revolution of the 1960s and 1970s came an increase in scientific research into sexual physiology and sexual dysfunctions. Masters and Johnson (1966, 1970) pioneered this work with their studies on human sexual response and the treatment of sexual dysfunctions. Spear (2001) reports:

> Sex therapy, the treatment of sexual disorders, has evolved from early studies on sexual behavior made over 50 years ago. During these 50 years, the approach to sex therapy has changed immensely. When William Masters and Virginia Johnson published *Human Sexual Inadequacy* in 1970, the sexual revolution, born in the 1960s, was not yet in full force. Due in part to the development of the oral contraceptive known as 'the pill' and the rise in the politics of feminism, society began to take a different, more open view of sexuality. The rise in sex therapy addressed [sexual] issues as they had never been addressed before, in the privacy of a doctor's office.

Sexual dysfunction consists of an impairment or disturbance in any of the phases of the sexual response cycle. No one knows exactly how many people experience sexual dysfunctions. Knowledge exists only about those who seek some kind of treatment for the problem, and they may be few in number compared with those who have a dysfunction but suffer quietly and never seek therapy.

In 1970, Masters and Johnson reported that 50 percent of all American couples suffered from some type of sexual dysfunction. In 1984, Robins and coworkers estimated that 24 percent of the U.S. population would experience a sexual dysfunction at some time in their lives. Data related to prevalence of sexual problems in the United States based on a recent survey are presented in Table 30-1. This survey included a total of 1,491 men and women ages 40 to 80, and less than 25 percent of the individuals had sought help for their sexual problem(s) from a health professional (Laumann, Glasser, Neves, & Moreira, 2009).

Types of Sexual Dysfunction

Erectile Disorder

Erectile disorder is characterized by marked difficulty in obtaining or maintaining an erection during sexual activity, or a decrease in erectile rigidity that interferes with sexual activity (APA, 2013). The problem has persisted for at least 6 months and causes the individual significant distress. *Primary erectile disorder* refers to cases in which the man has never been able to have intercourse; *secondary erectile disorder* refers to cases in which the man has difficulty getting or maintaining an erection but has been able to have vaginal or anal intercourse at least once.

Female Orgasmic Disorder

Female orgasmic disorder is defined by the *DSM-5* as a marked delay in, infrequency of, or absence of

TABLE 30-1	**Prevalence of Sexual Problems in Sexually Active Men and Women in the United States**	
DISORDER	MEN (%)	WOMEN (%)
Lack of sexual interest	18.1	33.2
Inability to reach orgasm	12.4	20.7
Pain during sex	3.1	12.7
Premature ejaculation	26.2	—
Erectile difficulties	22.5	—
Lubrication difficulties	—	21.5

Adapted from Laumann, E.O., Glasser, D.B., Neves, R.C.S., & Moreira, E.D. (2009). A population-based survey of sexual activity, sexual problems, and associated help-seeking behavior patterns in mature adults in the United States of America. *International Journal of Impotence Research, 21,* 171-178.

orgasm during sexual activity (APA, 2013). It may also be characterized by a reduced intensity of orgasmic sensation. The condition, which is sometimes referred to as **anorgasmia,** has lasted at least 6 months, and causes the individual significant distress. Women who can achieve orgasm through noncoital clitoral stimulation but are not able to experience it during coitus in the absence of manual clitoral stimulation are not necessarily categorized as anorgasmic.

A woman is considered to have *primary orgasmic disorder* when she has never experienced orgasm by any kind of stimulation. *Secondary orgasmic disorder* exists if the woman has experienced at least one orgasm, regardless of the means of stimulation, but no longer does so.

Delayed Ejaculation

Delayed ejaculation is characterized by marked delay in ejaculation or marked infrequency or absence of ejaculation during partnered sexual activity (APA, 2013). The condition has lasted for at least 6 months and causes the individual significant distress. With this disorder, the man is unable to ejaculate, even though he has a firm erection and has had more than adequate stimulation. The severity of the problem may range from only occasional problems ejaculating (*secondary disorder*) to a history of never having experienced an orgasm (*primary disorder*). In the most common version, the man cannot ejaculate during coitus but may be able to ejaculate as a result of other types of stimulation.

Premature (Early) Ejaculation

The *DSM-5* describes **premature (early) ejaculation** as persistent or recurrent ejaculation occurring within 1 minute of beginning partnered sexual activity and before the person wishes it (APA, 2013). The condition has lasted at least 6 months and causes the individual significant distress. The diagnosis should take into account factors that affect the duration of the excitement phase, such as the person's age, the uniqueness of the sexual partner, and frequency of sexual activity (Sadock & Sadock, 2007).

Premature (early) ejaculation is the most common sexual disorder for which men seek treatment. It is particularly common among young men who have a very high sex drive and have not yet learned to control ejaculation.

Female Sexual Interest/Arousal Disorder

This disorder is characterized by a reduced or absent interest or pleasure in sexual activity (APA, 2013). The individual typically does not initiate sexual activity, and is commonly unreceptive to partner's attempts to initiate. There is an absence of sexual thoughts or fantasies, and absent or reduced arousal in response to sexual or erotic cues. The condition has persisted for at least 6 months and causes the individual significant distress.

Male Hypoactive Sexual Desire Disorder

This disorder is defined by the *DSM-5* as a persistent or recurrent deficiency or absence of sexual fantasies and desire for sexual activity. In making the judgment of deficiency or absence, the clinician considers factors that affect sexual functioning, such as age and circumstances of the person's life (APA, 2013). The condition has persisted for at least 6 months and causes the individual significant distress.

An individual's absolute level of sexual desire may not be the problem; rather, the problem may be a discrepancy between the partners' levels. The conflict may occur if one partner wants to have sexual relations more often than the other does. Care must be taken not to label one partner as pathological when the problem actually lies in the discrepancy of sexual desire between the partners.

Genito-Pelvic Pain/Penetration Disorder

With this disorder, the individual experiences considerable difficulty with vaginal intercourse and attempts at penetration. Pain is felt in the vagina, around the vaginal entrance and clitoris, or deep in the pelvis. There is fear and anxiety associated with anticipation of pain or vaginal penetration. A tensing and tightening of the pelvic floor muscles occurs during attempted vaginal penetration (APA, 2013). The condition may be *lifelong* (present since the individual became sexually active) or *acquired* (began after a period of relatively normal sexual function). It has persisted for at least 6 months and causes the individual clinically significant distress.

Substance/Medication-Induced Sexual Dysfunction

With these disorders, the sexual dysfunction developed after substance intoxication or withdrawal or after exposure to a medication (APA, 2013). The dysfunction may involve pain, impaired desire, impaired arousal, or impaired orgasm. Some substances/medications that can interfere with sexual functioning include alcohol, amphetamines, cocaine, opioids, sedatives, hypnotics, anxiolytics, antidepressants, antipsychotics, antihypertensives, and others.

Predisposing Factors to Sexual Dysfunction

Biological Factors

Sexual Desire Disorders Studies have correlated decreased levels of serum testosterone with hypoactive sexual desire disorder in men. Evidence also exists that suggests a relationship between higher serum testosterone levels and increased female libido (Traish & Kim, 2006). Diminished libido has been observed in both men and women with elevated levels of serum prolactin (Nappi, Ferdeghini, & Polatti, 2006). Various

IMPLICATIONS OF RESEARCH FOR EVIDENCE-BASED PRACTICE

Bacon, C.G., Mittleman, M.A., Kawachi, I., Glovannucci, E., Glasser, D.B., & Rimm, E.B. (2003). Sexual function in men older than 50 years of age: Results from the health professionals follow-up study. *Annals of Internal Medicine, 139*(3), 161-168.

DESCRIPTION OF THE STUDY: The purpose of the Health Professionals Follow-up Study was to describe the association between age and several aspects of sexual functioning in men older than 50 years of age. Participants included 31,742 male dentists, optometrists, osteopaths, podiatrists, pharmacists, and veterinarians in the United States. The participants were mailed questionnaires every 2 years between 1986 and 2000. Age range of participants was 53 to 90 years. Measures of sexual function included ability to have and maintain an erection adequate for intercourse, sexual desire, and ability to reach orgasm. Independent modifiable health behaviors included physical activity, smoking, obesity, alcohol consumption, and sedentary lifestyle (measured by hours of TV viewing).

RESULTS OF THE STUDY: The results of this study reinforced those of previous studies that linked sexual dysfunction

to increasing age, certain disease processes (e.g., diabetes, cancer, stroke, and hypertension), and medications (e.g., antidepressants; beta-blockers). This study also addressed more specifically the correlation between sexual dysfunction and independent, modifiable risk factors. A higher risk for sexual dysfunction was associated with obesity, sedentary lifestyle, smoking, and excess alcohol consumption. Regular physical exercise (>32 metabolic equivalent hours per week), leanness, moderate alcohol consumption, and not smoking were statistically significant with decreased risk.

IMPLICATIONS FOR NURSING PRACTICE: This study has strong implications for nursing in terms of educating men over age 50 about contributing factors to sexual dysfunction. Establishing and conducting classes for weight reduction (including programs of regular exercise) and smoking cessation are well within the scope of nursing practice. Nurses can intervene to assist clients with behavior modification to achieve and/or maintain sexual wellness.

---

medications have also been implicated in the etiology of hypoactive sexual desire disorder. Some examples include antihypertensives, antipsychotics, antidepressants, anxiolytics, and anticonvulsants. Alcohol and cocaine have also been associated with impaired desire, especially after chronic use.

Sexual Arousal Disorders Postmenopausal women require a longer period of stimulation for lubrication to occur, and there is generally less vaginal transudate after menopause (Altman & Hanfling, 2003). Various medications, particularly those with antihistaminic and anticholinergic properties, may also contribute to decreased ability for arousal in women. Arteriosclerosis is a common cause of male erectile disorder as a result of arterial insufficiency (King, 2011). Various neurological disorders can contribute to erectile dysfunctions as well. The most common neurologically based cause may be diabetes, which places men at high risk for neuropathy (Kim & Brosman, 2013). Others include temporal lobe epilepsy and multiple sclerosis. Trauma (e.g., spinal cord injury, pelvic cancer surgery) can also result in erectile disorder. Several medications have been implicated in the etiology of this disorder, including antihypertensives, antipsychotics, antidepressants, and anxiolytics. Chronic use of alcohol has also been shown to be a contributing factor.

Orgasmic Disorders Some women report decreased ability to achieve orgasm following hysterectomy.

Conversely, some report increased sexual activity and decreased sexual dysfunction following hysterectomy (Rhodes, Kjerulff, Langenberg, & Guzinski, 1999). Studies of the use of transdermal testosterone for sexual dysfunction in women after hysterectomy have revealed mixed results (Nappi et al., 2005). Some medications (e.g., selective serotonin reuptake inhibitors) may inhibit orgasm. Medical conditions, such as depression, hypothyroidism, and diabetes mellitus, may cause decreased sexual arousal and orgasm.

Biological factors associated with delayed male orgasm include surgery of the genitourinary tract (e.g., prostatectomy), various neurological disorders (e.g., Parkinson's disease), and other diseases (e.g., diabetes mellitus). Medications that have been implicated include opioids, antihypertensives, antidepressants, and antipsychotics (Altman & Hanfling, 2003). Transient cases of the disorder may occur with excessive alcohol intake.

Although premature ejaculation is commonly caused by psychological factors, general medical conditions or substance use may also be contributing influences. Particularly in cases of secondary dysfunction, in which a man at one time had ejaculatory control but later lost it, physical factors may be involved. Examples include a local infection such as prostatitis or a degenerative neural disorder such as multiple sclerosis.

Sexual Pain Disorders A number of organic factors can contribute to painful intercourse in women, including intact hymen, episiotomy scar, vaginal or urinary tract infection, ligament injuries, endometriosis, or ovarian cysts or tumors. Painful intercourse in men may also be caused by various organic factors. For example, infection caused by poor hygiene under the foreskin of an uncircumcised man can cause pain. Phimosis, a condition in which the foreskin cannot be pulled back, can also cause painful intercourse. An allergic reaction to various vaginal spermicides or irritation caused by vaginal infections may be a contributing factor. Finally, various prostate problems may cause pain on ejaculation.

Psychosocial Factors

Sexual Desire Disorders Phillips (2000) has identified a number of individual and relationship factors that may contribute to hypoactive sexual desire disorder. Individual causes include religious orthodoxy; sexual identity conflicts; past sexual abuse; financial, family, or job problems; depression; and aging-related concerns (e.g., changes in physical appearance). Among the relationship causes are interpersonal conflicts; current physical, verbal, or sexual abuse; extramarital affairs; and desire or practices that differ from those of the partner.

Sexual Arousal Disorders A number of psychological factors have been cited as possible impediments to female arousal. They include doubt, guilt, fear, anxiety, shame, conflict, embarrassment, tension, disgust, irritation, resentment, grief, hostility toward partner, and a puritanical or moralistic upbringing. Sexual abuse has been identified as a significant risk factor for desire and arousal disorders in women.

Problems with male sexual arousal may be related to chronic stress, anxiety, or depression. Developmental factors that hinder the ability to be intimate, that lead to a feeling of inadequacy or distrust, or that develop a sense of being unloving or unlovable may also result in impotence. Relationship factors that may affect erectile functioning include lack of attraction to one's partner, anger toward one's partner, or being in a relationship that is not characterized by trust (Altman & Hanfling, 2003). Unfortunately, regardless of the etiology of the erectile dysfunction, once it occurs, the man may become increasingly anxious about his next sexual encounter. This anticipatory anxiety about achieving and maintaining an erection may then perpetuate the problem.

Orgasmic Disorders Numerous psychological factors are associated with inhibited female orgasm. They include fears of becoming pregnant or damage to the vagina, rejection by the sexual partner, hostility toward men, and feelings of guilt regarding sexual impulses (Sadock & Sadock, 2007). Negative cultural conditioning ("nice girls don't enjoy sex") may also influence the adult female's sexual response. Various developmental factors also have relevance to orgasmic dysfunction. Examples include childhood exposure to rigid religious orthodoxy, negative family attitudes toward nudity and sex, and traumatic sexual experiences during childhood or adolescence, such as incest or rape (Clayton, 2002; Phillips, 2000).

Psychological factors are also associated with inhibited male orgasm (delayed ejaculation). In the primary disorder (in which the man has never experienced orgasm), the man often comes from a rigid, puritanical background. He perceives sex as sinful and the genitals as dirty, and he may have conscious or unconscious incest wishes and guilt (Sadock & Sadock, 2007). In the case of secondary disorder (previously experienced orgasms that have now stopped), interpersonal difficulties are usually implicated. There may be some ambivalence about commitment, fear of pregnancy, or unexpressed hostility.

Premature (early) ejaculation may be related to a lack of physical awareness on the part of a sexually inexperienced man. The ability to control ejaculation occurs as a gradual maturing process with a sexual partner in which foreplay becomes more give-and-take "pleasuring," rather than strictly goal-oriented. The man becomes aware of the sensations and learns to delay the point of ejaculatory inevitability. Relationship problems such as a stressful marriage, negative cultural conditioning, anxiety over intimacy, and lack of comfort in the sexual relationship may also contribute to this disorder.

Sexual Pain Disorders Penetration disorders may occur in response to having experienced genito-pelvic pain for various organic reasons stated in the "Biological Factors" section. Involuntary constriction within the vagina occurs in response to anticipatory pain, making intercourse impossible. The diagnosis does not apply if the etiology is determined to be due to another medical condition. A variety of psychosocial factors have been implicated, including negative childhood conditioning of sex as dirty, sinful, and shameful. Early traumatic sexual experiences (e.g., rape or incest) may also cause penetration disorder. Other etiological factors that may be important include homosexual orientation, traumatic experience with an early pelvic examination, pregnancy phobia, STD phobia, or cancer phobia (Dreyfus, 2009; King, 2011; Leiblum, 1999; Phillips, 2000; Sadock & Sadock, 2007).

Transactional Model of Stress/Adaptation

The etiology of sexual dysfunction is most likely influenced by multiple factors. In Figure 30-2, a graphic depiction of the theory of multiple causation is presented in the Transactional Model of Stress/Adaptation.

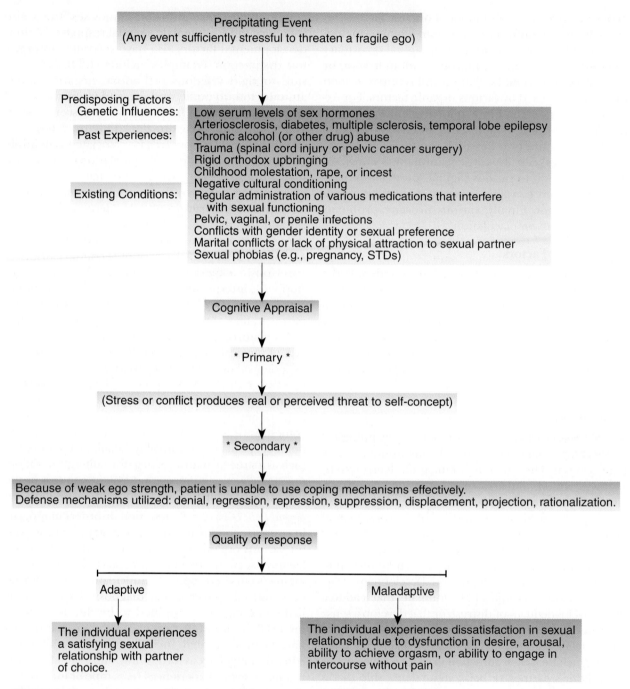

FIGURE 30–2 The dynamics of sexual dysfunction using the Transactional Model of Stress/Adaptation.

Application of the Nursing Process to Sexual Disorders

Assessment

Most assessment tools for taking a general nursing history contain some questions devoted to sexuality. Many nurses feel uncomfortable obtaining information about the subject. However, accurate data must be collected if problems are to be identified and resolutions attempted. Sexual health is an integral part of physical and emotional well-being. The nursing history is incomplete if items directed toward sexuality are not included.

Most nurses are not required to obtain a sexual history as in depth as the one presented in this chapter. However, for certain clients a more extensive sexual history is required than that which is included in the general nursing history. These include clients who have medical or surgical conditions that may affect their sexuality; clients with infertility problems, STDs, or complaints of sexual inadequacy; clients who are pregnant, or have gynecological problems; those seeking information on abortion or family planning; and individuals in premarital, marital, and psychiatric counseling.

The best approach for taking a sexual history is a nondirective one; that is, it is best to use the sexual history outline as a guideline but allow the interview to progress in a less restrictive manner than the outline permits (with one question immediately following the other). The order of the questions should be adjusted according to the client's needs as they are identified during the interview. A nondirective approach allows time for the client to interject information related to feelings or concerns about his or her sexuality.

The language used should be understandable to the client. If he or she uses terminology that is unfamiliar, ask for clarification. Take level of education and cultural influences into consideration.

The nurse's attitude must convey warmth, openness, honesty, and objectivity. Personal feelings, attitudes, and values should be clarified and should not interfere with acceptance of the client. The nurse must remain nonjudgmental. This is conveyed by listening in an interested matter-of-fact manner without overreacting to any information the client may present.

The content outline for a sexual history presented in Box 30-1 is not intended to be used as a rigid questionnaire but as a guideline from which the nurse may select appropriate topics for gathering information about the client's sexuality. The outline should be individualized according to client needs.

BOX 30-1 Sexual History: Content Outline

I. Identifying data
 A. Client
  1. Age
  2. Gender
  3. Marital status
 B. Parents
  1. Ages
  2. Dates of death and ages at death
  3. Birthplace
  4. Marital status
  5. Religion
  6. Education
  7. Occupation
  8. Congeniality
  9. Demonstration of affection
  10. Feelings toward parents
 C. Siblings (same information as above)
 D. Marital partner (same information as above)
 E. Children
  1. Ages
  2. Gender
  3. Strengths
  4. Identified problems

II. Childhood sexuality
 A. Family attitudes about sex
  1. Parents' openness about sex
  2. Parents' attitudes about nudity
 B. Learning about sex
  1. Asking parents about sex
  2. Information volunteered by parents
  3. At what age and how did client learn about: pregnancy, birth, intercourse, masturbation, nocturnal emissions, menstruation, homosexuality, STDs

 C. Childhood sex activity
  1. First sight of nude body
   a. Same gender
   b. Opposite gender
  2. First genital self-stimulation
   a. Age
   b. Feelings
   c. Consequences
  3. First sexual exploration at play with another child
   a. Age (of self and other child)
   b. Gender of other child
   c. Nature of the activity
   d. Feelings and consequences
  4. Sexual activity with older persons
   a. Age (of self and other person)
   b. Gender of other person
   c. Nature of the activity
   d. Client willingness to participate
   e. Feelings and consequences
 D. Did you ever see your parents (or others) having intercourse? Describe your feelings.
 E. Childhood sexual theories or myths:
  1. Thoughts about conception and birth.
  2. Roles of male/female genitals and other body parts in sexuality.

III. Onset of adolescence
 A. In girls
  1. Information about menstruation
   a. How received; from whom
   b. Age received
   c. Feelings

Continued

BOX 30-1 Sexual History: Content Outline—cont'd

2. Age
   a. Of first period
   b. When breasts began to develop
   c. At appearance of ancillary and pubic hair
3. Menstruation
   a. Regularity; discomfort; duration
   b. Feelings about first period
B. In boys
   1. Information about puberty
      a. How received; from whom
      b. Age received
      c. Feelings
   2. Age
      a. Of appearance of ancillary and pubic hair
      b. Change of voice
      c. First orgasm (with or without ejaculation); emotional reaction

IV. Orgastic experiences
A. Nocturnal emissions (male) or orgasms (female) during sleep.
   1. Frequency
B. Masturbation
   1. Age begun; ever punished?
   2. Frequency; methods used
   3. Marital partner's knowledge
   4. Practiced with others? Spouse?
   5. Emotional reactions
   6. Accompanying fantasies
C. Necking and petting ("making out")
   1. Age when begun
   2. Frequency
   3. Number of partners
   4. Types of activity
D. Premarital intercourse
   1. Frequency
   2. Relationship with and number of partners
   3. Contraceptives used
   4. Feelings
E. Orgasmic frequency
   1. Past
   2. Present

V. Feelings about self as masculine/feminine
A. The male client
   1. Does he feel masculine?
   2. Accepted by peers?
   3. Sexually adequate?
   4. Feelings/concerns about body
      a. Size
      b. Appearance
      c. Function
B. The female client
   1. Does she feel feminine?
   2. Accepted by peers?
   3. Sexually adequate?
   4. Feelings/concerns about body

a. Size
b. Appearance
c. Function

VI. Sexual fantasies and dreams
A. Nature of sex dreams
B. Nature of fantasies
   1. During masturbation
   2. During intercourse

VII. Dating
A. Age and feelings about
   1. First date
   2. First kissing
   3. First petting or "making out"
   4. First going steady

VIII. Engagement
A. Age
B. Sex activity during engagement period
   1. With fiancée
   2. With others

IX. Marriage
A. Date of marriage
B. Age at marriage: Spouse:
C. Spouse's occupation
D. Previous marriages: Spouse:
E. Reason for termination of previous marriages
   Client: Spouse:
F. Children from previous marriages
   Client: Spouse:
G. Wedding trip (honeymoon)
   1. Where? How long?
   2. Pleasant or unpleasant?
   3. Sexual considerations?
H. Sex in marriage
   1. General satisfaction/dissatisfaction.
   2. Thoughts about spouse's general satisfaction/dissatisfaction
I. Pregnancies
   1. Number: Ages of couple:
   2. Results (normal birth; cesarean delivery; miscarriage; abortion)
   3. Planned or unplanned
   4. Effects on sexual adjustment
   5. Sex of child wanted or unwanted

X. Extramarital sex
A. Emotional attachments
   1. Number; frequency; feelings
B. Sexual intercourse
   1. Number; frequency; feelings
C. Postmarital masturbation
   1. Frequency; feelings
D. Postmarital homosexuality
   1. Frequency; feelings
E. Multiple sex ("swinging")
   1. Frequency; feelings

BOX 30-1 Sexual History: Content Outline—cont'd

XI. Sex after widowhood, separation, or divorce
  A. Outlet
    1. Orgasms in sleep
    2. Masturbation
    3. Petting
    4. Intercourse
    5. Homosexuality
    6. Other
  B. Frequency; feelings

XII. Variation in sexual orientation
  A. Homosexuality
    1. First experience; describe circumstances.
    2. Frequency since adolescence

XIII. Paraphilias
  A. Sexual contact with animals
    1. First experience; describe nature of contact
    2. Frequency and recent contact
    3. Feelings
  B. Voyeurism
    1. Describe types of observation experienced
    2. Feelings
  C. Exhibitionism
    1. To whom? When?
    2. Feelings
  D. Fetishes; transvestitism
    1. Nature of fetish
    2. Nature of transvestite activity
    3. Feelings
  E. Sadomasochism
    1. Nature of activity
    2. Sexual response
    3. Frequency; recency
    4. Consequences
  F. Seduction and rape
    1. Has client seduced/raped another?
    2. Has client ever been seduced/raped?

G. Incest
    1. Nature of the sexual activity
    2. With whom?
    3. When occurred? Frequency; recency.
    4. Consequences

XIV. Prostitution
  A. Has client ever accepted/paid money for sex?
  B. Type of sexual activity engaged in
  C. Feelings about prostitution

XV. Certain effects of sex activities
  A. STDs
    1. Age at learning about STDs
    2. Type of STD contracted
    3. Age and treatment received
  B. Illegitimate pregnancy
    1. At what age(s)
    2. Outcome of the pregnancy(ies)
    3. Feelings
  C. Abortion
    1. Why performed?
    2. At what age(s)?
    3. How often?
    4. Before or after marriage?
    5. Circumstance: who, where, how?
    6. Feelings about abortion: at the time; in retrospect; anniversary reaction

XVI. Use of erotic material
  A. Personal response to erotic material
    1. Sexual pleasure—arousal
    2. Mild pleasure
    3. Disinterest; disgust
  B. Use in connection with sexual activity
    1. Type and frequency of use
    2. To accompany what type of sexual activity

Adapted from an outline prepared by the Group for Advancement of Psychiatry, based on the Sexual Performance Evaluation Questionnaire of the Marriage Council of Philadelphia. Used with permission.

Diagnosis/Outcome Identification

Nursing diagnoses are formulated from the data gathered during the assessment phase and with background knowledge regarding predisposing factors to the disorder. The following nursing diagnoses may be used for the client with sexual disorders:

■ Sexual dysfunction related to depression and conflict in relationship or certain biological or psychological contributing factors to the disorder evidenced by loss of sexual desire or ability to perform.

■ Ineffective sexuality pattern related to conflicts with sexual orientation or variant preferences, evidenced by expressed dissatisfaction with sexual behaviors.

Outcome Criteria

The following criteria may be used for measurement of outcomes in the care of the client with sexual disorders.

The client:

■ Can correlate stressful situations that decrease sexual desire
■ Can communicate with partner about sexual situation without discomfort
■ Can verbalize ways to enhance sexual desire
■ Verbalizes resumption of sexual activity at level satisfactory to self and partner
■ Can correlate variant behaviors with times of stress
■ Can verbalize fears about abnormality and inappropriateness of sexual behaviors

- Expresses desire to change variant sexual behavior
- Participates and cooperates with extended plan of behavior modification
- Expresses satisfaction with own sexuality pattern

Planning/Implementation

Following are nursing diagnoses commonly used with individuals experiencing alterations in sexual functioning. Short- and long-term goals and nursing interventions are presented for each.

Sexual Dysfunction

Sexual dysfunction is defined as "the state in which an individual experiences a change in sexual function during the sexual response phases of desire, excitation, and/or orgasm, which is viewed as unsatisfying, unrewarding, or inadequate" (NANDA International [NANDA-I], 2012, p. 323).

Client Goals

Outcome criteria include short- and long-term goals. Timelines are individually determined.

Short-Term Goals

- Client will identify stressors that may contribute to loss of sexual function within 1 week *OR*
- Client will discuss pathophysiology of disease process that contributes to sexual dysfunction within 1 week.
- (*For the client with permanent dysfunction due to disease process*): Client will verbalize willingness to seek professional assistance from a sex therapist in order to learn alternative ways of achieving sexual satisfaction with partner by (time is individually determined).

Long-Term Goal

- Client will resume sexual activity at a level satisfactory to self and partner by (time is individually determined).

Interventions

- Assess the client's sexual history and previous level of satisfaction in his or her sexual relationship. This history establishes a database from which to work and provides a foundation for goal setting.
- Assess the client's perception of the problem. The client's idea of what constitutes a problem may differ from that of the nurse. It is the client's perception on which the goals of care must be established.
- Help the client determine the timeline associated with the onset of the problem, and discuss what was happening in his or her life situation at that time. Stress in all areas of life will affect sexual functioning. The client may be unaware of the correlation between stress and sexual dysfunction.
- Assess the client's mood and level of energy. Depression and fatigue decrease desire and enthusiasm for participation in sexual activity.

- Review medication regimen; observe for side effects. Many medications can affect sexual functioning. Evaluation of the drug and the individual's response is important to ascertain whether the drug may be contributing to the problem.
- Encourage the client to discuss the disease process that may be contributing to sexual dysfunction. Ensure that the client is aware that alternative methods of achieving sexual satisfaction exist and can be learned through sex counseling if he or she and the partner desire to do so.
- Provide information regarding sexuality and sexual functioning. Increasing knowledge and correcting misconceptions can decrease feelings of powerlessness and anxiety and facilitate problem resolution.
- Make a referral for additional counseling or sex therapy, if required. Complex problems are likely to require assistance from an individual who is specially trained to treat problems related to sexuality. Client and partner may be somewhat embarrassed to seek this kind of assistance. Support from a trusted nurse can provide the impetus for them to pursue the help they need.

Ineffective Sexuality Pattern

Ineffective sexuality pattern is defined as "expressions of concern regarding own sexuality" (NANDA-I, 2012, p. 325).

Client Goals

Outcome criteria include short- and long-term goals. Timelines are individually determined.

Short-Term Goals

- Client will verbalize aspects about sexuality that he or she would like to change.
- Client and partner will communicate with each other ways in which each believes their sexual relationship could be improved.

Long-Term Goals

- Client will express satisfaction with own sexuality pattern.
- Client and partner will express satisfaction with sexual relationship.

Interventions

- Take a sexual history, noting the client's expression of areas of dissatisfaction with his or her sexual pattern. Knowledge of what the client perceives as the problem is essential for providing the type of assistance he or she may need.
- Assess areas of stress in the client's life and examine the relationship with his or her sexual partner. Variant sexual behaviors are often associated with added stress in the client's life. The relationship with his or her partner may deteriorate as the

individual eventually gains sexual satisfaction only from variant practices.

■ Note cultural, social, ethnic, racial, and religious factors that may contribute to conflicts regarding variant sexual practices. The client may be unaware of the influence these factors exert in creating feelings of discomfort, shame, and guilt regarding sexual attitudes and behavior.

■ Be accepting and nonjudgmental. Sexuality is a very personal and sensitive subject. The client is more likely to share this information if he or she does not fear being judged by the nurse.

■ Assist the therapist in a plan of behavior modification to help the client who desires to decrease variant sexual behaviors. Individuals with paraphilic disorders are treated by specialists who have experience in modifying variant sexual behaviors. Nurses can intervene by providing assistance with implementation of the plan for behavior modification.

■ If altered sexuality patterns are related to illness or medical treatment, provide information to the client and partner regarding the correlation between the illness and the sexual alteration. Explain possible modifications in usual sexual patterns that the client and partner may try in an effort to achieve a satisfying sexual experience in spite of the limitation. The client and his or her partner may be unaware of alternate possibilities for achieving sexual satisfaction, or anxiety associated with the limitation may interfere with rational problem solving.

■ Teach the client that sexuality is a normal human response and is not synonymous with any one sexual act; that it reflects the totality of the person and does not relate exclusively to the sex organs or sexual behavior. The client must understand that *sexual* feelings are *human* feelings.

■ If the client feels abnormal or very unlike everyone else, the self-concept is likely to be very low—even worthless. Helping him or her to understand that even though the behavior is variant, feelings and motivations are common, may help to increase feelings of self-worth and desire to change behavior.

Concept Care Mapping

The concept map care plan is an innovative approach to planning and organizing nursing care (see Chapter 9). It is a diagrammatic teaching and learning strategy that allows visualization of interrelationships between medical diagnoses, nursing diagnoses, assessment data, and treatments. An example of a concept map care plan for a client with a sexual disorder is presented in Figure 30-3.

Client/Family Education

The role of client teacher is important in the psychiatric area, as it is in all areas of nursing. A list of topics for client/family education relevant to sexual disorders is presented in Box 30-2.

Evaluation

Reassessment is necessary to determine if selected interventions have been successful in helping the client overcome problems with sexual functioning. Evaluation may be facilitated by gathering information using the following types of questions.

For the Client With Sexual Dysfunction:

■ Has the client identified life situations that promote feelings of depression and decreased sexual desire?

■ Can he or she verbalize ways to deal with this stress?

■ Can the client satisfactorily communicate with sexual partner about the problem?

■ Have the client and sexual partner identified ways to enhance sexual desire and the achievement of sexual satisfaction for both?

■ Are client and partner seeking assistance with relationship conflict?

■ Do both partners agree on what the major problem is? Do they have the motivation to attempt change?

■ Do client and partner verbalize an increase in sexual satisfaction?

For the Client With Variant Sexual Behaviors:

■ Can the client correlate an increase in variant sexual behavior to times of severe stress?

■ Has the client been able to identify those stressful situations and verbalize alternative ways to deal with them?

■ Does the client express a desire to change variant sexual behavior and a willingness to cooperate with extended therapy to do so?

■ Does the client express an understanding about the normalcy of sexual feelings, aside from the inappropriateness of his or her behavior?

■ Are expressions of increased self-worth evident?

Quality and Safety Education for Nurses (QSEN)

The Institute of Medicine (IOM), in its 2003 report, *Health Professions Education: A Bridge to Quality*, challenged faculties of medicine, nursing, and other health professions to ensure that their graduates have achieved a core set of competencies in order to meet the needs of the 21st-century health-care system. These competencies include *providing patient-centered care, working in interdisciplinary teams, employing evidence-based practice, applying quality improvement, ensuring safety,* and *utilizing informatics.* A QSEN teaching strategy is included in Box 30-3. The use of this type of activity is intended to arm the instructor and the student with guidelines for attaining the knowledge, skills, and attitudes necessary for achievement of quality and safety competencies in nursing.

Clinical Vignette: Harry (age 60) and Sally (age 58) have been married 35 years. They have come to the mental health clinic for couples therapy because they are having problems in their sexual relationship. They tell the psychiatric nurse practitioner that they once had an active, satisfying sexual relationship, but Sally admits that although she still loves Harry, she no longer has a desire for sex. She states that she must create sexual fantasies or view sexual videos to become aroused and that this makes her feel uncomfortable and "dirty." Harry desires sex with Sally but has lately developed some difficulties with erectile dysfunction. The nurse develops the following concept map care plan for Harry and Sally.

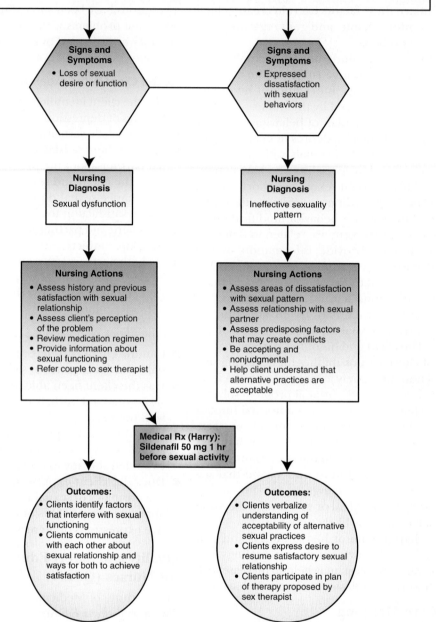

Signs and Symptoms
• Loss of sexual desire or function

Signs and Symptoms
• Expressed dissatisfaction with sexual behaviors

Nursing Diagnosis
Sexual dysfunction

Nursing Diagnosis
Ineffective sexuality pattern

Nursing Actions
• Assess history and previous satisfaction with sexual relationship
• Assess client's perception of the problem
• Review medication regimen
• Provide information about sexual functioning
• Refer couple to sex therapist

Nursing Actions
• Assess areas of dissatisfaction with sexual pattern
• Assess relationship with sexual partner
• Assess predisposing factors that may create conflicts
• Be accepting and nonjudgmental
• Help client understand that alternative practices are acceptable

Medical Rx (Harry): Sildenafil 50 mg 1 hr before sexual activity

Outcomes:
• Clients identify factors that interfere with sexual functioning
• Clients communicate with each other about sexual relationship and ways for both to achieve satisfaction

Outcomes:
• Clients verbalize understanding of acceptability of alternative sexual practices
• Clients express desire to resume satisfactory sexual relationship
• Clients participate in plan of therapy proposed by sex therapist

FIGURE 30–3 Concept map care plan for clients with sexual disorders.

BOX 30-2 **Topics for Client/Family Education Related to Sexual Disorders**

NATURE OF THE ILLNESS
1. The human sexual response cycle
2. What is "normal" and "abnormal?"
3. Types of sexual dysfunctions
4. Causes of sexual dysfunctions
5. Types of paraphilic disorders
6. Causes of paraphilic disorders
7. Symptoms associated with sexual dysfunctions and paraphilic disorders

MANAGEMENT OF THE DISORDER
1. Teach practices and ways of sexual expression.
2. Teach relaxation techniques.
3. Teach side effects of medications that may be contributing to sexual dysfunction.
4. Teach effects of alcohol consumption on sexual functioning.
5. Teach about STDs (see Table 30-2).

SUPPORT SERVICES
1. Provide appropriate referral for assistance from sex therapist.
2. One national association to which many qualified sex therapists belong is:

American Association of Sexuality Educators, Counselors and Therapists

> 1444 I Street NW, Suite 700
> Washington, D.C. 20005
> (202) 449-1099
> http://www.aasect.org

Treatment Modalities for Sexual Dysfunctions

Sexual Desire Disorders

Hypoactive Sexual Desire Disorder

Hypoactive sexual desire disorder has been treated in both men and women with the administration of testosterone. The masculinizing side effects make this approach unacceptable to women, and the evidence that it increases libido in men is inconclusive. Becker and Stinson (2008) describe the most effective treatment as a combination of cognitive therapy to deal with maladaptive beliefs; behavioral treatment, such as exercises to enhance sexual pleasuring and communication; and relationship therapy to deal with the individual's use of sex as a method of control.

Low sexual desire is often the result of partner incompatibility. If this is the case, the therapist may choose to shift from the sexual issue to helping a couple identify and deal with their incompatibility.

Sexual Arousal Disorders

Female Sexual Interest/Arousal Disorder

The goal of treatment for female sexual interest/arousal disorder is to reduce the anxiety associated with sexual activity. Masters and Johnson (1970) reported successful results using their behaviorally oriented **sensate focus** exercises to treat this disorder. The objective is to reduce the goal-oriented demands of intercourse on both partners, thus reducing

BOX 30-3 QSEN TEACHING STRATEGY

Assignment: Using a Capstone Cultural Diversity Paper for Program Outcomes Evaluation

Intervening With a Client of an Alternative Sexual Orientation

Competency Domain: Patient-Centered Care

Learning Objectives: Student will:
- Identify dimensions of the client's sexual orientation obtained through the nursing interview.
- Discuss common problems/concerns for the diverse group.
- Plan potential patient-centered interventions that promote wellness and demonstrate respect for the client's diversity.
- Identify how knowledge gained from this assignment will influence his/her future nursing care of clients with diverse sexual orientations.
- Recognize and analyze how culturally based attitudes, values, and beliefs impact nursing care.

Strategy Overview:
- **Part I. Client Interview Data**
  1. Using the Sexual History Assessment Tool in Box 30-1, conduct a sexual history of a client with a diverse sexual orientation.
  2. During the interview, identify the client's values, beliefs, practices, preferences, and expressed needs related to health care, communication, and sexual expression.

BOX 30-3 QSEN TEACHING STRATEGY—cont'd

• **Part II. Cultural Analysis and Health Care Needs Identification**

Submit a typed analysis of the client's diversity supported with in-text reference citations (minimum 3-4 pages). The paper should include the following information:

1. Using the client interview data and current literature, describe the traditional cultural health-care beliefs and practices, including interpersonal relationships and worldview beliefs for this diverse group.
2. Discuss any differences between what you have read in the literature and what your client told you. Include possible explanations for these differences.
3. Identify actual or potential health-care problems/concerns for the client and his/her diverse group.
4. Discuss potential therapeutic interventions for the client that promote wellness; that demonstrate respect for the client's diversity, rights, beliefs, values, and life experiences; and that incorporate professional values and practice standards.
5. Record your observations from the interview regarding verbal and nonverbal communication (such as eye contact, rate of speech, personal space, and touch) demonstrated by you and the client.

• **Part III. Personal Reflections**

Submit a paper describing personal reflections of how this knowledge might influence your nursing care of persons with diverse sexual orientations (minimum 2 pages). The paper should include the following information:

1. To what extent do your beliefs, prejudices, or bias influence your thinking and nursing care? Give several examples.
2. Discuss specifically how the knowledge from this assignment will influence your future nursing care of clients with different sexual orientations. Discuss several examples.

Adapted from teaching strategy submitted by Lisa Sue Flood, Associate Professor, Northern Michigan University, Marquette, MI. © 2009 QSEN; http://qsen.org. With permission.

performance pressures and anxiety associated with possible failure. Altman and Hanfling (2003) state:

> The cornerstone of sex therapy is a series of behavioral exercises called sensate focus exercises. These highly structured touching activities are designed to help overcome performance anxiety and increase comfort with physical intimacy. Initially, the couple agrees to refrain from intercourse or genital stimulation until the later stages of treatment. This helps dispel anxiety that's built up around sexual performance and allows establishment of new patterns of relating. (pp. 38-39)

The couple is instructed to take turns caressing each other's bodies. Initially, they are to avoid touching breasts and genitals, and to focus on the sensations of being touched. The caressing progresses to include touching of the breasts and genitals, to touching each other simultaneously, and eventually to include intercourse. These non-goal-oriented exercises promote the sensual side of sexual interaction in a nonpressured, nonevaluative way (Masters et al., 1995).

Erectile Disorder

Sensate focus has also been used effectively for erectile disorder in men. Clinicians widely agree that even when significant organic factors have been identified, psychological factors may also be present and must be considered in treatment.

Group therapy, hypnotherapy, and systematic desensitization have also been used successfully in reducing the anxiety that may contribute to erectile difficulties. Psychodynamic interventions may help alleviate intrapsychic conflicts contributing to performance anxiety (Becker & Stinson, 2008).

Various medications, including testosterone and yohimbine, have been used to treat erectile disorder. Penile injections of papaverine or prostaglandin have been used to produce an erection lasting from 1 to 4 hours. However, this treatment is unacceptable to many men because of pain of the injection and side effects, such as priapism and fibrotic nodules in the penis (Becker & Stinson, 2008).

Several other medications have been approved by the FDA for the treatment of erectile disorder. They include sildenafil (Viagra), tadalafil (Cialis), vardenafil (Levitra), and avanafil (Stendra). These newer impotence agents block the action of phosphodiesterase-5 (PDE5), an enzyme that breaks down cyclic guanosine monophosphate (cGMP), a compound that is required to produce an erection. This action only occurs, however, in the presence of nitric oxide (NO), which is released during sexual arousal. PDE5 inhibitors do not result in sexual arousal. They work to achieve penile erection in the presence of sexual arousal. Adverse effects include headache, facial flushing, indigestion, nasal congestion, dizziness, and visual changes (mild color tinges and blurred vision) (Vallerand & Sanoski, 2013). In 2005, the FDA ordered that the manufacturers of these medications add a warning to their labels. This action was taken in response to 43 cases of sudden vision loss by individuals taking the drugs. It is not possible to ascertain whether the medications are responsible for nonarteritic ischemic optic neuropathy (NAION), a condition in which blood flow to the optic nerve is blocked. More recently, the FDA has issued an additional warning associated with PDE5 inhibitors of risk of sudden hearing loss (Kim & Brosman, 2013). PDE5 inhibitors are contraindicated in concurrent use with nitrates.

Two other oral medications, apomorphine and phentolamine, are currently being investigated for use with erectile disorder. Phentolamine has been used in combination with papaverine in an injectable form that increases blood flow to the penis, resulting in an erection. Apomorphine acts directly on the dopamine receptors in the brain. This mode of stimulating dopamine in the brain is thought to enhance the sexual response.

For erectile disorder refractory to other treatment methods, penile prostheses may be implanted. Two basic types are currently available: a bendable silicone implant and an inflatable device. The bendable variety requires a relatively simple surgical technique for insertion of silicone rods into the erectile areas of the penis. This results in a perpetual state of semi-erection for the client. The inflatable penile prosthesis produces an erection only when it is desired, and the appearance of the penis in both the flaccid and erect states is completely normal. Potential candidates for penile implantation should undergo careful psychological and physical screening. Although penile implants do not enable the client to recover the ability to ejaculate or to have an orgasm, men with prosthetic devices have generally reported satisfaction with their subsequent sexual functioning.

Orgasmic Disorders

Female Orgasmic Disorder

Because anxiety may contribute to the lack of orgasmic ability in women, sensate focus is often advised to reduce anxiety, increase awareness of physical sensations, and transfer communication skills from the verbal to the nonverbal domain. Phillips (2000) provides the following description of therapy for the anorgasmic woman:

> Treatment relies on maximizing stimulation and minimizing inhibition. Stimulation may include masturbation with prolonged stimulation (initially up to one hour) and/or the use of a vibrator as needed, and muscular control of sexual tension (alternating contraction and relaxation of the pelvic muscles during high sexual arousal). The latter is similar to Kegal exercises. Methods to minimize inhibition include distraction by "spectatoring" (observing oneself from a third-party perspective), fantasizing, or listening to music (p. 135).

Treatment for secondary anorgasmia (in which the client has had orgasms in the past, but is now unable to achieve them) focuses on the couple and their relationship. Therapy with both partners is essential to the success of this disorder.

Delayed Ejaculation

Treatment for delayed ejaculation is very similar to that described for the anorgasmic woman. A combination of sensate focus and masturbatory training has been used with a high degree of success in the Masters and Johnson clinic. Treatment for male orgasmic disorder almost always includes the sexual partner.

Premature (Early) Ejaculation

Masters and associates (1995) advocate what they suggest is a highly successful technique for the treatment of premature ejaculation. Sensate focus is used, with progression to genital stimulation. When the man reaches the point of imminent ejaculation, his sexual partner is instructed to apply the "squeeze" technique: applying pressure at the base of the glans penis, using the thumb and first two fingers. Pressure is held for about 4 seconds and then released. This technique is continued until the man is no longer on the verge of ejaculating. This technique is practiced during subsequent periods of sexual stimulation.

No medication has been approved by the FDA for the treatment of premature ejaculation, but a number of studies have shown efficacy for this disorder with the selective serotonin reuptake inhibitors (SSRIs) (Benson, Ost, Noble, & Lakin, 2013). Some individuals may achieve positive results with single dosing prior to sexual relations, while others may require regular daily dosing to achieve an adequate blood level.

Genito-Pelvic Pain/Penetration Disorder

Treatment for the pain of intercourse begins with a thorough physical and gynecological examination. When organic pathology has been eliminated, the client's fears and anxieties underlying sexual functioning are investigated (Becker & Stinson, 2008). Systematic desensitization has been used successfully to decrease fears and anxieties associated with painful intercourse.

Treatment of penetration disorder begins with education of the woman and her sexual partner regarding the anatomy and physiology of the disorder (i.e., what exactly is occurring during the vaginal reflex and possible etiologies). The involuntary nature of the disorder is stressed in an effort to alleviate the sexual partner's perception that this occurrence is an act of willful withholding by the woman.

The second phase of treatment involves systematic desensitization. The client is taught a series of tensing and relaxing exercises aimed at relaxation of the pelvic musculature. Relaxation of the pelvic muscles is followed by a procedure involving the systematic insertion of dilators of graduated sizes until the woman is able to accept the penis into the vagina without discomfort. This physical therapy, combined with treatment of any identified relationship problems, has been used by the Masters and Johnson clinic with considerable success (Masters et al., 1995).

Gender Dysphoria

CORE CONCEPT
Gender
The condition of being either male or female.

Gender identity is the sense of knowing whether one is male or female—that is, the awareness of one's masculinity or femininity. Gender dysphoria occurs when there is incongruence between biological/assigned gender and one's experienced/expressed gender. The *DSM-5* categorizes diagnosis of the condition according to the client's current age: gender dysphoria in children and gender dysphoria in adolescents or adults. Although most cases of the condition begin in childhood, persons who present clinically with gender dysphoria may be of any age.

For purposes of this text, differentiation between the age groups will be discussed, but the major focus will be on the condition as it emerges in childhood. Nurses who work in areas of primary prevention with children can have the greatest effect in terms of treating this condition. Treatment aimed at reversal in behavior, if it is desired by the client, is considered cautiously optimistic if initiated in childhood. After establishment of a core gender identity, it is difficult later in life to instill attributes of an opposite identity, and most commonly, it is not desired by the individual.

There was much controversy in the psychiatric community about whether gender dysphoria should be included in the *DSM-5*. The transgender community expressed a great deal of concern, protesting to the psychiatric work group that, "different is not a disease." The work group attempted to address some of the concerns of the transgender community, taking into consideration the stigma associated with inclusion of the diagnosis, but also the need for inclusion in terms of access to adequate treatment and care. If the diagnosis was not included, those who chose to seek medical-surgical treatment may be denied third-party assistance. The term *gender dysphoria* was adopted to minimize the stigma that was connected to the previous label

(gender identity disorder), and to emphasize the emotional component associated with the condition.

Course and Epidemiology

The prevalence of gender dysphoria is estimated at 1 in 30,000 men and 1 in 100,000 women (Black & Andreasen, 2011). Most (approximately 75 percent) are biological males desiring reassignment to female gender (MTF), and the remaining 25 percent are females desiring to be male (FTM) (Martin, 2007). Some individuals with gender dysphoria choose to find ways of living with their cross-gender identity without altering their bodies. Others have a strong desire to change their physical body to reflect their core gender identity. It has been noted that gender dysphoria sometimes dissipates after early childhood; however, if it persists into adolescence, it appears to be irreversible (Dreger, 2009). King (2011) states:

> A recent study found that about 3 percent of 7-year-old boys and about 5 percent of girls showed cross-gender behavior. However, in a 10-year follow-up study, most were no longer displaying cross-gender behavior; this was true only in the most extreme cases. (p. 205)

Predisposing Factors
Biological Influences

Becker and Johnson (2008) report that studies of females with congenital adrenal hyperplasia (CAH) as a result of high levels of prenatal androgens suggest that there may be a relation between CAH and gender dysphoria. The data are still inconclusive, and further research in this area is indicated.

Several studies have been conducted to determine if sex hormone levels are abnormal in individuals with gender dysphoria. In some studies, decreased levels of testosterone were found in male transgendered individuals, and abnormally high levels of testosterone were found in female transgendered individuals, but the results have been inconsistent (Becker & Johnson, 2008). One large-scale study of cross-gender behavior in twins revealed that the similarity for cross-gender behavior was greater in monozygotic (identical) than in dizygotic (nonidentical) twin pairs, suggesting a possible genetic link (Beijsterveldt, Hudziak, & Boomsma, 2006).

Another study reported on possible effects of testosterone on brain differentiation (Zhou, Horman, Gooren, & Swaab, 1995). The researchers found that the red nucleus of the stria terminalis (a region of the hypothalamus) in male-to-female transsexuals corresponded to that of typical females, rather than that of typical males. This was the case whether the individual was heterosexual or homosexual, and was not accounted for by hormone therapy.

Family Dynamics

It appears that family dynamics may play an influential role in the etiology of gender dysphoria. Sadock and Sadock (2007) state, "Children usually develop a gender identity consonant with their sex of rearing (also known as *assigned sex*)" (p. 718). Gender roles are culturally determined, and parents encourage masculine or feminine behaviors in their children. Although "temperament" may play a role with certain behavioral characteristics being present at birth, mothers usually foster a child's pride in their gender. Sadock and Sadock (2007) state:

> The father's role is also important in the early years, and his presence normally helps the separation-individuation process. Without a father, mother and child may remain overly close. For a girl, the father is normally the prototype of future love objects; for a boy, the father is a model for male identification." (p. 719)

In a 2003 study, Zucker and associates found a high rate of psychopathology and family dysfunction in children with gender dysphoria. Maternal depression and bipolar disorder were frequently demonstrated, whereas fathers often exhibited depression and substance use disorders. The authors recommended that parental conflicts and psychopathology must be given careful consideration as an aspect in childhood gender dysphoria.

Psychoanalytic Theory

The psychoanalytic theory suggests that gender identity problems begin during the struggle of the Oedipal/Electra conflict. Problems may reflect both real family events and those created in the child's imagination. These conflicts, whether real or imagined, interfere with the child's loving of the opposite-gender parent and identifying with the same-gender parent, and ultimately with normal gender identity.

Application of the Nursing Process to Gender Dysphoria in Children

Background Assessment Data (Symptomatology)

Some children may resist wearing the clothing or playing with the toys that are typical for their assigned gender. This is often part of normal childhood behavior. But when these behaviors persist into later childhood and adolescence, they may progress into symptoms of gender dysphoria. Some of these symptoms include the following: the insistence of being of the opposite gender, disgust with one's own genitals, belief that one will grow up to become the opposite gender, refusal to wear clothing of the assigned gender, desirous of having the genitals of the opposite gender, and refusal to participate in the games and activities culturally associated with the assigned gender. These children may be subjected to teasing and rejection by their peers and disapproval from family members. This occurs early in childhood for boys, but often does not occur before adolescence in girls, because masculine behavior in girls is more culturally acceptable than feminine behavior in boys. Because of this rejection, interpersonal relationships are hampered. The condition is not common but occurs more frequently in boys than in girls. The *DSM-5* diagnostic criteria for gender dysphoria in children are presented in Box 30-4.

BOX 30-4 Diagnostic Criteria for Gender Dysphoria in Children

A. A marked incongruence between one's experienced/expressed gender and assigned gender, of at least 6 months' duration, as manifested by at least six of the following indicators (one of which must be Criterion A1):

1. A strong desire to be of the other gender or an insistence that he or she is the other gender (or some alternative gender different from one's assigned gender).
2. In boys (assigned gender), a strong preference for cross-dressing or simulating female attire; in girls (assigned gender), a strong preference for wearing only typical masculine clothing and a strong resistance to the wearing of typical feminine clothing.
3. A strong preference for cross-gender roles in make-believe or fantasy play.
4. A strong preference for the toys, games, or activities stereotypically used or engaged in by the other gender.
5. A strong preference for playmates of the other gender.
6. In boys (assigned gender), a strong rejection of typically masculine toys, games, and activities and a strong avoidance of rough-and-tumble play; or in girls (assigned gender), a strong rejection of typically feminine toys, games, and activities.
7. A strong dislike of one's sexual anatomy.
8. A strong desire for the primary and/or secondary sex characteristics that match one's experienced gender.

B. The condition is associated with clinically significant distress or impairment in social, occupational, or other important areas of functioning.

Specify if:

With a disorder of sex development (e.g., a congenital adrenogenital disorder such as congenital adrenal hyperplasia or androgen insensitivity syndrome).

Diagnosis/Outcome Identification

Based on the data collected during the nursing assessment, possible nursing diagnoses for the child with gender dysphoria may include the following:

■ Disturbed personal identity related to biological factors or parenting patterns that encourage culturally unacceptable behaviors for assigned gender

■ Impaired social interaction related to socially and culturally unacceptable behaviors

■ Low self-esteem related to rejection by peers

The following criteria may be used for measurement of outcomes in the care of the child with gender dysphoria.

The client:

■ Demonstrates trust in a therapist of the same gender

■ Demonstrates development of a close relationship with the parent of the same gender

■ Demonstrates a diminishment in the excessively close relationship with the parent of the opposite gender

■ Demonstrates behaviors that are culturally appropriate for assigned gender

■ Verbalizes and demonstrates comfort in, and satisfaction with, assigned gender role

■ Interacts appropriately with others demonstrating culturally acceptable behaviors

■ Verbalizes and demonstrates self-satisfaction with assigned gender role

Planning/Implementation

Following are nursing diagnoses commonly used with individuals experiencing gender dysphoria. Short- and long-term goals and nursing interventions are presented for each.

Disturbed Personal Identity

Disturbed personal identity is defined as the "inability to maintain an integrated and complete perception of self" (NANDA-I, 2012, p. 282).

Client Goals

Outcome criteria include short- and long-term goals. Timelines are individually determined.

Short-Term Goals

■ Client will verbalize knowledge of behaviors that are appropriate and culturally acceptable for assigned gender.

■ Client will verbalize desire for congruence between personal feelings and behavior and assigned gender.

Long-Term Goals

■ Client will demonstrate behaviors that are appropriate and culturally acceptable for assigned gender.

■ Client will express personal satisfaction and feelings of being comfortable in assigned gender.

Interventions

■ Spend time with the client and show positive regard. Trust and unconditional acceptance are essential to the establishment of a therapeutic nurse-client relationship.

■ Be aware of personal feelings and attitudes toward this client and his or her behavior. Attitudes influence behavior. The nurse must not allow negative attitudes to interfere with the effectiveness of interventions.

■ Allow the client to describe his or her perception of the problem. It is important to know how the client perceives the problem before attempting to correct misperceptions.

■ Discuss with the client the types of behaviors that are more culturally acceptable. Practice these behaviors through role-playing or with play therapy strategies (e.g., male and female dolls). Positive reinforcement or social attention may be given for use of appropriate behaviors. No response is given for stereotypical opposite-gender behaviors.

> **CLINICAL PEARL** The objective in working for behavioral change in a child who has gender dysphoria is to enhance culturally appropriate same-gender behaviors, but not necessarily to extinguish all coexisting opposite-gender behaviors.

■ Behavioral change is attempted with the child's best interests in mind. That is, to help him or her with cultural and societal integration, while maintaining individuality. To preserve self-esteem and enhance self-worth, the child must know that he or she is accepted unconditionally as a unique and worthwhile individual.

Impaired Social Interaction

Impaired social interaction is defined as "insufficient or excessive quantity or ineffective quality of social exchange" (NANDA-I, 2012, p. 320).

Client Goals

Outcome criteria include short- and long-term goals. Timelines are individually determined.

Short-Term Goal

■ Client will verbalize possible reasons for ineffective interactions with others.

Long-Term Goal

■ Client will interact with others using culturally acceptable behaviors.

Interventions

■ Once the client feels comfortable with the new behaviors in role playing or one-to-one nurse-client interactions, the new behaviors may be tried in group situations. If possible, remain with the client during initial interactions with others. The presence of a trusted individual provides security for the client in a new situation, and also provides the potential for feedback to the client about his or her behavior.

■ Observe client behaviors and the responses he or she elicits from others. Give social attention (e.g., smile, nod) to desired behaviors. Follow up these "practice" sessions with one-to-one processing of the interaction. Give positive reinforcement for efforts. Positive reinforcement encourages repetition of desirable behaviors. One-to-one processing provides time for discussing the appropriateness of specific behaviors and why they should or should not be repeated.

■ Offer support if client is feeling hurt from peer ridicule. Matter-of-factly discuss the behaviors that elicited the ridicule. Offer no personal reaction to the behavior. Personal reaction from the nurse would be considered judgmental. Validation of client's feelings is important, yet it is also important that client understand why his or her behavior was the subject of ridicule and how to avoid it in the future.

■ The goal is to create a trusting, nonthreatening atmosphere for the client in an attempt to change behavior and improve social interactions. Long-term studies have not yet revealed the significance of therapy with these children for psychosexual relationship development in adolescence or adulthood. One variable that must be considered is the evidence of psychopathology within the families of many of these children.

Low Self-Esteem

Low self-esteem is defined as "negative self-evaluating/feelings about self or self-capabilities" (NANDA-I, 2012, pp. 285-287).

Client Goals

Outcome criteria include short- and long-term goals. Timelines are individually determined.

Short-Term Goal

■ Client will verbalize positive statements about self, including past accomplishments and future prospects.

Long-Term Goal

■ Client will verbalize and demonstrate behaviors that indicate self-satisfaction with assigned gender,

ability to interact with others, and a sense of self as a worthwhile person.

Interventions

■ In an effort to enhance the child's self-esteem, encourage him or her to engage in activities in which he or she is likely to achieve success.

■ Help the child to focus on aspects of his or her life for which positive feelings exist. Discourage rumination about situations that are perceived as failures or over which the client has no control. Give positive feedback for these behaviors.

■ Help the client identify behaviors or aspects of life he or she would like to change. If realistic, assist the child in problem-solving ways to bring about the change. Having some control over his or her life may decrease feelings of powerlessness and increase feelings of self-worth and self-satisfaction.

■ Offer to be available for support to the child when he or she is feeling rejected by peers. Having an available support person who does not judge the child's behavior and who provides unconditional acceptance assists the child to progress toward acceptance of self as a worthwhile person.

Evaluation

The final step of the nursing process is to determine if the nursing interventions have been effective in achieving the intended outcomes. This evaluation process requires that the nurse reassess the client's behaviors and determine if the changes at which the interventions had been directed have occurred. For the child with gender dysphoria, this may be accomplished by using the following types of questions:

■ Does the client perceive that a problem existed that requires a change in behavior for resolution?

■ Does the client demonstrate use of behaviors that are culturally accepted for his or her assigned gender?

■ Can the client use these culturally accepted behaviors in interactions with others?

■ Is the client accepted by peers when same-gender behaviors are used?

■ If the client is refusing to change behaviors, what is the peer reaction?

■ What is the client's response to negative peer reaction?

■ Can the client verbalize positive statements about self?

■ Can the client discuss past accomplishments without dwelling on the perceived failures?

■ Has the client shown progress toward accepting self as a worthwhile person regardless of others' responses to his or her behavior?

Treatment Issues

Becker and Johnson (2008) stated:

> Treatment [of gender dysphoria in the child] has three goals: increasing peer support and acceptance, treating co-occurring mental health concerns, and reducing the likelihood of [gender dysphoria] in adulthood. (p. 737)

Treatment of children with gender dysphoria may be initiated when the behaviors cause significant distress and when the client desires it. Several controversial issues exist relative to treatment of these children. One type of treatment suggests that they should be encouraged to become satisfied with their assigned gender. Behavior modification therapy serves to help the child embrace the games and activities of his or her assigned gender and promotes development of friendships with same gender peers. A somewhat effeminate boy will not be forced to become an aggressive and competitive type, nor will a "tomboy" be expected to turn into a "girly-girl." The goal is acceptance of a culturally appropriate self-image without mental health concerns from discomfort associated with the assigned gender.

Another treatment model suggests that children who have problems with gender identity are dysphoric only because of their image within the culture. In this view, children should be accepted as they see themselves—different from their assigned gender—and supported in their efforts to live as the gender in which they feel most comfortable. Some professionals are recommending pubertal delay for adolescents aged 12 to 16 years who have suffered with extreme lifelong gender dysphoria, and who have supportive parents that encourage the child to pursue a desired change in gender (Gibson & Catlin, 2010). A gonadotropin-releasing hormone agonist is administered, which suppresses pubertal changes. The treatment is reversible if the adolescent decides later not to pursue the gender change. When the medication is withdrawn, external sexual development proceeds, and the individual has avoided permanent surgical intervention. If he or she decides as an adult to advance to the surgical intervention, the proponents of the hormonal treatment suggest that initiating pubertal delay at an early age will "most certainly result in high percentages of individuals who will more easily pass into the opposite gender role than when treatment commenced well after the development of secondary sexual characteristics" (Delemarre-van de Waal & Cohen-Kettenis, 2006).

The type of treatment one chooses for gender dysphoria (if any) is very individual and a matter of personal choice. However, issues associated with mental health concerns, such as depression, anxiety, social isolation, anger, self-esteem, and parental conflict, must be addressed, even if the client elects not to proceed with the behavior modification approach. Cohen-Kettenis and Pfäfflin (2003) reported that, in their clinic population, when the functional mental health problems within the family were resolved, the gender dysphoria often dissipated.

Behavior therapy of children with gender dysphoria typically occurs in outpatient clinics. Nurses working in these settings may encounter these clients from time to time, although the condition is not common. One-to-one nursing intervention may be provided by an advanced practice psychiatric clinical nurse specialist or nurse practitioner.

Gender Dysphoria in Adolescents or Adults

With this condition, an individual, despite having the anatomical characteristics of a given gender, has the self-perception of being of the opposite gender. Individuals with this disorder do not feel comfortable wearing the clothes of their assigned gender and often engage in cross-dressing. They may find their own genitals repugnant and may repeatedly submit requests to the health-care system for hormonal and surgical gender reassignment. Depression and anxiety are common and are often attributed by the individual to his or her inability to live in the desired gender role. (Refer to the previous section on gender dysphoria in children for predisposing factors to this condition.)

Treatment Issues

Intervention with adolescents and adults with gender dysphoria is difficult. Adolescents rarely have the desire or motivation to alter their cross-gender roles, and disruptive behaviors are not uncommon. Some adults seek therapy to learn how to cope with their altered sexual identity, while others have direct and immediate request for hormonal therapy and surgical sex reassignment. Treatment of the adult with gender dysphoria is a complex process. The true transgendered individual intensely desires to have the genitalia and physical appearance of the assigned gender changed to conform to his or her gender identity. This change requires a great deal more than surgical alteration of physical features. In most cases, the individual must undergo extensive psychological testing and counseling, as well as live in the role of the desired gender for up to 2 years before surgery.

Hormonal treatment is initiated during this period. Male clients receive estrogen, which results in a redistribution of body fat in a more "feminine" pattern, enlargement of the breasts, a softening of the skin, and reduction in body hair. Women receive testosterone, which also causes a redistribution of body fat, growth of facial and body hair, enlargement of the clitoris, and deepening of the voice (Becker & Johnson, 2008). Amenorrhea occurs within a few months.

Surgical treatment for male-to-female transgender reassignment involves removal of the penis and testes and creation of an artificial vagina. Care is taken to preserve sensory nerves in the area so that the individual may continue to experience sexual stimulation.

Surgical treatment for female-to-male transgender reassignment is more complex. A mastectomy and sometimes a hysterectomy are performed. A penis and scrotum are constructed from tissues in the genital and abdominal area, and the vaginal orifice is closed. A penile implant is used to attain erection.

Both men and women continue to receive maintenance hormone therapy following surgery. Satisfaction with the results is highest among clients who are emotionally healthy, have adequate social support, and attain reasonable cosmetic results (Martin, 2007). Black and Andreasen (2011) state, "Many patients will continue to benefit from psychotherapy following surgery to assist them in adjusting to their new gender role" (p. 340).

Nursing care of the post-gender-reassignment surgical client is similar to that of most other postsurgical clients. Particular attention is given to maintaining comfort, preventing infection, preserving integrity of the surgical site, maintaining elimination, and meeting nutritional needs. Psychosocial needs may have to do with body image, fears and insecurities about relating to others, and being accepted in the new gender role. Meeting these needs can begin with nursing in a nonthreatening, nonjudgmental healing atmosphere.

Variations in Sexual Orientation

Homosexuality

Homosexual activity occurs under some circumstances in probably all known human cultures and all mammalian species for which it has been studied. The term *homosexuality* is derived from the Greek root *homo* meaning "same," and refers to sexual preference for individuals of the same gender. It may be applied in a general way to homosexuals of both genders but is often used to specifically denote male homosexuality. The term *lesbianism*, used to identify female homosexuality, is traced to the Greek poet Sappho who lived on the island of Lesbos and is famous for the love poems she wrote to other women. Most homosexuals prefer the term "gay" because it

is less derogatory in its lack of emphasis on the sexual aspects of the orientation. A heterosexual is referred to as "straight."

Beginning in the late 1800s, homosexuality was classified as a mental illness. This remained the case until 1973 when the American Psychiatric Association removed the classification from the *DSM*. Homosexuality remained as a mental disorder in the World Health Organization's *International Classification of Diseases* until 1992. At one time, nearly all states had sodomy laws that forbade any sexual behavior that could not result in reproduction. In 2003, when these laws still remained in 13 states, the U.S. Supreme Court issued a broad-scoped decision that essentially invalided all sodomy laws (King, 2011). Attitudes change slowly, but they *are* changing.

In 1977, Americans were closely divided in their belief on the morality of homosexuality. At that time, 43 percent considered homosexual relations morally acceptable, and 43 percent stated they believed them to be morally wrong. A recent Gallup poll shows that the attitude toward homosexuality has taken a positive turn, with 63 percent indicating moral acceptability and only 31 percent believing it to be morally wrong (Gallup, 2012). Some experts believe that many Americans' attitudes toward homosexuals can best be described as homophobic. *Homophobia* is defined as a negative attitude toward or fear of homosexuality or homosexuals. It may be indicative of a deep-seated insecurity about one's own gender identity. Homophobic behaviors include extreme prejudice against, abhorrence of, and discomfort around homosexuals. These behaviors are usually rationalized by religious, moral, or legal considerations.

Relationship patterns are as varied among homosexuals as they are among heterosexuals. Some homosexuals may remain with one partner for an extended period of time, even for a lifetime, whereas others prefer not to make a commitment, and "play the field" instead.

No one knows for sure why people become homosexual or heterosexual. Various theories have been proposed regarding the issue, but no single etiological factor has consistently emerged. Many contributing factors likely influence the development of sexual orientation.

Predisposing Factors

Biological Theories

A study by Bailey and Pillard (1991) revealed a 52 percent concordance for homosexual orientation in monozygotic twins and 22 percent in dizygotic twins. Other studies have produced similar results (Kendler, Thornton, Gilman, & Kessler, 2000; Whitam, Diamond, & Martin, 1993). These data were significant to suggest the possibility of a heritable trait. Sadock and Sadock (2007) state:

> Gay men show a familial distribution; they have more brothers who are gay than do heterosexual men. One study found that 33 out of 40 pairs of gay brothers shared a genetic marker on the bottom half of the X chromosome. (p. 686)

A number of studies have been conducted to determine whether or not there is a hormonal influence in the etiology of homosexuality. It has been hypothesized that levels of testosterone may be lower and levels of estrogen higher in homosexual men than in heterosexual men. Results have been inconsistent. It has also been suggested that exposure to inappropriate levels of androgens during the critical fetal period of sexual differentiation may contribute to homosexual orientation. This hypothesis lacks definitive evidence, and conclusions regarding its validity remain tentative.

Psychosocial Theories

Freud (1930) believed that all humans are inherently bisexual, with the capacity for both heterosexual and homosexual behavior. He theorized that all individuals go through a homoerotic phase as children. Thus, if homosexuality occurs later in life, it is due to arrest of normal psychosexual development. He also believed homosexuality could occur as a result of pathological family relationships in which the child adopts a negative Oedipal position; that is, there is sexualized attachment to the parent of the same gender and identification with the parent of the opposite gender.

Some theories suggest that a dysfunctional family pattern may have an etiological influence in the development of homosexuality. These "nurture" theories focus on the parent-child relationship, and most specifically, the relationship with the same-gender parent. They suggest that gay men often have a dominant, supportive mother and a weak, remote, or hostile father. Lesbians may have had a dysfunctional mother-daughter relationship. Both subsequently try to meet their unmet same-gender needs through sexual relationships.

These theories of family dynamics have been disputed by some clinicians who believe that parents have very little influence on the outcome of their children's sexual-partner orientation. Others suggest there may not be one single answer—that sexual orientation may result from a complex interaction between biological and psychosocial factors, shaping the individual at an early age.

Special Concerns

People with homosexual preferences have problems that are similar to those of their heterosexual counterparts. Considerations of attractiveness, finding a partner, and concerns about sexual adequacy are common to both. STDs are epidemic among sexually active individuals of all sexual orientations. Of particular concern is acquired immunodeficiency syndrome (AIDS), which was considered a "gay disease" for the first few years of the epidemic. AIDS is a viral illness that, initially in the Western world, was indeed largely transmitted by male homosexual activity. Although AIDS is now known to spread through contaminated blood products, the sharing of needles by intravenous drug users, and heterosexual contact, some individuals still believe AIDS is God's way of punishing homosexuals. These societal attitudes are considered by many homosexuals to be their greatest burden.

Some homosexuals live in fear of the discovery of their sexual orientation; they fear being rejected by parents and significant others. They experience a great deal of cognitive dissonance related to the disparity between their overt behavior and their inner feelings. Social sanctions still exist in some areas for homosexuals in regard to employment, housing, and public accommodations. The Human Rights Commission protects homosexuals; however, discrimination is still widespread.

Another area of concern to the gay community is the issue of same-sex marriage. In the United States, same-sex marriage is legal in Connecticut, Iowa, New Hampshire, Washington, Maryland, Massachusetts, Vermont, New York, New Jersey, New Mexico, Maine, Delaware, Minnesota, Rhode Island, California, Hawaii, Illinois, Oregon, Pennsylvania, and Washington, DC. Same-sex marriage is also legal in Canada, Spain, the Netherlands, Belgium, Norway, Sweden, Argentina, Iceland, Portugal, Denmark, Brazil, France, New Zealand, and South Africa. Other U.S. states (e.g., Colorado, Nevada, and Wisconsin) and countries (e.g., Ecuador, Ireland, Mexico, Denmark, Germany, Austria, Luxembourg, Hungary, Switzerland, and United Kingdom) now recognize "civil unions" or "domestic partnerships," which allow same-sex couples various financial, insurance, and family benefits usually restricted to married heterosexual couples.

Opponents of same-sex marriage define marriage as an institution between one man and one woman. They argue that a gay relationship is not an optimal environment in which to raise children and that it goes against the traditional American value system. In addition, many people oppose homosexuality and same-sex marriage based on their religious beliefs, including the following: (1) that homosexuality is wrong because it involves sex that doesn't create life, (2) that homosexuality is "unnatural" (that God created men and women with the innate capacities for sexual relations that are distinctly absent from a same-sex relationship), and (3) that it is discouraged (or forbidden) by the Bible.

Proponents of same-sex marriage believe that the issue has to do with equality, pure and simple. They believe that all loving, consenting adult couples have the same rights under the law. They cite the real nature of marriage as a binding commitment (legally, socially, and personally) between two people, and they believe that individuals of the same gender have an equal right to make such a commitment to each other as do heterosexual couples. Regarding the rearing of children, research has suggested that having a gay or lesbian parent does not affect a child's social adjustment, school success, or sexual orientation (Wainright, Russell, & Patterson, 2004). The American Academy of Pediatrics (2013) has issued the following statement: "There is extensive research documenting that there is no causal relationship between parents' sexual orientation and children's emotional, psychosocial, and behavioral development."

Nurses must examine their personal attitudes and feelings about homosexuality. They must be able to recognize when negative feelings are compromising the care they give. Increasing numbers of homosexuals are being honest about their sexual orientation. Health-care workers must ensure that these individuals receive care with dignity, which is the right of all human beings. Nurses who have come to terms with their own feelings about homosexuality are better able to separate the person from the behavior. Unconditional acceptance of each individual is an essential component of compassionate nursing.

Bisexuality

A bisexual person is not exclusively heterosexual or homosexual; he or she engages in sexual activity with members of both genders. Bisexuals are also sometimes referred to as ambisexual.

Bisexuality is more common than exclusive homosexuality. Statistics suggest that approximately 75 percent of all men are exclusively heterosexual and only 2 percent are exclusively homosexual, leaving a relatively large percentage who have engaged in sexual activity with both men and women.

A diversity of sexual preferences exists among bisexuals. Some individuals prefer men and women equally, whereas others have a preference for one gender but also accept sexual activity with the other gender. Some bisexuals may alternate between homosexual and heterosexual activity for long periods; others may have both a male and a female lover at the same time. Whereas some individuals maintain their bisexual orientation throughout their lives, others may become exclusively homosexual or heterosexual.

Predisposing Factors

Little research exists on the etiology of bisexuality. As stated previously, Freud (1930) believed that all humans are inherently bisexual; that is, he believed that all individuals have the capacity for both heterosexual and homosexual interactions.

Much research on the development of homosexuality rests on the assumption that it is somehow determined by pathological conditions in childhood. Many heterosexual individuals, however, have their first homosexual encounter later in life. It is unlikely that an initial homosexual encounter that occurs in the 30s or 40s was determined by a pathological condition that occurred when the individual was 3 or 4 years old. Some encounters, too, are based solely on the situation, such as the heterosexual man who engages in homosexual behavior while in prison, and then returns to heterosexuality following his release. This behavior most likely was determined by circumstances rather than a pathological process that occurred in childhood.

Gender identity (determining whether one is male or female) is usually established by the age of 2 to 3 years. Sexual identity (determining whether one is heterosexual or homosexual or both) may continue to evolve throughout one's lifetime.

Sexually Transmitted Diseases

Sexually transmitted diseases (STDs) refer to infections that are contracted primarily through sexual activities or intimate contact with the genitals, mouth, or rectum of another individual. They may be transmitted from one person to another through heterosexual or homosexual contact, and external genital evidence of pathology may or may not be manifested.

STDs are at epidemic levels in the United States. Individuals are beginning an active sex life at an earlier age. More women are sexually active than ever before. The social changes that may have contributed to the increase in STDs are sometimes referred to as the three Ps: permissiveness, promiscuity, and the pill. The widespread knowledge that antibiotics were available to cure infections and the availability of oral contraceptives to prevent pregnancy resulted in significant increases in promiscuity and the subsequent exposure to and spread of STDs.

A primary nursing responsibility in STD control is education that is aimed at prevention of the disease. Nurses must know which diseases are most prevalent, how they are transmitted, their signs and symptoms, available treatment, and consequences of avoiding treatment (Table 30-2). They must teach this information to clients in hospitals and clinics and take an active role in programs of education in the community. Early education is important to decrease the spread of STDs.

STDs have a particularly emotive significance because they can be transmitted between sexual partners. Consequently, STDs carry strong connotations

TABLE 30–2 Sexually Transmitted Diseases

DISEASE	ORGANISM OF TRANSMISSION	METHOD OF TRANSMISSION	SIGNS AND SYMPTOMS	TREATMENT	POTENTIAL COMPLICATIONS
Gonorrhea	*Neisseria gonorrhoeae* (bacterium)	Vaginal sex, anal sex, genital-oral sex, via hand moistened with infected secretions and placed in contact with mucous membranes (e.g, the eyes)	Men: urethritis; dysuria, purulent discharge from urethra; proctitis; pharyngitis. Women: initially asymptomatic; progression to infection of cervix, urethra, and fallopian tubes	Combination therapy with ceftriaxone and azithromycin or doxycycline (CDC, 2012c)	Men: sterility from orchitis or epididymitis Women: chronic pelvic inflammatory disease, infertility, ectopic pregnancy, blindness from gonococcal conjunctivitis
Syphilis	*Treponema pallidum* (spirochete)	Vaginal sex, anal sex, genital-oral sex, via contact of infected secretions with intact mucous membranes or abraded skin	Primary stage: painless chancre on penis, vulva, vagina, mouth, anus, or other point of contact with mucous membranes or abraded skin Secondary stage: rash, headache, anorexia, weight loss, fever, sore throat, body aches, anemia	Long-acting penicillin G, tetracycline, erythromycin	Latent stage: lasts many years; no symptoms, but can be passed on to fetus Tertiary stage: blindness; heart disease; insanity; ulcerated lesions on skin, mucous membranes, or internal organs
Chlamydial infection	*Chlamydia trachomatis* (intracellular bacterium)	Vaginal sex, anal sex, via hand moistened with infected secretions and placed in contact with mucous membranes	Men: urethral discharge and dysuria Women: cervicitis (either asymptomatic or may have discharge, dysuria, soreness, bleeding)	Tetracycline; erythromycin; azithromycin	Scarring in the fallopian tubes, ectopic pregnancy, infertility
Genital herpes	Herpes simplex virus, type 1 or type 2	Vaginal sex, anal sex, genital-oral sex; skin-to-skin contact with infected areas, to newborn through vaginal delivery	Blistery lesions in the genital area causing pain, itching, burning; also vaginal or urethral discharge, fever, headache, malaise, and myalgias	No cure; treatment is palliative with acyclovir, valacyclovir, or famciclovir	Recurrences are possible; potential complications include meningitis, encephalitis, urethral strictures; possible risk of cervical cancer

Genital warts	*Condyloma acuminatum* (human papilloma virus)	Vaginal sex, anal sex, skin-to-skin contact with infected areas	Cauliflower-like warts that appear on penis or scrotum in men, and labia, vaginal walls, or cervix in women; mild itching may occur	Application of podofilox or podophyllin; cryotherapy; electrocautery; surgical removal	Recurrences possible; potential increased risk of cervical cancer
Hepatitis B	Hepatitis B virus	Vaginal sex, anal sex, genital-oral sex, contact with infectious blood or blood products, contact of infectious secretions with mucous membranes or abraded skin	Malaise, anorexia, nausea/vomiting, fever, headache, mild pain in right upper quadrant of abdomen, jaundice	No cure; treatment involves supportive care, bedrest for extended period; medications generally have not been found to be useful	Chronic hepatitis; cirrhosis; liver cancer
AIDS	Human immunodeficiency virus (HIV)	Exchange of body fluids via anal sex, vaginal sex, genital-oral sex Shared use of needles during drug use or accidental needle stick with infected needle Skin-to-skin contact when there are open sores on the skin Transfusion with contaminated blood Perinatal transmission: during delivery and through breast milk	May be asymptomatic for 10 years or longer following infection with HIV Early signs of AIDS include severe weight loss, diarrhea, fever, night sweats or the presence of a persistent opportunistic infection (e.g., herpes or candidiasis)	No cure; antiretroviral medication used to slow growth of the virus Other medications given for symptomatic relief and to treat opportunistic infections. The drug Truvada can be used as a preventive measure for people at high risk of acquiring HIV.	Regardless of treatment, AIDS is eventually fatal; new medications have dramatically increased the time from diagnosis to death, and research continues in drug treatments and vaccine development. One recent case of a baby who was born with HIV and treated with a combination of drugs for 18 months from birth has been pronounced free of the virus. This has provided optimism to the medical community that there is hope for a potential cure.

of illicit sex and considerable social stigma, as well as potentially disastrous medical consequences. Feelings of guilt in clients with STDs can be overwhelming. These individuals need strong support to overcome not only the physical difficulties but also the social and emotional ones associated with having this type of illness.

Prevention of STDs is the ideal goal, but early detection and appropriate treatment continue to be considered realistic objectives. Nurses are in an excellent position to provide the education required for prevention, as well as the physical treatment and social and emotional support to assist clients with STDs regain and maintain optimal wellness.

CASE STUDY AND SAMPLE CARE PLAN

NURSING HISTORY AND ASSESSMENT

Janet's obstetrician/gynecologist (OB/GYN) has referred her to the mental health clinic with what he has diagnosed as postpartum depression. Janet (age 30) tells Carol, the psychiatric nurse practitioner, that she and her husband Bert (age 32) have been married for 2 years, and that she gave birth 4 months ago to their first child, a boy they named Jason. Jason has been a difficult baby, was diagnosed with colic, and is wakeful and cries much of the time. Janet is sleep-deprived and continuously fatigued. Janet states, "I'm not depressed. I'm just exhausted! Bert is a computer analyst and is gone from home about 10 hours a day. When he gets home, we do what we can to put some dinner together and take care of Jason at the same time. By 9 o'clock, I'm ready to collapse, and Bert wants to go to bed and make love. I just don't have the energy. It's starting to cause a lot of friction in our marriage. Bert gets so angry when I refuse his advances. He also gets angry when I passively comply with his advances. To be honest, I'm just not interested in sex anymore. I certainly don't want to risk another pregnancy. But I also don't want to risk losing my husband. We used to have such a great sexual relationship, but that seems like another lifetime ago. I don't know what to do!"

NURSING DIAGNOSIS/OUTCOME IDENTIFICATION

From the assessment data, the nurse develops the following nursing diagnosis for Janet:

Sexual dysfunction related to extreme fatigue and depressed mood evidenced by loss of sexual desire.

a. **Short-Term Goals**
■ Client will identify ways to receive respite from child care.
■ Client will identify ways to devote time to regain satisfactory sexual relationship with husband.

b. **Long-Term Goal:** Client will resume sexual activity at a level satisfactory to herself and her husband.

PLANNING/IMPLEMENTATION

SEXUAL DYSFUNCTION
The following nursing interventions have been identified for Janet:
1. Take Janet's sexual history.
2. Determine the previous level of satisfaction in current sexual relationship.

3. Assess Janet's perception of the problem.
4. Suggest alternative strategies for resolution of the problem. (Because of Janet's fatigue and mild depression, she may not be able to adequately problem-solve the situation without assistance).
   a. Respite from child care (e.g., babysitting service, Mom's Day Out program, sharing babysitting with other mothers, grandparents).
   b. Schedule regular "date nights" with husband.
   c. Schedule periodic weekends away with husband.
5. Provide information regarding sexuality and sexual functioning.
6. Discuss with Janet her fear of pregnancy. Provide information about various methods of contraception.
7. Make referral to sex therapist, if Janet requests this service.

EVALUATION

The outcome criteria for Janet have been met. She was able to identify ways to receive respite from child care. She takes Jason to Mom's Day Out at her church every Friday morning. She now has an agreement with another new mother to trade one afternoon a week of babysitting duties. She inquired at the local community college in the department of early childhood education for names of students who would be interested in babysitting. Gina, a 19-year-old sophomore at the college, now babysits for Janet and Bert every Wednesday evening while they have a "date night." And one weekend a month, Bert's widowed mother stays with Jason while Janet and Bert have time away together. Her OB/GYN prescribed oral contraceptives, and Janet's fear of pregnancy has subsided. Janet's mood has lifted and she looks forward to her "free" time, and time alone with her husband. She reports that her sexual desire has increased, and that she and Bert now enjoy a satisfactory sexual relationship. She also states that she feels she is giving more quality care to Jason now that she has the periods of respite to which she looks forward every week.

Summary and Key Points

■ Paraphilic disorders are a group of behaviors involving sexual activity with nonhuman objects or nonconsenting partners or that involve suffering to others.

■ Types of paraphilic disorders include exhibitionistic disorder, fetishistic disorder, frotteuristic disorder, pedophilic disorder, sexual masochism disorder, sexual sadism disorder, transvestic disorder, and voyeuristic disorder.

■ Sexual dysfunctions are disturbances that occur in any of the phases of the normal human sexual response cycle.

■ Types of sexual dysfunctions include sexual desire disorders, sexual arousal disorders, orgasmic disorders, and sexual pain disorders.

■ Biological treatment of paraphilic disorders involves decreasing the level of circulating androgens.

■ Psychoanalytic treatment of paraphilic disorders focuses on helping the individual resolve early conflicts, thus relieving the anxiety that prevents him or her from forming appropriate sexual relationships.

■ Behavior therapy for paraphilic disorders includes use of aversion techniques, covert sensitization, and satiation.

■ Nurses may best become involved in the treatment of paraphilic disorders at the primary level of prevention.

■ Treatment of sexual dysfunction disorders involves a variety of techniques, including cognitive therapy, systematic desensitization, and sensate focus exercises.

■ Several medications are available for the treatment of erectile disorder. These include sildenafil (Viagra), tadalafil (Cialis), vardenafil (Levitra), and avanafil (Stendra). Others are currently under investigation.

■ Gender dysphoria occurs when there is incongruence between anatomical sex and the assigned gender role.

■ Individuals with gender dysphoria experience extreme discomfort in the assigned gender and desire to be, or insist that they are, the opposite gender.

■ Variations in sexual orientation include homosexuality and bisexuality.

■ Sexually transmitted diseases (STDs) refer to infections that are contracted primarily through sexual activities or intimate contact with the genitals, mouth, or rectum of another individual.

■ STDs are at epidemic levels in the United States. Prevention is the ideal goal, but early detection and appropriate treatment continue to be considered realistic objectives.

■ Nurses are in an excellent position to provide the education required for prevention, as well as the physical treatment and social and emotional support to assist clients with STDs regain and maintain optimal wellness.

■ Human sexuality influences all aspects of physical and mental health. Clients are becoming more open to discussing matters pertaining to sexuality, and it is therefore important for nurses to integrate information on sexuality into the care they give. This can be done by focusing on preventive, therapeutic, and educational interventions to assist individuals to attain, regain, or maintain sexual wellness.

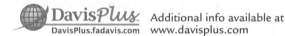

DavisPlus   Additional info available at
DavisPlus.fadavis.com   www.davisplus.com

Review Questions
Self-Examination/Learning Exercise

*Select the answer that is **most** appropriate for each of the following questions.*

1. Anne, age 24, and her husband are seeking treatment at the sex therapy clinic. They have been married for 3 weeks and have never had sexual intercourse together. Pain and vaginal tightness prevent penile entry. Sexual history reveals Anne was raped when she was 15 years old. The physician would most likely assign which of the following diagnoses to Anne?
    a. Female orgasmic disorder
    b. Genito-pelvic pain/penetration disorder
    c. Female sexual interest/arousal disorder
    d. Sexual aversion disorder

Continued

Review Questions—cont'd
Self-Examination/Learning Exercise

2. Anne, age 24, and her husband are seeking treatment at the sex therapy clinic. They have been married for 3 weeks and have never had sexual intercourse together. Pain and vaginal tightness prevent penile entry. Sexual history reveals Anne was raped when she was 15 years old. The most appropriate nursing diagnosis for Anne would be:
   a. Pain related to vaginal constriction
   b. Ineffective sexuality patterns related to inability to have vaginal intercourse
   c. Sexual dysfunction related to history of sexual trauma
   d. Complicated grieving related to loss of self-esteem because of rape

3. A client comes to the mental health clinic with a complaint of lack of sexual desire. In the initial interview, what assessments would the nurse make? (Select all that apply.)
   a. Mood
   b. Level of energy
   c. Medications being taken
   d. Previous level of sexual activity

4. Which of the following medications may be prescribed for early ejaculation?
   a. Paroxetine
   b. Tadalafil
   c. Diazepam
   d. Imipramine

5. Tom watches his neighbor through her window each night as she undresses for bed. Later he fantasizes about having sex with her. This is an example of which paraphilic disorder?
   a. Exhibitionistic disorder
   b. Voyeuristic disorder
   c. Frotteuristic disorder
   d. Pedophilic disorder

6. Frank drives his car up to a strange woman, stops, and asks her for directions. As she is explaining, he reveals his erect penis to her. This is an example of which paraphilic disorder?
   a. Sexual sadism disorder
   b. Sexual masochism disorder
   c. Frotteuristic disorder
   d. Exhibitionistic disorder

7. Tim, age 18, babysits for his 11-year-old neighbor, Jeff. Six months ago, Tim began fondling Jeff's genitals. They now engage in mutual masturbation each time they are together. This is an example of which paraphilic disorder?
   a. Fetishistic disorder
   b. Pedophilic disorder
   c. Exhibitionistic disorder
   d. Voyeuristic disorder

8. John is 32 years old. He buys women's clothing at the thrift shop. Sometimes he dresses as a woman and goes to a singles' bar. He becomes sexually excited as he fantasizes about men being attracted to him as a woman. This is an example of which paraphilic disorder?
   a. Sexual masochism disorder
   b. Voyeuristic disorder
   c. Exhibitionistic disorder
   d. Transvestic disorder

Review Questions—cont'd
Self-Examination/Learning Exercise

9. Fred rides a crowded subway every day. He stands beside a woman he views as very attractive. Just as the subway is about to stop, he places his hand on her breast and rubs his genitals against her buttock. As the door opens, he dashes out and away. Later he fantasizes she is in love with him. This is an example of which paraphilic disorder?
   a. Voyeuristic disorder
   b. Sexual sadism disorder
   c. Frotteuristic disorder
   d. Exhibitionistic disorder

10. A client with erectile disorder has a new prescription for sildenafil. The nurse who is providing education about this medication tells the client that which of the following are common side effects of this medication? (Select all that apply.)
    a. Headache
    b. Facial flushing
    c. Constipation
    d. Nasal congestion
    e. Indigestion

TEST YOUR CRITICAL THINKING SKILLS

Linda was hospitalized on the psychiatric unit for depression. During her nursing assessment interview, she stated, "According to my husband, I can't do anything right—not even have sex." When asked to explain further, Linda said she and her husband had been married for 17 years. She said that in the beginning, they had experienced a mutually satisfying sexual relationship and "made love" two or three times a week. Their daughter was born after they had been married 2 years, followed 2 years later by the birth of their son. They now have two teenagers (ages 15 and 13) who, by Linda's admission, require a great deal of her time and energy. She says, "I'm too tired for sex. And, besides, the kids might hear. I would be so embarrassed if they did. I walked in on my parents having sex once when I was a teenager, and I thought I would die! And my parents never mentioned it. It was just like it never happened! It was so awful! But sex is just so important to my husband, though, and we haven't had sex in months. We argue all the time about it. I'm afraid it's going to break us up."

Answer the following questions related to Linda.

1. Regarding her sexual relationship problem, what would be the nursing diagnosis for Linda?
2. What interventions for this problem might the nurse include in the treatment plan for Linda?
3. Regarding this problem, what would be a realistic goal for which Linda might strive?

References

Administration on Aging. (2014). *A profile of older Americans: 2013.* Washington, DC: U.S. Department of Health and Human Services.

Altman, A., & Hanfling, S. (2003). *Sexuality in midlife and beyond.* Boston, MA: Harvard Health Publications.

American Academy of Pediatrics. 2013). Policy statement: Promoting the well-being of children whose parents are gay or lesbian. *Pediatrics, 131*(4), 827-830.

American Psychiatric Association (APA). (2013). *Diagnostic and statistical manual of mental disorders* (5th ed.). Washington, DC: Author.

Bailey, J.M., & Pillard, R.C. (1991). A genetic study of male sexual orientation. *Archives of General Psychiatry, 48,* 1089-1096.

Becker, J.V., & Johnson, B.R. (2008). Gender identity disorders and paraphilias. In R.E. Hales, S.C. Yudofsky, & G.O. Gabbard (Eds.), *Textbook of psychiatry* (5th ed., pp. 729-753). Washington, DC: American Psychiatric Publishing.

Becker, J.V., & Stinson, J.D. (2008). Human sexuality and sexual dysfunction. In R.E. Hales, S.C. Yudofsky, & G.O. Gabbard (Eds.), *Textbook of psychiatry* (5th ed., pp. 711-728). Washington, DC: American Psychiatric Publishing.

Bednarczyk, R.A., Davis, R., Ault, K., Orenstein, W., & Omer, S.B. (2012). Sexual-activity related outcomes after human papillomavirus vaccination of 11- to 12-year-olds. *Pediatrics, 130*(5), 798-805.

Beijsterveldt, C.E.M., Hudziak, J.J., & Boomsma, D.I. (2006). Genetic and environmental influences on cross-gender behavior and relation to behavior problems: A study of Dutch twins at ages 7 and 10 years. *Archives of Sexual Behavior, 35*(6), 647-658.

Benson, A., Ost, L.B., Noble, M.J., & Lakin, M. (2013). Premature ejaculation. *MedscapeReference*. Retrieved from http://emedicine.medscape.com/article/435884-overview

Berman, J., & Berman, L. (2005). *For women only: A revolutionary guide to overcoming sexual dysfunction and reclaiming your sex life* (2nd ed.). New York, NY: Henry Holt.

Black, D.W., & Andreasen, N.C. (2011). *Introductory textbook of psychiatry* (5th ed.). Washington, DC: American Psychiatric Publishing.

Centers for Disease Control and Prevention (CDC). (2011). Recommendations on the use of quadrivalent human papillomavirus vaccine in males—Advisory Committee on Immunization Practices (ACIP), 2011. *Morbidity and Mortality Weekly Report, 60*(50), 1697-1728.

Centers for Disease Control and Prevention (CDC). (2012a). Human papillomavirus—Associated Cancers—United States, 2004-2008. *Morbidity and Mortality Weekly Report, 61*(15), 253-280.

Centers for Disease Control and Prevention (CDC). (2012b). *Trends in the prevalence of selected risk behaviors and obesity for all students national YRBS: 1991-2011.* Retrieved from www.cdc.gov/healthyyouth/yrbs/pdf/us_summary_all_trend_yrbs.pdf

Centers for Disease Control and Prevention (CDC). (2012c). Update to CDC's Sexually Transmitted Diseases Treatment Guidelines, 2010: Oral cephalosporins no longer a recommended treatment for gonococcal infections. *Morbidity and Mortality Weekly Report, 61*(31), 590-593.

Clayton, A.H. (2002). Sexual dysfunction. In S.G. Kornstein & A H. Clayton (Eds.), *Women's mental health.* New York, NY: The Guilford Press.

Cohen-Kettenis, P.T., & Pfäfflin, F. (2003). *Transgenderism and intersexuality in childhood and adolescence: Making choices.* Thousand Oaks, CA: Sage Publications.

Delemarre-van de Waal, H.A., & Cohen-Kettenis, P.T. (2006). Clinical management of gender identity disorder in adolescents: A protocol on psychological and pediatric endocrinology aspects. *European Journal of Endocrinology, 155*(1), 131-137.

Dreger, A. (2009). Gender identity disorder in childhood: Inconclusive advice to parents. *Hastings Center Report, 39*(1), 26-29.

Dreyfus, E.A. (2009). *Sexuality and sex therapy, Part II.* Retrieved from www.selfhelpmagazine.com/node/5025

Gallup. (2012). *Gay and lesbian rights.* Retrieved from www.gallup.com/poll/1651/gay-lesbian-rights.aspx

Gibson, B., & Catlin, A.J. (2010). Care of the child with the desire to change gender—Part I. *Pediatric Nursing, 36*(1), 53-59.

Institute of Medicine. (2003). *Health professions education: A bridge to quality.* Washington, DC: Author.

Kendler, K.S., Thornton, L.M., Gilman, S.E., & Kessler, R.C. (2000). Sexual orientation in a U.S. national sample of twin and nontwin sibling pairs. *American Journal of Psychiatry, 157,* 1843-1846.

Kim, E.D., & Brosman, S.A. (2013). Erectile dysfunction. Retrieved from http://emedicine.medscape.com/article/444220-overview

King, B.M. (2011). *Human sexuality today* (7th ed.). Upper Saddle River, NJ: Prentice Hall.

Laumann, E.O., Glasser, D.B., Neves, R.C.S., & Moreira, E.D. (2009). A population-based survey of sexual activity, sexual problems, and associated help-seeking behavior patterns in mature adults in the United States of America. *International Journal of Impotence Research, 21,* 171-178.

Leiblum, S.R. (1999). Sexual problems and dysfunction: Epidemiology, classification, and risk factors. *The Journal of Gender-Specific Medicine, 2*(5), 41-45.

Martin, K.A. (2007). Transsexualism: Clinical guide to gender identity disorder. *Current Psychiatry, 6*(2), 81-91.

Masters, W.H., Johnson, V.E., & Kolodny, R.C. (1995). *Human sexuality* (5th ed.). New York, NY: Addison Wesley Longman.

Murray, R.B., Zentner, J.P., & Yakimo, R. (2009). *Health promotion strategies through the life span* (8th ed.). Upper Saddle River, NJ: Prentice Hall.

NANDA International (NANDA-I). (2012). *Nursing diagnoses: Definitions and classification 2012-2014.* Hoboken, NJ: Wiley-Blackwell.

Nappi, R.E., Ferdeghini, F., & Polatti, F. (2006). Mechanisms involved in desire and arousal. In I. Goldstein, C.M. Meston, S.R. Davis, & A. Traish (Eds.), *Women's sexual function and dysfunction: Study, diagnosis, and treatment.* London, UK: Informa Healthcare.

Nappi, R.E., Salonia, A., Traish, A.M., vanLunsen, R.H.W., Vardi, Y., Kodiglu, A., & Goldstein, I. (2005). Clinical biologic pathophysiologies of women's sexual dysfunction. *Journal of Sexual Medicine, 2*(1), 4-25.

Phillips, N.A. (2000, July 1). Female sexual dysfunction: Evaluation and treatment. *American Family Physician, 62*(1), 127-136, 141-142.

Rhodes, J.C., Kjerulff, K.H., Langenberg, P.W., & Guzinski, G.M. (1999). Hysterectomy and sexual functioning. *Journal of the American Medical Association, 282*(20), 1934-1941.

Robins, L.N., Helzer, J.E., Weissman, M.M., Orvaschel, H., Gruenberg, E., Burke, J.D., & Regier, D.A. (1984). Lifetime prevalence of specific psychiatric disorders in three sites. *Archives of General Psychiatry, 41,* 949-958.

Sadock, B.J., & Sadock, V.A. (2007). *Synopsis of psychiatry: Behavioral sciences/clinical psychiatry* (10th ed.). Philadelphia, PA: Lippincott Williams & Wilkins.

Spear, J. (2001). Sex therapies. *Gale encyclopedia of psychology* (2nd ed.). Retrieved from http://www.encyclopedia.com/doc/1G2-3406000583.html

Traish, A., & Kim, N.N. (2006). Modulation of female genital sexual arousal by sex steroid hormones. In I. Goldstein, C.M. Meston, S.R. Davis, & A. Traish (Eds.), *Women's sexual function and dysfunction: Study, diagnosis, and treatment.* London, UK: Informa Healthcare.

Vallerand, A.H., & Sanoski, C.A. (2013). *Davis's drug guide for nurses* (13th ed.). Philadelphia, PA: F.A. Davis.

Wainright, J.L., Russell, S.T., & Patterson, C.J. (2004). Psychosocial adjustment, school outcomes, and romantic relationships of adolescents with same-sex parents. *Child Development, 75*(6), 1886-1898.

Whitam, F.L., Diamond, M., & Martin, J. (1993). Homosexual orientation in twins: A report on 61 pairs and three triplet sets. *Archives of Sexual Behavior, 22,* 187-205.

Zhou, J., Horman, M.A., Gooren, L.J., & Swaab, D.F. (1995). A sex difference in the human brain and its relation to transsexuality. *Nature, 378,* 68-70.

Zucker, K.J., Bradley, S.J., Ben-Dat, D.N., Ho, C., Johnson, L., & Owen, A. (2003). Psychopathology in the parents of boys with gender identity disorder. *Journal of the American Academy of Child and Adolescent Psychiatry, 42*(1), 2-4.

Classical References

Freud, S. (1930). *Three contributions to the theory of sex* (4th ed.). New York, NY: Nervous and Mental Disease Publishing.

Masters, W.H., & Johnson, V.E. (1966). *Human sexual response.* Boston, MA: Little, Brown.

Masters, W.H., & Johnson, V.E. (1970). *Human sexual inadequacy.* Boston, MA: Little, Brown.

@ INTERNET REFERENCES

• Additional information about sexual disorders and gender dysphoria may be located at the following websites:
  • http://www.sexualhealth.com
  • http://www.priory.com/sex.htm
  • http://emedicine.medscape.com/article/293890-overview
  • http://emedicine.medscape.com/article/291419-overview

• Additional information about sexually transmitted diseases may be located at the following websites:
  • http://www.cdc.gov/std
  • http://www3.niaid.nih.gov/topics/std

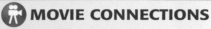

MOVIE CONNECTIONS

Mystic River (pedophilic disorder) • *Blue Velvet* (sexual masochism disorder) • *Looking for Mr. Goodbar* (sadism/masochism disorders) • *Normal* (transvestic disorder) • *TransAmerica* (gender dysphoria)

31 Eating Disorders

CHAPTER OUTLINE

KEY TERMS

amenorrhea

anorexia nervosa

anorexiants

binge-eating disorder

binging

bulimia nervosa

emaciated

obesity

purging

OBJECTIVES
After reading this chapter, the student will be able to:

1. Identify and differentiate among the various eating disorders.
2. Discuss epidemiological statistics related to eating disorders.
3. Describe symptomatology associated with anorexia nervosa, bulimia nervosa, and obesity, and use the information in client assessment.
4. Identify predisposing factors in the development of eating disorders.
5. Formulate nursing diagnoses and outcomes of care for clients with eating disorders.
6. Describe appropriate interventions for behaviors associated with eating disorders.
7. Identify topics for client and family teaching relevant to eating disorders.
8. Evaluate the nursing care of clients with eating disorders.
9. Discuss various modalities relevant to treatment of eating disorders.

HOMEWORK ASSIGNMENT
Please read the chapter and answer the following questions:

1. There is some speculation that anorexia nervosa may be associated with a primary dysfunction of which brain structure?
2. What is the level of body mass index (BMI) that is associated with the definition of obesity?
3. Individuals with anorexia nervosa have a "distorted body image." What does this mean?
4. What physiological signs may be associated with the excessive vomiting of the purging syndrome?

Nutrition is required to sustain life, and most individuals acquire nutrients from eating food; however, nutrition and life sustenance are not the only reasons most people eat food. Indeed, in an affluent culture, life sustenance may not even be a consideration. It is sometimes difficult to remember that many people within this affluent American culture, as well as all over the world, are starving from lack of food.

The hypothalamus contains the appetite regulation center within the brain. This complex neural system regulates the body's ability to recognize when it is hungry and when it has been sated. Halmi (2008) states:

> Eating behavior is now known to reflect an interaction between an organism's physiological state and environmental conditions. Salient physiological variables include the balance of various neuropeptides and neurotransmitters, metabolic state, metabolic rate, condition of the gastrointestinal tract, amount of storage tissue, and sensory receptors for taste and smell. Environmental conditions include features of the food such as taste, texture, novelty, accessibility, and nutritional composition, and other external conditions such as ambient temperature, presence of other people, and stress. (p. 971)

Society and culture have a great deal of influence on eating behaviors. Eating is a social activity; seldom does an event of any social significance occur without the presence of food. Yet, society and culture also influence how people (and in particular, women) must look. History reveals a regularity of fluctuation in what society has considered desirable in the human female body. Archives and historical paintings from the 16th and 17th centuries reveal that plump, full-figured women were considered fashionable and desirable. In the Victorian era, beauty was characterized by a slender, wan appearance that continued through the flapper era of the 1920s. During the Depression era and World War II, the full-bodied woman was again admired, only to be superseded in the late 1960s by the image of the superthin models propagated by the media, which remains the ideal of today. As it has been said, "A woman can't be too rich or too thin." Eating disorders, as we know them, can refute this concept.

This chapter explores the disorders associated with undereating and overeating. Because psychological or behavioral factors play a potential role in the presentation of these disorders, they fall well within the realm of psychiatry and psychiatric nursing. Epidemiological statistics are presented along with predisposing factors that have been implicated in the etiology of anorexia nervosa, bulimia nervosa, and obesity. An explanation of the symptomatology is presented as background knowledge for assessing the client with an eating disorder. Nursing care is described in the context of the nursing process. Various treatment modalities are explored.

Epidemiological Factors

Reports have indicated that the prevalence of **anorexia nervosa** has increased since the mid-20th century, both in the United States and in Western Europe (Halmi, 2008). Studies indicate a prevalence rate for anorexia nervosa among young women in the United States of approximately 1 percent (Black &

Andreasen, 2011). The disorder occurs predominantly in females 12 to 30 years of age. Fewer than 10 percent of the cases are male. Anorexia nervosa was once believed to be more prevalent in the higher socioeconomic classes, but evidence is lacking to support this hypothesis.

Bulimia nervosa is more prevalent than anorexia nervosa, with estimates up to 4 percent of young women (Black & Andreasen, 2011). Onset of bulimia nervosa occurs in late adolescence or early adulthood. Cross-cultural research suggests that bulimia nervosa occurs primarily in societies that place emphasis on thinness as the model of attractiveness for women and where an abundance of food is available.

Obesity has been defined as a body mass index (BMI) (weight/height^2) of 30 or greater. In the United States, statistics indicate that, among adults 20 years of age or older, 68.5 percent are overweight, with more than 35 percent of these in the obese range (Centers for Disease Control and Prevention [CDC], 2012). The percentage of obese individuals is higher in African Americans and Latino Americans than among the white population (CDC, 2012). The prevalence of obesity is greater among the lower socioeconomic group (Halmi, 2008), and there is an inverse relationship between obesity and level of education (CDC, 2012). The latest figures from the CDC indicate that 6.3 percent of the U.S. adult population may be categorized as *extremely* obese, which is defined by the National Institutes of Health as a BMI greater than 40 (CDC, 2012).

Application of the Nursing Process

Background Assessment Data (Anorexia Nervosa)

> ## CORE CONCEPT
> **Anorexia**
> Prolonged loss of appetite.

> ## CORE CONCEPT
> **Body Image**
> A subjective concept of one's physical appearance based on the personal perceptions of self and the reactions of others.

Anorexia nervosa is characterized by a morbid fear of obesity. Symptoms include gross distortion of body image, preoccupation with food, and refusal to eat. The term *anorexia* is actually a misnomer. It was initially believed that individuals with anorexia nervosa did not experience sensations of hunger. However, research indicates that they do indeed suffer from pangs of hunger, and it is only with food intake of less than 200 calories per day that hunger sensations actually cease.

The distortion in body image is manifested by the individual's perception of being "fat" when he or she is obviously underweight or even **emaciated** (excessively thin). Weight loss is usually accomplished by reduction in food intake and often extensive exercising. Self-induced vomiting and the abuse of laxatives or diuretics also may occur.

Weight loss is excessive. For example, the individual may present for health-care services weighing less than 85 percent of expected weight. Other symptoms include hypothermia, bradycardia, hypotension, edema, lanugo, and a variety of metabolic changes. **Amenorrhea** (absence of menstruation) usually follows weight loss, but sometimes it happens early on in the disorder, even before severe weight loss has occurred.

Individuals with anorexia nervosa may be obsessed with food. For example, they may hoard or conceal food, talk about food and recipes at great length, or prepare elaborate meals for others, only to restrict themselves to a limited amount of low-calorie food intake. Compulsive behaviors, such as hand washing, may also be present.

Age at onset is usually early to late adolescence and psychosexual development is often delayed. Feelings of depression and anxiety often accompany the disorder. In fact, some studies have suggested a possible interrelationship between eating disorders and affective disorders. Box 31-1 outlines the *Diagnostic and Statistical Manual of Mental Disorders, Fifth Edition (DSM-5)* (APA, 2013) diagnostic criteria for anorexia nervosa.

Background Assessment Data (Bulimia Nervosa)

> **CORE CONCEPT**
> **Bulimia**
> Excessive, insatiable appetite.

Bulimia nervosa is an episodic, uncontrolled, compulsive, rapid ingestion of large quantities of food over a short period of time (**binging**), followed by inappropriate compensatory behaviors to rid the body of the excess calories. The food consumed during a binge often has a high caloric content, a sweet taste, and a soft or smooth texture that can be eaten rapidly, sometimes even without being chewed (Sadock & Sadock, 2007). The binging episodes often occur in secret and are usually only terminated by abdominal discomfort, sleep, social interruption, or self-induced vomiting. Although the eating binges may bring pleasure while they are occurring, self-degradation and depressed mood commonly follow.

To rid the body of the excessive calories, the individual may engage in **purging** behaviors (self-induced vomiting, or the misuse of laxatives, diuretics, or enemas) or other inappropriate compensatory behaviors, such as fasting or excessive exercise. There is a persistent overconcern with personal appearance, particularly

---

BOX 31-1 **Diagnostic Criteria for Anorexia Nervosa**

A. Restriction of energy intake relative to requirements leading to a significantly low body weight in the context of age, sex, developmental trajectory, and physical health. *Significantly low weight* is defined as a weight that is less than minimally normal, or, for children and adolescents, less than that minimally expected.

B. Intense fear of gaining weight or becoming fat, or persistent behavior that interferes with weight gain, even though at a significantly low weight.

C. Disturbance in the way in which one's body weight or shape is experienced, undue influence of body weight or shape on self-evaluation, or persistent lack of recognition of the seriousness of the current low body weight.

Specify whether:

Restricting Type: During the last 3 months, the individual has not engaged in recurrent episodes of binge eating or purging behavior (i.e., self-induced vomiting or the misuse of laxatives, diuretics, or enemas). This subtype describes presentations in which weight loss is accomplished primarily through dieting, fasting, and/or excessive exercise.

Binge-Eating/Purging Type: During the last 3 months, the individual has engaged in recurrent episodes of binge eating or purging behavior (i.e., self-induced vomiting or the misuse of laxatives, diuretics, or enemas).

Specify if:
   In partial remission
   In full remission
Specify current severity:
   Mild: BMI ≥ 17 kg/m²   Severe: BMI 15-15.99 kg/m²
   Moderate: BMI 16-16.99 kg/m²   Extreme: BMI < 15 kg/m²

regarding how they believe others perceive them. Weight fluctuations are common because of the alternating binges and fasts. However, most individuals with bulimia nervosa are within a normal weight range— some slightly underweight, some slightly overweight.

Excessive vomiting and laxative or diuretic abuse may lead to problems with dehydration and electrolyte imbalance. Gastric acid in the vomitus also contributes to the erosion of tooth enamel. In rare instances, the individual may experience tears in the gastric or esophageal mucosa.

Some people with this disorder are subject to mood disorders, anxiety disorders, or substance abuse, most frequently involving central nervous central (CNS) stimulants or alcohol. The *DSM*-5 diagnostic criteria for bulimia nervosa are presented in Box 31-2.

Predisposing Factors Associated with Anorexia Nervosa and Bulimia Nervosa

Biological Influences

Genetics A hereditary predisposition to eating disorders has been hypothesized on the basis of family histories and an apparent association with other disorders for which the likelihood of genetic influences exists. In their study of monozygotic and dizygotic twins, Bulik and associates (2006) concluded that genetic factors account for 56 percent of the risk for developing anorexia nervosa. Other genetic studies have suggested possible linkage sites for anorexia nervosa on chromosomes 1, 2, and 13 (Halmi, 2008). Anorexia nervosa is more common among sisters and mothers of those with the disorder than among the general population. Several studies have reported a higher than expected frequency of mood and substance use disorders among first-degree biological relatives of individuals with eating disorders (Puri & Treasaden, 2011).

Neuroendocrine Abnormalities Some speculation has occurred regarding a primary hypothalamic dysfunction in anorexia nervosa. Studies consistent with this theory have revealed elevated cerebrospinal fluid cortisol levels and a possible impairment of dopaminergic regulation in individuals with anorexia nervosa (Halmi, 2008). Additional evidence in the etiological implication of hypothalamic dysfunction is gathered from the fact that many people with anorexia nervosa experience amenorrhea before the onset of starvation and significant weight loss.

Neurochemical Influences. Neurochemical influences in bulimia nervosa may be associated with the neurotransmitters serotonin and norepinephrine. This hypothesis has been supported by the positive response these individuals have shown to therapy with the selective serotonin reuptake inhibitors (SSRIs). Some studies have found high levels of endogenous opioids in the spinal fluid of clients with anorexia nervosa, promoting the speculation that these chemicals may contribute to denial of hunger (Sadock & Sadock, 2007). Some of these individuals have been shown to gain weight when given naloxone, an opioid antagonist.

Psychodynamic Influences

Psychodynamic theories suggest that eating disorders result from very early and profound disturbances in

---

BOX 31-2 Diagnostic Criteria for Bulimia Nervosa

A. Recurrent episodes of binge eating. An episode of binge eating is characterized by both of the following:
   1. Eating, in a discrete period of time (e.g., within any 2-hour period) an amount of food that is definitely larger than most individuals would eat during a similar period of time and under similar circumstances.
   2. A sense of lack of control over eating during the episode (e.g., a feeling that one cannot stop eating or control what or how much one is eating).
B. Recurrent inappropriate compensatory behaviors in order to prevent weight gain, such as self-induced vomiting; misuse of laxatives, diuretics, or other medications; fasting; or excessive exercise.
C. The binge eating and inappropriate compensatory behaviors both occur, on average, at least once a week for 3 months.
D. Self-evaluation is unduly influenced by body shape and weight.
E. The disturbance does not occur exclusively during episodes of anorexia nervosa.

   Specify if:
      In partial remission
      In full remission
   Specify current severity:
      Mild: An average of 1-3 episodes of inappropriate compensatory behaviors per week.
      Moderate: An average of 4-7 episodes of inappropriate compensatory behaviors per week.
      Severe: An average of 8-13 episodes of inappropriate compensatory behaviors per week.
      Extreme: An average of 14 or more episodes of inappropriate compensatory behaviors per week.

mother-infant interactions. The result is delayed ego development in the child and an unfulfilled sense of separation-individuation. This problem is compounded when the mother responds to the child's physical and emotional needs with food. Manifestations include a disturbance in body identity and a distortion in body image. When events occur that threaten the vulnerable ego, feelings of lack of control over one's body (self) emerge. Behaviors associated with food and eating serve to provide feelings of control over one's life.

Family Influences

Conflict Avoidance In the theory of the family as a system, psychosomatic symptoms, including anorexia nervosa, are reinforced in an effort to avoid spousal conflict. Parents are able to deny marital conflict by defining the sick child as the family problem. In these families, there is an unhealthy involvement between the members (enmeshment); the members strive at all costs to maintain "appearances"; and the parents endeavor to retain the child in the dependent position. Conflict avoidance may be a strong factor in the interpersonal dynamics of some families in which children develop eating disorders.

Elements of Power and Control The issue of control may become the overriding factor in the family of the client with an eating disorder. These families often consist of a passive father, a domineering mother, and an overly dependent child. A high value is placed on perfectionism in this family, and the child feels he or she must satisfy these standards. Parental criticism promotes an increase in obsessive and perfectionistic behavior on the part of the child, who continues to seek love, approval, and recognition. The child eventually begins to feel helpless and ambivalent toward the parents. In adolescence, these distorted eating patterns may represent a rebellion against the parents, viewed by the child as a means of gaining and remaining in control. The symptoms are often triggered by a stressor that the adolescent perceives as a loss of control in some aspect of his or her life.

Background Assessment Data (Obesity)

Obesity is not classified as a psychiatric disorder in the *DSM-5*, but because of the strong emotional factors and the potential serious health consequences associated with the condition, it may be considered under "Psychological Factors Affecting Medical Condition."

Binge-eating disorder (BED) is also described as an eating disorder in the *DSM-5* (APA, 2013). Obesity is a factor in BED because the individual binges on large amounts of food (as in bulimia nervosa) but does not engage in behaviors to rid the body of the excess calories. The *DSM-5* diagnostic criteria for BED are presented in Box 31-3.

BOX 31-3 **Diagnostic Criteria for Binge-Eating Disorder**

A. Recurrent episodes of binge eating. An episode of binge eating is characterized by both of the following:
  1. Eating, in a discrete period of time (e.g., within any 2-hour period), an amount of food that is definitely larger than what most people would eat in a similar period of time under similar circumstances
  2. A sense of lack of control over eating during the episode (e.g., a feeling that one cannot stop eating or control what or how much one is eating)
B. The binge-eating episodes are associated with 3 (or more) of the following:
  1. Eating much more rapidly than normal
  2. Eating until feeling uncomfortably full
  3. Eating large amounts of food when not feeling physically hungry
  4. Eating alone because of feeling embarrassed by how much one is eating
  5. Feeling disgusted with oneself, depressed, or very guilty after overeating
C. Marked distress regarding binge eating is present.
D. The binge eating occurs, on average, at least once a week for 3 months.
E. The binge eating is not associated with the recurrent use of inappropriate compensatory behavior as in bulimia nervosa and does not occur exclusively during the course of bulimia nervosa or anorexia nervosa.

Specify if:
  In partial remission
  In full remission
Specify current severity:
  Mild: 1-3 binge-eating episodes per week
  Moderate: 4-7 binge-eating episodes per week
  Severe: 8-13 binge-eating episodes per week
  Extreme: 14 or more binge-eating episodes per week

The following formula is used to determine extent of obesity in an individual:

$$\text{Body mass index} = \frac{\text{Weight (kg)}}{\text{Height (m)}^2}$$

The BMI range for normal weight is 20 to 24.9. Studies by the National Center for Health Statistics indicate that *overweight* is defined as a BMI of 25.0 to 29.9 (based on U.S. Dietary Guidelines for Americans). Based on criteria of the World Health Organization, *obesity* is defined as a BMI of 30.0 or greater. These guidelines, which were released by the National Heart, Lung, and Blood Institute in July 1998, markedly increased the number of Americans considered to be overweight. The average American woman has a BMI of 26, and fashion models typically have BMIs of 18. Anorexia nervosa is characterized by a BMI of 17.5 or lower (Black & Andreasen, 2011). Table 31-1 presents an example of some BMIs based on weight (in pounds) and height (in inches).

Individuals who are obese often present with hypertension and hyperlipidemia, particularly elevated triglyceride and cholesterol levels. They commonly have hyperglycemia and are at risk for developing diabetes mellitus. Osteoarthritis may be evident because of trauma to weight-bearing joints. Workload on the heart and lungs is increased, often leading to symptoms of angina or respiratory insufficiency.

Predisposing Factors Associated With Obesity

Biological Influences

Genetics Genetics have been implicated in the development of obesity in that 80 percent of offspring of two obese parents are obese (Halmi, 2008). Studies of twins and adoptees reared by normal and overweight parents have also supported this implication of heredity as a predisposing factor to obesity. Studies regarding the genetics of obesity are ongoing. Choquet and Meyre (2011) reported, "Recent discoveries in genetics have found that people differ in their perceptions of hunger and satiety on a genetic basis, and that predisposed subgroups of the population may be particularly vulnerable to obesity in 'obesogenic' societies with unlimited access to food" (p. 174).

Physiological Factors Lesions in the appetite and satiety centers in the hypothalamus may contribute to overeating and lead to obesity. Hypothyroidism is a problem that interferes with basal metabolism and may lead to weight gain. Weight gain can also occur in response to the decreased insulin production of diabetes mellitus and the increased cortisone production of Cushing's disease. Some evidence also exists to indicate that low levels of the neurotransmitter serotonin (5-hydroxytryptamine [5-HT]) may play a role in compulsive eating (Uceyler et al., 2010).

IMPLICATIONS OF RESEARCH FOR EVIDENCE-BASED PRACTICE

Long, J.D., and Stevens, K.R. (2004). Using technology to promote self-efficacy for healthy eating in adolescents. *Journal of Nursing Scholarship,* **36**(2), 134-139.

DESCRIPTION OF THE STUDY: Obesity and overweight have reached epidemic proportions and they are risk factors for the development of chronic disease. The purpose of this study was to test the effects of a classroom and World Wide Web (WWW) educational intervention on self-efficacy for healthy eating. The sample consisted of 63 adolescents in the participant group and 58 in the control group. The age range was between 12 and 16 years. The participant group received the intervention that consisted of 10 hours of classroom and 5 hours of Web-based nutrition education endorsed by the American Cancer Society and the National Cancer Institute. Information is included to encourage healthy eating behaviors that reduce the risk of cancer, obesity, heart disease and diabetes. Participants in the control group received the nutrition education integrated in the health, science, and home economics curriculum. All participants completed six questionnaires to measure dietary knowledge and eating behaviors. Pre- and post-tests were administered to both groups.

RESULTS OF THE STUDY: Although no difference in food consumption was found between groups during the month of intervention, the participant group had significantly higher scores related to knowledge of good nutrition and healthy eating behaviors. The study was limited to individual adolescents and did not attempt to initiate change in the home or school environment.

IMPLICATIONS FOR NURSING PRACTICE: Nurses, and especially school nurses, can become actively involved in nutrition education for children and adolescents. The authors report that 9 million young people are overweight—a number that more than doubled in the last 20 years. This has serious implications for nursing to assist in the educational process needed to reverse this unhealthy trend.

TABLE 31–1 Body Mass Index (BMI) Chart

BMI	19	20	21	22	23	24	25	26	27	28	29	30	31	32	33	34	35	36	37	38	39	40
HEIGHT (INCHES)												BODY WEIGHT (POUNDS)										
58	91	96	100	105	110	115	119	124	129	134	138	143	148	153	158	162	167	172	177	181	186	191
59	94	99	104	109	114	119	124	128	133	138	143	148	153	158	163	168	173	178	183	188	193	198
60	97	102	107	112	118	123	128	133	138	143	148	153	158	163	168	174	179	184	189	194	199	204
61	100	106	111	116	122	127	132	137	143	148	153	158	164	169	174	180	185	190	195	201	206	211
62	104	109	115	120	126	131	136	142	147	153	158	164	169	175	180	186	191	196	202	207	213	218
63	107	113	118	124	130	135	141	146	152	158	163	169	175	180	186	191	197	203	208	214	220	225
64	110	116	122	128	134	140	145	151	157	163	169	174	180	186	192	197	204	209	215	221	227	232
65	114	120	126	132	138	144	150	156	162	168	174	180	186	192	198	204	210	216	222	228	234	240
66	118	124	130	136	142	148	155	161	167	173	179	186	192	198	204	210	216	223	229	235	241	247
67	121	127	134	140	146	153	159	166	172	178	185	191	198	204	211	217	223	230	236	242	249	255
68	125	131	138	144	151	158	164	171	177	184	190	197	203	210	216	223	230	236	243	249	256	262
69	128	135	142	149	155	162	169	176	182	189	196	203	209	216	223	230	236	243	250	257	263	270
70	132	139	146	153	160	167	174	181	188	195	202	209	216	222	229	236	243	250	257	264	271	278
71	136	143	150	157	165	172	179	186	193	200	208	215	222	229	236	243	250	257	265	272	279	286
72	140	147	154	162	169	177	184	191	199	206	213	221	228	235	242	250	257	265	272	279	287	294
73	144	151	159	166	174	182	189	197	204	212	219	227	235	242	250	257	265	272	280	288	295	302
74	148	155	163	171	179	186	194	202	210	218	225	233	241	249	256	264	272	280	287	295	303	311
75	152	160	168	176	184	192	200	208	216	224	232	240	248	256	264	272	279	287	295	303	311	319
76	156	164	172	180	189	197	205	213	221	230	238	246	254	263	271	279	287	295	304	312	320	328

SOURCE: National Heart, Lung, and Blood Institute of the National Institutes of Health (2013).

Lifestyle Factors On a more basic level, obesity can be viewed as the ingestion of a greater number of calories than are expended. Weight gain occurs when caloric intake exceeds caloric output in terms of basal metabolism and physical activity. Many overweight individuals lead sedentary lifestyles, making it very difficult to burn off calories.

Psychosocial Influences

The psychoanalytic view of obesity proposes that obese individuals have unresolved dependency needs and are fixed in the oral stage of psychosexual development. The symptoms of obesity are viewed as depressive equivalents, attempts to regain "lost" or frustrated nurturance and caring. Depression and binge eating are strongly linked. As many as half of individuals with BED have a history of depression (Jaret, 2010). Depression may be a cause of binge eating when food provides comfort for the despondent mood. BED can also lead to depression, with respect to the feelings of disgust and despair that occur following episodes of binging.

Diagnosis/Outcome Identification

Nursing diagnoses are formulated from the data gathered during the assessment phase and with background knowledge regarding predisposing factors to the disorder. Table 31-2 presents a list of client behaviors and the NANDA nursing diagnoses that correspond to those behaviors, which may be used in planning care for clients with eating disorders.

Outcome Criteria

The following criteria may be used for measurement of outcomes in the care of the client with eating disorders:

The client:

■ Has achieved and maintained at least 80 percent of expected body weight.
■ Has vital signs, blood pressure, and laboratory serum studies within normal limits.
■ Verbalizes importance of adequate nutrition.
■ Verbalizes knowledge regarding consequences of fluid loss caused by self-induced vomiting (or laxative/diuretic abuse) and importance of adequate fluid intake.
■ Verbalizes events that precipitate anxiety and demonstrates techniques for its reduction.
■ Verbalizes ways in which he or she may gain more control of the environment and thereby reduce feelings of powerlessness.
■ Expresses interest in welfare of others and less preoccupation with own appearance.
■ Verbalizes that image of body as "fat" was misperception and demonstrates ability to take control of own life without resorting to maladaptive eating behaviors (anorexia nervosa).

TABLE 31–2 **Assigning Nursing Diagnoses to Behaviors Commonly Associated With Eating Disorders**	
BEHAVIORS	NURSING DIAGNOSES
Refusal to eat; abuse of laxatives, diuretics, and/or diet pills; loss of 15 percent of expected body weight; pale conjunctiva and mucous membranes; poor muscle tone; amenorrhea; poor skin turgor; electrolyte imbalances; hypothermia; bradycardia; hypotension; cardiac irregularities; edema	Imbalanced nutrition: Less than body requirements
Decreased fluid intake; abnormal fluid loss caused by self-induced vomiting; excessive use of laxatives, enemas, or diuretics; electrolyte imbalance; decreased urine output; increased urine concentration; elevated hematocrit; decreased blood pressure; increased pulse rate; dry skin; decreased skin turgor; weakness	Deficient fluid volume
Minimizes symptoms; unable to admit impact of disease on life pattern; does not perceive personal relevance of symptoms; does not perceive personal relevance of danger	Ineffective denial
Compulsive eating; excessive intake in relation to metabolic needs; sedentary lifestyle; weight 20 percent over ideal for height and frame; BMI of 30 or more	Imbalanced nutrition: More than body requirements
Distorted body image; views self as fat, even in the presence of normal body weight or severe emaciation; denies that problem with low body weight exists; difficulty accepting positive reinforcement; self-destructive behavior (self-induced vomiting, abuse of laxatives or diuretics, refusal to eat); preoccupation with appearance and how others perceive it *(anorexia nervosa, bulimia nervosa)* Verbalization of negative feelings about the way he or she looks and the desire to lose weight *(obesity)* Lack of eye contact; depressed mood *(all)*	Disturbed body image/Low self-esteem
Increased tension; increased helplessness; overexcited; apprehensive; fearful; restlessness; poor eye contact; increased difficulty taking oral nourishment; inability to learn	Anxiety (moderate to severe)

■ Has established a healthy pattern of eating for weight control, and weight loss toward a desired goal is progressing (obesity).

■ Verbalizes plans for future maintenance of weight control (obesity).

Planning/Implementation

In most instances, individuals with eating disorders are treated on an outpatient basis, but in some cases hospitalization becomes necessary. Reasons for hospitalization include the following: malnutrition (less than 85% of expected body weight), dehydration, severe electrolyte imbalance, cardiac arrhythmia, severe bradycardia, hypothermia, hypotension, suicidal ideation, or uncooperative outpatient treatment (Yager et al., 2006).

The following section presents a group of selected nursing diagnoses, with short- and long-term goals and nursing interventions for each.

Imbalanced Nutrition: Less Than Body Requirements/Deficient Fluid Volume (Risk for or Actual)

Imbalanced nutrition: less than body requirements is defined as "intake of nutrients insufficient to meet metabolic needs" (NANDA International [NANDA-I], 2012, p. 174). *Deficient fluid volume* is defined as "decreased intravascular, interstitial, and/or intracellular fluid" (NANDA-I, 2012, p. 186). Table 31-3 presents these nursing diagnoses in care plan format.

Client Goals

Outcome criteria include short- and long-term goals. Timelines are individually determined.

Short-Term Goals

■ The client will gain ___ pounds per week (amount to be established by client, nurse, and dietitian).

■ The client will drink 125 mL of fluid each hour during waking hours.

Long-Term Goal

■ By time of discharge from treatment, the client will exhibit no signs or symptoms of malnutrition or dehydration.

Interventions

■ For the client who is emaciated and is unable or unwilling to maintain an adequate oral intake, the physician may order a liquid diet to be administered via nasogastric tube. Without adequate nutrition, a life-threatening situation exists. Nursing care of the individual receiving tube feedings should be administered according to established hospital procedures.

■ For the client who is able and willing to consume an oral diet, the dietitian should determine the appropriate number of calories required to provide adequate nutrition and realistic (according to body structure and height) weight gain.

■ Explain the program of behavior modification to client and family. Explain that privileges and

---

Table 31-3 | CARE PLAN FOR CLIENT WITH EATING DISORDERS: ANOREXIA NERVOSA AND BULIMIA NERVOSA

NURSING DIAGNOSIS: IMBALANCED NUTRITION: LESS THAN BODY REQUIREMENTS/DEFICIENT FLUID VOLUME (RISK FOR OR ACTUAL)

RELATED TO: Refusal to eat/drink; self-induced vomiting; abuse of laxatives/diuretics

EVIDENCED BY: Loss of weight; poor muscle tone and skin turgor; lanugo; bradycardia; hypotension; cardiac arrhythmias; pale, dry mucous membranes

OUTCOME CRITERIA	NURSING INTERVENTIONS	RATIONALE
Short-Term Goals • Client will gain *x* pounds per week (amount to be established by client, nurse, and dietitian). • Client will drink 125 mL of fluid each hour during waking hours. **Long-Term Goal** • By time of discharge from treatment, client will exhibit no signs or symptoms of malnutrition or dehydration.	1. For the client who is emaciated and is unable or unwilling to maintain an adequate oral intake, the physician may order a liquid diet to be administered via nasogastric tube. Nursing care of the individual receiving tube feedings should be administered according to established hospital protocol. 2. For the client who is able and willing to consume an oral diet, the dietitian will determine the appropriate number of calories	1. Without adequate nutrition, a life-threatening situation exists. 2. Adequate calories are required to allow a weight gain of 2–3 pounds per week.

Table 31-3 | CARE PLAN FOR CLIENT WITH EATING DISORDERS: ANOREXIA NERVOSA AND BULIMIA NERVOSA—cont'd

OUTCOME CRITERIA	NURSING INTERVENTIONS	RATIONALE
	required to provide adequate nutrition and realistic weight gain.	
	3. Explain to the client that privileges and restrictions will be based on compliance with treatment and direct weight gain. Do not focus on food and eating.	3. The real issues have little to do with food or eating patterns. Focus on the control issues that have precipitated these behaviors.
	4. Weigh client daily, immediately upon arising and following first voiding. Always use same scale, if possible. Keep strict record of intake and output. Assess skin turgor and integrity regularly. Assess moistness and color of oral mucous membranes.	4. These assessments are important measurements of nutritional status and provide guidelines for treatment.
	5. Stay with client during established time for meals (usually 30 min) and for at least 1 hour following meals.	5. Lengthy mealtimes put excessive focus on food and eating and provide client with attention and reinforcement. The hour following meals may be used to discard food stashed from tray or to engage in self-induced vomiting.
	6. If weight loss occurs, enforce restrictions.	6. Restrictions and limits must be established and carried out consistently to avoid power struggles, to encourage client compliance with therapy, and to ensure client safety.
	7. Ensure that the client and family understand that if nutritional status deteriorates, tube feedings will be initiated. This is implemented in a matter-of-fact, nonpunitive way.	7. This intervention is carried out for the client's safety and protection from a life-threatening condition.
	8. Encourage the client to explore and identify the true feelings and fears that contribute to maladaptive eating behaviors.	8. Emotional issues must be resolved if these maladaptive responses are to be eliminated.

restrictions will be based on compliance with treatment and direct weight gain.

■ Do not focus on food and eating specifically. Instead, focus on the emotional issues that have precipitated these behaviors.

■ Do not discuss food or eating with the client once protocol has been established. Do, however, offer support and positive reinforcement for obvious improvements in eating behaviors.

■ Keep a strict record of intake and output. Weigh the client daily immediately on arising and following first voiding. Always use the same scale, if possible.

■ Assess skin turgor and integrity regularly. Assess moistness and color of oral mucous membranes. The condition of the skin and mucous membranes provides valuable data regarding client hydration. Discourage the client from bathing every day if the skin is very dry.

■ Sit with the client during mealtimes for support and to observe the amount ingested. A limit (usually 30 minutes) should be imposed on time allotted for meals. Without a time limit, meals can become lengthy, drawn-out sessions, providing the client with attention based on food and eating.

■ The client should be observed for at least 1 hour following meals. The client may use this time to discard food that has been stashed from the food tray or to engage in self-induced vomiting. He or she may need to be accompanied to the bathroom if self-induced vomiting is suspected.

■ If weight loss occurs, enforce restrictions. Restrictions and limits must be established and carried out consistently to avoid power struggles and to encourage client compliance with therapy.

■ Ensure that the client and family understand that if nutritional status deteriorates, tube feedings will be initiated. This is implemented in a matter-of-fact, nonpunitive way, for the client's safety and protection from a life-threatening condition.

■ Encourage the client to explore and identify the true feelings and fears that contribute to maladaptive eating behaviors. Emotional issues must be resolved if these maladaptive responses are to be eliminated.

Ineffective Denial

Ineffective denial is defined as a "conscious or unconscious attempt to disavow the knowledge or meaning of an event to reduce anxiety and/or fear, leading to the detriment of health" (NANDA-I, 2012, p. 358).

Client Goals

Outcome criteria include short- and long-term goals. Timelines are individually determined.

Short-Term Goal

■ The client will verbalize understanding of the correlation between emotional issues and maladaptive eating behaviors (within time deemed appropriate for individual client).

Long-Term Goal

■ By time of discharge from treatment, the client will demonstrate the ability to discontinue use of maladaptive eating behaviors and to cope with emotional issues in a more adaptive manner.

Interventions

■ Establish a trusting relationship with the client by being honest, accepting, and available, and by keeping all promises. Convey unconditional positive regard.

■ Acknowledge the client's anger at feelings of loss of control brought about by the established eating regimen associated with the program of behavior modification. Anger is a normal human response, and should be expressed in an appropriate manner. Feelings that are not expressed remain unresolved and add an additional component to an already serious situation.

■ Avoid arguing or bargaining with the client who is resistant to treatment. State matter-of-factly which behaviors are unacceptable and how privileges will be restricted for noncompliance. It is essential that all staff members are consistent with this intervention.

■ Encourage the client to verbalize feelings regarding his or her role within the family and issues related to dependence/independence, the intense need for achievement, and sexuality. Help the client recognize how maladaptive eating behaviors may be related to these emotional issues. Discuss ways in which he or she can gain control over these problematic areas of life without resorting to maladaptive eating behaviors.

Imbalanced Nutrition: More Than Body Requirements

Imbalanced nutrition: more than body requirements is defined as "intake of nutrients that exceeds metabolic needs" (NANDA-I, 2012, p. 175).

Client Goals

Outcome criteria include short- and long-term goals. Timelines are individually determined.

Short-Term Goal

■ Client will verbalize understanding of what must be done to lose weight.

Long-Term Goal

■ Client will demonstrate a change in eating patterns that results in a steady weight loss.

Interventions

■ Encourage the client to keep a diary of food intake. A food diary provides the opportunity for the client to gain a realistic picture of the amount of food ingested and provides a database on which to tailor the dietary program.

■ Discuss feelings and emotions associated with eating. This helps to identify when the client is eating to satisfy an emotional need rather than a physiological one.

■ With input from the client, formulate an eating plan that includes food from the required food groups with emphasis on low-fat intake. It is helpful to keep the plan as similar to the client's usual eating pattern as possible. The diet must eliminate calories while maintaining adequate nutrition. The client is more likely to stay on the eating plan if he or she is able to participate in its creation and it deviates as little as possible from usual types of foods.

■ Identify realistic incremental goals for weekly weight loss. Reasonable weight loss (1 to 2 pounds per week) results in more lasting effects. Excessive, rapid weight loss may result in fatigue and irritability and ultimately lead to failure in meeting goals for weight loss. Motivation is more easily sustained by meeting "stair-step" goals.

■ Plan a progressive exercise program tailored to individual goals and choice. Exercise may enhance weight loss by burning calories and reducing appetite, increasing energy, toning muscles, and enhancing sense of well-being and accomplishment. Walking is an excellent choice for overweight individuals.

■ Discuss the probability of reaching plateaus when weight remains stable for extended periods. The client should know this is likely to happen as changes in metabolism occur. Plateaus cause frustration, and the client may need additional support during these times to remain on the weight-loss program.

■ Provide instruction about medications to assist with weight loss if ordered by the physician. Appetite-suppressant drugs and others that have weight loss as a side effect may be helpful to someone who is severely overweight. They should be used for this purpose for only a short period while the individual attempts to adjust to the new pattern of eating.

Disturbed Body Image/Low Self-esteem

Disturbed body image is defined as "confusion in mental picture of one's physical self" (NANDA-I, 2012, p. 291). *Low self-esteem* is defined as "negative self-evaluating/feelings about self or self-capabilities" (NANDA-I, 2012, pp. 285-287).

Client Goals (for the Client With Anorexia Nervosa or Bulimia Nervosa)

Outcome criteria include short- and long-term goals. Timelines are individually determined.

Short-Term Goal

■ The client will verbally acknowledge misperception of body image as "fat" within specified time (depending on severity and chronicity of condition).

Long-Term Goal

■ By the time of discharge from treatment, client will demonstrate an increase in self-esteem as manifested by verbalizing positive aspects of self and exhibiting less preoccupation with own appearance as a more realistic body image is developed.

Client Goals (for the Client With Obesity)

Outcome criteria include short- and long-term goals. Timelines are individually determined.

Short-Term Goal

■ The client will begin to accept self based on self-attributes rather than on appearance.

Long-Term Goal

■ The client will pursue loss of weight as desired.

Interventions

For the client with anorexia nervosa or bulimia nervosa:

■ Help the client to develop a realistic perception of body image and relationship with food. Compare specific measurement of the client's body with the client's perceived calculations. There may be a large discrepancy between the actual body size and the client's perception of his or her body size. The client needs to recognize that the misperception of body image is unhealthy and that maintaining control through maladaptive eating behaviors is dangerous—even life threatening.

■ Promote feelings of control within the environment through participation and independent decision-making. Through positive feedback, help the client learn to accept self as is, including weaknesses as well as strengths. The client must come to understand that he or she is a capable, autonomous individual who can perform outside the family unit and who is not expected to be perfect. Control of his or her life must be achieved in other ways besides dieting and weight loss.

■ Help the client realize that perfection is unrealistic, and explore this need with him or her. As the client begins to feel better about self, identifies positive self-attributes, and develops the ability to accept certain personal inadequacies, the need for unrealistic achievement should diminish.

For the client with obesity:

■ Assess the client's feelings and attitudes about being obese. Obesity and compulsive eating behaviors may have deep-rooted psychological implications, such as compensation for lack of love and nurturing or a defense against intimacy.

■ Ensure that the client has privacy during self-care activities. The obese individual may be sensitive or self-conscious about his or her body.

■ Have the client recall coping patterns related to food in family of origin, and explore how these may affect current situation. Parents are role models for their children. Maladaptive eating behaviors are learned within the family system and are supported through positive reinforcement. Food may be substituted by the parent for affection and love, and eating is associated with a feeling of satisfaction, becoming the primary defense.

■ Determine the client's motivation for weight loss and set goals. The individual may harbor repressed feelings of hostility, which may be expressed inwardly on the self. Because of a poor self-concept, the person often has difficulty with relationships. When the motivation is to lose weight for someone else, successful weight loss is less likely to occur.

■ Help the client identify positive self-attributes. Focus on strengths and past accomplishments unrelated to physical appearance. It is important that self-esteem not be tied solely to size of the body. The client needs to recognize that obesity need not interfere with positive feelings regarding self-concept and self-worth.

■ Refer the client to a support or therapy group. Support groups can provide companionship, increase motivation, decrease loneliness and social ostracism, and give practical solutions to common problems. Group therapy can be helpful in dealing with underlying psychological concerns.

Concept Care Mapping

The concept map care plan is an innovative approach to planning and organizing nursing care (see Chapter 9). It is a diagrammatic teaching and learning strategy that allows visualization of interrelationships between medical diagnoses, nursing diagnoses, assessment data, and treatments. Examples of concept map care plans for clients with eating disorders are presented in Figures 31-1 and 31-2.

Client/Family Education

The role of client teacher is important in the psychiatric area, as it is in all areas of nursing. A list of topics

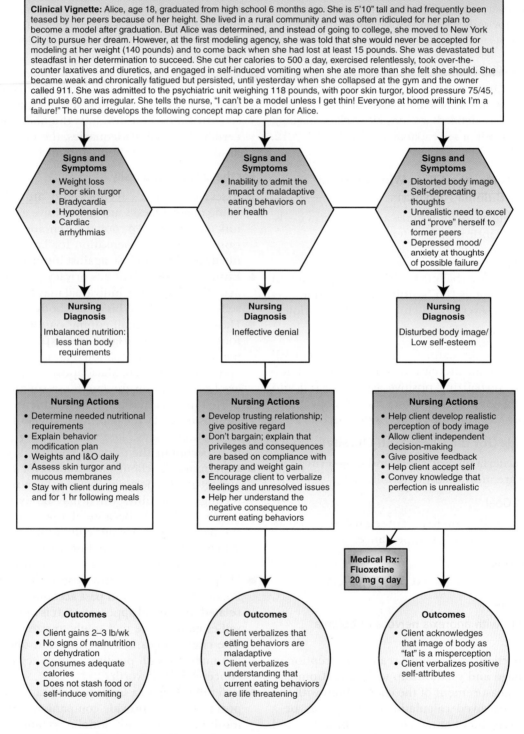

Clinical Vignette: Alice, age 18, graduated from high school 6 months ago. She is 5'10" tall and had frequently been teased by her peers because of her height. She lived in a rural community and was often ridiculed for her plan to become a model after graduation. But Alice was determined, and instead of going to college, she moved to New York City to pursue her dream. However, at the first modeling agency, she was told that she would never be accepted for modeling at her weight (140 pounds) and to come back when she had lost at least 15 pounds. She was devastated but steadfast in her determination to succeed. She cut her calories to 500 a day, exercised relentlessly, took over-the-counter laxatives and diuretics, and engaged in self-induced vomiting when she ate more than she felt she should. She became weak and chronically fatigued but persisted, until yesterday when she collapsed at the gym and the owner called 911. She was admitted to the psychiatric unit weighing 118 pounds, with poor skin turgor, blood pressure 75/45, and pulse 60 and irregular. She tells the nurse, "I can't be a model unless I get thin! Everyone at home will think I'm a failure!" The nurse develops the following concept map care plan for Alice.

Signs and Symptoms
- Weight loss
- Poor skin turgor
- Bradycardia
- Hypotension
- Cardiac arrhythmias

Signs and Symptoms
- Inability to admit the impact of maladaptive eating behaviors on her health

Signs and Symptoms
- Distorted body image
- Self-deprecating thoughts
- Unrealistic need to excel and "prove" herself to former peers
- Depressed mood/ anxiety at thoughts of possible failure

Nursing Diagnosis
Imbalanced nutrition: less than body requirements

Nursing Diagnosis
Ineffective denial

Nursing Diagnosis
Disturbed body image/ Low self-esteem

Nursing Actions
- Determine needed nutritional requirements
- Explain behavior modification plan
- Weights and I&O daily
- Assess skin turgor and mucous membranes
- Stay with client during meals and for 1 hr following meals

Nursing Actions
- Develop trusting relationship; give positive regard
- Don't bargain; explain that privileges and consequences are based on compliance with therapy and weight gain
- Encourage client to verbalize feelings and unresolved issues
- Help her understand the negative consequence to current eating behaviors

Nursing Actions
- Help client develop realistic perception of body image
- Allow client independent decision-making
- Give positive feedback
- Help client accept self
- Convey knowledge that perfection is unrealistic

Medical Rx: Fluoxetine 20 mg q day

Outcomes
- Client gains 2–3 lb/wk
- No signs of malnutrition or dehydration
- Consumes adequate calories
- Does not stash food or self-induce vomiting

Outcomes
- Client verbalizes that eating behaviors are maladaptive
- Client verbalizes understanding that current eating behaviors are life threatening

Outcomes
- Client acknowledges that image of body as "fat" is a misperception
- Client verbalizes positive self-attributes

FIGURE 31-1 Concept map care plan for a client with anorexia nervosa.

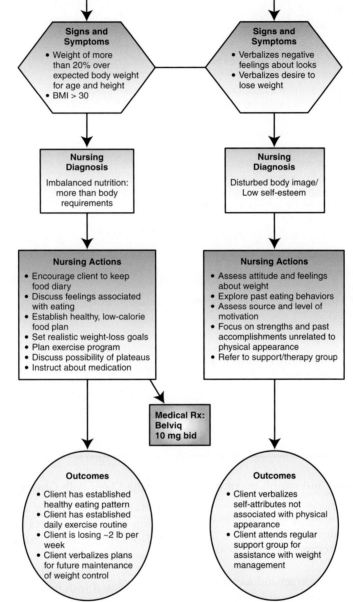

Clinical Vignette: Harriet, age 20, has been overweight since childhood. Her mother and sister were both of normal weight, but her mother always said, "Harriet took after her dad's side of the family." Through her teens, she tried innumerable times to lose weight, only to lose a few pounds and then gain back more. In college, out from under the watchful eye of her mother, she has gained even more weight. She has never had a date. Her sister is engaged to be married in 6 months and has asked Harriet to be her maid of honor. Harriet has come to the university student health center to seek assistance with weight loss. She is 5'4" tall and weighs 204 pounds. She tells the nurse, "I hate the way I look. I can't be in my sister's wedding looking like this!" The nurse develops the following concept map care plan for Harriet.

Signs and Symptoms
• Weight of more than 20% over expected body weight for age and height
• BMI > 30

Signs and Symptoms
• Verbalizes negative feelings about looks
• Verbalizes desire to lose weight

Nursing Diagnosis
Imbalanced nutrition: more than body requirements

Nursing Diagnosis
Disturbed body image/ Low self-esteem

Nursing Actions
• Encourage client to keep food diary
• Discuss feelings associated with eating
• Establish healthy, low-calorie food plan
• Set realistic weight-loss goals
• Plan exercise program
• Discuss possibility of plateaus
• Instruct about medication

Nursing Actions
• Assess attitude and feelings about weight
• Explore past eating behaviors
• Assess source and level of motivation
• Focus on strengths and past accomplishments unrelated to physical appearance
• Refer to support/therapy group

Medical Rx: Belviq 10 mg bid

Outcomes
• Client has established healthy eating pattern
• Client has established daily exercise routine
• Client is losing ~2 lb per week
• Client verbalizes plans for future maintenance of weight control

Outcomes
• Client verbalizes self-attributes not associated with physical appearance
• Client attends regular support group for assistance with weight management

FIGURE 31-2 Concept map care plan for a client with obesity.

for client/family education relevant to eating disorders is presented in Box 31-4.

Evaluation

Evaluation of the client with an eating disorder requires a reassessment of the behaviors for which the client sought treatment. Behavioral change will be required on both the part of the client and family members. The following types of questions may provide

assistance in gathering data required for evaluating whether the nursing interventions have been effective in achieving the goals of therapy.

For the Client With Anorexia Nervosa or Bulimia Nervosa:

■ Has the client steadily gained 2 to 3 pounds per week to at least 80 percent of body weight for age and size?

BOX 31-4 Topics for Client/Family Education Related to Eating Disorders

NATURE OF THE ILLNESS
1. Symptoms of anorexia nervosa
2. Symptoms of bulimia nervosa
3. Symptoms of BED
4. What constitutes obesity
5. Causes of eating disorders
6. Effects of the illness or condition on the body

MANAGEMENT OF THE ILLNESS
1. Principles of nutrition (foods for maintenance of wellness)
2. Ways client may feel in control of life (aside from eating)
3. Importance of expressing fears and feelings, rather than holding them inside
4. Alternative coping strategies (to maladaptive eating behaviors)
5. For the obese client:
   a. How to plan a reduced-calorie, nutritious diet
   b. How to read food content labels
   c. How to establish a realistic weight loss plan
   d. How to establish a planned program of physical activity
6. Correct administration of prescribed medications
7. Indication for and side effects of prescribed medications
8. Relaxation techniques
9. Problem-solving skills

SUPPORT SERVICES
1. Weight Watchers International
2. Overeaters Anonymous
3. National Association of Anorexia Nervosa and Associated Disorders (ANAD)
   800 East Diehl Road #160
   Naperville, IL 60563
   (630) 577-1330
   http://www.anad.org/
4. National Eating Disorders Association
   165 West 46th Street
   New York, NY 10036
   (212) 575-6200
   http://www.nationaleatingdisorders.org

■ Is the client free of signs and symptoms of malnutrition and dehydration?

■ Does the client consume adequate calories as determined by the dietitian?

■ Have there been any attempts to stash food from the tray to discard later?

■ Have there been any attempts to self-induce vomiting?

■ Has the client admitted that a problem exists and that eating behaviors are maladaptive?

■ Have behaviors aimed at manipulating the environment been discontinued?

■ Is the client willing to discuss the real issues concerning family roles, sexuality, dependence/independence, and the need for achievement?

■ Does the client understand how he or she has used maladaptive eating behaviors in an effort to achieve a feeling of some control over life events?

■ Has the client acknowledged that perception of body image as "fat" is incorrect?

For the Client With Obesity:

■ Has the client shown a steady weight loss since starting the new eating plan?

■ Does the client verbalize a plan to help stay on the new eating plan?

■ Does the client verbalize positive self-attributes not associated with body size or appearance?

For the Client With Anorexia, Bulimia, or Obesity:

■ Has the client been able to develop a more realistic perception of body image?

■ Has the client acknowledged that past self-expectations may have been unrealistic?

■ Does client accept self as less than perfect?

■ Has the client developed adaptive coping strategies to deal with stress without resorting to maladaptive eating behaviors?

Quality and Safety Education for Nurses (QSEN)

The Institute of Medicine (IOM), in its 2003 report, *Health Professions Education: A Bridge to Quality,* challenged faculties of medicine, nursing, and other health professions to ensure that their graduates have achieved a core set of competencies in order to meet the needs of the 21st-century health-care system.

These competencies include *providing patient-centered care, working in interdisciplinary teams, employing evidence-based practice, applying quality improvement, ensuring safety* and *utilizing informatics.* A QSEN teaching strategy is included in Box 31-5. The use of this type of activity is intended to arm the instructor and the student with guidelines for attaining the knowledge, skills, and attitudes necessary for achievement of quality and safety competencies in nursing.

IMPLICATIONS OF RESEARCH FOR EVIDENCE-BASED PRACTICE

Waller, T., Lampman, C., & Lupfer-Johnson, G. (2012). Assessing bias against overweight individuals among nursing and psychology students: An implicit association test. *Journal of Clinical Nursing, 21*(23-24), 3504-3512.

DESCRIPTION OF THE STUDY: Almost 69 percent of adults in the United States are overweight, and more than 35 percent of those are within the range of obesity. Obesity has become a leading health concern that impacts both physical and psychological health. Because attitudes can affect behaviors negatively, the authors undertook this study to determine the implicit or unconscious attitudes of nursing and psychology students toward overweight individuals in medical and non-medical contexts. Study participants included 90 students in upper division nursing and psychology programs at the University of Alaska Anchorage. Mean age was 25 years. The majority were white. Others reported their race as Alaska Native or American Indian, African American, Asian, Hispanic, and Filipino. Attitudes were measured using an implicit association test (IAT) that measures how readily a target concept and an attribute are associated by analyzing reaction times. Participants sat at computers with dominant hand on response pad with the following instructions: "Please press the *blue* key as quickly as possible if you see a *thin* or *normal weight* person, or if you see a *positive* attribute used to describe a person. Please press the *yellow* key if you see an *overweight* person, or if you see a *negative* attribute used to describe a person." Attitudes were measured according to rapidity of

response time in relation to associating images of overweight individuals with positive words and normal-weight or thin individuals with negative words (the inconsistent stereotype) as compared to associating positive words with thin or normal-weight individuals and negative words with obese or overweight individuals (the consistent stereotype). Scenarios exhibited individuals in both medical settings (patients) and non-medical settings.

RESULTS OF THE STUDY: Students enrolled in a Social Psychology class analyzed the data for a class assignment. Results indicated a statistically significant implicit bias toward overweight individuals by both the nursing students and the psychology students. A stronger weight bias was noted when the target stimulus in the scenario was female rather than male. No significant differences in degree of bias toward weight were found between nursing and psychology students or between subjects in medical versus non-medical settings.

IMPLICATIONS FOR NURSING PRACTICE: The authors suggest: "Providing education and support to overweight individuals is central to nursing practice in a society struggling to manage obesity. Negative stereotypes or beliefs about these individuals may result in poor patient care. Therefore, nurses and other healthcare professionals must be aware of personal biases and work to develop methods to address weight-related issues in a therapeutic manner." (p. 3504)

BOX 31-5 QSEN TEACHING STRATEGY

Assignment: Using Evidence to Address Clinical Problems
Intervention With a Client Who Fears Gaining Weight (Anorexia Nervosa)

Competency Domain: Evidence-Based Practice

Learning Objectives: Student will:
- Differentiate clinical opinion from research and evidence summaries.
- Explain the role of evidence in determining the best clinical practice for intervening with clients who do not want to eat.
- Identify gaps between what is observed in the treatment setting to what has been identified as best practice.
- Discriminate between valid and invalid reasons for modifying evidence-based clinical practice based on clinical expertise or other reasons.

Continued

BOX 31-5 QSEN TEACHING STRATEGY—cont'd

• Participate effectively in appropriate data collection and other research activities.
• Acknowledge own limitations in knowledge and clinical expertise before determining when to deviate from evidence-based best practices.

Strategy Overview:

1. Investigate the research related to intervening with a client who does not want to eat.
2. Identify best practices described in the literature. How were these best practices determined?
3. Compare and contrast staff intervention with best practices described in the literature.
4. Investigate staff perceptions related to intervening with a client who is refusing to eat. How have they developed these perceptions?
5. Do staff members view any problems associated with their practice versus best practice described in the literature? If so, how would they like to see the problem addressed?
6. Describe ethical issues associated with intervening with a client who does not want to eat.
7. What is your personal perception regarding the best evidence available to date related to intervening with a client who has anorexia nervosa? Are there situations that you can think of when you might deviate from the best practice model?
8. What questions do you have about intervening with a client who has anorexia nervosa that are not being addressed by current researchers?

Adapted from teaching strategy submitted by Pamela M. Ironside, Associate Professor, Indiana University School of Nursing, Indianapolis, IN. © 2009 QSEN; http://qsen.org. With permission.

Treatment Modalities

The immediate aim of treatment in eating disorders is to restore the client's nutritional status. Complications of emaciation, dehydration, and electrolyte imbalance can lead to death. Once the physical condition is no longer life-threatening, other treatment modalities may be initiated.

Behavior Modification

Efforts to change the maladaptive eating behaviors of clients with anorexia nervosa and bulimia nervosa have become the widely accepted treatment. The importance of instituting a behavior modification program with these clients is to ensure that the program does not "control" them. Issues of control are central to the etiology of these disorders, and in order for the program to be successful, the client must perceive that he or she is in control of the treatment.

Successes have been observed when the client with anorexia nervosa is allowed to contract for privileges based on weight gain. The client has input into the care plan and can clearly see what the treatment choices are. The client has control over eating, over

IMPLICATIONS OF RESEARCH FOR EVIDENCE-BASED PRACTICE

McIntosh, V.V.W., Jordan, J., Carter, F.A., Luty, S.E., McKenzie, J.M., Bulik, C.M., Frampton, C.M.A., and Joyce, P.R. (2005). Three psychotherapies for anorexia nervosa: A randomized, controlled trial. *American Journal of Psychiatry, 162*(4), 741-747.

DESCRIPTION OF THE STUDY: The objective of this study was to examine the efficacy of three types of therapies in treatment of anorexia nervosa. Fifty-six women (age range: 17 to 40 years) with anorexia nervosa were randomly assigned to one of three treatments. Two were specialized psychotherapies: cognitive-behavioral therapy (CBT) and interpersonal psychotherapy (IPT). The third (the intervention) included treatment combining clinical management and supportive psychotherapy (called nonspecific supportive clinical management). They participated in 20 therapy sessions over a minimum of 20 weeks. The intervention

consisted of education, care, and support, fostering a therapeutic relationship that promotes adherence to treatment. Emphasis was placed on resumption of normal eating and restoration of weight. Information on weight maintenance strategies, energy requirements, and relearning to eat normally were included. Outcomes were measured on a global anorexia nervosa measure using a 4-point ordinal scale:

4 = meets full criteria for the anorexia nervosa spectrum
3 = not full anorexia nervosa, but having a number of features of eating disorders
2 = few features of eating disorders
1 = no significant features of eating disorders

RESULTS OF THE STUDY: Of the participants who received nonspecific supportive clinical management, 56 percent received a score of 1 or 2 on the final outcome measure,

IMPLICATIONS OF RESEARCH FOR EVIDENCE-BASED PRACTICE–cont'd

compared with 32 percent and 10 percent of those receiving CBT and IPT, respectively. The authors suggest that IPT may not have been as successful because of the lack of symptom focus and relatively long time taken to decide on the problem area. They hypothesize that the CBT may have been less effective because of the large amount of psychoeducational material and extensive skills acquisition associated with this therapy, and the difficulty of anorexia clients to generate alternatives due to cognitive rigidity. These results were in direct opposition to the original hypothesis generated by the researchers in the beginning of the study.

IMPLICATIONS FOR NURSING PRACTICE: Nurses in advanced practice are usually trained to provide CBT and IPT. Often, generalist nurses do not have the theoretical background to perform these therapies. The interventions associated with nonspecific supportive clinical management are within the scope of nursing practice, and the results of this study indicate that they are superior to CBT and IPT in the treatment of anorexia nervosa. Nurses could become instrumental in establishing programs based on this type of treatment for individuals with anorexia nervosa.

the amount of exercise pursued, and even over whether or not to induce vomiting. Goals of therapy, along with the responsibilities of each for goal achievement, are agreed on by client and staff.

Staff and client also agree on a system of rewards and privileges that can be earned by the client, who is given ultimate control. He or she has a choice of whether or not to abide by the contract—a choice of whether or not to gain weight—thereby either earning the desired privilege or not.

This method of treatment gives a great deal of autonomy to the client. It must be understood, however, that these behavior modification techniques are helpful for weight restoration only. Concomitant individual and/or family psychotherapy are required to prevent or reduce further morbidity.

Some clinicians incorporate cognitive therapy concepts along with behavior modification techniques. Cognitive therapy helps the client to confront irrational thinking and strive to modify distorted and maladaptive cognitions about body image and eating behaviors. Halmi (2008) states, "Cognitive techniques such as cognitive restructuring and problem solving help the patient deal with distorted and overvalued beliefs about food and thinness and cope with life's stresses" (p. 981).

Cognitive-behavioral therapy (CBT) has also been shown to be helpful in treating clients with BED (Black & Andreasen, 2011; Wright, Thase, & Beck, 2008). The therapy serves to help normalize behavior by reducing the number of binging episodes. Some studies have shown CBT to be most beneficial in reducing binging, but it has not been consistently helpful in promoting weight loss in persons with BED (Wright et al., 2008).

Individual Therapy

Although individual psychotherapy is not the therapy of choice for eating disorders, it can be helpful when underlying psychological problems are contributing to the maladaptive behaviors. In supportive psychotherapy, the therapist encourages the client to explore unresolved conflicts and to recognize the maladaptive eating behaviors as defense mechanisms used to ease the emotional pain. The goals are to resolve the personal issues and establish more adaptive coping strategies for dealing with stressful situations.

Family Therapy

Kirkpatrick and Caldwell (2004) state:

Eating disorders have a profound effect on families. While these disorders can help bring families together, they always cause some level of distress. Stresses can cause a breakdown of the whole family unit if there isn't some form of intervention. Family therapy aims at finding solutions to help the healing process for everyone in the family. (pp. 159-160)

In many instances, eating disorders may be considered *family* disorders, and resolution cannot be achieved until dynamics within the family have improved. Family therapy deals with education of the members about the disorder's manifestations, possible etiology, and prescribed treatment. Support is given to family members as they deal with feelings of guilt associated with the perception that they may have contributed to the onset of the disorder. Support is also given as they deal with the social stigma of having a family member with emotional problems.

In some instances when the dysfunctional family dynamics are related to conflict avoidance, the family may be noncompliant with therapy, as they attempt to maintain equilibrium by keeping a member in the sick role. When this occurs, it is essential to focus on the functional operations within the family and to help them manage conflict and create change.

Referrals are made to local support groups for families of individuals with eating disorders. Resolution and growth can sometimes be achieved through interaction with others who are experiencing, or have experienced, the numerous problems of living with a family member with an eating disorder.

Psychopharmacology

There are no medications specifically indicated for eating disorders. Various medications have been prescribed for associated symptoms such as anxiety and depression. Halmi (2008) reported on success with fluoxetine (Prozac) and clomipramine (Anafranil) in clients with anorexia nervosa, and particularly those with depression or obsessive-compulsive symptoms. Cyproheptadine (Periactin), in its unlabeled use as an appetite stimulant, and the antipsychotic chlorpromazine (Thorazine) have also been used to treat this disorder in selected clients. Success has been reported in a controlled trial of olanzapine (Zyprexa) in clients with anorexia nervosa (Bissada, Tasca, Barber, & Bradwejn, 2008).

Fluoxetine (Prozac) has been found to be useful in the treatment of bulimia nervosa (Schatzberg, Cole, & DeBattista, 2010). A dosage of 60 mg/day (triple the usual antidepressant dosage) was found to be most effective. It is possible that fluoxetine, an SSRI, may decrease the craving for carbohydrates, thereby decreasing the incidence of binge eating, which is often associated with consumption of large amounts of carbohydrates. Other antidepressants, such as imipramine (Tofranil), desipramine (Norpramine), amitriptyline (Elavil), nortriptyline (Aventyl), and phenelzine (Nardil), also have been shown to be effective in controlled treatment studies (Halmi, 2008).

One study was conducted with the anticonvulsant topiramate (Topamax) in the long-term treatment of binge-eating disorder with obesity (McElroy et al., 2007). Dosage was titrated to 400 mg/day (or the maximum tolerated dose). Participants experienced a significant decline in mean weekly binge frequency and significant reduction in body weight. Nickel and associates (2005) also reported effective results with topiramate in clients with bulimia nervosa. Episodes of binging and purging were decreased. Clients lost weight and reported a significant improvement in health-related quality of life when compared with the placebo group.

Fluoxetine has been successful in treating clients who are overweight, possibly for the same reason that was explained for clients with bulimia. The effective dosage for promoting weight loss is 60 mg/day. Regarding the use of anorexiants, Sadock and Sadock (2007) state:

> Sympathomimetics are used in the treatment of obesity because of their anorexia-inducing effects. Because tolerance develops for the anorectic effects and because of the drugs' high abuse potential, their use for this indication is limited. (p. 1100)

Withdrawal from **anorexiants** may result in a rebound weight gain and, in some clients, a concomitant lethargy and depression. Two anorexiants that were once widely used, fenfluramine and dexfenfluramine, have been removed from the market because of their association with serious heart and lung disease. Other anorexiants currently on the market include phentermine, diethylpropion, benzphetamine, and phendimetrazine. All are indicated only for short-term weight loss.

A medication for treating obesity, called sibutramine (Meridia), was approved by the U.S. Food and Drug Administration (FDA) in 1998. It was indicated only for individuals who had a significant amount of weight to lose. The mechanism of action in the control of appetite appears to occur by inhibiting the neurotransmitters serotonin and norepinephrine. Some concern was expressed about possible cardiovascular disease associated with the use of sibutramine, and several deaths have been associated with its use by high-risk clients. Based on pressure from the FDA, the manufacturer issued a recall of the drug in October 2010.

Two new weight-loss drugs were approved by the FDA in 2012. Lorcaserin (Belviq) suppresses the appetite by altering various 5-HT2C serotonin receptors found within the hypothalamus, which is responsible for appetite and metabolism. Qsymia is a combined preparation of phentermine and topiramate in a timed-release capsule. Phentermine is a CNS stimulant that is thought to suppress appetite by triggering release of the neurotransmitter norepinephrine. Topiramate is an anticonvulsant medication that has weight loss as a side effect. It is also used in migraine prevention.

CASE STUDY AND SAMPLE CARE PLAN

NURSING HISTORY AND ASSESSMENT

When Connie fainted in history class, she was taken to the university health center by her roommate, Nan. Nan told the nurse that Connie had been taking a lot of over-the-counter laxatives and diuretics. She also said that Connie often self-induced vomiting when she felt that she had eaten too much. After an initial physical assessment, the nurse in the university health center referred Connie to the mental health clinic.

At the mental health clinic, Connie weighed 110 lbs, and measured 5'6" tall. She admitted to the psychiatric nurse, Kathy, that she tried to keep her weight down by dieting, but sometimes she got so hungry that she would overeat, and then she felt the need to self-induce vomiting to get rid

CASE STUDY AND SAMPLE CARE PLAN—cont'd

of the calories. "I really don't like doing it, but lots of the girls do. In fact, that is where I got the idea. I always thought I was too fat in high school, but the competition wasn't so great there. Here all the girls are so pretty . . . and so thin!! It's the only way I can keep my weight down!!"

Connie admitted to Kathy that she hoards food in her dorm room and that she eats when she is feeling particularly anxious and depressed (often during the night). She admitted to having eaten several bags of potato chips and whole packages of cookies in a single sitting. She sometimes drives to the local hamburger stand in the middle of the night, orders several hamburgers, fries, and milkshakes, and consumes them as she sits in her car alone. She stated that she feels so much better while she is eating these foods, but then feels panicky after they have been consumed. That is when she self-induces vomiting. "Then I feel more depressed, and the only thing that helps is eating! I feel so out of control!"

NURSING DIAGNOSES/OUTCOME IDENTIFICATION

From the assessment data, the nurse develops the following nursing diagnosis for Connie:

Ineffective coping related to feelings of helplessness, low self-esteem, and lack of control in life situation.

- **Short-Term Goal:** Client will identify and discuss fears and anxieties with the nurse.

- **Long-Term Goal:** Client will identify adaptive coping strategies that can be realistically incorporated into her lifestyle, thereby eliminating binging and purging in response to anxiety.

PLANNING/IMPLEMENTATION

INEFFECTIVE COPING

The following nursing interventions have been identified for Connie:

- Establish a trusting relationship with Connie. Be honest and accepting. Show unconditional positive regard.

- Help Connie identify the situations that produce anxiety and discuss how she coped with these situations before she began binging and purging.
- Help Connie identify the emotions that precipitate binging (e.g., fear, boredom, anger, loneliness).
- Once these high-risk situations have been identified, help her identify alternate behaviors, such as exercise, a hobby, or a warm bath.
- Encourage Connie to express feelings that have been suppressed because they were considered unacceptable. Help her identify healthier ways to express those feelings.
- Use role-play with Connie to deal with feelings and experiment with new behaviors.
- Explore the dynamics of Connie's family. Intrafamilial conflicts reinforce maladaptive eating behaviors.
- Teach the concepts of good nutrition, and the importance of healthy eating patterns in overall wellness.
- Consult with the physician about a prescription for fluoxetine for Connie.
- Help Connie find a support group for individuals with eating disorders. Encourage regular attendance in this group.

EVALUATION

The outcome criteria for Connie have been met. She discussed with the nurse the feelings that triggered binging episodes and the situations that precipitated those feelings. She has joined a support group of individuals with eating disorders and now has a "buddy" that she may call (even in the middle of the night) when she is feeling like binging. She has started riding her bicycle regularly and goes to the fitness center when she is feeling especially anxious. She still sees the mental health nurse weekly and continues to discuss her fears and anxieties. The urges to binge at stressful times have not disappeared completely. However, they have decreased in frequency, and Connie is now able to choose more adaptive strategies for dealing with stress.

Summary and Key Points

- The incidence of eating disorders has continued to increase since the middle of the 20th century.
- Individuals with anorexia nervosa, a disorder that is characterized by a morbid fear of obesity and a gross distortion of body image, literally can starve themselves to death.
- The individual with anorexia nervosa believes he or she is fat even when emaciated. The disorder is commonly accompanied by depression and anxiety.
- Bulimia nervosa is an eating disorder characterized by the consumption of huge amounts of food, usually in a short period of time, and often in secret.

- With bulimia nervosa, tension is relieved and pleasure felt during the time of the binge, but is soon followed by feelings of guilt and depression.
- Individuals with bulimia nervosa "purge" themselves of the excessive intake with self-induced vomiting or the misuse of laxatives, diuretics, or enemas. They also are subject to mood and anxiety disorders.
- Binge-eating disorder (BED) is characterized by the consumption of huge amounts of food by an individual who feels a lack of control over the eating behavior. BED differs from bulimia nervosa in that the individual does not engage in behaviors to rid the body of the excess calories.

- Compulsive eating can result in obesity, which is defined by the National Institutes of Health as a body mass index (BMI) of 30 or greater.
- Obesity predisposes the individual to many health concerns, and at the morbid level (a BMI of 40 or greater), the weight alone can contribute to increases in morbidity and mortality.
- Predisposing factors to eating disorders include genetics, physiological factors, family dynamics, and environmental and lifestyle factors.

- Treatment modalities for eating disorders include behavior modification, individual psychotherapy, cognitive-behavioral therapy, family therapy, and psychopharmacology.

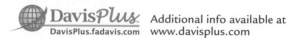 Additional info available at
DavisPlus.fadavis.com   www.davisplus.com

Review Questions
Self-Examination/Learning Exercise

*Select the answer that is **most** appropriate for each of the following questions.*

1. Some obese individuals take amphetamines to suppress appetite and help them lose weight. Which of the following is an adverse effect associated with use of amphetamines that makes this practice undesirable?
   a. Bradycardia
   b. Amenorrhea
   c. Tolerance
   d. Convulsions

2. Psychoanalytically, the theory of obesity relates to the individual's unconscious equation of food with:
   a. Nurturance and caring
   b. Power and control
   c. Autonomy and emotional growth
   d. Strength and endurance

3. From a physiological point of view, the most common cause of obesity is probably:
   a. Lack of nutritional education
   b. More calories consumed than expended
   c. Impaired endocrine functioning
   d. Low basal metabolic rate

4. Nancy, age 14, has just been admitted to the psychiatric unit for anorexia nervosa. She is emaciated and refusing to eat. What is the primary nursing diagnosis for Nancy?
   a. Complicated grieving
   b. Imbalanced nutrition: Less than body requirements
   c. Interrupted family processes
   d. Anxiety (severe)

5. Which of the following physical manifestations would you expect to assess in a client suffering from anorexia nervosa?
   a. Tachycardia, hypertension, hyperthermia
   b. Bradycardia, hypertension, hyperthermia
   c. Bradycardia, hypotension, hypothermia
   d. Tachycardia, hypotension, hypothermia

6. Nurse Jones is caring for a client who has been hospitalized with anorexia nervosa and is severely malnourished. The client continues to refuse to eat. What is the most appropriate response by the nurse?
   a. "You know that if you don't eat, you will die."
   b. "If you continue to refuse to take food orally, you will be fed through a nasogastric tube."
   c. "You might as well leave if you are not going to follow your therapy regimen."
   d. "You don't have to eat if you don't want to. It is your choice."

Review Questions—cont'd
Self-Examination/Learning Exercise

7. Which medication has been used with some success in clients with anorexia nervosa?
   a. Lorcaserin (Belviq)
   b. Diazepam (Valium)
   c. Fluoxetine (Prozac)
   d. Carbamazepine (Tegretol)

8. Jane is hospitalized on the psychiatric unit. She has a history and current diagnosis of bulimia nervosa. Which of the following symptoms would be congruent with Jane's diagnosis?
   a. Binging, purging, obesity, hyperkalemia
   b. Binging, purging, normal weight, hypokalemia
   c. Binging, laxative abuse, amenorrhea, severe weight loss
   d. Binging, purging, severe weight loss, hyperkalemia

9. A hospitalized client with bulimia nervosa has stopped vomiting in the hospital and tells the nurse she is afraid she is going to gain weight. Which is the most appropriate response by the nurse?
   a. "Don't worry. The dietitian will ensure you don't get too many calories in your diet."
   b. "Don't worry about your weight. We are going to work on other problems while you are in the hospital."
   c. "I understand that you are concerned about your weight, and we will talk about the importance of good nutrition; but for now I want you to tell me about your recent invitation to join the National Honor Society. That's quite an accomplishment."
   d. "You are not fat, and the staff will ensure that you do not gain weight while you are in the hospital, because we know that is important to you."

10. The binging episode is thought to involve:
    a. A release of tension, followed by feelings of depression
    b. Feelings of fear, followed by feelings of relief
    c. Unmet dependency needs and a way to gain attention
    d. Feelings of euphoria, excitement, and self-gratification

TEST YOUR CRITICAL THINKING SKILLS

Janice, a high school sophomore, wanted desperately to become a cheerleader. She practiced endlessly before tryouts, but she was not selected. A week later, her boyfriend, Roy, broke up with her to date another girl. Janice, who was 5'3" tall and weighed 110 pounds, decided it was because she was too fat. She began to exercise at every possible moment. She skipped meals, and tried to keep her daily consumption to no more than 300 calories. She lost a great deal of weight but became very weak. She felt cold all of the time and wore sweaters in the warm weather. She collapsed during her physical education class at school and was rushed to the emergency department. On admission, she weighed 90 pounds. She was emaciated and anemic. The physician admitted her with a diagnosis of anorexia nervosa.

Answer the following questions about Janice:

1. What will be the *primary* consideration in her care?
2. How will treatment be directed toward helping her gain weight?
3. How will the nurse know if Janice is using self-induced vomiting to rid herself of food consumed at meals?

References

American Psychiatric Association (APA). (2013). *Diagnostic and statistical manual of mental disorders* (5th ed.). Washington, DC: Author.

Bissada, H., Tasca, G., Barber, A.M., & Bradwejn, J. (2008). Olanzapine in the treatment of low body weight and obsessive thinking in women with anorexia nervosa: A randomized, double-blind, placebo-controlled trial. *American Journal of Psychiatry, 165*(10), 1281-1288.

Black, D.W., & Andreasen, N.C. (2011). *Introductory textbook of psychiatry* (5th ed.). Washington, DC: American Psychiatric Publishing.

Bulik, C.M., Sullivan, P.F., Tozzi, F., Furberg, H., Lichtenstein, P., & Pedersen, N.L. (2006). Prevalence, heritability, and prospective risk factors for anorexia nervosa. *Archives of General Psychiatry, 63*(3), 305-312.

Centers for Disease Control and Prevention (CDC). (2012). *Health, United States, 2011.* Retrieved from www.cdc.gov/nchs/data/hus/hus11.pdf

Choquet, H., & Meyre, D. (2011). Genetics of obesity: What have we learned? *Current Genomics, 12*(3), 169-179.

Halmi, K.A. (2008). Eating disorders: Anorexia nervosa, bulimia nervosa, and obesity. In R.E. Hales, S.C. Yudofsky, & G.O. Gabbard (Eds.), *Textbook of psychiatry* (5th ed., pp. 971-997). Washington, DC: American Psychiatric Publishing.

Institute of Medicine. (2003). *Health professions education: A bridge to quality.* Washington, DC: Author.

Jaret, P. (2010). *Eating disorders and depression.* Retrieved from www.webmd.com/depression/features/eating-disorders

Kirkpatrick, J., & Caldwell, P. (2004). *Eating disorders: Everything you need to know.* Buffalo, NY: Firefly Books.

McElroy, S.L., Hudson, J.I., Capece, J.A., Beyers, K., Fisher, A.C., & Rosenthal, N.R. (2007). Topiramate for the treatment of binge-eating disorder associated with obesity: A placebo-controlled study. *Biological Psychiatry, 61*(9), 1039-1048.

NANDA International (NANDA-I). (2012). *Nursing diagnoses: Definitions and classification 2012-2014.* Hoboken, NJ: Wiley-Blackwell.

National Heart, Lung, and Blood Institute. (2013). Clinical guidelines on the identification, evaluation, and treatment of overweight and obesity in adults: Body mass index tables. Retrieved from http://www.nhlbi.nih.gov/guidelines/obesity/bmi_tbl.htm

Nickel, C., Tritt, K., Muehlbacher, M., Pedrosa, F., Mitterlehner, F.O., Kaplan, P., et al., (2005). Topiramate treatment in bulimia nervosa patients: A randomized, double-blind, placebo-controlled trial. *International Journal of Eating Disorders, 38*(4), 295-300.

Puri, B.K., & Treasaden, I.H. (2011). *Textbook of psychiatry* (3rd ed.). Philadelphia, PA: Churchill Livingstone Elsevier.

Sadock, B.J., & Sadock, V.A. (2007). *Synopsis of psychiatry: Behavioral sciences/clinical psychiatry* (10th ed.). Philadelphia, PA: Lippincott Williams & Wilkins.

Schatzberg, A.F., Cole, J.O., & DeBattista, C. (2010). *Manual of clinical psychopharmacology* (7th ed.). Washington, DC: American Psychiatric Publishing.

Uceyler, N., Schutt, M., Palm, F., Vogel, C., Meier, M., Schmitt, A., Lesch, K.P., Mossner, R., & Sommer, C. (2010). Lack of serotonin transporter in mice reduces locomotor activity and leads to gender-dependent late onset obesity. *International Journal of Obesity, 34*(4), 701-711.

Wright, J.H., Thase, M.E., & Beck, A. T. (2008). Cognitive therapy. In R.E. Hales, S.C. Yudofsky, & G.O. Gabbard (Eds.), *Textbook of psychiatry* (5th ed., pp. 1211-1256). Washington, DC: American Psychiatric Publishing.

Yager, J., Devlin, M.J., Halmi, K.A., Herzog, D.B., Mitchell, J.E., Powers, P., & Zerbe, K.J. (2006). Practice guideline for the treatment of patients with eating disorders. *American Psychiatric Association practice guidelines for the treatment of psychiatric disorders, Compendium 2006.* Washington, DC: American Psychiatric Publishing.

 INTERNET REFERENCES

- Additional information about anorexia nervosa, bulimia nervosa, and binge-eating disorder (BED) may be located at the following websites:
  - http://www.anad.org
  - http://healthyminds.org
  - http://www.nationaleatingdisorders.org
  - http://www.mentalhealth.com/dis/p20-et01.html
  - http://www.mentalhealth.com/dis/p20-et02.html
  - http://www.nimh.nih.gov/health/publications/eating-disorders/complete-index.shtml
  - http://www.nlm.nih.gov/medlineplus/eatingdisorders.html
  - http://www.mayoclinic.com/health/binge-eating-disorder/DS00608
  - http://www.bedaonline.com
  - http://psychcentral.com/disorders/eating_disorders

- Additional information about obesity may be located at the following websites:
  - http://www.shapeup.org
  - http://www.obesity.org
  - http://www.nlm.nih.gov/medlineplus/obesity.html
  - http://www.asbp.org
  - http://win.niddk.nih.gov/publications/binge.htm

 MOVIE CONNECTIONS

The Best Little Girl in the World (anorexia nervosa) • *Kate's Secret* (bulimia nervosa) • *For the Love of Nancy* (anorexia nervosa) • *Super Size Me* (obesity)

Personality Disorders

32

CORE CONCEPT

personality

KEY TERMS

antisocial personality disorder

avoidant personality disorder

borderline personality disorder

dependent personality disorder

histrionic personality disorder

narcissistic personality disorder

object constancy

obsessive-compulsive personality disorder

paranoid personality disorder

schizoid personality disorder

schizotypal personality disorder

splitting

OBJECTIVES
After reading this chapter, the student will be able to:

1. Define *personality*.
2. Compare stages of personality development according to Sullivan, Erikson, and Mahler.
3. Identify various types of personality disorders.
4. Discuss historical and epidemiological statistics related to various personality disorders.
5. Describe symptomatology associated with borderline personality disorder and antisocial personality disorder, and use these data in client assessment.
6. Identify predisposing factors for borderline personality disorder and antisocial personality disorder.

7. Formulate nursing diagnoses and goals of care for clients with borderline personality disorder and antisocial personality disorder.
8. Describe appropriate nursing interventions for behaviors associated with borderline personality disorder and antisocial personality disorder.
9. Evaluate nursing care of clients with borderline personality disorder and antisocial personality disorder.
10. Discuss various modalities relevant to treatment of personality disorders.

HOMEWORK ASSIGNMENT
Please read the chapter and answer the following questions:

1. What are the primary psychosocial predisposing factors to avoidant personality disorder?
2. Monoamine oxidase inhibitors (MAOIs) have been shown to be effective in decreasing impulsivity and self-destructive acts in clients with borderline personality disorder. Why are they not commonly used?

3. How should a nurse care for the self-inflicted wounds of a client with borderline personality disorder?
4. What are some of the types of family dynamics that may predispose a person to antisocial personality disorder?

669

CORE CONCEPT

Personality

The totality of emotional and behavioral characteristics that are particular to a specific person and that remain somewhat stable and predictable over time.

The word *personality* is derived from the Greek term *persona*. It was originally used to describe the theatrical mask worn by some dramatic actors at the time. Over the years, it lost its connotation of pretense and illusion and came to represent the person behind the mask—the "real" person.

Personality *traits* may be defined as characteristics with which an individual is born or develops early in life. They influence the way in which he or she perceives and relates to the environment and are quite stable over time. Personality *disorders* occur when these traits become rigid and inflexible and contribute to maladaptive patterns of behavior or impairment in functioning. Virtually all individuals exhibit some behaviors associated with the various personality disorders from time to time. As previously stated, it is only when significant functional impairment occurs in response to these personality characteristics that the individual is thought to have a personality disorder.

Personality development occurs in response to a number of biological and psychological influences. These variables include (but are not limited to) heredity, temperament, experiential learning, and social interaction. A number of theorists have attempted to provide information about personality development. Most suggest that it occurs in an orderly, stepwise fashion. These stages overlap, however, as maturation occurs at different rates in different individuals. The theories of Sullivan (1953), Erikson (1963), and Mahler (Mahler, Pine, & Bergman, 1975) were presented at length in Chapter 3. The stages of personality development according to these three theorists are compared in Table 32-1. The nurse should understand "normal" personality development before learning about what is considered maladaptive.

TABLE 32–1 Comparison of Personality Development—Sullivan, Erikson, and Mahler

MAJOR DEVELOPMENTAL TASKS AND DESIGNATED AGES

SULLIVAN	ERIKSON	MAHLER
Birth to 18 months: Relief from anxiety through oral gratification of needs.	Birth to 18 months: To develop a basic trust in the mothering figure and be able to generalize it to others.	Birth to 1 month: Fulfillment of basic needs for survival and comfort.
18 months to 6 years: Learning to experience a delay in personal gratification without undue anxiety.	18 months to 3 years: To gain some self-control and independence within the environment.	1 to 5 months: Developing awareness of external source of need fulfillment.
6 to 9 years: Learning to form satisfactory peer relationships.	3 to 6 years: To develop a sense of purpose and the ability to initiate and direct own activities.	5 to 10 months: Commencement of a primary recognition of separateness from the mothering figure.
9 to 12 years: Learning to form satisfactory relationships with persons of the same gender; the initiation of feelings of affection for another person.	6 to 12 years: To achieve a sense of self-confidence by learning, competing, performing successfully, and receiving recognition from significant others, peers, and acquaintances.	10 to 16 months: Increased independence through locomotor functioning; increased sense of separateness of self.
12 to 14 years: Learning to form satisfactory relationships with persons of the opposite gender; developing a sense of identity.	12 to 20 years: To integrate the tasks mastered in the previous stages into a secure sense of self.	16 to 24 months: Acute awareness of separateness of self; learning to seek "emotional refueling" from mothering figure to maintain feeling of security.
14 to 21 years: Establishing self-identity; experiences satisfying relationships; working to develop a lasting, intimate opposite-gender relationship.	20 to 30 years: To form an intense, lasting relationship or a commitment to another person, a cause, an institution, or a creative effort.	24 to 36 months: Sense of separateness established; on the way to object constancy: able to internalize a sustained image of loved object/person

TABLE 32–1	**Comparison of Personality Development–Sullivan, Erikson, and Mahler–cont'd**	
MAJOR DEVELOPMENTAL TASKS AND DESIGNATED AGES		
SULLIVAN	ERIKSON	MAHLER
		when it is out of sight; resolution of separation anxiety.
	30 to 65 years: To achieve the life goals established for oneself, while also considering the welfare of future generations.	
	65 years to death: To review one's life and derive meaning from both positive and negative events, while achieving a positive sense of self-worth.	

Historical and epidemiological aspects of personality disorders are discussed in this chapter. Predisposing factors that have been implicated in the etiology of personality disorders are presented. Symptomatology is explained to provide background knowledge for assessing clients with personality disorders.

Individuals with personality disorders are not often treated in acute care settings for the personality disorder as their primary psychiatric diagnosis. However, many clients with other psychiatric and medical diagnoses manifest symptoms of personality disorders. Nurses are likely to encounter clients with these personality characteristics frequently in all health-care settings.

Nurses working in psychiatric settings are likely to encounter clients with borderline and antisocial personality characteristics. The behavior of clients with borderline personality disorder is very unstable, and hospitalization is often required as a result of attempts at self-injury. The client with antisocial personality disorder may enter the psychiatric arena as a result of judicially ordered evaluation. Psychiatric intervention may be an alternative to imprisonment for antisocial behavior if it is deemed potentially helpful.

Nursing care of clients with borderline personality disorder or antisocial personality disorder is presented in this chapter in the context of the nursing process. Various medical treatment modalities for personality disorders are explored.

Historical Aspects

The concept of a personality disorder has been described for thousands of years (Skodal & Gunderson, 2008). In the fourth century BC, Hippocrates concluded that all disease stemmed from an excess of or imbalance among four bodily humors: yellow bile, black bile, blood, and phlegm. Hippocrates identified four fundamental personality styles that he concluded stemmed from excesses in the four humors: the irritable and hostile choleric (yellow bile); the pessimistic melancholic (black bile); the overly optimistic and extraverted sanguine (blood); and the apathetic phlegmatic (phlegm).

The medical profession first recognized that personality disorders, apart from psychosis, were cause for their own special concern in 1801, with the recognition that an individual can behave irrationally even when the powers of intellect are intact. Nineteenth-century psychiatrists embraced the term *moral insanity*, the concept of which defines what we know today as personality disorders.

Historically, individuals with personality disorders have been labeled as "bad" or "immoral" and as deviants in the range of normal personality dimensions. The events and sequences that result in pathology of the personality are complicated and difficult to unravel. Continued study is needed to facilitate understanding of this complex behavioral phenomenon.

A major difficulty for psychiatrists has been the establishment of a classification of personality disorders. Ten specific types of personality disorders are identified in the *Diagnostic and Statistical Manual of Mental Disorders, Fifth Edition (DSM-5)* (American Psychiatric Association [APA], 2013). The APA has proposed a complex diagnostic system to identify impairments in personality functioning specifically related to the dimensions of *self* and *interpersonal relations* and to personality *trait domains and facets*. This diagnostic system is very specific and addresses symptoms that may differ not only among personality disorders, but also among individuals with the same personality disorder. This trait-specific diagnostic methodology is described in the *DSM-5* as an alternative approach to diagnosis of personality disorder, and is recommended for further study.

The current diagnostic system classifies the personality disorders into three clusters according to description of personality traits. These include the following:

1. **Cluster A:** Behaviors described as odd or eccentric.
   a. Paranoid personality disorder
   b. Schizoid personality disorder
   c. Schizotypal personality disorder
2. **Cluster B:** Behaviors described as dramatic, emotional, or erratic.
   a. Antisocial personality disorder
   b. Borderline personality disorder
   c. Histrionic personality disorder
   d. Narcissistic personality disorder
3. **Cluster C:** Behaviors described as anxious or fearful.
   a. Avoidant personality disorder
   b. Dependent personality disorder
   c. Obsessive-compulsive personality disorder

Types of Personality Disorders

Paranoid Personality Disorder

Definition and Epidemiological Statistics

Skodol and Gunderson (2008) define **paranoid personality disorder** as "a pervasive, persistent, and inappropriate mistrust of others. [Individuals with this disorder] are suspicious of others' motives and assume that others intend to exploit, harm, or deceive them" (p. 833). Prevalence of paranoid personality disorder has been estimated at 1 to 4 percent of the general population, and it is often only diagnosed when the individual seeks treatment for a mood or anxiety disorder (Black & Andreasen, 2011). The disorder is more commonly diagnosed in men than in women.

Clinical Picture

Individuals with paranoid personality disorder are constantly on guard, hypervigilant, and ready for any real or imagined threat. They appear tense and irritable. They have developed a hard exterior and become immune or insensitive to the feelings of others. They avoid interactions with other people, lest they be forced to relinquish some of their own power. They always feel that others are there to take advantage of them.

They are extremely oversensitive and tend to misinterpret even minute cues within the environment, magnifying and distorting them into thoughts of trickery and deception. Because they trust no one, they are constantly "testing" the honesty of others. Their intimidating manner provokes exasperation and anger in almost everyone with whom they come in contact.

Individuals with paranoid personality disorder maintain their self-esteem by attributing their shortcomings to others. They do not accept responsibility for their own behaviors and feelings and project this responsibility on to others. They are envious and hostile toward others who are highly successful and believe the only reason they are not as successful is because they have been treated unfairly. People who are paranoid are extremely vulnerable and constantly on the defensive. Any real or imagined threat can release hostility and anger that is fueled by animosities from the past. The desire for reprisal and vindication is so intense that a possible loss of control can result in aggression and violence. These outbursts are usually brief, and the paranoid person soon regains the external control, rationalizes the behavior, and reconstructs the defenses central to his or her personality pattern.

The *DSM-5* diagnostic criteria for paranoid personality disorder are presented in Box 32-1.

Predisposing Factors

Research has indicated a possible hereditary link in paranoid personality disorder. Studies have revealed a higher incidence of paranoid personality disorder

---

BOX 32-1 Diagnostic Criteria for Paranoid Personality Disorder

A. A pervasive distrust and suspiciousness of others such that their motives are interpreted as malevolent, beginning by early adulthood and present in a variety of contexts, as indicated by four (or more) of the following:
   1. Suspects, without sufficient basis, that others are exploiting, harming, or deceiving him or her
   2. Is preoccupied with unjustified doubts about the loyalty or trustworthiness of friends or associates
   3. Is reluctant to confide in others because of unwarranted fear that the information will be used maliciously against him or her
   4. Reads hidden demeaning or threatening meanings into benign remarks or events
   5. Persistently bears grudges (i.e., is unforgiving of insults, injuries, or slights)
   6. Perceives attacks on his or her character or reputation that are not apparent to others and is quick to react angrily or to counterattack
   7. Has recurrent suspicions, without justification, regarding fidelity of spouse or sexual partner
B. Does not occur exclusively during the course of schizophrenia, a bipolar disorder or depressive disorder with psychotic features, or another psychotic disorder and is not attributable to the physiological effects of another medical condition.

among relatives of clients with schizophrenia than among control subjects (Sadock & Sadock, 2007).

Psychosocially, people with paranoid personality disorder may have been subjected to parental antagonism and harassment. They likely served as scapegoats for displaced parental aggression and gradually relinquished all hope of affection and approval. They learned to perceive the world as harsh and unkind, a place calling for protective vigilance and mistrust. They entered the world with a "chip-on-the-shoulder" attitude and were met with many rebuffs and rejections from others. Anticipating humiliation and betrayal by others, the paranoid person learned to attack first.

Schizoid Personality Disorder

Definition and Epidemiological Statistics

Schizoid personality disorder is characterized primarily by a profound defect in the ability to form personal relationships or to respond to others in any meaningful way (Black & Andreasen, 2011). These individuals display a lifelong pattern of social withdrawal, and their discomfort with human interaction is apparent. The prevalence of schizoid personality disorder within the general population has been estimated at between 3 and 7.5 percent. Significant numbers of people with the disorder are never observed in a clinical setting. Gender ratio of the disorder is unknown, although it is diagnosed more frequently in men.

Clinical Picture

People with schizoid personality disorder appear cold, aloof, and indifferent to others. They prefer to work in isolation and are unsociable, with little need or desire for emotional ties. They are able to invest enormous affective energy in intellectual pursuits.

In the presence of others they appear shy, anxious, or uneasy. They are inappropriately serious about everything and have difficulty acting in a lighthearted manner. Their behavior and conversation exhibit little or no spontaneity. Typically they are unable to experience pleasure, and their affect is commonly bland and constricted.

The *DSM-5* diagnostic criteria for schizoid personality disorder are presented in Box 32-2.

Predisposing Factors

Although the role of heredity in the etiology of schizoid personality disorder is unclear, the feature of introversion appears to be a highly inheritable characteristic. Further studies are required before definitive statements can be made.

Psychosocially, the development of schizoid personality is probably influenced by early interactional patterns that the person found to be cold and unsatisfying. The childhoods of these individuals have often been characterized as bleak, cold, and notably lacking empathy and nurturing. A child brought up with this type of parenting may become a schizoid adult if that child possesses a temperamental disposition that is shy, anxious, and introverted. Skodol and Gunderson (2008) state:

> Clinicians have noted that schizoid personality disorder occurs in adults who experienced cold, neglectful, and ungratifying relationships in early childhood, which leads these persons to assume that relationships are not valuable or worth pursuing. (p. 836)

Schizotypal Personality Disorder

Definition and Epidemiological Statistics

Individuals with **schizotypal personality disorder** were once described as "latent schizophrenics." Their behavior is odd and eccentric but does not decompensate to the level of schizophrenia. Schizotypal personality is a graver form of the pathologically less severe schizoid personality pattern. Studies indicate

---

BOX 32-2 **Diagnostic Criteria for Schizoid Personality Disorder**

A. A pervasive pattern of detachment from social relationships and a restricted range of expression of emotions in interpersonal settings, beginning by early adulthood and present in a variety of contexts, as indicated by four (or more) of the following:
  1. Neither desires nor enjoys close relationships, including being part of a family
  2. Almost always chooses solitary activities
  3. Has little, if any, interest in having sexual experiences with another person
  4. Takes pleasure in few, if any, activities
  5. Lacks close friends or confidants other than first-degree relatives
  6. Appears indifferent to the praise or criticism of others
  7. Shows emotional coldness, detachment, or flattened affectivity
B. Does not occur exclusively during the course of schizophrenia, a bipolar disorder or depressive disorder with psychotic features, another psychotic disorder, or autism spectrum disorder and is not attributable to the physiological effects of another medical condition.

that schizotypal personality disorder has a prevalence of 1 to 2 percent (Black & Andreasen, 2011).

Clinical Picture

Individuals with schizotypal personality disorder are aloof and isolated and behave in a bland and apathetic manner. Magical thinking, ideas of reference, illusions, and depersonalization are part of their everyday world. Examples include superstitiousness; belief in clairvoyance, telepathy, or a "sixth sense"; and beliefs that "others can feel my feelings."

The speech pattern is sometimes bizarre. People with this disorder often cannot orient their thoughts logically and become lost in personal irrelevancies and in tangential asides that seem vague, digressive, and not pertinent to the topic at hand. This feature of their personality only further alienates them from others.

Under stress, these individuals may decompensate and demonstrate psychotic symptoms, such as delusional thoughts, hallucinations, or bizarre behaviors, but they are usually of brief duration (Sadock & Sadock, 2007). They often talk or gesture to themselves, as if "living in their own world." Their affect is bland or inappropriate, such as laughing at their own problems or at a situation that most people would consider sad.

The *DSM-5* diagnostic criteria for schizotypal personality disorder are presented in Box 32-3.

Predisposing Factors

Evidence suggests that schizotypal personality disorder is more common among the first-degree biological relatives of people with schizophrenia than among the general population. It is now considered as part of the genetic spectrum of schizophrenia (APA, 2013). Although speculative, other biogenic factors that may contribute to the development of this disorder include anatomical deficits or neurochemical dysfunctions resulting in diminished activation, minimal pleasure-pain sensibilities, and impaired cognitive functions. These biological etiological factors support the close link between schizotypal personality disorder and schizophrenia and were considered when classifying schizotypal personality disorder with schizophrenia rather than with the personality disorders in the *International Classification of Diseases (ICD-10)* (Skodol & Gunderson, 2008).

The early family dynamics of the individual with schizotypal personality disorder may have been characterized by indifference, impassivity, or formality, leading to a pattern of discomfort with personal affection and closeness. Early on, affective deficits made them unattractive and unrewarding social companions. They were likely shunned, overlooked, rejected, and humiliated by others, resulting in feelings of low self-esteem and a marked distrust of interpersonal relations. Having failed repeatedly to cope with these adversities, they began to withdraw and reduce contact with individuals and situations that evoked sadness and humiliation. Their new inner world provided them with a more significant and potentially rewarding existence than the one experienced in reality.

Antisocial Personality Disorder

Definition and Epidemiological Statistics

Antisocial personality disorder is a pattern of socially irresponsible, exploitative, and guiltless behavior that reflects a general disregard for the rights of others. These individuals exploit and manipulate others for personal gain and are unconcerned with obeying the law. They have difficulty sustaining consistent employment and in developing stable relationships.

BOX 32-3 **Diagnostic Criteria for Schizotypal Personality Disorder**

A. A pervasive pattern of social and interpersonal deficits marked by acute discomfort with, and reduced capacity for, close relationships as well as by cognitive or perceptual distortions and eccentricities of behavior, beginning by early adulthood and present in a variety of contexts, as indicated by five (or more) of the following:
  1. Ideas of reference (excluding delusions of reference)
  2. Odd beliefs or magical thinking that influences behavior and is inconsistent with subcultural norms (e.g., superstitiousness, belief in clairvoyance, telepathy, or "sixth sense;" in children and adolescents, bizarre fantasies or preoccupations)
  3. Unusual perceptual experiences, including bodily illusions
  4. Odd thinking and speech (e.g., vague, circumstantial, metaphorical, overelaborate, or stereotyped)
  5. Suspiciousness or paranoid ideation
  6. Inappropriate or constricted affect
  7. Behavior or appearance that is odd, eccentric, or peculiar
  8. Lack of close friends or confidants other than first-degree relatives
  9. Excessive social anxiety that does not diminish with familiarity and tends to be associated with paranoid fears rather than negative judgments about self
B. Does not occur exclusively during the course of schizophrenia, a bipolar disorder or depressive disorder with psychotic features, another psychotic disorder, or autism spectrum disorder.

Reprinted with permission from the *Diagnostic and Statistical Manual of Mental Disorders, Fifth Edition* (Copyright 2013). American Psychiatric Association.

It is one of the oldest and best researched of the personality disorders and has been included in all editions of the *Diagnostic and Statistical Manual of Mental Disorders*. In the United States, prevalence estimates range from 2 to 4 percent in men to about 1 percent in women (Black & Andreasen, 2011). The disorder is more common among the lower socioeconomic classes, particularly so among highly mobile inhabitants of impoverished urban areas. The *ICD-10* identifies this disorder as *dissocial personality disorder*.

> **NOTE:** The clinical picture, predisposing factors, nursing diagnoses, and interventions for care of clients with antisocial personality disorder are presented later in this chapter.

Borderline Personality Disorder

Definition and Epidemiological Statistics

Borderline personality disorder is characterized by a pattern of intense and chaotic relationships, with affective instability and fluctuating attitudes toward other people. These individuals are impulsive, are directly and indirectly self-destructive, and lack a clear sense of identity. Prevalence of borderline personality is estimated at 1 to 2 percent of the population. It is more common in women than in men, with female-to-male ratios being estimated as high as 4 to 1 (Lubit, 2011). The *ICD-10* identifies this disorder as *emotionally unstable personality disorder*.

> **NOTE:** The clinical picture, predisposing factors, nursing diagnoses, and interventions for care of clients with borderline personality disorder are presented later in this chapter.

Histrionic Personality Disorder

Definition and Epidemiological Statistics

Histrionic personality disorder is characterized by colorful, dramatic, and extroverted behavior in excitable, emotional people. They have difficulty maintaining long-lasting relationships, although they require constant affirmation of approval and acceptance from others. Prevalence of the disorder is thought to be about 2 to 3 percent, and it is more common in women than in men.

Clinical Picture

People with histrionic personality disorder tend to be self-dramatizing, attention seeking, overly gregarious, and seductive. They use manipulative and exhibitionistic behaviors in their demands to be the center of attention. People with histrionic personality disorder often demonstrate, in mild pathological form, what our society tends to foster and admire in its members: to be well liked, successful, popular, extroverted, attractive, and sociable. However, beneath these surface characteristics is a driven quality—an all-consuming need for approval and a desperate striving to be conspicuous and to evoke affection or attract attention at all costs. Failure to evoke the attention and approval they seek often results in feelings of dejection and anxiety.

Individuals with this disorder are highly distractible and flighty by nature. They have difficulty paying attention to detail. They can portray themselves as carefree and sophisticated on the one hand and as inhibited and naive on the other. They tend to be highly suggestible, impressionable, and easily influenced by others. They are strongly dependent.

Interpersonal relationships are fleeting and superficial. The person with histrionic personality disorder, having failed throughout life to develop the richness of inner feelings and lacking resources from which to draw, lacks the ability to provide another with genuinely sustained affection. Somatic complaints are not uncommon in these individuals, and fleeting episodes of psychosis may occur during periods of extreme stress.

The *DSM-5* diagnostic criteria for histrionic personality disorder are presented in Box 32-4.

Predisposing Factors

Neurobiological correlates have been proposed in the predisposition to histrionic personality disorder. Coccaro and Siever (2000) relate the characteristics of

---

BOX 32-4 **Diagnostic Criteria for Histrionic Personality Disorder**

A pervasive pattern of excessive emotionality and attention seeking, beginning by early adulthood and present in a variety of contexts, as indicated by five (or more) of the following:
1. Is uncomfortable in situations in which he or she is not the center of attention.
2. Interaction with others is often characterized by inappropriate sexually seductive or provocative behavior.
3. Displays rapidly shifting and shallow expression of emotions.
4. Consistently uses physical appearance to draw attention to self.
5. Has a style of speech that is excessively impressionistic and lacking in detail.
6. Shows self-dramatization, theatricality, and exaggerated expression of emotion.
7. Is suggestible (i.e., easily influenced by others or circumstances).
8. Considers relationships to be more intimate than they actually are.

enhanced sensitivity and reactivity to environmental stimuli to heightened noradrenergic activity in the individual with histrionic personality disorder. They suggested that the trait of impulsivity may be associated with decreased serotonergic activity.

Heredity also may be a factor because the disorder is apparently more common among first-degree biological relatives of people with the disorder than in the general population. Skodol and Gunderson (2008) report on research that suggests that the behavioral characteristics of histrionic personality disorder may be associated with a biogenetically determined temperament. From this perspective, histrionic personality disorder would arise out of "an extreme variation of temperamental disposition" (p. 844).

From a psychosocial perspective, learning experiences may contribute to the development of histrionic personality disorder. The child may have learned that positive reinforcement was contingent on the ability to perform parentally approved and admired behaviors. It is likely that the child rarely received either positive or negative feedback. Parental acceptance and approval came inconsistently and only when the behaviors met parental expectations. Millon (2004) states:

> Because nothing they do works consistently, such children experience frustration in getting their parents' attention and exaggerate behaviors basic to their gender stereotype to secure compliments and affection. Otherwise, they are ignored. Such children enter adolescence with a nearly insatiable thirst for attention and love. (p. 314)

Narcissistic Personality Disorder

Definition and Epidemiological Statistics

Persons with **narcissistic personality disorder** have an exaggerated sense of self-worth. They lack empathy, and are hypersensitive to the evaluation of others.

They believe that they have the inalienable right to receive special consideration and that their desire is sufficient justification for possessing whatever they seek.

This diagnosis appeared for the first time in the third edition of the *Diagnostic and Statistical Manual of Mental Disorders*. However, the concept of narcissism has its roots in the 19th century. It was viewed by early psychoanalysts as a normal phase of psychosexual development. The prevalence of narcissistic personality disorder is estimated at about 6 percent (Black & Andreasen, 2011). It is diagnosed more often in men than in women.

Clinical Picture

Individuals with narcissistic personality disorder appear to lack humility, being overly self-centered and exploiting others to fulfill their own desires. They often do not conceive of their behavior as being inappropriate or objectionable. Because they view themselves as "superior" beings, they believe they are entitled to special rights and privileges.

Although often grounded in grandiose distortions of reality, their mood is usually optimistic, relaxed, cheerful, and carefree. This mood can easily change, however, because of their fragile self-esteem. If they do not meet self-expectations, do not receive the positive feedback they expect from others, or draw criticism from others, they may respond with rage, shame, humiliation, or dejection. They may turn inward and fantasize rationalizations that convince them of their continued stature and perfection.

The exploitation of others for self-gratification results in impaired interpersonal relationships. In selecting a mate, narcissistic individuals frequently choose a person who will provide them with the praise and positive feedback that they require and who will not ask much from their partner in return.

The *DSM-5* diagnostic criteria for narcissistic personality disorder are presented in Box 32-5.

BOX 32-5 Diagnostic Criteria for Narcissistic Personality Disorder

A pervasive pattern of grandiosity (in fantasy or behavior), need for admiration, and lack of empathy, beginning by early adulthood and present in a variety of contexts, as indicated by five (or more) of the following:
1. Has a grandiose sense of self-importance (e.g., exaggerates achievements and talents, expects to be recognized as superior without commensurate achievements).
2. Is preoccupied with fantasies of unlimited success, power, brilliance, beauty, or ideal love.
3. Believes that he or she is "special" and unique and can only be understood by, or should associate with, other special or high-status people (or institutions).
4. Requires excessive admiration.
5. Has a sense of entitlement (i.e., unreasonable expectations of especially favorable treatment or automatic compliance with his or her expectations).
6. Is interpersonally exploitative (i.e., takes advantage of others to achieve his or her own ends).
7. Lacks empathy: is unwilling to recognize or identify with the feelings and needs of others.
8. Is often envious of others or believes that others are envious of him or her.
9. Shows arrogant, haughty behaviors or attitudes.

Predisposing Factors

Several psychodynamic theories exist regarding the predisposition to narcissistic personality disorder. Skodol and Gunderson (2008) suggest that, as children, these individuals had their fears, failures, or dependency needs responded to with criticism, disdain, or neglect. They grow up with contempt for these behaviors in themselves and others and are unable to view others as sources of comfort and support. They project an image of invulnerability and self-sufficiency that conceals their true sense of emptiness and contributes to their inability to feel deeply.

Martinez-Lewi (2008) suggests that the parents of individuals with narcissistic personality disorder were often narcissistic themselves. The parents were demanding, perfectionistic, and critical, and they placed unrealistic expectations on the child. Children model their parents' behavior, giving way to the adult narcissist. Some clinicians have suggested that the parents may have subjected the child to physical or emotional abuse or neglect.

Narcissism may also develop from an environment in which parents attempt to live their lives vicariously through their child. They expect the child to achieve the things they did not achieve, possess that which they did not possess, and have life better and easier than they did. The child is not subjected to the requirements and restrictions that may have dominated the parents' lives, and thereby grows up believing he or she is above that which is required for everyone else. Bosson and Prewitt-Freilino (2007) state:

> Some parents pamper and indulge their youngsters in ways that teach them that their every wish is a command, that they can receive without giving in return, and that they deserve prominence without even minimal effort. Consequently, these youngsters learn to associate the self with positive affect and develop extremely favorable implicit self-representations. [However, because] the world beyond home will not be so benign and accepting, in many cases of parental overindulgence, reality eventually intervenes—in the form of personal failures, humiliations,

weaknesses, and the like—and undermines the individual's explicit self-esteem. From this perspective, narcissists' tendencies toward entitlement and exploitativeness reflect the overblown implicit expectations their parents instilled in them, while their shame-proneness reflects their chronic perception of themselves as falling short of these expectations. (p. 414)

Avoidant Personality Disorder

Definition and Epidemiological Statistics

The individual with **avoidant personality disorder** is extremely sensitive to rejection and because of this may lead a very socially withdrawn life. It is not that he or she is asocial; in fact, there may be a strong desire for companionship. The extreme shyness and fear of rejection, however, create needs for unusually strong assurances of unconditional acceptance. Prevalence of the disorder in the general population is about 2.4 percent, and it appears to be equally common in men and women (APA, 2013).

Clinical Picture

Individuals with this disorder are awkward and uncomfortable in social situations. From a distance, others may perceive them as timid, withdrawn, or perhaps cold and strange. Those who have closer relationships with them, however, soon learn of their sensitivities, touchiness, evasiveness, and mistrustful qualities.

Their speech is usually slow and constrained, with frequent hesitations, fragmentary thought sequences, and occasional confused and irrelevant digressions. They are often lonely, and express feelings of being unwanted. They view others as critical, betraying, and humiliating. They desire to have close relationships but avoid them because of their fear of being rejected. Depression, anxiety, and anger at oneself for failing to develop social relations are commonly experienced.

The *DSM-5* diagnostic criteria for avoidant personality disorder are presented in Box 32-6.

BOX 32-6 Diagnostic Criteria for Avoidant Personality Disorder

A pervasive pattern of social inhibition, feelings of inadequacy, and hypersensitivity to negative evaluation, beginning by early adulthood and present in a variety of contexts, as indicated by four (or more) of the following:

1. Avoids occupational activities that involve significant interpersonal contact, because of fears of criticism, disapproval, or rejection.
2. Is unwilling to get involved with people unless certain of being liked.
3. Shows restraint within intimate relationships because of the fear of being shamed or ridiculed.
4. Is preoccupied with being criticized or rejected in social situations.
5. Is inhibited in new interpersonal situations because of feelings of inadequacy.
6. Views self as socially inept, personally unappealing, or inferior to others.
7. Is unusually reluctant to take personal risks or to engage in any new activities because they may prove embarrassing.

Reprinted with permission from the *Diagnostic and Statistical Manual of Mental Disorders, Fifth Edition* (Copyright 2013). American Psychiatric Association.

Predisposing Factors

There is no clear cause of avoidant personality disorder. Contributing factors are most likely a combination of biological, genetic, and psychosocial influences. Some infants who exhibit traits of hyperirritability, crankiness, tension, and withdrawal behaviors may possess a temperamental disposition toward an avoidant pattern.

The primary psychosocial predisposing influence to avoidant personality disorder is parental rejection and censure, which is often reinforced by peers (Millon, 2004). These children are often reared in families in which they are belittled, abandoned, and criticized, such that any natural optimism is extinguished and replaced with feelings of low self-worth and social alienation. They learn to be suspicious and to view the world as hostile and dangerous.

Dependent Personality Disorder

Definition and Epidemiological Statistics

Dependent personality disorder is characterized by "a pattern of relying excessively on others for emotional support" (Black & Andreasen, 2011, p. 312). This mode of behavior is evident in the tendency to allow others to make decisions, to feel helpless when alone, to act submissively, to subordinate needs to others, to tolerate mistreatment by others, to demean oneself to gain acceptance, and to fail to function adequately in situations that require assertive or dominant behavior.

The disorder is relatively common. Sadock and Sadock (2007) discuss the results of one study of personality disorders in which 2.5 percent of the sample were diagnosed with dependent personality disorder. It is more common in women than in men and more common in the youngest children of a family.

Clinical Picture

Individuals with dependent personality disorder have a notable lack of self-confidence that is often apparent in their posture, voice, and mannerisms. They are typically passive and acquiescent to the desires of others. They are overly generous and thoughtful and underplay their own attractiveness and achievements. They may appear to others to "see the world through rose-colored glasses," but when alone, they may feel pessimistic, discouraged, and dejected. Others are not made aware of these feelings; their "suffering" is done in silence.

Individuals with dependent personality disorder assume the passive and submissive role in relationships. They are willing to let others make their important decisions. Should the dependent relationship end, they feel fearful and vulnerable because they lack confidence in their ability to care for themselves. They may hastily and indiscriminately attempt to establish another relationship with someone they believe can provide them with the nurturance and guidance they need.

They avoid positions of responsibility and become anxious when forced into them. They have feelings of low self-worth and are easily hurt by criticism and disapproval. They will do almost anything, even if it is unpleasant or demeaning, to earn the acceptance of others.

The *DSM-5* diagnostic criteria for dependent personality disorder are presented in Box 32-7.

Predisposing Factors

An infant may be genetically predisposed to a dependent temperament. Twin studies measuring submissiveness have shown a higher correlation between identical twins than fraternal twins.

Psychosocially, dependency is fostered in infancy when stimulation and nurturance are experienced

---

BOX 32-7 Diagnostic Criteria for Dependent Personality Disorder

A pervasive and excessive need to be taken care of that leads to submissive and clinging behavior and fears of separation, beginning by early adulthood and present in a variety of contexts, as indicated by five (or more) of the following:

1. Has difficulty making everyday decisions without an excessive amount of advice and reassurance from others.
2. Needs others to assume responsibility for most major areas of his or her life.
3. Has difficulty expressing disagreement with others because of fear of loss of support or approval. (*Note*: Do not include realistic fears of retribution.)
4. Has difficulty initiating projects or doing things on his or her own (because of a lack of self-confidence in judgment or abilities rather than a lack of motivation or energy).
5. Goes to excessive lengths to obtain nurturance and support from others, to the point of volunteering to do things that are unpleasant.
6. Feels uncomfortable or helpless when alone because of exaggerated fears of being unable to care for himself or herself.
7. Urgently seeks another relationship as a source of care and support when a close relationship ends.
8. Is unrealistically preoccupied with fears of being left to take care of himself or herself.

exclusively from one source. The infant becomes attached to one source to the exclusion of all others. If this exclusive attachment continues as the child grows, the dependency is nurtured. A problem may arise when parents become overprotective and discourage independent behaviors on the part of the child. Parents who make new experiences unnecessarily easy for the child and refuse to allow him or her to learn by experience encourage their child to give up efforts at achieving autonomy. Dependent behaviors may be subtly rewarded in this environment, and the child may come to fear a loss of love or attachment from the parental figure if independent behaviors are attempted.

Obsessive-Compulsive Personality Disorder

Definition and Epidemiological Statistics

Individuals with **obsessive-compulsive personality disorder** are very serious and formal and have difficulty expressing emotions. They are overly disciplined, perfectionistic, and preoccupied with rules. They are inflexible about the way in which things must be done and have a devotion to productivity to the exclusion of personal pleasure. An intense fear of making mistakes leads to difficulty with decision-making. The disorder is relatively common and occurs more often in men than in women. Within the family constellation, it appears to be most common in oldest children.

Clinical Picture

Individuals with obsessive-compulsive personality disorder are inflexible and lack spontaneity. They are meticulous and work diligently and patiently at tasks that require accuracy and discipline. They are especially concerned with matters of organization and efficiency and tend to be rigid and unbending about rules and procedures.

Social behavior tends to be polite and formal. They are very "rank conscious," a characteristic that is reflected in their contrasting behaviors with "superiors" as opposed to "inferiors." They tend to be very solicitous to and ingratiating with authority figures. With subordinates, however, the compulsive person can become quite autocratic and condemnatory, often appearing pompous and self-righteous.

People with obsessive-compulsive personality disorder typify the "bureaucratic personality," the so-called company man. They see themselves as conscientious, loyal, dependable, and responsible, and are contemptuous of people whose behavior they consider frivolous and impulsive. Emotional behavior is considered immature and irresponsible.

Although on the surface these individuals appear to be calm and controlled, underneath this exterior lies a great deal of ambivalence, conflict, and hostility. Individuals with this disorder commonly use the defense mechanism of reaction formation. Not daring to expose their true feelings of defiance and anger, they withhold these feelings so strongly that the opposite feelings come forth. The defenses of isolation, intellectualization, rationalization, and undoing are also commonly evident.

The *DSM-5* diagnostic criteria for obsessive-compulsive personality disorder are presented in Box 32-8.

Predisposing Factors

In the psychoanalytical view, the parenting style in which the individual with obsessive-compulsive personality

---

BOX 32-8 Diagnostic Criteria for Obsessive-Compulsive Personality Disorder

A pervasive pattern of preoccupation with orderliness, perfectionism, and mental and interpersonal control, at the expense of flexibility, openness, and efficiency, beginning by early adulthood and present in a variety of contexts, as indicated by four (or more) of the following:

1. Is preoccupied with details, rules, lists, order, organization, or schedules to the extent that the major point of the activity is lost.
2. Shows perfectionism that interferes with task completion (e.g., is unable to complete a project because his or her own overly strict standards are not met).
3. Is excessively devoted to work and productivity to the exclusion of leisure activities and friendships (not accounted for by obvious economic necessity).
4. Is overconscientious, scrupulous, and inflexible about matters of morality, ethics, or values (not accounted for by cultural or religious identification).
5. Is unable to discard worn-out or worthless objects even when they have no sentimental value.
6. Is reluctant to delegate tasks or to work with others unless they submit to exactly his or her way of doing things.
7. Adopts a miserly spending style toward both self and others; money is viewed as something to be hoarded for future catastrophes.
8. Shows rigidity and stubbornness.

Reprinted with permission from the *Diagnostic and Statistical Manual of Mental Disorders, Fifth Edition* (Copyright 2013). American Psychiatric Association.

disorder was reared is one of overcontrol. These parents expect their children to live up to their imposed standards of conduct and condemn them if they do not. Praise for positive behaviors is bestowed on the child with much less frequency than punishment for undesirable behaviors. In this environment, individuals become experts in learning what they must *not* do to avoid punishment and condemnation rather than what they *can* do to achieve attention and praise. They learn to heed rigid restrictions and rules. Positive achievements are expected, taken for granted, and only occasionally acknowledged by their parents, whose comments and judgments are limited to pointing out transgressions and infractions of rules.

Application of the Nursing Process

Borderline Personality Disorder (Background Assessment Data)

Historically, there have been a group of clients who did not classically conform to the standard categories of neuroses or psychoses. The designation "borderline" was introduced to identify these clients who seemed to fall on the border between the two categories. Other terminology that has been used in an attempt to identify this disorder includes *ambulatory schizophrenia, pseudoneurotic schizophrenia,* and *emotionally unstable personality.* When the term *borderline* was first proposed for inclusion in the third edition of the *DSM,* some psychiatrists feared it might be used as a "wastebasket" diagnosis for difficult-to-treat clients. However, a specific set of criteria has been established for diagnosing what has been described as "a consistent and stable course of unstable behavior" (Box 32-9).

Clinical Picture

Individuals with borderline personality always seem to be in a state of crisis. Their affect is one of extreme intensity, and their behavior reflects frequent changeability. These changes can occur within days, hours, or even minutes. Often these individuals exhibit a single, dominant affective tone, such as depression, which may give way periodically to anxious agitation or inappropriate outbursts of anger.

Chronic Depression

Depression is so common in clients with this disorder that before the inclusion of borderline personality disorder in the *DSM,* many of these clients were diagnosed with depressive disorder. Depression occurs in response to feelings of abandonment by the mother in early childhood (see "Predisposing Factors"). Underlying the depression is a sense of rage that is sporadically turned inward on the self and externally on the environment. Seldom is the individual aware of the true source of these feelings until well into long-term therapy.

Inability to Be Alone

Because of this chronic fear of abandonment, clients with borderline personality disorder have little tolerance for being alone. They prefer a frantic search for companionship, no matter how unsatisfactory, to sitting with feelings of loneliness, emptiness, and boredom (Sadock & Sadock, 2007).

Patterns of Interaction

Clinging and Distancing

The client with borderline personality disorder commonly exhibits a pattern of interaction with others that is characterized by clinging and distancing behaviors.

BOX 32-9 Diagnostic Criteria for Borderline Personality Disorder

A pervasive pattern of instability of interpersonal relationships, self-image, and affects, and marked impulsivity beginning by early adulthood and present in a variety of contexts, as indicated by five (or more) of the following:

1. Frantic efforts to avoid real or imagined abandonment. (*Note:* Do not include suicidal or self-mutilating behavior covered in criterion 5.)
2. A pattern of unstable and intense interpersonal relationships characterized by alternating between extremes of idealization and devaluation.
3. Identity disturbance: markedly and persistently unstable self-image or sense of self.
4. Impulsivity in at least two areas that are potentially self-damaging (e.g., spending, sex, substance abuse, reckless driving, binge eating). (*Note:* Do not include suicidal or self-mutilating behavior covered in criterion 5.)
5. Recurrent suicidal behavior, gestures, or threats, or self-mutilating behavior.
6. Affective instability due to marked reactivity of mood (e.g., intense episodic dysphoria, irritability, or anxiety, usually lasting a few hours and only rarely more than a few days).
7. Chronic feelings of emptiness.
8. Inappropriate, intense anger or difficulty controlling anger (e.g., frequent displays of temper, constant anger, recurrent physical fights).
9. Transient, stress-related paranoid ideation or severe dissociative symptoms.

Reprinted with permission from the *Diagnostic and Statistical Manual of Mental Disorders, Fifth Edition* (Copyright 2013). American Psychiatric Association.

When clients are clinging to another individual, they may exhibit helpless, dependent, or even childlike behaviors. They overidealize a single individual with whom they want to spend all their time, with whom they express a frequent need to talk, or from whom they seek constant reassurance. Acting-out behaviors, even self-mutilation, may result when they cannot be with this chosen individual. Distancing behaviors are characterized by hostility, anger, and devaluation of others, arising from a feeling of discomfort with closeness. Distancing behaviors also occur in response to separations, confrontations, or attempts to limit certain behaviors. Devaluation of others is manifested by discrediting or undermining their strengths and personal significance.

Splitting

Splitting is a primitive ego defense mechanism that is common in people with borderline personality disorder. It arises from their lack of achievement of **object constancy** and is manifested by an inability to integrate and accept both positive and negative feelings. In their view, people—including themselves—and life situations are either all good or all bad. For example, if a caregiver is nurturing and supportive, he or she is lovingly idealized. Should the nurturing relationship be threatened in any way (e.g., the caregiver must move because of his or her job), suddenly the individual is devalued, and the idealized image changes from beneficent caregiver to one of hateful and cruel persecutor.

Manipulation

In their efforts to prevent the separation they so desperately fear, clients with this disorder become masters of manipulation. Virtually any behavior becomes an acceptable means of achieving the desired result: relief from separation anxiety. Playing one individual against another is a common ploy to allay these fears of abandonment.

Self-Destructive Behaviors

Repetitive, self-mutilative behaviors are classic manifestations of borderline personality disorder. Although these acts can be fatal, most commonly they are manipulative gestures designed to elicit a rescue response from significant others. Suicide attempts are quite common and often result from feelings of abandonment following separation from a significant other. The endeavor is commonly attempted, however, incorporating a measure of "safety" into the plan (e.g., swallowing pills in an area where the person will surely be discovered by others; or swallowing pills and making a phone call to report the deed to someone).

Other types of destructive behaviors include cutting, scratching, and burning. Various theories abound regarding why these individuals are able to inflict pain on themselves. One hypothesis suggests they may have higher levels of endorphins in their bodies than most people, thereby increasing their threshold for pain. Another theory relates to the individual's personal identity disturbance. It proposes that since many of the self-mutilating behaviors take place when the individual is in a state of depersonalization and derealization, he or she does not initially feel the pain. The mutilation continues until pain is felt in an attempt to counteract the feelings of unreality. Some clients with borderline personality disorder have reported that "to feel pain is better than to feel nothing." The pain validates their existence.

Impulsivity

Individuals with borderline personality disorder have poor impulse control based on primary process functioning. Impulsive behaviors associated with borderline personality disorder include substance abuse, gambling, promiscuity, reckless driving, and binging and purging. Many times these acting-out behaviors occur in response to real or perceived feelings of abandonment.

Predisposing Factors to Borderline Personality Disorder

Biological Influences

Biochemical Cummings and Mega (2003) have suggested a possible serotonergic defect in clients with borderline personality disorder. In positron emission tomography using α-[^{11}C] methyl-L-tryptophan (α-[^{11}C]MTrp), which reflects serotonergic synthesis capability, clients with borderline personality demonstrated significantly decreased α-[^{11}C]MTrp in medial frontal, superior temporal, and striatal regions of the brain. Cummings and Mega (2003) state:

> These functional imaging studies support a medial and orbitofrontal abnormality that may promote the impulsive aggression demonstrated by patients with the borderline personality disorder. (p. 230)

Genetic The decrease in serotonin also may have genetic implications for borderline personality disorder. Sadock and Sadock (2007) report that depression is common in the family backgrounds of clients with borderline personality disorder. They state:

> These patients have more relatives with mood disorders than do control groups, and persons with borderline personality disorder often have mood disorder as well. (p. 791)

Psychosocial Influences

Childhood Trauma Studies have shown that many individuals with borderline personality disorder were reared in families with chaotic environments. Lubit

(2011) states, "Risk factors [for borderline personality disorder] include family environments characterized by trauma, neglect, and/or separation; exposure to sexual and physical abuse; and serious parental psychopathology, such as substance abuse and antisocial personality disorder." Seventy percent of borderline personality disorder clients report a history of physical and/or sexual abuse (Gunderson, 2011). In some instances, this disorder has been likened to posttraumatic stress disorder in response to childhood trauma and abuse. Oldham and associates (2006) have stated:

> Even when full criteria for comorbid PTSD are not present, patients with borderline personality disorder may experience PTSD-like symptoms. For example, symptoms such as intrusion, avoidance, and hyperarousal may emerge during psychotherapy. Awareness of the trauma-related nature of these symptoms can facilitate both psychotherapeutic and pharmacological efforts in symptom relief. (p. 1267)

Developmental Factors

Theory of Object Relations According to Mahler's theory of object relations (Mahler et al., 1975), the infant passes through six phases from birth to 36 months, when a sense of separateness from the parenting figure is finally established. These phases include the following:

- **Phase 1 (Birth to 1 Month), Autistic Phase.** During this period, the baby spends most of his or her time in a half-waking, half-sleeping state. The main goal is fulfillment of needs for survival and comfort.
- **Phase 2 (1 to 5 Months), Symbiotic Phase.** At this time, there is a type of psychic fusion of mother and child. The child views the self as an extension of the parenting figure, although there is a developing awareness of external sources of need fulfillment.
- **Phase 3 (5 to 10 Months), Differentiation Phase.** The child is beginning to recognize that there is a separateness between the self and the parenting figure.
- **Phase 4 (10 to 16 Months), Practicing Phase.** This phase is characterized by increased locomotor functioning and the ability to explore the environment independently. A sense of separateness of the self is increased.
- **Phase 5 (16 to 24 Months), Rapprochement Phase.** Awareness of separateness of the self becomes acute. This is frightening to the child, who wants to regain some lost closeness but not return to symbiosis. The child wants the mother there as needed for "emotional refueling" and to maintain feelings of security.
- **Phase 6 (24 to 36 Months), On the Way to Object Constancy Phase.** In this phase, the child completes the individuation process and learns to relate to objects in an effective, constant manner. A sense of separateness is established, and the child is able to internalize a sustained image of the loved object or person when out of sight. Separation anxiety is resolved.

The individual with borderline personality disorder becomes fixed in the rapprochement phase of development. This occurs when the child shows increasing separation and autonomy. The mother, who feels secure in the relationship as long as the child is dependent, begins to feel threatened by the child's increasing independence. The mother may indeed be experiencing her own fears of abandonment. In response to separation behaviors, the mother withdraws the emotional support or "refueling" that is so vitally needed during this phase for the child to feel secure. Instead, the mother rewards clinging, dependent behaviors, and punishes (withholding emotional support) independent behaviors. With his or her sense of emotional survival at stake, the child learns to behave in a manner that satisfies the parental wishes. An internal conflict develops within the child, based on fear of abandonment. He or she wants to achieve independence common to this stage of development, but fears that mother will withdraw emotional support as a result. This unresolved fear of abandonment remains with the child into adulthood. Unresolved grief for the nurturing they failed to receive results in internalized rage that manifests itself in the depression so common in people with borderline personality disorder.

Diagnosis/Outcome Identification

Nursing diagnoses are formulated from the data gathered during the assessment phase and with background knowledge regarding predisposing factors to the disorder. Table 32-2 presents a list of client behaviors and the NANDA nursing diagnoses that correspond to these behaviors, which may be used in planning care for clients with borderline personality disorder.

Outcome Criteria

The following criteria may be used for measurement of outcomes in the care of clients with borderline personality disorder.

The client:

- Has not harmed self.
- Seeks out staff when desire for self-mutilation is strong.
- Is able to identify true source of anger.
- Expresses anger appropriately.
- Relates to more than one staff member.
- Completes activities of daily living independently.
- Does not manipulate one staff member against the other in order to fulfill own desires.

Planning/Implementation

The following section presents a group of selected nursing diagnoses common to clients with borderline

TABLE 32–2	Assigning Nursing Diagnoses to Behaviors Commonly Associated With Borderline Personality Disorder	
BEHAVIORS	**NURSING DIAGNOSES**
Risk factors: History of self-injurious behavior; history of inability to plan solutions; impulsivity; irresistible urge to damage self; feels threatened with loss of significant relationship	Risk for self-mutilation
Risk factors: History of suicide attempts; suicidal ideation; suicidal plan; impulsiveness; childhood abuse; fears of abandonment; internalized rage	Risk for self-directed violence; Risk for suicide
Risk factors: Body language (e.g., rigid posture, clenching of fists and jaw, hyperactivity, pacing, breathlessness, threatening stances); history of childhood abuse; impulsivity; transient psychotic symptomatology	Risk for other-directed violence
Depression; persistent emotional distress; rumination; separation distress; traumatic distress; verbalizes feeling empty; inappropriate expression of anger	Complicated grieving
Alternating clinging and distancing behaviors; staff splitting; manipulation	Impaired social interaction
Feelings of depersonalization and derealization	Disturbed personal identity
Transient psychotic symptoms (disorganized thinking; misinterpretation of the environment); increased tension; decreased perceptual field	Anxiety (severe to panic)
Dependent on others; excessively seeks reassurance; manipulation of others; inability to tolerate being alone	Chronic low self-esteem

personality disorder, with short- and long-term goals and nursing interventions for each.

Risk for Self-Mutilation/Risk for Self-Directed or Other-Directed Violence

Risk for self-mutilation is defined as "at risk for deliberate self-injurious behavior causing tissue damage with the intent of causing nonfatal injury to attain relief of tension" (NANDA International [NANDA-I], 2012, p. 451). *Risk for self-directed or other-directed violence* is defined as "at risk for behaviors in which an individual demonstrates that he or she can be physically, emotionally, and/or sexually harmful to self or others" (NANDA-I, 2012, pp. 447, 448).

Client Goals

Outcome criteria include short- and long-term goals. Timelines are individually determined.

Short-Term Goals

■ The client will seek out staff member if feelings of harming self or others emerge.
■ The client will not harm self or others.

Long-Term Goal

■ The client will not harm self or others.

Interventions

■ Observe the client's behavior frequently. Do this through routine activities and interactions; avoid appearing watchful and suspicious. Close observation is required so that intervention can occur if required to ensure client's (and others') safety.
■ Secure a verbal contract from the client that he or she will seek out a staff member when the urge for self-mutilation is experienced. Discussing feelings of self-harm with a trusted individual provides some relief to the client. A contract gets the subject out in the open and places some of the responsibility for his or her safety with the client. An attitude of acceptance of the client as a worthwhile individual is conveyed.

■ If self-mutilation occurs, care for the client's wounds in a matter-of-fact manner. Do not give positive reinforcement to this behavior by offering sympathy or additional attention. Lack of attention to the maladaptive behavior may decrease repetition of its use.
■ Encourage the client to talk about feelings he or she was having just before this behavior occurred. To problem-solve the situation with the client, knowledge of the precipitating factors is important.
■ Act as a role model for the appropriate expression of angry feelings, and give positive reinforcement to the client when attempts to conform are made. It is vital that the client expresses angry feelings because suicide and other self-destructive behaviors are often viewed as a result of anger turned inward on the self.
■ Remove all dangerous objects from the client's environment so that he or she may not purposefully or inadvertently use them to inflict harm to self or others.
■ Try to redirect violent behavior with physical outlets for the client's anxiety (e.g., punching bag, jogging). Physical exercise is a safe and effective way of relieving pent-up tension.

■ Have sufficient staff available to indicate a show of strength to the client if it becomes necessary. This conveys to the client evidence of control over the situation and provides some physical security for staff.

■ Administer tranquilizing medications as ordered by the physician or obtain an order if necessary. Monitor the client for effectiveness of the medication and for the appearance of adverse side effects. Tranquilizing medications such as anxiolytics or antipsychotics may have a calming effect on the client and may prevent aggressive behaviors.

■ If client is not calmed by "talking down" or by medication, use of mechanical restraints may be necessary. The avenue of the "least restrictive alternative" must be selected when planning interventions for a violent client. Restraints should be used only as a last resort, after all other interventions have been unsuccessful, and the client is clearly at risk of harm to self or others.

■ If restraint is deemed necessary, ensure that sufficient staff is available to assist. Follow protocol established by the institution. The Joint Commission requires that an in-person evaluation by a physician or other licensed independent practitioner (LIP) be conducted within 1 hour of the initiation of the restraint or seclusion (The Joint Commission, 2010). The physician or LIP must reissue a new order for restraints every 4 hours for adults and every 1 to 2 hours for children and adolescents.

■ The Joint Commission requires that the client in restraints be observed at least every 15 minutes to ensure that circulation to extremities is not compromised (check temperature, color, pulses); to assist the client with needs related to nutrition, hydration, and elimination; and to position the client so that comfort is facilitated and aspiration is prevented. Some institutions may require continuous one-to-one monitoring of restrained clients, particularly those who are highly agitated, and for whom there is a high risk of self- or accidental injury.

■ As agitation decreases, assess the client's readiness for restraint removal or reduction. Remove one restraint at a time while assessing the client's response. This minimizes the risk of injury to client and staff.

■ If warranted by high acuity of the situation, staff may need to be assigned on a one-to-one basis. Because of their extreme fear of abandonment, clients with borderline personality disorder should not be left alone at a stressful time as it may cause an acute rise in anxiety and agitation levels.

Complicated Grieving

Complicated grieving is defined as "a disorder that occurs after the death of a significant other [or any other loss of significance to the individual], in which the experience of distress accompanying bereavement fails to follow normative expectations and manifests in functional impairment" (NANDA-I, 2012, p. 365). Table 32-3 presents this nursing diagnosis in care plan format.

Table 32-3 | CARE PLAN FOR THE CLIENT WITH BORDERLINE PERSONALITY DISORDER

NURSING DIAGNOSIS: COMPLICATED GRIEVING

RELATED TO: Maternal deprivation during rapprochement phase of development (internalized as a loss, with fixation in anger stage of grieving process); possible childhood physical or sexual abuse

EVIDENCED BY: Depressed mood, acting-out behaviors

OUTCOME CRITERIA	NURSING INTERVENTIONS	RATIONALE
Short-Term Goal • Within 5 days, the client will discuss with nurse or therapist maladaptive patterns of expressing anger. **Long-Term Goal** • By time of discharge from treatment, the client will be able to identify the true source of angry feelings,	1. Convey an accepting attitude—one that creates a nonthreatening environment for the client to express feelings. Be honest and keep all promises. 2. Identify the function that anger, frustration, and rage serve for the client. Allow him or her to express these feelings within reason. 3. Encourage client to discharge pent-up anger through participation in large motor activities (e.g., brisk walks, jogging,	1. An accepting attitude conveys to the client that you believe he or she is a worthwhile person. Trust is enhanced. 2. Verbalization of feelings in a nonthreatening environment may help client come to terms with unresolved issues. 3. Physical exercise provides a safe and effective method for discharging pent-up tension.

Table 32-3	CARE PLAN FOR THE CLIENT WITH BORDERLINE PERSONALITY DISORDER—cont'd		
OUTCOME CRITERIA	**NURSING INTERVENTIONS**	**RATIONALE**
accept ownership of these feelings, and express them in a socially acceptable manner, in an effort to satisfactorily progress through the grieving process.	physical exercises, volleyball, punching bag, exercise bike).	
	4. Explore with client the true source of the anger. This is a painful therapy that often leads to regression as the client deals with the feelings of early abandonment or issues of abuse.	4. Reconciliation of the feelings associated with this stage is necessary before progression through the grieving process can continue.
	5. As anger is displaced onto the nurse or therapist, caution must be taken to guard against the negative effects of countertransference. These are very difficult clients who have the capacity for eliciting a whole array of negative feelings from the therapist.	5. The existence of negative feelings by the nurse or therapist must be acknowledged, but they must not be allowed to interfere with the therapeutic process.
	6. Explain the behaviors associated with the normal grieving process. Help the client recognize his or her position in this process.	6. Knowledge of the acceptability of the feelings associated with normal grieving may help to relieve some of the guilt that these responses generate.
	7. Help the client understand appropriate ways to express anger. Give positive reinforcement for behaviors used to express anger appropriately. Act as a role model. It is important to let the client know when he or she has done something that has generated angry feelings in you.	7. Positive reinforcement enhances self-esteem and encourages repetition of desirable behaviors. Role modeling ways to express anger in an appropriate manner is a powerful learning tool.
	8. Set limits on acting-out behaviors and explain consequences of violation of those limits. Be supportive, yet consistent and firm in caring for this client.	8. Client lacks sufficient self-control to limit maladaptive behaviors, so assistance is required. Without consistency on the part of all staff members working with this client, a positive outcome will not be achieved.

Client Goals

Outcome criteria include short- and long-term goals. Timelines are individually determined.

Short-Term Goal

■ Within 5 days, the client will discuss with nurse or therapist maladaptive patterns of expressing anger.

Long-Term Goal

■ By the time of discharge from treatment, the client will be able to identify the true source of angry feelings, accept ownership of these feelings, and express them in a socially acceptable manner, in an effort to satisfactorily progress through the grieving process.

Interventions

■ Convey an accepting attitude—one that creates a nonthreatening environment for the client to express feelings. Be honest and keep all promises. An accepting attitude conveys to the client that you believe he or she is a worthwhile person. Trust is enhanced.

■ Identify the function that anger, frustration, and rage serve for the client. Allow him or her to express these feelings within reason. Verbalization of feelings in a nonthreatening environment may help the client come to terms with unresolved issues.

■ Encourage the client to discharge pent-up anger through participation in large motor activities (e.g., brisk walks, jogging, physical exercises, volleyball, punching bag, exercise bike). Physical exercise provides a safe and effective method for discharging pent-up tension.

■ Explore with the client the true source of anger. This is painful therapy that often leads to regression as the client deals with feelings of early abandonment or abuse. It seems that sometimes the client must "get worse before he or she can get better." Reconciliation of the feelings associated with this stage is necessary before progression through the grieving process can continue.

■ As anger is displaced onto the nurse or therapist, caution must be taken to guard against the negative effects of countertransference (see Chapter 7). These are very difficult clients who have the capacity for eliciting a whole array of negative feelings from the therapist. The existence of negative feelings by the nurse or therapist must be acknowledged, but they must not be allowed to interfere with the therapeutic process.

■ Explain the behaviors associated with the normal grieving process. Help the client recognize his or her position in this process. Knowledge of the acceptability of the feelings associated with normal grieving may help to relieve some of the guilt that these responses generate.

■ Help the client understand appropriate ways of expressing anger. Give positive reinforcement for behaviors used to express anger appropriately. Act as a role model. It is appropriate to let the client know when he or she has done something that has generated angry feelings in you. Role modeling ways to express anger in an appropriate manner is a powerful learning tool.

■ Set limits on acting-out behaviors and explain the consequences of violation of those limits. Be supportive, yet consistent and firm, in caring for this client. The client lacks sufficient self-control to limit maladaptive behaviors, so assistance is required. Without consistency on the part of all staff members working with this client, a positive outcome will not be achieved.

Impaired Social Interaction

Impaired social interaction is defined as "insufficient or excessive quantity or ineffective quality of social exchange" (NANDA-I, 2012, p. 320).

Client Goals

Outcome criteria include short- and long-term goals. Timelines are individually determined.

Short-Term Goal

■ Within 5 days, client will discuss with nurse or therapist behaviors that impede the development of satisfactory interpersonal relationships.

Long-Term Goal

■ By the time of discharge from treatment, client will interact appropriately with others in the therapy setting in both social and therapeutic activities (evidencing a discontinuation of splitting and clinging and distancing behaviors).

Interventions

■ Encourage the client to examine these behaviors (to recognize that they are occurring). He or she may be unaware of splitting or of clinging and distancing pattern of interaction with others. Recognition must take place before change can occur.

■ Help the client understand that you will be available, without reinforcing dependent behaviors. Knowledge of your availability may provide needed security.

■ Rotate staff members who work with the client in order to avoid his or her developing a dependence on particular individuals. The client must learn to relate to more than one staff member in an effort to decrease the use of splitting and to diminish fears of abandonment.

■ With the client, explore feelings that relate to fears of abandonment and engulfment. Help him or her to understand that clinging and distancing behaviors are engendered by these fears. Exploration of feelings with a trusted individual may help the client come to terms with unresolved issues.

■ Help the client understand how these behaviors interfere with satisfactory relationships. He or she may be unaware of how others perceive these behaviors and why they are not acceptable.

■ Assist the client to work toward achievement of object constancy. Be available, without promoting dependency. Give positive reinforcement for independent behaviors. The client must resolve fears of abandonment in the process toward developing the ability to establish satisfactory intimate relationships.

> **CLINICAL PEARL** Recognize when the client is playing one staff member against another. Remember that splitting is the primary defense mechanism of these individuals, and the impressions they have of others as either "good" or "bad" are a manifestation of this defense. Do not listen as the client tries to degrade other staff members. Suggest that the client discuss the problem directly with the staff person involved.

Concept Care Mapping

The concept map care plan is an innovative approach to planning and organizing nursing care (see Chapter 9). It is a diagrammatic teaching and learning strategy that allows visualization of interrelationships between medical diagnoses, nursing diagnoses, assessment data, and treatments. An example of a concept map care plan for a client with borderline personality disorder is presented in Figure 32-1.

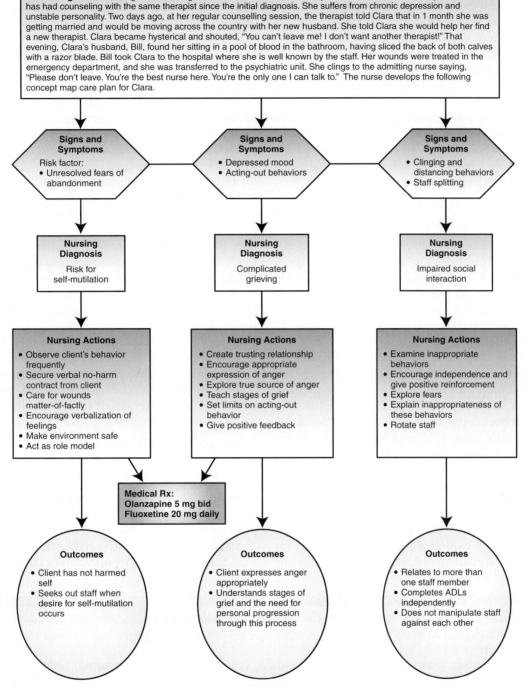

Clinical Vignette: Clara, age 37, was diagnosed with Borderline Personality Disorder when she was 22 years old. She has had counseling with the same therapist since the initial diagnosis. She suffers from chronic depression and unstable personality. Two days ago, at her regular counselling session, the therapist told Clara that in 1 month she was getting married and would be moving across the country with her new husband. She told Clara she would help her find a new therapist. Clara became hysterical and shouted, "You can't leave me! I don't want another therapist!" That evening, Clara's husband, Bill, found her sitting in a pool of blood in the bathroom, having sliced the back of both calves with a razor blade. Bill took Clara to the hospital where she is well known by the staff. Her wounds were treated in the emergency department, and she was transferred to the psychiatric unit. She clings to the admitting nurse saying, "Please don't leave. You're the best nurse here. You're the only one I can talk to." The nurse develops the following concept map care plan for Clara.

Signs and Symptoms

Risk factor:
• Unresolved fears of abandonment

Signs and Symptoms

• Depressed mood
• Acting-out behaviors

Signs and Symptoms

• Clinging and distancing behaviors
• Staff splitting

Nursing Diagnosis

Risk for self-mutilation

Nursing Diagnosis

Complicated grieving

Nursing Diagnosis

Impaired social interaction

Nursing Actions

• Observe client's behavior frequently
• Secure verbal no-harm contract from client
• Care for wounds matter-of-factly
• Encourage verbalization of feelings
• Make environment safe
• Act as role model

Nursing Actions

• Create trusting relationship
• Encourage appropriate expression of anger
• Explore true source of anger
• Teach stages of grief
• Set limits on acting-out behavior
• Give positive feedback

Nursing Actions

• Examine inappropriate behaviors
• Encourage independence and give positive reinforcement
• Explore fears
• Explain inappropriateness of these behaviors
• Rotate staff

Medical Rx:
Olanzapine 5 mg bid
Fluoxetine 20 mg daily

Outcomes

• Client has not harmed self
• Seeks out staff when desire for self-mutilation occurs

Outcomes

• Client expresses anger appropriately
• Understands stages of grief and the need for personal progression through this process

Outcomes

• Relates to more than one staff member
• Completes ADLs independently
• Does not manipulate staff against each other

FIGURE 32–1 Concept map care plan for a client with borderline personality disorder.

Evaluation

Reassessment is conducted to determine if the nursing actions have been successful in achieving the objectives of care. Evaluation of the nursing actions for the client with borderline personality disorder may be facilitated by gathering information using the following types of questions:

■ Has the client been able to seek out staff when feeling the desire for self-harm?

■ Has the client avoided self-harm?
■ Can the client correlate times of desire for self-harm to times of elevation in level of anxiety?
■ Can the client discuss feelings with staff (particularly feelings of depression and anger)?
■ Can the client identify the true source toward which the anger is directed?
■ Can the client verbalize understanding of the basis for his or her anger?

- Can the client express anger appropriately?
- Can the client function independently?
- Can the client relate to more than one staff member?
- Can the client verbalize the knowledge that the staff members will return and are not abandoning the client when leaving for the day?
- Can the client separate from the staff in an appropriate manner?
- Can the client delay gratification and refrain from manipulating others in order to fulfill own desires?
- Can the client verbalize resources within the community from whom he or she may seek assistance in times of extreme stress?

Antisocial Personality Disorder (Background Assessment Data)

In the *DSM-I*, antisocial behavior was categorized as a "sociopathic or psychopathic" reaction that was symptomatic of any of several underlying personality disorders. The *DSM-II* represented it as a separate personality type, a distinction that has been retained in subsequent editions. The *DSM-5* diagnostic criteria for antisocial personality disorder are presented in Box 32-10.

Individuals with antisocial personality disorder are seldom seen in most clinical settings, and when they are, it is commonly a way to avoid legal consequences. Sometimes they are admitted to the health-care system by court order for psychological evaluation. Most frequently, however, these individuals may be encountered in prisons, jails, and rehabilitation services.

Clinical Picture

Antisocial personality disorder is a pattern of socially irresponsible, exploitative, and guiltless behavior that reflects a general disregard for the rights of others. These individuals exploit and manipulate others for personal gain and are unconcerned with obeying the law. They have difficulty sustaining consistent employment and in developing stable relationships. They appear cold and callous, often intimidating others with their brusque and belligerent manner. They tend to be argumentative and, at times, cruel and malicious. They lack warmth and compassion and are often suspicious of these qualities in others.

Individuals with antisocial personality have a very low tolerance for frustration, act impetuously, and are unable to delay gratification. They are restless and easily bored, often taking chances and seeking thrills, as if they were immune to danger.

When things go their way, individuals with this disorder act cheerful, even gracious and charming. Because of their low tolerance for frustration, this pleasant exterior can change very quickly. When what they desire at the moment is challenged, they are likely to become furious and vindictive. Easily provoked to attack, their first inclination is to demean and dominate. They believe that "good guys come in last," and show contempt for the weak and underprivileged. They exploit others to fulfill their own desires, showing no trace of shame or guilt for their behavior.

Individuals with antisocial personalities see themselves as victims, using projection as the primary ego defense mechanism. They do not accept responsibility for the consequences of their behavior. Gorman and Sultan (2008) state:

> Manipulative individuals have come to suspect that any person or institution may try to control them, rendering them powerless and vulnerable to attack. (p. 195)

In their own minds, this perception justifies their malicious behavior, lest they be the recipient of unjust persecution and hostility from others.

Satisfying interpersonal relationships are not possible because individuals with antisocial personalities

---

BOX 32-10 Diagnostic Criteria for Antisocial Personality Disorder

A. A pervasive pattern of disregard for and violation of the rights of others occurring since age 15 years, as indicated by three (or more) of the following:
  1. Failure to conform to social norms with respect to lawful behaviors as indicated by repeatedly performing acts that are grounds for arrest.
  2. Deceitfulness, as indicated by repeated lying, use of aliases, or conning others for personal profit or pleasure.
  3. Impulsivity or failure to plan ahead.
  4. Irritability and aggressiveness, as indicated by repeated physical fights or assaults.
  5. Reckless disregard for safety of self or others.
  6. Consistent irresponsibility, as indicated by repeated failure to sustain consistent work behavior or honor financial obligations.
  7. Lack of remorse, as indicated by being indifferent to or rationalizing having hurt, mistreated, or stolen from another.
B. Individual is at least 18 years.
C. There is evidence of conduct disorder with onset before age 15 years.
D. The occurrence of antisocial behavior is not exclusively during the course of schizophrenia or bipolar disorder.

have learned to place their trust only in themselves. They have a philosophy that "it's every man for himself," and that one should stop at nothing to avoid being manipulated by others.

One of the most distinctive characteristics of individuals with antisocial personality is their tendency to ignore conventional authority and rules. They act as though established social norms and guidelines for self-discipline and cooperative behavior do not apply to them. They are flagrant in their disrespect for the law and for the rights of others.

Predisposing Factors to Antisocial Personality Disorder

Biological Influences

Antisocial personality is more common among first-degree biological relatives of those with the disorder than among the general population (Tharp, 2009). Twin and adoptive studies have implicated the role of genetics in antisocial personality disorder (Skodol & Gunderson, 2008). These studies of families of individuals with the disorder show higher numbers of relatives with antisocial personality or alcoholism than are found in the general population. The studies have also shown that children of parents with antisocial behavior are more likely to be diagnosed with antisocial personality, even when they are separated at birth from their biological parents and reared by individuals without the disorder.

Characteristics associated with temperament in the newborn may be significant in the predisposition to antisocial personality disorder. Parents who bring their children with behavior disorders to clinics often report that the child displayed temper tantrums from infancy and would become furious when awaiting a bottle or a diaper change. As these children mature, they commonly develop a bullying attitude toward other children. Parents report that they are undaunted by punishment and generally quite unmanageable. They

are daring and foolhardy in their willingness to chance physical harm, and they seem unaffected by pain.

Fischer, Barkley, Smallish, and Fletcher (2002) identified attention-deficit/hyperactivity disorder and conduct disorder during childhood and adolescence as predisposing factors to antisocial personality disorder.

Although these biogenetic influences may describe some familial pattern to the development of antisocial personality disorder, no basic pathological process has yet been determined as an etiological factor. Bienenfeld (2013) states:

> Low levels of behavioral inhibition may be mediated by serotonergic dysregulation in the septohippocampal system. There may also be developmental or acquired abnormalities in the prefrontal brain systems and reduced autonomic activity in antisocial personality disorder. This may underlie the low arousal, poor fear conditioning, and decision-making deficits described in antisocial personality disorder.

Family Dynamics

Antisocial personality disorder frequently arises from a chaotic home environment. Parental deprivation during the first 5 years of life appears to be a critical predisposing factor in the development of antisocial personality disorder. Separation due to parental delinquency appears to be more highly correlated with the disorder than is parental loss from other causes. The presence or intermittent appearance of inconsistent impulsive parents, not the loss of a consistent parent, is environmentally *most* damaging.

Studies have shown that individuals with antisocial personality disorder often have been severely physically abused in childhood. The abuse contributes to the development of antisocial behavior in several ways. First, it provides a model for behavior. Second, it may result in injury to the child's central nervous system, thereby

---

IMPLICATIONS OF RESEARCH FOR EVIDENCE-BASED PRACTICE

Dekovic, M., Janssens, J.A.M., & Van As, N.M.C. (2003). Family predictors of antisocial behavior in adolescence. *Family Process, 42*(2), 223-235.

DESCRIPTION OF THE STUDY: The objective of this study was to examine the combined and unique ability of different aspects of family functioning to predict involvement in antisocial behavior in a large community (nonclinical) sample of adolescents. The aspects of family functioning that were measured included:

1. *Proximal factors*: parental child-rearing behaviors and the quality of the parent-adolescent relationship.

2. *Distal factors:* parental characteristics (e.g., depression; parental confidence in his or her competence as a parent)

3. *Contextual factors:* family characteristics (e.g., family cohesion, quality of the marital relationship; involvement between members)

4. *Global factors:* family socioeconomic status; family composition (e.g., single-parent family)

The researchers hypothesized that proximal factors would play a stronger role in future antisocial behavior than the

Continued

IMPLICATIONS OF RESEARCH FOR EVIDENCE-BASED PRACTICE—cont'd

other three variables. The sample included 508 families with an adolescent between 12 and 18 years. There were 254 females and 254 males. The parent sample consisted of 969 parents (502 mothers and 467 fathers). Ninety-one percent of the families were intact families, 7 percent of the parents were divorced or separated, and 2 percent were widowed. There was a wide range of socioeconomic and educational backgrounds, although the parents with low educational and occupational levels were slightly underrepresented. Data were gathered in the subjects' homes through a battery of questionnaires administered individually to adolescents, mothers, and fathers.

RESULTS OF THE STUDY: Results showed that proximal factors were significant predictors of antisocial behavior, independent of their shared variance with other factors. Also consistent with the hypothesized model, the effects of distal and contextual factors appear to be mostly indirect: after their association with proximal factors was taken into account, these factors were no longer significantly related to antisocial behavior. Global indicators of family functioning (socioeconomic status and family composition) were unrelated to adolescent antisocial behavior. This study showed that supportive parents, parents who use more subtle

means of guidance (i.e., supervision rather than punitive strategies), and parents who are consistent in their behavior toward adolescents, have a lower risk that their child would become involved in antisocial behavior. Adolescents who are exposed to coercive and hostile parenting probably adopt this aggressive style of interacting with others. The parent-adolescent relationship that was characterized by elevated levels of conflict and a lack of closeness and acceptance emerged as a risk factor for involvement in antisocial behavior. Parental depression, conflict in the marital dyad, and lack of cohesion between members were also found to influence adolescent antisocial behavior, but less directly than the proximal factors.

IMPLICATIONS FOR NURSING PRACTICE: Nurses may use this information to design and implement effective parenting programs. Nurses can become actively involved in teaching parents, in inpatient, outpatient, and community education programs. The researchers state, "The findings of this study suggest that, when designing interventions that focus on family factors, in addition to teaching parents adequate child-rearing skills, more attention should be given to finding methods to improve the general *quality* of the parent-adolescent relationship."

impairing the child's ability to function appropriately. Finally, it engenders rage in the victimized child, which is then displaced onto others in the environment.

A number of factors associated with disordered family functioning have been implicated in the development of antisocial personality (Hill, 2003; Ramsland, 2013; Skodol & Gunderson, 2008). The following circumstances may influence the predisposition to antisocial personality disorder:

■ Absence of parental discipline
■ Extreme poverty
■ Removal from the home
■ Growing up without parental figures of both genders
■ Erratic and inconsistent methods of discipline
■ Being "rescued" each time they are in trouble (never having to suffer the consequences of one's own behavior)
■ Maternal deprivation

Diagnosis/Outcome Identification

Nursing diagnoses are formulated from the data gathered during the assessment phase and with background knowledge regarding predisposing factors to the disorder. Table 32-4 presents a list of client behaviors and the NANDA nursing diagnoses that correspond to those behaviors, which may be used in planning care for clients with antisocial personality disorder.

Outcome Criteria

The following criteria may be used for measurement of outcomes in the care of the client with antisocial personality disorder.

The client:

■ Discusses angry feelings with staff and in group sessions.
■ Has not harmed self or others.
■ Can rechannel hostility into socially acceptable behaviors.
■ Follows rules and regulations of the therapy environment.
■ Can verbalize which of his or her behaviors are not acceptable.
■ Shows regard for the rights of others by delaying gratification of own desires when appropriate.
■ Does not manipulate others in an attempt to increase feelings of self-worth.
■ Verbalizes understanding of knowledge required to maintain basic health needs.

Planning/Implementation

The following section presents a group of selected nursing diagnoses common to clients with antisocial personality disorder, with short- and long-term goals and nursing interventions for each.

TABLE 32–4 Assigning Nursing Diagnoses to Behaviors Commonly Associated With Antisocial Personality Disorder

BEHAVIORS	NURSING DIAGNOSES
Risk factors: Body language (e.g., rigid posture, clenching of fists and jaw, hyperactivity, pacing, breathlessness, threatening stances); cruelty to animals; rage reactions; history of childhood abuse; history of violence against others; impulsivity; substance abuse; negative role-modeling; inability to tolerate frustration	Risk for other-directed violence
Disregard for societal norms and laws; absence of guilty feelings; inability to delay gratification; denial of obvious problems; grandiosity; hostile laughter; projection of blame and responsibility; ridicule of others; superior attitude toward others	Defensive coping
Manipulation of others to fulfill own desires; inability to form close, personal relationships; frequent lack of success in life events; passive-aggressiveness; overt aggressiveness (hiding feelings of low self-esteem)	Chronic low self-esteem
Inability to form a satisfactory, enduring, intimate relationship with another; dysfunctional interaction with others; use of unsuccessful social interaction behaviors	Impaired social interaction
Demonstration of inability to take responsibility for meeting basic health practices; history of lack of health-seeking behavior; demonstrated lack of knowledge regarding basic health practices; lack of expressed interest in improving health behaviors	Ineffective health maintenance

Risk for Other-Directed Violence

Risk for other-directed violence is defined as "at risk for behaviors in which an individual demonstrates that he or she can be physically, emotionally, and/or sexually harmful to others" (NANDA-I, 2012, p. 447).

Client Goals

Outcome criteria include short- and long-term goals. Timelines are individually determined.

Short-Term Goals

■ Within 3 days, client will discuss angry feelings and situations that precipitate hostility.
■ Client will not harm others.

Long-Term Goal

■ Client will not harm others.

Interventions

■ Convey an accepting attitude toward this client. Feelings of rejection are undoubtedly familiar to him or her. Work on development of trust. Be honest, keep all promises, and convey the message to the client that it is not *him* or *her*, but the *behavior* that is unacceptable. An attitude of acceptance promotes feelings of self-worth. Trust is the basis of a therapeutic relationship.
■ Maintain a low level of stimuli in the client's environment (low lighting, few people, simple decor, low noise level). A stimulating environment may increase agitation and promote aggressive behavior.
■ Observe the client's behavior frequently. Do this through routine activities and interactions; avoid appearing watchful and suspicious. Close observation is required so that intervention can occur

if needed to ensure the client's (and others') safety.
■ Remove all dangerous objects from the client's environment so that he or she may not purposefully or inadvertently use them to inflict harm to self or others.
■ Help the client identify the true object of his or her hostility (e.g., "You seem to be upset with . . ."). Because of weak ego development, the client may be misusing the defense mechanism of displacement. Helping him or her recognize this in a nonthreatening manner may help reveal unresolved issues so that they may be confronted.
■ Encourage the client to gradually verbalize hostile feelings. Verbalization of feelings in a nonthreatening environment may help client come to terms with unresolved issues.
■ Explore with the client alternative ways of handling frustration (e.g., large motor skills that channel hostile energy into socially acceptable behavior). Physically demanding activities help to relieve pent-up tension.
■ The staff should maintain and convey a calm attitude toward the client. Anxiety is contagious and can be transferred from staff to client. A calm attitude provides the client with a feeling of safety and security.
■ Have sufficient staff available to present a show of strength to the client if necessary. This conveys to the client evidence of control over the situation and provides some physical security for the staff.
■ Administer tranquilizing medications as ordered by the physician or obtain an order if necessary. Monitor

the client for effectiveness of the medication as well as for appearance of adverse side effects. Antianxiety agents (e.g., lorazepam, chlordiazepoxide, oxazepam) produce a calming effect and may help to allay hostile behaviors. (**NOTE:** Medications are not often prescribed for clients with antisocial personality disorder because of these individuals' strong susceptibility to addictions.)

■ If client is not calmed by "talking down" or by medication, use of mechanical restraints may be necessary. The avenue of the "least restrictive alternative" must be selected when planning interventions for a violent client. Restraints should be used only as a last resort, after all other interventions have been unsuccessful, and the client is clearly at risk of harm to self or others.

■ If restraint is deemed necessary, ensure that sufficient staff is available to assist. Follow protocol established by the institution. The Joint Commission requires that an in-person evaluation by a physician or other licensed independent practitioner (LIP) be conducted within 1 hour of the initiation of the restraint or seclusion (The Joint Commission, 2010). The physician or LIP must reissue a new order for restraints every 4 hours for adults and every 1 to 2 hours for children and adolescents.

■ The Joint Commission requires that the client in restraints be observed at least every 15 minutes to ensure that circulation to extremities is not compromised (check temperature, color, pulses); to assist the client with needs related to nutrition, hydration, and elimination; and to position the client so that comfort is facilitated and aspiration is prevented. Some institutions may require continuous one-to-one monitoring of restrained clients, particularly those who are highly agitated, and for whom there is a high risk of self- or accidental injury.

■ As agitation decreases, assess the client's readiness for restraint removal or reduction. Remove one restraint at a time while assessing the client's response. This minimizes the risk of injury to client and staff.

Defensive Coping

Defensive coping is defined as "repeated projection of falsely positive self-evaluation based on a self-protective pattern that defends against underlying perceived threats to positive self-regard" (NANDA-I, 2012, p. 346).

Client Goals

Outcome criteria include short- and long-term goals. Timelines are individually determined.

Short-Term Goals

■ Within 24 hours after admission, client will verbalize understanding of treatment setting rules and regulations and the consequences for violation of them.

■ Client will verbalize personal responsibility for difficulties experienced in interpersonal relationships within (time period reasonable for client).

Long-Term Goals

■ By the time of discharge from treatment, the client will be able to cope more adaptively by delaying gratification of own desires and following rules and regulations of the treatment setting.

■ By the time of discharge from treatment, the client will demonstrate ability to interact with others without becoming defensive, rationalizing behaviors, or expressing grandiose ideas.

Interventions

■ From the onset, the client should be made aware of which behaviors are acceptable and which are not. Explain consequences of violation of the limits. A consequence must involve something of value to the client. All staff must be consistent in enforcing these limits. Consequences should be administered in a matter-of-fact manner immediately following the infraction. Because the client cannot (or will not) impose own limits on maladaptive behaviors, these behaviors must be delineated and enforced by staff. Undesirable consequences may help to decrease repetition of these behaviors.

■ The ideal goal would be for this client to eventually internalize societal norms, beginning with a step-by-step, "either/or" approach on the unit (*either* you do [don't do] this, *or* this will occur). Explanations must be concise, concrete, and clear, with little or no capacity for misinterpretation.

CLINICAL PEARL 💬

Do not attempt to coax or convince the client to do the "right thing." Do not use the words "You should (or shouldn't) . . ."; instead, use the words "You will be expected to . . ."

■ Provide positive feedback or reward for acceptable behaviors. Positive reinforcement enhances self-esteem and encourages repetition of desirable behaviors.

■ In an attempt to assist the client to delay gratification, begin to increase the length of time requirement for acceptable behavior in order to achieve the reward. For example, 2 hours of acceptable behavior may be exchanged for a phone call; 4 hours of acceptable behavior for 2 hours of television; 1 day of acceptable behavior for a recreational therapy bowling activity; 5 days of acceptable behavior for a weekend pass.

■ A milieu unit provides the appropriate environment for the client with antisocial personality. The democratic approach, with specific rules and regulations, community meetings, and group therapy sessions emulates the type of societal situation in which the client must learn to live. Feedback from peers is often more effective than confrontation from an authority figure. The client learns to follow the rules of the group as a positive step in the progression toward internalizing the rules of society.

■ Help the client to gain insight into his or her own behavior. Often, these individuals rationalize to such an extent that they deny that their behavior is inappropriate. For example, thinking may be reflected in statements such as: "The owner of this store has so much money, he'll never miss the little bit I take. He has everything, and I have nothing. It's not fair! I deserve to have some of what he has." The client must come to understand that certain behaviors will not be tolerated within the society and that severe consequences will be imposed on those individuals who refuse to comply. The client must *want* to become a productive member of society before he or she can be helped.

■ Talk about past behaviors with the client. Discuss which behaviors are acceptable by societal norms and which are not. Help the client identify ways in which he or she has exploited others. Encourage the client to explore how he or she would feel if the circumstances were reversed. An attempt may be made to enlighten the client to the sensitivity of others by promoting self-awareness in an effort to help the client gain insight into his or her own behavior.

■ Throughout the relationship with the client, maintain an attitude of "It is not *you*, but *your behavior*, that is unacceptable." An attitude of acceptance promotes feelings of dignity and self-worth.

Concept Care Mapping

The concept map care plan is an innovative approach to planning and organizing nursing care (see Chapter 9). It is a diagrammatic teaching and learning strategy that allows visualization of interrelationships between medical diagnoses, nursing diagnoses, assessment data, and treatments. An example of a concept map care plan for a client with antisocial personality disorder is presented in Figure 32-2.

Evaluation

Reassessment is conducted to determine if the nursing actions have been successful in achieving the objectives of care. Evaluation of the nursing actions for the client with antisocial personality disorder may be facilitated by gathering information using the following types of questions:

■ Does the client recognize when anger is getting out of control?
■ Can the client seek out staff instead of expressing anger in an inappropriate manner?
■ Can the client use other sources for rechanneling anger (e.g., physical activities)?
■ Has harm to others been avoided?
■ Can the client follow rules and regulations of the therapeutic milieu with little or no reminding?
■ Can the client verbalize which behaviors are appropriate and which are not?
■ Does the client express a desire to change?
■ Can the client delay gratifying own desires in deference to those of others when appropriate?
■ Does the client refrain from manipulating others to fulfill own desires?
■ Does the client fulfill activities of daily living willingly and independently?
■ Can the client verbalize methods of achieving and maintaining optimal wellness?
■ Can the client verbalize community resources from which he or she can seek assistance with daily living and healthcare needs when required?

Treatment Modalities

Few would argue that treatment of individuals with personality disorders is difficult and, in some instances, may even seem impossible. Personality characteristics are learned very early in life and perhaps may even be genetic. It is not surprising, then, that these enduring patterns of behavior may take years to change, if change occurs. Skodol and Gunderson (2008) state:

> Because personality disorders have been thought to consist of deeply ingrained attitudes and behavior patterns that consolidate during development and have endured since early adulthood, they have traditionally been believed to be very resistant to change. Moreover, treatment efforts are further confounded by the degree to which patients with personality disorders do not recognize their maladaptive personality traits as undesirable or in need of change. (p. 831)

Most clinicians believe it best to strive for lessening the inflexibility of the maladaptive traits and reducing their interference with everyday functioning and meaningful relationships. Little research exists to guide the decision of which therapy is most appropriate in the treatment of personality disorders. Selection of intervention is generally based on the area of greatest dysfunction, such as cognition, affect, behavior, or interpersonal relations. Following is a brief

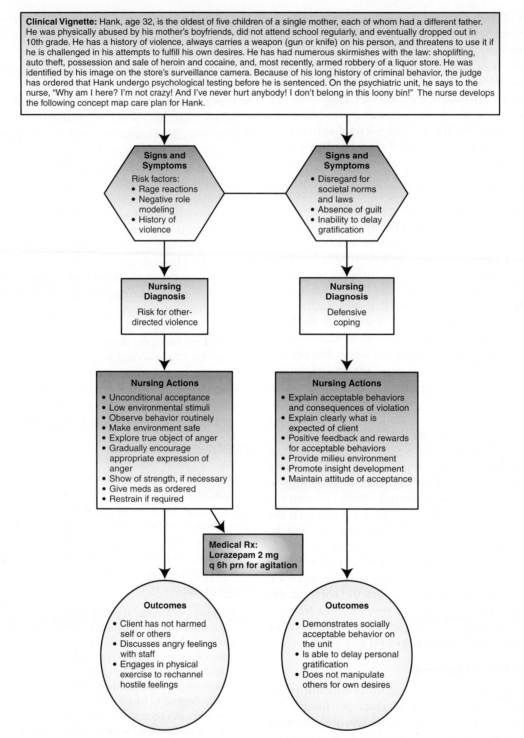

Clinical Vignette: Hank, age 32, is the oldest of five children of a single mother, each of whom had a different father. He was physically abused by his mother's boyfriends, did not attend school regularly, and eventually dropped out in 10th grade. He has a history of violence, always carries a weapon (gun or knife) on his person, and threatens to use it if he is challenged in his attempts to fulfill his own desires. He has had numerous skirmishes with the law: shoplifting, auto theft, possession and sale of heroin and cocaine, and, most recently, armed robbery of a liquor store. He was identified by his image on the store's surveillance camera. Because of his long history of criminal behavior, the judge has ordered that Hank undergo psychological testing before he is sentenced. On the psychiatric unit, he says to the nurse, "Why am I here? I'm not crazy! And I've never hurt anybody! I don't belong in this loony bin!" The nurse develops the following concept map care plan for Hank.

Signs and Symptoms

Risk factors:
• Rage reactions
• Negative role modeling
• History of violence

Signs and Symptoms

• Disregard for societal norms and laws
• Absence of guilt
• Inability to delay gratification

Nursing Diagnosis

Risk for other-directed violence

Nursing Diagnosis

Defensive coping

Nursing Actions

• Unconditional acceptance
• Low environmental stimuli
• Observe behavior routinely
• Make environment safe
• Explore true object of anger
• Gradually encourage appropriate expression of anger
• Show of strength, if necessary
• Give meds as ordered
• Restrain if required

Nursing Actions

• Explain acceptable behaviors and consequences of violation
• Explain clearly what is expected of client
• Positive feedback and rewards for acceptable behaviors
• Provide milieu environment
• Promote insight development
• Maintain attitude of acceptance

Medical Rx:
Lorazepam 2 mg
q 6h prn for agitation

Outcomes

• Client has not harmed self or others
• Discusses angry feelings with staff
• Engages in physical exercise to rechannel hostile feelings

Outcomes

• Demonstrates socially acceptable behavior on the unit
• Is able to delay personal gratification
• Does not manipulate others for own desires

FIGURE 32–2 Concept map care plan for a client with antisocial personality disorder.

description of various types of therapies and the disorders to which they are customarily suited.

Interpersonal Psychotherapy

Depending on the therapeutic goals, interpersonal psychotherapy with personality disorders is brief and time-limited, or it may involve long-term exploratory psychotherapy. Interpersonal psychotherapy may be

particularly appropriate because personality disorders largely reflect problems in interpersonal style.

Long-term psychotherapy attempts to understand and modify the maladjusted behaviors, cognition, and affects of clients with personality disorders that dominate their personal lives and relationships. The core element of treatment is the establishment of an empathic therapist-client relationship based on collaboration and guided discovery in which the therapist functions as a role model for the client.

Interpersonal psychotherapy is suggested for clients with paranoid, schizoid, schizotypal, borderline, dependent, narcissistic, and obsessive-compulsive personality disorders.

Psychoanalytical Psychotherapy

The treatment of choice for individuals with histrionic personality disorder has been psychoanalytical psychotherapy (Skodol & Gunderson, 2008). Treatment focuses on the unconscious motivation for seeking total satisfaction from others and for being unable to commit oneself to a stable, meaningful relationship.

Milieu or Group Therapy

This treatment is especially appropriate for individuals with antisocial personality disorder, who respond more adaptively to support and feedback from peers. In milieu or group therapy, feedback from peers is more effective than in one-to-one interaction with a therapist.

Group therapy—particularly homogenous supportive groups that emphasize the development of social skills—may be helpful in overcoming social anxiety and developing interpersonal trust and rapport in clients with avoidant personality disorder.

Feminist consciousness-raising groups can be useful in helping dependent clients struggling with social-role stereotypes.

Cognitive/Behavioral Therapy

Behavioral strategies offer reinforcement for positive change. Social skills training and assertiveness training teach alternative ways to deal with frustration. Cognitive strategies help the client recognize and correct inaccurate internal mental schemata. This type of therapy may be useful for clients with obsessive-compulsive, antisocial, and avoidant personality disorders.

Dialectical Behavior Therapy

Dialectical behavior therapy (DBT) is a type of psychotherapy that was originally developed by Marsha Linehan, PhD, as a treatment for the chronic self-injurious and parasuicidal behavior of clients with borderline personality disorder (Sadock & Sadock, 2007). It is a complex, eclectic treatment that combines the concepts of cognitive, behavioral, and interpersonal therapies with Eastern mindfulness practices (Dimeff & Linehan, 2001). Dimeff and Linehan (2001) identify the following five functions of DBT:

1. To enhance behavioral capabilities
2. To improve motivation to change
3. To ensure that new capabilities generalize to the natural environment

4. To structure the treatment environment such that client and therapist capabilities are supported and effective behaviors are reinforced
5. To enhance therapist capabilities and motivation to treat clients effectively

The four primary modes of treatment in DBT include the following:

1. **Group skills training.** In these groups, clients are taught skills considered relevant to the particular problems experienced by people with borderline personality disorder, such as core mindfulness skills, interpersonal effectiveness skills, emotion modulation skills, and distress tolerance skills (Kiehn & Swales, 2013).
2. **Individual psychotherapy.** Weekly sessions in which dysfunctional behavioral patterns, personal motivation, and skills strengthening are addressed.
3. **Telephone contact.** The therapist is available to the client by telephone, usually on a 24-hour per day basis, but according to limits set by the therapist. Kiehn and Swales (2013) state, "Telephone contact is to give the patient help and support in applying the skills that she is learning to her real life situation between sessions and to help her find ways of avoiding self-injury."
4. **Therapist consultation/team meeting.** Therapists meet regularly to review their work with their clients. These meetings are focused specifically on providing support for each other, keeping the therapists motivated, and providing effective treatment to their clients (Dimeff & Linehan, 2001).

In controlled studies, DBT has been shown to diminish self-destructive behaviors in clients with borderline personality disorder. Additionally, DBT has shown to decrease the drop-out rate from treatment and the number of hospitalizations. Improvement has also been shown in reducing anger and in global and social adjustment scores (Dimeff & Linehan, 2001). This method of treatment is now being used with other disorders, including substance use disorders, eating disorders, schizophrenia, and post-traumatic stress disorder (Sadock & Sadock, 2007).

Psychopharmacology

Psychopharmacology may be helpful in some instances. Although these drugs have no effect in the direct treatment of the disorder itself, some symptomatic relief can be achieved. Antipsychotic medications are helpful in the treatment of psychotic decompensations experienced by clients with paranoid, schizotypal, and borderline personality disorders (Skodol & Gunderson, 2008).

A variety of pharmacological interventions have been used with borderline personality disorder. The

IMPLICATIONS OF RESEARCH FOR EVIDENCE-BASED PRACTICE

Nickel, M.K., Muehlbacher, M., Nickel, C., Kettler, C., Gil, F.P., Bachler, E., Buschmann, W., Rother, N., Fartacek, R., Egger, C., Anvar, J., Rother, W.K., Loew, T.H., & Kaplan, P. (2006). Aripiprazole in the treatment of patients with borderline personality disorder: A double-blind, placebo-controlled study. *American Journal of Psychiatry,* 163(5), 833-838.

DESCRIPTION OF THE STUDY: The purpose of this study was to determine whether aripiprazole is effective in the treatment of several domains of symptoms of borderline personality disorder (BPD). Subjects included 43 women and 9 men who met the DSM criteria for BPD. Subjects were randomly assigned to 15 mg/day of aripiprazole or placebo for 8 weeks. Outcome measures included changes in scores on the symptom checklist (SCL-90-R), the Hamilton Depression Rating Scale (HAM-D), the Hamilton Anxiety Rating Scale (HAM-A), and the State-Trait Anger Expression Inventory. Test results were assessed weekly, along with side effects and self-injury reports using a non-validated questionnaire.

RESULTS OF THE STUDY: Aripiprazole was associated with a significantly greater rate of improvement than the placebo group on most of the SCL-90-R scales (with the exception of somatization), as well as on the HAM-D and HAM-A, and on all of the State-Trait Anger Expression Inventory scales. Self-injury occurred during the course of the 8-week trial, but only 2 episodes occurred in the aripiprazole group, compared with 7 in the placebo group. The most commonly reported side effects of aripiprazole included headache, insomnia, nausea, numbness, constipation, and anxiety. No significant weight changes were observed, and no serious side effects or suicidal attempts occurred during the study.

IMPLICATIONS FOR NURSING PRACTICE: The authors state, "Aripiprazole appears to be a safe and effective agent for improving not only the symptoms of borderline personality disorder but also the associated health-related quality of life and interpersonal problems." Nurses who work with individuals who have BPD should be familiar with this medication and understand the nursing implications associated with its administration. The implications of this study are particularly significant for nurses who have prescriptive authority and treat clients with BPD.

selective serotonin reuptake inhibitors (SSRIs) and monoamine oxidase inhibitors (MAOIs) have been successful in decreasing impulsivity and self-destructive acts in these clients. The MAOIs are not commonly used, however, because of concerns about violations of dietary restrictions and the higher risk of fatality with overdose. The combination of an SSRI and an atypical antipsychotic has been successful in treating dysphoria, mood instability, and impulsivity in clients with borderline personality disorder (Schatzberg, Cole, & DeBattista, 2010). Antipsychotics have resulted in improvement in illusions, ideas of reference, paranoid thinking, anxiety, and hostility in some clients.

Lithium carbonate and propranolol (Inderal) may be useful for the violent episodes observed in clients with antisocial personality disorder (Coccaro & Siever, 2000). Caution must be given to prescribing medications outside the structured setting because of the high risk for substance abuse by these individuals.

For the client with avoidant personality disorder, anxiolytics are sometimes helpful whenever previously avoided behavior is being attempted. The mere possession of the medication may be reassurance enough to help the client through the stressful period. Antidepressants, such as sertraline (Zoloft) and paroxetine (Paxil), may be useful with these clients if panic disorder develops.

CASE STUDY AND SAMPLE CARE PLAN

NURSING HISTORY AND ASSESSMENT

Anthony, age 34, has been admitted to the psychiatric unit with a diagnosis of antisocial personality disorder. He was recently arrested and convicted for armed robbery of a convenience store, and attempted murder of the store clerk. Due to the actions of the store clerk, who quickly alerted police, and to the store surveillance camera, Anthony was identified and apprehended within hours of the crime. The judge has ordered physical, neurological, and psychiatric evaluations before sentencing Anthony.

Anthony was physically and psychologically abused as a child by his alcoholic father. He was suspended from high school because of failing grades and habitual truancy. He has a long history of arrests, beginning with shoplifting at age 7, and progressing in adolescence to burglary, auto theft, and sexual assault, and finally to armed robbery, and attempted murder. He was out on probation when he committed his latest crime.

On the psychiatric unit, Anthony is loud, belligerent, and uncooperative. When Carol, his admitting nurse, arrives to

CASE STUDY AND SAMPLE CARE PLAN

work the evening shift on Anthony's second hospital day, he says to her, "I'm so glad you are finally here. You are the best nurse on the unit. I can't talk to anyone but you. These people are nothing but a bunch of loonies around here . . . and that includes staff as well as patients! Maybe you and I could walk down to the coffee shop together later. Are you married? I'd sure like to get to know you better after I get out of this nut house!"

NURSING DIAGNOSES/OUTCOME IDENTIFICATION

From the assessment data, the nurse develops the following nursing diagnoses for Anthony:

1. **Risk for other-directed violence** related to history of violence against others and history of childhood abuse.
   a. **Short-Term Goals:** Client will discuss angry feelings and situations that precipitate hostility. Client will not harm others.
   b. **Long-Term Goal:** Client will not harm others.

2. **Defensive coping** related to low self-esteem, dysfunctional nuclear family, underdeveloped ego and superego, evidenced by absence of guilt feelings, disregard for societal laws and norms, inability to delay gratification, superior attitude toward others, denial of problems, and projection of blame and responsibility.
   a. **Short-Term Goals:** Client will verbalize understanding of unit rules and regulations and consequences for violation of them.
   b. **Long-Term Goal:** Client will be able to delay gratification and follow rules and regulations of the unit. Client will verbalize personal responsibility for own actions and behaviors.

PLANNING/IMPLEMENTATION

RISK FOR OTHER-DIRECTED VIOLENCE
The following nursing interventions have been identified for Anthony.

1. Develop a trusting relationship with Anthony by conveying an accepting attitude. Ensure that he understands it is not *him* but *his behavior* that is unacceptable.
2. Try to keep excess stimuli out of the environment. Speak to Anthony in a calm quiet voice.
3. Observe Anthony's behavior regularly. Do this through routine activity so that he doesn't become suspicious and angry about being watched. This is important so that if hostile and aggressive behaviors are observed, intervention may prevent harm to Anthony, staff members, and/or other patients.
4. Sit with Anthony and encourage him to talk about his anger and hostile feelings. Help him understand where

these feelings originate and who is the true target of the hostility.
5. Help him develop adaptive ways of dealing with frustration, such as exercise and other physical activities.
6. Administer tranquilizing medication, as ordered by the physician.
7. If Anthony should become out of control and mechanical restraints become necessary, ensure that sufficient staff is available to intervene. Do not use restraints as a punishment, but only as a protective measure for Anthony and the other patients.

DEFENSIVE COPING
The following nursing interventions have been identified for Anthony.

1. Explain to Anthony which of his behaviors are acceptable on the unit and which are not. Simply state that unacceptable behaviors will not be tolerated.
2. Determine appropriate consequences for violation of these limits (e.g., no TV or movies; no phone calls; time-out room). Ensure that all staff members follow through with these consequences.
3. Don't be taken in by this "charmer." Compliments from Anthony are another form of manipulative behavior. Explain to Anthony that you will not accept these types of comments from him, and if they continue, impose consequences.
4. Encourage Anthony to talk about his past misdeeds. Try to help him understand how he would feel if someone treated him in the manner that he has treated others.

EVALUATION

The outcome criteria for Anthony have only partially been met. Personality characteristics such as those of Anthony's are deep-rooted and enduring. He is not likely to change. Unless testing reveals a serious medical problem, Anthony will no doubt go to prison for most of the rest of his life. During his time on the psychiatric unit, harm to self and others has been avoided. He has discussed his anger and hostile feelings with Carol and other staff members. He continues to become belligerent when told that he cannot smoke on the unit and must wait for someone to escort him to the smoking area. He yells at the other patients and calls them "nut cases." He refuses to take responsibility for his actions and blames negative behavioral outcomes on others. He has begun a regular exercise program in the fitness room, and receives positive feedback from the staff for this attempt to integrate healthier coping strategies.

Summary and Key Points

■ Clients with personality disorders are undoubtedly some of the most difficult ones health-care workers are likely to encounter.

■ Personality characteristics are formed very early in life and are difficult, if not impossible, to change. In fact, some clinicians believe the therapeutic approach is not to try to change the characteristics but rather to decrease the inflexibility of the maladaptive traits and reduce their interference with everyday functioning and meaningful relationships.

■ The concept of a personality disorder has been present throughout the history of medicine. Problems have arisen in the attempt to establish a classification system for these disorders.

■ The *DSM-5* identifies ten individual personality disorders: antisocial, avoidant, borderline, histrionic, dependent, narcissistic, obsessive-compulsive, paranoid, schizoid, and schizotypal.

■ Nursing care of the client with a personality disorder is accomplished using the steps of the nursing process.

■ Other treatment modalities include interpersonal psychotherapy, psychoanalytical psychotherapy, milieu or group therapy, cognitive/behavioral therapy, dialectical behavior therapy, and psychopharmacology.

■ Individuals with borderline personality disorder may enter the health-care system because of their instability and frequent attempts at self-destructive behavior.

■ The individual with antisocial personality disorder may become part of the health-care system to avoid legal consequences or because of a court order for psychological evaluation.

■ Nurses who work in all types of clinical settings should be familiar with the characteristics associated with personality disorders.

■ Nurses working in psychiatry must be knowledgeable about appropriate intervention with these clients, for it is unlikely that they will encounter a greater professional challenge than these clients present.

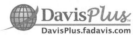 **DavisPlus** Additional info available at
DavisPlus.fadavis.com www.davisplus.com

Review Questions
Self-Examination/Learning Exercise

Select the answer that is most appropriate for each of the following questions.

1. Kim has a diagnosis of borderline personality disorder. She often exhibits alternating clinging and distancing behaviors. The most appropriate nursing intervention with this type of behavior would be to:
   a. Encourage Kim to establish trust in one staff person, with whom all therapeutic interaction should take place.
   b. Secure a verbal contract from Kim that she will discontinue these behaviors.
   c. Withdraw attention if these behaviors continue.
   d. Rotate staff members who work with Kim so that she will learn to relate to more than one person.

2. Kim, a client diagnosed with borderline personality disorder, manipulates the staff in an effort to fulfill her own desires. All of the following may be examples of manipulative behaviors in the borderline client *except*:
   a. Refusal to stay in room alone, stating, "It's so lonely."
   b. Asking Nurse Jones for cigarettes after 30 minutes, knowing the assigned nurse has explained she must wait 1 hour.
   c. Stating to Nurse Jones, "I really like having you for my nurse. You're the best one around here."
   d. Cutting arms with razor blade after discussing dismissal plans with physician.

3. "Splitting" by the client with borderline personality disorder denotes:
   a. Evidence of precocious development
   b. A primitive defense mechanism in which the client sees objects as all good or all bad
   c. A brief psychotic episode in which the client loses contact with reality
   d. Two distinct personalities within the borderline client

Review Questions—cont'd
Self-Examination/Learning Exercise

4. According to Margaret Mahler, predisposition to borderline personality disorder occurs when developmental tasks go unfulfilled in which of the following phases?
   a. Autistic phase, during which the child's needs for security and comfort go unfulfilled
   b. Symbiotic phase, during which the child fails to bond with the mother
   c. Differentiation phase, during which the child fails to recognize a separateness between self and mother
   d. Rapprochement phase, during which the mother withdraws emotional support in response to the child's increasing independence

5. Jack is a new client on the psychiatric unit with a diagnosis of antisocial personality disorder. Which of the following characteristics would you expect to assess in Jack?
   a. Lack of guilt for wrongdoing
   b. Insight into his own behavior
   c. Ability to learn from past experiences
   d. Compliance with authority

6. Milieu therapy is a good choice for clients with antisocial personality disorder because it:
   a. Provides a system of punishment and rewards for behavior modification
   b. Emulates a social community in which the client may learn to live harmoniously with others
   c. Provides mostly one-to-one interaction between the client and therapist
   d. Provides a very structured setting in which the clients have very little input into the planning of their care

7. In evaluating the progress of Jack, a client diagnosed with antisocial personality disorder, which of the following behaviors would be considered the most significant indication of positive change?
   a. Jack got angry only once in group this week.
   b. Jack was able to wait a whole hour for a cigarette without verbally abusing the staff.
   c. On his own initiative, Jack sent a note of apology to a man he had injured in a recent fight.
   d. Jack stated that he would no longer start any more fights.

8. Which of the following behavioral patterns is characteristic of individuals with narcissistic personality disorder?
   a. Overly self-centered and exploitative of others
   b. Suspicious and mistrustful of others
   c. Rule conscious and disapproving of change
   d. Anxious and socially isolated

9. Carol is a new nursing graduate being oriented on a medical/surgical unit by the head nurse, Mrs. Carey. When Carol describes a new technique she has learned for positioning immobile clients, Mrs. Carey states, "What are you trying to do . . . tell me how to do my job? We have always done it this way on this unit, and we will continue to do it this way until I say differently!" This is an example of which type of personality characteristic?
   a. Antisocial
   b. Paranoid
   c. Passive-aggressive
   d. Obsessive-compulsive

10. Which of the following behavioral patterns is characteristic of individuals with schizotypal personality disorder?
    a. Belittling themselves and their abilities
    b. A lifelong pattern of social withdrawal
    c. Suspicious and mistrustful of others
    d. Overreacting inappropriately to minor stimuli

TEST YOUR CRITICAL THINKING SKILLS

Lana, age 32, was diagnosed with borderline personality disorder when she was 26 years old. Her husband took her to the emergency department when he walked into the bathroom and found her cutting her legs with a razor blade. At that time, assessment revealed that Lana had a long history of self-mutilation, which she had carefully hidden from her husband and others. Lana began long-term psychoanalytical psychotherapy on an outpatient basis. Therapy revealed that Lana had been physically and sexually abused as a child by both her mother and her father, both now deceased. She admitted to having chronic depression, and her husband related episodes of rage reactions. Lana has been hospitalized on the psychiatric unit for a week because of suicidal ideations. After making a no-suicide contract with the staff, she is allowed to leave the unit on pass to keep a dental appointment that she made a number of weeks ago. She has just returned to the unit and says to her nurse, "I just took 20 Desyrel while I was sitting in my car in the parking lot."

Answer the following questions related to Lana:

1. The nurse is well acquainted with Lana and believes this is a manipulative gesture. How should the nurse handle this situation?
2. What is the priority nursing diagnosis for Lana?
3. Lana likes to "split" the staff into "good guys" and "bad guys." What is the most important intervention for splitting by a person with borderline personality disorder?

Communication Exercises

1. Nathan, age 37, has been admitted to the hospital for a psychiatric evaluation after being arrested for armed robbery of a convenience store. He has a history of encounters with law enforcement since early adolescence. He has been diagnosed with antisocial personality disorder. Nathan says to the nurse, "Hey pretty lady! Where have you been all my life?"

   • How would the nurse respond appropriately to this statement by Nathan?

2. "I really got a bum rap! I had no intentions of hurting anyone. The gun only had one bullet in it! I just wanted to scare that clerk into giving me a few bucks! Just my bad luck an off-duty cop had to walk in about that time."

   • How would the nurse respond appropriately to this statement by Nathan?

3. "You're really cute. Are you married? I'm pretty sure my lawyer can get me out of this rap, and I'll be a free man! Why don't you give me your phone number and I'll call you sometime. We could go out and have some fun!"

   • How would the nurse respond appropriately to this statement by Nathan?

References

American Psychiatric Association. (2013). *Diagnostic and statistical manual of mental disorders* (5th ed.). Washington, DC: Author.

Bienenfeld, D. (2013). Personality disorders. Retrieved from http://emedicine.medscape.com/article/294307-overview

Black, D.W., & Andreasen, N.C. (2011). *Introductory textbook of psychiatry* (5th ed.). Washington, DC: American Psychiatric Publishing.

Bosson, J.K., & Prewitt-Freilino, J.L. (2007). Overvalued and ashamed: Considering the roles of self-esteem and self-conscious emotions in covert narcissism. In J.L. Tracy, R.W. Robins, & J.P. Tangney (Eds.), *The self-conscious emotions: Theory and research.* New York, NY: Guilford Press.

Coccaro, E.F., & Siever, L.J. (2000). The neuropsychopharmacology of personality disorders. *Psychopharmacology: The fourth generation of progress.* The American College of Neuropsychopharmacology. Retrieved from www.acnp.org/G4/GN401000152/CH148.html

Cummings, J.L., & Mega, M.S. (2003). *Neuropsychiatry and behavioral neuroscience.* New York, NY: Oxford University Press.

Dimeff, L., & Linehan, M.M. (2001). Dialectical behavior therapy in a nutshell. *The California Psychologist, 34,* 10-13.

Fischer, M., Barkley, R.A., Smallish, L., & Fletcher, K. (2002). Young adult follow-up of hyperactive children: Self-reported psychiatric disorders, comorbidity, and the role of childhood conduct problems and teen CD. *Journal of Abnormal Child Psychology, 30*(5), 463-475.

Gorman, L., & Sultan, D.F. (2008). *Psychosocial nursing for general patient care* (3rd ed.). Philadelphia, PA: F.A. Davis.

Gunderson, J.G. (2011). An introduction to borderline personality disorder: Diagnosis, origins, course, and treatment. *National Education Alliance—Borderline Personality Disorder.* Retrieved from www.borderlinepersonalitydisorder.com/understading-bpd/a-bpd-brief/

Hill, J. (2003). Early identification of individuals at risk for antisocial personality disorder. *British Journal of Psychiatry, 182*(Suppl. 44), s11-s14.

Kiehn, B., & Swales, M. (2013). An overview of dialectical behaviour therapy in the treatment of borderline personality disorder. *Psychiatry Online.* Retrieved from http://www.priory.com/dbt.htm

Lubit, R.H. (2011). Borderline personality disorder. *eMedicine Psychiatry.* Retrieved from http://emedicine.medscape.com/article/913575-overview

Martinez-Lewi, L. (2008). *Freeing yourself from the narcissist in your life.* New York, NY: Penguin Group.

Millon, T. (2004). *Personality disorders in modern life* (2nd ed.). Hoboken, NJ: John Wiley and Sons.

Oldham, J.M., Gabbard, G.O., Goin, M.K., Gunderson, J., Soloff, P., Spiegel, D., Stone, M., & Phillips, K.A. (2006). Practice guideline for the treatment of patients with borderline personality disorder. In *The American Psychiatric Association Practice Guidelines for the Treatment of Psychiatric Disorders, Compendium 2006.* Washington, DC: American Psychiatric Publishing.

Ramsland, K. (2013). *The childhood psychopath: Bad seed or bad parents?* Retrieved from http://www.trutv.com/library/crime/criminal_mind/psychology/psychopath/2.html

Sadock, B.J., & Sadock, V.A. (2007). *Synopsis of psychiatry: Behavioral sciences/clinical psychiatry* (10th ed.). Philadelphia, PA: Lippincott Williams & Wilkins.

Skodol, A.E., & Gunderson, J.G. (2008). Personality disorders. In R.E. Hales, S.C. Yudofsky, & G.O. Gabbard (Eds.), *Textbook of psychiatry* (5th ed.). Washington, DC: American Psychiatric Publishing.

Schatzberg, A.F., Cole, J.O., & DeBattista, C. (2010). *Manual of clinical Psychopharmacology* (7th ed.). Washington, DC: American Psychiatric Publishing.

Tharp, D.T. (2009). Antisocial personality disorder. *Stonebriar Psychiatric Services News & Views, 5*(6), 1-2.

The Joint Commission. (2010). *The comprehensive accreditation manual for hospitals: The official handbook* (January, 2010). Oakbrook Terrace, IL: Joint Commission Resources.

Classical References

Erikson, E. (1963). *Childhood and society* (2nd ed.). New York, NY: WW Norton.

Mahler, M., Pine, F., & Bergman, A. (1975). *The psychological birth of the human infant.* New York, NY: Basic Books.

Sullivan, H.S. (1953). *The interpersonal theory of psychiatry.* New York, NY: WW Norton.

 MOVIE CONNECTIONS

Taxi Driver (schizoid personality) • *One Flew Over the Cuckoo's Nest* (antisocial) • *The Boston Strangler* (antisocial) • *Just Cause* (antisocial) • *The Dream Team* (antisocial) • *Goodfellas* (antisocial) • *Fatal Attraction* (borderline) • *Play Misty for Me* (borderline) • *Girl, Interrupted* (borderline) • *Gone With the Wind* (histrionic) • *Wall Street* (narcissistic) • *The Odd Couple* (obsessive-compulsive) • *As Good As It Gets* (obsessive-compulsive)

@ INTERNET REFERENCES

- Additional information about personality disorders may be located at the following websites:
  - http://www.mentalhealth.com/dis/p20-pe01.html
  - http://www.mentalhealth.com/dis/p20-pe02.html
  - http://www.mentalhealth.com/dis/p20-pe03.html
  - http://www.mentalhealth.com/dis/p20-pe04.html
  - http://www.mentalhealth.com/dis/p20-pe05.html
  - http://www.mentalhealth.com/dis/p20-pe06.html
  - http://www.mentalhealth.com/dis/p20-pe07.html
  - http://www.mentalhealth.com/dis/p20-pe08.html
  - http://www.mentalhealth.com/dis/p20-pe09.html
  - http://www.mentalhealth.com/dis/p20-pe10.html
  - http://www.mentalhealth.com/p13.html#Per
  - http://www.ncbi.nlm.nih.gov/pubmedhealth/PMH0001935/
  - http://www.mayoclinic.com/health/personality-disorders/DS00562

Psychiatric/Mental Health Nursing of Special Populations

33

Children and Adolescents

OBJECTIVES
After reading this chapter, the student will be able to:

1. Identify psychiatric disorders that most commonly have their onset in infancy, childhood, or adolescence.
2. Discuss predisposing factors implicated in the etiology of intellectual disability, autism spectrum disorder, attention-deficit/hyperactivity disorder, conduct disorder, oppositional defiant disorder, Tourette's disorder, and separation anxiety disorder.
3. Identify symptomatology and use the information in the assessment of clients with the aforementioned disorders.
4. Identify nursing diagnoses common to clients with these disorders and select appropriate nursing interventions for each.
5. Discuss relevant criteria for evaluating nursing care of clients with selected infant, childhood, and adolescent psychiatric disorders.
6. Describe treatment modalities relevant to selected disorders of infancy, childhood, and adolescence.

HOMEWORK ASSIGNMENT
Please read the chapter and answer the following questions:

1. What maternal prenatal activity has been associated with attention-deficit/hyperactivity disorder (ADHD) in children?
2. What antidepressant medication has been used with some success in treating ADHD?
3. Neuroimaging brain studies in children with Tourette's disorder have been consistent in finding dysfunction in what area of the brain?
4. What are some family behaviors that have been implicated as influential in the development of separation anxiety disorder?

This chapter examines various disorders in which the symptoms usually first become evident during infancy, childhood, or adolescence. That is not to say that some of the disorders discussed in this chapter do not appear later in life or that symptoms associated with other disorders, such as major depressive disorder or bipolar disorder, do not appear in childhood or adolescence. These disorders, with consideration of the variances in age and developmental level, are discussed in Chapters 25 and 26.

Developmental theories were discussed in Chapter 3. All nurses working with children or adolescents should be knowledgeable about "normal" stages of growth and development. At best, the developmental process is one that is fraught with frustrations and difficulties. Behavioral responses are individual and idiosyncratic. They are, indeed, *human* responses.

Whether or not a child's behavior indicates emotional problems is often difficult to determine. Guidelines for making such a determination should consider appropriateness of the behavior regarding age and cultural norms and whether the behavior interferes with adaptive functioning. This chapter focuses on the nursing process in care of clients with intellectual disability, autism spectrum disorder, attention-deficit/hyperactivity disorder, conduct disorder, oppositional defiant disorder, Tourette's disorder, and separation anxiety disorder. Additional treatment modalities are included.

Neurodevelopmental Disorders

Intellectual Disability (Intellectual Developmental Disorder)

The *Diagnostic and Statistical Manual of Mental Disorders, Fifth Edition (DSM-5)* (American Psychiatric Association [APA], 2013) defines intellectual disability as a "disorder with onset during the developmental period that includes both intellectual and adaptive functioning deficits in conceptual, social, and practical domains" (p. 33). Onset of intellectual and adaptive deficits occurs during the developmental period. Level of severity (mild, moderate, severe, or profound) is based on adaptive functioning within the three domains. General intellectual functioning is measured by both clinical assessment and an individual's performance on intelligence quotient (IQ) tests. Adaptive functioning refers to the person's ability to adapt to the requirements of daily living and the expectations of his or her age and cultural group. The *DSM-5* diagnostic criteria for intellectual disability are presented in Box 33-1.

Predisposing Factors

The etiology of intellectual disability may be primarily biological, primarily psychosocial, a combination of both, or in some instances, unknown. Black and Andreasen (2011) state that intellectual disability "is a syndrome that represents a final common pathway produced by a variety of factors that injure the brain and affect its normal development" (p. 411).

Genetic Factors

Genetic factors are implicated as the cause of intellectual disability in approximately 5 percent of the cases. These factors include inborn errors of metabolism, such as Tay-Sachs disease, phenylketonuria, and hyperglycinemia. Also included are chromosomal disorders, such as Down syndrome and Klinefelter's syndrome, and single-gene abnormalities, such as tuberous sclerosis and neurofibromatosis.

Disruptions in Embryonic Development

Conditions that result in early alterations in embryonic development account for approximately 30 percent of

---

BOX 33-1 Diagnostic Criteria for Intellectual Disability (Intellectual Developmental Disorder)

Intellectual disability (intellectual developmental disorder) is a disorder with onset during the developmental period that includes both intellectual and adaptive functioning deficits in conceptual, social, and practical domains. The following three criteria must be met:

A. Deficits in intellectual functions, such as reasoning, problem solving, planning, abstract thinking, judgment, academic learning, and learning from experience, confirmed by both clinical assessment and individualized, standardized intelligence testing.

B. Deficits in adaptive functioning that result in failure to meet developmental and sociocultural standards for personal independence and social responsibility. Without ongoing support the adaptive deficits limit functioning in one or more activities of daily life, such as communication, social participation, and independent living, across multiple environments, such as home, school, work, and community.

C. Onset of intellectual and adaptive deficits during the developmental period.

Specify current severity:

Mild
Moderate
Severe
Profound

intellectual disability cases. Damages may occur in response to toxicity associated with maternal ingestion of alcohol or other drugs. Maternal illnesses and infections during pregnancy (e.g., rubella, cytomegalovirus) and complications of pregnancy (e.g., toxemia, uncontrolled diabetes) also can result in congenital intellectual disability (Sadock & Sadock, 2007).

Pregnancy and Perinatal Factors

Approximately 10 percent of cases of intellectual disability are the result of circumstances that occur during pregnancy (e.g., fetal malnutrition, viral and other infections, and prematurity) or during the birth process. Examples of the latter include trauma to the head incurred during the process of birth, placenta previa or premature separation of the placenta, and prolapse of the umbilical cord.

General Medical Conditions Acquired in Infancy or Childhood

General medical conditions acquired during infancy or childhood account for approximately 5 percent of cases of intellectual disability. They include infections, such as meningitis and encephalitis; poisonings, such as from insecticides, medications, and lead; and

physical trauma, such as head injuries, asphyxiation, and hyperpyrexia (Sadock & Sadock, 2007).

Sociocultural Factors and Other Mental Disorders

Between 15 and 20 percent of cases of intellectual disability may be attributed to deprivation of nurturance and social stimulation and to impoverished environments associated with poor prenatal and perinatal care and inadequate nutrition. Additionally, severe mental disorders, such as autism spectrum disorder, can result in intellectual disability.

Recognition of the cause and period of inception provides information regarding what to expect in terms of behavior and potential. However, each child is different, and consideration must be given on an individual basis in every case.

Application of the Nursing Process to Intellectual Disability

Background Assessment Data (Symptomatology)

The degree of severity of intellectual disability may be measured by the client's IQ level. Four levels have been delineated: mild, moderate, severe, and profound. The various behavioral manifestations and abilities associated with each of these levels of severity are outlined in Table 33-1.

TABLE 33–1	Developmental Characteristics of Intellectual Disability by Degree of Severity			
LEVEL (IQ)	**ABILITY TO PERFORM SELF-CARE ACTIVITIES**	**COGNITIVE/EDUCATIONAL CAPABILITIES**	**SOCIAL/COMMUNICATION CAPABILITIES**	**PSYCHOMOTOR CAPABILITIES**
Mild (50–70)	Capable of independent living, with assistance during times of stress.	Capable of academic skills to sixth-grade level. As adult can achieve vocational skills for minimum self-support.	Capable of developing social skills. Functions well in a structured, sheltered setting.	Psychomotor skills usually not affected, although may have some slight problems with coordination.
Moderate (35–49)	Can perform some activities independently. Requires supervision.	Capable of academic skill to second-grade level. As adult may be able to contribute to own support in sheltered workshop.	May experience some limitation in speech communication. Difficulty adhering to social convention may interfere with peer relationships.	Motor development is fair. Vocational capabilities may be limited to unskilled gross motor activities.
Severe (20–34)	May be trained in elementary hygiene skills. Requires complete supervision.	Unable to benefit from academic or vocational training. Profits from systematic habit training.	Minimal verbal skills. Wants and needs often communicated by acting-out behaviors.	Poor psychomotor development. Able to perform only simple tasks under close supervision.
Profound (below 20)	No capacity for independent functioning. Requires constant aid and supervision.	Unable to profit from academic or vocational training. May respond to minimal training in self-help if presented in the close context of a one-to-one relationship.	Little, if any, speech development. No capacity for socialization skills.	Lack of ability for both fine and gross motor movements. Requires constant supervision and care. May be associated with other physical disorders.

SOURCES: Adapted from Black & Andreasen (2011); Sadock & Sadock (2007); Ursano, Kartheiser, & Barnhill (2008).

Nurses should assess and focus on each client's strengths and individual abilities. Knowledge regarding level of independence in the performance of self-care activities is essential to the development of an adequate plan for the provision of nursing care.

Nursing Diagnosis

Selection of appropriate nursing diagnoses for the client with intellectual disability depends largely on the degree of severity of the condition and the client's capabilities. Possible nursing diagnoses include the following:

- Risk for injury related to altered physical mobility or aggressive behavior
- Self-care deficit related to altered physical mobility or lack of maturity
- Impaired verbal communication related to developmental alteration
- Impaired social interaction related to speech deficiencies or difficulty adhering to conventional social behavior
- Delayed growth and development related to isolation from significant others, inadequate environmental stimulation, genetic factors
- Anxiety (moderate to severe) related to hospitalization and absence of familiar surroundings
- Defensive coping related to feelings of powerlessness and threat to self-esteem
- Ineffective coping related to inadequate coping skills secondary to developmental delay

Outcome Identification

Outcome criteria include short- and long-term goals. Timelines are individually determined. The following criteria may be used for measurement of outcomes in the care of the client with intellectual disability.

The client:

- Has experienced no physical harm.
- Has had self-care needs fulfilled.
- Interacts with others in a socially appropriate manner.
- Has maintained anxiety at a manageable level.
- Is able to accept direction without becoming defensive.
- Demonstrates adaptive coping skills in response to stressful situations.

Planning/Implementation

Table 33-2 provides a plan of care for the child with intellectual disability using selected nursing diagnoses, outcome criteria, and appropriate nursing interventions and rationales.

Although this plan of care is directed toward the individual client, it is essential that family members or primary caregivers participate in the ongoing care of the client with intellectual disability. They need to receive information regarding the scope of the condition, realistic expectations and client potentials, methods for modifying behavior as required, and community resources from which they may seek assistance and support.

Table 33-2 | CARE PLAN FOR THE CHILD WITH INTELLECTUAL DISABILITY

NURSING DIAGNOSIS: RISK FOR INJURY

RELATED TO: Altered physical mobility or aggressive behavior

OUTCOME CRITERIA	NURSING INTERVENTIONS	RATIONALE
Short- and Long-Term Goal • Client will not experience injury.	1. Create a safe environment for the client.	1-5. Client safety is a nursing priority.
	2. Ensure that small items are removed from area where client will be ambulating and that sharp items are out of reach.	
	3. Store items that client uses frequently within easy reach.	
	4. Pad side rails and headboard of client with history of seizures.	
	5. Prevent physical aggression and acting out behaviors by learning to recognize signs that client is becoming agitated.	

Continued

Table 33-2 | CARE PLAN FOR THE CHILD WITH INTELLECTUAL DISABILITY—cont'd

NURSING DIAGNOSIS: SELF-CARE DEFICIT

RELATED TO: Altered physical mobility or lack of maturity

OUTCOME CRITERIA	NURSING INTERVENTIONS	RATIONALE
Short-Term Goal • Client will be able to participate in aspects of self-care. **Long-Term Goal** • Client will have all self-care needs met.	1. Identify aspects of self-care that may be within the client's capabilities. Work on one aspect of self-care at a time. Provide simple, concrete explanations. Offer positive feedback for efforts. 2. When one aspect of self-care has been mastered to the best of the client's ability, move on to another. Encourage independence but intervene when client is unable to perform.	1. Positive reinforcement enhances self-esteem and encourages repetition of desirable behaviors. 2. Client comfort and safety are nursing priorities.

NURSING DIAGNOSIS: IMPAIRED VERBAL COMMUNICATION

RELATED TO: Developmental alteration

OUTCOME CRITERIA	NURSING INTERVENTIONS	RATIONALE
Short-Term Goal • Client will establish trust with caregiver and a means of communication of needs. **Long-Term Goal** • Client's needs are being met through established means of communication. • If client cannot speak or communicate by other means, needs are met by caregiver's anticipation of client's needs.	1. Maintain consistency of staff assignment over time. 2. Anticipate and fulfill client's needs until satisfactory communication patterns are established. Learn (from family, if possible) special words client uses that are different from the norm. Identify nonverbal gestures or signals that client may use to convey needs if verbal communication is absent. Practice these communications skills repeatedly.	1. Consistency of staff assignments facilitates trust and the ability to understand client's actions and communications. 2. Some children with intellectual disability, particularly at the severe level, can learn only by systematic habit training.

NURSING DIAGNOSIS: IMPAIRED SOCIAL INTERACTION

RELATED TO: Speech deficiencies or difficulty adhering to conventional social behavior

OUTCOME CRITERIA	NURSING INTERVENTIONS	RATIONALE
Short-Term Goal • Client will attempt to interact with others in the presence of trusted caregiver. **Long-Term Goal** • Client will be able to interact with others using behaviors that are socially acceptable and appropriate to developmental level.	1. Remain with client during initial interactions with others on the unit. 2. Explain to other clients the meaning behind some of the client's nonverbal gestures and signals. Use simple language to explain to client which behaviors are acceptable and which are not. Establish a procedure for behavior modification with rewards for appropriate behaviors and aversive reinforcement for inappropriate behaviors.	1. Presence of a trusted individual provides a feeling of security. 2. Positive, negative, and aversive reinforcements can contribute to desired changes in behavior. These privileges and penalties are individually determined as staff learns the likes and dislikes of the client.

Evaluation

Evaluation of care given to the client with intellectual disability should reflect positive behavioral changes. Evaluation is accomplished by determining if the goals of care have been met through implementation of the nursing actions selected. The nurse reassesses the plan and makes changes as required. Reassessment data may include information gathered by asking the following questions:

- Have nursing actions providing for the client's safety been sufficient to prevent injury?
- Have all of the client's self-care needs been fulfilled? Can he or she fulfill some of these needs independently?
- Has the client been able to communicate needs and desires so that he or she can be understood?
- Has the client learned to interact appropriately with others?
- When regressive behaviors surface, can the client accept constructive feedback and discontinue the inappropriate behavior?
- Has anxiety been maintained at a manageable level?
- Has the client learned new coping skills through behavior modification? Does the client demonstrate evidence of increased self-esteem because of the accomplishment of these new skills and adaptive behaviors?
- Have primary caregivers been taught realistic expectations of the client's behavior and methods for attempting to modify unacceptable behaviors?
- Have primary caregivers been given information regarding various resources from which they can seek assistance and support within the community?

CORE CONCEPT

Autism Spectrum Disorder

A disorder that is characterized by impairment in social interaction skills and interpersonal communication and a restricted repertoire of activities and interests (Black & Andreasen, 2011).

Autism Spectrum Disorder

Clinical Findings

In the *Diagnostic and Statistical Manual of Mental Disorders, Fourth Edition, Text Revision (DSM-IV-TR)* (APA, 2000), the category of Autism Spectrum Disorders encompassed a broad spectrum of diagnoses that included autistic disorder, Rett's disorder, childhood disintegrative disorder, pervasive developmental disorder not otherwise specified, and Asperger's disorder. The *DSM-5* groups these disorders into a single diagnostic category—**autism spectrum disorder** (ASD). The diagnosis is adapted to each individual by clinical specifiers (e.g., level of severity, verbal abilities) and associated features (e.g., known genetic disorders, epilepsy, intellectual disability) (APA, 2013). ASD is characterized by a withdrawal of the child into the self and into a fantasy world of his or her own creation. The child has markedly abnormal or impaired development in social interaction and communication and a markedly restricted repertoire of activity and interests, some of which may be considered somewhat bizarre.

Epidemiology and Course

A study by the Autism and Developmental Disabilities Monitoring (ADDM) Network and funded by the Centers for Disease Control and Prevention (CDC) determined the prevalence of ASD in the United States to be about 11.3 per 1,000 (1 in 88) children (CDC, 2012b). It occurs about 4.5 times more often in boys than in girls. Onset of the disorder occurs in early childhood, and in most cases it runs a chronic course, with symptoms persisting into adulthood.

Predisposing Factors

Neurological Implications

Imaging studies have revealed a number of alterations in major brain structures of individuals with ASD. In one recent study, the investigators found a disproportionate enlargement in temporal lobe white matter and an increase in surface area in the temporal, frontal, and parieto-occipital lobes (Hazlett et al., 2011). Other imaging studies have revealed an overall impairment in brain connectivity networks associated with attention, consciousness, and self-awareness (Black & Andreasen, 2011). The role of neurotransmitters, such as serotonin, dopamine, and epinephrine, is currently under investigation.

Physiological Implications

Ursano, Kartheiser, and Barnhill (2008) listed a number of medical conditions that may be implicated in the predisposition to ASD. These include tuberous sclerosis, fragile X syndrome, maternal rubella, congenital hypothyroidism, phenylketonuria, Down syndrome, neurofibromatosis, and Angelman syndrome. Ursano and associates stated, "In the vast majority of cases (likely greater than 90 percent), there is no readily identifiable cause for autism" (p. 879).

Genetics

Research has revealed strong evidence that genetic factors play a significant role in the etiology of ASD. Studies have shown that parents who have one child with ASD are at increased risk for having more than one child with the disorder. Other studies with both monozygotic and dizygotic twins also have provided evidence of a genetic involvement. Research into how genetic factors influence the development of ASD is ongoing. A number of linkage studies have implicated areas on several chromosomes in the development of the disorder, most notably chromosomes 2, 7, 15, 16, and 17 (Brkanac, Raskind, & King, 2008; Shriber, 2012; Ursano et al., 2008). The results of a study by the Autism Genome Project Consortium, which was funded by the U.S. National Institutes of Health, have implicated a region on chromosome 11 and aberrations in a brain-development gene called *neurexin 1* (Autism Genome Project Consortium, 2007). The researchers stress that these findings strongly suggest the need for further study in this area.

Perinatal Influences

In a study by researchers at Kaiser Permanente in Oakland, California, it was found that women who suffered from asthma and/or allergies around the time of pregnancy were at increased risk of having a child affected by ASD (Croen, Grether, Yoshida, Odouli, & Van dewater, 2005). Women with asthma and allergies recorded during the second trimester had a greater than twofold elevated risk of having a child affected by the disorder. The researchers have postulated that this may be due to maternal immune response during pregnancy, or that asthma and allergy may share environmental risk factors with ASD.

Application of the Nursing Process to Autism Spectrum Disorder

Background Assessment Data (Symptomatology)

The symptomatology presented here is common among children with ASD. This information, as well as knowledge about predisposing factors associated with the disorder, is important in creating an accurate plan of care for the client. Because ASD is a *spectrum* disorder, the symptomatology described here would be observed on a degree-of-gravity continuum from mild to more severe.

Impairment in Social Interaction Children with ASD have difficulty forming interpersonal relationships with others. They show little interest in people and often do not respond to others' attempts at interaction. As infants they may have an aversion to affection and physical contact. As toddlers, the attachment to a significant adult may be either absent or manifested as exaggerated adherence behaviors. In childhood, there is failure to develop cooperative play, imaginative play, and friendships. Those children with minimal handicaps may eventually progress to the point of recognizing other children as part of their environment, if only in a passive manner.

Impairment in Communication and Imaginative Activity Both verbal and nonverbal skills are affected. Language may be totally absent or characterized by immature structure or idiosyncratic utterances whose meaning is clear only to those who are familiar with the child's past experiences. Nonverbal communication, such as facial expression or gestures, is often absent or socially inappropriate. The pattern of imaginative play is often restricted and stereotypical.

Restricted Activities and Interests Even minor changes in the environment are often met with resistance or sometimes with hysterical responses. Attachment to, or extreme fascination with, objects that move or spin (e.g., fans) is common. Routine may become an obsession, with minor alterations in routine leading to marked distress. Stereotyped body movements (hand-clapping, rocking, whole-body swaying) and verbalizations (repetition of words or phrases) are typical. Diet abnormalities may include eating only a few specific foods or consuming an excessive amount of fluids. Behaviors that are self-injurious, such as head banging or biting the hands or arms, may be evident.

The *DSM-5* diagnostic criteria for ASD are presented in Box 33-2. The criteria specify a range of behaviors, thus addressing the spectrum of symptomatology associated with this diagnosis.

Nursing Diagnosis

Based on data collected during the nursing assessment, possible nursing diagnoses for the client with ASD include the following:

■ Risk for self-mutilation related to neurological alterations; history of self-mutilative behaviors; hysterical reactions to changes in the environment

■ Impaired social interaction related to inability to trust; neurological alterations, evidenced by lack of responsiveness to, or interest in, people

■ Impaired verbal communication related to withdrawal into the self; neurological alterations, evidenced by inability or unwillingness to speak; lack of nonverbal expression

■ Disturbed personal identity related to neurological alterations; delayed developmental stage, evidenced by difficulty separating own physiological and emotional needs and personal boundaries from those of others

Outcome Identification

Outcome criteria include short- and long-term goals. Timelines are individually determined. The following criteria may be used for measurement of outcomes in the care of the client with ASD.

The client:

■ Exhibits no evidence of self-harm.
■ Interacts appropriately with at least one staff member.

BOX 33-2 Diagnostic Criteria for Autism Spectrum Disorder

A. Persistent deficits in social communication and social interaction across multiple contexts, as manifested by the following, currently or by history (examples are illustrative, not exhaustive):

1. Deficits in social-emotional reciprocity, ranging, for example, from abnormal social approach and failure of normal back-and-forth conversation; to reduced sharing of interests, emotions, or affect; to failure to initiate or respond to social interactions.
2. Deficits in nonverbal communicative behaviors used for social interaction, ranging, for example, from poorly integrated verbal and nonverbal communication; to abnormalities in eye contact and body language or deficits in understanding and use of gestures; to a total lack of facial expressions and nonverbal communication.
3. Deficits in developing, maintaining, and understanding relationships, ranging, for example, from difficulties adjusting behavior to suit various social contexts; to difficulties in sharing imaginative play or in making friends; to absence of interest in peers.

Specify current severity:

Severity is based on social communication impairments and restricted, repetitive patterns of behavior.

B. Restricted, repetitive patterns of behavior, interests, or activities, as manifested by at least two of the following, currently or by history (examples are illustrative, not exhaustive):

1. Stereotyped or repetitive motor movements, use of objects, or speech (e.g., simple motor stereotypies, lining up toys or flipping objects, echolalia, idiosyncratic phrases).
2. Insistence on sameness, inflexible adherence to routines, or ritualized patterns of verbal or nonverbal behavior (e.g., extreme distress at small changes, difficulties with transitions, rigid thinking patterns, greeting rituals, need to take same route or eat same food every day).

3. Highly restricted, fixated interests that are abnormal in intensity or focus (e.g., strong attachment to or preoccupation with unusual objects, excessively circumscribed or perseverative interests).
4. Hyper- or hypo-reactivity to sensory input or unusual interest in sensory aspects of environment (e.g., apparent indifference to pain/temperature, adverse response to specific sounds or textures, excessive smelling or touching of objects, visual fascination with lights or movement).

Specify current severity:

Severity is based on social communication impairments and restricted, repetitive patterns of behavior.

C. Symptoms must be present in the early developmental period (but may not become fully manifest until social demands exceed limited capacities, or may be masked by learned strategies in later life).
D. Symptoms cause clinically significant impairment in social, occupational, or other important areas of current functioning.
E. These disturbances are not better explained by intellectual disability (intellectual developmental disorder) or global developmental delay. Intellectual disability and autism spectrum disorder frequently co-occur; to make comorbid diagnoses of autism spectrum disorder and intellectual disability, social communication should be below that expected for general developmental level.

Specify if:

With or without accompanying intellectual impairment
With or without accompanying language impairment
Associated with a known medical or genetic condition or environmental factor
Associated with another neurodevelopmental, mental, or behavioral disorder
With catatonia

Reprinted with permission from the Diagnostic and Statistical Manual of Mental Disorders, Fifth Edition *(Copyright 2013). American Psychiatric Association.*

■ Demonstrates trust in at least one staff member.
■ Is able to communicate so that he or she can be understood by at least one staff member.
■ Demonstrates behaviors that indicate he or she has begun the separation/individuation process.

Planning/Implementation

Table 33-3 provides a plan of care for the child with ASD, including selected nursing diagnoses, outcome criteria, and appropriate nursing interventions and rationales.

Evaluation

Evaluation of care for the child with ASD reflects whether the nursing actions have been effective in

achieving the established goals. The nursing process calls for reassessment of the plan. Questions for gathering reassessment data may include the following:

■ Has the child been able to establish trust with at least *one* caregiver?
■ Have the nursing actions directed toward preventing mutilative behaviors been effective in protecting the client from self-harm?
■ Has the child attempted to interact with others? Has he or she received positive reinforcement for these efforts?
■ Has eye contact improved?

Table 33-3 | CARE PLAN FOR THE CHILD WITH AUTISM SPECTRUM DISORDER

NURSING DIAGNOSIS: RISK FOR SELF-MUTILATION

RELATED TO: Neurological alterations; history of self-mutilative behaviors; hysterical reactions to changes in the environment

OUTCOME CRITERIA	NURSING INTERVENTIONS	RATIONALE
Short-Term Goal • Client will demonstrate alternative behavior (e.g., initiating interaction between self and nurse) in response to anxiety within specified time. (Length of time required for this objective will depend on severity and chronicity of the disorder.) **Long-Term Goal** • Client will not harm self.	1. Work with the child on a one-to-one basis. 2. Try to determine if the self-mutilative behavior occurs in response to increasing anxiety, and if so, to what the anxiety may be attributed. 3. Try to intervene with diversion or replacement activities and offer self to the child as anxiety level starts to rise. 4. Protect the child when self-mutilative behaviors occur. Devices such as a helmet, padded hand mitts, or arm covers may provide protection when the risk for self-harm exists.	1. One-to-one interaction facilitates trust. 2. Mutilative behaviors may be averted if the cause can be determined and alleviated. 3. Diversion and replacement activities may provide needed feelings of security and substitute for self-mutilative behaviors. 4. Client safety is a priority nursing intervention.

NURSING DIAGNOSIS: IMPAIRED SOCIAL INTERACTION

RELATED TO: Inability to trust; neurological alterations

EVIDENCED BY: Lack of responsiveness to, or interest in, people

OUTCOME CRITERIA	NURSING INTERVENTIONS	RATIONALE
Short-Term Goal • Client will demonstrate trust in one caregiver (as evidenced by facial responsiveness and eye contract) within specified time (depending on severity and chronicity of disorder). **Long-Term Goal** • Client will initiate social interactions (physical, verbal, nonverbal) with caregiver by time of discharge from treatment.	1. Assign a limited number of caregivers to the child. Ensure that warmth, acceptance, and availability are conveyed. 2. Provide child with familiar objects, such as familiar toys or a blanket. Support child's attempts to interact with others. 3. Give positive reinforcement for eye contact with something acceptable to the child (e.g., food, familiar object). Gradually replace with social reinforcement (e.g., touch, smiling, hugging).	1. Warmth, acceptance, and availability, along with consistency of assignment, enhance the establishment and maintenance of a trusting relationship. 2. Familiar objects and presence of a trusted individual provide security during times of distress. 3. Being able to establish eye contact is essential to the child's ability to form satisfactory interpersonal relationships.

Table 33-3 | CARE PLAN FOR THE CHILD WITH AUTISM SPECTRUM DISORDER–cont'd

NURSING DIAGNOSIS: IMPAIRED VERBAL COMMUNICATION

RELATED TO: Withdrawal into the self; neurological alterations

EVIDENCED BY: Inability or unwillingness to speak; lack of nonverbal expression

OUTCOME CRITERIA	NURSING INTERVENTIONS	RATIONALE
Short-Term Goal • Client will establish trust with one caregiver (as evidenced by facial responsiveness and eye contact) by specified time (depending on severity and chronicity of disorder). **Long-Term Goal** • Client will establish a means of communicating needs and desires to others.	1. Maintain consistency in assignment of caregivers. 2. Anticipate and fulfill the child's needs until communication can be established. 3. Seek clarification and validation. 4. Give positive reinforcement when eye contact is used to convey nonverbal expressions.	1. Consistency facilitates trust and enhances the caregiver's ability to understand the child's attempts to communicate. 2. Anticipating needs helps to minimize frustration while the child is learning communication skills. 3. Validation ensures that the intended message has been conveyed. 4. Positive reinforcement increases self-esteem and encourages repetition.

NURSING DIAGNOSIS: DISTURBED PERSONAL IDENTITY

RELATED TO: Neurological alterations; delayed developmental stage

EVIDENCED BY: Difficulty separating own physiological and emotional needs and personal boundaries from those of others

OUTCOME CRITERIA	NURSING INTERVENTIONS	RATIONALE
Short-Term Goal • Client will name own body parts as separate and individual from those of others. **Long-Term Goal** • Client will develop ego identity (evidenced by ability to recognize physical and emotional self as separate from others) by time of discharge from treatment.	1. Assist child to recognize separateness during self-care activities, such as dressing and feeding. 2. Assist the child in learning to name own body parts. This can be facilitated by the use of mirrors, drawings, and pictures of the child. Encourage appropriate touching of, and being touched by, others.	1. Recognition of body parts during dressing and feeding increases the child's awareness of self as separate from others. 2. All of these activities may help increase the child's awareness of self as separate from others.

■ Has the child established a means of communicating his or her needs and desires to others? Have all self-care needs been met?

■ Does the child demonstrate an awareness of self as separate from others? Can he or she name own body parts and body parts of caregiver?

■ Can he or she accept touch from others? Does he or she willingly and appropriately touch others?

Psychopharmacological Intervention for ASD

The U.S. Food and Drug Administration (FDA) has approved two medications for the treatment of irritability associated with ASD: risperidone (Risperdal; in children and adolescents 5 to 16 years) and aripiprazole (Abilify; in children and adolescents 6 to 17 years). The behavior symptoms for which these medications are targeted include:

■ Aggression
■ Deliberate self-injury
■ Temper tantrums
■ Quickly changing moods

Dosage of risperidone for ASD is based on weight of the child and the clinical response. In clinical trials, children weighing between 15 and 45 kg received 2.5 mg per day, and those weighing more than 45 kg received 3.5 mg per day. The most common side effects were drowsiness, mild to moderate increase in appetite, nasal congestion, fatigue, constipation, drooling, dizziness, and weight gain. Although some reports of "abnormal movements" were described, no cases of tardive dyskinesia were reported in clinical studies (Research Units on Pediatric Psychopharmacology Autism Network, 2002, 2005). When administering risperidone, caution must be maintained concerning less common but more serious possible side effects, including neuroleptic malignant syndrome, tardive dyskinesia, hyperglycemia, and diabetes.

In clinical studies with aripiprazole, the most frequently reported adverse events included sedation, fatigue, weight gain, vomiting, somnolence, and tremor. The most common reasons for discontinuation of aripiprazole were sedation, drooling, tremor, vomiting, and extrapyramidal disorder.

Dosage with aripiprazole for irritability in ASD is initiated at 2 mg/day. Dosage may be increased by 5 mg/day at intervals of no less than 1 week, up to a maximum of 15 mg/day. The efficacy of maintenance therapy with aripiprazole has not been evaluated, and clients should be periodically reassessed to determine the need for continued treatment.

CORE CONCEPT

Hyperactivity

Excessive psychomotor activity that may be purposeful or aimless, accompanied by physical movements and verbal utterances that are usually more rapid than normal. Inattention and distractibility are common with hyperactive behavior.

Attention-Deficit/Hyperactivity Disorder

Clinical Findings, Epidemiology, and Course

The essential behavior pattern of a child with attention-deficit/hyperactivity disorder (ADHD) is one of inattention and/or hyperactivity and **impulsivity.** These children are highly distractible and unable to contain their responses to stimuli. Motor activity is excessive, and movements are random and impulsive. Onset of the disorder is difficult to diagnose in children younger than age 4 years because their characteristic behavior is much more variable than that of older children. Frequently the disorder is not recognized until the child enters school. It is more common in boys than in girls by a ratio of approximately 3:1 and may occur in as many as 9 percent of school-age children (CDC, 2011). In about 60 to 70 percent

of the cases, ADHD persists into young adulthood, and about 25 percent will subsequently meet the criteria for antisocial personality disorder as adults (Black & Andreasen, 2011).

In making the diagnosis of ADHD, the *DSM-5* criteria are further specified according to current clinical presentation. These subtypes include a combined presentation (meeting the criteria for both inattention and hyperactivity/impulsivity), a predominantly inattentive presentation, and a predominantly hyperactive/impulsive presentation.

CORE CONCEPT

Impulsiveness

The trait of acting without reflection and without thought to the consequences of the behavior. An abrupt inclination to act (and the inability to resist acting) on certain behavioral urges.

Predisposing Factors

Biological Influences

Genetics A number of studies have revealed supportive evidence of genetic influences in the etiology of ADHD. Results have indicated that a large number of parents of hyperactive children showed signs of hyperactivity during their own childhood; that hyperactive children are more likely than other children to have siblings who are also hyperactive; and that when one twin of an identical twin pair has the disorder, the other is likely to have it too (Kollins, 2008). Adoption studies reveal that biological parents of children with ADHD have more psychopathology than the adoptive parents.

One research study of genetic evidence for ADHD found copy number variants on a specific region of chromosome 16 (Williams et al., 2010). The researchers also found that copy number variants overlap with chromosomal regions previously linked to ASD and schizophrenia.

Biochemical Theory Although it is believed that certain neurotransmitters—particularly dopamine, norepinephrine, and possibly serotonin—are involved in producing the symptoms associated with ADHD, their involvement is still under investigation. Abnormal levels of these neurotransmitters may be associated with the symptoms of inattention, hyperactivity, impulsivity, mood, and **aggression** often observed in individuals with the disorder (Faraone, 2006; Hunt, 2006). (See Fig. 33-1).

Anatomical Influences Some studies have implicated alterations in specific areas of the brain in individuals with ADHD. These regions include the prefrontal

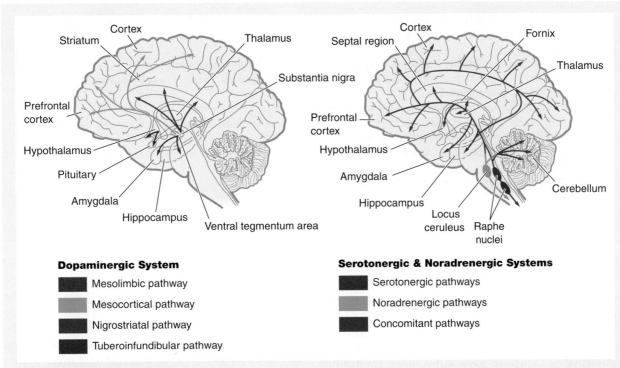

FIGURE 33-1 Neurobiology of attention-deficit/hyperactivity disorder.

NEUROTRANSMITTERS

The major neurotransmitters implicated in the pathophysiology of ADHD are dopamine, norepinephrine, and possibly serotonin. Dopamine and norepinephrine appear to be depleted in ADHD. Serotonin in ADHD has been studied less extensively, but recent evidence suggests that it also is reduced in children with ADHD.

NEUROTRANSMITTER FUNCTIONS

- Norepinephrine is thought to play a role in the ability to perform executive functions, such as analysis and reasoning, and in the cognitive alertness essential for processing stimuli and sustaining attention and thought (Hunt, 2006).
- Dopamine is thought to play a role in sensory filtering, memory, concentration, controlling emotions, locomotor activity, and reasoning.
- Deficits in norepinephrine and dopamine have both been implicated in the inattention, impulsiveness, and hyperactivity associated with ADHD.
- Serotonin appears to play a role in ADHD, although possibly less significant than norepinephrine and dopamine. It has been suggested that alterations in serotonin may be related to the disinhibition and impulsivity observed in children with ADHD. It may play a role in mood disorders, particularly depression, which is a common comorbid disorder associated with ADHD.

FUNCTIONAL AREAS OF THE BRAIN AFFECTED

- **Prefrontal cortex:** Associated with maintaining attention, organization, and executive function. Also serves to modulate behavior inhibition, with serotonin as the predominant central inhibiting neurotransmitter for this function.
- **Basal ganglia** (particularly the caudate nucleus and globus pallidus): Involved in the regulation of high-level movements. In association with its connecting circuits to the prefrontal cortex, may also be important in cognition. Interruptions in these circuits may result in inattention or impulsivity.
- **Hippocampus:** Plays an important role in learning and memory.
- **Limbic system** (composed of the amygdala, hippocampus, mammillary body, hypothalamus, thalamus, fornix, cingulate gyrus and septum pallucidum): Regulation of emotions. A neurotransmitter deficiency in this area may result in restlessness, inattention, or emotional volatility.
- **Reticular activating system** (composed of the reticular formation [located in the brain stem] and its connections): It is the major relay system among the many pathways that enter and leave the brain. It is thought to be the center of arousal and motivation and is crucial for maintaining a state of consciousness.

MEDICATIONS FOR ADHD

CNS Stimulants

- Amphetamines (dextroamphetamine, lisdexamfetamine, methamphetamine, and mixtures): cause the release of norepinephrine from central noradrenergic neurons. At higher doses, dopamine may be released in the mesolimbic system.
- Methylphenidate and dexmethylphenidate: block the reuptake of norepinephrine and dopamine into the presynaptic neuron and increase the release of these monoamines into the extraneuronal space.

Continued

Side effects of CNS stimulants include restlessness, insomnia, headache, palpitations, weight loss, suppression of growth in children (with long-term use), increased blood pressure, abdominal pain, anxiety, tolerance, and physical and psychological dependence.

Others

• Atomoxatine: selectively inhibits the reuptake of norepinephrine by blocking the presynaptic transporter.

Side effects include headache, upper abdominal pain, nausea and vomiting, anorexia, cough, dry mouth, constipation, increase in heart rate and blood pressure, and fatigue.

• Bupropion: inhibits the reuptake of norepinephrine and dopamine into presynaptic neurons.

Side effects include headache, dizziness, insomnia or sedation, tachycardia, increased blood pressure, dry mouth, nausea and vomiting, weight gain or loss, and seizures (dose dependent).

• Alpha agonists (clonidine, guanfacine): stimulate central alpha-adrenoreceptors in the brain resulting in reduced sympathetic outflow from the CNS.

Side effects include palpitations, bradycardia, constipation, dry mouth, and sedation.

lobes, basal ganglia, caudate nucleus, globus pallidus, and cerebellum (Ursano et al., 2008).

Prenatal, Perinatal, and Postnatal Factors Maternal smoking during pregnancy has been linked to hyperkinetic-impulsive behavior in offspring (Linnet et al., 2005; Rizwan, Manning, & Brabin, 2007). Intrauterine exposure to toxic substances, including alcohol, can produce effects on behavior. Fetal alcohol syndrome includes hyperactivity, impulsivity, and inattention, as well as physical anomalies (see Chapter 23).

Perinatal influences that may contribute to ADHD are prematurity or low birth weight, signs of fetal distress, precipitated or prolonged labor, and perinatal asphyxia and low Apgar scores (Bhat, Grizenko, Ben-Amor, & Joober, 2005). Postnatal factors that have been implicated include cerebral palsy, seizures, and other central nervous system (CNS) abnormalities resulting from trauma, infections, or other neurological disorders (Ben-Amor et al., 2005; Popper, Gammon, West, & Bailey, 2003).

Environmental Influences

Environmental Lead Studies continue to provide evidence of the adverse effects of elevated body levels of lead on cognitive and behavioral development in children (Braun, Kahn, Froehlich, Auinger, & Lanphear, 2006; Nigg, Nikolas, Knottnerus, Cavanagh, & Friderici, 2010). The government has placed tighter restrictions on the substance in recent years, making exposure to toxic levels less prevalent than it once was. However, reports indicate that at least 4 million households in the United States have children living in them who are being exposed to lead, and that approximately 500,000 U.S. children ages 1 to 5 have blood lead levels above 5 micrograms per deciliter, the reference level at which the initiation of public health actions are recommended (CDC, 2012a).

Diet Factors The possible link between food dyes and additives, such as artificial flavorings and preservatives, was introduced in the mid-1970s. Studies on the effect of food and food-additive allergies remain controversial, largely because of the inconsistencies in the results. Striking improvement in behavior has been reported by some parents and teachers when hyperactive children are placed on a diet free of dyes and additives. Researchers in Great Britain reported on a study that revealed significant hyperactive behavior in 3-, 8-, and 9-year-old children who were given fruit drinks with food additives compared with children who received a placebo drink (McCann et al., 2007). Further study in this area is still required.

Another diet factor that has received much attention in its possible link to ADHD is sugar. A number of studies have been conducted in an effort to determine the effect of sugar on hyperactive behavior, and the results strongly suggest that sugar plays no role in hyperactivity.

Psychosocial Influences

Disorganized or chaotic environments or a disruption in family equilibrium may contribute to ADHD in some individuals. A high degree of psychosocial stress, maternal mental disorder, paternal criminality, low socioeconomic status, living in poverty, growing up in an institution, and unstable foster care have been shown to increase the risk of ADHD in predisposed individuals (Dopheide & Pliszka, 2009; Voeller, 2004).

Application of the Nursing Process to ADHD

Background Assessment Data (Symptomatology)

A major portion of the hyperactive child's problems relate to difficulties in performing age-appropriate tasks. Hyperactive children are highly distractible and have extremely limited attention spans. They often shift from one uncompleted activity to another. Impulsivity, or deficit in inhibitory control, is also common.

Hyperactive children have difficulty forming satisfactory interpersonal relationships. They demonstrate behaviors that inhibit acceptable social interaction. They are disruptive and intrusive in group endeavors. They have difficulty complying with social norms. Some children with ADHD are very aggressive or oppositional, whereas others exhibit more regressive and immature behaviors. Low frustration tolerance and outbursts of temper are common.

Children with ADHD have boundless energy, exhibiting excessive levels of activity, restlessness, and fidgeting. They have been described as "perpetual motion machines," continuously running, jumping, wiggling, or squirming. They experience a greater than average number of accidents, from minor mishaps to more serious incidents that may lead to physical injury or the destruction of property. The *DSM-5* diagnostic criteria for ADHD are presented in Box 33-3.

BOX 33-3 Diagnostic Criteria for Attention-Deficit/Hyperactivity Disorder

A. A persistent pattern of inattention and/or hyperactivity-impulsivity that interferes with functioning or development, as characterized by (1) and/or (2):

1. **Inattention:** Six (or more) of the following symptoms have persisted for at least 6 months to a degree that is inconsistent with developmental level and that negatively impacts directly on social and academic/occupational activities. *Note:* The symptoms are not solely a manifestation of oppositional behavior, defiance, hostility, or failure to understand tasks or instructions. For older adolescents and adults (age 17 and older), at least five symptoms are required.
   a. Often fails to give close attention to details or makes careless mistakes in schoolwork, at work, or during other activities (e.g., overlooks or misses details, work is inaccurate).
   b. Often has difficulty sustaining attention in tasks or play activities (e.g., has difficulty remaining focused during lectures, conversations, or reading lengthy reading).
   c. Often does not seem to listen when spoken to directly (e.g., mind seems elsewhere, even in the absence of any obvious distraction).
   d. Often does not follow through on instructions and fails to finish schoolwork, chores, or duties in the workplace (e.g., starts tasks but quickly loses focus and is easily sidetracked).
   e. Often has difficulty organizing tasks and activities (e.g., difficulty managing sequential tasks; difficulty keeping materials and belongings in order; messy, disorganized, work; has poor time management; fails to meet deadlines).
   f. Often avoids, dislikes, or is reluctant to engage in tasks that require sustained mental effort (e.g., schoolwork or homework; for older adolescents and adults, preparing reports, completing forms, reviewing lengthy papers).
   g. Often loses things necessary for tasks or activities (e.g., school materials, pencils, books, tools, wallets, keys, paperwork, eyeglasses, or mobile telephones).
   h. Is often easily distracted by extraneous stimuli (for older adolescents and adults, may include unrelated thoughts).
   i. Is often forgetful in daily activities (e.g., chores, running errands; for older adolescents and adults, returning calls, paying bills, keeping appointments).

2. **Hyperactivity and Impulsivity:** Six (or more) of the following symptoms have persisted for at least 6 months to a degree that is inconsistent with developmental level and that negatively impacts directly on social and academic/occupational activities. *Note:* The symptoms are not solely a manifestation of oppositional behavior, defiance, hostility, or a failure to understand tasks or instructions. For older adolescents and adults (age 17 and older), at least five symptoms are required.
   a. Often fidgets with or taps hands or feet or squirms in seat.
   b. Often leaves seat in situations when remaining seated is expected (e.g., leaves his or her place in the classroom, in the office or other workplace, or in other situations that require remaining in place).
   c. Often runs about or climbs in situations where it is inappropriate. (*Note:* In adolescents or adults, may be limited to feeling restless).
   d. Often unable to play or engage in leisure activities quietly.
   e. Is often "on the go," acting as if "driven by a motor" (e.g., is unable to be or uncomfortable being still for extended time, as in restaurants, meetings; may be experienced by others as being restless and difficult to keep up with).
   f. Often talks excessively.
   g. Often blurts out an answer before a question has been completed (e.g., completes people's sentences; cannot wait for turn in conversation).
   h. Often has difficulty waiting his or her turn (e.g., while waiting in line).
   i. Often interrupts or intrudes on others (e.g., butts into conversations, games, or activities; may start using other people's things without asking or receiving permission; for adolescents or adults, may intrude into or take over what others are doing).

B. Several inattentive or hyperactive-impulsive symptoms were present prior to age 12 years.

C. Several inattentive or hyperactive-impulsive symptoms are present in two or more settings (e.g., at home, school or work; with friends or relatives; in other activities).

D. There is clear evidence that the symptoms interfere with or reduce the quality of social, academic, or occupational functioning.

Continued

BOX 33-3 Diagnostic Criteria for Attention-Deficit/Hyperactivity Disorder–cont'd

E. The symptoms do not occur exclusively during the course of schizophrenia or another psychotic disorder and are not better explained by another mental disorder (e.g., mood disorder, anxiety disorder, dissociative disorder, personality disorder, substance intoxication or withdrawal).

Specify whether:

1. **Combined presentation:** If both Criterion A1 (inattention) and Criterion A2 (hyperactivity-impulsivity) are met for the past 6 months.

2. **Predominantly inattentive presentation:** If Criterion A1 (inattention) is met but Criterion A2 (hyperactivity-impulsivity) is not met for the past 6 months.

3. **Predominantly hyperactive/impulsive presentation:** If Criterion A2 (hyperactivity-impulsivity) is met and Criterion A1 (inattention) is not met for the past 6 months.

Specify if: **In partial remission**
Specify current severity: **Mild, Moderate, Severe**

Reprinted with permission from the Diagnostic and Statistical Manual of Mental Disorders, Fifth Edition *(Copyright 2013). American Psychiatric Association.*

Comorbidity The prevalence of comorbid psychiatric disorders with ADHD may be as high as 84 percent (Ferguson-Noyes & Wilkinson, 2008). Those commonly identified include oppositional defiant disorder, conduct disorder, anxiety, depression, bipolar disorder, and substance abuse. It is extremely important to identify and treat any comorbid psychiatric conditions in a child with ADHD. In some instances, as with anxiety and depression, the comorbid disorders may be treated concurrently with the symptoms of ADHD. Jenson (2005) suggests that comorbid depression and ADHD may respond to bupropion or atomoxetine as a single agent, and individuals with comorbid anxiety and ADHD may benefit from treatment with atomoxetine (Dopheide & Pliszka, 2009).

Other disorders may require separate treatment. Wilens and Upadhyaya (2007) state, "In patients with coexisting substance use disorders and ADHD, the priority is to stabilize the addiction before treating the ADHD." Because stimulants can exacerbate mania, it is suggested that medication for ADHD be initiated only after bipolar symptoms have been controlled with a mood stabilizer (Dopheide & Pliszka, 2009). Types of conditions often seen with ADHD and their rate of comorbidity are presented in Table 33-4.

Nursing Diagnosis

Based on the data collected during the nursing assessment, possible nursing diagnoses for the child with ADHD include the following:

■ Risk for injury related to impulsive and accident-prone behavior and the inability to perceive self-harm

■ Impaired social interaction related to intrusive and immature behavior

■ Low self-esteem related to dysfunctional family system and negative feedback

TABLE 33–4 Type and Frequency of Comorbidity With Attention-Deficit/Hyperactivity Disorder

COMORBIDITY	RATES
Oppositional defiant disorder	Up to 50%
Conduct disorder	~33%
Learning disorders	20%–30%
Anxiety	25%–35%
Depression	~26%
Bipolar disorder	11%–20%
Substance use	13%–26%

SOURCES: Dopheide & Pliszka (2009); Ferguson-Noyes & Wilkinson (2008); Jenson (2005); and Robb (2006).

■ Noncompliance with task expectations related to low frustration tolerance and short attention span

Outcome Identification

Outcome criteria include short- and long-term goals. Timelines are individually determined. The following criteria may be used for measurement of outcomes in the care of the child with ADHD.

The client:

■ Has experienced no physical harm.
■ Interacts with others appropriately.
■ Verbalizes positive aspects about self.
■ Demonstrates fewer demanding behaviors.
■ Cooperatives with staff in an effort to complete assigned tasks.

Planning/Implementation

Table 33-5 provides a plan of care for the child with ADHD using nursing diagnoses common to the

Table 33-5 | CARE PLAN FOR THE CHILD WITH ATTENTION-DEFICIT/HYPERACTIVITY DISORDER

NURSING DIAGNOSIS: RISK FOR INJURY

RELATED TO: Impulsive and accident-prone behavior and the inability to perceive self-harm

OUTCOME CRITERIA	NURSING INTERVENTIONS	RATIONALE
Short- and Long-Term Goal • Client will be free of injury.	1. Ensure that client has a safe environment. Remove objects from immediate area on which client could injure self as a result of random, hyperactive movements.	1. Objects that are appropriate to the normal living situation can be hazardous to the child whose motor activities are out of control.
	2. Identify deliberate behaviors that put the child at risk for injury. Institute consequences for repetition of this behavior.	2. Behavior can be modified with aversive reinforcement.
	3. If there is risk of injury associated with specific therapeutic activities, provide adequate supervision and assistance, or limit client's participation if adequate supervision is not possible.	3. Client safety is a nursing priority.

NURSING DIAGNOSIS: IMPAIRED SOCIAL INTERACTION

RELATED TO: Intrusive and immature behavior

OUTCOME CRITERIA	NURSING INTERVENTIONS	RATIONALE
Short-Term Goal • Client will interact in age-appropriate manner with nurse in one-to-one relationship within 1 week. **Long-Term Goal** • Client will observe limits set on intrusive behavior and will demonstrate ability to interact appropriately with others.	1. Develop a trusting relationship with the child. Convey acceptance of the child separate from the unacceptable behavior.	1. Unconditional acceptance increases feelings of self-worth.
	2. Discuss with client those behaviors that are and are not acceptable. Describe in a matter-of-fact manner the consequences of unacceptable behavior. Follow through.	2. Aversive reinforcement can alter undesirable behaviors.
	3. Provide group situations for client.	3. Appropriate social behavior is often learned from the positive and negative feedback of peers.

NURSING DIAGNOSIS: LOW SELF-ESTEEM

RELATED TO: Dysfunctional family system and negative feedback

OUTCOME CRITERIA	NURSING INTERVENTIONS	RATIONALE
Short-Term Goal • Client will independently direct own care and activities of daily living within 1 week.	1. Ensure that goals are realistic.	1. Unrealistic goals set up client for failure, which diminishes self-esteem.
	2. Plan activities that provide opportunities for success.	2. Success enhances self-esteem.

Continued

Table 33-5 | CARE PLAN FOR THE CHILD WITH ATTENTION-DEFICIT/HYPERACTIVITY DISORDER—cont'd

OUTCOME CRITERIA	NURSING INTERVENTIONS	RATIONALE
Long-Term Goal • Client will demonstrate increased feelings of self-worth by verbalizing positive statements about self and exhibiting fewer demanding behaviors.	3. Convey unconditional acceptance and positive regard. 4. Offer recognition of successful endeavors and positive reinforcement for attempts made. Give immediate positive feedback for acceptable behavior.	3. Affirmation of client as worthwhile human being may increase self-esteem. 4. Positive reinforcement enhances self-esteem and may increase the desired behaviors.

NURSING DIAGNOSIS: NONCOMPLIANCE (WITH TASK EXPECTATIONS)

RELATED TO: Low frustration tolerance and short attention span

OUTCOME CRITERIA	NURSING INTERVENTIONS	RATIONALE
Short-Term Goal • Client will participate in and cooperate during therapeutic activities. **Long-Term Goal** • Client will be able to complete assigned tasks independently or with a minimum of assistance.	1. Provide an environment for task efforts that is as free of distractions as possible. 2. Provide assistance on a one-to-one basis, beginning with simple, concrete instructions. 3. Ask client to repeat instructions to you. 4. Establish goals that allow client to complete a part of the task, rewarding each step-completion with a break for physical activity. 5. Gradually decrease the amount of assistance given, while assuring the client that assistance is still available if deemed necessary.	1. Client is highly distractible and is unable to perform in the presence of even minimal stimulation. 2. Client lacks the ability to assimilate information that is complicated or has abstract meaning. 3. Repetition of the instructions helps to determine client's level of comprehension. 4. Short-term goals are not so overwhelming to one with such a short attention span. The positive reinforcement (physical activity) increases self-esteem and provides incentive for client to pursue the task to completion. 5. This encourages the client to perform independently while providing a feeling of security with the presence of a trusted individual.

disorder, outcome criteria, and appropriate nursing interventions and rationales.

Concept Care Mapping

The concept map care plan is an innovative approach to planning and organizing nursing care (see Chapter 9). It is a diagrammatic teaching and learning strategy that allows visualization of interrelationships between medical diagnoses, nursing diagnoses, assessment data, and treatments. An example of a concept map care plan for a client with ADHD is presented in Figure 33-2.

Evaluation

Evaluation of the care of a client with ADHD involves examining client behaviors following implementation of the nursing actions to determine if the goals of therapy have been achieved. Collecting data by using the following types of questions may provide appropriate information for evaluation.

■ Have the nursing actions directed at client safety been effective in protecting the child from injury?
■ Has the child been able to establish a trusting relationship with the primary caregiver?

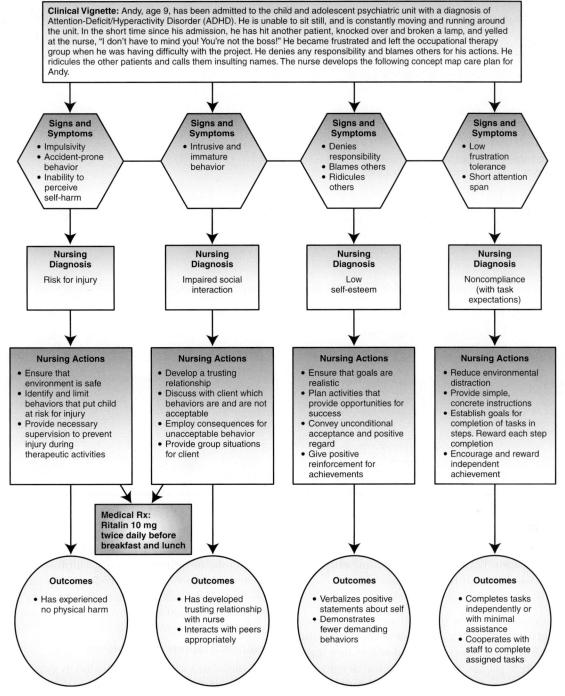

Clinical Vignette: Andy, age 9, has been admitted to the child and adolescent psychiatric unit with a diagnosis of Attention-Deficit/Hyperactivity Disorder (ADHD). He is unable to sit still, and is constantly moving and running around the unit. In the short time since his admission, he has hit another patient, knocked over and broken a lamp, and yelled at the nurse, "I don't have to mind you! You're not the boss!" He became frustrated and left the occupational therapy group when he was having difficulty with the project. He denies any responsibility and blames others for his actions. He ridicules the other patients and calls them insulting names. The nurse develops the following concept map care plan for Andy.

Signs and Symptoms
- Impulsivity
- Accident-prone behavior
- Inability to perceive self-harm

Signs and Symptoms
- Intrusive and immature behavior

Signs and Symptoms
- Denies responsibility
- Blames others
- Ridicules others

Signs and Symptoms
- Low frustration tolerance
- Short attention span

Nursing Diagnosis
Risk for injury

Nursing Diagnosis
Impaired social interaction

Nursing Diagnosis
Low self-esteem

Nursing Diagnosis
Noncompliance (with task expectations)

Nursing Actions
- Ensure that environment is safe
- Identify and limit behaviors that put child at risk for injury
- Provide necessary supervision to prevent injury during therapeutic activities

Nursing Actions
- Develop a trusting relationship
- Discuss with client which behaviors are and are not acceptable
- Employ consequences for unacceptable behavior
- Provide group situations for client

Nursing Actions
- Ensure that goals are realistic
- Plan activities that provide opportunities for success
- Convey unconditional acceptance and positive regard
- Give positive reinforcement for achievements

Nursing Actions
- Reduce environmental distraction
- Provide simple, concrete instructions
- Establish goals for completion of tasks in steps. Reward each step completion
- Encourage and reward independent achievement

Medical Rx: Ritalin 10 mg twice daily before breakfast and lunch

Outcomes
- Has experienced no physical harm

Outcomes
- Has developed trusting relationship with nurse
- Interacts with peers appropriately

Outcomes
- Verbalizes positive statements about self
- Demonstrates fewer demanding behaviors

Outcomes
- Completes tasks independently or with minimal assistance
- Cooperates with staff to complete assigned tasks

FIGURE 33–2 Concept map care plan for a client with attention-deficit/hyperactivity disorder.

■ Is the client responding to limits set on unacceptable behaviors?

■ Is the client able to interact appropriately with others?

■ Is the client able to verbalize positive statements about self?

■ Is the client able to complete tasks independently or with a minimum of assistance? Can he or she follow through after listening to simple instructions?

■ Is the client able to apply self-control to decrease motor activity?

Psychopharmacological Intervention for ADHD

Indications

Examples of commonly used agents for ADHD are presented in Table 33-6. The medications discussed in this section are used for ADHD in children and adults. Amphetamines are also used in the treatment of narcolepsy and exogenous obesity. Bupropion is

TABLE 33–6 Medications for Attention-Deficit/Hyperactivity Disorder

CHEMICAL CLASS	GENERIC (TRADE) NAME	DAILY DOSAGE RANGE (mg)	CONTROLLED CATEGORIES	PREGNANCY CATEGORIES/ HALF-LIFE (hr)
CNS STIMULANTS	Dextroamphetamine sulfate (Dexedrine; Dextrostat)	2.5–40	C-II	C/ ~12
Amphetamines	Methamphetamine (Desoxyn)	5–25	C-II	C/ 4–5
	Lisdexamfetamine (Vyvanse)	20–70	C-II	C/< 1
Amphetamine Mixtures	Dextroamphetamine/ amphetamine (Adderall; Adderall XR)	2.5–40	C-II	C/ 9–13
Miscellaneous	Methylphenidate (Ritalin; Ritalin-SR; Ritalin LA; Methylin; Methylin ER; Metadate ER; Metadate CD; Concerta; Daytrana)	10–60	C-II	C/ 2–4
	Dexmethylphenidate (Focalin)	5–20	C-II	C/ 2.2
ALPHA AGONISTS	Clonidine (Catapres)	0.05–0.3	—	C/ 12–16
	Guanfacine (Tenex; Intuniv)	1–4	—	B/ 10–30
MISCELLANEOUS	Atomoxetine (Strattera)	>70 kg: 40–100; ≤ 70 kg: 0.5– 1.4 mg/kg (or 100 mg– whichever is less)	—	C/ 5.2 (metabolites 6–8)
	Bupropion (Wellbutrin; Wellbutrin SR; Wellbutrin XL)	3 mg/kg (ADHD); 100–300 (depression)	—	C/ 8–24

used in the treatment of major depression and for smoking cessation (Zyban only). Clonidine and guanfacine are used to treat hypertension.

Action

CNS stimulants increase levels of neurotransmitters (probably norepinephrine, dopamine, and serotonin) in the CNS. They produce CNS and respiratory stimulation, dilated pupils, increased motor activity and mental alertness, diminished sense of fatigue, and brighter spirits. The CNS stimulants discussed in this section include dextroamphetamine sulfate, methamphetamine, lisdexamfetamine, amphetamine mixtures, methylphenidate, and dexmethylphenidate. Action in the treatment of ADHD is unclear. However, recent research indicates that their effectiveness in the treatment of hyperactivity disorders is based on the activation of dopamine D4 receptors in the basal ganglia and thalamus, which depress, rather than enhance, motor activity (Erlij et al, 2012).

Atomoxetine inhibits the reuptake of norepinephrine, and bupropion blocks the neuronal uptake of serotonin, norepinephrine, and dopamine. Clonidine and guanfacine stimulate central alpha-adrenoreceptors in the brain resulting in reduced sympathetic outflow from the CNS. The exact mechanism by which these nonstimulant drugs produce the therapeutic effect in ADHD is unclear.

Contraindications/Precautions

CNS stimulants are contraindicated in individuals with hypersensitivity to sympathomimetic amines. They should not be used in advanced arteriosclerosis, cardiovascular disease, hypertension, hyperthyroidism, glaucoma, agitated or hyperexcitability states; in clients with a history of drug abuse; during or within 14 days of receiving therapy with monoamine oxidase inhibitors (MAOIs); in children younger than 3 years of age; and in pregnancy and lactation. Atomoxetine and bupropion are contraindicated in clients with hypersensitivity to the drugs or their components; in lactation; and in concomitant use with, or within 2 weeks of using MAOIs. Atomoxetine is contraindicated in clients with narrow-angle glaucoma. Bupropion is contraindicated in individuals with known or suspected seizure disorder, in the acute phase of myocardial infarction, and in clients with bulimia or anorexia nervosa. Alpha agonists are contraindicated in clients with known hypersensitivity to the drugs.

Caution is advised in using CNS stimulants in children with psychosis; in Tourette's disorder; in clients with anorexia or insomnia; in elderly, debilitated, or asthenic clients; and in clients with a history of suicidal or homicidal tendencies. Prolonged use may result in tolerance and physical or psychological dependence. Atomoxetine and bupropion should be used cautiously in clients with urinary retention; hypertension; hepatic, renal, or cardiovascular disease; suicidal clients; pregnancy; and elderly and debilitated clients. Alpha agonists should be used with caution in clients with coronary insufficiency, recent myocardial infarction, or cerebrovascular disease; in chronic renal or hepatic failure; in the elderly; and in pregnancy and lactation.

Interactions

CNS Stimulants (Amphetamines) Effects of amphetamines are increased with furazolidone or urinary alkalinizers. Hypertensive crisis may occur with concomitant use of (and up to several weeks after discontinuing) MAOIs. Increased risk of serotonin syndrome occurs with coadministration of selective serotonin reuptake inhibitors (SSRIs). Decreased effects of amphetamines occur with urinary acidifiers, and decreased hypotensive effects of guanethidine occur with amphetamines.

Dexmethylphenidate and Methylphenidate Effects of antihypertensive agents and pressor agents (e.g., dopamine, epinephrine, phenylephrine) are decreased with concomitant use of the methylphenidates. Effects of coumarin anticoagulants, anticonvulsants (e.g., phenobarbital, phenytoin, primidone), tricyclic antidepressants, and SSRIs are increased with the methylphenidates. Hypertensive crisis may occur with coadministration of MAOIs.

Atomoxetine Effects of atomoxetine are increased with concomitant use of cytochrome P450 isozyme 2D6 (CYP2D6) inhibitors (e.g., paroxetine, fluoxetine, quinidine). Potentially fatal reactions may occur with concurrent use of (or within 2 weeks of discontinuation of) MAOIs. Risk of cardiovascular effects is increased with concomitant use of albuterol or vasopressors.

Bupropion Effects of bupropion are increased with amantadine, levodopa, or ritonavir. Effects of bupropion are decreased with carbamazepine. There is increased risk of acute toxicity with MAOIs. Increased risk of hypertension may occur with nicotine replacement agents, and adverse neuropsychiatric events may occur with

alcohol. Increased anticoagulant effects of warfarin, as well as increased effects of drugs metabolized by CYP2D6 (e.g., nortriptyline, imipramine, desipramine, paroxetine, fluoxetine, sertraline, haloperidol, risperidone, thioridazine, metoprolol, propafenone, and flecainide), occur with concomitant use.

Alpha Agonists Synergistic pharmacologic and toxic effects, possibly causing atrioventricular (AV) block, bradycardia, and severe hypotension, may occur with concomitant use of calcium channel blockers or beta blockers. Additive sedation occurs with CNS depressants, including alcohol, antihistamines, opioid analgesics, and sedative/hypnotics. Effects of clonidine may be decreased with concomitant use of tricyclic antidepressants and prazosin. Decreased effects of levodopa may occur with clonidine, and effects of guanfacine are decreased with barbiturates or phenytoin.

Side Effects

The plan of care should include monitoring for the following side effects from agents for ADHD. Nursing implications related to each side effect are designated by an asterisk (*).

■ Overstimulation, restlessness, insomnia (with CNS stimulants)
  *Assess mental status for changes in mood, level of activity, degree of stimulation, and aggressiveness.
  *Ensure that the client is protected from injury.
  *Keep stimuli low and environment as quiet as possible to discourage overstimulation.
  *To prevent insomnia, administer the last dose at least 6 hours before bedtime. Administer sustained-release forms in the morning.

■ Palpitations, tachycardia (with CNS stimulants; atomoxetine; bupropion; clonidine) or bradycardia (with clonidine and guanfacine)
  *Monitor and record vital signs at regular intervals (two or three times a day) throughout therapy. Report significant changes to the physician immediately.

NOTE: The FDA has issued warnings associated with CNS stimulants and atomoxetine of the risk for sudden death in patients who have cardiovascular disease. A careful personal and family history of heart disease, heart defects, or hypertension should be obtained before these medications are prescribed. Careful monitoring of cardiovascular function during administration must be ongoing.

■ Anorexia, weight loss (with CNS stimulants, atomoxetine, and bupropion)
  *To reduce anorexia, the medication may be administered immediately after meals. The client should be weighed regularly (at least weekly) when receiving therapy with CNS stimulants, atomoxetine, or

bupropion because of the potential for anorexia and weight loss, and temporary interruption of growth and development.

■ Tolerance, physical and psychological dependence (with CNS stimulants)

*Tolerance develops rapidly.

*In children with ADHD, a drug "holiday" should be attempted periodically under the supervision of the physician to determine the effectiveness of the medication and the need for continuation.

*The drug should not be withdrawn abruptly. To do so could initiate the following syndrome of symptoms: nausea, vomiting, abdominal cramping, headache, fatigue, weakness, mental depression, suicidal ideation, increased dreaming, and psychotic behavior.

■ Nausea and vomiting (with atomoxetine and bupropion)

*May be taken with food to minimize GI upset.

■ Constipation (with atomoxetine, bupropion, clonidine, and guanfacine)

*Increase fiber and fluid in diet, if not contraindicated.

■ Dry mouth (with clonidine and guanfacine)

*Offer the client sugarless candy, ice, frequent sips of water.

*Strict oral hygiene is very important.

■ Sedation (with clonidine and guanfacine)

*Warn client that this effect is increased by concomitant use of alcohol and other CNS drugs.

*Warn clients to refrain from driving or performing hazardous tasks until response has been established.

■ Potential for seizures (with bupropion)

*Protect client from injury if seizure should occur. Instruct family and significant others of clients on bupropion therapy how to protect client during a seizure if one should occur. Ensure that doses of the immediate release medication are administered at least 4 to 6 hours apart and doses of the sustained release medication at least 8 hours apart.

■ Severe liver damage (with atomoxetine)

*Monitor for the following side effects and report to physician immediately: itching, dark urine, right upper quadrant pain, yellow skin or eyes, sore throat, fever, malaise.

■ New or worsened psychiatric symptoms (with CNS stimulants and atomoxetine)

*Monitor for psychotic symptoms (e.g., hearing voices, paranoid behaviors, delusions).

*Monitor for manic symptoms, including aggressive and hostile behaviors.

■ Rebound syndrome (with clonidine and guanfacine)

*Client should be instructed not to discontinue therapy abruptly. To do so may result in symptoms of nervousness, agitation, headache, tremor, and a rapid rise in blood pressure. Dosage should be tapered gradually under the supervision of the physician.

Tourette's Disorder

Clinical Findings, Epidemiology, and Course

Tourette's disorder is characterized by the presence of multiple motor tics and one or more vocal tics, which may appear simultaneously or at different periods during the illness (APA, 2013). The disturbance may cause distress or interfere with social, occupational, or other important areas of functioning. The age at onset of Tourette's disorder can be as early as 2 years, but the disorder occurs most commonly during childhood (around age 6 to 7 years). Prevalence of the disorder is estimated at from 3 to 8 per 1,000 in school-age children (APA, 2013). It is more common in boys than in girls. Although the disorder can be lifelong, the symptoms usually diminish during adolescence and adulthood, and in some cases, disappear altogether by early adulthood (Leckman, Bloch, Scahill, & King, 2006).

Predisposing Factors

Biological Factors

Genetics Tics are noted in two-thirds of relatives of Tourette's disorder clients (Popper et al., 2003). Twin studies with both monozygotic and dizygotic twins suggest an inheritable component. Evidence suggests that Tourette's disorder may be transmitted in an autosomal pattern intermediate between dominant and recessive (Sadock & Sadock, 2007). Singer, Leffler, and Murray (2008) state:

> The precise gene and mechanism of inheritance remain undetermined. A complex genetic mechanism is likely, perhaps one associated with multiple genes or an epigenetic effect, i.e., an environmental exposure influencing gene expression.

Biochemical Factors Abnormalities in levels of dopamine, serotonin, dynorphin, gamma-aminobutyric acid (GABA), acetylcholine, and norepinephrine have been associated with Tourette's disorder (Popper et al., 2003). Neurotransmitter pathways through the basal ganglia, globus pallidus, and subthalamic regions appear to be involved.

Structural Factors Neuroimaging brain studies have been consistent in finding dysfunction in the area of the basal ganglia. One study found a correlation between smaller size of corpus callosum and Tourette's disorder in children (Plessen et al., 2007). Peterson and associates (2007) found larger volumes in subregions of the hippocampus and amygdala in children with Tourette's disorder.

Environmental Factors

Additional retrospective findings may be implicated in the etiology of Tourette's disorder. Complications of pregnancy (e.g., severe nausea and vomiting or excessive stress), low birth weight, head trauma, carbon monoxide poisoning, and encephalitis are thought to be associated with the onset of nongenetic Tourette's disorder. Tourette's disorder may also arise as a result of a postinfection autoimmune phenomenon induced by childhood streptococcal infection (Black & Andreasen, 2011).

Application of the Nursing Process to Tourette's Disorder

Background Assessment Data (Symptomatology)

The motor tics of Tourette's disorder may involve the head, torso, and upper and lower limbs. Initial symptoms may begin with a single motor tic, most commonly eye blinking, or with multiple symptoms. Simple motor tics include movements such as eye blinking, neck jerking, shoulder shrugging, and facial grimacing. The more complex motor tics include squatting, hopping, skipping, tapping, and retracing steps.

Vocal tics include various words or sounds such as squeaks, grunts, barks, sniffs, snorts, coughs and, in rare instances, a complex vocal tic involving the uttering of obscenities. Vocal tics may include repeating certain words or phrases out of context, repeating one's own sounds or words (**palilalia**), or repeating what others say (**echolalia**).

The movements and vocalizations are experienced as compulsive and irresistible, but they can be suppressed for varying lengths of time. They are exacerbated by stress and attenuated during periods in which the individual becomes totally absorbed by an activity. In most cases, tics are diminished during sleep (Singer et al., 2008).

Comorbid disorders common with Tourette's disorder include ADHD, obsessive-compulsive disorder, depression, and anxiety. Episodic outbursts and school difficulties may also be observed. In severe cases, self-injurious behaviors may be exhibited (Singer et al., 2008).

The *DSM-5* diagnostic criteria for Tourette's disorder are presented in Box 33-4.

Nursing Diagnosis

Based on data collected during the nursing assessment, possible nursing diagnoses for the client with Tourette's disorder include the following:

■ Risk for self-directed or other-directed violence related to low tolerance for frustration
■ Impaired social interaction related to impulsiveness and oppositional and aggressive behavior

---

> ## BOX 33-4 Diagnostic Criteria for Tourette's Disorder
>
> A. Both multiple motor and one or more vocal tics have been present at some time during the illness, although not necessarily concurrently.
> B. The tics may wax and wane in frequency but have persisted for more than 1 year since first tic onset.
> C. Onset is before age 18 years.
> D. The disturbance is not attributable to the physiological effects of a substance (e.g., cocaine) or another medical condition (e.g., Huntington's disease, postviral encephalitis).

Reprinted with permission from the Diagnostic and Statistical Manual of Mental Disorders, Fifth Edition *(Copyright 2013). American Psychiatric Association.*

■ Low self-esteem related to embarrassment associated with tic behaviors

Outcome Identification

Outcome criteria include short- and long-term goals. Timelines are individually determined. The following criteria may be used for measurement of outcomes in the care of the client with Tourette's disorder.

The client:

■ Has not harmed self or others.
■ Interacts with staff and peers in an appropriate manner.
■ Demonstrates self-control by managing tic behavior.
■ Follows rules of the unit without becoming defensive.
■ Verbalizes positive aspects about self.

Planning/Implementation

Table 33-7 provides a plan of care for the child or adolescent with Tourette's disorder using selected nursing diagnoses, outcome criteria, and appropriate nursing interventions and rationales.

Evaluation

Evaluation of care for the child with Tourette's disorder reflects whether or not the nursing actions have been effective in achieving the established goals. The nursing process calls for reassessment of the plan. Questions for gathering reassessment data may include the following:

■ Has the client refrained from causing harm to self or others during times of increased tension?
■ Has the client developed adaptive coping strategies for dealing with frustration to prevent resorting to self-destruction or aggression to others?
■ Is the client able to interact appropriately with staff and peers?
■ Is the client able to suppress tic behaviors when he or she chooses to do so?

Table 33-7 | CARE PLAN FOR THE CHILD OR ADOLESCENT WITH TOURETTE'S DISORDER

NURSING DIAGNOSIS: RISK FOR SELF-DIRECTED OR OTHER-DIRECTED VIOLENCE

RELATED TO: Low tolerance for frustration

OUTCOME CRITERIA	NURSING INTERVENTIONS	RATIONALE
Short-Term Goal • Client will seek out staff or support person at any time if thoughts of harming self or others should occur. **Long-Term Goal** • Client will not harm self or others.	1. Observe client's behavior frequently through routine activities and interactions. Become aware of behaviors that indicate a rise in agitation. 2. Monitor for self-destructive behavior and impulses. A staff member may need to stay with the client to prevent self-mutilation. 3. Provide hand coverings and other restraints that prevent the client from self-mutilative behaviors. 4. Redirect violent behavior with physical outlets for frustration.	1. Stress commonly increases tic behaviors. Recognition of behaviors that precede the onset of aggression may provide the opportunity to intervene before violence occurs. 2. Client safety is a nursing priority. 3. For the client's protection, provide immediate external controls against self-aggressive behaviors. 4. Excess energy is released through physical activities and a feeling of relaxation is induced.

NURSING DIAGNOSIS: IMPAIRED SOCIAL INTERACTION

RELATED TO: Impulsiveness; oppositional and aggressive behavior

OUTCOME CRITERIA	NURSING INTERVENTIONS	RATIONALE
Short-Term Goal • Client will develop a one-to-one relationship with a nurse or support person within 1 week. **Long-Term Goal** • Client will be able to interact with staff and peers using age-appropriate, acceptable behaviors.	1. Develop a trusting relationship with the client. Convey acceptance of the person separate from the unacceptable behavior. 2. Discuss with client which behaviors are and are not acceptable. Describe in matter-of-fact manner the consequences of unacceptable behavior. Follow through. 3. Provide group situations for client.	1. Unconditional acceptance increases feelings of self-worth. 2. Aversive reinforcement can alter undesirable behaviors. 3. Appropriate social behavior is often learned from the positive and negative feedback of peers.

NURSING DIAGNOSIS: LOW SELF-ESTEEM

RELATED TO: Embarrassment associated with tic behaviors

OUTCOME CRITERIA	NURSING INTERVENTIONS	RATIONALE
Short-Term Goal • Client will verbalize positive aspects about self not associated with tic behaviors.	1. Convey unconditional acceptance and positive regard.	1. Communicating a perception of the client as a worthwhile human being may increase self-esteem.

Table 33-7 | CARE PLAN FOR THE CHILD OR ADOLESCENT WITH TOURETTE'S DISORDER—cont'd

OUTCOME CRITERIA	NURSING INTERVENTIONS	RATIONALE
Long-Term Goal • Client will exhibit increased feeling of self-worth as evidenced by verbal expression of positive aspects about self, past accomplishments, and future prospects.	2. Set limits on manipulative behavior. Take caution not to reinforce manipulative behaviors by providing desired attention. Identify the consequences of manipulation. Administer consequences matter-of-factly when manipulation occurs.	2. Aversive consequences may work to decrease unacceptable behaviors.
	3. Help client understand that he or she uses manipulation to try to increase own self-esteem. Interventions should reflect other actions to accomplish this goal.	3. When client feels better about self, the need to manipulate others will diminish.
	4. If client chooses to suppress tics in the presence of others, provide a specified "tic time," during which he or she "vents" tics, feelings, and behaviors (alone or with staff).	4. Allows for release of tics and assists in sense of control and management of symptoms.
	5. Ensure that client has regular one-to-one time with nursing staff.	5. One-to-one time gives the nurse the opportunity to provide the client with information about the illness and healthy ways to manage it. Exploring feelings about the illness helps the client incorporate the illness into a healthy sense of self.

■ Does the client set a time for "release" of the suppressed tic behaviors?

■ Does the client verbalize positive aspects about self, particularly as they relate to his or her ability to manage the illness?

■ Does the client comply with treatment in a nondefensive manner?

Psychopharmacological Intervention for Tourette's Disorder

Pharmacotherapy is often not recommended to treat Tourette's disorder unless it is causing significant functional impairment or physical discomfort, or is interfering with the individual's overall quality of life or psychological adjustment (Singer et al., 2008; Ursano et al., 2008). Pharmacotherapy is most effective when it is combined with psychosocial therapy, such as behavioral therapy, individual counseling or psychotherapy, and/or family therapy. Medications that are used in the treatment of Tourette's disorder include antipsychotics and alpha agonists.

Antipsychotics

The conventional antipsychotics, haloperidol (Haldol) and pimozide (Orap), have been approved by the FDA for control of tics and vocal utterances associated with Tourette's disorder. These drugs have been widely investigated and have proved to be highly effective in alleviating these symptoms. They are often not the first-line choice of therapy, however, because of their propensity for severe adverse effects, such as extrapyramidal symptoms (EPS), neuroleptic malignant syndrome, tardive dyskinesia, and electrocardiographic changes. Haloperidol is not recommended for children younger than 3 years of age, and pimozide should not be administered to children younger than 12 years.

Although not presently approved by the FDA for use in Tourette's disorder, some clinicians prefer to prescribe the atypical antipsychotics, such as risperidone (Risperdal), olanzapine (Zyprexa), or ziprasidone (Geodon), because of their more favorable side-effect profiles. In clinical trials, these medications have been shown to be effective in treating the symptoms of Tourette's disorder. These medications have a lower incidence of neurological side effects than the typical antipsychotics, although EPS has been observed with risperidone. Common side effects include weight gain and sedation. Ziprasidone has been associated with increased risk of QTc interval prolongation. Hyperglycemia has also been reported in some patients taking atypical antipsychotics.

Alpha Agonists

Clonidine (Catapres) and guanfacine (Tenex; Intuniv) are alpha-adrenergic agonists that are approved for use as antihypertensive agents. The extended-release forms have been approved by the FDA for the treatment of ADHD. These medications are often the first-line choice for treatment of Tourette's disorder because of their favorable side-effect profile and because they are often effective for comorbid symptoms of ADHD, anxiety, and insomnia (Zinner, 2004). Common side effects include dry mouth, sedation, headaches, fatigue, and dizziness or postural hypotension. Guanfacine is longer lasting and less sedating than clonidine. Alpha agonists should not be prescribed for children and adolescents with pre-existing cardiac or vascular disease. They should not be discontinued abruptly; to do so could result in symptoms of nervousness, agitation, tremor, and a rapid rise in blood pressure.

Disruptive Behavior Disorders

Oppositional Defiant Disorder

Clinical Findings, Epidemiology, and Course

Oppositional defiant disorder (ODD) is characterized by a persistent pattern of angry mood and defiant behavior that occurs more frequently than is usually observed in individuals of comparable age and developmental level, and interferes with social, educational, occupational, or other important areas of functioning (APA, 2013). The disorder typically begins by 8 years of age and usually not later than early adolescence. Prevalence estimates range from 2 to 12 percent, and common comorbid disorders include ADHD and anxiety and mood disorders (Ursano et al., 2008). It is more prevalent in boys than in girls before puberty, but the rates are more closely equal after puberty. In some cases of ODD, there may be a progression to conduct disorder (Lubit, 2011).

Predisposing Factors

Biological Influences

What role, if any, genetics, temperament, or biochemical alterations play in the etiology of ODD is still being investigated. A study by Comings and associates (2000) suggests the genes for metabolism of dopamine, serotonin, and norepinephrine may be contributing factors in the development of ODD.

Family Influences

Opposition during various developmental stages is both normal and healthy. Children first exhibit oppositional behaviors at around 10 or 11 months of age, again as toddlers between 18 and 36 months of age, and finally during adolescence. Pathology is considered only when the developmental phase is prolonged, or when there is overreaction in the child's environment to his or her behavior.

Some children exhibit these behaviors in a more intense form than others. Sadock and Sadock (2007) report, "Epidemiological studies of negativistic traits in nonclinical populations found such behavior in 16 to 22 percent of school-age children" (p. 1218).

Some parents interpret average or increased level of developmental oppositional behavior as hostility and a deliberate effort on the part of the child to be in control. If power and control are issues for parents, or if they exercise authority for their own needs, a power struggle can be established between the parents and the child that sets the stage for the development of ODD. Lubit (2011) suggested the following pattern of family dynamics:

■ There is the combination of a strong-willed child with a reactive and high-energy temperament and parents who are authoritarian rather than authoritative.

■ The parents become frustrated with the strong-willed child who does not obey and increase their attempts to enforce authority.

■ The child reacts to the excessive parental control with anger and increased self-assertion.

Lubit (2011) stated:

A downward spiral occurs, with the parent trying to control the child and the child feeling he or she must refuse to give in and must defend his or her autonomy. Both parties become angry and increasingly rigid in their stances as they try to defend their self-esteem. The child's negative behaviors may be inadvertently rewarded by attention, which, even though may be negative, is still desired.

Application of the Nursing Process to ODD

Background Assessment Data (Symptomatology)

ODD is characterized by passive-aggressive behaviors such as stubbornness, procrastination, disobedience, carelessness, **negativism**, testing of limits, resistance to directions, deliberately ignoring the communication of others, and unwillingness to compromise. Other symptoms that may be evident are running away, school avoidance, school underachievement, temper tantrums, fighting, and argumentativeness.

Initially, the oppositional attitude is directed toward the parents, but in time, relationships with peers and teachers become affected. These impairments in social interaction often lead to depression, anxiety, and additional problematic behavior (Lubit, 2011).

Usually these children do not see themselves as being oppositional but view the problem as arising from others whom they believe are making unreasonable demands on them. These children are often friendless, perceiving human relationships as negative and unsatisfactory. School performance is usually poor because of their refusal to participate and their resistance to external demands.

The *DSM-5* (APA, 2013) diagnostic criteria for ODD are presented in Box 33-5.

Nursing Diagnosis

Based on the data collected during the nursing assessment, possible nursing diagnoses for the client with ODD include the following:

■ Noncompliance with therapy related to negative temperament, denial of problems, underlying hostility

■ Defensive coping related to retarded ego development, low self-esteem, unsatisfactory parent/child relationship

■ Low self-esteem related to lack of positive feedback, retarded ego development

■ Impaired social interaction related to negative temperament, underlying hostility, manipulation of others

Outcome Identification

Outcome criteria include short- and long-term goals. Timelines are individually determined. The following criteria may be used for measurement of outcomes in the care of the client with ODD.

The client:

■ Complies with treatment by participating in therapies without negativism.

■ Accepts responsibility for his or her part in the problem.

■ Takes direction from staff without becoming defensive.

■ Does not manipulate other people.

BOX 33-5 Diagnostic Criteria for Oppositional Defiant Disorder

A. A pattern of angry/irritable mood, argumentative/defiant behavior, or vindictiveness lasting at least 6 months as evidenced by at least four symptoms from any of the following categories, and exhibited during interaction with at least one individual that is not a sibling.

Angry/Irritable Mood

1. Often loses temper.
2. Is often touchy or easily annoyed.
3. Is often angry and resentful.

Argumentative/Defiant Behavior

4. Often argues with authority figures or, for children and adolescents, with adults.
5. Often actively defies or refuses to comply with requests from authority figures or with rules.
6. Often deliberately annoys others.
7. Often blames others for his or her mistakes or misbehavior.

Vindictiveness

8. Has been spiteful or vindictive at least twice within the past 6 months.

Note: The persistence and frequency of these behaviors should be used to distinguish a behavior that is within normal limits from a behavior that is symptomatic. For children younger than 5 years, the behavior should occur on most days for a period of at least 6 months unless otherwise noted (Criterion A8). For individuals 5 years or older, the behavior should occur at least once per week for at least 6 months, unless otherwise noted (Criterion A8). While these frequency criteria provide guidance on a minimal level of frequency to define symptoms, other factors should also be considered, such as whether the frequency and intensity of the behaviors are outside a range that is normative for the individual's developmental level, gender, and culture.

B. The disturbance in behavior is associated with distress in the individual or others in his or her immediate social context (e.g., family, peer group, work colleagues), or it impacts negatively on social, educational, occupational, or other important areas of functioning.

C. The behaviors do not occur exclusively during the course of a psychotic, substance use, depressive, or bipolar disorder. Also, the criteria are not met for disruptive mood dysregulation disorder.

Specify current severity:

Mild: Symptoms are confined to only one setting (e.g., at home, at school, at work, with peers).

Moderate: Some symptoms are present in at least two settings.

Severe: Some symptoms are present in three or more settings.

Reprinted with permission from the Diagnostic and Statistical Manual of Mental Disorders, Fifth Edition *(Copyright 2013). American Psychiatric Association.*

■ Verbalizes positive aspects about self.
■ Interacts with others in an appropriate manner.

Planning/Implementation

Table 33-8 provides a plan of care for the child with ODD using nursing diagnoses common to the disorder,

outcome criteria, and appropriate nursing interventions and rationales.

Evaluation

The evaluation step of the nursing process calls for reassessment of the plan of care to determine if the

---

Table 33-8 | CARE PLAN FOR THE CHILD/ADOLESCENT WITH OPPOSITIONAL DEFIANT DISORDER

NURSING DIAGNOSIS: NONCOMPLIANCE WITH THERAPY

RELATED TO: Negative temperament; denial of problems; underlying hostility

OUTCOME CRITERIA	NURSING INTERVENTIONS	RATIONALE
Short-Term Goal • Client will participate in and cooperate during therapeutic activities. **Long-Term Goal** • Client will complete assigned tasks willingly and independently or with a minimum of assistance.	1. Set forth a structured plan of therapeutic activities. Start with minimum expectations and increase as client begins to manifest evidence of compliance. 2. Establish a system of rewards for compliance with therapy and consequences for noncompliance. Ensure that the rewards and consequences are concepts of value to the client. 3. Convey acceptance of the client separate from the undesirable behaviors being exhibited. ("It is not *you*, but your *behavior*, that is unacceptable").	1. Structure provides security and one or two activities may not seem as overwhelming as the whole schedule of activities presented at one time. 2. Positive, negative, and aversive reinforcements can contribute to desired changes in behavior. 3. Unconditional acceptance enhances self-worth and may contribute to a decrease in the need for passive-aggression toward others.

NURSING DIAGNOSIS: DEFENSIVE COPING

RELATED TO: Retarded ego development; low self-esteem; unsatisfactory parent/child relationship

OUTCOME CRITERIA	NURSING INTERVENTIONS	RATIONALE
Short-Term Goal • Client will verbalize personal responsibility for difficulties experienced in interpersonal relationships within (time period reasonable for client). **Long-Term Goal** • Client will accept responsibility for own behaviors and interact with others without becoming defensive.	1. Help client recognize that feelings of inadequacy provoke defensive behaviors, such as blaming others for problems, and the need to "get even." 2. Provide immediate, nonthreatening feedback for passive-aggressive behavior. 3. Help identify situations that provoke defensiveness and practice through role-play more appropriate responses. 4. Provide immediate positive feedback for acceptable behaviors.	1. Recognition of the problem is the first step toward initiating change. 2. Because client denies responsibility for problems, he or she is denying the inappropriateness of behavior. 3. Role-playing provides confidence to deal with difficult situations when they actually occur. 4. Positive feedback encourages repetition, and immediacy is significant for these children who respond to immediate gratification.

Table 33-8 | CARE PLAN FOR THE CHILD/ADOLESCENT WITH OPPOSITIONAL DEFIANT DISORDER–cont'd

NURSING DIAGNOSIS: LOW SELF-ESTEEM

RELATED TO: Lack of positive feedback; retarded ego development

OUTCOME CRITERIA	NURSING INTERVENTIONS	RATIONALE
Short-Term Goal • Client will participate in own self-care and discuss with nurse aspects of self about which he or she feels good. **Long-Term Goal** • Client will demonstrate increased feelings of self-worth by verbalizing positive statements about self and exhibiting fewer manipulative behaviors.	1. Ensure that goals are realistic. 2. Plan activities that provide opportunities for success. 3. Convey unconditional acceptance and positive regard. 4. Set limits on manipulative behavior. Take caution not to reinforce manipulative behaviors by providing desired attention. Identify the consequences of manipulation. Administer consequences matter-of-factly when manipulation occurs. 5. Help client understand that he or she uses this behavior to try to increase own self-esteem. Interventions should reflect other actions to accomplish this goal.	1. Unrealistic goals set up client for failure, which diminishes self-esteem. 2. Success enhances self-esteem. 3. Affirmation of client as a worthwhile human being may increase self-esteem. 4. Aversive reinforcement may work to decrease unacceptable behaviors. 5. When client feels better about self, the need to manipulate others will diminish.

NURSING DIAGNOSIS: IMPAIRED SOCIAL INTERACTION

RELATED TO: Negative temperament; underlying hostility; manipulation of others

OUTCOME CRITERIA	NURSING INTERVENTIONS	RATIONALE
Short-Term Goal • Client will interact in age-appropriate manner with nurse in one-to-one relationship within 1 week. **Long-Term Goal** • Client will be able to interact with staff and peers using age-appropriate, acceptable behaviors.	1. Develop a trusting relationship with the client. Convey acceptance of the person separate from the unacceptable behavior. 2. Explain to the client about passive-aggressive behavior. Explain how these behaviors are perceived by others. Describe which behaviors are not acceptable and role-play more adaptive responses. Give positive feedback for acceptable behaviors. 3. Provide peer group situations for the client.	1. Unconditional acceptance increases feelings of self-worth and may serve to diminish feelings of rejection that have accumulated over a long period. 2. Role-playing is a way to practice behaviors that do not come readily to the client, making it easier when the situation actually occurs. Positive feedback enhances repetition of desirable behaviors. 3. Appropriate social behavior is often learned from the positive and negative feedback of peers. Groups also provide an atmosphere for using the behaviors rehearsed in role-play.

nursing actions have been effective in achieving the goals of therapy. The following questions can be used with the child or adolescent with ODD to gather information for the evaluation:

■ Is the client cooperating with schedule of therapeutic activities? Is level of participation adequate?
■ Is the client's attitude toward therapy less negative?
■ Is the client accepting responsibility for problem behavior?
■ Is the client verbalizing the unacceptability of his or her passive-aggressive behavior?
■ Is he or she able to identify which behaviors are unacceptable and substitute more adaptive behaviors?
■ Is the client able to interact with staff and peers without defending behavior in an angry manner?
■ Is the client able to verbalize positive statements about self?
■ Is increased self-worth evident with fewer manifestations of manipulation?
■ Is the client able to make compromises with others when issues of control emerge?
■ Is anger and hostility expressed in an appropriate manner? Can the client verbalize ways of releasing anger adaptively?
■ Is he or she able to verbalize true feelings instead of allowing them to emerge through use of passive-aggressive behaviors?

Conduct Disorder

Clinical Findings, Epidemiology, and Course

With conduct disorder, there is a repetitive and persistent pattern of behavior in which the basic rights of others or major age-appropriate societal norms or rules are violated (APA, 2013). Physical aggression is common, and peer relationships are disturbed. In general population studies, prevalence of the disorder has been estimated at 1 to 10 percent, with a male predominance ranging from 2:1 to 4:1 (Ursano et al., 2008). There is a higher male predominance among those with the child-onset subtype. A number of comorbidities are common with conduct disorder, including ADHD, mood disorders, learning disorders, and substance use disorders. When the disorder begins in childhood, there is more likely to be a history of ODD and a greater likelihood of antisocial personality disorder in adulthood than if the disorder is diagnosed in adolescence. Black and Andreasen (2011) report that an estimated 40 percent of boys and 25 percent of girls with conduct disorder will develop adult antisocial personality disorder.

> ## CORE CONCEPT
> **Temperament**
> Personality characteristics that define an individual's mood and behavioral tendencies. The sum of physical, emotional, and intellectual components that affect or determine a person's actions and reactions.

Predisposing Factors

Biological Influences

Genetics   Family, twin, and adoptive studies have revealed a significantly higher number of individuals with conduct disorder among those who have family members with the disorder (Black & Andreasen, 2011). Although genetic factors appear to be involved in the etiology of conduct disorder, little is yet known about the actual mechanisms involved in genetic transmission. One study found that regions on chromosomes 19 and 2 may contain genes conferring risk to conduct disorder (Dick et al., 2004). In this study, the same region on chromosome 2 was also linked to alcohol dependence. These researchers reported that childhood conduct disorder is known to be associated with the susceptibility to future alcohol problems. They concluded that these findings suggest that some of the genes contributing to alcohol dependence in adulthood may also contribute to conduct disorder in childhood.

Temperament   The term *temperament* refers to personality traits that become evident very early in life and may be present at birth. Evidence suggests a genetic component in temperament and an association between temperament and behavioral problems later in life. Studies have shown that, without appropriate intervention, difficult temperament at age 3 has significant links to conduct disorder and movement into care or institutional life at age 17 (Bagley & Mallick, 2000).

Biochemical Factors   Researchers have investigated various chemicals as biological markers. Alterations in the neurotransmitters norepinephrine and serotonin have been suggested by some studies (Comings et al., 2000; Searight, Rottnek, & Abby, 2001). Some investigators have examined the possibility of testosterone association with violence. One study correlates higher levels of testosterone in pubertal boys with social dominance and association with deviant peers (Rowe, Maughan, Worthman, Costello, & Angold, 2004).

Psychosocial Influences

Peer Relationships   Social groups have a significant impact on a child's development. Peers play an essential role in the socialization of interpersonal competence, and skills acquired in this manner affect the child's long-term adjustment. Studies have shown that poor peer relations during childhood were consistently implicated in the etiology of later deviance (Ladd, 1999). Aggression was found to be the principal cause of peer rejection, thus contributing to a cycle of maladaptive behavior.

Family Influences

The following factors related to family dynamics have been implicated as contributors in the predisposition to conduct disorder (Foley et al., 2004; Sadock & Sadock, 2007; Ursano et al., 2008):

- Parental rejection
- Inconsistent management with harsh discipline
- Early institutional living
- Frequent shifting of parental figures
- Large family size
- Absent father
- Parents with antisocial personality disorder and/or alcohol dependence
- Marital conflict and divorce
- Inadequate communication patterns
- Parental permissiveness

Application of the Nursing Process to Conduct Disorder

Background Assessment Data (Symptomatology)

The classic characteristic of conduct disorder is the use of physical aggression in the violation of the rights of others. The behavior pattern manifests itself in virtually all areas of the child's life (home, school, with peers, and in the community). Stealing, lying, and truancy are common problems. The child lacks feelings of guilt or remorse.

The use of tobacco, liquor, or nonprescribed drugs, as well as the participation in sexual activities, occurs earlier than at the expected age for the peer group. Projection is a common defense mechanism.

Low self-esteem is manifested by a "tough guy" image. Characteristics include poor frustration tolerance, irritability, and frequent temper outbursts. Symptoms of anxiety and depression are not uncommon.

Level of academic achievement may be low in relation to age and IQ. Manifestations associated with ADHD (e.g., attention difficulties, impulsiveness, and hyperactivity) are common in children with conduct disorder.

The *DSM-5* diagnostic criteria for conduct disorder are presented in Box 33-6.

Nursing Diagnosis

Based on the data collected during the nursing assessment, possible nursing diagnoses for the client with conduct disorder include the following:

- Risk for other-directed violence related to characteristics of temperament, peer rejection, negative parental role models, dysfunctional family dynamics
- Impaired social interaction related to negative parental role models, impaired peer relations leading to inappropriate social behaviors

---

BOX 33-6 **Diagnostic Criteria for Conduct Disorder**

A. A repetitive and persistent pattern of behavior in which the basic rights of others or major age-appropriate societal norms or rules are violated, as manifested by the presence of at least three of the following 15 criteria in the past 12 months from any of the categories below, with at least one criterion present in the past 6 months:

Aggression to People and Animals

1. Often bullies, threatens, or intimidates others.
2. Often initiates physical fights.
3. Has used a weapon that can cause serious physical harm to others (e.g., a bat, brick, broken bottle, knife, gun).
4. Has been physically cruel to people.
5. Has been physically cruel to animals.
6. Has stolen while confronting a victim (e.g., mugging, purse snatching, extortion, armed robbery).
7. Has forced someone into sexual activity.

Destruction of Property

8. Has deliberately engaged in fire setting with the intention of causing serious damage.
9. Has deliberately destroyed others' property (other than by fire setting).

Deceitfulness or Theft

10. Has broken into someone else's house, building, or car.
11. Often lies to obtain goods or favors or to avoid obligations (i.e., "cons" others).
12. Has stolen items of nontrivial value without confronting a victim (e.g., shoplifting, but without breaking and entering; forgery).

Serious Violations of Rules

13. Often stays out at night despite parental prohibitions, beginning before age 13 years.

Continued

BOX 33-6 Diagnostic Criteria for Conduct Disorder—cont'd

14. Has run away from home overnight at least twice while living in parental or parental surrogate home, or once without returning for a lengthy period.
15. Is often truant from school, beginning before age 13 years.

B. The disturbance in behavior causes clinically significant impairment in social, academic, or occupational functioning.

C. If the individual is age 18 years or older, criteria are not met for antisocial personality disorder.

Specify whether:

Childhood-Onset Type: Individuals show at least one symptom characteristic of conduct disorder prior to age 10 years.

Adolescent-Onset Type: Individuals show no symptom characteristic of conduct disorder prior to age 10 years.

Unspecified Onset: Criteria for a diagnosis of conduct disorder are met, but there is not enough information available to determine whether the onset of the first symptom was before or after age 10 years.

Specify if:

With limited prosocial emotions

Specify current severity:

Mild
Moderate
Severe

Reprinted with permission from the Diagnostic and Statistical Manual of Mental Disorders, Fifth Edition *(Copyright 2013). American Psychiatric Association.*

■ Defensive coping related to low self-esteem and dysfunctional family system
■ Low self-esteem related to lack of positive feedback and unsatisfactory parent-child relationship.

Outcome Identification

Outcome criteria include short- and long-term goals. Timelines are individually determined. The following criteria may be used for measurement of outcomes in the care of the client with conduct disorder.

The client:

■ Has not harmed self or others.
■ Interacts with others in a socially appropriate manner.
■ Accepts direction without becoming defensive.
■ Demonstrates evidence of increased self-esteem by discontinuing exploitative and demanding behaviors toward others.

Planning/Implementation

Table 33-9 provides a plan of care for the child with conduct disorder using nursing diagnoses common to the disorder, outcome criteria, and appropriate nursing interventions and rationales.

Evaluation

Following the planning and implementation of care, evaluation is made of the behavioral changes in the child with conduct disorder. This is accomplished by determining if the goals of therapy have been achieved. Reassessment, the next step in the nursing process, may be initiated by gathering information using the following questions:

■ Have the nursing actions directed toward managing the client's aggressive behavior been effective?

■ Have interventions prevented harm to others or others' property?
■ Is the client able to express anger in an appropriate manner?
■ Has the client developed more adaptive coping strategies to deal with anger and feelings of aggression?
■ Does the client demonstrate the ability to trust others? Is he or she able to interact with staff and peers in an appropriate manner?
■ Is the client able to accept responsibility for his or her own behavior? Is there less blaming of others?
■ Is the client able to accept feedback from others without becoming defensive?
■ Is the client able to verbalize positive statements about self?
■ Is the client able to interact with others without engaging in manipulation?

Anxiety Disorders

Separation Anxiety Disorder
Clinical Findings, Epidemiology, and Course

Separation anxiety disorder is characterized by excessive fear or anxiety concerning separation from those to whom the individual is attached (APA, 2013). The anxiety is beyond that which would be expected for the individual's developmental level and interferes with social, academic, occupational, or other areas of functioning. Onset may occur any time before age 18 years but is most commonly diagnosed around age 5 or 6, when the child goes to school. Prevalence estimates for the disorder average about 4 percent in children and young adults, and it is more common in girls than in boys. Most children grow out of it, but in some instances the symptoms can persist into adulthood

Table 33-9 | CARE PLAN FOR CHILD/ADOLESCENT WITH CONDUCT DISORDER

NURSING DIAGNOSIS: RISK FOR OTHER-DIRECTED VIOLENCE

RELATED TO: Characteristics of temperament, peer rejection, negative parental role models, dysfunctional family dynamics

OUTCOME CRITERIA	NURSING INTERVENTIONS	RATIONALE
Short-Term Goal • Client will discuss feelings of anger with nurse or therapist. **Long-Term Goal** • Client will not harm others or others' property.	1. Observe client's behavior frequently through routine activities and interactions. Become aware of behaviors that indicate a rise in agitation. 2. Redirect violent behavior with physical outlets for suppressed anger and frustration. 3. Encourage client to express anger and act as a role model for appropriate expression of anger. 4. Ensure that a sufficient number of staff is available to indicate a show of strength if necessary. 5. Administer tranquilizing medication, if ordered, or use mechanical restraints or isolation room only if situation cannot be controlled with less restrictive means.	1. Recognition of behaviors that precede the onset of aggression may provide the opportunity to intervene before violence occurs. 2. Excess energy is released through physical activities, inducing a feeling of relaxation. 3. Discussion of situations that create anger may lead to more effective ways of dealing with them. 4. This conveys evidence of control over the situation and provides physical security for staff and others. 5. It is the client's right to expect the use of techniques that ensure safety of the client and others by the least restrictive means.

NURSING DIAGNOSIS: IMPAIRED SOCIAL INTERACTION

RELATED TO: Negative parental role models; impaired peer relations leading to inappropriate social behavior

OUTCOME CRITERIA	NURSING INTERVENTIONS	RATIONALE
Short-Term Goal • Client will interact in age-appropriate manner with nurse in one-to-one relationship within 1 week. **Long-Term Goal** • Client will be able to interact with staff and peers using age-appropriate, acceptable behaviors.	1. Develop a trusting relationship with the client. Convey acceptance of the person separate from the unacceptable behavior. 2. Discuss with client which behaviors are and are not acceptable. Describe in matter-of-fact manner the consequence of unacceptable behavior. Follow through. 3. Provide group situations for client.	1. Unconditional acceptance increases feeling of self-worth. 2. Aversive reinforcement can alter or extinguish undesirable behaviors. 3. Appropriate social behavior is often learned from the positive and negative feedback of peers.

NURSING DIAGNOSIS: DEFENSIVE COPING

RELATED TO: Low self-esteem and dysfunctional family system

OUTCOME CRITERIA	NURSING INTERVENTIONS	RATIONALE
Short-Term Goal • Client will verbalize personal responsibility for difficulties experienced in interpersonal relationships within a time period reasonable for client.	1. Explain to client the correlation between feelings of inadequacy and the need for acceptance from others and how these feelings provoke defensive behaviors, such as blaming others for own behaviors.	1. Recognition of the problem is the first step in the change process toward resolution.

Continued

Table 33-9 | CARE PLAN FOR CHILD/ADOLESCENT WITH CONDUCT DISORDER–cont'd

OUTCOME CRITERIA	NURSING INTERVENTIONS	RATIONALE
Long-Term Goal • Client will accept responsibility for own behaviors and interact with others without becoming defensive.	2. Provide immediate, matter-of-fact, nonthreatening feedback for unacceptable behaviors. 3. Help identify situations that provoke defensiveness and practice through role-play more appropriate responses. 4. Provide immediate positive feedback for acceptable behaviors.	2. Client may not realize how these behaviors are being perceived by others. 3. Role-playing provides confidence to deal with difficult situations when they actually occur. 4. Positive feedback encourages repetition, and immediacy is significant for these children, who respond to immediate gratification.

NURSING DIAGNOSIS: LOW SELF-ESTEEM

RELATED TO: Lack of positive feedback and unsatisfactory parent/child relationship

OUTCOME CRITERIA	NURSING INTERVENTIONS	RATIONALE
Short-Term Goal • Client will participate in own self-care and discuss with nurse aspects of self about which he or she feels good. **Long-Term Goal** • Client will demonstrate increased feelings of self-worth by verbalizing positive statements about self and exhibiting fewer manipulative behaviors.	1. Ensure that goals are realistic. 2. Plan activities that provide opportunities for success. 3. Convey unconditional acceptance and positive regard. 4. Set limits on manipulative behavior. Take caution not to reinforce manipulative behaviors by providing desired attention. Identify the consequences of manipulation. Administer consequences matter-of-factly when manipulation occurs. 5. Help client understand that he or she uses this behavior in order to try to increase own self-esteem. Interventions should reflect other actions to accomplish this goal.	1. Unrealistic goals set client up for failure, which diminishes self-esteem. 2. Success enhances self-esteem. 3. Communicating that client is a worthwhile human being helps to increase self-esteem. 4. Aversive consequences may work to decrease unacceptable behaviors. 5. When the client feels better about self, the need to manipulate others will diminish.

(Harvard Medical School, 2007). Separation anxiety disorder can be a precursor to adult panic disorder (Black & Andreasen, 2011).

Predisposing Factors

Biological Influences

Genetics Studies have been conducted in which the children of adult clients diagnosed as having separation anxiety disorder were studied. A second method, studying parents and other relatives of children diagnosed as having separation anxiety disorder, has also been used. The results have shown that a greater number of children with relatives who manifest anxiety problems develop anxiety disorders themselves than do children with no such family patterns. The results are significant enough to speculate that there is a hereditary influence in the development of separation anxiety disorder, but the mode of genetic transmission has not been determined. Sadock and Sadock (2007) state:

> Current consensus on the genetics of anxiety disorders suggests that what is inherited is a general predisposition toward anxiety, with resulting heightened levels of arousability, emotional reactivity, and increased negative affect, all of which increase the risk for the development of separation anxiety disorder [and other anxiety disorders]. (p. 1278)

Temperament It is well established that children differ from birth, or shortly thereafter, on a number of temperamental characteristics. Shamir-Essakow, Ungerer, and Rapee (2005) state:

> A temperament construct termed "behavioral inhibition to the unfamiliar" is characterized by the predisposition to be irritable as an infant, unusually shy and fearful as a toddler, and quiet, cautious, and withdrawn in the preschool and early school age years, with marked behavioral restraint and physiological arousal in unfamiliar situations. Integrated models propose that environmental factors, such as parent-child attachment, may combine with temperament to increase the risk for the development of childhood anxiety. (p. 131)

Individual differences in temperaments may be related to the acquisition of fear and anxiety disorders in childhood. This may be referred to as *anxiety proneness* or *vulnerability* and may denote an inherited "disposition" toward developing anxiety disorders.

Environmental Influences

Stressful Life Events Studies have shown a relationship between life events and the development of anxiety disorders (Sadock & Sadock, 2007). It is thought that perhaps children who already are vulnerable or predisposed to developing anxiety disorders may be affected significantly by stressful life events. More research is needed before firm conclusions can be drawn.

Family Influences

Various theories expound on the idea that anxiety disorders in children are related to an overattachment to the mother. Attachment theorists attribute the major determinants of anxiety disorders to transactions relating to separation issues between mother (or mothering figure) and child (Shamir-Essakow et al., 2005).

Some parents may instill anxiety in their children by overprotecting them from expectable dangers or by exaggerating the dangers of the present and the future (Sadock & Sadock, 2007). Some parents may also transfer their fears and anxieties to their children through role modeling. For example, a parent who becomes fearful in the presence of a small, harmless dog and retreats with dread and apprehension teaches the young child by example that this is an appropriate response.

Application of the Nursing Process to Separation Anxiety Disorder

Background Assessment Data (Symptomatology)

Age at onset of this disorder may be as early as preschool age; it rarely begins as late as adolescence. In most cases, the child has difficulty separating from the mother. Occasionally the separation reluctance is directed toward the father, siblings, or other significant individual to whom the child is attached. Anticipation of separation may result in tantrums, crying, screaming, complaints of physical problems, and **clinging** behaviors.

Reluctance or refusal to attend school is especially common in adolescence. Younger children may "shadow" or follow around the person from whom they are afraid to be separated. During middle childhood or adolescence they may refuse to sleep away from home (e.g., at a friend's house or at camp). Interpersonal peer relationships are usually not a problem with these children. They are generally well liked by their peers and are reasonably socially skilled.

Worrying is common and relates to the possibility of harm coming to self or to the attachment figure. Younger children may even have nightmares to this effect.

Specific phobias are not uncommon (e.g., fear of the dark, ghosts, animals). Depressed mood is frequently present and often precedes the onset of the anxiety symptoms, which commonly occur following a major stressor. The *DSM-5* diagnostic criteria for separation anxiety disorder are presented in Box 33-7.

Nursing Diagnosis

Based on the data collected during the nursing assessment, possible nursing diagnoses for the client with separation anxiety disorder include the following:

- Anxiety (severe) related to family history, temperament, overattachment to parent, negative role modeling
- Ineffective coping related to unresolved separation conflicts and inadequate coping skills evidenced by numerous somatic complaints
- Impaired social interaction related to reluctance to be away from attachment figure

Outcome Identification

Outcome criteria include short- and long-term goals. Timelines are individually determined. The following criteria may be used for measurement of outcomes in the care of the client with separation anxiety disorder.

BOX 33-7 Diagnostic Criteria for Separation Anxiety Disorder

A. Developmentally inappropriate and excessive fear or anxiety concerning separation from those to whom the individual is attached, as evidenced by at least three of the following:
  1. Recurrent excessive distress when anticipating or experiencing separation from home or major attachment figures.
  2. Persistent and excessive worry about losing major attachment figures or about possible harm to them, such as illness, injury, disasters, or death.
  3. Persistent and excessive worry about experiencing an untoward event (e.g., getting lost, being kidnapped, having an accident, becoming ill) that causes separation from a major attachment figure.
  4. Persistent reluctance or refusal to go out, away from home, to school, to work, or elsewhere because of fear of separation.
  5. Persistent and excessive fear of or reluctance about being alone or without major attachment figures at home or in other settings.
  6. Persistent reluctance or refusal to sleep away from home or to go to sleep without being near a major attachment figure.

  7. Repeated nightmares involving the theme of separation.
  8. Repeated complaints of physical symptoms (e.g., headaches, stomachaches, nausea, vomiting) when separation from major attachment figures occurs or is anticipated.
B. The fear, anxiety, or avoidance is persistent, lasting at least 4 weeks in children and adolescents and typically 6 months or more in adults.
C. The disturbance causes clinically significant distress or impairment in social, academic, occupational, or other important areas of functioning.
D. The disturbance is not better accounted for by another mental disorder, such as refusing to leave home because of excessive resistance to change in autism spectrum disorder; delusions or hallucinations concerning separation in psychotic disorders; refusal to go outside without a trusted companion in agoraphobia; worries about ill health or other harm befalling significant others in generalized anxiety disorder; or concerns about having an illness in illness anxiety disorder.

Reprinted with permission from the Diagnostic and Statistical Manual of Mental Disorders, Fifth Edition *(Copyright 2013). American Psychiatric Association.*

The client:

■ Is able to maintain anxiety at manageable level.
■ Demonstrates adaptive coping strategies for dealing with anxiety when separation from attachment figure is anticipated.
■ Interacts appropriately with others and spends time away from attachment figure to do so.

Planning/Implementation

Table 33-10 provides a plan of care for the child or adolescent with separation anxiety, using nursing diagnoses common to this disorder, outcome criteria, and appropriate nursing interventions and rationales.

Evaluation

Evaluation of the child or adolescent with separation anxiety disorder requires reassessment of the behaviors for which the family sought treatment. Both the client and the family members will have to change their behavior. The following types of questions may provide assistance in gathering data required for evaluating whether the nursing interventions have been effective in achieving the goals of therapy:

■ Is the client able to maintain anxiety at a manageable level (i.e., without temper tantrums, screaming, or clinging)?
■ Have complaints of physical symptoms diminished?

■ Has the client demonstrated the ability to cope in more adaptive ways in the face of escalating anxiety?
■ Have the parents identified their role in the separation conflict? Are they able to discuss more adaptive coping strategies?
■ Does the client verbalize an intention to return to school?
■ Have nightmares and fears of the dark subsided?
■ Is the client able to interact with others away from the attachment figure?
■ Has the precipitating stressor been identified? Have strategies for coping more adaptively to similar stressors in the future been established?

Quality and Safety Education for Nurses (QSEN)

The Institute of Medicine (IOM), in its 2003 report, *Health Professions Education: A Bridge to Quality*, challenged faculties of medicine, nursing, and other health professions to ensure that their graduates have achieved a core set of competencies in order to meet the needs of the 21st-century health-care system. These competencies include *providing patient-centered care, working in interdisciplinary teams, employing evidence-based practice, applying quality improvement, ensuring safety,* and *utilizing informatics.* A QSEN teaching strategy is presented in Box 33-8. The use of this type of

Table 33-10 | CARE PLAN FOR THE CLIENT WITH SEPARATION ANXIETY DISORDER

NURSING DIAGNOSIS: ANXIETY (SEVERE)

RELATED TO: Family history; temperament; overattachment to parent; negative role modeling

OUTCOME CRITERIA	NURSING INTERVENTIONS	RATIONALE
Short-Term Goal • Client will discuss fears of separation with trusted individual. **Long-Term Goal** • Client will maintain anxiety at no higher than moderate level in the face of events that formerly have precipitated panic.	1. Establish an atmosphere of calmness, trust, and genuine positive regard. 2. Assure client of his or her safety and security. 3. Explore the child or adolescent's fears of separating from the parents. Explore with the parents possible fears they may have of separation from the child. 4. Help parents and child initiate realistic goals (e.g., child to stay with sitter for 2 hours with minimal anxiety; or, child to stay at friend's house without parents until 9 p.m. without experiencing panic anxiety). 5. Give, and encourage parents to give, positive reinforcement for desired behaviors.	1. Trust and unconditional acceptance are necessary for satisfactory nurse-client relationship. Calmness is important because anxiety is easily transmitted from one person to another. 2. Symptoms of panic anxiety are very frightening. 3. Some parents may have an underlying fear of separation from the child, of which they are unaware and which they are unconsciously transferring to the child. 4. Parents may be so frustrated with child's clinging and demanding behaviors that assistance with problem-solving may be required. 5. Positive reinforcement encourages repetition of desirable behaviors.

NURSING DIAGNOSIS: INEFFECTIVE COPING

RELATED TO: Unresolved separation conflicts and inadequate coping skills

EVIDENCED BY: Numerous somatic complaints

OUTCOME CRITERIA	NURSING INTERVENTIONS	RATIONALE
Short-Term Goal • Client will verbalize correlation of somatic symptoms to fear of separation. **Long-Term Goal** • Client will demonstrate use of more adaptive coping strategies (than physical symptoms) in response to stressful situations.	1. Encourage child or adolescent to discuss specific situations in life that produce the most distress and describe his or her response to these situations. Include parents in the discussion. 2. Help the child or adolescent who is perfectionistic to recognize that self-expectations may be unrealistic. Connect times of unmet self-expectations to the exacerbation of physical symptoms. 3. Encourage parents and child to identify more adaptive coping strategies that the child could use in the face of anxiety that feels overwhelming. Practice through role-play.	1. Client and family may be unaware of the correlation between stressful situations and the exacerbation of physical symptoms. 2. Recognition of maladaptive patterns is the first step in the change process. 3. Practice facilitates the use of the desired behavior when the individual is actually faced with the stressful situation.

Continued

Table 33-10 | CARE PLAN FOR THE CLIENT WITH SEPARATION ANXIETY DISORDER—cont'd

NURSING DIAGNOSIS: IMPAIRED SOCIAL INTERACTION

RELATED TO: Reluctance to be away from attachment figure

OUTCOME CRITERIA	NURSING INTERVENTIONS	RATIONALE
Short-Term Goal • Client will spend time with staff or other support person, without presence of attachment figure, without excessive anxiety. **Long-Term Goal** • Client will be able to spend time with others (without presence of attachment figure) without excessive anxiety.	1. Develop a trusting relationship with client. 2. Attend groups with the child and support efforts to interact with others. Give positive feedback. 3. Convey to the child the acceptability of his or her not participating in group in the beginning. Gradually encourage small contributions until client is able to participate more fully. 4. Help client set small personal goals (e.g., "Today I will speak to one person I don't know").	1. This is the first step in helping the client learn to interact with others. 2. Presence of a trusted individual provides security during times of distress. Positive feedback encourages repetition. 3. Small successes will gradually increase self-confidence and decrease self-consciousness, so that client will feel less anxious in the group situation. 4. Simple, realistic goals provide opportunities for success that increase self-confidence and may encourage the client to attempt more difficult objectives in the future.

BOX 33-8 QSEN TEACHING STRATEGY

Assignment: Patient-Centered Care: Kleinman's Mini-Ethnography
Interviewing Families of Children With Psychiatric Disorders

Competency Domain: Patient-Centered Care

Learning Objectives: Student will:
• Demonstrate skills in hearing patients' and family members' stories of living with the disorder.
• Identify their own explanatory models of the disorder.
• Demonstrate attitudes that reflect a desire to cultivate cultural humility and cultural competence in nursing practice.

Strategy Overview:
1. Read the article, "Anthropology in the Clinic: The Problem of Cultural Competency and How to Fix It," by A. Kleinman and P. Benson. The article is available online at www.plosmedicine.org/article/info:doi/10.1371/journal.pmed. 0030294
2. Based on the "mini ethnography" described by Kleinman and Benson, interview a family member of a child with a psychiatric disorder and elicit a narrative of his or her experience in living with the disorder.
3. Drawing on notes from the interview, write one paper that is the narrative of the illness from the perspective of the interviewee and another paper that describes the student's own explanatory model.

SOURCE: Adapted from teaching strategy submitted by Lisa Day, Assistant Clinical Professor, UCSF, School of Nursing, San Francisco, CA. © 2009 QSEN; http://qsen.org. With permission.

activity is intended to arm the instructor and the student with guidelines for attaining the knowledge, skills, and attitudes necessary for achievement of quality and safety competencies in nursing.

General Therapeutic Approaches

Behavior Therapy

Behavior therapy is based on the concepts of classical conditioning and operant conditioning. Behavior therapy is a common and effective treatment with disruptive behavior disorders such as ADHD, ODD, and conduct disorder. With this approach, rewards are given for appropriate behaviors and withheld when behaviors are disruptive or otherwise inappropriate. The principle behind behavior therapy is that positive reinforcements encourage repetition of desirable behaviors and aversive reinforcements (punishments) discourage repetition of undesirable behaviors. Behavior modification techniques—the system of rewards and consequences—can be taught to parents to be used in the home environment. Consistency is an essential component.

In the treatment setting, individualized behavior modification programs are designed for each client. A case study example, based on a token economy, is presented in Chapter 18.

Family Therapy

Children cannot be separated from their family. Therapy for children and adolescents must involve the entire family if problems are to be resolved. Parents should be involved in designing and implementing the treatment plan for the child and should be involved in all aspects of the treatment process.

The genogram can be used to identify problem areas between family members (see Chapter 11). It provides an overall picture of the life of the family over several generations, including roles that various family members play and emotional distance between specific individuals. Areas for change can be easily identified.

The impact of family dynamics on disruptive behavior disorders has been identified. The impact of disruptive behavior on family dynamics cannot be ignored. Family coping can become severely compromised by the chronic stress of dealing with a child with a behavior disorder. It is therefore imperative that the treatment plan for the identified client be instituted within the context of family-centered care.

Group Therapy

Group therapy provides children and adolescents with the opportunity to interact within an association of their peers. This can be both gratifying and overwhelming, depending on the child.

Group therapy provides a number of benefits. Appropriate social behavior often is learned from the positive and negative feedback of peers. Opportunity is provided to learn to tolerate and accept differences in others, to learn that it is acceptable to disagree, to learn to offer and receive support from others, and to practice these new skills in a safe environment. It is a way to learn from the experiences of others.

Group therapy with children and adolescents can take several forms. Music therapy groups allow clients to express feelings through music, often when they are unable to express themselves in any other way. Art and activity/craft therapy groups allow individual expression through artistic means.

Group play therapy is the treatment of choice for many children between the ages of 3 and 9 years. Landreth and Bratton (2007) state:

> Play therapy is to children what counseling or psychotherapy is to adults. Play provides children with a means of expressing their inner world. The use of toys enables children to transfer anxieties, fears, fantasies, and guilt to objects rather than people. In the process, children are safe from their own feelings and reactions because play enables children to distance themselves from traumatic events and experiences. For children, play therapy changes what may be unmanageable in reality into manageable situations through symbolic representation. This provides children with opportunities for learning to cope.

Psychoeducational groups are very beneficial for adolescents. The only drawback to this type of group is that it works best when the group is closed-ended; that is, once the group has been formed, no one is allowed to join until the group has reached its preestablished closure. Members are allowed to propose topics for discussion. The leader serves as teacher much of the time and facilitates discussion of the proposed topic. Members may from time to time be presenters and serve as discussion leaders. Sometimes, psychoeducation groups evolve into traditional therapy discussion groups.

Psychopharmacology

Several of the disorders presented in this chapter are treated with medications. The appropriate pharmacology was presented following the section in which the disorder was discussed. Medication should never be the sole method of treatment. It is undeniable that medication can and does improve quality of life for families of children and adolescents with these disorders. However, research has indicated that medication alone is not as effective as a combination of medication and psychosocial therapy. It is important for families to understand that there is no way to "give him a pill and make him well." The importance of the psychosocial therapies cannot be overstressed. Some clinicians will not prescribe medications for a client unless he or she also participates in concomitant psychotherapy sessions. The beneficial effects of the medications promote improved coping ability, which in turn enhances the intent of the psychosocial therapy.

Summary and Key Points

- Intellectual disability is defined by deficits in general intellectual functioning and adaptive functioning.
- Four levels of intellectual disability—mild, moderate, severe, and profound—are associated with various behavioral manifestations and abilities.
- Autism spectrum disorder (ASD) is characterized by a withdrawal of the child into the self and into a fantasy world of his or her own creation.
- It is generally accepted that ASD is caused by abnormalities in brain structures or functions. Genetic factors are also thought to play a significant role in ASD.
- Children with attention-deficit/hyperactivity disorder (ADHD) may exhibit symptoms of inattention or hyperactivity and impulsiveness or a combination of the two.
- Genetics plays a role in the etiology of ADHD. Neurotransmitters that have been implicated include dopamine, norepinephrine, and serotonin. Maternal smoking during pregnancy has been linked to hyperactive behavior in offspring.
- CNS stimulants, alpha agonists, atomoxetine, and bupropion are commonly used to treat ADHD.

- The essential feature of Tourette's disorder is the presence of multiple motor tics and one or more vocal tics.
- Common medications used with Tourette's disorder include haloperidol, pimozide, clonidine, guanfacine, and atypical antipsychotics such as risperidone, olanzapine, and ziprasidone.
- Oppositional defiant disorder is characterized by a pattern of negativistic, defiant, disobedient, and hostile behavior toward authority figures that occurs more frequently than is usually observed in individuals of comparable age and developmental level.
- With conduct disorder, there is a repetitive and persistent pattern of behavior in which the basic rights of others or major age-appropriate societal norms or rules are violated.
- The essential feature of separation anxiety disorder is excessive anxiety concerning separation from the home or from those to whom the person is attached.
- Children with separation anxiety disorder may have temperamental characteristics present at birth that predispose them to the disorder.
- General therapeutic approaches for child and adolescent psychiatric disorders include behavior therapy, family therapy, group therapies (including music, art, crafts, play, and psychoeducation), and psychopharmacology.

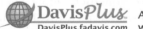 **DavisPlus** DavisPlus.fadavis.com Additional info available at www.davisplus.com

Review Questions
Self-Examination/Learning Exercise

*Select the answer that is **most** appropriate for each of the following questions.*

1. In an effort to help the child with mild to moderate intellectual developmental disorder develop satisfying relationships with others, which of the following nursing interventions is most appropriate?
   a. Interpret the child's behavior for others.
   b. Set limits on behavior that is socially inappropriate.
   c. Allow the child to behave spontaneously, for he or she has no concept of right or wrong.
   d. This child is not capable of forming social relationships.

2. The child with autism spectrum disorder (ASD) has difficulty with trust. With this in mind, which of the following nursing actions would be most appropriate?
   a. Encourage all staff to hold the child as often as possible, conveying trust through touch.
   b. Assign a different staff member each day so the child will learn that everyone can be trusted.
   c. Assign the same staff person as often as possible to promote feelings of security and trust.
   d. Avoid eye contact, because this is extremely uncomfortable for the child, and may even discourage trust.

Review Questions—cont'd
Self-Examination/Learning Exercise

3. Which of the following nursing diagnoses would be considered the *priority* in planning care for the child with ASD?
   a. Risk for self-mutilation evidenced by banging head against wall.
   b. Impaired social interaction evidenced by unresponsiveness to people.
   c. Impaired verbal communication evidenced by absence of verbal expression.
   d. Disturbed personal identity evidenced by inability to differentiate self from others.

4. Which of the following activities would be most appropriate for the child with attention-deficit/hyperactivity disorder (ADHD)?
   a. Monopoly
   b. Volleyball
   c. Pool
   d. Checkers

5. Which of the following groups is most commonly used for drug management of the child with ADHD?
   a. CNS depressants (e.g., diazepam [Valium])
   b. CNS stimulants (e.g., methylphenidate [Ritalin])
   c. Anticonvulsants (e.g., phenytoin [Dilantin])
   d. Major tranquilizers (e.g., haloperidol [Haldol])

6. The child with ADHD has a nursing diagnosis of impaired social interaction. Which of the following nursing interventions are appropriate for this child? (Select all that apply.)
   a. Socially isolate the child when interactions with others are inappropriate.
   b. Set limits with consequences on inappropriate behaviors.
   c. Provide rewards for appropriate behaviors.
   d. Provide group situations for the child.

7. The nursing history and assessment of an adolescent with a conduct disorder might reveal all of the following behaviors *except*:
   a. Manipulation of others for fulfillment of own desires
   b. Chronic violation of rules
   c. Feelings of guilt associated with the exploitation of others
   d. Inability to form close peer relationships

8. Certain family dynamics often predispose adolescents to the development of conduct disorder. Which of the following patterns is thought to be a contributing factor?
   a. Parents who are overprotective
   b. Parents who have high expectations for their children
   c. Parents who consistently set limits on their children's behavior
   d. Parents who are alcohol dependent

9. Which of the following is *least* likely to predispose a child to Tourette's disorder?
   a. Absence of parental bonding
   b. Family history of the disorder
   c. Abnormalities of brain neurotransmitters
   d. Structural abnormalities of the brain

10. Which of the following medications is used to treat Tourette's disorder?
    a. Methylphenidate (Ritalin)
    b. Haloperidol (Haldol)
    c. Imipramine (Tofranil)
    d. Phenytoin (Dilantin)

IMPLICATIONS OF RESEARCH FOR EVIDENCE-BASED PRACTICE

Frame, K., Kelly, L., & Bayley, E. (2003). Increasing perceptions of self-worth in preadolescents diagnosed with ADHD. *Journal of Nursing Scholarship, 35*(3), 225-229.

DESCRIPTION OF THE STUDY: The theoretical framework for this study was based on the Roy adaptation model. The sample in this study consisted of 65 preadolescents diagnosed with ADD or ADHD in an upper-middle class community in the United States. Participants were randomly assigned to either the control group or the experimental group, and all completed the Harter's Self-Perception Profile for Children instrument at the beginning of the study and 4 weeks later. This tool was designed to measure perceptions of scholastic competence, social acceptance, athletic competence, physical appearance, behavioral conduct, and global self-worth. Children in the experimental group participated in a school-nurse facilitated support group that met twice weekly for 4 weeks. In the group, the participants were assisted to learn strategies for effective interactions with their peers, teachers, and families. Interventions served to promote adaptive self-evaluations and to address the unfavorable self-perceptions of many children with ADHD.

RESULTS OF THE STUDY: On post-testing, participants in the support group scored significantly higher than controls on each of the six subscales, with significant increases on four of the subscales, including perceived social acceptance, perceived athletic competence, perceived physical appearance, and perceived global self-worth.

IMPLICATIONS FOR NURSING PRACTICE: This study has implications for nurses who work with children, and particularly those who work with children diagnosed with ADHD. Because preadolescence is a time when children compare themselves, either positively or negatively, with their peers, group interaction is an especially significant intervention. The authors stated, "The support group, with children helping children, enabled participants to engage in creative problem-solving and to develop solutions to their difficulties." This intervention was shown to promote positive perceptions and behaviors among children with ADD and ADHD. It is especially appropriate for the role of school nurse, but it is also consistent with the role of any nurse who interacts directly with children or adolescents who have similar problems.

IMPLICATIONS OF RESEARCH FOR EVIDENCE-BASED PRACTICE

Hall, L.A., Rayens, M.K., & Peden, A.R. (2008). Maternal factors associated with child behavior. *Journal of Nursing Scholarship, 40*(2), 124-130.

DESCRIPTION OF THE STUDY: The purpose of this study was to identify maternal predictors of children's internalizing behaviors (e.g., anxiety, depression, withdrawal, and somatic complaints) and externalizing behaviors (e.g., impulsivity, disruptiveness, and aggression). The sample included 205 low-income, single mothers with children between 2 and 6 years of age. Other criteria for inclusion in the study sample were not being in psychiatric care or counseling, not taking antidepressant medication, not being suicidal, not being pregnant, and having no children younger than 1 year of age. Maternal variables were measured as follows: The Beck Depression Inventory was used to measure depressive symptoms; negative thinking was measured using the Crandell Cognitions Inventory; self-worth and self-acceptance were measured on the Rosenberg Self-esteem Scale; and chronic stress was measured on the Everyday Stressors Index, which assesses common problems faced daily by mothers with young children. Surveys were conducted using in-home interviews with the mothers.

RESULTS OF THE STUDY: Maternal stress exerted the largest total effects on children's internalizing and externalizing behaviors. Depressive symptoms had the second largest total effect, followed by negative thinking. Mothers' self-esteem displayed the weakest total effect on both child outcomes. Other studies have shown that maternal depression is associated with their children's poor school performance, slow cognitive and motor development, and elevated cortisol levels. Very young children with behavior problems are at risk for continuation of these problems into school age and adolescence.

IMPLICATIONS FOR NURSING PRACTICE: The authors suggest that the types of stressors faced by low-income women need to be identified and attempts made at alleviation by intervention or referral to social services for support. Treatment of the mother's depression with antidepressant medication and cognitive-behavioral strategies to reduce negative thinking may also provide positive benefits for their children. The authors state:

> The findings of this study indicate that a focus on decreasing mothers' negative thinking may provide a way to reduce their depressive symptoms and result in fewer behavior problems among their young children. Nurses working in primary care and community-based setting are in key positions to address this problem and improve the mental health of low-income mothers and positively affect the behavior of their children.

TEST YOUR CRITICAL THINKING SKILLS

Jimmy, age 9, has been admitted to the child psychiatric unit with a diagnosis of attention-deficit/hyperactivity disorder. He has been unmanageable at school and at home, and has had several suspensions from school for continuous disruption of his class. He refuses to sit in his chair or do his work. He yells out in class, interrupts the teacher and the other students, and lately has become physically aggressive when he cannot have his way. Most recently, he was suspended after hitting his teacher when she asked him to return to his seat.

Jimmy's mother describes him as a restless and demanding baby, who grew into a restless and demanding toddler. He has never gotten along well with his peers. Even as a small child, he would take his friends' toys away from them or bite them if they tried to hold their own with him. His 5-year-old sister is afraid of him and refuses to be alone with him.

During the nurse's intake assessment, Jimmy paced the room or rocked in his chair. He talked incessantly on a superficial level and jumped from topic to topic. He told the nurse that he did not know why he was there. He acknowledged that he had some problems at school but said that was only because the other kids picked on him and the teacher did not like him. He said he got into trouble at home sometimes but that was because his parents liked his little sister better than they liked him.

The physician has ordered methylphenidate 5 mg twice a day for Jimmy. His response to this order is, "I'm not going to take drugs. I'm not sick!"

Answer the following questions related to Jimmy:

1. What are the pertinent assessment data to be noted by the nurse?
2. What is the primary nursing diagnosis for Jimmy?
3. Aside from client safety, to what problems would the nurse want to direct intervention with Jimmy?

References

American Psychiatric Association (APA). (2000). *Diagnostic and statistical manual of mental disorders* (4th ed., text rev.) Washington, DC: Author.

American Psychiatric Association. (2013). *Diagnostic and statistical manual of mental disorders* (5th ed.). Washington, DC: Author.

Autism Genome Project Consortium. (2007). Mapping autism risk loci using genetic linkage and chromosomal rearrangements. *Nature Genetics, 39*(3), 319-328.

Bagley, C., & Mallick, K. (2000). Spiraling up and spiraling down: Implications of a long-term study of temperament and conduct disorder for social work with children. *Child & Family Social Work, 5*(4), 291-301.

Ben-Amor, L., Grizenko, N., Schwartz, G., Lageix, P., Baron, C., Ter-Stepanian, M., Zappitelli, M., Mbekou, V., & Joober, R. (2005). Perinatal complications in children with attention-deficit hyperactivity disorder and their unaffected siblings. *Journal of Psychiatry & Neuroscience, 30*(2), 120-126.

Bhat, M., Grizenko, N., Ben-Amor, L., & Joober, R. (2005). Obstetric complications in children with attention deficit/hyperactivity disorder and learning disability. *McGill Journal of Medicine, 8*(2), 109-113.

Black, D.W., & Andreasen, N.C. (2011). *Introductory textbook of psychiatry* (5th ed.). Washington, DC: American Psychiatric Publishing.

Braun, J., Kahn, R.S., Froehlich, T., Auinger, P., & Lanphear, B.P. (2006). Exposures to environmental toxicants and attention-deficit/hyperactivity disorder in U.S. children. *Environmental Health Perspectives, 114*(12), 1904-1909.

Brkanac, Z., Raskind, W.H., & King, B.H. (2008). Pharmacology and genetics of autism: Implications for diagnosis and treatment. *Personalized Medicine, 5*(6), 599-607.

Centers for Disease Control and Prevention (CDC). (2011, August). Attention deficit hyperactivity disorder among children aged 5-17 in the United States 1998-2009. *NCHS Data Brief, 70*. Hyattsville, MD: National Center for Health Statistics.

Centers for Disease Control and Prevention. (CDC). (2012a). *Childhood lead poisoning data, statistics, and surveillance.* Retrieved from http://www.cdc.gov/nceh/lead

Centers for Disease Control and Prevention. (CDC). (2012b). Prevalence of Autism Spectrum Disorders—Autism and Developmental Disabilities Monitoring Network, 14 Sites, United States, 2008. *Morbidity and Mortality Weekly Report, 61*(3), 1-24.

Comings, D.E., Gade-Andavolu, R., Gonzalez, N., Wu, S., Mahleman, D., Blake, H., Dietz, G., Saucier, G., & MacMurray, J.P. (2000). Comparison of the role of dopamine, serotonin, and noradrenaline genes in ADHD, ODD, and conduct disorder: Multivariate regression analysis of 20 genes. *Clinical Genetics, 57*(3), 178-196.

Croen, L.A., Grether, J.K., Yoshida, C.K., Odouli, R., & Van dewater, J. (2005). Maternal autoimmune diseases, asthma and allergies, and childhood autism spectrum disorders. *Archives of Pediatrics and Adolescent Medicine, 159*(2), 151-157.

Dick, D.M., Li, T-K, Edenberg, H.J., Hesselbrock, V., Kramer, J., Kuperman, S., Porjesz, B., Bucholz, K., Goate, A., Nurnberger, J., & Foroud, T. (2004). A genome-wide screen for genes influencing conduct disorder. *Molecular Psychiatry, 9*(1), 81-86.

Dopheide, J.A., & Pliszka, S.R. (2009). Attention deficit/hyperactivity disorder: An Update. *Pharmacotherapy, 29*(6), 656-679.

Erlij, D., Acosta-Garcia, J., Rojas-Marquez, M., Gonzalez-Hernandez, B., Escartin-Perez, E., Aceves, J., & Floran, B. (2012). Dopamine D4 receptor stimulation in GABAergic projections of the globus pallidus to the reticular thalamic nucleus and the substantia nigra reticulate of the rat decreases locomotor activity. *Neuropharmacology, 62*(2), 1111-1118.

Faraone, S.V. (2006). The genetics of attention deficit/hyperactivity disorder: Current status and clinical implications. *Medscape Psychiatry & Mental Health, 11*(2). Retrieved from http://www.medscape.com/viewarticle/546469

Ferguson-Noyes, N., & Wilkinson, A.M. (2008). Caring for individuals with ADHD throughout the lifespan: An introduction to ADHD. *Psychiatric Nurse Counseling Points, 1*(1), 1-15.

Foley, D.L., Eaves, L.J., Wormley, B., Silberg, J.L., Maes, H.H., Kuh, J., & Riley, B.(2004). Childhood adversity, monoamine oxidase A genotype, and risk for conduct disorder. *Archives of General Psychiatry, 61*(7), 738-744.

Harvard Medical School. (2007). Separation anxiety. *Harvard Mental Health Letter, 23*(7), 1-3.

Hazlett, H.C., Poe, M.D., Gerig, G., Styner, M., Chappell, C., Smith, R.G., Vachet, C., & Piven, J. (2011). Early brain overgrowth in autism associated with an increase in cortical surface area before age 2 years. *Archives of General Psychiatry, 68*(5), 467-476.

Hunt, R.D. (2006). The neurobiology of ADHD. *Medscape Psychiatry & Mental Health, 11*(2). Retrieved from http://www.medscape.com/viewarticle/541543

Institute of Medicine. (2003). *Health professions education: A bridge to quality.* Washington, DC: Institute of Medicine.

Jenson, J. (2005, Fall). Attention-deficit/hyperactivity disorder: Treatment update. *Pediatric Rounds: Newsletter of the Children's Specialty Group.* Milwaukee, WI: Medical College of Wisconsin.

Kollins, S.H. (2008). ADHD genetics, neurobiology, and neuropharmacology. *Medscape Psychiatry.* Retrieved from http://www.medscape.com/viewprogram/17290

Ladd, G.W. (1999). Peer relationships and social competence during early and middle childhood. *Annual Review of Psychology, 50*(1), 333-359.

Landreth, G., & Bratton, S. (2007). Play therapy. *ERIC Digests.* Retrieved from http://www.ericdigests.org/2000-1/play.html

Leckman, J.F., Bloch, M.H., Scahill, L., & King, R.A. (2006). Tourette syndrome: The self under siege. *Journal of Child Neurology, 21*(8), 642-649.

Linnet, K.M., Wisborg, K., Obel, C., Secher, N.J., Thomsen, P.H., Agerbo, E., &, Henriksen, T.B. (2005). Smoking during pregnancy and the risk for hyperkinetic disorder in offspring. *Pediatrics, 116*(2), 462-467.

Lubit, R.H. (2011). Oppositional defiant disorder. Retrieved from http://emedicine.medscape.com/article/918095-overview

McCann, D., Barrett, A., Cooper, A., Crumpler, D., Dalen, L., Grimshaw, K., Kitchin, E., Lok, K., Porteous, L., Prince, E., Sonuga-Barke, E., Warner, J.O., & Stevenson, J. (2007, November 3). Food additives and hyperactive behaviour in 3-year-old and 8/9-year-old children in the community: A randomized double-blinded, placebo-controlled trial. *Lancet, 370*(9598), 1560-1567.

Nigg, J.T., Nikolas, M., Knottnerus, G.M., Cavanagh, K., & Friderici, K. (2010). Confirmation and extension of association of blood lead with attention-deficit/hyperactivity disorder (ADHD) and ADHD symptom domains at population-typical exposure levels. *Journal of Child Psychology and Psychiatry, 51*(1), 58-65.

Peterson, B.S., Choi, H.A., Hao, X., Amat, J.A., Zhu, H., Whiteman, R., Liu, J., Xu, D., & Bansal, R. (2007). Morphologic features of the amygdala and hippocampus in children and adults with Tourette syndrome. *Archives of General Psychiatry, 65*(11), 1281-1291.

Plessen, K.J., Lundervold, A., Grunner, R., Hammar, A., Lundervold, A., Peterson, B.S., & Hugdahl, K. (2007). Functional brain asymmetry, attentional modulation, and interhemispheric transfer in boys with Tourette syndrome. *Neuropsychologia, 45*(4), 767-774.

Popper, C.W., Gammon, G.D., West, S.A., & Bailey, C.E. (2003). Disorders usually first diagnosed in infancy, childhood, or adolescence. In R.E. Hales & S.C. Yudofsky, (Eds.), *Textbook of clinical psychiatry* (4th ed., pp. 833-974). Washington, DC: American Psychiatric Publishing.

Research Units on Pediatric Psychopharmacology Autism Network. (2002). Risperidone in children with autism and serious behavioral problems. *New England Journal of Medicine, 347*(5), 314-321.

Research Units on Pediatric Psychopharmacology Autism Network. (2005). Risperidone treatment of autistic disorder: Longer-term benefits and blinded discontinuation after 6 months. *American Journal of Psychiatry, 162*(7), 1361-1369.

Rizwan, S., Manning, J.T., & Brabin, B.J. (2007). Maternal smoking during pregnancy and possible effects of in utero testosterone: Evidence from the 2D:4D finger length ratio. *Early Human Development, 83*(2), 87-90.

Robb, A.S. (2006). Managing ADHD in a patient with substance use disorder. *Medscape Psychiatry & Mental Health CME.* Retrieved from http://cme.medscape.com/viewarticle/549218

Rowe, R., Maughan, B., Worthman, C.M., Costello, E.J., & Angold, A. (2004). Testosterone, antisocial behavior, and social dominance in boys: Pubertal development and biosocial interaction. *Biological Psychiatry, 55*(5), 546-552.

Sadock, B.J., & Sadock, V.A. (2007). Synopsis of psychiatry: Behavioral sciences/clinical psychiatry (10th ed.). Philadelphia, PA: Lippincott Williams & Wilkins.

Searight, H.R., Rottnek, F., & Abby, S.L. (2001). Conduct disorder: Diagnosis and treatment in primary care. *American Family Physician, 63*(8), 1579-1588.

Shamir-Essakow, G., Ungerer, J.A., & Rapee, R. (2005). Attachment, behavioral inhibition, and anxiety in preschool children. *Journal of Abnormal Child Psychology, 33*(2), 131-143.

Shriber, L. (2012). Autism: A neurological and sensory based perspective. *International Encyclopedia of Rehabilitation.* Retrieved from http://cirrie.buffalo.edu/encyclopedia/en/article/285

Singer, H.S., Leffler, J.B., & Murray, C.F. (2008). Tics and Tourette syndrome: A clinical review. *MedscapePsychiatry CME.* Retrieved from http://cme.medscape.com/viewarticle/574198

Ursano, A.M., Kartheiser, P.H., & Barnhill, L.J. (2008). Disorders usually first diagnosed in infancy, childhood, or adolescence. In R.E. Hales, S.C. Yudofsky, & G.O. Gabbard (Eds.), *Textbook of psychiatry* (5th ed., pp. 861-920). Washington, DC: American Psychiatric Publishing.

Voeller, K.K.S. (2004). Attention-deficit hyperactivity disorder (ADHD). *Journal of Child Neurology, 19*(10), 798-814.

Wilens, T.E., & Upadhyaya, H.P. (2007). ADHD and substance abuse: A frequent—and risky—combination. *Medscape Psychiatry & Mental Health CME.* Retrieved from http://www.medscape.com/viewprogram/6506

Williams, N.M., Zaharieva, I., Martin, A., Langley, K., Mantripragada, K., Fossdal, R., et al. (2010). Rare chromosomal deletions and duplications in attention-deficit hyperactivity disorder: A genome-wide analysis. *Lancet, 376*(9750), 1401-1408.

Zinner, S.H. (2004). Tourette syndrome—much more than tics. *Contemporary Pediatrics, 21*(8), 38-49.

@ INTERNET REFERENCES

- Additional information about ADHD may be located at the following websites:
  - http://www.chadd.org
  - http://www.nimh.nih.gov/health/topics/attention-deficit-hyperactivity-disorder-adhd/index.shtml

- Additional information about ASD may be located at the following websites:
  - http://www.autism-society.org
  - http://www.nimh.nih.gov/health/topics/autism-spectrum-disorders-asd/index.shtml

- Additional information about Tourette's disorder may be located at the following websites:
  - http://www.ninds.nih.gov/disorders/tourette/detail_tourette.htm
  - http://www.tsa-usa.org

- Additional information about medications to treat ADHD and Tourette's disorder may be located at the following websites:
  - http://www.drugs.com
  - http://www.nlm.nih.gov/medlineplus/druginformation.html

MOVIE CONNECTIONS

Bill (intellectual disability) • *Bill, On His Own* (intellectual disability) • *Sling Blade* (intellectual disability) • *Forrest Gump* (intellectual disability) • *Rain Man* (autism spectrum disorder [ASD]) • *Mercury Rising* (ASD) • *Niagara, Niagara* (Tourette's disorder) • *Toughlove* (conduct disorder)

The Aging Individual

34

KEY TERMS

attachment

bereavement overload

disengagement theory

geriatrics

gerontology

geropsychiatry

"granny-bashing"

"granny-dumping"

long-term memory

Medicaid

Medicare

menopause

osteoporosis

reminiscence therapy

short-term memory

OBJECTIVES

After reading this chapter, the student will be able to:

1. Discuss societal perspectives on aging.
2. Describe an epidemiological profile of aging in the United States.
3. Discuss various theories of aging.
4. Describe biological, psychological, sociocultural, and sexual aspects of the normal aging process.
5. Discuss retirement as a special concern to the aging individual.
6. Explain personal and sociological perspectives of long-term care of the aging individual.
7. Describe the problem of elder abuse as it exists in today's society.
8. Discuss the implications of the increasing number of suicides among the elderly population.
9. Apply the steps of the nursing process to the care of aging individuals.

HOMEWORK ASSIGNMENT

Please read the chapter and answer the following questions:

1. Which theory of aging postulates that life span and longevity changes are predetermined?
2. How is the ability to learn affected by aging?
3. What is the most common cause of psychopathology in the elderly?
4. What are some factors that are thought to contribute to elder abuse?

What is it like to grow old? It is not likely that many people in the American culture would state that it is something they want to do. Most would agree, however, that it is "better than the alternative."

Roberts (1991) tells the following often-told tale of Supreme Court Justice Oliver Wendell Holmes, Jr. In the year before he retired at age 91 as the oldest justice ever to sit on the Supreme Court of the United States, Holmes and his close friend Justice Louis Brandeis, then a mere 74 years old, were out for one of their frequent walks on Washington's Capitol Hill. On this particular day, the justices spotted a very attractive young woman approaching them. As she passed, Holmes paused, sighed, and said to Brandeis, "Oh, to be 70 again!" Obviously, being old is relative to the individual experiencing it.

Growing old has not been popular among the youth-oriented American culture. However, with 66 million "baby-boomers" reaching their 65th birthdays by the year 2030, greater emphasis is being placed on the needs of an aging population. The disciplines of **gerontology** (the study of the aging process), **geriatrics** (the branch of clinical medicine specializing in problems of the elderly), and **geropsychiatry** (the branch of clinical medicine specializing in psychopathology of the elderly population) are expanding rapidly in response to this predictable demand.

Growing old in a society that has been obsessed with youth may have a critical impact on the mental health of many people. This situation has serious implications for psychiatric nursing.

What is it like to grow old? More and more people will be able to answer this question as the 21st century progresses. Perhaps they will also be asking the question that Roberts (1991) asks: "How did I get here so fast?"

This chapter focuses on physical and psychological changes associated with the aging process, as well as special concerns of the elderly population, such as retirement, long-term care, elder abuse, and high suicide rates. The nursing process is presented as the vehicle for delivery of nursing care to elderly individuals.

How Old Is *Old*?

The concept of "old" has changed drastically over the years. Our prehistoric ancestors probably had a life span of 40 years, with the average individual living around 18 years. As civilization developed, mortality rates remained high as a result of periodic famine and frequent malnutrition. An improvement in the standard of living was not truly evident until about the middle of the 17th century. Since that time, assured food supply, changes in food production, better housing conditions, and more progressive medical and sanitation facilities have contributed to population growth, declining mortality rates, and substantial increases in longevity.

In 1900, the average life expectancy in the United States was 47 years, and only 4 percent of the population was age 65 or over. By 2011, the average life expectancy at birth was 78.7 years (76.3 years for men and 81.1 years for women) (National Center for Health Statistics [NCHS], 2012a).

The U.S. Census Bureau has created a system for classification of older Americans:

■ Older: 55 through 64 years
■ Elderly: 65 through 74 years
■ Aged: 75 through 84 years
■ Very old: 85 years and older

Some gerontologists have elected to use a simpler classification system:

■ Young old: 60 through 74 years
■ Middle old: 75 through 84 years
■ Old old: 85 years and older

So how old is *old*? Obviously the term cannot be defined by a number. Myths and stereotypes of aging have long obscured our understanding of the aged and the process of aging. Ideas that all elderly individuals are sick, depressed, obsessed with death, senile, and incapable of change affect the way elderly people are treated. They even shape the pattern of aging of the people who believe them. They can become self-fulfilling prophecies—people start to believe they should behave in certain ways and, therefore, act according to those beliefs. Generalized assumptions can be demeaning and interfere with the quality of life for older individuals.

Just as there are many differences in individual adaptation at earlier stages of development, so it is in the elderly population. Erikson (1963) has suggested that the mentally healthy older person possesses a sense of ego integrity and self-acceptance that will help in adapting to the ambiguities of the future with a sense of security and optimism.

Murray, Zentner, and Yakimo (2009) stated:

> [Having accomplished the earlier developmental tasks], the person accepts life as his or her own and as the only life for the self. He or she would wish for none other and would defend the meaning and the dignity of the lifestyle. The person has further refined the characteristics of maturity described for the middle-aged adult, achieving both wisdom and an enriched perspective about life and people. (p. 662)

Everyone, particularly health-care workers, should see aging people as individuals, each with specific needs and abilities, rather than as a stereotypical group. Some individuals may seem "old" at 40, whereas others may not seem "old" at 70. Variables such as attitude, mental health, physical health, and degree of independence strongly influence how an individual perceives himself or herself. Surely, in the final analysis, whether one is considered "old" must be self-determined.

Epidemiological Statistics

The Population

In 1980, Americans 65 years of age or older numbered 25.5 million. By 2012, these numbers had increased to 43.1 million, representing 13.7 percent of the population (Administration on Aging [AoA], 2014). This trend is expected to continue, with a projection for 2040 at about 79.7 million, or 21 percent of the population.

Marital Status

In 2013, of individuals age 65 and older, 71 percent of men and 45 percent of women were married (AoA, 2014). Thirty-six percent of all women in this age group were widowed. There were over three times as many widows as widowers, because women live longer than men and tend to marry men older than themselves.

Living Arrangements

The majority of individuals age 65 or older live alone, with a spouse, or with relatives (AoA, 2014). At any one time, fewer than 5 percent of people in this age group live in institutions. This percentage increases dramatically with age, ranging from 1 percent for persons 65 to 74 years, to 3 percent for persons 75 to 84 years, and 10 percent for persons 85 and older. See Figure 34-1 for a distribution of living arrangements for noninstitutionalized persons age 65 and older.

Economic Status

More than 3.9 million persons age 65 or older were below the poverty level in 2012 (AoA, 2014). Older women had a higher poverty rate than older men, and older Hispanic women living alone had the highest poverty rate. Poor people who have worked all their lives can expect to become poorer in old age, and others will become poor only after becoming old. However, there are a substantial number of affluent and middle-income older persons who enjoy a high quality of life.

Of individuals in this age group, 81 percent owned their own homes in 2011 (AoA, 2014). However, the housing of this population of Americans is usually older and less adequate than that of the younger population; therefore, a higher percentage of income must be spent on maintenance and repairs.

Employment

With the passage of the Age Discrimination in Employment Act in 1967, forced retirement has been virtually eliminated in the workplace. Evidence suggests that involvement in purposeful activity is vital to successful adaptation and perhaps even to survival. In 2013, 8.1 million Americans age 65 and older were in the labor force (working or actively seeking work) (AoA, 2014).

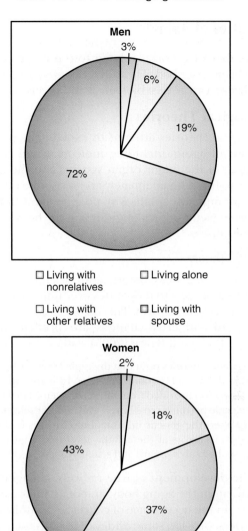

FIGURE 34-1 Living arrangements of noninstitutionalized persons age 65 and older (NCHS, 2012c).

Health Status

The number of days in which usual activities are restricted because of illness or injury increases with age. The National Council on Aging (NCOA) (2012) reports that approximately 92 percent of older adults have at least one chronic condition, and 77 percent have at least two. The most commonly occurring conditions among the elderly population are hypertension, arthritis, heart disease, cancer, and diabetes (AoA, 2014).

Emotional and mental illnesses increase over the life cycle. Depression is particularly prevalent, and suicide is a serious problem among elderly Americans. Neurocognitive disorders increase dramatically in old age.

Theories of Aging*

A number of theories related to the aging process have been described. These theories are grouped into two broad categories: biological and psychosocial.

Biological Theories

Biological theories attempt to explain the physical process of aging, including molecular and cellular changes in the major organ systems and the body's ability to function adequately and resist disease. They also attempt to explain why people age differently and what factors affect longevity and the body's ability to resist disease.

Genetic Theory

According to genetic theory, aging is an involuntarily inherited process that operates over time to alter cellular or tissue structures. This theory suggests that life span and longevity changes are predetermined. Stanley, Blair, and Beare (2005) state:

> [Genetic] theories posit that the replication process at the cellular level becomes deranged by inappropriate information provided from the cell nucleus. The DNA molecule becomes cross-linked with another substance that alters the genetic information. This cross-linking results in errors at the cellular level that eventually cause the body's organs and systems to fail. (p. 12)

The development of free radicals, collagen, and lipofuscin in the aging body, and of an increased frequency in the occurrence of cancer and autoimmune disorders, provide some evidence for this theory and the proposition that error or mutation occurs at the molecular and cellular level.

Wear-and-Tear Theory

Proponents of this theory believe that the body wears out on a scheduled basis. Free radicals, which are the waste products of metabolism, accumulate and cause damage to important biological structures. Free radicals are molecules with unpaired electrons that exist normally in the body; they also are produced by ionizing radiation, ozone, and chemical toxins. According to this theory, these free radicals cause DNA damage, cross-linkage of collagen, and the accumulation of age pigments.

Environmental Theory

According to this theory, factors in the environment (e.g., industrial carcinogens, sunlight, trauma, and infection) bring about changes in the aging process.

---

*This section was adapted from M. Stanley, K.A. Blair, & P.G. Beare (2005). *Gerontological nursing: Promoting successful aging with older adults* (3rd ed.). Philadelphia, PA: F.A. Davis, with permission.

Although these factors are known to accelerate aging, the impact of the environment is a secondary rather than a primary factor in aging. Science is only beginning to uncover the many environmental factors that affect aging.

Immunity Theory

The immunity theory describes an age-related decline in the immune system. As people age, their ability to defend against foreign organisms decreases, resulting in susceptibility to diseases such as cancer and infection. Along with the diminished immune function, a rise in the body's autoimmune response occurs, leading to the development of autoimmune diseases such as rheumatoid arthritis and allergies to food and environmental agents.

Neuroendocrine Theory

This theory proposes that aging occurs because of a slowing of the secretion of certain hormones that have an impact on reactions regulated by the nervous system. This is most clearly demonstrated in the pituitary gland, thyroid, adrenals, and the glands of reproduction. Although research has given some credence to a predictable biological clock that controls fertility, there is much more to be learned from the study of the neuroendocrine system in relation to a systemic aging process that is controlled by a "clock."

Psychosocial Theories

Psychosocial theories focus on social and psychological changes that accompany advancing age, as opposed to the biological implications of anatomic deterioration. Several theories have attempted to describe how attitudes and behavior in the early phases of life affect people's reactions during the late phase. This work is called the process of "successful aging."

Personality Theory

Personality theories address aspects of psychological growth without delineating specific tasks or expectations of older adults. Some evidence suggests that personality characteristics in old age are highly correlated with early life characteristics. Murray and associates (2009) state:

> No specific personality changes occur as a result of aging. The older person becomes more of what he or she was. The older person continues to develop emotionally and in personality and adds on characteristics instead of making drastic changes. (p. 663)

In extreme old age, however, people show greater similarity in certain characteristics, probably because of similar declines in biological functioning and societal opportunities.

In a classic study by Reichard, Livson, and Peterson (1962), the personalities of older men were classified into the following five major categories according to their patterns of adjustment to aging.

1. *Mature men* are considered well-balanced persons who maintain close personal relationships. They accept both the strengths and weaknesses of their age, finding little to regret about retirement and approaching most problems in a relaxed or convivial manner without continually having to assess blame.

2. *"Rocking chair" personalities* are found in passive-dependent individuals who are content to lean on others for support, to disengage, and to let most of life's activities pass them by.

3. *Armored men* have well-integrated defense mechanisms, which serve as adequate protection. Rigid and stable, they present a strong silent front and often rely on activity as an expression of their continuing independence.

4. *Angry men* are bitter about life, themselves, and other people. Aggressiveness is common, as is suspicion of others, especially of minorities or women. With little tolerance for ambiguity or frustration, they have always shown some instability in work and their personal lives, and now feel extremely threatened by old age.

5. *Self-haters* are similar to angry men, except that most of their animosity is turned inward on themselves. Seeing themselves as dismal failures, being old only depresses them all the more.

The investigators identified the mature, "rocking chair," and armored categories as characteristic of healthy, adjusted individuals and the angry and self-hater categories as less successful at aging. In all cases, the evidence suggested that the personalities of the subjects, although distinguished by age-specific criteria, had not changed appreciably throughout most of adulthood.

In a more recent study of personality traits, Srivastava, John, Gosling, and Potter (2003) examined the "big five" personality trait dimensions in a large sample to determine how personality changes over the life span. Age range of the subjects was from 21 to 60. The personality traits tested included conscientiousness, agreeableness, neuroticism, openness, and extraversion. They found that conscientiousness (being organized and disciplined) increased throughout the age range studied, with the biggest increases during the 20s. Agreeableness (being warm, generous, and helpful) increased most during a person's 30s. Neuroticism (being anxious and emotionally labile) declined with age for women, but did not decline for men. Openness (being acceptable to new experiences) showed small declines with age for both men and women. Extroversion (being outwardly expressive and interested in the environment) declined for women but did not show changes in men. This study contradicts the view that personality traits tend to stop changing in early adulthood. These researchers suggest that personality traits change gradually but systematically throughout the life span.

Developmental Task Theory

Developmental tasks are the activities and challenges that one must accomplish at specific stages in life to achieve successful aging. Erikson (1963) described the primary task of old age as being able to see one's life as having been lived with integrity. In the absence of achieving that sense of having lived well, the older adult is at risk for becoming preoccupied with feelings of regret or despair.

Disengagement Theory

Disengagement theory describes the process of withdrawal by older adults from societal roles and responsibilities. According to the theory, this withdrawal process is predictable, systematic, inevitable, and necessary for the proper functioning of a growing society. Older adults were said to be happy when social contacts diminished and responsibilities were assumed by a younger generation. The benefit to the older adult is thought to be in providing time for reflecting on life's accomplishments and for coming to terms with unfulfilled expectations. The benefit to society is thought to be an orderly transfer of power from old to young.

There have been many critics of this theory, and the postulates have been challenged. For many healthy and productive older individuals, the prospect of a slower pace and fewer responsibilities is undesirable.

Activity Theory

In direct opposition to the disengagement theory is the activity theory of aging, which holds that the way to age successfully is to stay active. Multiple studies have validated the positive relationship between maintaining meaningful interaction with others and physical and mental well-being.

Sadock and Sadock (2007) suggested that social integration is the prime factor in determining psychosocial adaptation in later life. Social integration refers to how the aging individual is included and takes part in the life and activities of his or her society. This theory holds that the maintenance of activities is important to most people as a basis for deriving and sustaining satisfaction, self-esteem, and health.

Continuity Theory

This theory, also known as the developmental theory, is a follow-up to the disengagement and activity theories. It emphasizes the individual's previously established coping abilities and personal character traits as a basis for predicting how the person will adjust to the changes of aging. Basic lifestyle characteristics are likely to remain stable in old age, barring physical or other types of complications that necessitate change. A person who has enjoyed the company of others and an active social life will continue to enjoy this lifestyle into old age. One who has preferred solitude and a limited number of activities will probably find satisfaction in a continuation of this lifestyle.

Maintenance of internal continuity is motivated by the need for preservation of self-esteem, ego integrity, cognitive function, and social support. As they age, individuals maintain their self-concept by reinterpreting their current experiences so that old values can take on new meanings in keeping with present circumstances. Internal self-concepts and beliefs are not readily vulnerable to environmental change, and external continuity in skills, activities, roles, and relationships can remain remarkably stable into the 70s. Physical illness or death of friends and loved ones may preclude continued social interaction (Sadock & Sadock, 2007).

The Normal Aging Process

Biological Aspects of Aging

Individuals are unique in their physical and psychological aging processes, as influenced by their predisposition or resistance to illness; the effects of their external environment and behaviors; their exposure to trauma, infections, and past diseases; and the health and illness practices they have adopted during their life span. As the individual ages, there is a quantitative loss of cells and changes in many of the enzymatic activities within cells, resulting in a diminished responsiveness to biological demands made on the body. Age-related changes occur at different rates for different individuals, although in actuality, when growth stops, aging begins. This section presents a brief overview of the normal biological changes that occur with the aging process.

Skin

One of the most dramatic changes that occurs in aging is the loss of elastin in the skin. This effect, as well as changes in collagen, causes aged skin to wrinkle and sag. Excessive exposure to sunlight compounds these changes and increases the risk of developing skin cancer.

Fat redistribution results in a loss of the subcutaneous cushion of adipose tissue. Thus, older people lose "insulation" and are more sensitive to extremes of ambient temperature than are younger people (Stanley, Blair, & Beare, 2005). A diminished supply of blood vessels to the skin results in a slower rate of healing.

Cardiovascular System

The age-related decline in the cardiovascular system is thought to be the major determinant of decreased tolerance for exercise and loss of conditioning and the overall decline in energy reserve. The aging heart is characterized by modest hypertrophy and loss of pacemaker cells, resulting in a decrease in maximal heart rate and diminished cardiac output (Blair, 2012). This results in a decrease in response to work demands and some diminishment of blood flow to the brain, kidneys, liver, and muscles. Heart rate also slows with time. If arteriosclerosis is present, cardiac function is further compromised.

Respiratory System

Thoracic expansion is diminished by an increase in fibrous tissue and loss of elastin. Pulmonary vital capacity decreases, and the amount of residual air increases. Scattered areas of fibrosis in the alveolar septa interfere with exchange of oxygen and carbon dioxide. These changes are accelerated by the use of cigarettes or other inhaled substances. Cough and laryngeal reflexes are reduced, causing decreased ability to defend the airway. Decreased pulmonary blood flow and diffusion ability result in reduced efficiency in responding to sudden respiratory demands.

Musculoskeletal System

Skeletal aging involving the bones, muscles, ligaments, and tendons probably generates the most frequent limitations on activities of daily living experienced by aging individuals. Loss of muscle mass is significant, although this occurs more slowly in men than in women. Demineralization of the bones occurs at a rate of about 1 percent per year throughout the life span in both men and women. However, this increases to approximately 10 percent in women around **menopause**, making them particularly vulnerable to **osteoporosis**.

Individual muscle fibers become thinner and less elastic with age. Muscles become less flexible following disuse. There is diminished storage of muscle glycogen, resulting in loss of energy reserve for increased activity. These changes are accelerated by nutritional deficiencies and inactivity.

Gastrointestinal System

In the oral cavity, the teeth show a reduction in dentine production, shrinkage and fibrosis of root pulp, gingival retraction, and loss of bone density in the alveolar ridges. There is some loss of peristalsis in the stomach and intestines, and gastric acid production decreases. Levels of intrinsic factor may also decrease, resulting in vitamin B_{12} malabsorption in some aging individuals. A significant decrease in absorptive surface area of the small intestine may be associated with some decline in nutrient absorption. Motility slowdown of the large intestine, combined with poor dietary habits, dehydration, lack of exercise, and some medications, may give rise to problems with constipation.

There is a modest decrease in size and weight of the liver resulting in losses in enzyme activity required to deactivate certain medications by the liver. These age-related changes can influence the metabolism and excretion of these medications. These changes, along with the pharmacokinetics of the drug, must be considered when giving medications to aging individuals.

Endocrine System

A decreased level of thyroid hormones causes a lowered basal metabolic rate. Decreased amounts of adrenocorticotropic hormone may result in less efficient stress response.

Impairments in glucose tolerance are evident in aging individuals. Studies of glucose challenges show that insulin levels are equivalent to or slightly higher than those from younger challenged individuals, although peripheral insulin resistance appears to play a significant role in carbohydrate intolerance. The observed glucose clearance abnormalities and insulin resistance in older people may be related to many factors other than biological aging (e.g., obesity, family history of diabetes) and may be influenced substantially by diet or exercise.

Genitourinary System

Age-related declines in renal function occur because of a steady attrition of nephrons and sclerosis within the glomeruli over time. Vascular changes affect blood flow to the kidneys, which results in reduced glomerular filtration and tubular function. Elderly people are prone to develop the syndrome of inappropriate antidiuretic hormone secretion, and levels of blood urea nitrogen and creatinine may be elevated slightly. The overall decline in renal functioning has serious implications for physicians who prescribe medications for elderly individuals.

In men, enlargement of the prostate gland is common as aging occurs. Prostatic hypertrophy is associated with an increased risk for urinary retention and may also be a cause of urinary incontinence (Johnston, Harper, & Landefeld, 2013). Loss of muscle and sphincter control, as well as the use of some medications, may cause urinary incontinence in women. Not only is this problem a cause of social stigma, but also, if left untreated, it increases the risk of urinary tract infection and local skin irritation. Normal changes in the genitalia are discussed in the section "Sexual Aspects of Aging."

Immune System

Aging results in changes in both cell-mediated and antibody-mediated immune responses. The size of the thymus gland declines continuously from just beyond puberty to about 15 percent of its original size at age 50. The consequences of these changes include a greater susceptibility to infections and a diminished inflammatory response that results in delayed healing. There is also evidence of an increase in various autoantibodies as a person ages, increasing the risk of autoimmune disorders, such as rheumatoid arthritis (National Institutes of Health [NIH], 2012).

Because of the overall decrease in efficiency of the immune system, the proliferation of abnormal cells is facilitated in the elderly individual. Cancer is the best example of aberrant cells allowed to proliferate due to the ineffectiveness of the immune system.

Nervous System

With aging, there is an absolute loss of neurons, which correlates with decreases in brain weight of about 10 percent by age 90 (Murray et al., 2009). Gross morphological examination reveals gyral atrophy in the frontal, temporal, and parietal lobes; widening of the sulci; and ventricular enlargement. However, it must be remembered that these changes have been identified in careful study of adults with normal intellectual function.

The brain has enormous reserve, and little cerebral function is lost over time, although greater functional decline is noted in the periphery (Stanley et al., 2005). There appears to be a disproportionately greater loss of cells in the cerebellum, the locus coeruleus, the substantia nigra, and olfactory bulbs, accounting for some of the more characteristic aging behaviors such as mild gait disturbances, sleep disruptions, and decreased smell and taste perception.

Some of the age-related changes within the nervous system may be due to alterations in neurotransmitter release, uptake, turnover, catabolism, or receptor functions (Beers & Jones, 2004; Blair, 2012). A great deal of attention is being given to brain biochemistry and in particular to the neurotransmitters acetylcholine, dopamine, norepinephrine, and epinephrine. These biochemical changes may be responsible for the altered responses of many older persons to stressful events and some biological treatments.

Sensory Systems

Vision

Visual acuity begins to decrease in midlife. Presbyopia (blurred near vision) is the standard marker of aging of the eye. It is caused by a loss of elasticity of the crystalline lens, and results in compromised accommodation.

Cataract development is inevitable if the individual lives long enough for the changes to occur. Cataracts occur when the lens of the eye becomes less resilient (due to compression of fibers) and increasingly opaque (as proteins lump together), ultimately resulting in a loss of visual acuity.

The color in the iris may fade, and the pupil may become irregular in shape. A decrease in production of secretions by the lacrimal glands may cause dryness and result in increased irritation and infection. The pupil may become constricted, requiring an increase in the amount of light needed for reading.

Hearing

Hearing changes significantly with the aging process. Gradually over time, the ear loses its sensitivity to discriminate sounds because of damage to the hair cells of the cochlea. The most dramatic decline appears to be in perception of high-frequency sounds.

Age-related hearing loss, called *presbycusis*, is common and affects more than half of all adults by age 75 years (Blevins, 2013). It is more common in men than it is in women, a fact that may be related to differences in levels of lifetime noise exposure.

Taste and Smell

Taste sensitivity decreases over the life span. Taste discrimination decreases, and bitter taste sensations predominate. Sensitivity to sweet and salty tastes is diminished.

The deterioration of the olfactory bulbs is accompanied by loss of smell acuity. The aromatic component of taste perception diminishes.

Touch and Pain

Organized sensory nerve receptors on the skin continue to decrease throughout the life span; thus, the touch threshold increases with age (Pietraniec-Shannon, 2007). The ability to feel pain also decreases in response to these changes, and the ability to perceive and interpret painful stimuli changes. These changes have critical implications for the elderly in their potential inability to use sensory warnings to escape serious injury.

Psychological Aspects of Aging

Memory Functioning

Age-related memory deficiencies have been extensively reported in the literature. Although **short-term memory** seems to deteriorate with age, perhaps because of poorer sorting strategies, **long-term memory** does not show similar changes. However, in nearly every instance, well-educated, mentally active people do not exhibit the same decline in memory functioning as their age peers who lack similar opportunities to flex their minds. Nevertheless, with few exceptions, the time required for memory scanning is longer for both recent and remote recall among older people. This can sometimes be attributed to social or health factors (e.g., stress, fatigue, illness), but it can also occur because of certain normal physical changes associated with aging (e.g., decreased blood flow to the brain).

Intellectual Functioning

There appears to be a high degree of regularity in intellectual functioning across the adult age span. Crystallized abilities, or knowledge acquired in the course of the socialization process, tend to remain stable over the adult life span. Fluid abilities, or abilities involved in solving novel problems, tend to decline gradually from young to old adulthood. In other words, intellectual abilities of older people do not decline but do become obsolete. The age of their formal educational experiences is reflected in their intelligence scoring.

Learning Ability

The ability to learn is not diminished by age. Studies, however, have shown that some aspects of learning do change with age. The ordinary slowing of reaction time with age for nearly all tasks or the over-arousal of the central nervous system may account for lower performance levels on tests requiring rapid responses. Under conditions that allow for self-pacing by the participant, differences in accuracy of performance diminish. Ability to learn continues throughout life, although strongly influenced by interests, activity, motivation, health, and experience. Adjustments do need to be made in teaching methodology and time allowed for learning.

Adaptation to the Tasks of Aging

Loss and Grief

Individuals experience losses from the very beginning of life. By the time individuals reach their 60s and 70s, they have experienced numerous losses, and mourning has become a lifelong process. Unfortunately, with the aging process comes a convergence of losses, the timing of which makes it impossible for the aging individual to complete the grief process in response to one loss before another occurs. Because grief is cumulative, this can result in **bereavement overload**, which has been implicated in the predisposition to depression in the elderly.

Attachment to Others

Many studies have confirmed the importance of interpersonal relationships at all stages in the life cycle. Murray and associates (2009) state:

> [Social networks] contribute to well-being of the elder by (a) promoting socialization and companionship, (b) elevating morale and life satisfaction, (c) buffering the effects of stressful events, (d) providing a confidant, and (e) facilitating coping skills and mastery. (p. 620)

This need for **attachment** is consistent with the activity theory of aging that correlates the importance of social integration with successful adaptation in later life.

Maintenance of Self-Identity

Self-concept and self-image appear to remain stable over time. Factors that have been shown to favor good psychosocial adjustment in later life are sustained family relationships, maturity of ego defenses, absence of alcoholism, and absence of depressive disorder (Vaillant, 2003). Studies show that the elderly have a strong need for and remarkable capability of retaining a persistent self-concept in the face of the many changes that contribute to instability in later life.

Dealing With Death

Death anxiety among the aging is apparently more of a myth than a reality. Studies have not supported the negative view of death as an overriding psychological factor in the aging process. Various investigators who have worked with dying persons report that it is not death itself, but abandonment, pain, and confusion that are feared. What many desire most is someone to talk with, to show them their life's meaning is not shattered merely because they are about to die (Kübler-Ross, 1969; Murray et al., 2009).

Psychiatric Disorders in Later Life

The later years constitute a time of especially high risk for emotional distress. Sadock and Sadock (2007) state:

> Several psychosocial risk factors predispose older people to mental disorders. These risk factors include loss of social roles, loss of autonomy, the deaths of friends and relatives, declining health, increased isolation, financial constraints, and decreased cognitive functioning. (p. 1353)

Neurocognitive Disorder

Neurocognitive disorders (NCDs) are the most common causes of psychopathology in the elderly. About half of these disorders are of the Alzheimer's type, which is characterized by an insidious onset and a gradually progressive course of cognitive impairment. No curative treatment is currently available. Symptomatic treatments, including pharmacological interventions,

attention to the environment, and family support, can help to maximize the client's level of functioning.

Delirium

Delirium is one of the most common and critical forms of psychopathology in later life. A number of factors have been identified that predispose elderly people to delirium, including structural brain disease, reduced capacity for homeostatic regulation, impaired vision and hearing, a high prevalence of chronic disease, reduced resistance to acute stress, and age-related changes in the pharmacokinetics and pharmacodynamics of drugs. Delirium needs to be recognized and the underlying condition treated as soon as possible. A high mortality rate is associated with this condition.

Depression

Depressive disorders are the most common affective illnesses occurring after the middle years. The incidence of increased depression among elderly people is influenced by the variables of physical illness, functional disability, cognitive impairment, and loss of a spouse (Lang, 2012). Somatic symptoms are common in the depressed elderly. Symptomatology often mimics that of NCD, a condition that is referred to as *pseudodementia*. (See Table 22-1 for a comparison of the symptoms of NCD and pseudodementia.) Suicide is prevalent in the elderly, with declining health and decreased economic status being considered important influencing factors. Treatment of depression in the elderly individual is with psychotropic medications or electroconvulsive therapy.

Schizophrenia

Schizophrenia and delusional disorders may continue into old age or may manifest themselves for the first time only during senescence (Blazer, 2008). In most instances, individuals who manifest psychotic disorders early in life show a decline in psychopathology as they age. Late-onset schizophrenia (after age 60) is not common, but when it does occur, it often is characterized by delusions or hallucinations of a persecutory nature. The course is chronic, and treatment is with neuroleptics and supportive psychotherapy.

IMPLICATIONS OF RESEARCH FOR EVIDENCE-BASED PRACTICE

Helmes, E. & Wiancko, D.C. (2006). Effects of music in reducing disruptive behavior in a general hospital. *Journal of the American Psychiatric Nurses Association, 12*(1), 37-44.

DESCRIPTION OF THE STUDY: In settings where cognitively impaired elderly individuals reside, it is not uncommon for loud, disruptive vocalizations such as shouting and the

banging of objects to be heard. Studies have shown that music can alleviate the tension and reduce the disruptive vocalizations of some individuals with dementia. Most reports on the effect of music on these disruptive outbursts have been conducted in residential care facilities. Because there are few studies about the prevalence of disruptive behaviors or the method of dealing with them in the acute

Continued

IMPLICATIONS FOR EVIDENCE BASED PRACTICE—cont'd

care setting, the authors sought to determine if soothing music found to be effective in residential settings could be generalized to acute care environments.

RESULTS OF THE STUDY: The study sample included 7 women and 2 men ranging in age from 68 to 95 years. Diagnoses were varied, including diabetes, pneumonia, alcoholic dementia, depression, Alzheimer's disease, Parkinson's dementia, stroke, and congestive heart failure. Length of hospital stays ranged from 1 day to 54 days. All exhibited disruptive behaviors, such as shouting and banging of objects within reach, such as tray tables or bed rails. The intervention included the playing of baroque music in the client's room at a comfortable volume for the listener. Each of the participants was observed for a minimum of four 30-minute periods on a minimum of 3 successive days. Control trials with each participant were also conducted in a randomized order to have at least two observations from each condition. Observations were made

unobtrusively, and routine activity of staff and visitors was not minimized during the course of the study. With all participants, the music intervention resulted in a decrease in frequency of noisy disruptive behaviors, with reductions ranging from 30 to 90 percent, when compared with the control trials.

IMPLICATIONS FOR NURSING PRACTICE: The use of music for its soothing and calming effect is a simple intervention well within the scope and capability of nursing practice. This study did not pursue whether the benefits carry over after the music has stopped, and whether more extensive use of music would retain its effectiveness. The authors concluded, "The use of music to reduce disruptive noise in an acute care setting appears to be as effective as other such interventions have been in residential care facilities." One additional benefit was reported. The authors stated, "Nurses on the two units noted positive effects for them in the form of increased pleasant affect that seemed to be independent of the effects of reduced disruptive noise from the participants."

Anxiety Disorders

Most anxiety disorders begin in early to middle adulthood, but some appear for the first time after age 60. Because the autonomic nervous system is more fragile in older persons, the response to a major stressor is often quite intense. The presence of physical disability frequently compounds the situation, resulting in a more severe post-traumatic stress response than is commonly observed in younger persons. In older adults, symptoms of anxiety and depression often accompany each other, making it difficult to determine which disorder is dominant.

Personality Disorders

Personality disorders are uncommon in the elderly population. The incidence of personality disorders among individuals over age 65 is less than 5 percent. Most elderly people with personality disorder have likely manifested the symptomatology for many years.

Sleep Disorders

Sleep disorders are very common in the aging individual. Sleep disturbances affect 50 percent of people age 65 and older who live at home and 66 percent of those who live in long-term care facilities (Stanley et al., 2005). Some common causes of sleep disturbances among elderly people include age-dependent decreases in the ability to sleep ("sleep decay"); increased prevalence of sleep apnea; depression; NCD; anxiety; pain; impaired mobility; medications; and psychosocial factors such as loneliness, inactivity, and boredom. Sedative-hypnotics, along with nonpharmacological

approaches, are often used as sleep aids with the elderly. Changes in aging associated with metabolism and elimination must be considered when maintenance medications are administered for chronic insomnia in the aging client.

Sociocultural Aspects of Aging

Old age brings many important socially induced changes, some of which have the potential for negative effect on both the physical and mental well-being of older persons. In American society, old age is defined arbitrarily as being 65 years or older because that is the age when most people have been able to retire with full Social Security and other pension benefits. Recent legislation has increased the age beyond 65 years for full Social Security benefits. Currently, the age increases yearly (based on year of birth) until 2027, when the age for full benefits will be 67 years for all individuals.

Elderly people in virtually all cultures share some basic needs and interests. There is little doubt that most individuals choose to live the most satisfying life possible until their demise. They want protection from hazards and release from the weariness of everyday tasks. They want to be treated with the respect and dignity that is deserving of individuals who have reached this pinnacle in life; and they want to die with the same respect and dignity.

From the beginning of human culture, the aged have had a special status in society. Even today, in some cultures the aged are the most powerful, the most engaged, and the most respected members of the society. This has not been the case in the modern industrial societies, although trends in the status of the aged differ widely between one industrialized country and another. For example, the status and integration of the aged in Japan have remained relatively high when compared with other industrialized nations, such as the United States. There are subcultures in the United States, however, in which the elderly are afforded a higher degree of status than they receive in the mainstream population. Examples include Latino Americans, Asian Americans, and African Americans. The aged are awarded a position of honor in cultures that place emphasis on family cohesiveness. In these cultures, the aged are revered for their knowledge and wisdom gained through their years of life experiences (Purnell, 2013).

Many negative stereotypes color the perspective on aging in the United States. Ideas that elderly individuals are always tired or sick, slow and forgetful, isolated and lonely, unproductive, and angry determine the way younger individuals relate to the elderly in this society. Increasing disregard for the elderly has resulted in a type of segregation, as aging individuals voluntarily seek out or are involuntarily placed in special residences for the aged.

Assisted living centers, retirement apartment complexes, and even entire retirement communities intended solely for individuals over age 50 are becoming more and more common. In 2012, more than half (59 percent) of persons age 65 and older lived in 12 states, with the largest numbers in California, Florida, New York, Texas, and Pennsylvania (AoA, 2014). It is important for elderly individuals to feel part of an integrated group, and they are migrating to these areas in an effort to achieve this integration. This phenomenon provides additional corroboration for the activity theory of aging, and the importance of attachment to others.

Employment is another area in which the elderly experience discrimination. Although compulsory retirement has been virtually eliminated, discrimination still exists in hiring and promotion practices. Many employers are not eager to retain or hire older workers. It is difficult to determine how much of the failure to hire and promote results from discrimination based on age alone and how much of it is related to a realistic and fair appraisal of the aged employee's ability and efficiency. It is true that some elderly individuals are no longer capable of doing as good a job as a younger worker; however, there are many who likely can do a *better* job than their younger counterparts, if given the opportunity. Nevertheless, surveys have shown that some employers accept the negative stereotypes about elderly individuals and believe that older workers are hard to please, set in their ways, less productive, frequently absent, and involved in more accidents.

The status of the elderly may improve with time and as their numbers increase with the aging of the "baby boomers." As older individuals gain political power, the benefits and privileges designed for the elderly will increase. There is power in numbers, and the 21st century promises power for people age 65 and older.

Sexual Aspects of Aging

Sexuality and the sexual needs of elderly people are frequently misunderstood, condemned, stereotyped, ridiculed, repressed, and ignored. Americans have grown up in a society that has liberated sexual expression for all other age groups, but still retains certain Victorian standards regarding sexual expression by the elderly. Negative stereotyped notions concerning sexual interest and activity of the elderly are common. Some of these include ideas that older people have no sexual interests or desires; that they are sexually undesirable; or that they are too fragile or too ill to engage in sexual activity. Some people even believe it is disgusting or comical to consider elderly individuals as sexual beings.

These cultural stereotypes undoubtedly play a large part in the misperception many people hold regarding sexuality of the aged, and they may be reinforced by the common tendency of the young to deny the inevitability of aging. With reasonable good health and an interesting and interested partner, there is no inherent reason why individuals should not enjoy an active sexual life well into late adulthood (King, 2012).

Physical Changes Associated With Sexuality

Many of the changes in sexuality that occur in later years are related to the physical changes that are taking place at that time of life.

Changes in Women

Menopause may begin anytime during the 40s or early 50s. During this time there is a gradual decline in the functioning of the ovaries and the subsequent production of estrogen, which results in a number of changes. The walls of the vagina become thin and inelastic, the vagina itself shrinks in both width and length, and the amount of vaginal lubrication decreases noticeably. Orgasmic uterine contractions may become spastic. All of these changes can result in painful penetration, vaginal burning, pelvic aching, or irritation on urination. In some women, the discomfort may be severe enough to result in an avoidance of intercourse. Paradoxically, these symptoms are more likely to occur with infrequent intercourse of only one time a month or less. Regular and more frequent sexual activity results in a greater capacity for sexual performance (King, 2012). Other symptoms that are associated with menopause in some women include hot flashes, night sweats, sleeplessness, irritability, mood swings, migraine headaches, urinary incontinence, and weight gain.

Some menopausal women elect to take hormone replacement therapy for relief of these changes and symptoms. With estrogen therapy, the symptoms of menopause are minimized or do not occur at all. However, some women choose not to take the hormone because of an increased risk of breast cancer, and when given alone, an increased risk of endometrial cancer. To combat this latter effect, many women also take a second hormone, progesterone. Taken for 7 to 10 days during the month, progesterone decreases the risk of estrogen-induced endometrial cancer. Some physicians prescribe a low dose of progesterone that is taken, along with estrogen, for the entire month. A combination pill, taken in this manner, is also available.

Results of the Women's Health Initiative (WHI), as reported in the *Journal of the American Medical Association,* indicated that the combination pill is associated with an increased risk of cardiovascular disease and breast cancer. Benefits related to colon cancer and osteoporosis were reported; however, investigators stopped this arm of the study and suggested discontinuation of this type of therapy. In a 3-year follow-up study of the participants, the results showed that the increased risk for cardiovascular disease dissipated with discontinuation of the hormone therapy (Heiss et al., 2008).

Changes in Men

Testosterone production declines gradually over the years, beginning between ages 40 and 60. A major change resulting from this hormone reduction is that erections occur more slowly and require more direct genital stimulation to achieve. There may also be a modest decrease in the firmness of the erection in men older than age 60. The refractory period lengthens with age, increasing the amount of time following orgasm before the man may achieve another erection. The volume of ejaculate gradually decreases, and the force of ejaculation lessens. The testes become somewhat smaller, but most men continue to produce viable sperm well into old age. Prolonged control over ejaculation in middle-aged and elderly men may bring increased sexual satisfaction for both partners.

Sexual Behavior in the Elderly

Coital frequency in early marriage and the overall quantity of sexual activity between ages 20 and 40 correlate significantly with frequency patterns of sexual activity during aging (Masters, Johnson, & Kolodny, 1995). Although sexual interest and behavior do appear to decline somewhat with age, studies show that significant numbers of elderly men and women have active and satisfying sex lives well into their 80s. A survey commissioned by the American Association of Retired Persons (AARP) provided some revealing information regarding the sexual attitudes and behavior of senior citizens. Some statistics from the survey are summarized in Table 34-1. The information from this survey clearly indicates that sexual activity can and does continue well past the 70s for healthy active individuals who have regular opportunities for sexual expression. King (2012) states: "For healthy men and women with healthy partners, sexual activity will probably continue throughout life if they had a positive attitude about sex when they were younger" (p. 268).

TABLE 34–1 **Sexuality at Midlife and Beyond**			
	AGES	MEN (%)	WOMEN (%)
Have sex at least once a week	45–49	50	26
	50–59	41	32
	60–69	24	24
	70+	15	5
Report very satisfied with physical relationship	45–49	60	48
	50–59	50	40
	60–69	52	41
	70+	26	27
Report very satisfied with emotional relationship	45–49	26	37
	50–59	32	23
	60–69	28	29
	70+	20	24
Report sexual activity is important to their overall quality of life	45–49	69	33
	50–59	65	28

TABLE 34-1 Sexuality at Midlife and Beyond—cont'd			
	AGES	MEN (%)	WOMEN (%)
	60–69	55	33
	70+	46	12
Believe non–marital sex is okay	45–49	88	86
	50–59	91	75
	60–69	80	71
	70+	68	61
Describe their partners as physically attractive	45–49	50	60
	50–59	53	48
	60–69	58	58
	70+	51	48
Report always or usually having an orgasm with sexual intercourse	45–49	95	70
	50–59	88	64
	60–69	91	59
	70+	82	61
Report being impotent	45–49	6	
	50–59	16	
	60–69	29	
	70+	48	
Report having used medicine, hormones, or other treatments to improve sexual functioning	45–49	7	9
	50–59	12	16
	60–69	14	14
	70+	13	13
What would most improve your sex life?	All	Better health for self; partner initiates sex more often; less stress	Less stress; better health for self and partner; finding a partner

Adapted from American Association of Retired Persons. (2010). *Sex, romance, and relationships: AARP survey of midlife and older adults.* Washington, DC: Author.

Special Concerns of the Elderly Population

Retirement

Statistics reflect that a larger percentage of Americans are living longer and that many of them are retiring earlier. Reasons often given for the increasing pattern of early retirement include health problems, Social Security and other pension benefits, attractive "early out" packages offered by companies, and long-held plans (e.g., turning a hobby into a money-making situation).

Studies show that about 10 to 20 percent of individuals reenter the workforce following retirement (Cahill, Giandrea, & Quinn, 2011). Reentry is more common among men than women, and among those individuals who are at a younger age and in good health at the time of their retirement. Some reasons people give for returning to work following retirement include negative reactions to being retired, feelings of being unproductive, economic hardship, and loneliness. Recent downturns in economic conditions have forced many retired people to seek employment to augment dwindling retirement resources.

About 8.1 million older Americans were in the labor force (working or actively seeking work) in 2013. These included 4.5 million men and 3.6 million women, and constituted 5 percent of the U.S. labor force (AoA, 2014).

Retirement has both social and economic implications for elderly individuals. The role is fraught with a great deal of ambiguity and is one that requires many adaptations on the part of those involved.

Social Implications

Retirement is often anticipated as an achievement in principle, but met with mixed feelings when it actually occurs. Our society places a great deal of importance on productivity, making as much money as possible, and doing it at as young an age as possible. These types of values contribute to the ambiguity associated with retirement. Although leisure has been acknowledged as a legitimate reward for workers, leisure during retirement historically has lacked the same social value. Adjustment to this life-cycle event becomes more difficult in the face of societal values that are in direct conflict with the new lifestyle.

Historically, many women have derived a good deal of their self-esteem from their families—birthing them, rearing them, and being a "good mother." Likewise, many men have achieved self-esteem through work-related activities—creativity, productivity, and earning money. With the termination of these activities may come a loss of self-worth, resulting in depression in some individuals who are unable to adapt satisfactorily. Well-being in retirement is linked to factors such as stable health status and access to health-care services, adequate income, the ability to pursue new goals or activities, extended social network of family and friends, and satisfaction with current living arrangements (Murray et al., 2009).

American society often identifies an individual by his or her occupation. This is reflected in the conversation of people who are meeting each other for the first time. Undoubtedly, most everyone has either asked or been asked at some point in time, "What do you do?" or "Where do you work?" Occupation determines status, and retirement represents a significant change in status. The basic ambiguity of retirement occurs in an individual's or society's definition of this change. Is it undertaken voluntarily or involuntarily? Is it desirable or undesirable? Is one's status made better or worse by the change?

In looking at the trend of the past 2 decades, we may presume that retirement is becoming, and will continue to become, more accepted by societal standards. With many individuals retiring earlier and living longer, a growing number of aging people will spend a significantly longer time in retirement. It is a major life event that requires planning and realistic expectations of life changes.

Economic Implications

Because retirement is generally associated with a 20 to 40 percent reduction in personal income, the standard of living after retirement may be adversely affected. Most older adults derive post-retirement income from a combination of Social Security benefits, public and private pensions, and income from savings or investments.

In 2012, the median income in households containing families headed by persons 65 or older was $48,957 and more than 3.9 million elderly people were below the poverty level (AoA, 2014). The rate of those living in poverty was higher among women than men and higher among African Americans and Latino Americans than whites.

The Social Security Act of 1935 promised assistance with financial security for the elderly. Since then, the original legislation has been modified, yet the basic philosophy remains intact. Its effectiveness, however, is now being questioned. Faced with deficits, the program is forced to pay benefits to those currently retired from both the reserve funds and monies being collected at present. There is genuine concern about future generations, when there may be no reserve funds from which to draw. Because many of the programs that benefit older adults depend on contributions from the younger population, the growing ratio of older Americans to younger people may affect society's ability to supply the goods and services necessary to meet this expanding demand.

Medicare and **Medicaid** were established by the government to provide medical care benefits for elderly and indigent Americans. The Medicaid program is jointly funded by state and federal governments, and coverage varies significantly from state to state. Medicare covers only a percentage of health-care costs; therefore, to reduce risk related to out-of-pocket expenditures, many older adults purchase private "medigap" policies designed to cover charges in excess of those approved by Medicare.

The magnitude of retirement earnings depends almost entirely on pre-retirement income. The poor will remain poor and the wealthy are unlikely to lower their status during retirement; however, for many in the middle classes, the relatively fixed income sources may be inadequate, possibly forcing them to face financial hardship for the first time in their lives.

Long-Term Care

Stanley and associates (2005) stated, "The concept of long-term care covers a broad spectrum of comprehensive health care that addresses both illness and wellness and the support services necessary to provide the physical, social, spiritual, and economic needs of persons with chronic illnesses, including disabilities" (p. 94). Long-term care facilities are defined by the level of care they provide. They may be skilled nursing facilities, intermediate care facilities, or a combination of the two. Some institutions provide convalescent care for individuals recovering from acute illness or injury, some provide long-term care for individuals with chronic illness or disabilities, and still others provide both types of assistance.

Most elderly individuals prefer to remain in their own homes or in the homes of family members for as long as this can meet their needs without deterioration of family or social patterns. Many elderly individuals are placed in institutions as a last resort only after heroic efforts have been made to keep them in their own or a relative's home. The increasing emphasis on home health care has extended the period of independence for aging individuals.

Fewer than 5 percent of the population ages 65 and older live in nursing homes. The percentage increases dramatically with age, ranging from 1 percent for persons aged 65 to 74, to 3 percent for persons aged 75 to 84, and to 10 percent for persons aged 85 and older (AoA, 2014). A profile of the "typical" elderly nursing home resident is about 80 years of age, white, female, widowed, with multiple chronic health conditions.

Risk Factors for Institutionalization

In determining who in our society will need long-term care, several factors have been identified that appear to place people at risk. The following risk factors are taken into consideration to predict potential need for services and to estimate future costs.

Age

Because people grow older in very different ways, and the range of differences becomes greater with the passage of time, age is becoming a less relevant characteristic than it was historically. However, because of the high prevalence of chronic health conditions and disabilities, as well as the greater chance of diminishing social supports associated with advancing age, the 65-and-older population is often viewed as an important long-term care target group.

Health

Level of functioning, as determined by ability to perform various behaviors or activities—such as bathing, eating, mobility, meal preparation, handling finances, judgment, and memory—is a measurable risk factor. The need for ongoing assistance from another person is critical in determining the need for long-term care.

Mental Health Status

Mental health problems are risk factors in assessing need for long-term care. Many of the symptoms associated with certain mental disorders (especially neurocognitive disorders), such as memory loss, impaired judgment, impaired intellect, and disorientation, would render the individual incapable of meeting the demands of daily living independently.

Socioeconomic and Demographic Factors

Low income generally is associated with greater physical and mental health problems among the elderly. Because many elderly individuals have limited finances, they are less able to purchase care resources available outside of institutions (e.g., home health care), although Medicare and Medicaid now contribute a limited amount to this type of noninstitutionalized care.

Women are at greater risk of being institutionalized than men, not because they are less healthy but because they tend to live longer and, thus, reach the age at which more functional and cognitive impairments

occur. They are also more likely to be widowed. Whites have a higher rate of institutionalization than nonwhites. This may be related to cultural and financial influences.

Marital Status, Living Arrangement, and the Informal Support Network

Individuals who are married and live with a spouse are the least likely of all disabled people to be institutionalized. Those who live alone without resources for home care and with few or no relatives living nearby to provide informal care are at higher risk for institutionalization.

Attitudinal Factors

Many people dread the thought of even visiting a nursing home, let alone moving to one or placing a relative in one. Negative perceptions exist of nursing homes as "places to go to die." The media picture and subsequent reputation of nursing homes has not been positive. Stories of substandard care and patient abuse have scarred the industry, making it difficult for those facilities that are clean, well-managed, and that provide innovative, quality care to their residents to rise above the stigma.

State and national licensing boards perform periodic inspections to ensure that standards set forth by the federal government are being met. These standards address quality of patient care as well as adequacy of the nursing home facility. Yet, many elderly individuals and their families perceive nursing homes as a place to go to die, and the fact that many of these institutions are poorly equipped, understaffed, and disorganized keeps this societal perception alive. There are, however, many excellent nursing homes that strive to go beyond the minimum federal regulations for Medicaid and Medicare reimbursement. In addition to medical, nursing, rehabilitation, and dental services, social and recreational services are provided to increase the quality of life for elderly people living in nursing homes. These activities include playing cards, bingo, and other games; parties; church activities; books; television; movies; and arts, crafts, and other classes. Some nursing homes provide occupational and professional counseling. These facilities strive to enhance opportunities for improving quality of life and for becoming "places to live," rather than "places to die."

Elder Abuse

Abuse of elderly individuals, which at times has been referred to in the media as "**granny-bashing**," is a serious form of family violence. Statistics regarding the prevalence of elder abuse are difficult to determine. It is estimated that annually up to 2 million older adults in the United States are victims of abuse

(Stark, 2012). However, the data suggest that only about 84 percent of these cases are reported to authorities. The abuser is often a relative who lives with the elderly person and may be the assigned caregiver. Typical caregivers who are likely to be abusers of the elderly were described by Murray and associates (2009) as being under economic stress, substance abusers, themselves the victims of previous family violence, and exhausted and frustrated by the caregiver role. Identified risk factors for victims of abuse included being a white female age 70 or older, being mentally or physically impaired, being unable to meet daily self-care needs, and having care needs that exceeded the caretaker's ability.

Abuse of elderly individuals may be psychological, physical, or financial. Neglect may be intentional or unintentional. Psychological abuse includes yelling, insulting, harsh commands, threats, silence, and social isolation. Physical abuse is described as striking, shoving, beating, or restraint. Financial abuse refers to misuse or theft of finances, property, or material possessions. Neglect implies failure to fulfill the physical needs of an individual who cannot do so independently. Unintentional neglect is inadvertent, whereas intentional neglect is deliberate. In addition, elderly individuals may be the victims of sexual abuse, which is sexual intimacy between two persons that occurs without the consent of one of the persons involved. Another type of abuse, which has been called "**granny-dumping**" by the media, involves abandoning elderly individuals at emergency departments, nursing homes, or other facilities—literally leaving them in the hands of others when the strain of caregiving becomes intolerable. Types of elder abuse are summarized in Box 34-1.

Elder victims often minimize the abuse or deny that it has occurred. The elderly person may be unwilling to disclose information because of fear of retaliation, embarrassment about the existence of abuse in the family, protectiveness toward a family member, or unwillingness to institute legal action. Adding to this unwillingness to report is the fact that infirm elders are often isolated so their mistreatment is less likely to be noticed by those who might be alert to symptoms of abuse. For these reasons, detection of abuse in the elderly is difficult at best.

Factors That Contribute to Abuse

A number of contributing factors have been implicated in the abuse of elderly individuals.

Longer Life

The 65-and-older age group has become the fastest growing segment of the population. Within this segment, the number of elderly older than age 75 has increased most rapidly. This trend is expected to continue well into the 21st century. The 75-and-older age group is the one most likely to be physically or mentally impaired, requiring assistance and care from family members. This group also is the most vulnerable to abuse from caregivers.

Dependency

Dependency appears to be the most common precondition in domestic abuse. Changes associated with normal aging or induced by chronic illness often result in loss of self-sufficiency in the elderly person, requiring that they become dependent on another for assistance with daily functioning. Long life may also consume finances to the point that the elderly

---

BOX 34-1 Examples of Elder Abuse

PHYSICAL ABUSE
Striking, hitting, beating
Shoving
Bruising
Cutting
Restraining

PSYCHOLOGICAL ABUSE
Yelling
Insulting, name-calling
Harsh commands
Threats
Ignoring, silence, social isolation
Withholding of affection

NEGLECT (INTENTIONAL OR UNINTENTIONAL)
Withholding food and water
Inadequate heating

Unclean clothes and bedding
Lack of needed medication
Lack of eyeglasses, hearing aids, false teeth

FINANCIAL ABUSE OR EXPLOITATION
Misuse of the elderly person's income by the caregiver
Forcing the elderly person to sign over financial affairs to another person against his or her will or without sufficient knowledge about the transaction

SEXUAL ABUSE
Sexual molestation; rape
Any type of sexual intimacy against the elderly person's will

SOURCES: Murray, Zentner, & Yakimo (2009), Sadock & Sadock (2007); and Stanley, Blair, & Beare (2005).

individual becomes financially dependent on another as well. This type of dependency also increases the elderly person's vulnerability to abuse.

Stress

The stress inherent in the caregiver role is a factor in most abuse cases. Some clinicians believe that elder abuse results from individual or family psychopathology. Others suggest that even psychologically healthy family members can become abusive as the result of the exhaustion and acute stress caused by overwhelming caregiving responsibilities. This is compounded in an age group that has been dubbed the "sandwich generation"—those individuals who elected to delay childbearing so that they are now at a point in their lives when they are "sandwiched" between providing care for their children and providing care for their aging parents.

Learned Violence

Children who have been abused or witnessed abusive and violent parents are more likely to evolve into abusive adults. In some families, abusive behavior is the normal response to tension or conflict, and this type of behavior can be transmitted from one generation to another. There may be some unresolved family conflicts or retaliation for previous maltreatment that foster and promote abuse of the elderly person.

Identifying Elder Abuse

Because so many elderly individuals are reluctant to report personal abuse, health-care workers need to be able to detect signs of mistreatment when they are in a position to do so. Box 34-1 listed a number of *types* of elder abuse. The following *manifestations* of the various categories of abuse have been identified (Koop, 2012; Murray et al., 2009; Stanley et al., 2005):

- Indicators of psychological abuse include a broad range of behaviors such as the symptoms associated with depression, withdrawal, anxiety, sleep disorders, and increased confusion or agitation.
- Indicators of physical abuse may include bruises, welts, lacerations, burns, punctures, evidence of hair pulling, and skeletal dislocations and fractures.
- Neglect may be manifested as consistent hunger, poor hygiene, inappropriate dress, consistent lack of supervision, consistent fatigue or listlessness, unattended physical problems or medical needs, or abandonment.
- Sexual abuse may be suspected when the elderly person is presented with pain or itching in the genital area; bruising or bleeding in external genitalia, vaginal, or anal areas; or unexplained sexually transmitted disease.
- Financial abuse may be occurring when there is an obvious disparity between assets and satisfactory living conditions or when the elderly person complains of a sudden lack of sufficient funds for daily living expenses.

Health-care workers often feel intimidated when confronted with cases of elder abuse. In these instances, referral to an individual experienced in management of victims of such abuse may be the most effective approach to evaluation and intervention. Health-care workers are responsible for reporting any suspicions of elder abuse. An investigation is then conducted by regulatory agencies, whose job it is to determine if the suspicions are corroborated. Every effort must be made to ensure the client's safety, but it is important to remember that a competent elderly person has the right to choose his or her health-care options. As inappropriate as it may seem, some elderly individuals choose to return to the abusive situation. In this instance, he or she should be provided with names and phone numbers to call for assistance if needed. A follow-up visit by an adult protective services representative should be conducted.

Increased efforts need to be made to ensure that health-care providers have comprehensive training in the detection of and intervention in elder abuse. More research is needed to increase knowledge and understanding of the phenomenon of elder abuse and ultimately to effect more sophisticated strategies for prevention, intervention, and treatment.

Suicide

Although persons ages 65 and older comprise only 13.7 percent of the population, they represent a disproportionately high percentage of individuals who commit suicide. Of all suicides, more than 15 percent are committed by this age group (NCHS, 2012b). The group especially at risk appears to be white men. Predisposing factors include loneliness, financial problems, physical illness, loss, and depression (Sadock & Sadock, 2007).

Although the rate of suicide among the elderly remains high, the numbers of suicides among this age group dropped steadily from 1930 to 1980. Investigators who study these trends surmise that this decline was due to increases in services for older people and an understanding of their problems in society. Statistics show that from 1980 to 1986, the number of suicides among people ages 65 and older increased by 25 percent, which suggests that there are other contributing factors to the problem. However, since 1987, there has been a gradual decline in the number of elderly suicides.

It has been suggested that increased social isolation may be a contributing factor to suicide among the elderly. The number of elderly individuals who are divorced, widowed, or otherwise living alone has increased. Men

IMPLICATIONS OF RESEARCH FOR EVIDENCE-BASED PRACTICE

Turvey, C.L., Conwell, Y., Jones, M.P., Phillips, C., Simonsick, E., Pearson, J.L., & Wallace, R. (2002). **Risk factors for late-life suicide: A prospective, community-based study.** *American Journal of Geriatric Psychiatry,* 10(4), 398-406.

DESCRIPTION OF THE STUDY: Studies have suggested that a negative or depressive mental outlook, being widowed or divorced, sleeping more than 9 hours per day, and drinking more than three alcoholic beverages per day were risk factors for late-life suicide. The primary aim of this study was to examine the relationship between completed suicide in late life and physical health, disability, and social support. The participants were 14,456 individuals selected from a general population of elderly subjects age 65 and older. Control subjects were a group of 420 individuals who were matched by age and sex. It was a 10-year longitudinal study beginning in 1981. Variables were assessed at baseline, year 3, and year 6, with a 10-year mortality follow-up. Baseline variables included sleep quality, social support, alcohol use, medical illness, physical impairment, cognitive impairment, and depressive symptoms.

RESULTS OF THE STUDY: The 10-year mortality follow-up indicated that 75 percent of the control subjects had died, but none had died from suicide. Twenty-one of the 14,456 participants committed suicide within the follow-up period. Twenty of the 21 suicide victims were male. Average age was 78.6 years, with a range from 67 to 90 years. The most common means was gunshot. Other means included hanging, cutting, overdose, drowning, carbon monoxide inhalation, and one participant jumped to his death. In this study, presence of friends or relatives to confide in was negatively associated with suicide. Likewise, regular church attendance was more common in control subjects than in the participant sample, indicating an even wider range of community support. Those who committed suicide had reported more depressive symptoms than those who did not, but they did not consume more alcohol (inconsistent with previous studies). Poor sleep quality was positively correlated with suicide in this study, but no specific physical illness was identified as a predisposition. The authors identify the small suicide sample as a limitation of this study.

IMPLICATIONS FOR NURSING PRACTICE: This study identified depression, poor sleep quality, and limited social support as important variables in the potential for elderly suicide. Sleep disturbance may be an important indicator of depression, whereas limited social support may be a contributing factor. The study provides reinforcement for the U.S. Department of Health and Human Services (USDHHS) recommendation in their *National Strategy for Suicide Prevention: Goals and Objectives for Action* (2001). The USDHHS recommends detection and treatment of depression as a strategy to prevent late-life suicide. The authors stated, "Because both depression and social support are amenable to intervention, this study provides further evidence for the possible effectiveness of such strategies to reduce suicides among older adults." Nurses can become actively involved in assessing for these risk factors, as well as planning, implementing, and evaluating the effectiveness of strategies for preventing suicide in the elderly population.

---

seem especially vulnerable after the loss of a spouse, with a relative risk three times that of married men (O'Connell, Chin, Cunningham, & Lawlor, 2004).

The National Institute of Mental Health [NIMH] (2010) suggests that major depression is a significant predictor of suicide in older adults. Unfortunately, it is widely underrecognized and undertreated by the medical community. The NIMH (2010) states:

> Studies show that many older adults who die by suicide—up to 75 percent—visited a physician within a month before death. These findings point to the urgency of improving detection and treatment of depression to reduce suicide risk among older adults.

Many elderly individuals express symptoms associated with depression that are never recognized as such. Any sign of helplessness or hopelessness should elicit a supportive intervening response. Stanley and associates (2005) suggest that, in assessing suicide intention, while using concern and compassion, direct questions such as the following should be asked:

■ Have you thought life is not worth living?
■ Have you considered harming yourself?

■ Do you have a plan for hurting yourself?
■ Have you ever acted on that plan?
■ Have you ever attempted suicide?

Components of intervention with a suicidal elderly person should include demonstrations of genuine concern, interest, and caring; indications of empathy for their fears and concerns; and help in identifying, clarifying, and formulating a plan of action to deal with the unresolved issue. If the elderly person's behavior seems particularly lethal, additional family or staff coverage and contact should be arranged to prevent isolation.

Application of the Nursing Process

Assessment

Assessment of the elderly individual may follow the same framework used for all adults, but with consideration of the possible biological, psychological, sociocultural, and sexual changes that occur in the normal aging process described previously in this chapter. In no other area of nursing is it more important for nurses to practice holistic nursing than with the elderly. Older adults are likely to have multiple physical problems that contribute to problems in other areas of their lives. Obviously, these components cannot be addressed as separate entities. Nursing the elderly is a multifaceted, challenging process because of the multiple changes occurring at this time in the life cycle and the way in which each change affects every aspect of the individual.

Several considerations are unique to assessment of the elderly. Assessment of the older person's thought processes is a primary responsibility. Knowledge about the presence and extent of disorientation or confusion will influence the way in which the nurse approaches elder care.

Information about sensory capabilities is also extremely important. Because hearing loss is common, the nurse should lower the pitch and loudness of his or her voice when addressing the older person. Looking directly into the face of the older person when talking facilitates communication. Questions that require a declarative sentence in response should be asked; in this way, the nurse is able to assess the client's ability to use words correctly. Visual acuity can be determined by assessing adaptation to the dark, color matching, and the perception of color contrast. Knowledge about these aspects of sensory functioning is essential in the development of an effective care plan.

The nurse should be familiar with the normal physical changes associated with the aging process. Examples of some of these changes include the following:

■ Less effective response to changes in environmental temperature, resulting in hypothermia.
■ Decreases in oxygen use and the amount of blood pumped by the heart, resulting in cerebral anoxia or hypoxia.
■ Skeletal muscle wasting and weakness, resulting in difficulty in physical mobility.
■ Limited cough and laryngeal reflexes, resulting in risk of aspiration.
■ Demineralization of bones, resulting in spontaneous fracturing.
■ Decrease in gastrointestinal motility, resulting in constipation.
■ Decrease in the ability to interpret painful stimuli, resulting in risk of injury.

Common psychosocial changes associated with aging include the following:

■ Prolonged and exaggerated grief, resulting in depression.
■ Physical changes, resulting in disturbed body image.
■ Changes in status, resulting in loss of self-worth.

This list is by no means exhaustive. The nurse should consider many other alterations in his or her assessment of the client. Knowledge of the client's functional capabilities is essential for determining the physiological, psychological, and sociological needs of the elderly individual. Age alone does not preclude the occurrence of all these changes. The aging process progresses at a wide range of variance, and each client must be assessed as a unique individual.

Diagnosis/Outcome Identification

Virtually any nursing diagnosis may be applicable to the aging client, depending on individual needs for assistance. Based on normal changes that occur in the elderly, the following nursing diagnoses may be considered:

Physiologically Related Diagnoses

■ Risk for trauma related to confusion, disorientation, muscular weakness, spontaneous fractures, falls
■ Hypothermia related to loss of adipose tissue under the skin, evidenced by increased sensitivity to cold and body temperature below 98.6°F
■ Decreased cardiac output related to decreased myocardial efficiency secondary to age-related changes, evidenced by decreased tolerance for activity and decline in energy reserve
■ Ineffective breathing pattern related to increase in fibrous tissue and loss of elasticity in lung tissue, evidenced by dyspnea and activity intolerance
■ Risk for aspiration related to diminished cough and laryngeal reflexes
■ Impaired physical mobility related to muscular wasting and weakness, evidenced by need for assistance in ambulation
■ Imbalanced nutrition, less than body requirements, related to inefficient absorption from gastrointestinal tract, difficulty chewing and swallowing, anorexia, difficulty in feeding self, evidenced by wasting syndrome, anemia, weight loss
■ Constipation related to decreased motility; inadequate diet; insufficient activity or exercise, evidenced by decreased bowel sounds; hard, formed stools; or straining at stool
■ Stress urinary incontinence related to degenerative changes in pelvic muscles and structural supports associated with increased age, evidenced by reported or observed dribbling with increased abdominal pressure or urinary frequency
■ Urinary retention related to prostatic enlargement, evidenced by bladder distention, frequent voiding of small amounts, dribbling, or overflow incontinence
■ Disturbed sensory perception related to age-related alterations in sensory transmission, evidenced by decreased visual acuity, hearing loss, diminished sensitivity to taste and smell, or increased touch threshold. (This diagnosis has been retired by NANDA-I but retained in this text because of its appropriateness to the specific behaviors described.)

- Insomnia related to age-related cognitive decline, decrease in ability to sleep ("sleep decay"), or medications, evidenced by interrupted sleep, early awakening, or falling asleep during the day
- Chronic pain related to degenerative changes in joints, evidenced by verbalization of pain or hesitation to use weight-bearing joints
- Self-care deficit (specify) related to weakness, confusion, or disorientation, evidenced by inability to feed self, maintain hygiene, dress/groom self, or toilet self without assistance
- Risk for impaired skin integrity related to alterations in nutritional state, circulation, sensation, or mobility

Psychosocially Related Diagnoses

- Disturbed thought processes related to age-related changes that result in cerebral anoxia, evidenced by short-term memory loss, confusion, or disorientation. (This diagnosis has been retired by NANDA-I but retained in this text because of its appropriateness to the specific behaviors described.)
- Complicated grieving related to bereavement overload, evidenced by symptoms of depression
- Risk for suicide related to depressed mood and feelings of low self-worth
- Powerlessness related to lifestyle of helplessness and dependency on others, evidenced by depressed mood, apathy, or verbal expressions of having no control or influence over life situation
- Low self-esteem related to loss of pre-retirement status, evidenced by verbalization of negative feelings about self and life
- Fear related to nursing home placement, evidenced by symptoms of severe anxiety and statements such as, "Nursing homes are places to go to die."
- Disturbed body image related to age-related changes in skin, hair, and fat distribution, evidenced by verbalization of negative feelings about body
- Ineffective sexuality pattern related to pain associated with vaginal dryness, evidenced by reported dissatisfaction with decrease in frequency of sexual intercourse
- Sexual dysfunction related to medications (e.g., antihypertensives) evidenced by inability to achieve an erection
- Social isolation related to total dependence on others, evidenced by expression of inadequacy in or absence of significant purpose in life
- Risk for trauma (elder abuse) related to caregiver role strain
- Caregiver role strain related to severity and duration of the care receiver's illness; lack of respite and recreation for the caregiver, evidenced by feelings of stress in relationship with care receiver; feelings of depression and anger; or family conflict around issues of providing care

Outcome Criteria

The following criteria may be used for measurement of outcomes in the care of the elderly client.

The client:

- Has not experienced injury.
- Maintains reality orientation consistent with cognitive level of functioning.
- Manages own self-care with assistance.
- Expresses positive feelings about self, past accomplishments, and hope for the future.
- Compensates adaptively for diminished sensory perception.

Caregivers:

- Can problem-solve effectively regarding care of the elderly client.
- Demonstrate adaptive coping strategies for dealing with stress of caregiver role.
- Openly express feelings.
- Express desire to join a support group of other caregivers.

Planning/Implementation

In Table 34-2, selected nursing diagnoses are presented for the elderly client. Outcome criteria are included, along with appropriate nursing interventions and rationale for each.

Reminiscence therapy is especially helpful with elderly clients. This therapeutic intervention is highlighted in Box 34-2.

Evaluation

Reassessment is conducted to determine if the nursing actions have been successful in achieving the objectives of care. Evaluation of the nursing actions for the elderly client may be facilitated by gathering information using the following types of questions:

- Has the client escaped injury from falls, burns, or other means to which he or she is vulnerable because of age?
- Can caregivers verbalize means of providing a safe environment for the client?
- Does the client maintain reality orientation at an optimum for his or her cognitive functioning?
- Can the client distinguish between reality-based and non-reality-based thinking?
- Can caregivers verbalize ways in which to orient client to reality, as needed?

Table 34-2 | CARE PLAN FOR THE ELDERLY CLIENT

NURSING DIAGNOSIS: RISK FOR TRAUMA

RELATED TO: Confusion, disorientation, muscular weakness, spontaneous fractures, falls

OUTCOME CRITERIA	NURSING INTERVENTIONS	RATIONALE

Short-Term Goals
• Client will call for assistance when ambulating or carrying out other activities.
• Client will not experience injury.
 	
Long-Term Goal
• Client will not experience injury.
	1. The following measures may be instituted:
	  a. Arrange furniture and other items in the room to accommodate client's disabilities.
	  b. Store frequently used items within easy access.
	  c. Keep bed in unelevated position. Pad side rails and headboard if client has history of seizures. Keep bed rails up when client is in bed (if permitted by institutional policy).
	  d. Assign room near nurses' station; observe frequently.
	  e. Assist client with ambulation.
	  f. Keep a dim light on at night.
	  g. If client is a smoker, cigarettes and lighter or matches should be kept at the nurses' station and dispensed only when someone is available to stay with client while he or she is smoking.
	  h. Frequently orient client to place, time, and situation.
	  i. Soft restraints may be required if client is very disoriented and hyperactive.
		1. To ensure client safety.

NURSING DIAGNOSIS: DISTURBED THOUGHT PROCESSES

RELATED TO: Age-related changes that result in cerebral anoxia

EVIDENCED BY: Short-term memory loss, confusion, or disorientation

OUTCOME CRITERIA	NURSING INTERVENTIONS	RATIONALE
Short-Term Goal • Client will accept explanations of inaccurate interpretations of the environment within (time to be determined based on client condition). **Long-Term Goal** • Client will interpret the environment accurately and maintain reality orientation to the best of his or her cognitive ability.	1. Frequently orient client to reality. Use clocks and calendars with large numbers that are easy to read. Notes and large, bold signs may be useful as reminders. Allow client to have personal belongings. 2. Keep explanations simple. Use face-to-face interaction. Speak slowly and do not shout. 3. Discourage rumination of delusional thinking. Talk about real events and real people. 4. Monitor for medication side effects.	1. To help maintain orientation and aid in memory and recognition. 2. To facilitate comprehension. Shouting may create discomfort, and in some instances, may provoke anger. 3. Rumination promotes disorientation. Reality orientation increases sense of self-worth and personal dignity. 4. Physiological changes in the elderly can alter the body's response to certain medications. Toxic effects may intensify altered thought processes.

Continued

Table 34-2 | CARE PLAN FOR THE ELDERLY CLIENT–cont'd

NURSING DIAGNOSIS: SELF-CARE DEFICIT (SPECIFY)

RELATED TO: Weakness, disorientation, confusion, or memory deficits

EVIDENCED BY: Inability to fulfill activities of daily living (ADLs)

OUTCOME CRITERIA	NURSING INTERVENTIONS	RATIONALE

Short-Term Goal
• Client will participate in ADLs with assistance from caregiver.
 	
Long-Term Goals
• Client will accomplish activities of daily living to the best of his or her ability.
• Unfulfilled needs will be met by caregivers.
	1. Provide a simple, structured environment:
	  a. Identify self-care deficits and provide assistance as required. Promote independent actions as able.
	  b. Allow plenty of time for client to perform tasks.
	  c. Provide guidance and support for independent actions by talking the client through the task one step at a time.
	  d. Provide a structured schedule of activities that do not change from day to day.
	  e. ADLs should follow home routine as closely as possible.
	  f. Allow consistency in assignment of daily caregivers.
		1. To minimize confusion.

NURSING DIAGNOSIS: CAREGIVER ROLE STRAIN

RELATED TO: Severity and duration of the care receiver's illness; lack of respite and recreation for the caregiver

EVIDENCED BY: Feelings of stress in relationship with care receiver; feelings of depression and anger; family conflict around issues of providing care

OUTCOME CRITERIA	NURSING INTERVENTIONS	RATIONALE
Short-Term Goal • Caregivers will verbalize understanding of ways to facilitate the caregiver role. **Long-Term Goal** • Caregivers will achieve effective problem-solving skills and develop adaptive coping mechanisms to regain equilibrium.	1. Assess prospective caregivers' ability to anticipate and fulfill client's unmet needs. Provide information to assist caregivers with this responsibility. Ensure that caregivers are aware of available community support systems from which they can seek assistance when required. Examples include adult day-care centers, housekeeping and homemaker services, respite care services, or a local chapter of the Alzheimer's Association. This organization sponsors a nationwide 24-hour hotline to provide information and link families who need assistance with nearby chapters and affiliates. The hotline number is 800-272-3900. 2. Encourage caregivers to express feelings, particularly anger.	1. Caregivers require relief from the pressures and strain of providing 24-hour care for their loved one. Studies have shown that elder abuse arises out of caregiving situations that place overwhelming stress on the caregivers. 2. Release of these emotions can serve to prevent psychopathology, such as depression or psychophysiological disorders, from occurring.

Table 34-2 | CARE PLAN FOR THE ELDERLY CLIENT—cont'd

OUTCOME CRITERIA	NURSING INTERVENTIONS	RATIONALE
	3. Encourage participation in support groups composed of members with similar life situations.	3. Hearing others who are experiencing the same problems discuss ways in which they have coped may help caregiver adopt more adaptive strategies. Individuals with similar life experiences provide empathy and support for each other.

NURSING DIAGNOSIS: LOW SELF-ESTEEM

RELATED TO: Loss of pre-retirement status; early stages of cognitive decline

EVIDENCED BY: Verbalization of negative feelings about self and life

OUTCOME CRITERIA	NURSING INTERVENTIONS	RATIONALE

Short-Term Goal
• Client will verbalize positive aspects of self and past accomplishments.
 	
Long-Term Goal
• Client will participate in group activities in which he or she can experience a feeling of enjoyment and accomplishment (to the best of his or her ability).
	1. Encourage client to express honest feelings in relation to loss of prior status. Acknowledge pain of loss. Support client through process of grieving.
	
	2. If lapses in memory are occurring, devise methods for assisting client with memory deficit. Examples:
	  a. Name sign on door identifying client's room.
	  b. Identifying sign on outside of dining room door.
	  c. Identifying sign on outside of restroom door.
	  d. Large clock, with oversized numbers and hands, appropriately placed.
	  e. Large calendar, indicating one day at a time, with month, day, and year in bold print.
	  f. Printed, structured daily schedule, with one copy for client and one posted on unit wall.
	  g. "News board" on unit wall where current news of national and local interest may be posted.
	
	3. Encourage client's attempts to communicate. If verbalizations are not understandable, express to client what you think he or she intended to say. It may be necessary to reorient client frequently.
	
	4. Encourage reminiscence and discussion of life review (see Box 34-2). Sharing picture albums, if possible, is especially good. Also discuss present-day events.
	
	5. Encourage participation in group activities. May need to accompany
		1. Client may be fixed in anger stage of grieving process, which is turned inward on the self, resulting in diminished self-esteem.
		
		2. These aids may assist client to function more independently, thereby increasing self-esteem.
		
		3. The ability to communicate effectively with others may enhance self-esteem.
		
		4. Reminiscence and life review help client resume progression through the grief process associated with disappointing life events and increase self-esteem as successes are reviewed.
		
		5. Positive feedback from group members will increase self-esteem.

Continued

Table 34-2 | CARE PLAN FOR THE ELDERLY CLIENT—cont'd

OUTCOME CRITERIA	NURSING INTERVENTIONS	RATIONALE
	client at first, until he or she feels secure that the group members will be accepting, regardless of limitations in verbal communication.	
	6. Encourage client to be as independent as possible in self-care activities. Provide written schedule of tasks to be performed. Intervene in areas where client requires assistance.	6. The ability to perform independently preserves self-esteem.

NURSING DIAGNOSIS: DISTURBED SENSORY PERCEPTION

RELATED TO: Age-related alterations in sensory transmission

EVIDENCED BY: Decreased visual acuity, hearing loss, diminished sensitivity to taste and smell, and increased touch threshold

OUTCOME CRITERIA	NURSING INTERVENTIONS*	RATIONALE

Short-Term Goal
• Client will not experience injury due to diminished sensory perception.
 	
Long-Term Goals
• Client will attain optimal level of sensory stimulation.
 	
• Client will not experience injury due to diminished sensory perception.
	1. The following nursing strategies are indicated:
	  a. Provide meaningful sensory stimulation to all special senses through conversation, touch, music, or pleasant smells.
	  b. Encourage wearing of glasses, hearing aids, prostheses, and other adaptive devices.
	  c. Use bright, contrasting colors in the environment.
	  d. Provide large-print reading materials, such as books, clocks, calendars, and educational materials.
	  e. Maintain room lighting that distinguishes day from night and that is free of shadows and glare.
	  f. Teach client to scan the environment to locate objects.
	  g. Help client to locate food on plate using "clock" system, and describe food if client is unable to visualize; assist with feeding as needed.
	  h. Arrange physical environment to maximize functional vision.
	  i. Place personal items and call light within client's field of vision.
	  j. Teach client to watch the person who is speaking.
	  k. Reinforce wearing of hearing aid; if client does not have an aid, may consider a communication device (e.g., amplifier).
	  l. Communicate clearly, distinctly, and slowly, using a low-pitched voice and facing client; avoid over-articulation.
	  m. Remove as much unnecessary background noise as possible.
	  n. Do not use slang or extraneous words.
		1. To assist client with diminished sensory perception and because client safety is a nursing priority.

Table 34-2 | CARE PLAN FOR THE ELDERLY CLIENT—cont'd

OUTCOME CRITERIA	NURSING INTERVENTIONS	RATIONALE
	o. As speaker, position self at eye level and no farther than 6 feet away. p. Get the client's attention before speaking. q. Avoid speaking directly into the client's ear. r. If the client does not understand what is being said, rephrase the statement rather than simply repeating it. s. Help client select foods from the menu that will ensure discrimination between various tastes and smells. t. Ensure that food has been properly cooled so that client with diminished pain threshold is not burned. u. Ensure that bath or shower water is appropriate temperature. v. Use backrubs and massage as therapeutic touch to stimulate sensory receptors.	

*The interventions for this nursing diagnosis were adapted from Rogers-Seidl, F.F. (1997). *Geriatric nursing care plans* (2nd ed). St. Louis, MO: Mosby Year Book.

BOX 34-2 Reminiscence Therapy and Life Review With the Elderly

Stanley, Blair, and Beare (2005) stated:

> Stimulation of life memories helps older adults to work through their losses and maintain self-esteem. Life review provides older adults with an opportunity to come to grips with guilt and regrets, and to emerge feeling good about themselves. (p. 268)

Studies have indicated that *reminiscence*, or thinking about the past and reflecting on it, may promote better mental health in old age. *Life review* is related to reminiscence, but differs from it in that it is a more guided or directed cognitive process that constructs a history or story in an autobiographical way (Murray et al., 2009).

Elderly individuals who spend time thinking about the past experience an increase in self-esteem and are less likely to suffer depression. Some psychologists believe that life review may help some people adjust to memories of an unhappy past. Others view reminiscence and life review as ways to bolster feelings of well-being, particularly in older people who can no longer remain active.

Reminiscence therapy can take place on a one-to-one basis or in a group setting. In reminiscence groups, elderly individuals share significant past events with peers. The nurse leader facilitates the discussion of topics that deal with specific life transitions, such as childhood, adolescence, marriage, childbearing, grandparenthood, and retirement. Members share both positive and negative aspects, including personal feelings, about these life-cycle events.

Reminiscence on a one-to-one basis can provide a way for elderly individuals to work through unresolved issues from the past. Painful issues may be too difficult to discuss in the group setting. As the individual reviews his or her life process, the nurse can validate feelings and help the elderly client come to terms with painful issues that may have been long suppressed. This process is necessary if the elderly individual is to maintain (or attain) a sense of positive identity and self-esteem and ultimately achieve the goal of ego integrity as described by Erikson (1963).

A number of creative measures can be used to facilitate life review with the elderly individual. Having the client keep a journal for sharing may be a way to stimulate discussion (as well as providing a permanent record of past events for significant others). Pets, music, and special foods have a way of provoking memories from the client's past. Photographs of family members and past significant events are an excellent way of guiding the elderly client through his or her autobiographical review.

Care must be taken in the life review to assist clients to work through unresolved issues. Anxiety, guilt, depression, and despair may result if the individual is unable to work through the problems and accept them. Life review can work in a negative way if the individual comes to believe that his or her life was meaningless. However, it can be a very positive experience for the person who can take pride in past accomplishments and feel satisfied with his or her life, resulting in a sense of serenity and inner peace in the older adult.

■ Is the client able to accomplish self-care activities independently to his or her optimum level of functioning?

■ Does the client seek assistance for aspects of self-care that he or she is unable to perform independently?

■ Does the client express positive feelings about himself or herself?

■ Does the client reminisce about accomplishments that have occurred in his or her life?

■ Does the client express some hope for the future?

■ Does the client wear eyeglasses or a hearing aid, if needed, to compensate for sensory deficits?

■ Does the client consistently look at others in the face to facilitate hearing when they are talking to him or her?

■ Does the client use helpful aids, such as signs identifying various rooms, to help maintain orientation?

■ Can the caregivers work through problems and make decisions regarding care of the elderly client?

■ Do the caregivers include the elderly client in the decision-making process, if appropriate?

■ Can the caregivers demonstrate adaptive coping strategies for dealing with the strain of long-term caregiving?

■ Are the caregivers open and honest in expression of feelings?

■ Can the caregivers verbalize community resources to which they can go for assistance with their caregiving responsibilities?

■ Have the caregivers joined a support group?

Summary and Key Points

■ Care of the aging individual presents one of the greatest challenges for nursing.

■ The growing population of individuals aged 65 and older suggests that the challenge will progress well into the 21st century.

■ America is a youth-oriented society. It is not desirable to be old in this culture.

■ In some cultures, the elderly are revered and hold a special place of honor within the society, but in highly industrialized countries such as the United States, status declines with the decrease in productivity and participation in the mainstream of society.

■ Individuals experience many changes as they age. Physical changes occur in virtually every body system.

■ Psychologically, there may be age-related memory deficiencies, particularly for recent events.

■ Intellectual functioning does not decline with age, but length of time required for learning increases.

■ Aging individuals experience many losses, potentially leading to bereavement overload. They are vulnerable to depression and to feelings of low self-worth.

■ The elderly population represents a disproportionately high percentage of individuals who commit suicide.

■ Neurocognitive disorders are the most frequent causes of psychopathology in the elderly. Sleep disorders are very common.

■ The need for sexual expression by the elderly is often misunderstood within our society. Although many physical changes occur at this time of life that alter an individual's sexuality, if he or she has reasonably good health and a willing partner, sexual activity can continue well past the 70s for most people.

■ Retirement has both social and economic implications for elderly individuals. Society often equates an individual's status with occupation, and loss of employment may result in the need for adjustment in the standard of living because retirement income may be reduced by 20 to 40 percent of preretirement earnings.

■ Less than 5 percent of the population ages 65 and older live in nursing homes. A profile of the typical elderly nursing home resident is a white woman about 80 years old, widowed, with multiple chronic health conditions. Much stigma is attached to what some still call "rest homes" or "old age homes," and many elderly people still equate them with a place "to go to die."

■ The strain of the caregiver role has become a major dilemma in our society. Elder abuse is sometimes inflicted by caregivers for whom the role has become overwhelming and intolerable. There is an intense need to find assistance for these people, who must provide care for their loved ones on a 24-hour basis. Home health care, respite care, support groups, and financial assistance are needed to ease the burden of this role strain.

■ Caring for elderly individuals requires a special kind of inner strength and compassion. The poem that follows conveys a vital message for nurses.

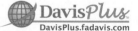 Additional info available at
DavisPlus.fadavis.com www.davisplus.com

What Do You See, Nurse?

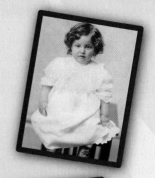

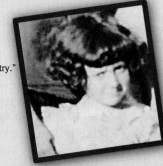

What do you see, nurse, what do you see?
    What are you thinking when you look at me?
A crabbed old woman, not very wise,
    Uncertain of habit, with faraway eyes.
Who dribbles her food and makes no reply
    When you say in a loud voice, "I do wish you'd try."
Who seems not to notice the things that you do
    And forever is losing a stocking or shoe.
Who unresisting or not, lets you do as you will
    With bathing and feeding, the long day to fill.
Is that what you're thinking, is that what you see?
    Then open your eyes, you're not looking at me.
I'll tell you who I am as I sit there so still.
    As I move at your bidding, as I eat at your will.
I'm a small child of ten with a father and a mother,
    Brothers and sisters who love one another.

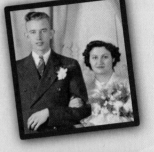

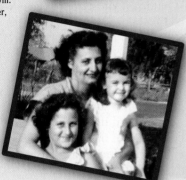

A young girl at sixteen with wings on her feet
    Dreaming that soon now a lover she'll meet.
A bride soon at twenty—my heart gives a leap
    Remembering the vows that I promised to keep.
At twenty-five, now, I have young of my own
    Who need me to build a secure happy home.
A woman of thirty, my young now grow fast
    Bound to each other with ties that should last.

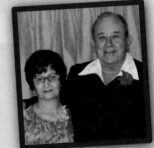

At forty my young will now soon be gone,
    But my man stays beside me to see I don't mourn.
At fifty once more babies play round my knee.
    Again we know children, my loved one and me.

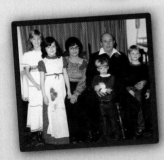

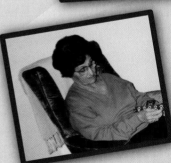

Dark days are upon me, my husband is dead.
    I look at the future, I shudder with dread.
For my young are all busy rearing young of their own.
    And I think of the years and the love I have known.

I'm an old woman now and nature is cruel.
    Tis her jest to make old age look like a fool.
The body it crumbles, grace and vigor depart.
    There is now just a stone where I once had a heart.
But inside this old carcass a young girl still dwells.
    And now and again my battered heart swells.

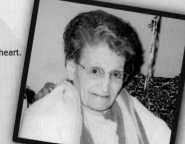

I remember the joys, I remember the pain.
    And I'm loving and living life all over again.
I think of the years all too few—gone so fast.
    And accept the stark fact that nothing can last.
So open your eyes, nurse, open and see.
    Not a crabbed old woman—look closer—SEE ME.

Author Unknown

Review Questions
Self-Examination/Learning Exercise

*Select the answer that is **most** appropriate for each of the following questions.*

1. Stanley, age 72, is admitted to the hospital for depression. His son reports that he has periods of confusion and forgetfulness. In her admission assessment, the nurse notices an open sore on Stanley's arm. When she questions him about it, he says, "I scraped it on the fence 2 weeks ago. It's smaller than it was." How might the nurse analyze these data?
   a. Consider that Stanley may have been attempting self-harm.
   b. The delay in healing may indicate that Stanley has developed skin cancer.
   c. A diminished inflammatory response in the elderly increases healing time.
   d. Age-related skin changes and distribution of adipose tissue delay healing in the elderly.

2. What is the most appropriate way to communicate with an elderly person who is deaf in his right ear?
   a. Speak loudly into his left ear.
   b. Speak to him from a position on his left side.
   c. Speak face-to-face in a high-pitched voice.
   d. Speak face-to-face in a low-pitched voice.

3. Why is it important for the nurse to check the temperature of the water before an elderly individual gets into the shower?
   a. The client may catch cold if the water temperature is too low.
   b. The client may burn himself because of a higher pain threshold.
   c. Elderly clients have difficulty discriminating between hot and cold.
   d. The water must be exactly 98.6°F.

4. Mr. B, age 79, is admitted to the psychiatric unit for depression. He has lost weight and has become socially isolated. His wife died 5 years ago and his son tells the nurse, "He did very well when Mom died. He didn't even cry." Which would be the priority nursing diagnosis for Mr. B?
   a. Complicated grieving
   b. Imbalanced nutrition: less than body requirements
   c. Social isolation
   d. Risk for injury

5. Mr. B, age 79, is admitted to the psychiatric unit for depression. He has lost weight and has become socially isolated. His wife died 5 years ago and he lives alone. A suicide assessment is conducted. Why is Mr. B at high risk for suicide?
   a. All depressed people are at high risk for suicide.
   b. Mr. B is in the age group in which the highest percentage of suicides occur.
   c. Mr. B is a white man, recently bereaved, living alone.
   d. His son reports that Mr. B owns a gun.

6. Mr. B, age 79, is admitted to the psychiatric unit for depression. He has lost weight and has become socially isolated. His wife died 5 years ago and his son tells the nurse, "He did very well when Mom died. He didn't even cry." Which would be the priority nursing intervention for Mr. B?
   a. Take blood pressure once each shift.
   b. Ensure that Mr. B attends group activities.
   c. Encourage Mr. B to eat all of the food on his food tray.
   d. Encourage Mr. B to talk about his wife's death.

7. In group exercise, Mr. B, a 79-year-old man with major depression, becomes tired and short of breath very quickly. This is most likely due to:
   a. Age-related changes in the cardiovascular system
   b. A sedentary lifestyle
   c. The effects of pathological depression
   d. Medication the physician has prescribed for depression

Review Questions—cont'd
Self-Examination/Learning Exercise

8. Clara, an 80-year-old woman, says to the nurse, "I'm all alone now. My husband is gone. My best friend is gone. My daughter is busy with her work and family. I might as well just go, too." Which is the best response by the nurse?
   a. "Are you thinking that you want to die, Clara?"
   b. "You have lots to live for, Clara."
   c. "Cheer up, Clara. You have so much to be thankful for."
   d. "Tell me about your family, Clara."

9. An elderly client says to the nurse, "I don't want to go to that crafts class. I'm too old to learn anything." Based on knowledge of the aging process, which of the following is a true statement?
   a. Memory functioning in the elderly most likely reflects loss of long-term memories of remote events.
   b. Intellectual functioning declines with advancing age.
   c. Learning ability remains intact, but time required for learning increases with age.
   d. Cognitive functioning is rarely affected in aging individuals.

10. According to the literature, which of the following is most important for individuals to maintain a healthy, adaptive old age?
   a. To remain socially interactive
   b. To disengage slowly in preparation of the last stage of life
   c. To move in with family
   d. To maintain total independence and accept no help from anyone

TEST YOUR CRITICAL THINKING SKILLS

Mrs. M, age 76, is seeing her primary physician for her regular 6-month physical exam. Mrs. M's husband died 2 years ago, at which time she sold her home in Kansas and came to live in California with her only child, a daughter. The daughter is married and has three children (one in college and two teenagers at home). The daughter reports that her mother is becoming increasingly withdrawn, stays in her room, and eats very little. She has lost 13 pounds since her last 6-month visit. The primary physician refers Mrs. M to a psychiatrist who hospitalizes her for evaluation. He diagnoses Mrs. M with major depressive disorder.

Mrs. M tells the nurse, "I didn't want to leave my home, but my daughter insisted. I would have been all right. I miss my friends and my church. Back home I drove my car everywhere. But there's too much traffic out here. They sold my car and I have to depend on my daughter or grandkids to take me places. I hate being so dependent! I miss my husband so much. I just sit and think about him and our past life all the time. I don't have any interest in meeting new people. I want to go home!!"

Mrs. M admits to having some thoughts of dying, although she denies feeling suicidal. She denies having a plan or means for taking her life. "I really don't want to die, but I just can't see much reason for living. My daughter and her family are so busy with their own lives. They don't need me—or even have time for me!"

Answer the following questions about Mrs. M:

1. What would be the *primary* nursing diagnosis for Mrs. M?
2. Formulate a short-term goal for Mrs. M.
3. From the assessment data, identify the major problem that may be a long-term focus of care for Mrs. M.

References

Administration on Aging (AoA). (2014). *A profile of older Americans: 2013.* Washington, DC: U.S. Department of Health and Human Services.

American Association of Retired Persons (AARP). (2010). *Sex, romance, and relationships: AARP survey of midlife and older adults.* Washington, DC: American Association of Retired Persons.

Beers, M.H., & Jones, T.V. (Eds.). (2004). *The Merck manual of health & aging.* Whitehouse Station, NJ: Merck Research Laboratories.

Blair, K. (2012). Assessing the older adult: What's different? In J.W. Lange (Ed.), *The nurse's role in promoting optimal health of older adults* (pp. 149-160). Philadelphia, PA: F.A. Davis.

Blazer, D. (2008). Treatment of seniors. In R.E. Hales, S.C. Yudofsky, & G.O. Gabbard (Eds.), *Textbook of psychiatry* (5th ed., pp. 1449-1469). Washington, DC: American Psychiatric Publishing.

Blevins, N.H. (2013). Presbycusis. *Wolters Kluwer Health.* Retrieved from http://www.uptodate.com/contents/presbycusis

Cahill, K.E., Giandrea, M.D., & Quinn, J.F. (2011). Reentering the labor force after retirement. Bureau of Labor Statistics. *Monthly Labor Review, June 2011,* 34-42.

Heiss, G., Wallace, R., Anderson, G.L., Aragak, A., Beresford, S.A.A., Brzyski, R., Chlebowski, R.T., Gass, M., LaCroix, A., Manson, J.E., Prentice, R.L., Rossouw, J., and Stefanick, M.L. (2008). Health risks and benefits three years after stopping randomized treatment with estrogen and progestin. *Journal of the American Medical Association, 299*(9), 1036-1045.

Johnston, C.B., Harper, G.M., & Landefeld, C.S. (2013). Geriatric disorders. In S.J. McPhee & M.A. Papadakis (Eds.), *Current medical diagnosis and treatment* (pp. 57-73). New York, NY: McGraw Hill Medical.

King, B.M. (2012). *Human sexuality today* (7th ed.). Upper Saddle River, NJ: Pearson Prentice Hall.

Koop, P.M. (2012). Older adults as caregivers and care recipients. In J.W. Lange (Ed.), *The nurse's role in promoting optimal health of older adults* (pp. 295-305). Philadelphia, PA: F.A. Davis.

Lang, R. (2012). Challenges to mental wellness. In J.W. Lange (Ed.), *The nurse's role in promoting optimal health of older adults* (pp. 339-370). Philadelphia, PA: F.A. Davis.

Masters, W.H., Johnson, V.E., & Kolodny, R.C. (1995). *Human sexuality* (5th ed.). New York, NY: Addison-Wesley Longman.

Murray, R.B., Zentner, J.P., & Yakimo, R. (2009). *Health promotion strategies through the life span* (8th ed.). Upper Saddle River, NJ: Prentice Hall.

National Center for Health Statistics (NCHS). (2012a, October 10). Deaths: Preliminary data for 2011. *National Vital Statistics Reports, 61*(6), 1-52.

National Center for Health Statistics (NCHS). (2012b, November 12). Deaths, percent of total deaths, and death rates for the 15 leading causes of death in 5-year age groups, by race and sex: United States, 2010. Retrieved from http://www.cdc.gov/nchs/data/dvs/lcwk1_2010.pdf

National Center for Health Statistics (NCHS). (2012c). *Older Americans 2012: Key indicators of well-being.* Federal Interagency Forum on Aging-Related Statistics. Washington, DC: U.S. Government Printing Office.

National Council on Aging (NCOA). (2012). *Healthy aging.* Retrieved from http://www.ncoa.org/assets/files/pdf/FactSheet_HealthyAging.pdf

National Institutes of Health (NIH). (2012). *Aging changes in immunity.* Retrieved from http://www.nlm.nih.gov/medlineplus/ency/article/004008.htm

National Institute of Mental Health [NIMH]. (2010). *Older adults: Depression and suicide facts.* Retrieved from http://www.nimh.nih.gov/health/publications/older-adults-depression-and-suicide-facts-fact-sheet/index.shtml

O'Connell, H., Chin, A.V., Cunningham, C., & Lawlor, B.A. (2004). Recent developments: Suicide in older people. *British Medical Journal, 329,* 895-899.

Pietraniec-Shannon, M. (2007). Nursing care of older adult patients. In L.S. Williams & P.D. Hopper (Eds.), *Understanding medical-surgical nursing* (3rd ed.). Philadelphia, PA: F.A. Davis.

Purnell, L.D. (2013). *Transcultural health care: A culturally competent approach* (4th ed.). Philadelphia, PA: F.A. Davis.

Roberts, C.M. (1991). *How did I get here so fast?* New York, NY: Warner Books.

Rogers-Seidl, F.F. (1997). *Geriatric nursing care plans* (2nd ed.). St. Louis, MO: Mosby Year Book.

Sadock, B.J., & Sadock, V.A. (2007). *Synopsis of psychiatry: Behavioral sciences/clinical psychiatry* (10th ed.). Philadelphia, PA: Lippincott Williams & Wilkins.

Srivastava, S., John, O.P., Gosling, S.D., & Potter, J. (2003). Development of personality in early and middle adulthood: Set like plaster or persistent change? *Journal of Personality and Social Psychology, 84*(5), 1041-1053.

Stanley, M., Blair, K.A., & Beare, P.G. (2005). *Gerontological nursing: Promoting successful aging with older adults* (3rd ed.). Philadelphia, PA: F.A. Davis.

Stark, S. (2012). Elder abuse: Screening, intervention, and prevention. *Nursing2012, 42*(10), 24-29.

Vaillant, G.E. (2003). *Aging well: Surprising guideposts to a happier life from the landmark Harvard study of adult development.* New York, NY: Little, Brown, & Company.

Classical References

Erikson, E.H. (1963). *Childhood and society* (2nd ed.). New York, NY: WW Norton.

Kübler-Ross, E. (1969). *On death and dying.* New York, NY: Macmillan.

Reichard, S., Livson, F., & Peterson, P.G. (1962). *Aging and personality.* New York, NY: John Wiley & Sons.

@ INTERNET REFERENCES

- Additional sources related to aging may be located at the following websites:
  - http://www.4woman.org/Health/Menopause.htm
  - http://www.aarp.org
  - http://www.ssa.gov
  - http://www.nih.gov/nia
  - http://www.medicare.gov
  - http://www.seniorlaw.com
  - http://www.growthhouse.org/cesp.html
  - http://www.aoa.gov
  - http://www.nsclc.org

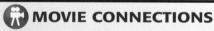 MOVIE CONNECTIONS

The Hiding Place • *On Golden Pond* • *To Dance With the White Dog*

Survivors of Abuse or Neglect

35

CORE CONCEPTS

abuse

battering

incest

neglect

rape

KEY TERMS

child sexual abuse	emotional abuse	safe house or shelter
compounded rape reaction	emotional neglect	sexual exploitation of a child
controlled response pattern	expressed response pattern	silent rape reaction
cycle of battering	marital rape	statutory rape
date (acquaintance) rape	physical neglect	

OBJECTIVES
After reading this chapter, the student will be able to:

1. Describe epidemiological statistics associated with intimate partner violence, child abuse, and sexual assault.
2. Discuss characteristics of victims and victimizers.
3. Identify predisposing factors to abusive behaviors.
4. Describe physical and psychological effects on the survivors of intimate partner violence, child abuse, and sexual assault.
5. Identify nursing diagnoses, goals of care, and appropriate nursing interventions for care of survivors of intimate partner violence, child abuse, and sexual assault.
6. Evaluate nursing care of survivors of intimate partner violence, child abuse, and sexual assault.
7. Discuss various modalities relevant to treatment of survivors of abuse.

HOMEWORK ASSIGNMENT
Please read the chapter and answer the following questions:

1. What neurotransmitters have been implicated in the etiology of aggression and violence?
2. What is the most common reason that women give for staying in an abusive relationship?
3. Describe a compounded rape reaction.
4. What are some adult manifestations of childhood sexual abuse?

CORE CONCEPT
Abuse
The maltreatment of one person by another.

Abuse is on the rise in this society. Books, newspapers, movies, and television inundate their readers and viewers with stories of "man's inhumanity to man" (no gender bias intended).

Nearly 3 in 10 women and 1 in 10 men in the United States report having been the victim of intimate partner violence (Centers for Disease Control and Prevention [CDC], 2012a). More injuries are attributed to intimate partner violence than to all rapes, muggings, and automobile accidents combined.

Rape is vastly underreported in the United States. Because many of these attacks occurring daily go unreported and unrecognized, sexual assault is often considered a silent-violent epidemic. In the United States, 1 in 5 women and 1 in 71 men report having been raped at some time in their lives (CDC, 2012b).

An increase in the incidence of child abuse and related fatalities has also been documented. In 2011, an estimated 3.7 million cases of possible child abuse or neglect were reported to child protective services, and about one-fifth of these cases were substantiated (U.S. Department of Health and Human Services [USD-HHS], 2012). An estimated 1,545 children died from causes related to abuse or neglect in 2011.

Abuse affects all populations equally. It occurs among all races, religions, economic classes, ages, and educational backgrounds. The phenomenon is cyclical in that many abusers were themselves victims of abuse as children.

Family violence is not a new problem; in fact, it is probably as old as humankind, and has been documented as far back as biblical times. Child abuse became a mandatory reportable occurrence in the United States in 1968. Responsibility for the protection of elders from abuse rests primarily with the states. In 1987, Congress passed amendments to the Older Americans Act of 1965 that provide for state Area Agencies on Aging to assess the need for elder abuse prevention services. These events have made it possible for individuals who once felt powerless to stop the abuse against them, to come forward and seek advice, support, and protection.

Aside from the individual physical, psychological, and social devastation that violence incurs, there are economic implications as well. The annual cost of intimate partner violence, measured in terms of medical care and lost productivity, is close to $6 billion (CDC, 2013).

This chapter discusses intimate partner violence, child abuse (including neglect), and sexual assault. Elder abuse is discussed in Chapter 34. Factors that predispose individuals to commit acts of abuse against others, as well as the physical and psychological effects on the survivors, are examined.

Nursing of individuals who have experienced abusive behavior from others is presented within the context of the nursing process. Various treatment modalities are described.

Predisposing Factors

What predisposes individuals to be abusive? Although no one really knows for sure, several theories have been espoused. A brief discussion of ideas associated with biological, psychological, and sociocultural views is presented here.

Biological Theories

Neurophysiological Influences

Various components of the neurological system in both humans and animals have been implicated in both the facilitation and inhibition of aggressive impulses. Areas of the brain that may be involved include the temporal lobe, the limbic system, and the amygdaloid nucleus (Tardiff, 2003).

Biochemical Influences

Studies show that various neurotransmitters—in particular norepinephrine, dopamine, and serotonin—may play a role in the facilitation and inhibition of aggressive impulses (Hollander, Berlin, & Stein, 2008). This theory is consistent with the "fight or flight" arousal described by Selye (1956) in his theory of the response to stress (see Chapter 1). An explanation of these biochemical influences on violent behavior is presented in Figure 35-1.

Genetic Influences

Various genetic components related to aggressive behavior have been investigated. Some studies have linked increased aggressiveness with selective inbreeding in mice, suggesting the possibility of a direct genetic link. Another genetic characteristic that was once thought to have some implication for aggressive behavior was the genetic karyotype XYY. The XYY syndrome has been found to contribute to aggressive behavior in a small percentage of cases (Sadock & Sadock, 2007). The evidence linking this chromosomal aberration to aggressive and deviant behavior has not been firmly established.

Disorders of the Brain

Organic brain syndromes associated with various cerebral disorders have been implicated in the predisposition to aggressive and violent behavior (Cummings & Mega, 2003; Sadock & Sadock, 2007; Tardiff, 2003). Brain tumors, particularly in the areas of the limbic system and the temporal lobes; trauma to the brain, resulting in cerebral changes; and diseases, such as encephalitis (or medications that may effect this

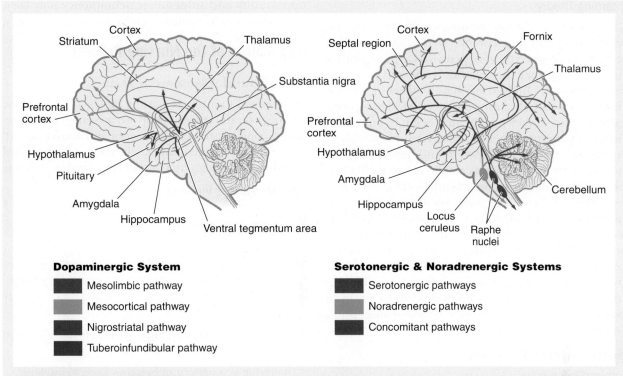

FIGURE 35–1   Neurobiology of violence.

NEUROTRANSMITTERS

Neurotransmitters that have been implicated in the etiology of aggression and violence include decreases in serotonin and increases in norepinephrine and dopamine (Hollander et al., 2008; Tardiff, 2003).

ASSOCIATED AREAS OF THE BRAIN

• Limbic structures: Emotional alterations
• Prefrontal & frontal cortices: Modulation of social judgment
• Amygdala: Anxiety, rage, fear
• Hypothalamus: Stimulates sympathetic nervous system in "fight-or-flight" response
• Hippocampus: Learning and memory

MEDICATIONS USED TO MODULATE AGGRESSION

1. Studies have suggested that selective serotonin reuptake inhibitors (SSRIs) may reduce irritability and aggression consistent with the hypothesis of reduced serotonergic activity in aggression.
2. Mood stabilizers that dampen limbic irritability may be important in reducing the susceptibility to react to provocation or threatening stimuli by overactivation of limbic system structures such as the amygdala (Siever, 2002). Carbamazepine (Tegretol), phenytoin (Dilantin), and divalproex sodium (Depakote) have yielded positive results. Lithium has also been used effectively in violent individuals (Schatzberg, Cole, & DeBattista, 2010).
3. Anti-adrenergic agents such as beta-blockers (e.g., propranolol) have been shown to reduce aggression in some individuals, presumably by dampening excessive noradrenergic activity (Schatzberg et al., 2010).
4. In their ability to modulate excessive dopaminergic activity, antipsychotics—both typical and atypical—have been helpful in the control of aggression and violence, particularly in individuals with co-morbid psychosis.

syndrome) and epilepsy, particularly temporal lobe epilepsy, have all been implicated.

Psychological Theories

Psychodynamic Theory

The psychodynamic theorists imply that unmet needs for satisfaction and security result in an underdeveloped ego and a weak superego. It is thought that when frustration occurs, aggression and violence supply this individual with a dose of power and prestige that boosts the self-image and validates a significance to his or her life that is lacking. The immature ego cannot prevent dominant id behaviors from occurring, and the weak superego is unable to produce feelings of guilt.

Learning Theory

Children learn to behave by imitating their role models, which are usually their parents. Models are more likely to be imitated when they are perceived as prestigious or influential, or when the behavior is followed by positive reinforcement. Children may have an idealistic perception of their parents during the very early developmental stages but, as they mature, may begin to imitate the behavior patterns of their teachers, friends, and others. Individuals who were abused as children or who witnessed domestic violence as a child are more likely to behave in an abusive manner as adults (Hornor, 2005).

Adults and children alike model many of their behaviors after individuals they observe on television and in movies. Unfortunately, modeling can result in maladaptive as well as adaptive behavior, particularly when children view heroes triumphing over villains by using violence. It is also possible that individuals who have a biological predisposition toward aggressive behavior may be more susceptible to negative role modeling.

Sociocultural Theories

Societal Influences

Although they agree that perhaps some biological and psychological aspects are influential, social scientists believe that aggressive behavior is primarily a product of one's culture and social structure.

American society essentially was founded on a general acceptance of violence as a means of solving problems. The concept of relative deprivation has been shown to have a profound effect on collective violence within a society. Kennedy and associates (1998) have stated:

> Studies have shown that poverty and income are powerful predictors of homicide and violent crime. The effect of the growing gap between the rich and poor is mediated through an undermining of social cohesion, or social capital, and decreased social capital is in turn associated with increased firearm homicide and violent crime. (p. 7)

Indeed, the United States was populated by the violent actions of one group of people over another. Since that time, much has been said and written, and laws have been passed, regarding the civil rights of all people. However, to this day many people would agree that the statement "All men are created equal" is hypocritical in our society.

Societal influences may contribute to violence when individuals realize that their needs and desires are not being met relative to other people (Tardiff, 2003). When poor and oppressed people find that they have limited access through legitimate channels, they are more likely to resort to delinquent behaviors in an effort to obtain desired ends. This lack of opportunity and subsequent delinquency may even contribute to a subculture of violence within a society.

Application of the Nursing Process

Background Assessment Data

Data related to intimate partner violence, child abuse and neglect, and sexual assault are presented in this section. Characteristics of both victim and abuser are addressed. This information may be used as background knowledge in designing plans of care for these clients.

Intimate Partner Violence

> ## CORE CONCEPT
> **Battering**
> A pattern of coercive control founded on and supported by physical and/or sexual violence or threat of violence of an intimate partner.

The National Coalition Against Domestic Violence (2013) states:

> Battering is a pattern of behavior used to establish power and control over another person with whom an intimate relationship is or has been shared through fear and intimidation, often including the threat or use of violence. Battering happens when one person believes that they are entitled to control another.

The U.S. Department of Justice (2012) defines *intimate partner violence* as:

> A pattern of abusive behavior that is used by an intimate partner to gain or maintain power and control over the other intimate partner. [Intimate partner] violence can be physical, sexual, emotional, economic, or psychological actions or threats of actions that influence another person. This includes any behaviors that intimidate, manipulate, humiliate, isolate, frighten, terrorize, coerce, threaten, blame, hurt, injure, or wound someone.

Physical abuse between domestic partners may be known as spouse abuse, domestic or family violence, wife or husband battering, or intimate partner violence (IPV). Data from the U.S. Bureau of Justice Statistics (2012) reflect the following: (1) 82 percent of victims of intimate violence were women, (2) women ages 25 to 34 experienced the highest per capita rates of intimate violence, and (3) intimate partners committed 2 percent of the nonfatal violence against men. Many of the victimizations are not reported to the police, and the main reason given for not reporting is that it was "considered a personal matter."

Profile of the Victim

Battered women represent all age, racial, religious, cultural, educational, and socioeconomic groups.

They may be married or single, housewives or business executives. Many women who are battered have low self-esteem, commonly adhere to feminine sex-role stereotypes, and often accept the blame for the batterer's actions. Feelings of guilt, anger, fear, and shame are common. They may be isolated from family and support systems.

Some women who are in violent relationships grew up in abusive homes and may have left those homes, even gotten married, at a very young age in order to escape the abuse. The battered woman views her relationship as male dominant, and as the battering continues, her ability to see the options available to her and to make decisions concerning her life (and possibly those of her children) decreases. The phenomenon of *learned helplessness* may be applied to the woman's progressing inability to act on her own behalf. Learned helplessness occurs when an individual comes to understand that regardless of his or her behavior, the outcome is unpredictable and usually undesirable.

Profile of the Victimizer

Men who batter usually are characterized as persons with low self-esteem. Pathologically jealous, they present a "dual personality," one to the partner and one to the rest of the world (Meskill & Conner, 2010). They are often under a great deal of stress, but have limited ability to cope with the stress. The typical abuser is very possessive and perceives his spouse as a possession. He becomes threatened when she shows any sign of independence or attempts to share herself and her time with others. Small children are often ignored by the abuser; however, they may also become the targets of abuse as they grow older, particularly if they attempt to protect their mother from abuse. The abuser also may use threats of taking the children away as a tactic of emotional abuse.

The abusing man typically wages a continuous campaign of degradation against his female partner. He insults and humiliates her and everything she does at every opportunity. He strives to keep her isolated from others and totally dependent on him. He demands to know where she is at every moment, and when she tells him he challenges her honesty. He achieves power and control through intimidation.

The Cycle of Battering

In her classic studies of battered women and their relationships, Walker (1979) identified a cycle of predictable behaviors that are repeated over time. The behaviors can be divided into three distinct phases that vary in time and intensity both within the same relationship and among different couples. Figure 35-2 depicts a graphic representation of the **cycle of battering.**

Phase I: The Tension-Building Phase During this phase, the woman senses that the man's tolerance for frustration is declining. He becomes angry with little

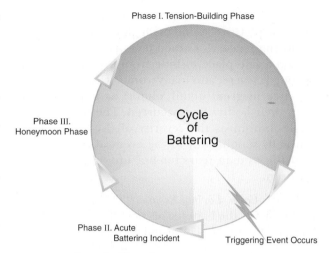

FIGURE 35-2   The cycle of battering.

provocation but, after lashing out at her, may be quick to apologize. The woman may become very nurturing and compliant, anticipating his every whim in an effort to prevent his anger from escalating. She may just try to stay out of his way.

Minor battering incidents may occur during this phase, and in a desperate effort to avoid more serious confrontations, the woman accepts the abuse as legitimately directed toward her. She denies her anger and rationalizes his behavior (e.g., "I need to do better"; "He's under so much stress at work"; "It's the alcohol. If only he didn't drink"). She assumes the guilt for the abuse, even reasoning that perhaps she *did* deserve the abuse, just as her aggressor suggests.

The minor battering incidents continue, and the tension mounts as the woman waits for the impending explosion. The abuser begins to fear that his partner will leave him. His jealousy and possessiveness increase, and he uses threats and brutality to keep her in his captivity. Battering incidents become more intense, after which the woman becomes less and less psychologically capable of restoring equilibrium. She withdraws from him, which he misinterprets as rejection, further escalating his anger toward her. Phase I may last from a few weeks to many months or even years.

Phase II: The Acute Battering Incident This phase is the most violent and the shortest, usually lasting up to 24 hours. It most often begins with the batterer justifying his behavior to himself. By the end of the incident, however, he cannot understand what has happened, only that in his rage he has lost control over his behavior.

This incident may begin with the batterer wanting to "just teach her a lesson." In some instances, the woman may intentionally provoke the behavior. Having come to a point in phase I in which the tension is unbearable, long-term battered women know that once the acute phase is behind them, things will be better.

During phase II, women feel their only option is to find a safe place to hide from the batterer. The beating is severe, and many women can describe the violence in great detail, almost as if dissociation from their bodies had occurred. The batterer generally minimizes the severity of the abuse. Help is usually sought only in the event of severe injury or if the woman fears for her life or those of her children.

Phase III: Calm, Loving, Respite ("Honeymoon") Phase
In this phase, the batterer becomes extremely loving, kind, and contrite. He promises that the abuse will never recur and begs her forgiveness. He is afraid she will leave him and uses every bit of charm he can muster to ensure this does not happen. He believes he now can control his behavior, and because now that he has "taught her a lesson," he believes she will not "act up" again.

He plays on her feelings of guilt, and she desperately wants to believe him. She wants to believe that he *can* change, and that she will no longer have to suffer abuse. During this phase the woman relives her original dream of ideal love and chooses to believe that *this* is what her partner is *really* like.

This loving phase becomes the focus of the woman's perception of the relationship. She bases her reason for remaining in the relationship on this "magical" ideal phase and hopes against hope that the previous phases will not be repeated. This hope is evident even in those women who have lived through a number of horrendous cycles.

Although phase III usually lasts somewhere between the lengths of time associated with phases I and II, it can be so short as to almost pass undetected. In most instances, the cycle soon begins again with renewed tensions and minor battering incidents. In an effort to "steal" a few precious moments of the phase III kind of loving, the battered woman becomes a collaborator in her own abusive lifestyle. Victim and batterer become locked together in an intense, symbiotic relationship.

Why Does She Stay?

Probably the most common response that battered women give for staying is that they fear for their life and/or the lives of their children. As the battering progresses, the man gains power and control through intimidation and instilling fear with threats such as, "I'll kill you and the kids if you try to leave." Challenged by these threats, and compounded by her low self-esteem and sense of powerlessness, the woman sees no way out. In fact, she may try to leave only to return when confronted by her partner and the psychological power he holds over her.

Women have been known to stay in an abusive relationship for many reasons, some of which include the following (Crisis Intervention Center, 2013; Meskill & Conner, 2010; Mouradian, 2004):

- **Fear of retaliation:** Her partner may have told her that if she leaves he will find her and kill her and the children.
- **For the children:** She may fear losing custody of the children if she leaves.
- **For financial reasons:** She may have no financial resources, access to the resources, or job skills.
- **Lack of a support network:** She may be under pressure from family members to stay in the marriage and try to work things out.
- **Religious reasons:** She may have religious convictions against divorce, believing that she must save the marriage at all costs.
- **Hopefulness:** She remembers good times and love in the relationship and has hope that her partner will change his behavior and they can have good times again.

Child Abuse

Erik Erikson (1963) stated, "The worst sin is the mutilation of a child's spirit." Children are vulnerable and relatively powerless, and the effects of maltreatment are infinitely deep and long lasting. Child maltreatment typically includes physical or emotional injury, physical or emotional neglect, or sexual acts inflicted upon a child by a caregiver. The Child Abuse Prevention and Treatment Act (CAPTA), as amended and reauthorized in 2003, identifies a minimum set of acts or behaviors that characterize maltreatment (Child Welfare Information Gateway [CWIG], 2013). States may use these as foundations on which to establish state legislation.

Physical Abuse

Physical abuse of a child includes "any nonaccidental physical injury (ranging from minor bruises to severe fractures or death) as a result of punching, beating, kicking, biting, shaking, throwing, stabbing, choking, hitting (with a hand, stick, strap, or other object), burning, or any other method that is inflicted by a parent, caregiver, or other person who has responsibility for the child" (American Psychiatric Association [APA], 2013, p. 717). Maltreatment is considered whether or not the caretaker intended to cause harm, or even if the injury resulted from over-discipline or physical punishment. The most obvious way to detect it is by outward physical signs. However, behavioral indicators also may be evident.

Signs of Physical Abuse Indicators of physical abuse may include any of the following (CWIG, 2013). The child:

- Has unexplained burns, bites, bruises, broken bones, or black eyes.
- Has fading bruises or other marks noticeable after an absence from school.

■ Seems frightened of the parents and protests or cries when it is time to go home.

■ Shrinks at the approach of adults.

■ Reports injury by a parent or another adult caregiver.

■ Abuses animals or pets.

Physical abuse may be suspected when the parent or other adult caregiver (CWIG, 2013):

■ Offers conflicting, unconvincing, or no explanation for the child's injury.

■ Describes the child as "evil," or in some other very negative way.

■ Uses harsh physical discipline with the child.

■ Has a history of abuse as a child.

■ Has a history of abusing animals or pets.

Emotional Abuse

Emotional abuse involves a pattern of behavior on the part of the parent or caretaker that results in serious impairment of the child's social, emotional, or intellectual functioning. Examples of emotional injury include belittling or rejecting the child, ignoring the child, blaming the child for things over which he or she has no control, isolating the child from normal social experiences, and using harsh and inconsistent discipline. Behavioral indicators of emotional injury may include (CWIG, 2013):

■ Shows extremes in behavior, such as overly compliant or demanding behavior, extreme passivity, or aggression

■ Is either inappropriately adult (e.g., parenting other children) or inappropriately infantile (e.g., frequently rocking or head-banging)

■ Is delayed in physical or emotional development

■ Has attempted suicide

■ Reports a lack of attachment to the parent

Emotional abuse may be suspected when the parent or other adult caregiver (CWIG, 2013):

■ Constantly blames, belittles, or berates the child.

■ Is unconcerned about the child and refuses to consider offers of help for the child's problems.

■ Overtly rejects the child.

Physical and Emotional Neglect

> ## CORE CONCEPT
>
> **Neglect**
>
> *Physical neglect* of a child includes refusal of or delay in seeking health care, abandonment, expulsion from the home or refusal to allow a runaway to return home, and inadequate supervision.
>
> *Emotional neglect* refers to a chronic failure by the parent or caretaker to provide the child with the hope, love, and support necessary for the development of a sound, healthy personality.

Indicators of Neglect The possibility of neglect may be considered when the child (CWIG, 2013):

■ Is frequently absent from school.

■ Begs or steals food or money.

IMPLICATIONS OF RESEARCH FOR EVIDENCE-BASED PRACTICE

Sachs, B., Hall, L.A., Lutenbacher, M., and Rayens, M.K. (1999). Potential for abusive parenting by rural mothers with low-birth-weight children. *Image: Journal of Nursing Scholarship, 31*(1), 21-25.

DESCRIPTION OF THE STUDY: The purpose of this study was to describe factors influencing the potential for abusive parenting by rural mothers of low-birth-weight (LBW) children. The convenience sample in this study included 48 mothers of LBW children, ranging in age from 18 to 39 years, all living in a rural area of the state, and all living with their LBW infant at the time of the study. Average length of the children's hospitalization after birth was 6 weeks, and the average age at time of the study was 9 months. In-home interviews were conducted using structured questionnaires to assess the mothers' everyday stressors, depressive symptoms, functional social support, quality of family relationships, and child abuse potential.

RESULTS OF THE STUDY: According to the questionnaires used for measurement, 54 percent of the mothers indicated a high level of depressive symptoms and 63 percent indicated a high potential for physical child abuse. No significant differences were noted in depressive symptoms

and potential for child abuse by birth weight, health status of the child, or time since hospital discharge. Mothers with high child abuse potential reported more everyday stressors and depressive symptoms, less functional social support, and poorer family functioning. Because in this study everyday stressors and the two social support systems (functional social support and quality of family relationships) were examined as predictors of depressive symptoms, it is suggested that everyday stressors exert both a direct and an indirect effect on mothers' potential for child abuse. The strongest predictor of child abuse potential was mothers' depressive symptoms.

IMPLICATIONS FOR NURSING PRACTICE: The researchers conclude that rural mothers of LBW children are at risk for abusive parenting. This study demonstrated the adverse effects of everyday stressors, minimal social resources, and depressive symptoms on mothers' potential for abusive parenting. Nurses should provide attention to the mental health of mothers living in isolated, rural areas. Information should be made available to these mothers regarding community resources that offer social support and child-care assistance. Nurses could establish and conduct educational programs to improve parenting skills and promote more positive child health outcomes.

■ Lacks needed medical or dental care, immunizations, or glasses.
■ Is consistently dirty and has severe body odor.
■ Lacks sufficient clothing for the weather.
■ Abuses alcohol or other drugs.
■ States that there is no one at home to provide care.

The possibility of neglect may be considered when the parent or other adult caregiver (CWIG, 2013):

■ Appears to be indifferent to the child.
■ Seems apathetic or depressed.
■ Behaves irrationally or in a bizarre manner.
■ Is abusing alcohol or other drugs.

Sexual Abuse of a Child

Various definitions of **child sexual abuse** are available in the literature. CAPTA defines *sexual abuse* as:

> Employment, use, persuasion, inducement, enticement, or coercion of any child to engage in, or assist any other person to engage in, any sexually explicit conduct or simulation of such conduct for the purpose of producing any visual depiction of such conduct; or the rape, and in cases of caretaker or inter-familial relationships, statutory rape, molestation, prostitution, or other form of sexual exploitation of children, or incest with children. (CWIG, 2013)

Included in the definition is **sexual exploitation of a child**, in which a child is induced or coerced into engaging in sexually explicit conduct for the purpose of promoting any performance, and child sexual abuse, in which a child is being used for the sexual pleasure of an adult (parent or caretaker) or any other person.

CORE CONCEPT

Incest

The occurrence of sexual contacts or interaction between, or sexual exploitation of, close relatives, or between participants who are related to each other by a kinship bond that is regarded as a prohibition to sexual relations (e.g., caretakers, stepparents, stepsiblings) (Sadock & Sadock, 2007).

Indicators of Sexual Abuse Child abuse may be considered a possibility when the child (CWIG, 2013):

■ Has difficulty walking or sitting.
■ Suddenly refuses to change for gym or to participate in physical activities.
■ Reports nightmares or bedwetting.
■ Experiences a sudden change in appetite.
■ Demonstrates bizarre, sophisticated, or unusual sexual knowledge or behavior.

■ Becomes pregnant or contracts a venereal disease, particularly if under age 14.
■ Runs away.
■ Reports sexual abuse by a parent or another adult caregiver.

Sexual abuse may be considered a possibility when the parent or other adult caregiver (CWIG, 2013):

■ Is unduly protective of the child or severely limits the child's contact with other children, especially of the opposite sex.
■ Is secretive and isolated.
■ Is jealous or controlling with family members.

Characteristics of the Abuser

A number of factors have been associated with adults who abuse or neglect their children. Sadock & Sadock (2007) report that 90 percent of parents who abuse their children were severely physically abused by their own mothers or fathers. Murray, Zentner, and Yakimo (2009) identify the following as additional characteristics that may be associated with abusive parents:

■ Experiencing a stressful life situation (e.g., unemployment; poverty)
■ Having few, if any, support systems; commonly isolated from others
■ Lacking understanding of child development or care needs
■ Lacking adaptive coping strategies; angers easily; has difficulty trusting others
■ Expecting the child to be perfect; may exaggerate any mild difference the child manifests from the "usual"

Flaherty and Stirling (2010) identify a number of factors that place a child at risk for maltreatment. They cite certain characteristics of the child, the parent, and the environment. These characteristics are presented in Box 35-1. When multiple factors coexist, the risk of child abuse increases.

The Incestuous Relationship

A great deal of attention has been given to the study of father-daughter incest. In these cases there is usually an impaired sexual relationship between the parents. Communication between the parents is ineffective, which prevents them from correcting their problems. Typically, the father is domineering, impulsive, and physically abusing; whereas the mother is passive and submissive, and denigrates her role as wife and mother. She is often aware of, or at least strongly suspects, the incestuous behavior between the father and daughter but may believe in or fear her husband's absolute authority over the family. She may deny that her daughter is being harmed and may actually be grateful that her husband's sexual demands are being met by someone other than herself.

Onset of the incestuous relationship typically occurs when the daughter is 8 to 10 years of age and

BOX 35-1 **Factors and Characteristics That Place a Child at Risk for Maltreatment**		
CHILD	**PARENT**	**ENVIRONMENT (COMMUNITY AND SOCIETY)**
Emotional/behavioral difficulties	Low self-esteem	Social isolation
Chronic illness	Poor impulse control	Poverty
Physical disabilities	Substance abuse/alcohol abuse	Unemployment
Developmental disabilities	Young maternal or paternal age	Low educational achievement
Preterm birth	Abused as a child	Single-parent home
Unwanted	Depression or other mental illness	Non-biologically related male
Unplanned	Poor knowledge of child development or unrealistic expectations of the child	living in the home
	Negative perception of normal child behavior	Family or intimate partner violence

SOURCE: Flaherty, E.G., & Stirling, J., et al. (2010). *Clinical report—The pediatrician's role in child maltreatment prevention.* Pediatrics, 126(4), 833-841. Reprinted with permission.

commonly begins with genital touching and fondling. In the beginning, the child may accept the sexual advances from her father as signs of affection. As the incestuous behavior continues and progresses, the daughter usually becomes more bewildered, confused, and frightened, never knowing whether her father will be paternal or sexual in his interactions with her.

The relationship may become a love-hate situation on the part of the daughter. She continues to strive for the ideal father-daughter relationship but is fearful and hateful of the sexual demands he places on her. The mother may be alternately caring and competitive as she witnesses her husband's possessiveness and affections directed toward her daughter. Out of fear that his daughter may expose their relationship, the father may attempt to interfere with her normal peer relationships (Sadock & Sadock, 2007).

It has been suggested that some fathers who participate in incestuous relationships may have unconscious homosexual tendencies and have difficulty achieving a stable heterosexual orientation. On the other hand, some men have frequent sex with their wives and several of their own children but are unwilling to seek sexual partners outside the nuclear family because of a need to maintain the public facade of a stable and competent patriarch. Although the oldest daughter in a family is most vulnerable to becoming a participant in father-daughter incest, some fathers form sequential relationships with several daughters. If incest has been reported with one daughter, it should be suspected with all of the other daughters (Murray et al., 2009).

The Adult Survivor of Incest

Several common characteristics have been identified in adults who have experienced incest as children. Basic to these characteristics is a fundamental lack of trust resulting from an unsatisfactory parent-child relationship, which causes low self-esteem and a poor sense of identity. Children of incest often feel trapped, for they have been admonished not to talk about the experience and may be afraid, or even fear for their lives, if they are exposed. If they do muster the courage to report the incest, particularly to the mother, they sometimes are not believed. This is confusing to the child, who is then left with a sense of self-doubt and the inability to trust his or her own feelings. The child develops feelings of guilt with the realization over the years that the parents are using him or her in an attempt to solve their own problems.

Childhood sexual abuse commonly distorts the development of a normal association of pleasure with sexual activity (Reeves, 2003). Peer relationships are often delayed, altered, inhibited, or perverted. In some instances, individuals who were sexually abused as children completely retreat from sexual activity and avoid all close interpersonal relationships throughout life. Other adult manifestations of childhood sexual abuse in women include diminished libido, pain/penetration disorder, nymphomania, and promiscuity. In male survivors of childhood sexual abuse, erectile disorder, premature ejaculation, exhibitionistic disorder, and compulsive sexual conquests may occur. Lerner (2005) suggested that adult survivors of incest are at risk for experiencing symptoms of posttraumatic stress disorder, sexual dysfunction, somatic symptom disorders, compulsive sexual behaviors, depression, anxiety, eating disorders, substance disorders, and intolerance of or constant search for intimacy.

The conflicts associated with pain (either physical or emotional) and sexual pleasure experienced by children who are sexually abused are commonly manifested symbolically in adult relationships. Women who were abused as children commonly enter into relationships with men who abuse them physically, sexually, or emotionally (Bensley, VanEenwyk, & Wynkoop, 2003).

Adult survivors of incest who decide to come forward with their stories usually are estranged from nuclear family members. They are blamed by family members for disclosing the "family secret" and often accused of overreacting to the incest. Frequently the estrangement becomes permanent when family members continue to deny the behavior and the individual is accused of lying. In recent years, a number of celebrities have come forward with stories of their childhood sexual abuse. Some have chosen to make the disclosure only after the death of their parents. Revelation of these past activities can be one way of contributing to the healing process for which incest survivors so desperately strive.

Sexual Assault

> ### CORE CONCEPT
> **Rape**
> The expression of power and dominance by means of sexual violence, most commonly by men over women, although men may also be rape victims.

Sexual assault is viewed as any type of sexual act in which an individual is threatened or coerced, or forced to submit against his or her will. Rape, a type of sexual assault, occurs over a broad spectrum of experiences ranging from the surprise attack by a stranger to insistence on sexual intercourse by an acquaintance or spouse. Regardless of the defining source, one common theme always emerges: Rape is an act of aggression, not one of passion.

Acquaintance rape (called **date rape** if the encounter is a social engagement agreed to by the victim) is a term applied to situations in which the rapist is acquainted with the victim. They may be out on a first date, may have been dating for a number of months, or merely may be acquaintances or schoolmates. College campuses are the location for a staggering number of these types of rapes, a great many of which go unreported. An increasing number of colleges and universities are establishing programs for rape prevention and counseling for survivors of rape.

Marital rape, which has been recognized only in recent years as a legal category, is the case in which a spouse may be held liable for sexual abuse directed at a marital partner against that person's will. Historically, with societal acceptance of the concept of women as marital property, the legal definition of rape held an exemption within the marriage relationship. In 1993, marital rape became a crime in all 50 states, under at least one section of the sexual offenses code. In 17 states and the District of Columbia, there are no exemptions from rape prosecution granted to husbands. However, in 33 states, there are still some exemptions given to husbands from rape prosecution.

Statutory rape is defined as unlawful intercourse between a person who is over the age of consent and a person who is under the age of consent. The legal age of consent varies from state to state, ranging from age 14 to 18 (King, 2012). An adult who has intercourse with a person who is under the age of consent can be arrested for statutory rape, although the interaction may have occurred between consenting individuals.

Profile of the Victimizer

Older profiles of the individual who rapes were described by Abrahamsen (1960) and Macdonald (1971), who identified the rapist's childhood as "mother-dominated" and the mother as "seductive but rejecting." The behavior of the mother toward the son was described as overbearing, with seductive undertones. Mother and son shared little secrets, and she rescued him when his delinquent acts created problems with others. However, she was quick to withdraw her love and attention when he went against her wishes, a rejection that was powerful and unyielding. She was domineering and possessive of the son, a dominance that often continued into his adult life. Macdonald (1971) stated:

> The seductive mother arouses overwhelming anxiety in her son with great anger, which may be expressed directly toward her but more often is displaced onto other women. When this seductive behavior is combined with parental encouragement of assaultive behavior, the setting is provided for personality development in the child which may result in sadistic, homicidal sexual attacks on women in adolescence or adult life.

Many rapists report growing up in abusive homes (McCormack, 2002). Even when the parental brutality is discharged by the father, the anger may be directed toward the mother who did not protect her child from physical assault. More recent feminist theories suggest that the rapist displaces this anger on the rape victim because he cannot directly express it toward other men (Sadock & Sadock, 2007). Another feminist view suggests that rape is most common in societies that encourage aggressiveness in males, that have distinct gender roles, and in which men regard women's roles as inferior (King, 2012).

Statistics show that the greatest number of rapists are between the ages of 25 and 44. Of rapists, 54 percent are white, 32 percent are African-American, and the remainder are of other races, mixed race, or of unknown race (U.S. Bureau of Justice Statistics, 2011). Many are either married or cohabiting at the time of their offenses. For those with previous criminal activity, the majority of their convictions are for crimes against property rather than against people. Most rapists do not have histories of mental illness.

The Victim

Rape can occur at any age; however, the most recent statistics suggest that the highest-risk age group is 16 to 34 years (U.S. Bureau of Justice Statistics, 2011).

Most sexual assault victims are single women, and the attack frequently occurs in or close to the victim's own neighborhood.

Scully (1994), in a study of a prison sample of rapists, found that in "stranger rapes," victims were not chosen for any reason having to do with appearance or behavior, but simply because the individual happened to be in a certain place at a certain time. Scully stated:

> The most striking and consistent factor in all the stranger rapes, whether committed by a lone assailant or a group, is the unfortunate fact that the victim was "just there" in a location unlikely to draw the attention of a passerby. Almost every one of these men said exactly the same thing, "It could have been any woman," and a few added that because it was dark, they could not even see what their victim looked like very well. (p. 175)

In her study, Scully found that 62 percent of the rapists used a weapon, most frequently a knife. Most suggested that they used the weapon to terrorize and subdue the victim but not to inflict serious injury. The presence of a weapon (real or perceived) appears to be the principal measure of the degree to which a woman resists her attacker.

Rape survivors who present themselves for care shortly after the crime has occurred likely may be experiencing an overwhelming sense of violation and helplessness that began with the powerlessness and intimidation experienced during the rape. Burgess (2010) identified two emotional patterns of response that may occur within hours after a rape and with which health-care workers may be confronted in the emergency department or rape crisis center. In the **expressed response pattern**, the survivor expresses feelings of fear, anger, and anxiety through such behaviors as crying, sobbing, restlessness, and tension. In the **controlled response pattern**, the feelings are masked or hidden, and a calm, composed, or subdued affect is seen.

The following manifestations may be evident in the days and weeks after the attack (Burgess, 2010):

- Contusions and abrasions about various parts of the body
- Headaches, fatigue, sleep pattern disturbances
- Stomach pains, nausea and vomiting
- Vaginal discharge and itching, burning upon urination, rectal bleeding and pain
- Rage, humiliation, embarrassment, desire for revenge, and self-blame
- Fear of physical violence and death

The long-term effects of sexual assault depend largely on the individual's ego strength, social support system, and the way he or she was treated as a victim (Burgess, 2010). Various long-term effects include increased restlessness, dreams and nightmares, and phobias (particularly those having to do with sexual interaction). Some women report that it takes years to get over the experience; they describe a sense of vulnerability and a loss of control over their own lives during this period. They feel defiled and unable to wash themselves clean, and some women are unable to remain living alone in their home or apartment.

Some survivors develop a **compounded rape reaction**, in which additional symptoms such as depression and suicide, substance abuse, and even psychotic behaviors may be noted (Burgess, 2010). Another variation has been called the **silent rape reaction**, in which the survivor tells no one about the assault. Anxiety is suppressed and the emotional burden may become overwhelming. The unresolved sexual trauma may not be revealed until the woman is forced to face another sexual crisis in her life that reactivates the previously unresolved feelings.

Diagnosis/Outcome Identification

Nursing diagnoses are formulated from the data gathered during the assessment phase and with background knowledge regarding predisposing factors to the situation. Some common nursing diagnoses for survivors of abuse include:

- Rape-trauma syndrome related to sexual assault evidenced by verbalizations of the attack; bruises and lacerations over areas of body; severe anxiety.
- Powerlessness related to cycle of battering evidenced by verbalizations of abuse; bruises and lacerations over areas of body; fear for her safety and that of her children; verbalizations of no way to get out of the relationship.
- Risk for delayed development related to abusive family situation.

Outcome Criteria

The following criteria may be used to measure outcomes in the care of abuse survivors:

The client who has been sexually assaulted:

- Is no longer experiencing panic anxiety.
- Demonstrates a degree of trust in the primary nurse.
- Has received immediate attention to physical injuries.
- Has initiated behaviors consistent with the grief response.

The client who has been physically battered:

- Has received immediate attention to physical injuries.
- Verbalizes assurance of his or her immediate safety.
- Discusses life situation with primary nurse.
- Can verbalize choices from which he or she may receive assistance.

The child who has been abused:

- Has received immediate attention to physical injuries.
- Demonstrates trust in primary nurse by discussing abuse through the use of play therapy.
- Is demonstrating a decrease in regressive behaviors.

Planning/Implementation

Table 35-1 provides a plan of care for the client who is a survivor of abuse. Nursing diagnoses are presented, along with outcome criteria, appropriate nursing interventions, and rationales for each.

Concept Care Mapping

The concept map care plan is an innovative approach to planning and organizing nursing care (see Chapter 9). It is a diagrammatic teaching and learning strategy that allows visualization of interrelationships between medical diagnoses, nursing diagnoses, assessment data, and treatments. An example of a concept map care plan for a client who is a survivor of abuse is presented in Figure 35-3.

Evaluation

Evaluation of nursing actions to assist survivors of abuse must be considered on both a short- and a long-term basis.

Short-term evaluation may be facilitated by gathering information using the following types of questions:

■ Has the individual been reassured of his or her safety?

Table 35-1 | CARE PLAN FOR SURVIVORS OF ABUSE

NURSING DIAGNOSIS: RAPE-TRAUMA SYNDROME
RELATED TO: Sexual assault
EVIDENCED BY: Verbalizations of the attack; bruises and lacerations over areas of body; severe anxiety

OUTCOME CRITERIA	NURSING INTERVENTIONS	RATIONALE
Short-Term Goal • Client's physical wounds will heal without complication. **Long-Term Goal** • Client will begin a healthy grief resolution, initiating the process of physical and psychological healing (time to be individually determined).	1. It is important to communicate the following to the individual who has been sexually assaulted: • You are safe here. • I'm sorry that it happened. • I'm glad you survived. • It's not your fault. No one deserves to be treated this way. • You did the best that you could.	1. The woman who has been sexually assaulted fears for her life and must be reassured of her safety. She may also be overwhelmed with self-doubt and self-blame, and these statements instill trust and validate self-worth.
	2. Explain every assessment procedure that will be conducted and why it is being conducted. Ensure that data collection is conducted in a caring, nonjudgmental manner.	2. This may serve to decrease fear/anxiety and increase trust.
	3. Ensure that the client has adequate privacy for all immediate post-crisis interventions. Try to have as few people as possible providing the immediate care or collecting immediate evidence.	3. The post-trauma client is extremely vulnerable. Additional people in the environment increase this feeling of vulnerability and serve to escalate anxiety.
	4. Encourage the client to give an account of the assault. Listen, but do not probe.	4. Nonjudgmental listening provides an avenue for catharsis that the client needs to begin healing. A detailed account may be required for legal follow-up, and a caring nurse, as client advocate, may help to lessen the trauma of evidence collection.
	5. Discuss with the client whom to call for support or assistance. Provide information about referrals for aftercare.	5. Because of severe anxiety and fear, the client may need assistance from others during this immediate post-crisis period. Provide referral information in writing for later reference (e.g., psychotherapist, mental health clinic, community advocacy group).

Table 35-1 | CARE PLAN FOR SURVIVORS OF ABUSE—cont'd

NURSING DIAGNOSIS: POWERLESSNESS
RELATED TO: Cycle of battering
EVIDENCED BY: Verbalizations of abuse; bruises and lacerations over areas of body; fear for own safety and that of children; verbalizations of no way to get out of the relationship

OUTCOME CRITERIA	NURSING INTERVENTIONS	RATIONALE
Short-Term Goal • Client will recognize and verbalize choices available, thereby perceiving some control over life situation. **Long-Term Goal** • Client will exhibit control over life situation by making decision about what to do regarding living with cycle of abuse.	1. In collaboration with physician, ensure that all physical wounds, fractures, and burns receive immediate attention. Take photographs if the individual will permit. 2. Take the client to a private area to do the interview. 3. If she has come alone or with her children, assure her of her safety. Encourage her to discuss the battering incident. Ask questions about whether this has happened before, whether the abuser takes drugs, whether the woman has a safe place to go, and whether she is interested in pressing charges. 4. Ensure that "rescue" efforts are not attempted by the nurse. Offer support, but remember that the final decision must be made by the client. 5. Stress to the individual the importance of safety. She must be made aware of the variety of resources that are available to her. These may include crisis hotlines, community groups for women who have been abused, shelters, counseling services, and information regarding the victim's rights in the civil and criminal justice system. Following a discussion of these available resources, the woman may choose for herself. If her decision is to return to the marriage and home, this choice also must be respected.	1. Client safety is a nursing priority. Photographs may be called in as evidence if charges are filed. 2. If the client is accompanied by the person who did the battering, she is not likely to be truthful about the injuries. 3. Some women will attempt to keep secret how their injuries occurred in an effort to protect the partner or because they are fearful that the partner will kill them if they tell. 4. Making her own decision will give the client a sense of control over her life situation. Imposing judgments and giving advice are nontherapeutic. 5. Knowledge of available choices decreases the individual's sense of powerlessness, but true empowerment comes only when she chooses to use that knowledge for her own benefit.

Continued

Table 35-1 | CARE PLAN FOR SURVIVORS OF ABUSE—cont'd

NURSING DIAGNOSIS: RISK FOR DELAYED DEVELOPMENT
RELATED TO: Abusive family situation

OUTCOME CRITERIA	NURSING INTERVENTIONS	RATIONALE
Short-Term Goal • Client will develop trusting relationship with nurse and report how evident injuries were sustained. **Long-Term Goal** • Client will demonstrate behaviors consistent with age-appropriate growth and development.	1. Perform complete physical assessment of the child. Take particular note of bruises (in various stages of healing), lacerations, and client complaints of pain in specific areas. Do not overlook or discount the possibility of sexual abuse. Assess for nonverbal signs of abuse: aggressive conduct, excessive fears, extreme hyperactivity, apathy, withdrawal, age-inappropriate behaviors.	1. An accurate and thorough physical assessment is required to provide appropriate care for the client.
	2. Conduct an in-depth interview with the parent or adult who accompanies the child. Consider: If the injury is being reported as an accident, is the explanation reasonable? Is the injury consistent with the explanation? Is the injury consistent with the child's developmental capabilities?	2. Fear of imprisonment or loss of child custody may place the abusive parent on the defensive. Discrepancies may be evident in the description of the incident, and lying to cover up involvement is a common defense that may be detectable in an in-depth interview.
	3. Use games or play therapy to gain child's trust. Use these techniques to assist in describing his or her side of the story.	3. Establishing a trusting relationship with an abused child is extremely difficult. He or she may not even want to be touched. These types of play activities can provide a nonthreatening environment that may enhance the child's attempt to discuss these painful issues.
	4. Determine whether the nature of the injuries warrants reporting to authorities. Specific state statutes must enter into the decision of whether to report suspected child abuse. Individual state statutes regarding what constitutes child abuse and neglect may be found at http://www.childwelfare.gov/systemwide/laws_policies/state/	4. A report is commonly made if there is reason to suspect that a child has been injured as a result of physical, mental, emotional, or sexual abuse. "Reason to suspect" exists when there is evidence of a discrepancy or inconsistency in explaining a child's injury. Most states require that the following individuals report cases of suspected child abuse: all health-care workers, all mental health therapists, teachers, child-care providers, firefighters, emergency medical personnel, and law enforcement personnel. Reports are made to the Department of Health and Human Services or a law enforcement agency.

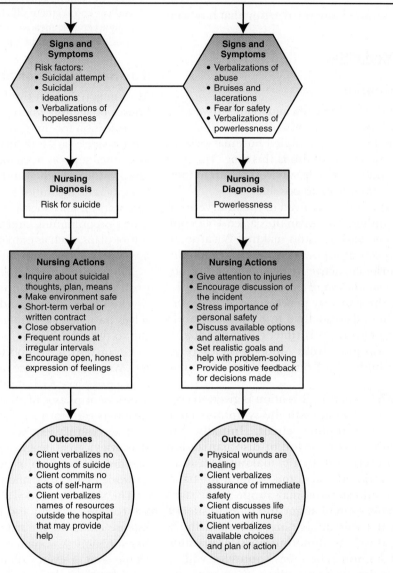

Clinical Vignette: Annette and Charles, both 21, have been dating for two years. Charles has always been jealous and gets very angry when Annette even talks to another man. He has hit her several times, hard enough to produce bruises, but never on her face, and she is able to hide the abuse from others. Tonight at a party, Annette danced with another man, and Charles became violent. He punched the man in the face and dragged Annette out to the parking lot. She yelled at him, "This is it! We are through! I don't ever want to see you again!" He started beating her around the face and upper body, and yelled, "You can't break up with me! I won't allow it! You belong to me, and no one else!" He left her lying in the parking lot. She felt powerless, and, in her despondency, opened her purse and swallowed half a bottle of acetaminophen. When she told her girlfriend, Dana, what had happened, Dana called 911, and Annette was taken to the hospital. She was treated for the overdose, and her wounds were cleaned and dressed. Following physical stability, she was transferred to the psychiatric unit. She tells the nurse, "I can't live like this. He won't let me go! I don't know what to do!" The nurse develops the following concept map care plan for Annette.

Signs and Symptoms

Risk factors:
• Suicidal attempt
• Suicidal ideations
• Verbalizations of hopelessness

Signs and Symptoms

• Verbalizations of abuse
• Bruises and lacerations
• Fear for safety
• Verbalizations of powerlessness

Nursing Diagnosis

Risk for suicide

Nursing Diagnosis

Powerlessness

Nursing Actions

• Inquire about suicidal thoughts, plan, means
• Make environment safe
• Short-term verbal or written contract
• Close observation
• Frequent rounds at irregular intervals
• Encourage open, honest expression of feelings

Nursing Actions

• Give attention to injuries
• Encourage discussion of the incident
• Stress importance of personal safety
• Discuss available options and alternatives
• Set realistic goals and help with problem-solving
• Provide positive feedback for decisions made

Outcomes

• Client verbalizes no thoughts of suicide
• Client commits no acts of self-harm
• Client verbalizes names of resources outside the hospital that may provide help

Outcomes

• Physical wounds are healing
• Client verbalizes assurance of immediate safety
• Client discusses life situation with nurse
• Client verbalizes available choices and plan of action

FIGURE 35-3 Concept map care plan for a client with physical abuse.

■ Is this evidenced by a decrease in panic anxiety?
■ Have wounds been properly cared for and provision made for follow-up care?
■ Have emotional needs been attended to?
■ Has trust been established with at least one person to whom the client feels comfortable relating the abusive incident?
■ Have available support systems been identified and notified?
■ Have options for immediate circumstances been presented?

Long-term evaluation may be conducted by healthcare workers who have contact with the individual long after the immediate crisis has passed.

■ Is the individual able to conduct activities of daily living satisfactorily?
■ Have physical wounds healed properly?
■ Is the client appropriately progressing through the behaviors of grieving?
■ Is the client free of sleep disturbances (nightmares, insomnia); psychosomatic symptoms (headaches, stomach pains, nausea/vomiting); regressive behaviors

(enuresis, thumb sucking, phobias); and psycho-sexual disturbances?
■ Is the individual free from problems with interpersonal relationships?
■ Has the individual considered the alternatives for change in his or her personal life?
■ Has a decision been made relative to the choices available?
■ Is he or she satisfied with the decision that has been made?

Treatment Modalities

Crisis Intervention

The focus of the initial interview and follow-up with the client who has been sexually assaulted is on the rape incident alone. Problems identified but unassociated with the rape are not dealt with at this time. The goal of crisis intervention is to help survivors return to their previous lifestyle as quickly as possible.

The client should be involved in the intervention from the beginning. This promotes a sense of competency, control, and decision making. Because an overwhelming sense of powerlessness accompanies the rape experience, active involvement by the survivor is both a validation of personal worth and the beginning of the recovery process. Crisis intervention is time limited—usually 6 to 8 weeks. If problems resurface beyond this time, the individual is referred for assistance from other agencies (e.g., long-term psychotherapy from a psychiatrist or mental health clinic).

During the crisis period, attention is given to coping strategies for dealing with the symptoms common to the post-trauma client. Initially the individual undergoes a period of disorganization during which there is difficulty making decisions, extreme or irrational fears, and general mistrust. Observable manifestations may range from stark hysteria, to expression of anger and rage, to silence and withdrawal. Guilt and feelings of responsibility for the rape, as well as numerous physical manifestations, are common. The crisis counselor will attempt to help the individual draw upon previous successful coping strategies to regain control over his or her life.

If the client is a victim of domestic violence, the counselor ensures that various resources and options are made known to the individual so that she may make a personal decision regarding what she wishes to do with her life. Support groups provide a valuable forum for reducing isolation and learning new strategies for coping with the aftermath of physical or sexual abuse. Particularly for the survivor of rape, the peer support group provides a therapeutic forum for reducing the sense of isolation she may feel in the aftermath of predictable social and interpersonal responses to her experience.

Sadock and Sadock (2007) state:

Few women emerge from the assault completely unscathed. The manifestations and the degree of damage depend on the violence of the attack itself, the vulnerability of the woman, and the support system available to her immediately after the attack. A rape victim fares best when she receives immediate support and can ventilate her fear and rage to loving family members, sympathetic physicians, and law enforcement officials. Knowing that she has socially acceptable means of recourse, such as the arrest and conviction of the rapist, can help a rape victim. (p. 884)

The Safe House or Shelter

Most major cities in the United States now have **safe houses or shelters** where women can go to be assured of protection for them and their children. These shelters provide a variety of services, and the women receive emotional support from staff and each other. Most shelters provide individual and group counseling; help with bureaucratic institutions such as the police, legal representation, and social services; child care and children's programming; and aid for the woman in making future plans, such as employment counseling and linkages with housing authorities.

The shelters are usually run by a combination of professional and volunteer staff, including nurses, psychologists, lawyers, and others. Women who themselves have been previously abused are often among the volunteer staff members.

Group work is an important part of the service of shelters. Women in residence range from those in the immediate crisis phase to those who have progressed through a variety of phases of the grief process. Those newer members can learn a great deal from the women who have successfully resolved similar problems. Length of stay varies a great deal from individual to individual, depending on a number of factors, such as outside support network, financial situation, and personal resources.

The shelter provides a haven of physical safety for the battered woman and promotes expression of the intense emotions she may be experiencing regarding her situation. A woman often exhibits depression, extreme fear, or even violent expressions of anger and rage. In the shelter, she learns that these feelings are normal and that others have also experienced these same emotions in similar situations. She is allowed to grieve for what has been lost and for what was expected but not achieved. Help is provided in overcoming the tremendous guilt associated with self-blame. This is a difficult step for someone who has accepted responsibility for another's behavior over a long period.

New arrivals at the shelter are given time to experience the relief from the safety and security provided. Making decisions is discouraged during the period of immediate crisis and disorganization. Once the woman's emotions have become more stable, planning for the future begins. Through information

IMPLICATIONS OF RESEARCH FOR EVIDENCE-BASED PRACTICE

Humphreys, J. (2000). Spirituality and distress in sheltered battered women. *Image: Journal of Nursing Scholarship, 32*(3), 273-278.

DESCRIPTION OF THE STUDY: The purpose of this study was to examine the relationship between spiritual beliefs and psychological distress in sheltered battered women. The convenience sample in this study included 50 women, ages ranging from 19 to 60, who had resided for at least 21 days in one of 4 battered women's shelters in the San Francisco Bay Area. Ethnicity included 20 African Americans, 11 European Americans, 11 Latino Americans, 5 Asian Americans, 1 Native American, and 2 other (mixed or not given). All had been abused by a husband or partner. Psychological distress was measured using the Symptom Checklist-90-Revised (SCL-90), a test that is scored and interpreted for 9 primary symptom dimensions: somatization, obsessive-compulsiveness, interpersonal sensitivity, depression, anxiety, hostility, phobic anxiety, paranoid ideation, and psychoticism. Spirituality was measured using the Spiritual Perspectives Scale (SPS), a 10-item scale that measures the extent to which one holds certain spiritual views and engages in spiritually related interactions. In the instructions, spirituality is referred to as "an awareness of one's inner self and a sense of connection to a higher being, nature, others, or to some purpose greater than oneself."

RESULTS OF THE STUDY: The women in this study suffered significant psychological distress that was highly correlated with the frequency and severity of battering they had experienced. However, participants who scored higher on the SPS experienced fewer and less intense symptoms in the obsessive-compulsive, interpersonal sensitivity, and hostility dimensions of the SCL-90. Eighty percent of the participants indicated a belief in God or a "higher power," and that their spirituality was a significant part of their lives. Some indicated that they strongly relied on their spiritual support for survival in their stressful life situation. Eighty-two percent reported that they thought forgiveness was an important part of their spirituality.

IMPLICATIONS FOR NURSING PRACTICE: The results of this study indicate that spirituality among battered women is a means of reducing psychological stress by a connection with powers beyond oneself. The author cited research studies, which concluded that "the role of nurses is not to solve the spiritual problems of clients but to provide an environment where spirituality can be expressed." Suggested nursing interventions include (1) spiritual assessment, (2) identification of resources that have been a source of spiritual support, (3) offering compassionate presence and support, (4) open and honest communication, (5) listening, (6) fostering caring relationships with significant other people in clients' lives, and (7) encouraging prayer and meditation. The author concludes, "Encouraging battered women to consider personal resources that have been helpful to them in the past, including their spiritual beliefs, may provide benefit to these women who face tremendous demands with limited external resource."

from staff and peers, she learns what resources are available to her within the community. Feedback is provided, but the woman makes her own decision about "where she wants to go from here." She is accepted and supported in whatever she chooses to do.

Family Therapy

The focus of therapy with families who use violence is to help them develop democratic ways of solving problems. Studies show that the more a family uses the democratic means of conflict resolution, the less likely they are to engage in physical violence. Families need to learn to deal with problems in ways that can produce mutual benefits for all concerned, rather than engaging in power struggles among family members.

Parents also need to learn more effective methods of disciplining children, aside from physical punishment. Time-out techniques and methods that emphasize the importance of positive reinforcement for acceptable behavior can be very effective. Family members must be committed to consistent use of this behavior modification technique for it to be successful.

Teaching parents about expectations for various developmental levels may alleviate some of the stress that accompanies these changes. Knowing what to expect from individuals at various stages of development may provide needed anticipatory guidance to deal with the crises commonly associated with these stages.

Therapy sessions with all family members together may focus on problems with family communication. Members are encouraged to express honest feelings in a manner that is nonthreatening to other family members. Active listening, assertiveness techniques, and respecting the rights of others are taught and encouraged. Barriers to effective communication are identified and resolved.

Referrals to agencies that promote effective parenting skills (e.g., parent effectiveness training) may be made. Alternative agencies that may relieve the stress of parenting (e.g., "Mom's Day Out" programs, sitter-sharing organizations, and day-care institutions) also may be considered. Support groups for abusive parents may also be helpful, and assistance in locating or initiating such a group may be provided.

Summary and Key Points

- Abuse is the maltreatment of one person by another.
- Intimate partner violence, child abuse, and sexual assault are widespread, and all populations are equally affected.

- Various factors have been theorized as influential in the predisposition to violent behavior. Physiological and biochemical influences within the brain have been suggested, as has the possibility of a direct genetic link.
- Organic brain syndromes associated with various cerebral disorders have been implicated in the predisposition to aggressive and violent behavior.
- Psychoanalytical theorists relate the predisposition to violent behavior to underdeveloped ego and a poor self-concept.
- Learning theorists suggest that children imitate the abusive behavior of their parents. This theory has been substantiated by studies that show that individuals who were abused as children or whose parents disciplined them with physical punishment are more likely to be abusive as adults.
- Societal influences, such as general acceptance of violence as a means of solving problems, also have been implicated.
- Women who are battered often take blame for their situation. They may have been reared in abusive families and have come to expect this type of behavior.
- Battered women commonly see no way out of their present situation and may be encouraged by their social support network to remain in the abusive relationship.

- Child abuse includes physical and emotional abuse, physical and emotional neglect, and sexual abuse of a child.
- A child may experience many years of abuse without reporting it because of fear of retaliation by the abuser.
- Some children report incest experiences to their mothers, only to be rebuffed by her and told to remain secretive about the abuse.
- Adult survivors of incest often experience a number of physical and emotional manifestations relating back to the incestuous relationship.
- Sexual assault is identified as an act of aggression, not passion.
- Many rapists report growing up in abusive homes, and some theorists relate the predisposition to rape to a "seductive, but rejecting, mother."
- Rape is a traumatic experience, and many women experience flashbacks, nightmares, rage, physical symptoms, depression, and thoughts of suicide for many years after the occurrence.
- Treatment modalities for survivors of abuse include crisis intervention with the sexual assault victim, safe shelter for battered women, and therapy for families who use violence.

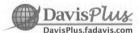 **DavisPlus** Additional info available at
DavisPlus.fadavis.com www.davisplus.com

Review Questions
Self-Examination/Learning Exercise

*Select the answer that is **most** appropriate for each of the following questions.*

1. Sharon, a woman with multiple cuts and abrasions, arrives at the emergency department (ED) with her three small children. She tells the nurse her husband inflicted these wounds on her. She says, "I didn't want to come. I'm really okay. He only does this when he has too much to drink. I just shouldn't have yelled at him." The best response by the nurse is:
   a. "How often does he drink too much?"
   b. "It is not your fault. You did the right thing by coming here."
   c. "How many times has he done this to you?"
   d. "He is not a good husband. You have to leave him before he kills you."

2. Sharon, a woman with multiple cuts and abrasions, arrives at the ED with her three small children. She tells the nurse her husband inflicted these wounds on her. In the interview, Sharon tells the nurse, "He's been getting more and more violent lately. He's been under a lot of stress at work the last few weeks, so he drinks a lot when he gets home. He always gets mean when he drinks. I was getting scared. So I just finally told him I was going to take the kids and leave. He got furious when I said that and began beating me with his fists." With knowledge about the cycle of battering, what does this situation represent?
   a. Phase I; Sharon was desperately trying to stay out of his way and keep everything calm.
   b. Phase I; a minor battering incident for which Sharon assumes all the blame.
   c. Phase II; the acute battering incident that Sharon provoked with her threat to leave.
   d. Phase III; the honeymoon phase where the husband believes that he has "taught her a lesson and she won't act up again."

Review Questions—cont'd
Self-Examination/Learning Exercise

3. A battered woman presents to the ED with multiple cuts and abrasions. Her right eye is swollen shut. She says that her husband did this to her. The *priority* nursing intervention is:
   a. Tending to the immediate care of her wounds
   b. Providing her with information about a safe place to stay
   c. Administering the prn tranquilizer ordered by the physician
   d. Explaining how she may go about bringing charges against her husband

4. A woman who has a long history of being battered by her husband is staying at the woman's shelter. She has received emotional support from staff and peers and has been made aware of the alternatives open to her. Nevertheless, she decides to return to her home and marriage. The best response by the nurse to the woman's decision is:
   a. "I just can't believe you have decided to go back to that horrible man."
   b. "I'm just afraid he will kill you or the children when you go back."
   c. "What makes you think things have changed with him?"
   d. "I hope you have made the right decision. Call this number if you need help."

5. Jana, age 5, is sent to the school nurse's office with an upset stomach. She has vomited and soiled her blouse. When the nurse removes her blouse, she notices that Jana has numerous bruises on her arms and torso, in various stages of healing. She also notices some small scars. Jana's abdomen protrudes on her small, thin frame. From the objective physical assessment, the nurse suspects that:
   a. Jana is experiencing physical and sexual abuse.
   b. Jana is experiencing physical abuse and neglect.
   c. Jana is experiencing emotional neglect.
   d. Jana is experiencing sexual and emotional abuse.

6. A school nurse notices bruises and scars on a child's body, but the child refuses to say how she received them. Another way in which the nurse can get information from the child is to:
   a. Have her evaluated by the school psychologist.
   b. Tell her she may select a "treat" from the treat box (e.g., sucker, balloon, junk jewelry) if she answers the nurse's questions.
   c. Explain to her that if she answers the questions, she may stay in the nurse's office and not have to go back to class.
   d. Use a "family" of dolls to role-play the child's family with her.

7. A school nurse notices bruises and scars on a child's body. The nurse suspects that the child is being physically abused. How should the nurse proceed with this information?
   a. As a health-care worker, report the suspicion to the Department of Health and Human Services.
   b. Check Jana again in a week and see if there are any new bruises.
   c. Meet with Jana's parents and ask them how Jana got the bruises.
   d. Initiate paperwork to have Jana placed in foster care.

8. Kate is an 18-year-old freshman at the state university. She was extremely flattered when Don, a senior star football player, invited her to a party. On the way home, he parked the car in a secluded area by the lake. He became angry when she refused his sexual advances. He began to beat her and finally raped her. She tried to fight him, but his physical strength overpowered her. He dumped her in the dorm parking lot and left. The dorm supervisor rushed Kate to the emergency department. Kate says to the nurse, "It's all my fault. I shouldn't have allowed him to stop at the lake." The nurse's best response is:
   a. "Yes, you're right. You put yourself in a very vulnerable position when you allowed him to stop at the lake."
   b. "You are not to blame for his behavior. You obviously made some right decisions, because you survived the attack."
   c. "There's no sense looking back now. Just look forward, and make sure you don't put yourself in the same situation again."
   d. "You'll just have to see that he is arrested so he won't do this to anyone else."

Continued

Review Questions—cont'd
Self-Examination/Learning Exercise

9. A young woman who has just undergone a sexual assault is brought into the ED by a friend. The *priority* nursing intervention would be:
   a. Help her to bathe and clean herself up.
   b. Provide physical and emotional support during evidence collection.
   c. Provide her with a written list of community resources for survivors of rape.
   d. Discuss the importance of a follow-up visit to evaluate for sexually transmitted diseases.

10. A woman who was sexually assaulted 6 months ago by a man with whom she was acquainted has since been attending a support group for survivors of rape. From this group, she has learned that the most likely reason the man raped her was:
    a. Because he had been drinking, he was not in control of his actions.
    b. He had not had sexual relations with a girl in many months.
    c. He was predisposed to become a rapist by virtue of the poverty conditions under which he was reared.
    d. He was expressing power and dominance by means of sexual aggression and violence.

TEST YOUR CRITICAL THINKING SKILLS

Sandy is a psychiatric RN who works at the Safe House for battered women. Lisa has just been admitted with her two small children after she was treated in the emergency department. She had been beaten severely by her husband while he was intoxicated last night. She escaped with her children after he passed out in their bedroom.

In her initial assessment, Sandy learns from Lisa that she has been battered by her husband for 5 years, beginning shortly after their marriage. She explained that she "knew he drank quite a lot before we were married, but thought he would stop after we had kids." Instead, the drinking has increased. Sometimes he doesn't even get home from work until 11 o'clock or midnight, after stopping to drink at the bar with his buddies.

Lately, he has begun to express jealousy and a lack of trust in Lisa, accusing her of numerous infidelities and indiscretions, none of which is true. Lisa says, "If only he wasn't under so much stress on his job, then maybe he wouldn't drink so much. Maybe if I tried harder to make everything perfect for him at home—I don't know. What do you think I should do to keep him from acting this way?"

Answer the following questions related to Lisa:

1. What is an appropriate response to Lisa's question?
2. Identify the priority psychosocial nursing diagnosis for Lisa.
3. What must the nurse ensure that Lisa learns from this experience?

Communication Exercises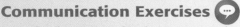

1. Sarah is being treated in the emergency department for wounds inflicted by her husband. Sandy says to the nurse, "He's really not a bad person. He's just under so much stress right now. His company is laying people off, and he thinks he will be next. He drinks a lot when he comes home from work. I just need to make things easier for him at home. I shouldn't have asked him to mow the lawn."
   • How would the nurse respond appropriately to this statement by Sarah?

2. "I don't know what to do. I'm afraid he will hurt the kids."
   • How would the nurse respond appropriately to this statement by Sarah?

3. "I don't want to press charges. I just want to go home!"
   • How would the nurse respond appropriately to this statement by Sarah?

References

American Psychiatric Association (APA). (2013). *Diagnostic and Statistical Manual of Mental Disorders* (5th ed.). Washington, DC: American Psychiatric Publishing.

Bensley, L., VanEenwyk, J., & Wynkoop, K.S. (2003). Childhood family violence history and women's risk for intimate partner violence and poor health. *American Journal of Preventive Medicine, 25*(1), 38-44.

Burgess, A. (2010). *Rape violence.* Gannett Education Course #60025. Retrieved from http://ce.nurse.com/60025/Rape-Violence

Centers for Disease Control and Prevention (CDC). (2012a). *Understanding intimate partner violence.* Retrieved from http://www.cdc.gov/violenceprevention/pdf/IPV_factsheet-a.pdf

Centers for Disease Control and Prevention (CDC). (2012b). *Understanding sexual violence.* Retrieved from http://www.cdc.gov/violenceprevention/pdf/SV_factsheet-a.pdf

Centers for Disease Control and Prevention (CDC). (2013). *Costs of intimate partner violence against women in the United States.* Retrieved from http://www.cdc.gov/violenceprevention/pub/IPV_cost.html

Child Welfare Information Gateway (CWIG). (2013). *What is child abuse and neglect? Recognizing signs and symptoms.* Retrieved from http://www.childwelfare.gov/pubs/factsheets/whatiscan.pdf

Crisis Intervention Center. (2013). *Why do people stay in abusive relationships?* Retrieved from http://www.crisisinterventioncenter.org/index.php?option=com_content&view=article&id=95:why-do-they-stay&catid=36:dv&Itemid=76

Cummings, J.L., & Mega, M.S. (2003). *Neuropsychiatry and behavioral neuroscience.* New York, NY: Oxford University Press.

Flaherty, E.G., Stirling, J., & The Committee on Child Abuse and Neglect. (2010). The pediatrician's role in child maltreatment prevention. *Pediatrics, 126*(4), 833-841.

Hollander, E., Berlin, H.A., & Stein, D.J. (2008). Impulse-control disorders not elsewhere classified. In R.E. Hales, S.C. Yudofsky, & G.O. Gabbard (Eds.), *Textbook of psychiatry* (5th ed., pp. 777-820). Washington, DC: American Psychiatric Publishing.

Hornor, G. (2005). Domestic violence and children. *Journal of Pediatric Health Care, 19*(4), 206-212.

Kennedy, B.P., Kawachi, I., Prothrow, S.D., Lochner, K., and Gupta, V. (1998). Social capital, income inequality, and firearm violent crime. *Social Science and Medicine, 47*(1), 7-17.

King, B.M. (2012). *Human sexuality today* (7th ed.). Upper Saddle River, NJ: Prentice Hall.

Lerner, M. (2005). *Adult manifestations of childhood sexual abuse.* New York, NY: The American Academy of Experts in Traumatic Stress.

McCormack, J. (2002, May). Sexual offenders' perceptions of their early interpersonal relationships: An attachment perspective. *Journal of Sex Research, 39*(2), 85-93.

Meskill, J., & Conner, M. (2010). *Understanding and dealing with domestic violence against women.* Retrieved from http://www.oregoncounseling.org/Handouts/DomesticViolenceWomen.htm

Mouradian, V.E. (2004). Battered women: What goes into the stay-leave decision? *Wellesley Centers for Women.* Retrieved from http://www.wcwonline.org/Past-years/battered-women-what-goes-into-the-stay-leave-decision

Murray, R.B., Zentner, J.P., & Yakimo, R. (2009). *Health promotion strategies through the life span* (8th ed.). Upper Saddle River, NJ: Pearson Education.

National Coalition Against Domestic Violence. (2013). *What is battering?* Retrieved from http://www.ncadv.org/learn/TheProblem.php

Reeves, C.R. (2003). *Childhood: It should not hurt.* Huntersville, NC: LTI Publishing.

Sadock, B.J., & Sadock, V.A. (2007). *Synopsis of psychiatry: Behavioral sciences/clinical psychiatry* (10th ed.). Philadelphia, PA: Lippincott Williams & Wilkins.

Schatzberg, A.F., Cole, J.O., & DeBattista, C. (2010). *Manual of clinical psychopharmacology* (7th ed.). Washington, DC: American Psychiatric Publishing.

Scully, D. (1994). *Understanding sexual violence: A study of convicted rapists.* New York, NY: Routledge.

Siever, L.J. (2002, August). Neurobiology of impulsive aggressive personality disordered patients. *Psychiatric Times, 19*(8). Retrieved from http://www.psychiatrictimes.com/display/article/10168/47131

Tardiff, K.J. (2003). Violence. In R.E. Hales & S.C. Yudofsky (Eds.), *Textbook of clinical psychiatry* (4th ed., pp. 1485-1509). Washington, DC: The American Psychiatric Publishing.

U.S. Bureau of Justice Statistics (2011). *Criminal victimization in the United States—Statistical Tables Index.* Retrieved from http://bjs.ojp.usdoj.gov/content/pub/html/cvus/index.cfm

U.S. Bureau of Justice Statistics (2012). *Intimate partner violence, 1993-2010.* Retrieved from http://bjs.ojp.usdoj.gov/index.cfm?ty=pbdetail&iid=4536

U.S. Department of Health and Human Services (USDHHS). (2012). *Child maltreatment 2011.* Retrieved from http://www.acf.hhs.gov/programs/cb/resource/child-maltreatment-2011

U.S. Department of Justice. (2012). *Areas of focus.* Retrieved from http://www.ovw.usdoj.gov/areas-focus.html

Classical References

Abrahamsen D. (1960). *The psychology of crime.* New York, NY: John Wiley & Sons.

Erikson, E.H. (1963). *Childhood and society* (2nd ed.). New York, NY: W.W. Norton & Co.

Macdonald, J.M. (1971). *Rape: Offenders and their victims.* Springfield, IL: Charles C. Thomas.

Selye, H. (1956). *The stress of life.* New York, NY: McGraw-Hill.

Walker, L.E. (1979). *The battered woman.* New York, NY: Harper & Row.

@ INTERNET REFERENCES

- Additional information related to child abuse may be located at the following websites:
  - http://www.childwelfare.gov
  - http://www.child-abuse.com
  - http://www.nlm.nih.gov/medlineplus/childabuse.html

- Additional information related to sexual assault may be located at the following websites:
  - http://www.nsvrc.org
  - http://www.nlm.nih.gov/medlineplus/sexualassault.html

- Additional information related to intimate partner violence may be located at the following websites:
  - http://www.thehotline.org
  - http://www.nursingworld.org/MainMenuCategories/ANAMarketplace/ANAPeriodicals/OJIN/TableofContents/Volume72002/No1Jan2002/DomesticViolenceChallenge.html
  - http://www.cdc.gov/ViolencePrevention/intimatepartnerviolence/index.html
  - http://www.nursingworld.org/MainMenuCategories/ANAMarketplace/ANAPeriodicals/OJIN/TableofContents/Volume72002/No1Jan2002/IntimatePartnerViolence.html

MOVIE CONNECTIONS

The Burning Bed (domestic violence) • *Life With Billy* (domestic violence) • *Two Story House* (child abuse) • *The Prince of Tides* (domestic violence) • *Radio Flyer* (child abuse) • *Flowers in the Attic* (child abuse) • *A Case of Rape* (sexual assault) • *The Accused* (sexual assault)

36 Community Mental Health Nursing

KEY TERMS

case management
case manager
deinstitutionalization

diagnosis-related groups
    (DRGs)
mobile outreach units

prospective payment
shelters
storefront clinics

OBJECTIVES
After reading this chapter, the student will be able to:

1. Discuss the changing focus of care in the field of mental health.
2. Define the concepts of care associated with the public health model.
3. Discuss primary prevention of mental illness within the community.
4. Identify populations at risk for mental illness within the community.
5. Discuss nursing intervention in primary prevention of mental illness within the community.
6. Discuss secondary prevention of mental illness within the community.
7. Describe treatment alternatives related to secondary prevention within the community.

8. Discuss tertiary prevention of mental illness within the community as it relates to the seriously mentally ill and homeless mentally ill.
9. Relate historical and epidemiological factors associated with caring for the seriously mentally ill and homeless mentally ill within the community.
10. Identify treatment alternatives for care of the seriously mentally ill and homeless mentally ill within the community.
11. Apply steps of the nursing process to care of the seriously mentally ill and homeless mentally ill within the community.

HOMEWORK ASSIGNMENT
Please read the chapter and answer the following questions:

1. What are *diagnosis-related groups* (DRGs)?
2. Describe and differentiate how interventions at the primary, secondary, and tertiary prevention levels are implemented.
3. Name three common client populations that benefit from psychiatric home health nursing.

4. What is the most common psychiatric diagnosis among homeless people with mental illness?

This chapter explores the concepts of primary and secondary prevention of mental illness within communities. Additional focus is placed on tertiary prevention of mental illness: treatment with community resources of those who suffer from severe and persistent mental illness and homeless persons with mental illness. Emphasis is given to the role of the psychiatric nurse in the various treatment alternatives within the community setting.

The Changing Focus of Care

Before 1840, there was no known treatment for individuals with mental illness. Because mental illness was perceived as incurable, the only "reasonable" intervention was thought to be removing these individuals from the community to a place where they would do no harm to themselves or others.

In 1841, Dorothea Dix, a former schoolteacher, began a personal crusade across the land on behalf of institutionalized individuals with mental illness. Her efforts resulted in more humane treatment of these clients and the establishment of a number of psychiatric hospitals.

After the movement initiated by Dix, the number of hospitals for persons with mental illness increased, although unfortunately not as rapidly as did the population with mental illness. The demand soon outgrew the supply, and hospitals became overcrowded and understaffed, with conditions that would have sorely distressed Dorothea Dix.

The community mental health movement had its impetus in the 1940s. With establishment of the National Mental Health Act of 1946, the U.S. government awarded grants to the states to develop mental health programs outside of state hospitals. Outpatient clinics and psychiatric units in general hospitals were inaugurated. Then, in 1949, as an outgrowth of the National Mental Health Act, the National Institute of Mental Health (NIMH) was established. The U.S. government has charged this agency with the responsibility for mental health in the United States.

In 1955, the Joint Commission on Mental Health and Illness was established by Congress to identify the nation's mental health needs and to make recommendations for improvement in psychiatric care. In 1961, the Joint Commission published the report, *Action for Mental Health,* in which recommendations were made for treatment of clients with mental illness, training for caregivers, and improvements in education and research on mental illness. With consideration given to these recommendations, Congress passed the Mental Retardation Facilities and Community Mental Health Centers Construction Act (often called the Community Mental Health Centers Act) of 1963. This act called

for the construction of comprehensive community mental health centers, the cost of which would be shared by federal and state governments. The **deinstitutionalization** movement (the closing of state mental hospitals and discharging of individuals with mental illness) had begun.

Unfortunately, many state governments did not have the capability to match the federal funds required for the establishment of these mental health centers. Some communities found it difficult to follow the rigid requirements for services required by the legislation that provided the grant.

In 1980 the Community Mental Health Systems Act, which was to have played a major role in renovation of mental health care, was established. Funding was authorized for community mental health centers, for services to high-risk populations, and for rape research and services. Approval was also granted for the appointment of an associate director for minority concerns at NIMH. However, before this plan could be enacted, the newly inaugurated administration set forth its intention to diminish federal involvement. Budget cuts reduced the number of mandated services, and federal funding for community mental health centers was terminated in 1984.

Meanwhile, costs of care for hospitalized psychiatric clients continued to rise. The problem of the "revolving door" began to intensify. Individuals with severe and persistent mental illness had no place to go when their symptoms exacerbated, except back to the hospital. Individuals without support systems remained in the hospital for extended periods because of lack of appropriate community services. Hospital services were paid for by cost-based, retrospective reimbursement: Medicaid, Medicare, and private health insurance. Retrospective reimbursement encouraged hospital expenditure; the more services provided, the more payment received.

This system of delivery of health care was interrupted in 1983 with the advent of **prospective payment**—the Reagan administration's proposal of cost containment. It was directed at control of Medicare costs by setting forth preestablished amounts that would be reimbursed for specific diagnoses, or **diagnosis-related groups (DRGs)**. Since that time, prospective payment has also been integrated by the states (Medicaid) and by some private insurance companies, drastically affecting the amount of reimbursement for health-care services.

Mental health services have been influenced by prospective payment. General hospital services to psychiatric clients have been severely restricted. Clients who present with acute symptoms, such as acute psychosis, suicidal ideations or attempts, or manic exacerbations, constitute the largest segment of the psychiatric hospital census. Clients with less serious illnesses (e.g., moderate depression or adjustment disorders) may be hospitalized, but length of stay has been shortened considerably by the reimbursement guidelines. Clients are being discharged from the hospital with a greater need for aftercare than in the past, when hospital stays were longer.

Deinstitutionalization continues to be the changing focus of mental health care in the United States. Care for the client in the hospital has become cost prohibitive, whereas care for the client in the community is cost effective. The reality of the provision of health-care services today is often more of a political and funding issue than providers would care to admit. Decisions about how to treat are rarely made without consideration of cost and method of payment.

Provision of outpatient mental health services not only is the wave of the future, it is the reality of today. We must serve the consumer by providing the essential services to assist with health promotion or prevention, to initiate early intervention, and to ensure rehabilitation or prevention of long-term disability.

The Public Health Model

The premise of the model of public health is based largely on the concepts set forth by Gerald Caplan (1964) during the initial community mental health movement. They include primary prevention, secondary prevention, and tertiary prevention. These concepts no longer have relevance only to mental health; rather, they have been widely adapted as guiding principles in many clinical and community settings over a range of medical and nursing specialties.

CORE CONCEPT

Primary Prevention

Services aimed at reducing the incidence of mental disorders within the population.

Primary prevention targets both individuals and the environment. Emphasis is twofold:

1. Assisting individuals to increase their ability to cope effectively with stress.
2. Targeting and diminishing harmful forces (stressors) within the environment.

Nursing in primary prevention is focused on the targeting of groups at risk and the provision of educational programs. Examples include:

■ Teaching parenting skills and child development to prospective new parents
■ Teaching physical and psychosocial effects of alcohol/drugs to elementary school students
■ Teaching techniques of stress management to virtually anyone who desires to learn
■ Teaching groups of individuals ways to cope with the changes associated with various maturational stages
■ Teaching concepts of mental health to various groups within the community
■ Providing education and support to unemployed or homeless individuals
■ Providing education and support to other individuals in various transitional periods (e.g., widows and widowers, new retirees, and women entering the workforce in middle life)

These are only a few examples of the types of services nurses provide in primary prevention. Such services can be offered in a variety of settings that are convenient for the public (e.g., churches, schools, colleges, community centers, YMCAs and YWCAs, workplaces of employee organizations, meetings of women's groups, or civic or social organizations such as parent-teacher associations, health fairs, and community shelters).

CORE CONCEPT

Secondary Prevention

Interventions aimed at minimizing early symptoms of psychiatric illness and directed toward reducing the prevalence and duration of the illness.

Secondary prevention is accomplished through early identification of problems and prompt initiation of effective treatment. Nursing in secondary prevention focuses on recognition of symptoms and provision of, or referral for, treatment. Examples include:

■ Ongoing assessment of individuals at high risk for illness exacerbation (e.g., during home visits, day care, community health centers, or in any setting where screening of high-risk individuals might occur)
■ Provision of care for individuals in whom illness symptoms have been assessed (e.g., individual or group counseling, medication administration, education and support during period of increased stress [crisis intervention], staffing rape crisis centers, suicide hotlines, homeless shelters, shelters for abused persons, or mobile mental health units)
■ Referral for treatment of individuals in whom illness symptoms have been assessed. Referrals may come from support groups, community mental health centers, emergency services, psychiatrists or psychologists, and day or partial hospitalization. Inpatient therapy on a psychiatric unit of a general hospital or in a private psychiatric hospital may be necessary. Psychopharmacology and various adjunct therapies may be initiated as part of the treatment.

Secondary prevention has been addressed extensively in Unit 4 of this text. Nursing assessment, diagnosis/outcome identification, planning/implementation, and evaluation were discussed for many of the mental illnesses identified in the *Diagnostic and Statistical Manual of Mental Disorders, Fifth Edition* (DSM-5) (American Psychiatric Association [APA], 2013). These concepts may be applied in any setting where nursing is practiced.

CORE CONCEPT

Tertiary Prevention

Services aimed at reducing the residual defects that are associated with severe and persistent mental illness.

Tertiary prevention is accomplished in two ways:

1. Preventing complications of the illness
2. Promoting rehabilitation that is directed toward achievement of each individual's maximum level of functioning

Historically, individuals with severe and persistent mental illness often experienced long hospitalizations that resulted in loss of social skills and increased dependency. With deinstitutionalization, many of these individuals may never have experienced hospitalization, but they still do not possess adequate skills to live productive lives within the community.

Nursing in tertiary prevention focuses on helping clients learn or relearn socially appropriate behaviors so that they may achieve a satisfying role within the community. Examples include:

■ Consideration of the rehabilitation process at the time of initial diagnosis and treatment planning
■ Teaching the client daily living skills and encouraging independence to his or her maximum ability
■ Referring clients for various aftercare services (e.g., support groups, day treatment programs, partial hospitalization programs, psychosocial rehabilitation programs, group home or other transitional housing)
■ Monitoring effectiveness of aftercare services (e.g., through home health visits or follow-up appointments in community mental health centers)
■ Making referrals for support services when required (e.g., some communities have programs linking individuals with serious mental disorders to volunteers who serve to develop friendships with the individuals and who may assist with household chores, shopping, and other activities of daily living with which the individual is having difficulty, in addition to participating in social activities with the individual)

Nursing care at the tertiary level of prevention can be administered on an individual or group basis and in a variety of settings, such as inpatient hospitalization, day or partial hospitalization, group home or halfway house, shelters, home health care, nursing homes, and community mental health centers.

The Community as Client

Primary Prevention

CORE CONCEPT

Community

A group, population, or cluster of people with at least one common characteristic, such as geographic location, occupation, ethnicity, or health concern (Langley, 2002).

Primary prevention within communities encompasses the twofold emphasis defined earlier in this chapter. These include:

1. Identifying stressful life events that precipitate crises and targeting the relevant populations at high risk.

IMPLICATIONS OF RESEARCH FOR EVIDENCE-BASED PRACTICE

McDevitt, J., Snyder, M., Miller, A., & Wilbur, J. (2006). Perceptions of barriers and benefits to physical activity among outpatients in psychiatric rehabilitation. *Journal of Nursing Scholarship, 38*(1), 50-55.

DESCRIPTION OF THE STUDY: The purpose of this study was to explore perceived barriers and benefits to physical activity in people with serious and persistent mental illness (SPMI) who were enrolled in community-based psychiatric rehabilitation. The sample included 34 participants (16 men and 18 women) aged 18 to 50 from two community-based psychiatric rehabilitation centers in a large Midwestern urban area. Ethnic breakdown included 24 African Americans, 7 Whites, and 3 of Hispanic or unknown ethnicity. Four focus groups lasting 50 minutes each were held over a 3-week period, with 7 to 9 participants in each group. Themes of the focus groups included barriers and benefits of physical activity.

RESULTS OF THE STUDY: Barriers to physical activity identified by the study participants included symptoms of the mental illness itself, being medicated, gaining weight, being in a

Continued

rehabilitation program, and living in urban neighborhoods. They cited symptoms of lethargy and lack of initiative (from either the medication or the illness) and weight gain from the medications interfering with physical activity. Neighborhood safety concerns and being identified as a person with a mental disorder were also identified. Benefits of physical activity cited included feeling more energetic, less stressed, and improved sleep. Keeping busy and providing distraction from problems were also recognized. Both men and women suggested they would appreciate exercise and activities for same-gender groups.

IMPLICATIONS FOR NURSING PRACTICE: Several recommendations from the participants emerged from the focus groups. Some of these included the following:

• Need a good leader who encourages, but does not coerce; provides participants with choices

• Groups that provide relevant information that pertains to client health concerns, such as weight gain, and how to address these concerns
• Offer group support, but provide individual options as well.
• Offer a choice of different types of activities, to reduce boredom

The authors of this study stated, "Confronting how attitudes and barriers specific to this population can affect activity and reframing program compliance to include the independent initiation of activity as part of improving health should assist clients of mental health services to become more active" (p. 55).

2. Intervening with these high-risk populations to prevent or minimize harmful consequences.

Populations at Risk

One way to view populations at risk is to focus on types of crises that individuals experience in their lives. Two broad categories are maturational crises and situational crises.

Maturational Crises

Maturational crises are crucial experiences that are associated with various stages of growth and development. Erikson (1963) described eight stages of the life cycle during which individuals struggle with developmental "tasks." Crises can occur during any of these stages, although several developmental periods and life-cycle events have been recognized as having increased crisis potential: adolescence, marriage, parenthood, midlife, and retirement.

Adolescence The task for adolescence according to Erikson (1963) is *identity versus role confusion*. This is the time in life when individuals ask questions such as "Who am I?" "Where am I going?" and "What is life all about?"

Adolescence is a transition into young adulthood. It is a very volatile time in most families. Commonly, there is conflict over issues of control. Parents sometimes have difficulty relinquishing even a minimal amount of the control they have had throughout their child's infancy, toddler, and school-age years, at this time when the adolescent is seeking increased independence. It may seem that the adolescent is 25 years old one day and 5 years old the next. An often-quoted definition of an

adolescent, by an anonymous author, is: "A toddler with hormones and wheels."

At this time, adolescents are "trying out their wings," although they possess an essential need to know that the parents (or surrogate parents) are available if support is required. Mahler, Pine, and Bergman (1975) have termed this vital concept "emotional refueling," and although they were referring to toddlers when they coined the term, it is highly applicable to adolescents as well. In fact, it is believed that the most frequent immediate precipitant to adolescent suicide is loss, or threat of loss, or abandonment by parents or closest peer relationship.

Adolescents have many issues to deal with and many choices to make. Some of these include issues that relate to self-esteem and body image (in a body that is undergoing rapid changes), peer relationships (with both genders), education and career selection, establishing a set of values and ideals, sexuality and sexual experimentation (including issues of birth control and prevention of sexually transmitted diseases), drug and alcohol use, and physical appearance.

Nursing interventions with adolescents at the primary level of prevention focus on providing support and accurate information to ease the difficult transition they are undergoing. Educational offerings can be presented in schools, churches, youth centers, or any location in which groups of teenagers gather. Types of programs may include (but are not limited to):

■ Alateen groups for adolescents with alcoholic parent(s)
■ Other support groups for teenagers who are in need of assistance to cope with stressful situations (e.g., children dealing with divorce of their

parents, pregnant teenagers, teenagers coping with abortion, adolescents coping with the death of a parent)

■ Educational programs that inform about and validate bodily changes and emotions about which there may be some concerns

■ Educational programs that inform about nutritional needs specific for this age group

■ Educational programs that inform about sexuality, pregnancy, contraception, and sexually transmitted diseases

■ Educational programs that inform about the use of alcohol and other drugs

Marriage The "American dream" of the 1950s—especially that of the American woman—was to marry, have two or three children, buy a house in the suburbs, and drive a station wagon. To not be at least betrothed by their mid-20s caused many women to fear becoming an "old maid." Living together without the benefit of marriage was an unacceptable and rarely considered option.

Times have changed considerably since the middle of the 20th century. Today's young women are choosing to pursue careers before entering into marriage, to continue their careers after marriage, or to not marry at all. Many couples are deciding to live together without being married, and, as with most trends, the practice now receives more widespread societal acceptance than it once did.

Why is marriage considered one of the most common maturational crises? Sheehy (1976), in her classic volume about life's passages, wrote:

> No two people can possibly coordinate all their developmental crises. The timing of outside opportunities will almost never be the same. But more importantly, each one has an inner life structure with its own idiosyncrasies. Depending on what has gone before, each one will alternate differently between times of feeling full of certainty, hope, and heightened potential and times of feeling vulnerable, unfocused, and scared. (p. 138)

Additional conflicts sometimes also arise when the marriage is influenced by crossovers in religion, ethnicity, social status, or race, although these types of differences have become more individually and societally acceptable than they once were.

Nursing interventions at the primary level of prevention with individuals in this stage of development involve education regarding what to expect at various stages in the marriage. Many high schools now offer courses in marriage and family living in which students role-play through anticipatory marriage and family situations. Nurses could offer these kinds of classes within the community to individuals considering marriage. Too many people enter marriage with the

notion that, as sure as the depth of their love, their soon-to-be husband or wife will discontinue his or her "undesirable" traits and change into the perceived ideal spouse. Primary prevention with these individuals involves:

■ Encouraging honest communication

■ Determining what each person expects from the relationship

■ Ascertaining whether or not each individual can accept compromise

This type of intervention can be effective in individual or couple's therapy and in support or educational groups of couples experiencing similar circumstances.

Parenthood Murray, Zentner, and Yakimo (2009) state:

> The coming of the child is a developmental and sometimes situational crisis, a turning point in the couple's life in which old patterns of living must be changed for new ways of living and new values. With the advent of parenthood, a couple is embarking on a journey from which there is no return. To put it simply, parents cannot quit. The child's birth brings finality to many privileges and a permanence of responsibilities. (p. 249)

There is perhaps no developmental stage that creates an upheaval equal to that of the arrival of a child. Even when the child is desperately wanted and pleasurably anticipated, his or her arrival usually results in some degree of chaos within the family.

Because the family operates as a system, the addition of a new member influences all parts of the system as a whole. If it is a first child, the relationship between the spouses is likely to be affected by the demands of caring for the infant on a 24-hour basis. If there are older children, they may resent the attention showered on the new arrival and show their resentment in a variety of creative ways.

The concept of having a child (particularly the first one) is often romanticized, with little or no consideration given to the realities and responsibilities that accompany this "bundle of joy." Many young parents are shocked to realize that such a tiny human can create so many changes in so many lives. It is unfortunate that although parenting is one of the most important positions an individual will hold in life, it is one for which he or she is often least prepared.

Nursing intervention at the primary level of prevention with those in the developmental stage of parenthood must begin long before the child is even born. How do we prepare individuals for parenthood? *Anticipatory guidance* is the term used to describe the interventions used to help new parents know what they might expect. Volumes have been written on the subject, but it is also important for expectant parents to have a support person or network with whom they can talk, express feelings, excitement, and fears. Nurses can provide the following type of information to help ease the transition into parenthood (Mandleco, 2004; Murray et al., 2009; Spock, 2012).

■ **Prepared childbirth classes:** These classes present what most likely will happen, but with additional information about possible variations from that which is expected.

■ **Information about what to expect after the baby arrives:**

  ■ *Parent-infant bonding.* Expectant parents should know that it is common for parent-infant bonding not to occur immediately. The strong attachment will occur as parent and infant get to know each other.

  ■ *Changing husband-wife relationships.* The couple should be encouraged to engage in open honest communication and role-playing of typical situations that are likely to arise after the baby becomes a part of the family.

  ■ *Clothing and equipment.* Expectant parents need to know what is required to care for a newborn child. Family economics, space available, and lifestyle should be considered.

  ■ *Feeding.* Advantages and disadvantages of breastfeeding and formula feeding should be presented. The couple should be supported in whatever method is chosen. Anticipatory guidance related to technique should be provided for one or both methods, as the expectant parents request.

  ■ *Other expectations.* It is important for expectant parents to receive anticipatory guidance about the infant's sleeping and crying patterns, bathing the infant, care of the circumcision and cord, toys that provide stimulation of the newborn's senses, aspects of providing a safe environment, and when to call the physician.

■ **Stages of growth and development:** It is very important for parents to understand what behaviors should be expected at what stage of development. It is also important to know that their child may not necessarily follow the age guidelines associated with these stages. However, a substantial deviation from these guidelines should be reported to their physician.

Midlife What is middle age? A colleague once remarked that upon turning 50 years of age she stated, "Now I can say I am officially middle aged . . . until I began thinking about how few individuals I really knew who were 100!"

Midlife crises are not defined by a specific number. Various sources in the literature identify these conflicts as occurring anytime between age 35 and 65.

What is a midlife crisis? This, too, is very individual, but a number of patterns have been identified within three broad categories:

1. **An alteration in perception of the self.** One's perception of self may occur slowly. One may suddenly become aware of being "old" or "middle aged." Murray and associates (2009) stated:

   Now the person looks in the mirror and sees changes that others may have noticed some time ago. Gray, thinning hair, wrinkles, coarsening features, decreased muscular tone, weight gain, varicosities, and capillary breakage may be the first signs of impending age. (p. 569)

   Other biological changes that occur naturally with the aging process may also affect the crises that occur at this time. In women, a gradual decrease in the production of estrogen initiates the menopause, which results in a variety of physical and emotional symptoms. Some physical symptoms include "hot flashes," vaginal dryness, cessation of menstruation, loss of reproductive ability, night sweats, insomnia, headaches, and minor memory disturbances. Emotional symptoms include anxiety, depression, crying for no reason, and temper outbursts.

   Although the menopausal period in men is not as evident as it is in women, most clinicians subscribe to the belief that men undergo a climacteric experience related to the gradual decrease in production of testosterone. Although sperm production diminishes with advancing age, there is usually no complete cessation, as there is of ovum production in women at menopause (Scanlon & Sanders, 2011). Some men experience hot flashes, sweating, chills, dizziness, and heart palpitations (Murray et al., 2009), whereas others may experience severe depression and an overall decline in physical vigor (Sadock & Sadock, 2007). An alteration in sexual functioning is not uncommon (see Chapter 34).

2. **An alteration in perception of others.** A change in relationship with adult children requires a sensitive shift in caring. Wright and Leahey (2013) state:

   The family of origin must relinquish the primary roles of parent and child. They must adapt to the new roles of parent and adult child. This involves renegotiation of emotional and financial commitments. The key emotional process during this stage is for family members to deal with a multitude of exits from and entries into the family system. (p. 107)

These experiences are particularly difficult when parents' values conflict with the relationships and types of lifestyles their children choose. An alteration in perception of one's parents also begins to occur during this time. Having always looked to parents for support and comfort, the middle-aged individual may suddenly find that the roles are beginning to reverse. Aging parents may look to their children for assistance with making decisions regarding their everyday lives and for assistance with chores that they have previously accomplished independently. When parents die, middle-aged individuals must come to terms with their own mortality. The process of recognition and resolution of one's own finitude begins in earnest at this time.

3. **An alteration in perception of time.** Middle age has been defined as the end of youth and the beginning of old age. Individuals often experience a sense that time is running out: "I haven't done all I want to do or accomplished all I intended to accomplish!" Depression and a sense of loss may occur as individuals realize that some of the goals established in their youth may go unmet.

The term "empty nest syndrome" has been used to describe the adjustment period parents experience when the last child leaves home to establish an independent residence. The crisis is often more profound for the mother who has devoted her life to nurturing her family. As the last child leaves, she may perceive her future as uncertain and meaningless.

Some women who have devoted their lives to rearing their children decide to develop personal interests and pursue personal goals once the children are grown. This occurs at a time when many husbands have begun to decrease what may have been a compulsive drive for occupational security during the earlier years of their lives. This disparity in common goals may create conflict between husband and wife. At a time when she is experiencing more value in herself and her own life, he may begin to feel less valued. This may also relate to a decrease in the amount of time and support from the wife to which the husband has become accustomed. This type of role change will require numerous adaptations on the part of both spouses.

Finally, an alteration in one's perception of time may be related to the societal striving for eternal youth. The individual may try to delay the external changes that come with aging by the use of cosmetics, hormone creams, or even surgery. This yearning for youth may take the form of sexual promiscuity or extramarital affairs with much younger individuals, in an effort to prove that one "still has what it takes." Some individuals reach for the trappings of youth with regressive-type behaviors, such as the middle-aged man who buys a motorcycle and joins a motorcycle club, and the 50-year-old woman who wears miniskirts and flirts with her daughter's boyfriends. These individuals may be denying their own past and experience. With a negative view of self, they strongly desire to relive their youth.

Nursing intervention at the primary level of prevention with those in the developmental stage of midlife involves providing accurate information regarding changes that occur during this time of life and support for adapting to these changes effectively. These interventions might include:

■ Nutrition classes to inform individuals in this age group about the essentials of diet and exercise. Educational materials on how to avoid obesity or reduce weight can be included, along with the importance of good nutrition.

■ Assistance with ways to improve health (e.g., quit smoking, cease or reduce alcohol consumption, reduce fat intake).

■ Discussions of the importance of having regular physical examinations, including Pap and breast examinations for women and prostate examinations for men. Monthly breast self-examinations should be taught and yearly mammograms encouraged.

■ Classes on menopause should be given. Provide information about what to expect. Myths that abound regarding this topic should be expelled. Support groups for women (and men) undergoing the menopausal experience could be formed.

■ Support and information related to physical changes occurring in the body during this time of life. Assist with the grief response that some individuals will experience in relation to loss of youth, "empty nest," and sense of identity.

■ Support and information related to care of aging parents should be given. Individuals should be referred to community resources for respite and assistance before strain of the caregiver role threatens to disrupt the family system.

Retirement Retirement, which is often anticipated as an achievement in principle, may be met with a great deal of ambivalence when it actually occurs. Our society places a great deal of importance on productivity and on earning as much money as possible at as young an age as possible. These types of values contribute to the ambivalence associated with retirement. Although leisure has been acknowledged as a legitimate reward for workers, leisure during retirement has never been accorded the same social value. Adjustment to this life-cycle event becomes more difficult in the face of societal values that are in direct conflict with the new lifestyle.

Historically, many women have derived much of their self-esteem from having children, rearing children, and being a "good mother." Likewise, many men have achieved self-esteem through work-related activities—creativity, productivity, and earning money. Termination of these activities can result in a loss of self-worth, and individuals who are unable to adapt satisfactorily may become depressed.

It would appear that retirement is becoming, and will continue to become, more accepted by societal standards. With more and more individuals retiring earlier and living longer, the growing number of aging persons will spend a significantly longer time in retirement. At present, retirement has become more of an institutionalized expectation, and there appears to be increasing acceptance of it as a social status.

Nursing intervention at the primary level of prevention with the developmental task of retirement involves providing information and support to individuals who have retired or are considering retirement. Support can be on a one-to-one basis to assist these individuals to sort out their feelings regarding retirement. Well-being in retirement is linked to factors such as stable health status and access to health-care services, adequate income, the ability to pursue new goals or activities, extended social network of family and friends, and satisfaction with current living arrangements (Murray et al., 2009).

Support can also be provided in a group environment. Support groups of individuals undergoing the same types of experiences can be extremely helpful. Nurses can form and lead these types of groups to assist retiring individuals through this critical period. These groups can also serve to provide information about available resources that offer assistance to individuals in or nearing retirement, such as information concerning Medicare, Social Security, and Medicaid; information related to organizations that specialize in hiring retirees; and information regarding ways to use newly acquired free time constructively.

Situational Crises

Situational crises are acute responses that occur as a result of an external circumstantial stressor. The number and types of situational stressors are limitless and may be real or exist only in the perception of the individual. Some types of situational crises that put individuals at risk for mental illness include the following.

Poverty A number of studies have identified poverty as a direct correlation to emotional illness. This may have to do with the direct consequences of poverty, such as inadequate and crowded living conditions,

nutritional deficiencies, medical neglect, unemployment, or being homeless.

High Rate of Life Change Events Miller and Rahe (1997) found that frequent changes in life patterns due to a large number of significant events occurring in close proximity tend to decrease a person's ability to deal with stress, and physical or emotional illness may be the result. These include life change events such as death of a loved one, divorce, being fired from a job, a change in living conditions, a change in place of employment or residence, physical illness, or a change in body image caused by the loss of a body part or function.

Environmental Conditions Environmental conditions can create situational crises. Tornados, floods, hurricanes, and earthquakes have wreaked devastation on thousands of individuals and families in recent years.

Trauma Individuals who have encountered traumatic experiences must be considered at risk for emotional illness. These include traumatic experiences usually considered outside the range of usual human experience, such as rape, war, physical attack, torture, or natural or manmade disaster.

Nursing intervention at the primary level of prevention with individuals experiencing situational crises is aimed at maintaining the highest possible level of functioning while offering support and assistance with problem solving during the crisis period. Interventions for nursing of clients in crisis include the following:

■ Use a reality-oriented approach. The focus of the problem is on the here and now.

■ Remain with the individual who is experiencing panic anxiety.

■ Establish a rapid working relationship by showing unconditional acceptance, by active listening, and by attending to immediate needs.

■ Discourage lengthy explanations or rationalizations of the situation; promote an atmosphere for verbalization of true feelings.

■ Set firm limits on aggressive, destructive behaviors. At high levels of anxiety, behavior is likely to be impulsive and regressive. Establish at the outset what is acceptable and what is not, and maintain consistency.

■ Clarify the problem that the individual is facing. The nurse does this by describing his or her perception of the problem and comparing it with the individual's perception of the problem.

■ Help the individual determine what he or she believes precipitated the crisis.

■ Acknowledge feelings of anger, guilt, helplessness, and powerlessness, while taking care not to provide positive feedback for these feelings.

■ Guide the individual through a problem-solving process by which he or she may move in the direction of positive life change:

  ■ Help the individual confront the source of the problem that is creating the crisis response.

  ■ Encourage the individual to discuss changes he or she would like to make. Jointly determine whether desired changes are realistic.

  ■ Encourage exploration of feelings about aspects that cannot be changed, and explore alternative ways of coping more adaptively in these situations.

  ■ Discuss alternative strategies for creating change in situations that can realistically be changed.

  ■ Weigh benefits and consequences of each alternative.

  ■ Assist the individual to select alternative coping strategies that will help alleviate future crises.

■ Identify external support systems and new social networks from which the individual may seek assistance in times of stress.

Nursing at the level of primary prevention focuses largely on education of the client to prevent initiation or exacerbation of mental illness. An example of just one type of teaching plan for use in primary prevention situations is presented in Table 36-1.

Secondary Prevention

Populations at Risk

Secondary prevention within communities relates to using early detection and prompt intervention with individuals experiencing mental illness symptoms. The same maturational and situational crises that were presented in the previous section on primary prevention are used to discuss intervention at the secondary level of prevention.

Maturational Crises

Adolescence The need for intervention at the secondary level of prevention in adolescence occurs when disruptive and age-inappropriate behaviors become the norm, and the family can no longer cope adaptively with the situation. All levels of dysfunction are considered—from dysfunctional family coping to the need for hospitalization of the adolescent.

Nursing intervention with the adolescent at the secondary level of prevention may occur in the community setting at community mental health centers, physician's offices, schools, public health departments, and crisis intervention centers. Nurses may work with families to problem-solve and improve coping and communication skills, or they may work on a one-to-one basis with the adolescent in an attempt to modify behavior patterns.

Adolescents may be hospitalized for a variety of problems, including (but not limited to) conduct disorders, adjustment disorders, eating disorders, substance-related disorders, depression, and anxiety disorders. Inpatient care is determined by severity of symptomatology. Nursing care of adolescents in the hospital setting focuses on problem identification and stabilizing a crisis situation. Once stability has been achieved, clients are commonly discharged to outpatient care. If an adolescent's home situation has been deemed unsatisfactory, the state may take custody and the child is then discharged to a group or foster home. Care plans for intervention with the adolescent at the secondary level of prevention can be found in Chapter 33 and in other chapters that address the specific diagnoses.

Marriage Problems in a marriage are as far-reaching as the individuals who experience them. Problems that are not uncommon to the disruption of a marriage relationship include substance abuse on the part of one or both partners and disagreements on issues of sex, money, children, gender roles, and infidelity, among others. Murray and associates (2009) state:

> Marriage to one person and living with the frustrations, conflicts, and boredom that is part of any close and lengthy relationship requires constant work by both parties. (p. 504)

Nursing intervention at the secondary level of prevention with individuals encountering marriage problems may include one or more of the following:

■ Counseling with the couple or with one of the spouses on a one-to-one basis

■ Referral to a couples' support group

■ Identification of the problem and possible solutions; support and guidance as changes are undertaken

■ Referral to a sex therapist

■ Referral to a financial advisor

■ Referral to parent effectiveness training

Murray and associates (2009) state:

> When marriage fails and bonds are broken, aloneness, anger, mistrust, hostility, guilt, shame, a sense of betrayal, fear, disappointment, loss of identity, anxiety, and depression, alone or in combination, may appear both in the divorcee and the one initiating the divorce. (p. 547)

In Miller and Rahe's (1997) life change questionnaire, only death of a spouse or other family member scored higher than divorce in severity of stress experienced. This is an area in which nurses can intervene to help ease the transition and prevent emotional breakdown. In community health settings, nurses can lead support groups for newly divorced individuals. They can also provide one-to-one counseling for individuals experiencing the emotional chaos engendered by the dissolution of a marriage relationship.

TABLE 36–1 Client Education for Primary Prevention: Drugs of Abuse

CLASS OF DRUGS	EFFECTS	SYMPTOMS OF OVERDOSE	TRADE NAMES	COMMON NAMES	EFFECTS ON THE BODY (CHRONIC OR HIGH-DOSE USE)
CNS DEPRESSANTS					
Alcohol	Relaxation, loss of inhibitions, lack of concentration, drowsiness, slurred speech, sleep	Nausea, vomiting; shallow respirations; cold, clammy skin; weak, rapid pulse; coma; possible death	Ethyl alcohol, beer, gin, rum, vodka, bourbon, whiskey, liqueurs, wine, brandy, sherry, champagne	Booze, alcohol, liquor, drinks, cocktails, highballs, nightcaps, moonshine, white lightning, firewater	Peripheral nerve damage, skeletal muscle wasting, encephalopathy, psychosis, cardiomyopathy, gastritis, esophagitis, pancreatitis, hepatitis, cirrhosis of the liver, leukopenia, thrombocytopenia, sexual dysfunction
Other (barbiturates and non-barbiturates)	Same as alcohol	Anxiety, fever, agitation, hallucinations, disorientation, tremors, delirium, convulsions, possible death	Seconal Nembutal Amytal Valium Librium Chloral hydrate Miltown	Red birds Yellow birds Blue birds Blues/yellows Green & whites Mickies Downers	Decreased REM sleep, respiratory depression, hypotension, possible kidney or liver damage, sexual dysfunction
CNS STIMULANTS					
Amphetamines and related drugs	Hyperactivity, agitation, euphoria, insomnia, loss of appetite	Cardiac arrhythmias, headache, convulsions, hypertension, rapid heart rate, coma, possible death	Dexedrine, Didrex, Tenuate, Bontril, Ritalin, Focalin, Provigil	Uppers, pep pills, wakeups, bennies, eyeopeners, speed, black beauties, sweet A's	Aggressive, compulsive behavior, paranoia; hallucinations; hypertension
Cocaine	Euphoria, hyperactivity, restlessness, talkativeness, increased pulse, dilated pupils	Hallucinations, convulsions, pulmonary edema, respiratory failure, coma, cardiac arrest, possible death	Cocaine hydrochloride	Coke, flake, snow, dust, happy dust, gold dust, girl, Cecil, C, toot, blow, crack	Pulmonary hemorrhage, myocardial infarction, ventricular fibrillation
Synthetic stimulants	Agitation, insomnia, irritability, dizziness, decreased ability to think clearly, increased heart rate, chest pains	Depression, paranoia, delusions, suicidal thoughts, seizures, panic attacks, nausea, vomiting, heart attack, stroke	Mephedrone, MDPV (3-4 methylenedioxypyrovalerone)	Bath salts, bliss, vanilla sky, ivory wave, purple wave	Increased heart rate, increased blood pressure, nosebleeds, hallucinations, aggressive behavior

Category	Intoxication effects	Overdose	Drug	Street names	Long-term/withdrawal effects
OPIOIDS	Euphoria, lethargy, drowsiness, lack of motivation, constricted pupils	Shallow breathing, slowed pulse, clammy skin, pulmonary edema, respiratory arrest, convulsions, coma, possible death	Heroin Morphine Codeine Dilaudid Demerol Dolophine Percodan Talwin Opium	Snow, stuff, H, Harry, horse M, morph, Miss Emma Schoolboy Lords Doctors Dollies Perkies T's Big O, black stuff	Respiratory depression, constipation, fecal impaction, hypotension, decreased libido, retarded ejaculation, impotence, orgasm failure
HALLUCINOGENS	Visual hallucinations, disorientation, confusion, paranoid delusions, euphoria, anxiety, panic, increased pulse	Agitation, extreme hyperactivity, violence, hallucinations, psychosis, convulsions, possible death	LSD PCP Mescaline DMT STP, DOM MDMA Ketamine	Acid, cube, big D Angel dust, hog, peace pill Mesc Businessman's trip Serenity and peace Ecstasy, XTC Special K, Vitamin K, Kit Kat	Panic reaction, acute psychosis, flashbacks
CANNABINOLS	Relaxation, talkativeness, lowered inhibitions, euphoria, mood swings	Fatigue, paranoia, delusions, hallucinations, possible psychosis	Cannabis Hashish	Marijuana, pot, grass, joint, Mary Jane, MJ Hash, rope, Sweet Lucy	Tachycardia, orthostatic hypotension, chronic bronchitis, problems with infertility, amotivational syndrome

Divorce also has an impact on the children involved. Nurses can intervene with the children of divorce in an effort to prevent dysfunctional behaviors associated with the break-up of a marriage.

Parenthood Intervention at the secondary level of prevention with parents can be required for a number of reasons. A few of these include:

■ Physical, emotional, or sexual abuse of a child
■ Physical or emotional neglect of a child
■ Birth of a child with special needs
■ Diagnosis of a terminal illness in a child
■ Death of a child

Nursing intervention at the secondary level of prevention includes being able to recognize the physical and behavioral signs that indicate possible abuse of a child. The child may be cared for in the emergency department or as an inpatient on the pediatric unit or child psychiatric unit of a general hospital.

Nursing intervention with parents may include teaching effective methods of disciplining children, aside from physical punishment. Methods that emphasize the importance of positive reinforcement for acceptable behavior can be very effective. Family members must be committed to consistent use of this behavior modification technique for it to be successful.

Parents should also be informed about behavioral expectations at the various levels of development. Knowledge of what to expect from children at these various stages may provide needed anticipatory guidance to deal with the crises commonly associated with each stage.

Therapy sessions with all family members together may focus on problems with family communications. Members are encouraged to express honest feelings in a manner that is nonthreatening to other family members. Active listening, assertiveness techniques, and respect for the rights of others are taught and encouraged. Barriers to effective communication are identified and resolved.

Referrals to agencies that promote effective parenting skills may be made (e.g., parent effectiveness training). Alternative agencies that may provide relief from the stress of parenting may also be considered (e.g., "Mom's Day Out" programs, sitter-sharing organizations, and day-care institutions). Support groups for abusive parents may also be helpful and assistance in locating or initiating such a group may be provided.

The nurse can assist parents who are grieving the loss of a child or the birth of a child with special needs by helping them to express their true feelings associated with the loss. Feelings such as shock, denial, anger, guilt, powerlessness, and hopelessness need to be expressed in order for the parents to progress through the grief response.

Home health-care assistance can be provided for the family of a child with special needs. This can be done by making referrals to other professionals, such as speech, physical, and occupational therapists; medical social workers; psychologists; and nutritionists. If the child with special needs is hospitalized, the home health nurse can provide specific information to hospital staff that may be helpful in providing continuity of care for the client and help in the transition for the family.

Nursing intervention also includes providing assistance in the location of and referral to support groups that deal with loss of a child or birth of a child with special needs. Some nurses may serve as leaders of these types of groups in the community.

Midlife Nursing care at the secondary level of prevention during midlife becomes necessary when the individual is unable to integrate all of the changes that are occurring during this period. An inability to accept the physical and biological changes, the changes in relationships between themselves and their adult children and aging parents, and the loss of the perception of youth may result in depression for which the individual may require help to resolve.

Retirement Retirement can also result in depression for individuals who are unable to satisfactorily grieve for the loss of this aspect of their lives. This is more likely to occur if the individuals have not planned for retirement and if they have derived most of their self-esteem from their employment.

Nursing intervention at the secondary level of prevention with depressed individuals takes place in both inpatient and outpatient settings. Severely depressed clients with suicidal ideations will need close observation in the hospital setting, whereas those with mild to moderate depression may be treated in the community. A plan of care for the client with depression is found in Chapter 25. These concepts apply to the secondary level of prevention and may be used in all nursing care settings.

The physician may elect to use pharmacotherapy with antidepressants. Nurses may intervene by providing information to the client about what to expect from the medication, possible side effects, adverse effects, and how to self-administer the medication.

Situational Crises

Nursing care at the secondary level of prevention with clients undergoing situational crises occurs only if crisis intervention at the primary level failed and the individual is unable to function socially or occupationally. Exacerbation of mental illness symptoms requires intervention at the secondary level of prevention.

These disorders were addressed extensively in Unit 4. Nursing assessment, diagnosis and outcome identification, planning, and implementation, and evaluation were discussed for many of the mental illnesses identified in the *DSM-5* (APA, 2013). These skills may be applied in any setting where nursing is practiced.

A case study situation of nursing care at the secondary level of prevention in a community setting is presented in Box 36-1.

Tertiary Prevention

Individuals With Severe and Persistent Mental Illness

Severe and persistent mental illness is characterized by a functional impairment that interferes with vocational capacity, creates serious interpersonal difficulties, or is associated with a suicide plan or attempt (Jans, Stoddard, & Kraus, 2004). These disorders are identified by criteria listed in the *DSM-5*. Diagnoses include schizophrenia and related disorders, bipolar disorder, autism spectrum disorder, major depressive disorder, panic disorder, obsessive-compulsive disorder, posttraumatic stress disorder, borderline personality disorder, and attention-deficit/hyperactivity disorder (Jans et al., 2004; National Alliance on Mental Illness [NAMI], 2012). Severe and persistent mental disorders affect 5 to 10 million adults and 3 to 5 million children in the United States.

BOX 36-1 Secondary Prevention Case Study: Parenthood

The identified patient was a petite, doll-like 4-year-old girl named Tanya. She was the older of two children in a Latino American family. The other child was a boy named Joseph, aged 2. The mother was 5 months pregnant with their third child. The family had been referred to the nurse after Tanya was placed in foster care following a report to the Department of Health and Human Services by her nursery school teacher that the child had marks on her body suspicious of child abuse.

The parents, Paulo and Annette, were in their mid-20s. Paulo had lost his job at an aircraft plant 3 months ago and had been unable to find work since. Annette brought in a few dollars from cleaning houses for other people, but the family was struggling to survive.

Paulo and Annette were angry at having to see the nurse. After all, "Parents have the right to discipline their children." The nurse did not focus on the *intent* of the behavior, but instead looked at factors in the family's life that could be viewed as stressors. This family had multiple stressors: poverty, the father's unemployment, the age and spacing of the children, the mother's chronic fatigue from work at home and in other people's homes, and finally, having a child removed from the home against the parents' wishes.

During therapy with this family, the nurse discussed the behaviors associated with various developmental levels. She also discussed possible deviations from these norms and when they should be reported to the physician. The nurse and the family discussed Tanya's behavior, and how it compared with the norms.

The parents also discussed their own childhoods. They were able to relate some of the same types of behaviors that they observed in Tanya. But they both admitted that they came from families whose main method of discipline was physical punishment. Annette had been the oldest child in her large family and had been expected to "keep the younger ones in line." When she had not done so, she was punished with her father's belt. She expressed anger toward her father, although she had never been allowed to express it at the time.

Paulo's father had died when he was a small boy, and Paulo had been expected to be the "man of the family." From the time he was very young, he worked at odd jobs to bring money into the home. Because of this, he had little time for the usual activities of childhood and adolescence. He held much resentment toward the young men who "had everything and never had to work for it."

Paulo and Annette had high expectations for Tanya. In effect, they expected her to behave in a manner well beyond her developmental level. These expectations were based on the reflections of their own childhoods. They were uncomfortable with the spontaneity and playfulness of childhood because they had had little personal experience with these behaviors. When Tanya balked and expressed the verbal assertions common to early childhood, Paulo and Annette interpreted these behaviors as defiance toward them and retaliated with anger in the manner in which they had been parented.

With the parents, the nurse explored feelings and behaviors from their past so that they were able to understand the correlation to their current behaviors. They learned to negotiate ways to deal with Tanya's age-appropriate behaviors. In combined therapy with Tanya, they learned how to relate to her childishness, and even how to enjoy playing with both of their children.

The parents ceased blaming each other for the family's problems. Annette had spent a good deal of her time deprecating Paulo for his lack of support of his family, and Paulo blamed Annette for being "unable to control her daughter." Communication patterns were clarified, and life in the family became more peaceful.

Without a need to "prove himself" to his wife, Paulo's efforts to find employment met with success because he no longer felt the need to turn down jobs that he believed his wife would perceive to be beneath his capabilities. Annette no longer works outside the home, and both she and Paulo participate in the parenting chores. Tanya and her siblings continue to demonstrate age-appropriate developmental progression.

Historical and Epidemiological Aspects

In 1955, more than half a million individuals resided in public mental hospitals. Estimates suggest that this number is fewer than 100,000 today.

Deinstitutionalization of persons with serious mental illness began in the 1960s as national policy change and with a strong belief in the individual's right to freedom. Other considerations included the deplorable conditions of some of the state asylums, the introduction of psychotropic medications, and the cost-effectiveness of caring for these individuals in the community setting.

Deinstitutionalization began to occur rapidly and without sufficient planning for the needs of these individuals as they reentered the community. Those who were fortunate enough to have support systems to provide assistance with living arrangements and sheltered employment experiences most often received the outpatient treatment they required. Those without adequate support, however, either managed to survive on a meager existence or were forced to join the ranks of the homeless. Some ended up in nursing homes meant to provide care for individuals with physical disabilities.

Certain segments of our population with severe and persistent mental illness have been left untreated: the elderly, the "working poor," the homeless, and those individuals previously covered by funds that have been cut by various social reforms. These circumstances have promoted in individuals with severe and persistent mental illness a greater number of crisis-oriented emergency department visits and hospital admissions, and repeated confrontations with law enforcement officials.

In 2002, President George W. Bush established the New Freedom Commission on Mental Health. This commission was charged with the task of conducting a comprehensive study of the United States mental health service delivery system. They were to identify unmet needs and barriers to services and recommend steps for improvement in services and support for individuals with serious mental illness. In July 2003, the commission presented its final report to the President (President's New Freedom Commission on Mental Health, 2003). The Commission identified the following five barriers:

1. **Fragmentation and gaps in care for children.** About 7 to 9 percent of all children (ages 9 to 17) have a serious emotional disturbance (SED). The Commission found that services for children are even more fragmented than those for adults, with more uncoordinated funding and differing eligibility requirements. Only a fraction of children with SED appear to have access to school-based or school-linked mental health services. Children with SED who are identified for special education services have higher levels of absenteeism, higher drop-out rates, and lower levels of academic achievement than students with other disabilities.

2. **Fragmentation and gaps in care for adults with serious mental illness.** The commission expressed concern that so many adults with serious mental illness are homeless, dependent on alcohol or drugs, unemployed, and go without treatment. According to the World Health Organization (WHO), neuropsychiatric conditions account for 13 percent of the total Disability Adjusted Life Years (DALYs) lost due to all disease and injuries in the world, and are expected to increase by 15 percent by the year 2020 (WHO, 2004). The Commission identified public attitudes and the stigma associated with mental illness as major barriers to treatment. Stigma is often internalized by individuals with mental illness, leading to hopelessness, lower self-esteem, and isolation. Stigma deprives these individuals of the support they need to recover.

3. **High unemployment and disability for people with serious mental illness.** Undetected, untreated, and poorly treated mental disorders interrupt careers, leading many individuals into lives of disability, poverty, and long-term dependence. The commission found a 90 percent unemployment rate among adults with serious mental illness—the worst level of employment of any group of people with disabilities. Some surveys have shown that many individuals with serious mental illness *want* to work, and could, with modest assistance. However, the largest "program" of assistance the United States has for people with mental illness is disability payments. Sadly, societal stigma is also reflected in employment discrimination against people with mental illness.

4. **Older adults with mental illnesses are not receiving care.** The commission reported that about 5 to 10 percent of older adults have major depression, yet most are not properly recognized and treated. The report stated:

   Older people are reluctant to get care from specialists. They feel more comfortable going to their primary care physician. Still, they are often more sensitive to the stigma of mental illness, and do not readily bring up their sadness and despair. If they acknowledge problems, they are more likely than young people to describe physical symptoms. Primary care doctors may see their suffering as "natural" aging, or treat their reported physical distress instead of the underlying mental disorder. What is often missed is the deep impact of depression on older people's capacity to function in ways that are seemingly effortless for others.

5. **Mental health and suicide prevention are not yet national priorities.** The fact that the United States has failed to prioritize mental health puts many lives at stake. Families struggle to maintain equilibrium while communities strain (and often fail) to provide needed assistance for adults and children who suffer from mental illness. Over 30,000 lives are lost annually to suicide. About 90 percent of those who take their life have a mental disorder. Many individuals who commit suicide have not had the care in the months before their death that would help them to affirm life. Both the American Psychiatric Association and the National Mental Health Association have called on the U.S. Congress to pass parity legislation. Lack of equal access to insurance coverage is conspicuous evidence of the low priority placed on mental health treatment.

The Commission outlined the following goals and recommendations for mental health reform:

Goal 1. Americans will understand that mental health is essential to overall health.

Commission recommendations:

- Advance and implement a national campaign to reduce the stigma of seeking care and a national strategy for suicide prevention.
- Address mental health with the same urgency as physical health.

Goal 2. Mental health care will be consumer and family driven.

Commission recommendations:

- Develop an individualized plan of care for every adult with a serious mental illness and child with a serious emotional disturbance.
- Involve consumers and families fully in orienting the mental health system toward recovery.
- Align relevant federal programs to improve access and accountability for mental health services.
- Create a comprehensive state mental health plan.
- Protect and enhance the rights of people with mental illness.

Goal 3. Disparities in mental health services will be eliminated.

Commission recommendations:

- Improve access to quality care that is culturally competent.
- Improve access to quality care in rural and geographically remote areas.

Goal 4. Early mental health screening, assessment, and referral to services will be common practice.

Commission recommendations:

- Promote the mental health of young children.
- Improve and expand school mental health programs.
- Screen for co-occurring mental and substance use disorders and link with integrated treatment strategies.
- Screen for mental disorders in primary health care, across the life span, and connect to treatment and supports.

Goal 5. Excellent mental health care will be delivered and research will be accelerated.

Commission recommendations:

- Accelerate research to promote recovery and resilience, and ultimately to cure and prevent mental illnesses.
- Advance evidence-based practices using dissemination and demonstration projects, and create a public-private partnership to guide their implementation.
- Improve and expand the workforce providing evidence-based mental health services and supports.
- Develop the knowledge base in four understudied areas: mental health disparities, long-term effects of medications, trauma, and acute care.

Goal 6. Technology will be used to access mental health care and information.

Commission recommendations:

- Use health technology and telehealth to improve access and coordination of mental health care, especially for Americans in remote areas or in underserved populations.
- Develop and implement integrated electronic health record and personal health information systems.

Since the release of this report, a number of organizations have released plans for implementing some of these recommendations. Von Esenwein and associates (2005) conducted a follow-up survey of organizations represented at the 19th annual Rosalynn Carter Symposium on Mental Health Policy (which was held in 2003 just following release of the report). In this survey, nearly half of the respondents reported that at least one change had been made in their organization in response to the commission's report. Von Esenwein and associates (2005) reported:

> Factors most consistently identified as contributing to successful implementation of the recommendations of the New Freedom Commission were willingness to change within the organization, partnerships with community agencies, and availability of public funding. The most common barriers cited were financial constraints, other competing priorities within the organization, and lack of local political support. (p. 606)

The Substance Abuse and Mental Health Services Administration (SAMHSA), in collaboration with a number of other federal agencies, has outlined a plan to implement the New Freedom Commission's proposals. They have stated, "This *Federal Mental Health Action Agenda* represents the first 'to do list' of a multiyear effort to alter the form and function of the mental health system from the top down and from the bottom up" (SAMHSA, 2009). This report delineates a number of principles and action items designed to "help adults with serious mental illnesses and children with serious emotional disturbances achieve recovery to live, work, learn, and participate fully in their communities."

If the proposals outlined by the President's New Freedom Commission on Mental Health became reality, it would surely mean improvement in the care of individuals with severe and persistent mental illness. Many nurse leaders see this period of healthcare reform as an opportunity for nurses to expand their roles and assume key positions in education, prevention, assessment, and referral. Nurses are, and will continue to be, in key positions to assist individuals with severe and persistent mental illness to remain as independent as possible, to manage their illness within the community setting, and to strive to minimize the number of hospitalizations required.

Treatment Alternatives

Community Mental Health Centers The goal of community mental health centers in caring for individuals with severe and persistent mental illness is to improve coping ability and prevent exacerbation of acute symptoms. A major obstacle in meeting this goal has been the lack of advocacy or sponsorship for clients who require services from a variety of sources. This has placed responsibility for health care on an individual with mental illness who is often barely able to cope with everyday life. **Case management** (which was discussed in Chapter 9 of this text) has become a recommended method of treatment for individuals with severe and persistent mental illness. Ling and Ruscin (2013) state:

> Nurses may be uniquely qualified to be case managers because of their holistic and broad-based background, understanding of health care, and role in patient education and referrals. Case management is an area of practice that offers nurses an opportunity to build on their clinical knowledge, communication, and nursing process skills to function in an expanded patient care role.

Ling and Ruscin (2013) identify six essential activities and nursing role functions that blend with the steps of the nursing process to form a framework for nursing case management. The essential activities include:

■ **Assessment.** During the assessment process, the nurse gathers pertinent information about a client's situation and ability to function. Information may be obtained through physical examination, client interview, medical records, and reports from significant others. Ling and Ruscin state, "The case manager's goal is to obtain accurate information about the patient's status and identify factors that may significantly affect the patient's recovery and care."

■ **Planning.** A service care plan is devised with client participation. The plan should include mutually agreed-on goals, specific actions directed toward goal achievement, and selection of essential resources and services through collaboration among health care professionals, the client, and the family or significant others.

■ **Implementation.** In this phase, the client receives the needed services from the appropriate providers. In some instances the nursing **case manager** is also a provider of care, whereas in others, he or she is only the coordinator of care.

■ **Coordination.** The case manager organizes, secures, integrates, and modifies the resources necessary to accomplish the case management goals (Case Management Society of America [CMSA], 2010). This coordination effort involves the client, the physician, any other pertinent health-care providers, and family members or significant others concerned with the client's care. The case manager ensures that all tests and treatments are conducted according to schedule, and maintains close communication with all health-care providers to ensure that client care is proceeding according to the plan.

■ **Monitoring.** The case manager monitors the effectiveness of the care plan by gathering pertinent information from various sources at regular intervals to determine the client's response and progress (CMSA, 2010). If problems are identified, immediate adjustments are made.

■ **Evaluation.** The case manager evaluates the client's responses to interventions and progress toward preestablished goals. Regular contact is maintained with client, family or significant others, and direct service providers. Ongoing coordination of care continues until outcomes have been achieved. If the expected outcomes are not achieved, the case manager reevaluates the plan to determine the reason, and takes steps to intervene and modify the existing plan.

A case study of nursing case management within a community mental health center is presented in Box 36-2.

Program of Assertive Community Treatment (PACT) NAMI (2013) defines PACT as a service-delivery model that provides comprehensive, locally based treatment to people with serious and persistent mental illnesses. PACT is a type of case-management program that provides highly individualized services directly to

BOX 36-2 Nursing Case Management in the Community Mental Health Center: A Case Study

Michael, 73 years old with a history of multiple psychiatric admissions, has lived in various adult foster homes and boarding houses for the past 10 years. He was originally diagnosed as having schizophrenia, but he was recently rediagnosed as having bipolar I disorder. His symptoms are well controlled with lithium 300 mg three times a day, which is prescribed by the outpatient psychiatrist.

The nurse practitioner/case manager in the outpatient clinic coordinates Michael's care, advocates for his needs, and counsels him regarding his health problems, She orders routine blood tests to assess his lithium levels. When Michael experienced visual disturbances, she referred him for an emergency eye evaluation. He was found to have a retinal detachment and was sent to a local Veteran's Administration (VA) hospital for emergency surgery. After his eye surgery, the nurse practitioner arranged transportation to his follow-up visits with the eye doctor and instructed him about his eye care and instillation of his eye drops. Michael did not like putting eye drops in his eye and tended to neglect doing it. Because he also had glaucoma and required ongoing treatment with pilocarpine and timolol maleate eye drops twice daily, he needed a great deal of education and reassurance to continue using the eye drops.

In addition to routine quarterly visits for ongoing case management, the nurse practitioner also performs his annual health assessment consisting of history, review of systems, mental status exam, and physical assessment. During Michael's last physical exam, the nurse practitioner

detected a thyroid mass and referred him for a complete evaluation including thyroid function tests, a thyroid scan, and evaluation by a surgeon and an endocrinologist. She discussed his thyroid problem with the surgeon and the endocrinologist, and they determined that Michael would best benefit from thyroid replacement (i.e., levothyroxine sodium 0.1 mg daily).

Because Michael eats all of his meals in restaurants, the nurse was concerned about his diet. A brief diet review revealed that his diet was low in vitamin C. He was then instructed in which foods and juices he should include in his daily menu. The nurse practitioner discussed ways that Michael could get the best nutrition for the least cost.

Michael currently is living in a boarding house and is totally responsible for taking his own medication, attending to his activities of daily living, and managing his own money. He has very limited income and depends on donations for many of his clothing needs.

Despite his age, he is quite active and alert. He attends many VA-sponsored social activities and does daily volunteer work at the VA, such as pushing wheelchairs, running errands, and escorting other veterans to clinic appointments. His nurse case manager arranged for him to receive free lunches as a reward for some of his volunteer activities.

Nursing case management has helped this elderly gentleman with severe and persistent psychiatric illness and many years of hospitalization to live independently within the community setting.

From Pittman, D.C. (1989). Nursing case management: Holistic care for the deinstitutionalized chronically mentally ill. Journal of Psychosocial Nursing, 27(11), 23-27, with permission.

consumers. It is a team approach, and includes members from psychiatry, social work, nursing, and substance abuse and vocational rehabilitation. The PACT team provides these services 24 hours a day, 7 days a week, 365 days a year.

NAMI (2013) identifies the primary goals of PACT as follows:

■ To lessen or eliminate the debilitating symptoms of mental illness each individual client experiences

■ To minimize or prevent recurrent acute episodes of the illness

■ To meet basic needs and enhance quality of life

■ To improve functioning in adult social and employment roles

■ To enhance an individual's ability to live independently in his or her own community

■ To lessen the family's burden of providing care

The PACT team provides treatment, rehabilitation, and support services to individuals with severe and persistent mental illness who are unable on their own to receive treatment from a traditional model of case management. The team is usually able to provide most services with minimal referrals to other mental health

programs or providers. Services are provided within community settings, such as a person's home, local restaurants, parks, nearby stores, and any other place that the individual requires assistance with living skills.

Studies have shown that PACT clients spend significantly less time in hospitals and more time in independent living situations, have less time unemployed, earn more income from competitive employment, experience more positive social relationships, express greater satisfaction with life, and are less symptomatic (NAMI, 2013). Only about half of the states currently have PACT programs established or under pilot testing. NAMI (2013) states:

> Despite the documented treatment success of PACT, only a fraction of those with the greatest needs have access to this uniquely effective program. In the United States, adults with severe and persistent mental illnesses constitute one-half to 1 percent of the adult population. It is estimated that 10 to 20 percent of this group could be helped by the PACT model if it were available.

Day-Evening Treatment/Partial Hospitalization Programs

Day or evening treatment programs (also called partial hospitalization) are designed to prevent institutionalization or to ease the transition from in-patient hospitalization to community living. Various types of treatment are offered. Many include therapeutic community (milieu) activities; individual, group, and family therapies; psychoeducation; alcohol and drug education; crisis intervention; therapeutic recreational activities; and occupational therapy. Many programs offer medication administration and monitoring as part of their care. Some programs have established medication clinics for individuals on long-term psychopharmacological therapy. These clinics may include educational classes and support groups for individuals with similar conditions and treatments.

Partial hospitalization programs generally offer a comprehensive treatment plan formulated by an inter-disciplinary team of psychiatrists, psychologists, nurses, occupational and recreational therapists, and social workers. Nurses take a leading role in the administration of partial hospitalization programs. They lead groups, provide crisis intervention, conduct individual counseling, act as role models, and make necessary referrals for specialized treatment. Use of the nursing process provides continual evaluation of the program, and modifications can be made as necessary.

Partial hospitalization programs have proven to be an effective method of preventing hospitalization for many individuals with severe and persistent mental illness. They are a way of transitioning these individuals from the acute care setting back into the mainstream of the community. For some individuals who have been deinstitutionalized, they provide structure, support, opportunities for socialization, and an improvement in their overall quality of life.

Community Residential Facilities Community residential facilities for persons with severe and persistent mental illness are known by many names: group homes, halfway houses, foster homes, boarding homes, sheltered care facilities, transitional housing, independent living programs, social rehabilitation residences, and others. These facilities differ by the purpose for which they exist and the activities that they offer.

Some of these facilities provide food, shelter, housekeeping, and minimal supervision and assistance with activities of daily living. Others may also include a variety of therapies and serve as a transition between hospital and independent living. In addition to the basics, services might include individual and group counseling, medical care, job training or employment assistance, and leisure-time activities.

A wide variety of personnel staff these facilities. Some facilities have live-in professionals who are available at all times, some have professional staff who are on call for intervention during crisis situations, and some are staffed by volunteers and individuals with

little knowledge or background for understanding and treating persons with severe and persistent mental illness.

The concept of transitional housing for individuals with serious mental illness is sound and has proved in many instances to be a successful means of therapeutic support and intervention for maintaining them within the community. However, without guidance and planning, transition to the community can be futile. These individuals may be ridiculed and rejected by the community. They may be targets of unscrupulous individuals who take advantage of their inability to care for themselves satisfactorily. These behaviors may increase maladaptive responses to the demands of community living and exacerbate the mental illness. A period of structured reorientation to the community in a living situation that is supervised and monitored by professionals is more likely to result in a successful transition for the individual with severe and persistent mental illness.

Psychiatric Home Health Care For the individual with serious mental illness who no longer lives in a structured, supervised setting, home health care may be the element that helps to keep him or her living independently. To receive home health care, individuals must validate their homebound status for the prospective payer (Medicare, Medicaid, most insurance companies, and Department of Veterans Affairs [VA] benefits). An acute psychiatric diagnosis is not enough to qualify for the service. The client must show that he or she is unable to leave the home without considerable difficulty or the assistance of another person. The plan of treatment and subsequent charting must explain why the client's psychiatric disorder keeps him or her at home and justify the need for home services.

Homebound clients most often have a diagnosis of depressive disorder, neurocognitive disorder, anxiety disorder, bipolar disorder, or schizophrenia. Many elderly clients are homebound because of medical conditions that impair mobility and necessitate home care.

Nurses who provide psychiatric home care must have an in-depth knowledge of psychopathology, psychopharmacology, and how medical and physical problems can be influenced by psychiatric impairments. These nurses must be highly adept at performing biopsychosocial assessments. They must be sensitive to changes in behavior that signal that the client is decompensating psychiatrically or medically so that early intervention may be implemented.

Another important job of the psychiatric home health nurse is monitoring the client's adherence to the regimen of psychotropic medications. Some clients who are receiving injectable medications remain on home health care only until they can be placed on oral medications. Those clients receiving oral medications require close monitoring for adherence and assistance with the uncomfortable side effects of some of these drugs. Lack of adherence to the medication regimen is responsible for approximately two-thirds of psychiatric hospital readmissions. Home health nurses can assist clients with this problem by helping them to see the relationship between control of their psychiatric symptoms and adherence to their medication regimen.

Client populations that benefit from psychiatric home health nursing include:

■ **Elderly clients.** These individuals may not have a psychiatric diagnosis, but they may be experiencing emotional difficulties that have arisen from medical, sociocultural, or developmental factors. Depressed mood and social isolation are common.

■ **Persons with severe and persistent mental illness.** These individuals have a history of psychiatric illness and hospitalization. They require long-term medications and continual supportive care. Common diagnoses include recurrent major depressive disorder, schizophrenia, and bipolar disorder.

■ **Individuals in acute crisis situations.** These individuals are in need of crisis intervention and/or short-term psychotherapy.

The American Nurses Association (ANA) (2008) defines home health nursing as:

> . . . nursing practice applied to patients of all ages in the patient's residences, which may include private homes, assisted living, or personal care facilities. Patients and their families and other caregivers are the focus of home health nursing practice. The goal of care is to maintain or improve the quality of life for patients and their families and other caregivers, or to support patients in their transition to end of life. (p. 3)

Medicare requires that psychiatric home nursing care be provided by "psychiatrically trained nurses," which they define as, ". . . nurses who have special training and/or experience beyond the standard curriculum required for a registered nurse" (Centers for Medicare & Medicaid Services [CMS], 2011).

The guidelines that cover psychiatric nursing services are not well defined by the CMS. This has presented some reimbursement problems for psychiatric nurses in the past. The CMS statement regarding psychiatric nursing services is presented in Box 36-3.

Preparation for psychiatric home health nursing, in addition to the registered nurse licensure, should include several years of psychiatric inpatient treatment experience. It is also recommended that the nurse have medical-surgical nursing experience, because of

---

BOX 36-3 CMS Guidelines for Psychiatric Home Nursing Care

PSYCHIATRIC EVALUATION, THERAPY, AND TEACHING

The evaluation, psychotherapy, and teaching needed by a patient suffering from a diagnosed psychiatric disorder that requires active treatment by a psychiatrically trained nurse and the costs of the psychiatric nurse's services may be covered as a skilled nursing service. Psychiatrically trained nurses are nurses who have special training and/or experience beyond the standard curriculum required for a registered nurse. The services of the psychiatric nurse are to be provided under a plan of care established and reviewed by a physician.

From Centers for Medicare & Medicaid Services. (2011). Medicare benefit policy manual. Baltimore, MD: Author.

---

common client physical co-morbidity and the holistic nursing perspective. Additional training and experience in psychotherapy is viewed as an asset. However, psychotherapy is not the primary focus of psychiatric home nursing care. In fact, most reimbursement sources do not pay for exclusively insight-oriented therapy. Crisis intervention, client education, and hands-on care are common interventions in psychiatric home nursing care.

The psychiatric home health nurse provides comprehensive nursing care, incorporating interventions for physical and psychosocial problems into the treatment plan. The interventions are based on the client's mental and physical health status, cultural influences, and available resources. The nurse is accountable to the client at all times during the therapeutic relationship. Nursing interventions are carried out with appropriate knowledge and skill, and referrals are made when the need is outside the scope of nursing practice. Continued collaboration with other members of the health-care team (e.g., psychiatrist, social worker, psychologist, occupational therapist, and/or physical therapist) is essential for maintaining continuity of care.

A case study of psychiatric home health care and the nursing process is presented in Box 36-4. A plan of care for Mrs. C (the client in the case study) is presented in Table 36-2. Nursing diagnoses are presented, along with outcome criteria, appropriate nursing interventions, and rationale for each.

Care for the Caregivers Another aspect of psychiatric home health care is to provide support and assistance to primary caregivers. When family is the provider of care on a 7-day-a-week, 24-hour-a-day schedule for a loved one with a severe and persistent mental disorder,

BOX 36-4 Psychiatric Home Health Care and the Nursing Process: A Case Study

ASSESSMENT

Mrs. C, aged 76, has been living alone in her small apartment for 6 months since the death of her husband, to whom she had been married for 51 years. Mrs. C had been an elementary school teacher for 40 years, retiring at age 65 with an adequate pension. She and her husband had no children. A niece looks in on Mrs. C regularly. It was she who contacted Mrs. C's physician when she observed that Mrs. C was not eating properly, was losing weight, and seemed to be isolating herself more and more. She had not left her apartment in weeks. Her physician referred her to psychiatric home health care.

On her initial visit, Carol, the psychiatric home health nurse, conducted a preliminary assessment revealing the following information about Mrs. C:

1. Blood pressure 90/60 mm Hg.
2. Height 5'5"; weight 102 lb.
3. Poor skin turgor; dehydration.
4. Subjective report of occasional dizziness.
5. Subjective report of loss of 20 pounds since the death of her husband.
6. Oriented to time, place, person, and situation.
7. Memory (remote and recent) intact.
8. Flat affect.
9. Mood is dysphoric and tearful at times, but client is cooperative.
10. Denies thoughts to harm self, but states, "I feel so alone; so useless."
11. Subjective report of difficulty sleeping.
12. Subjective report of constipation.

DIAGNOSIS/OUTCOME IDENTIFICATION

The following nursing diagnoses were formulated for Mrs. C:

1. Complicated grieving related to death of husband evidenced by symptoms of depression such as withdrawal, anorexia, weight loss, difficulty sleeping, dysphoric/tearful mood.
2. Risk for injury related to dizziness and weakness from lack of activity, low blood pressure, and poor nutritional status.
3. Social isolation related to depressed mood and feelings of worthlessness, evidenced by staying home alone, refusing to leave her apartment.

Outcome Criteria

The following criteria were selected as measurement of outcomes in the care of Mrs. C:

1. Experiences no physical harm/injury.
2. Is able to discuss feelings about husband's death with nurse.

3. Sets realistic goals for self.
4. Is able to participate in problem solving regarding her future.
5. Eats a well-balanced diet with snacks to restore nutritional status and gain weight.
6. Drinks adequate fluid daily.
7. Sleeps at least 6 hours per night and verbalizes feeling well rested.
8. Shows interest in personal appearance and hygiene, and is able to accomplish self-care independently.
9. Seeks to renew contact with previous friends and acquaintances.
10. Verbalizes interest in participating in social activities.

PLAN/IMPLEMENTATION

A plan of care for Mrs. C is presented in Table 36-2.

EVALUATION

Mrs. C started the second week taking trazodone (Desyrel) 150 mg at bedtime. Her sleep was enhanced and within 2 weeks she showed a noticeable improvement in mood. She began to discuss how angry she felt about being all alone in the world. She admitted that she had felt anger toward her husband but experienced guilt and tried to suppress that anger. As she was assured that these feelings were normal, they became easier for her to express.

The nurse arranged for a local teenager to do some weekly grocery shopping for Mrs. C and contacted the local Meals on Wheels program, which delivered her noon meal to her every day. Mrs. C began to eat more and slowly to gain a few pounds. She still has an occasional problem with constipation but verbalizes improvement with the addition of vegetables, fruit, and a daily stool softener prescribed by her physician.

Mrs. C used her walker until she felt she was able to ambulate without assistance. She reports that she no longer experiences dizziness, and her blood pressure has stabilized at around 100/70 mm Hg.

Mrs. C has joined a senior citizens group and attends activities weekly. She has renewed previous friendships and formed new acquaintances. She sees her physician monthly for medication management and visits a local adult day health center for regular blood pressure and weight checks. Her niece still visits regularly, but her favorite relationship is the one she has formed with her constant canine companion, Molly, whom Mrs. C rescued from the local animal shelter and who continually demonstrates her unconditional love and gratitude.

Table 36-2 | CARE PLAN FOR PSYCHIATRIC HOME HEALTH CARE OF DEPRESSED ELDERLY (MRS. C)

NURSING DIAGNOSIS: COMPLICATED GRIEVING

RELATED TO: Death of husband

EVIDENCED BY: Symptoms of depression such as withdrawal, anorexia, weight loss, difficulty sleeping, and dysphoric/tearful mood

OUTCOME CRITERIA	NURSING INTERVENTIONS	RATIONALE
Short-Term Goal • Mrs. C will discuss any angry feelings she has about the loss of her husband. **Long-Term Goal** • Mrs. C will demonstrate adaptive grieving behaviors and evidence of progression toward resolution.	1. Assess Mrs. C's position in the grief process. 2. Develop a trusting relationship by showing empathy and caring. Be honest and keep all promises. Show genuine positive regard. 3. Explore feelings of anger and help Mrs. C direct them toward the source. Help her understand it is appropriate and acceptable to have feelings of anger and guilt about her husband's death. 4. Encourage Mrs. C to review honestly the relationship she had with her husband. With support and sensitivity, point out reality of the situation in areas where misrepresentations may be expressed. 5. Determine if Mrs. C has spiritual needs that are going unfulfilled. If so, contact spiritual leader for intervention with Mrs. C. 6. Refer Mrs. C to physician for medication evaluation.	1. Accurate baseline data are required to plan accurate care for Mrs. C. 2. These interventions provide the basis for a therapeutic relationship 3. Knowledge of acceptability of the feelings associated with normal grieving may help to relieve some of the guilt that these responses generate. 4. Mrs. C must give up an idealized perception of her husband. Only when she is able to see both positive and negative aspects about the relationship will the grieving process be complete. 5. Recovery may be blocked if spiritual distress is present and care is not provided. 6. Antidepressant therapy may help Mrs. C to function while confronting the dynamics of her depression.

NURSING DIAGNOSIS: RISK FOR INJURY

RELATED TO: Dizziness and weakness from lack of activity, low blood pressure, and poor nutritional status

OUTCOME CRITERIA	NURSING INTERVENTIONS	RATIONALE
Short-Term Goals • Mrs. C will use walker when ambulating. • Mrs. C will not experience physical harm or injury. **Long-Term Goal** • Mrs. C will not experience physical harm or injury.	1. Assess vital signs at every visit. Report to physician should they fall below baseline. 2. Encourage Mrs. C to use walker until strength has returned. 3. Visit Mrs. C during mealtimes and sit with her while she eats. Encourage her niece to do the same. Ensure that easy to prepare, nutritious foods for meals and snacks are available in the house and that they are items that Mrs. C likes.	1. Client safety is a nursing priority. 2. The walker will help prevent Mrs. C from falling. 3. She is more likely to eat what is convenient and what she enjoys.

Continued

Table 36-2 | CARE PLAN FOR PSYCHIATRIC HOME HEALTH CARE OF DEPRESSED ELDERLY (MRS. C)–cont'd

OUTCOME CRITERIA	NURSING INTERVENTIONS	RATIONALE
	4. Contact local meal delivery service (e.g., Meals on Wheels) to deliver some of Mrs. C's meals.	4. This would ensure that she receives at least one complete and nutritious meal each day.
	5. Weigh Mrs. C each week.	5. Weight gain is a measurable, objective means of assessing whether Mrs. C is eating.
	6. Ensure that diet contains sufficient fluid and fiber.	6. Adequate dietary fluid and fiber will help to alleviate constipation. She may also benefit from a daily stool softener.

NURSING DIAGNOSIS: SOCIAL ISOLATION

RELATED TO: Depressed mood and feelings of worthlessness

EVIDENCED BY: Staying home alone, refusing to leave apartment

OUTCOME CRITERIA	NURSING INTERVENTIONS	RATIONALE
Short-Term Goal • Mrs. C will discuss with nurse feelings about past social relationships and those she may like to renew. **Long-Term Goal** • Mrs. C will renew contact with friends and participate in social activities.	1. As nutritional status is improving and strength is gained, encourage Mrs. C to become more active. Take walks with her; help her perform simple tasks around her house.	1. Increased activity enhances both physical and mental status.
	2. Assess lifelong patterns of relationships.	2. Basic personality characteristics will not change. Mrs. C will very likely keep the same style of relationship development that she had in the past.
	3. Help her identify present relationships that are satisfying and activities that she considers interesting.	3. She is the person who truly knows what she likes, and these personal preferences will facilitate success in reversing social isolation.
	4. Consider the feasibility of a pet.	4. There are many documented studies of the benefits to elderly individuals of companion pets.
	5. Suggest possible alternatives that Mrs. C may consider as she seeks to participate in social activities. These may include foster grandparent programs, senior citizens centers, church activities, craft groups, and volunteer activities. Help her to locate individuals with whom she may attend some of these activities.	5. She is more likely to attend and participate if she does not have to do so alone.

it can be very exhausting and very frustrating. A care plan for primary caregivers is presented in Table 36-3.

The Homeless Population

Historical and Epidemiological Aspects

In 1993, Dr. Richard Lamb, a recognized expert in the field of severe and persistent mental illness, wrote:

> Alec Guinness, in his memorable role as a British Army colonel in *Bridge on the River Kwai*, exclaims at the end of the film when he finally realizes he has been working to help the enemy, "What have I done?" As a vocal advocate and spokesman for deinstitutionalization and community treatment of severely mentally ill patients for well over two decades, I often find myself asking that same question (p. 1209).

The number of homeless in the United States has been estimated at somewhere between 250,000 and 4 million. It is difficult to determine the true scope of the problem because even the statisticians who collect

---

Table 36-3 | CARE PLAN FOR PRIMARY CAREGIVER OF CLIENT WITH SEVERE AND PERSISTENT MENTAL ILLNESS

NURSING DIAGNOSIS: CAREGIVER ROLE STRAIN

RELATED TO: Severity and duration of the care receiver's illness and lack of respite and recreation for the caregiver

EVIDENCED BY: Feelings of stress in relationship with care receiver, feelings of depression and anger, family conflict around issues of providing care

OUTCOME CRITERIA	NURSING INTERVENTIONS	RATIONALE
Short-Term Goal • Caregivers will verbalize understanding of ways to facilitate the caregiver role. **Long-Term Goal** • Caregivers will demonstrate effective problem-solving skills and develop adaptive coping mechanisms to regain equilibrium.	1. Assess caregivers' abilities to anticipate and fulfill client's unmet needs. Provide information to assist caregivers with this responsibility. Ensure that caregivers encourage client to be as independent as possible.	1. Caregivers may be unaware of what the client can realistically accomplish. They may be unaware of the nature of the illness.
	2. Ensure that caregivers are aware of available community support systems from which they may seek assistance when required. Examples include respite care services, day treatment centers, and adult day-care centers.	2. Caregivers require relief from the pressures and strain of providing 24-hour care for their loved one. Studies have shown that abuse arises out of caregiving situations that place overwhelming stress on the caregivers.
	3. Encourage caregivers to express feelings, particularly anger.	3. Release of these emotions can serve to prevent psychopathology, such as depression or psychophysiological disorders, from occurring.
	4. Encourage participation in support groups comprised of members with similar life situations. Provide information about support groups that may be helpful: a. National Alliance on Mental Illness (NAMI) (800) 950-NAMI b. American Association on Intellectual and Developmental Disabilities (AAIDD) (800) 424-3688 c. Alzheimer's Association (800) 272-3900	4. Hearing others who are experiencing the same problems discuss ways in which they have coped may help caregiver adopt more adaptive strategies. Individuals who are experiencing similar life situations provide empathy and support for each other.

the data have difficulty defining homeless persons. They have sometimes been identified as, "those people who sleep in shelters or public spaces." This approach results in underestimates because available shelter services are insufficient to meet the numbers of homeless people (U.S. Conference of Mayors [USCM], 2012).

According to the Stewart B. McKinney Act, a person is considered homeless who:

> lacks a fixed, regular, and adequate night-time residence; and . . . has a primary night-time residency that is: (A) a supervised publicly or privately operated shelter designed to provide temporary living accommodations, (B) an institution that provides a temporary residence for individuals intended to be institutionalized, or (C) a public or private place not designed for, or ordinarily used as, a regular sleeping accommodation for human beings. (National Coalition for the Homeless [NCH], 2009d)

Two methods of counting the homeless are commonly used (NCH, 2009c). The *point-in-time* method attempts to count all the people who are literally homeless on a given day or during a given week. The second method (called *period prevalence counts*) examines the number of people who are homeless over a given period of time. This second method may result in a more accurate count because the extended time period would allow for including the people who are homeless one day (or week) but find employment and affordable housing later, removing them from the homeless count. At the same time during this extended period, others would lose housing and become homeless.

Who Are the Homeless?

The homeless are increasingly a heterogeneous group. The NCH (2009d) provided the following demographics:

Age Studies have produced a variety of statistics related to age of the homeless: 39 percent are younger than 18 years of age; individuals between the ages of 25 and 34 make up 25 percent; and 6 percent are ages 55 to 64.

Gender Statistics for 2010 indicated that 62 percent of homeless individuals were male and 38 percent were female (SAMHSA, 2011).

Families Families with children are among the fastest growing segments of the homeless population. They make up 23 percent of the homeless population, but research indicates that this number is higher in rural areas, where families, single mothers, and children account for the largest group of homeless people.

Ethnicity The homeless population is estimated to be 37 percent African American, 41 percent Caucasian,

10 percent Hispanic, 5 percent of other single races, and 7 percent of multiple races (SAMHSA, 2011). The ethnic makeup of homeless populations varies according to geographic location.

Mental Illness and Homelessness

The USCM (2012) survey revealed that approximately 30 percent of the homeless population suffers from some form of mental illness. Who are these individuals, and why are they homeless? Some blame the deinstitutionalization movement. Persons with mental illness who were released from state and county mental hospitals and who did not have families with whom they could reside sought residence in board-and-care homes of varying quality. Halfway houses and supportive group living arrangements were helpful but scarce. Many of those with families returned to their homes, but because families received little if any instruction or support, the consequences of their mentally ill loved one returning to live at home were often turbulent, resulting in the individual frequently leaving home.

Types of Mental Illness Among the Homeless A number of studies have been conducted, primarily in large, urban areas, that have addressed the most common types of mental illness identified among homeless individuals. Schizophrenia is frequently described as the most common diagnosis. Other prevalent disorders include bipolar disorder, substance addiction, depression, personality disorders, and neurocognitive disorders. Many exhibit psychotic symptoms, many are former residents of long-term care institutions for the mentally ill, and many have such a strong desire for independence that they isolate themselves in an effort to avoid being identified as a part of the mental health system. Many of them are clearly a danger to themselves or others, yet they often do not even see themselves as ill.

Contributing Factors to Homelessness Among Individuals With Mental Illness

Deinstitutionalization As previously stated, deinstitutionalization is frequently implicated as a contributing factor to homelessness among individuals with mental illness. Deinstitutionalization began out of expressed concern by mental health professionals and others who described the "deplorable conditions" under which mentally ill individuals were housed.

The advent of psychotropic medications and the community mental health movement began a growing philosophical view that individuals with mental illness receive better and more humanitarian treatment in the community than in state hospitals far removed from their homes. It was believed that commitment and institutionalization in many ways deprived these individuals of their civil rights. Not the least of the motivating factors for deinstitutionalization was the financial burden these clients placed on state governments.

In fact, deinstitutionalization has not failed completely. About 50 percent of the mentally ill population—those who have insight into their illness and need for medication—have done reasonably well. It is individuals from the other 50 percent, those who lack such insight and who frequently stop taking their medication, that often end up on the streets.

However, because the vast increases in homelessness did not occur until the 1980s, the release of severely mentally ill people from institutions cannot be solely to blame. A number of other factors have been implicated.

Poverty Cuts in various government entitlement programs have depleted the allotments available for individuals with severe and persistent mental illness living in the community. The job market is prohibitive for individuals whose behavior is incomprehensible or even frightening to many. The stigma and discrimination associated with mental illness may be diminishing slowly, but it is highly visible to those who suffer from its effects.

A Scarcity of Affordable Housing The National Coalition for the Homeless (NCH, 2009e) states:

> A lack of affordable housing and the limited scale of housing assistance programs have contributed to the current housing crisis and to homelessness. The lack of affordable housing has led to high rent burdens (rents which absorb a high proportion of income), overcrowding, and substandard housing. These phenomena, in turn, have not only forced many people to become homeless; they have put a large and growing number of people at risk of becoming homeless. Recently, [a rise in the percentage of housing] foreclosures has increased the number of people who experience homelessness.

In addition, the number of single-room-occupancy (SRO) hotels has diminished drastically. These SRO hotels provided a means of relatively inexpensive housing, and although some people believe that these facilities nurtured isolation, they provided adequate shelter from the elements for their occupants. So many individuals currently frequent the shelters of our cities that there is concern that the shelters are becoming mini-institutions for individuals with serious mental illness.

Other Factors Several other factors that may contribute to homelessness have been identified (NCH, 2009e). They include the following:

■ **Lack of affordable health care.** For families barely able to scrape together enough money to pay for

day-to-day living, a catastrophic illness can create the level of poverty that starts the downward spiral to homelessness.

■ **Domestic Violence.** The NCH (2009e) reports that domestic violence is a primary cause of homelessness, with approximately 63 percent of homeless women having experienced domestic violence in their adult lives. Battered women are often forced to choose between an abusive relationship and homelessness.

■ **Addiction Disorders.** For individuals with alcohol or drug addictions, in the absence of appropriate treatment, the chances increase for being forced into life on the street. The following have been cited as obstacles to addiction treatment for homeless persons: lack of health insurance, lack of documentation, waiting lists, scheduling difficulties, daily contact requirements, lack of transportation, ineffective treatment methods, lack of supportive services, and cultural insensitivity.

Community Resources for the Homeless

Interfering Factors Among the many issues that complicate service planning for homeless individuals with mental illness is this population's penchant for mobility. Frequent relocation confounds service delivery and interferes with providers' efforts to ensure appropriate care. Some individuals with serious mental illness may be affected by homelessness only temporarily or intermittently. These individuals are sometimes called the "episodically homeless." Others move around within neighborhoods or cities as needs change and based on whether or not they can obtain needed services. A large number of the homeless mentally ill population exhibits continuous unbounded movement over wide geographical areas.

Not all homeless individuals with mental illness are mobile. Some studies have indicated that a large percentage remains in the same location over a number of years. Health-care workers must identify movement patterns of homeless people in their area to at least try to bring the best care possible to this unique population. This may indeed mean delivering services to those individuals who do not seek out services on their own.

Health Issues Life as a homeless person can have severe consequences in terms of health. Exposure to the elements, poor diet, sleep deprivation, risk of violence, injuries, and little or no health care lead to a precarious state of health and exacerbate any preexisting illnesses. One of the major afflictions is alcoholism. It has been estimated that about 40 percent of homeless individuals abuse alcohol. Compared to other homeless individuals, those who abuse alcohol are at greater risk for neurological impairment, heart disease and hypertension, chronic lung disease, gastrointestinal (GI) disorders, hepatic dysfunction, and trauma.

Thermoregulation is a health problem for all homeless individuals because of their exposure to all kinds of weather. It is a compounded problem for the homeless alcoholic who spends much time in an altered level of consciousness.

It is difficult to determine whether mental illness is a cause or an effect of homelessness. Some behaviors that may seem deviant to some people may in actuality be adaptations to life on the street. It has been suggested that some homeless individuals may even seek hospitalization in psychiatric institutions in an attempt to get off the streets for a while.

Outbreaks of tuberculosis among homeless persons continue to challenge public control efforts (Centers for Disease Control and Prevention [CDC], 2013). Crowded **shelters** provide ideal conditions for spread of respiratory infections among their inhabitants. The risk of acquiring tuberculosis is also increased by the prevalence of alcoholism, drug addiction, HIV infection, and poor nutrition among homeless individuals.

Dietary deficiencies are a continuing problem for homeless individuals. Not only is the homeless person commonly in a poor nutritional state, but also the condition itself exacerbates a number of other health problems. Homeless people suffer from higher mortality rates and a greater number of serious disorders than their counterparts in the general population.

Sexually transmitted diseases (STDs), such as gonorrhea and syphilis, are a serious problem for the homeless. One of the most serious STDs prevalent among homeless individuals is HIV infection. Street life is precarious for individuals whose systems are immunosuppressed by the HIV. Rummaged food scraps are often spoiled, and exposure to the elements is a continuous threat. Individuals with HIV disease who stay in shelters often are exposed to the infectious diseases of others, which can be life threatening in their vulnerable condition.

HIV disease is a serious problem among the homeless population. The NCH (2009a) reported that an estimated 3.4 percent of the homeless population are HIV-positive, compared to 0.4 percent within the general population. It is estimated that up to 50 percent of persons living with HIV disease are expected to need housing assistance of some kind during their lifetimes.

Homeless children have special health needs. The NCH (2009b) reports that children without a home have higher rates of asthma, ear infections, stomach problems, and speech problems than their counterparts who are not homeless. They also experience more mental health problems, such as anxiety, depression, and withdrawal. They are twice as likely to experience hunger and four times as likely to have delayed development.

IMPLICATIONS OF RESEARCH FOR EVIDENCE-BASED PRACTICE

Rew, L., Fouladi, R.T., & Yockey, R.D. (2002). Sexual health practices of homeless youth. *Journal of Nursing Scholarship, 34*(2), 139-145.

DESCRIPTION OF THE STUDY: The purpose of this study was to describe the sexual health practices of homeless adolescents, examine relationships among variables in a conceptual model of sexual health practices, and determine direct and indirect effects of population characteristics, cognitive-perceptual factors, and behavioral factors on sexual health practices among homeless adolescents. A survey was administered to a convenience sample of 414 homeless young men (244) and women (170) aged 16 to 20 years, the majority of whom were Anglo American. Likert-scale questionnaires were administered seeking information regarding sexually transmitted diseases (STDs), knowledge about AIDS, self-efficacy to use condoms, future time perspective, intentions to use condoms, social support, sexual health practices, assertive communication, and background information.

RESULTS OF THE STUDY: Thirty-five percent of the sample reported homosexual or bisexual orientation, and sexual orientation was reported as a reason for leaving home. Over half reported a history of sexual abuse and nearly 1 in 4 had been treated for gonorrhea. Seven percent had been treated for HIV, 8 percent for chlamydia, 3.6 percent for syphilis, and 32 percent had received one or more immunizations to prevent hepatitis B. Future time perspective scores were low, a finding that was not surprising, knowing the daily challenges of living on the street. Perceived social support scores were also low, again being an expected finding, due to lack of socially supportive environments of homes, parents, and schools. The mean safe-sex behavior score was higher than those in a study of university males. The authors speculated that this may indicate that participants were exposed to safe-sex messages more frequently at the street outreach center than were the university males. Those participants who had higher scores in perceived social support and assertive communication also had higher scores in self-efficacy to use condoms.

IMPLICATIONS FOR NURSING PRACTICE: The authors suggest that the correlation of self-efficacy to use condoms with social support and assertive communication may indicate that an intervention directed at the enhancement of assertive communication skills and social support might result in

IMPLICATIONS OF RESEARCH FOR EVIDENCE-BASED PRACTICE–cont'd

increased self-efficacy, which could in turn increase safe-sex behaviors. The authors state:

> The relationship of intention to use condoms with future time perspective, social connectedness, and self-efficacy to use condoms, but also with sexual health responsibility indicates yet another domain in which to intervene with homeless adolescents. Interventions that focus on enhancing sexual health

responsibility (e.g., seeking health care services if one suspects an STD or refusing to engage in sexual intercourse with someone known to have HIV) could have positive effects on these youth. (p. 144)

This study provides information that can be used by nurses who work with the homeless population, in an effort to change risky behavior and promote positive health-care habits under frequently unfavorable conditions.

Types of Resources Available

Homeless Shelters The system of shelters for the homeless in the United States varies widely, from converted warehouses that provide cots or floor space on which to sleep overnight to significant operations that provide a multitude of social and health-care services. They are run by volunteers and paid professionals and are sponsored by churches, community governments, and a variety of social agencies.

It is impossible, then, to describe a "typical" shelter. One profile may be described as the provision of lodging, food, and clothing to individuals who are in need of these services. Some shelters also provide medical and psychiatric evaluations, first aid and other health-care services, and referral for case management services by nurses or social workers.

Individuals who seek services from the shelter are generally assigned a bed or cot, issued a set of clean linen, provided a place to shower, shown laundry facilities, and offered a meal in the shelter kitchen or dining hall. Most shelters attempt to separate dormitory areas for men and women, with various consequences for those who violate the rules.

Shelters cover expenses through private and corporate donations, church sponsorships, and government grants. From the outset, shelters were conceptualized as "temporary" accommodations for individuals who needed a place to spend the night. Realistically, they have become permanent lodging for homeless individuals with little hope for improving their situation. Some individuals use shelters for their mailing address.

Shelters provide a safe and supportive environment for homeless individuals who have no other place to go. Some homeless people who inhabit shelters use the resources offered to improve their lot in life, whereas others become hopelessly dependent on the shelter's provisions. To a few, the availability of a shelter may even mean the difference between life and death.

Health-Care Centers and Storefront Clinics Some communities have established "street clinics" to serve the homeless population. Many of these clinics are operated by nurse practitioners who work in consultation with physicians in the area. In recent years, some of these clinics have provided clinical sites for nursing students in their community health rotation. Some have been staffed by faculties of nursing schools that have established group practices in the community setting.

A wide variety of services are offered at these clinics, including administering medications, assessing vital signs, screening for tuberculosis and other communicable diseases, giving immunizations and flu shots, changing dressings, and administering first aid. Physical and psychosocial assessments, health education, and supportive counseling are also frequent interventions.

Nursing in **storefront clinics** for the homeless provides many special challenges, not the least of which is poor working conditions. These clinics often operate under severe budgetary constraints with inadequate staffing, supplies, and equipment, in rundown facilities located in high-crime neighborhoods. Frustration is often high among nurses who work in these clinics, as they are seldom able to see measurable progress in their homeless clients. Maintenance of health management is virtually impossible for many individuals who have no resources outside the health-care setting. When return appointments for preventive care are made, the lack of follow-through is high.

Mobile Outreach Units Outreach programs literally reach out to the homeless in their own environment in an effort to provide health care. Volunteers and paid professionals form teams to drive or walk around and seek out homeless individuals who are in need of assistance. They offer coffee, sandwiches, and blankets in an effort to show concern and establish trust. If assistance can be provided at the site, it is done so. If not, every effort is made to ensure that the individual is linked with a source that can provide the necessary services.

Mobile outreach units provide assistance to homeless individuals who are in need of physical or psychological care. The emphasis of outreach programs is to accommodate the homeless who refuse to seek treatment elsewhere. Most target the mentally ill segment of the population. When trust has been established, and the individual agrees to come to the team's office, medical and psychiatric treatment is initiated. Involuntary hospitalization is initiated when an individual is deemed harmful to self or others, or otherwise meets the criteria for being considered "gravely disabled."

The Homeless Client and the Nursing Process

A case study demonstrating the nursing process with a homeless client is presented in Box 36-5.

BOX 36-5 Case Study: Nursing Process With a Homeless Client

ASSESSMENT

Joe, age 68, is brought to the Community Health Clinic by two of his peers, who report: "He just had a fit. He needs a drink bad!" Joe is dirty and unkempt, has visible tremors of the upper extremities, and is weak enough to require assistance when ambulating. He is cooperative as the nurse completes the intake assessment. He is coherent, although thought processes are slow. He is disoriented to time and place. He appears somewhat frightened as he scans the unfamiliar surroundings. He is unable to tell the nurse when he had his last drink. He reports no physical injury, and none is observable.

Joe carries a small bag with a few personal items inside, including a Department of Veterans Affairs (VA) benefit card, identifying him as a veteran of the Vietnam War. The nurse finds a cot for Joe to lie down, ensures that his vital signs are stable, and telephones the number on the VA card. The clinic nurse discovers that Joe is well known to the admissions personnel at the VA. He has a 35-year history of schizophrenia, with numerous hospitalizations. At the time of his last discharge, he was taking fluphenazine (Prolixin) 10 mg twice a day. He told the clinic nurse that he took the medication for a few months after he got out of the hospital but then did not have the prescription refilled. He could not remember when he had last taken fluphenazine.

Joe also has a long history of alcohol-related disorders and has participated in the VA substance rehabilitation program three times. He has no home address and receives his VA disability benefit checks at a shelter address. He reports that he has no family. The nurse makes arrangements for VA personnel to drive Joe from the clinic to the VA hospital, where he is admitted for detoxification. She sets up a case management file for Joe and arranges with the hospital to have Joe return to the clinic after discharge.

DIAGNOSIS/OUTCOME IDENTIFICATION

The following nursing diagnosis was formulated for Joe:

Ineffective health maintenance related to ineffective coping skills evidenced by abuse of alcohol, lack of follow-through with antipsychotic medication, and lack of personal hygiene.

Ongoing criteria were selected as outcomes for Joe. They include:

• Follows the rules of the group home and maintains his residency status.
• Attends weekly sessions of group therapy at the VA day treatment program.

• Attends weekly sessions of Alcoholics Anonymous and maintains sobriety.
• Reports regularly to the health clinic for injections of fluphenazine.
• Volunteers at the VA hospital 3 days a week.
• Secures and retains permanent employment.

PLAN/IMPLEMENTATION

During Joe's hospitalization, the clinic nurse remained in contact with his case. Joe received complete physical and dental examinations and treatment during his hospital stay. The clinic nurse attended the treatment team meeting for Joe as his outpatient case manager. It was decided at the meeting to try giving Joe injections of fluphenazine decanoate because of his history of lack of adherence to his daily oral medication regimen. The clinic nurse would administer the injection every 4 weeks.

At Joe's follow-up clinic visit the nurse explains to Joe that she has found a group home where he may live with others who have personal circumstances similar to his. At the group home, meals will be provided and the group home manager will ensure that Joe's basic needs are fulfilled. A criterion for remaining at the residence is for Joe to remain alcohol free. Joe is agreeable to these living arrangements.

With Joe's concurrence, the clinic nurse also performs the following interventions:

• Goes shopping with Joe to purchase some new clothing, allowing Joe to make decisions as independently as possible.
• Helps Joe move into the group home and introduces him to the manager and residents.
• Helps Joe change his address from the shelter to the group home so that he may continue to receive his VA benefits.
• Enrolls Joe in the weekly group therapy sessions of the day treatment facility connected with the VA hospital.
• Helps Joe locate the nearest Alcoholics Anonymous group and identifies a sponsor who will ensure that Joe gets to the meetings.
• Sets up a clinic appointment for Joe to return in 4 weeks for his fluphenazine injection; telephones Joe 1 day in advance to remind him of his appointment.
• Instructs Joe to return to or call the clinic if any of the following symptoms occur: sore throat, fever, nausea and vomiting, severe headache, difficulty urinating, tremors, skin rash, or yellow skin or eyes.
• Assists Joe in securing transportation to and from appointments.

BOX 36-5 Case Study: Nursing Process With a Homeless Client—cont'd

- Encourages Joe to set realistic goals for his life and offers recognition for follow-through.
- When Joe is ready, discusses employment alternatives with him; suggests the possibility of starting with a volunteer job (perhaps as a VA hospital volunteer).

EVALUATION

Evaluation of the nursing process with homeless individuals who have mental illness must be highly individualized. Statistics show that chances for relapse with this population are high. Therefore, it is extremely important that outcome criteria be realistic so as not to set up the client for failure.

Summary and Key Points

- The trend in psychiatric care is shifting from that of inpatient hospitalization to a focus of outpatient care within the community. This trend is largely due to the need for greater cost-effectiveness in the provision of medical care to the masses.
- The community mental health movement began in the 1960s with the closing of state hospitals and the deinstitutionalization of many individuals with severe and persistent mental illness.
- Mental health care within the community targets primary prevention (reducing the incidence of mental disorders within the population), secondary prevention (reducing the prevalence of psychiatric illness by shortening the course of the illness), and tertiary prevention (reducing the residual defects that are associated with severe and persistent mental illness).
- Primary prevention focuses on identification of populations at risk for mental illness, increasing their ability to cope with stress, and targeting and diminishing harmful forces within the environment.

- The focus of secondary prevention is accomplished through early identification of problems and prompt initiation of effective treatment.
- Tertiary prevention focuses on preventing complications of the illness and promoting rehabilitation that is directed toward achievement of the individual's maximum level of functioning.
- Registered nurses serve as providers of psychiatric/mental health care in the community setting.
- Nurses provide outpatient care for individuals with severe and persistent mental illness in community mental health centers, in day and evening treatment programs, in partial hospitalization programs, in community residential facilities, and with psychiatric home health care.
- Homeless persons with mental illness provide a special challenge for the community mental health nurse. Care is provided within homeless shelters, at health-care centers or storefront clinics, and through mobile outreach programs.

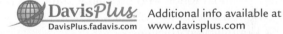

DavisPlus Additional info available at
DavisPlus.fadavis.com   www.davisplus.com

Review Questions
Self-Examination/Learning Exercise

*Select the answer that is **most** appropriate for each of the following questions.*

1. Which of the following represents a nursing intervention at the primary level of prevention?
   a. Teaching a class in parent effectiveness training
   b. Leading a group of adolescents in drug rehabilitation
   c. Referring a married couple for sex therapy
   d. Leading a support group for battered women

2. Which of the following represents a nursing intervention at the secondary level of prevention?
   a. Teaching a class about menopause to middle-aged women
   b. Providing support in the emergency room to a rape victim
   c. Leading a support group for women in transition
   d. Making monthly visits to the home of a client with schizophrenia to ensure medication compliance

Continued

Review Questions—cont'd
Self-Examination/Learning Exercise

3. Which of the following represents a nursing intervention at the tertiary level of prevention?
   a. Serving as case manager for a mentally ill homeless client
   b. Leading a support group for newly retired men
   c. Teaching prepared childbirth classes
   d. Caring for a depressed widow in the hospital

4. John, a homeless person, has just come to live in the shelter. The shelter nurse is assigned to his care. Which of the following is a *priority* intervention on the part of the nurse?
   a. Referring John to a social worker
   b. Developing a plan of care for John
   c. Conducting a behavioral and needs assessment on John
   d. Helping John apply for Social Security benefits

5. John, a homeless person, has a history of schizophrenia and nonadherence to his medication regimen. Which of the following medications might be the best choice for John?
   a. Haldol
   b. Navane
   c. Lithium carbonate
   d. Prolixin decanoate

6. Ann is a psychiatric home health nurse. She has just received an order to begin regular visits to Mrs. W, a 78-year-old widow who lives alone. Mrs. W's primary-care physician has diagnosed her as depressed. Which of the following criteria would qualify Mrs. W for home health visits?
   a. Mrs. W never learned to drive and has to depend on others for her transportation.
   b. Mrs. W is physically too weak to travel without risk of injury.
   c. Mrs. W refuses to seek assistance as suggested by her physician, "because I don't have a psychiatric problem."
   d. Mrs. W says she would prefer to have home visits than go to the physician's office.

7. Ann is a psychiatric home health nurse. She has just received an order to begin regular visits to Mrs. W, a 78-year-old widow who lives alone. Mrs. W's primary-care physician has diagnosed her as depressed. Based on a needs assessment, which of the following problems would Ann address during her first visit?
   a. Complicated grieving
   b. Social isolation
   c. Risk for injury
   d. Sleep pattern disturbance

8. Mrs. W (a 78-year-old depressed widow) says to her home health nurse, "What's the use? I don't have anything to live for anymore." Which is the best response on the part of the nurse?
   a. "Of course you do, Mrs. W. Why would you say such a thing?"
   b. "You seem so sad. I'm going to do my best to cheer you up."
   c. "Let's talk about why you are feeling this way."
   d. "Have you been thinking about harming yourself in any way?"

9. The physician orders trazadone (Desyrel) for Mrs. W (a 78-year-old widow with depression), 150 mg to take at bedtime. Which of the following statements about this medication would be appropriate for the home health nurse to make in teaching Mrs. W about trazadone?
   a. "You may feel dizzy when you stand up, so go slowly when you get up from sitting or lying down."
   b. "You must be sure and not eat any chocolate while you are taking this medicine."
   c. "We will need to draw a sample of blood to send to the lab every month while you are on this medication."
   d. "If you don't feel better right away with this medicine, the doctor can order a different kind for you."

10. Three predominant client populations have been identified as benefiting most from psychiatric home health care. Which of the following is not included among this group?
    a. Elderly individuals
    b. Individuals living in poverty
    c. Individuals with severe and persistent mental illness
    d. Individuals in acute crisis situations

References

American Nurses Association (ANA) (2008). *Home health nursing: Scope and standards of practice.* Silver Spring, MD: Author.

American Psychiatric Association. (2013). *Diagnostic and statistical manual of mental disorders* (5th ed.). Washington, DC: Author.

Case Management Society of America (CMSA). (2010). *Standards of practice for case management.* Little Rock, AR: CMSA.

Centers for Disease Control and Prevention (CDC). (2013, March 22). Trends in tuberculosis—United States, 2012. *Morbidity and Mortality Weekly, 62*(11), 201-205.

Centers for Medicare & Medicaid Services (CMS). (2011). *Medicare benefit policy manual.* Baltimore, MD: CMS.

Jans, L., Stoddard, S., & Kraus, L. (2004). *Chartbook on mental health and disability in the United States.* An InfoUse Report. Washington, DC: U.S. Department of Education, National Institute on Disability and Rehabilitation Research.

Lamb, H.R. (1993). Perspectives on effective advocacy for homeless mentally ill persons. *Hospital and Community Psychiatry, 43*(12), 1209-1212.

Langley, C. (2002). Community-based nursing practice: An overview in the United States. In J.M. Sorrell & G.M. Redmond (Eds.), *Community-based nursing practice: Learning through students' stories* (pp. 3-19). Philadelphia, PA: F.A. Davis.

Ling, C., & Ruscin, C. (2013). *Case management basics.* Gannett Education Course #60102. Retrieved from http://ce.nurse.com/60102/Case-Management-Basics

Mandleco, B.L. (2004). *Growth & development handbook: Newborn through adolescent.* New York, NY: Delmar Learning.

Miller, M.A., & Rahe, R.H. (1997). Life changes scaling for the 1990s. *Journal of Psychosomatic Research, 43*(3), 279-292.

Murray, R.B., Zentner, J.P., & Yakimo, R. (2009). *Health promotion strategies through the life span* (8th ed.). Upper Saddle River, NJ: Prentice Hall.

National Alliance on Mental Illness (NAMI). (2012). *NAMI public policy platform* (10th ed.). Arlington, VA: Author.

National Alliance on Mental Illness (NAMI). (2013). *PACT: Program of assertive community treatment.* Retrieved from http://www.nami.org

National Coalition for the Homeless (NCH). (2009a). *HIV/AIDS and homelessness.* Retrieved from http://www.nationalhomeless.org

National Coalition for the Homeless (NCH). (2009b). *Homeless families with children.* Retrieved from http://www.nationalhomeless.org

National Coalition for the Homeless (NCH). (2009c). *How many people experience homelessness?* Retrieved from http://www.nationalhomeless.org

National Coalition for the Homeless (NCH). (2009d). *Who is homeless?* Retrieved from http://www.nationalhomeless.org

National Coalition for the Homeless (NCH). (2009e). *Why are people homeless?* Retrieved from http://www.nationalhomeless.org

Pittman, D.C. (1989). Nursing case management: Holistic care for the deinstitutionalized chronically mentally ill. *Journal of Psychosocial Nursing, 27*(11), 23-27.

President's New Freedom Commission on Mental Health. (2003). *Achieving the promise: Transforming mental health care in America.* Retrieved from http://govinfo.library.unt.edu/mentalhealthcommission/reports/reports.htm

Sadock, B.J., & Sadock, V.A. (2007). *Synopsis of psychiatry: Behavioral sciences/clinical psychiatry* (10th ed.). Philadelphia, PA: Lippincott Williams & Wilkins.

Scanlon, V.C., & Sanders, T. (2011). *Essentials of anatomy and physiology* (6th ed.). Philadelphia, PA: F.A. Davis.

Spock, B. (2012). *Baby and child care* (9th ed.). New York, NY: Gallery Books.

Substance Abuse & Mental Health Services Administration (SAMHSA). (2009). *Transforming mental health care in America: The Federal Action Agenda First Steps.* Retrieved from http://www.samhsa.gov/Federalactionagenda/NFC_TOC.aspx

Substance Abuse and Mental Health Services Administration (SAMHSA). (2011). *Current statistics on the prevalence and characteristics of people experiencing homelessness in the United States.* Retrieved from http://homeless.samhsa.gov/ResourceFiles/hrc_factsheet.pdf

U.S. Conference of Mayors (USCM). (2012). *A status report on hunger and homelessness in America's cities: 2012.* Washington, DC: Author.

Von Esenwein, S.A., Bornemann, T., Ellingson, L., Palpant, R., Randolph, L., & Druss, B.G. (2005). A survey of mental health leaders one year after the President's New Freedom Commission Report. *Psychiatric Services, 56*(5), 605-607.

World Health Organization (WHO). (2004). *Prevention of mental disorders: Effective interventions and policy options.* Retrieved from http://www.who.int/mental_health/evidence/en/prevention_of_mental_disorders_sr.pdf

Wright, L.M., & Leahey, M. (2013). *Nurses and families: A guide to family assessment and intervention* (6th ed.). Philadelphia, PA: F.A. Davis.

Classical References

Caplan, G. (1964). *Principles of preventive psychiatry.* New York, NY: Basic Books.

Erikson, E. (1963). *Childhood and society* (2nd ed.). New York, NY: W.W. Norton.

Mahler, M., Pine, F., & Bergman, A. (1975). *The psychological birth of the human infant.* New York, NY: Basic Books.

Sheehy, G. (1976). *Passages: Predictable crises of adult life.* New York, NY: Bantam Books.

37

The Bereaved Individual

CHAPTER OUTLINE

KEY TERMS

OBJECTIVES
After reading this chapter, the student will be able to:

1. Describe various types of loss that trigger the grief response in individuals.
2. Discuss theoretical perspectives of grieving as proposed by Elisabeth Kübler-Ross, John Bowlby, George Engel, and J. William Worden.
3. Differentiate between normal and maladaptive responses to loss.
4. Discuss grieving behaviors common to individuals at various stages across the life span.
5. Describe customs associated with grief in individuals of various cultures.
6. Formulate nursing diagnoses and goals of care for individuals experiencing the grief response.
7. Describe appropriate nursing interventions for individuals experiencing the grief response.
8. Identify relevant criteria for evaluating nursing care of individuals experiencing the grief response.
9. Describe the concept of hospice care for people who are dying and their families.
10. Discuss the use of advance directives for individuals to provide directions about their future medical care.

HOMEWORK ASSIGNMENT
Please read the chapter and answer the following questions:

1. What type of maladaptive response to loss occurs when an individual becomes fixed in the anger stage of grief? What clinical disorder is associated with this occurrence?
2. Describe the phenomenon of bereavement overload.
3. With what types of behaviors is grief manifested in school-age children?
4. According to Engel, when is the grief response thought to be resolved?

CORE CONCEPT

Loss

The experience of separation from something of personal importance.

Loss is anything that is perceived as such by the individual. The separation from loved ones or the giving up of treasured possessions, for whatever reason; the experience of failure, either real or perceived; or life events that create change in a familiar pattern of existence—all can be experienced as loss, and all can trigger behaviors associated with the grieving process. Loss and bereavement are universal events encountered by all beings that experience emotions. Following are examples of some notable forms of loss:

■ A significant other (person or pet), through death, divorce, or separation for any reason.

■ Illness or debilitating conditions. Examples include (but are not limited to) diabetes, stroke, cancer, rheumatoid arthritis, multiple sclerosis, Alzheimer's disease, hearing or vision loss, and spinal cord or head injuries. Some of these conditions not only incur a loss of physical and/or emotional wellness, but may also result in the loss of personal independence.

■ Developmental/maturational changes or situations, such as menopause, andropause, infertility, "empty nest," aging, impotence, or hysterectomy.

■ A decrease in self-esteem due to inability to meet self-expectations or the expectations of others (even if these expectations are only perceived by the individual as unfulfilled). This includes a loss of potential hopes and dreams.

■ Personal possessions that symbolize familiarity and security in a person's life. Separation from these familiar and personally valued external objects represents a loss of material extensions of the self.

CORE CONCEPT

Grief

Deep mental and emotional anguish that is a response to the subjective experience of loss of something significant.

Some texts differentiate the terms **mourning** and grief by describing mourning as the psychological process (or stages) through which the individual passes on the way to successful adaptation to the loss of a valued object. Grief may be viewed as the subjective states that accompany mourning, or the emotional work involved in the mourning process. For purposes of this text, grief work and the process of mourning are collectively referred to as the *grief response*.

This chapter examines human responses to the experience of loss. Care of bereaved individuals is presented in the context of the nursing process.

Theoretical Perspectives on Loss and Bereavement

Stages of Grief

Behavior patterns associated with the grief response include many individual variations. However, sufficient similarities have been observed to warrant characterization of grief as a syndrome that has a predictable course with an expected resolution. Early theorists, including Kübler-Ross (1969), Bowlby (1961), and Engel (1964), described behavioral stages through which individuals advance in their progression toward resolution. A number of variables influence one's progression through the grief process. Some individuals may reach acceptance, only to revert back to an earlier stage; some may never complete the sequence; and some may never progress beyond the initial stage.

A more contemporary grief specialist, J. William Worden (2009), offers a set of tasks that must be processed in order to complete the grief response. He suggests that it is possible for a person to accomplish some of these tasks and not others, resulting in an incomplete bereavement, and thus impairing further growth and development. A comparison of the similarities among these four models is presented in Table 37-1.

Elisabeth Kübler-Ross

The following well-known stages of the grief process were identified by Kübler-Ross in her extensive work with dying patients. Behaviors associated with each of these stages can be observed in individuals experiencing the loss of any concept of personal value.

■ **Stage I: Denial.** In this stage the individual has difficulty believing that the loss has occurred. He or she may say, "No, it can't be true!" or "It's just not possible." This stage may protect the individual against the psychological pain of reality.

■ **Stage II: Anger.** This is the stage when reality sets in. Feelings associated with this stage include sadness, guilt, shame, helplessness, and hopelessness. Self-blame or blaming of others may lead to feelings of anger toward the self and others. The anxiety level may be elevated, and the individual may experience confusion and a decreased ability to function independently. He or she may be preoccupied with an idealized image of what has been lost. Numerous somatic complaints are common.

TABLE 37–1 Stages and Tasks of the Normal Grief Response: A Comparison of Models by Elisabeth Kübler-Ross, John Bowlby, George Engel, and William Worden

KÜBLER-ROSS	BOWLBY	ENGEL	WORDEN	POSSIBLE TIME DIMENSION	BEHAVIORS
I. Denial	I. Numbness/protest	I. Shock/disbelief	I. Accepting the reality of the loss	Occurs immediately on experiencing the loss. Usually lasts no more than a few weeks.	Individual has difficulty believing that the loss has occurred.
II. Anger	II. Disequilibrium	II. Developing awareness		In most cases begins within hours of the loss. Peaks within a few weeks.	Anger is directed toward self or others. Ambivalence and guilt may be felt toward the lost entity.
III. Bargaining					The individual fervently seeks alternatives to improve current situation.
		III. Restitution			Attends to various rituals associated with the culture in which the loss has occurred.
IV. Depression	III. Disorganization and despair	IV. Resolution of the loss	II. Processing the pain of grief	Very individual. Commonly 6 to 12 months. Longer for some.	The actual work of grieving. Preoccupation with the lost entity. Feelings of helplessness and loneliness occur in response to realization of the loss. Feelings associated with the loss are confronted.
			III. Adjusting to a world without the lost entity.	Ongoing	How the environment changes depends on the roles the lost entity played in the life of the bereaved person. Adaptations will have to be made as the changes are presented in daily life. New coping skills will have to be developed.
V. Acceptance	IV. Reorganization	V. Recovery	IV. Finding an enduring connection with the lost entity in the midst of embarking on a new life.		Resolution is complete. The bereaved person experiences a reinvestment in new relationships and new goals. The lost entity is not purged or replaced, but relocated in the life of the bereaved. At this stage, terminally ill persons express a readiness to die.

■ **Stage III: Bargaining.** At this stage in the grief response, the individual attempts to strike a bargain with God for a second chance, or for more time. The person acknowledges the loss, or impending loss, but holds out hope for additional alternatives, as evidenced by statements such as, "If only I could . . . ." or "If only I had . . . ."

■ **Stage IV: Depression.** In this stage, the individual mourns for that which has been or will be lost. This is a very painful stage, during which the individual must confront feelings associated with having lost someone or something of value (called *reactive* depression). An example might be the individual who is mourning a change in body image. Feelings associated with an impending loss (called *preparatory* depression) are also confronted. Examples include permanent lifestyle changes related to the altered body image or even an impending loss of life itself. Regression, withdrawal, and social isolation may be observed behaviors with this stage. Therapeutic intervention should be available, but not imposed, and with guidelines for implementation based on client readiness.

■ **Stage V: Acceptance.** At this time, the individual has worked through the behaviors associated with the other stages and accepts or is resigned to the loss. Anxiety decreases, and methods for coping with the loss have been established. The client is less preoccupied with what has been lost and increasingly interested in other aspects of the environment. If this is an impending death of self, the individual is ready to die. The person may become very quiet and withdrawn, seemingly devoid of feelings. These behaviors are an attempt to facilitate the passage by slowly disengaging from the environment.

John Bowlby

John Bowlby hypothesized four stages in the grief process. He implies that these behaviors can be observed in all individuals who have experienced the loss of something or someone of value, even in babies as young as 6 months of age.

■ **Stage I: Numbness or Protest.** This stage is characterized by a feeling of shock and disbelief that the loss has occurred. Reality of the loss is not acknowledged.

■ **Stage II: Disequilibrium.** During this stage, the individual has a profound urge to recover what has been lost. Behaviors associated with this stage include a preoccupation with the loss, intense weeping and expressions of anger toward the self and others, and feelings of ambivalence and guilt associated with the loss.

■ **Stage III: Disorganization and Despair.** Feelings of despair occur in response to realization that the loss has occurred. Activities of daily living become increasingly disorganized, and behavior is characterized by restlessness and aimlessness. Efforts to regain productive patterns of behavior are ineffective and the individual experiences fear, helplessness, and hopelessness. Somatic complaints are common. Perceptions of visualizing or being in the presence of that which has been lost may occur. Social isolation is common, and the individual may feel a great deal of loneliness.

■ **Stage IV: Reorganization.** The individual accepts or becomes resigned to the loss. New goals and patterns of organization are established. The individual begins a reinvestment in new relationships and indicates a readiness to move forward within the environment. Grief subsides and recedes into valued remembrances.

George Engel

■ **Stage I: Shock and Disbelief.** The initial reaction to a loss is a stunned, numb feeling and refusal by the individual to acknowledge the reality of the loss. Engel states that this stage is an attempt by the individual to protect the self "against the effects of the overwhelming stress by raising the threshold against its recognition or against the painful feelings evoked thereby."

■ **Stage II: Developing Awareness.** This stage begins within minutes to hours of the loss. Behaviors associated with this stage include excessive crying and regression to a state of helplessness and a childlike manner. Awareness of the loss creates feelings of emptiness, frustration, anguish, and despair. Anger may be directed toward the self or toward others in the environment who are held accountable for the loss.

■ **Stage III: Restitution.** In this stage, the various rituals associated with loss within a culture are performed. Examples include funerals, wakes, special attire, a gathering of friends and family, and religious practices customary to the spiritual beliefs of the bereaved. Participation in these rituals is thought to assist the individual to accept the reality of the loss and to facilitate the recovery process.

■ **Stage IV: Resolution of the Loss.** This stage is characterized by a preoccupation with the loss. The concept of the loss is idealized, and the individual may even imitate admired qualities of the lost entity. Preoccupation with the loss gradually decreases over a year or more, and the individual eventually begins to reinvest feelings in others.

■ **Stage V: Recovery.** Obsession with the loss has ended, and the individual is able to go on with his or her life.

J. William Worden

Worden views the bereaved person as active and self-determining rather than a passive participant in the grief process. He proposes that bereavement includes a set of tasks that must be reconciled in order to complete the grief process. Worden's four tasks of mourning include the following:

■ **Task I: Accepting the Reality of the Loss.** When something of value is lost, it is common for individuals to refuse to believe that the loss has occurred. Behaviors include misidentifying individuals in the environment for their lost loved one, retaining possessions of the lost loved one as though he or she has not died, and removing all reminders of the lost loved one so as not to have to face the reality of the loss. Worden (2009) stated:

Coming to an acceptance of the reality of the loss takes time since it involves not only an intellectual acceptance but also an emotional one. The bereaved person may be intellectually aware of the finality of the loss long before the emotions allow full acceptance of the information as true. (p. 42)

Belief and denial are intermittent while grappling with this task. It is thought that traditional rituals such as the funeral help some individuals move toward acceptance of the loss.

■ **Task II: Processing the Pain of Grief.** Pain associated with a loss includes both physical pain and emotional pain. This pain must be acknowledged and worked through. To avoid or suppress it serves only to delay or prolong the grieving process. People do this by refusing to allow themselves to think painful thoughts, by idealizing or avoiding reminders of lost entity, and by using alcohol or drugs. The intensity of the pain and the manner in which it is experienced are different for all individuals. However, the commonality is that it *must* be experienced. Failure to do so generally results in some form of depression that commonly requires therapy, which then focuses on working through the pain of grief that the individual failed to work through at the time of the loss. In this very difficult Task II, individuals must "allow themselves to process the pain—to feel it and to know that one day it will pass" (Worden, 2009, p. 45).

■ **Task III: Adjusting to a World Without the Lost Entity.** It usually takes a number of months for a bereaved person to realize what his or her world will be like without the lost entity. In the case of a lost loved one, how the environment changes will depend on the types of roles that person fulfilled in life. In the case of a changed lifestyle, the individual will be required to make adaptations to his or her environment in terms of the changes as they are presented in daily life. In addition, those individuals who had defined their identity through the lost entity will require an adjustment to their own sense of self. Worden (2009) states:

The coping strategy of redefining the loss in such a way that it can redound to the benefit of the survivor is often part of the successful completion of Task III. (p. 47)

If the bereaved person experiences failures in his or her attempt to adjust in an environment without the lost entity, feelings of low self-esteem may result. Regressed behaviors and feelings of helplessness and inadequacy are not uncommon. Worden (2009) states:

[Another] area of adjustment is to one's sense of the world. Loss through death can challenge one's fundamental life values and philosophical beliefs—beliefs that are influenced by our families, peers, education, and religion as well as life experiences. The bereaved person searches for meaning in the loss and its attendant life changes in order to make sense of it and to regain some control of his or her life. (pp. 48-49)

To be successful in Task III, bereaved individuals must develop new skills to cope and adapt to their new environment without the lost entity. Successful achievement of this task determines the outcome of the mourning process—that of continued growth or a state of arrested development.

■ **Task IV: Finding an Enduring Connection With the Lost Entity in the Midst of Embarking on a New Life.** This task allows for the bereaved person to identify a special place for the lost entity. Individuals need not purge from their history or find a replacement for that which has been lost. Instead, there is a kind of continued presence of the lost entity that only becomes *relocated* in the life of the bereaved. Successful completion of Task IV involves letting go of past attachments and forming new ones. However, there is also the recognition that although the relationship between the bereaved and what has been lost is changed, it is nonetheless still a relationship. Worden (2009) suggested that one never loses memories of a significant relationship. He states:

For many people, Task IV is the most difficult one to accomplish. They get stuck at this point in their grieving and later realize that their life in some way stopped at the point the loss occurred. (p. 52)

Worden (2009) related the story of a teenaged girl who had a difficult time adjusting to the death of her father. After 2 years, when she began to finally fulfill some of the tasks associated with successful grieving, she wrote these words that express rather clearly what bereaved people in Task IV are struggling with: "There are other people to be loved, and it doesn't mean that I love Dad any less" (p. 52).

Length of the Grief Response

Stages of grief allow bereaved persons an orderly approach to the resolution of mourning. Each stage presents tasks that must be overcome through a painful experiential process. Engel (1964) has stated that successful resolution of the grief response is thought to have occurred when a bereaved individual is able "to remember comfortably and realistically both the pleasures and disappointments of [that which is lost]." The length of the grief process depends on the individual and can last for a number of years without being maladaptive. The acute phase of normal grieving usually lasts about 6 to 8 weeks—longer in older adults—but complete resolution of the grief response may take much longer. Sadock and Sadock (2007) stated:

> Ample evidence suggests that the bereavement process does not end within a prescribed interval; certain aspects persist indefinitely for many otherwise high-functioning, normal individuals. Common manifestations of protracted grief occur intermittently. Most grief does not fully resolve or permanently disappear; rather grief becomes circumscribed and submerged only to reemerge in response to certain triggers. (p. 64)

A number of factors influence the eventual outcome of the grief response. The grief response can be more difficult if:

■ The bereaved person was strongly dependent on or perceived the lost entity as an important means of physical and/or emotional support.
■ The relationship with the lost entity was highly ambivalent. A love-hate relationship may instill feelings of guilt that can interfere with the grief work.
■ The individual has experienced a number of recent losses. Grief tends to be cumulative, and if previous losses have not been resolved, each succeeding grief response becomes more difficult.

■ The loss is that of a young person. Grief over loss of a child is often more intense than it is over the loss of an elderly person.
■ The state of the person's physical or psychological health is unstable at the time of the loss.
■ The bereaved person perceives (whether real or imagined) some responsibility for the loss.

The grief response may be facilitated if:

■ The individual has the support of significant others to assist him or her through the mourning process.
■ The individual has the opportunity to prepare for the loss. Grief work is more intense when the loss is sudden and unexpected. The experience of *anticipatory grieving* is thought to facilitate the grief response that occurs at the time of the actual loss.

Worden (2009) states:

> There is a sense in which mourning can be finished, when people regain an interest in life, feel more hopeful, experience gratification again, and adapt to new roles. There is also a sense in which mourning is never finished. [People must understand] that mourning is a long-term process and that the culmination will not be a pre-grief state. (p. 77)

Anticipatory Grief

Anticipatory grieving is the experiencing of the feelings and emotions associated with the normal grief response before the loss actually occurs. One dissimilar aspect relates to the fact that conventional grief tends to diminish in intensity with the passage of time. Anticipatory grief can become more intense as the expected loss becomes imminent.

Although anticipatory grief is thought to facilitate the actual mourning process following the loss, there may be some problems. In the case of a dying person, difficulties can arise when the family members complete the process of anticipatory grief, and detachment from the dying person occurs prematurely. The person who is dying experiences feelings of loneliness and isolation as the psychological pain of imminent death is faced without family support. Another example of difficulty associated with premature completion of the grief response is one that can occur on the return of persons long absent and presumed dead (e.g., soldiers missing in action or prisoners of war). In this instance, resumption of the previous relationship may be difficult for the bereaved person.

Anticipatory grieving may serve as a defense for some individuals to ease the burden of loss when it actually occurs. It may prove to be less functional for others who, because of interpersonal, psychological, or sociocultural variables, are unable in advance of the actual loss to express the intense feelings that accompany the grief response.

IMPLICATIONS OF RESEARCH FOR EVIDENCE-BASED PRACTICE

Bratcher, J.R. (2010). How do critical care nurses define a "good death" in the intensive care unit? *Critical Care Nursing Quarterly, 33*(1), 87-99.

DESCRIPTION OF THE STUDY: The purpose of this study was to explore and describe the characteristics of a good death as defined by critical care nurses working in the intensive care unit (ICU). The number of deaths in the ICU is likely to increase as the population ages and the use of life-prolonging technologies expands. Research has indicated a growing awareness of inadequacies with end-of-life (EOL) care in the ICU. The author states, "Findings from the Committee on Care at the End of Life demonstrated that people suffer needlessly at the EOL; physicians and nurses lack basic training necessary to provide EOL care; economic, cultural, and organizational structures in the US healthcare system encumbers the delivery of good EOL care; and knowledge to guide care for patients at the EOL is deficient" (p. 87).

RESULTS OF THE STUDY: The study group consisted of 15 registered nurses (5 males; 10 females) working in the medical/surgical ICU at a Veteran's Administration hospital in a mid-sized urban city. Ages ranged from 36 to 59, and years in nursing ranged from 3 to 26. Eight participants had associate degrees and 7 had baccalaureate degrees. Personal interviews were conducted by the author and lasted up to 60 minutes. Interviews were taped and transcribed verbatim. Each interview started with the question, "How do you define a good death in the ICU?" Nurses were encouraged to recall personal situations with specific patients whom they believed had experienced a good death. A great deal of diversity was revealed in the participants'

descriptions of a good death. Following are various themes that emerged. The number in parentheses indicates the number of nurses who identified each theme in their interview.

- Patient does not die alone (11) (includes allowing patient's pet)
- Patient does not suffer (10) (includes those who suggested patient's death is quick)
- Acceptance of death by patient and/or loved ones (8)
- Patient dies with dignity (3) (implying with solemnity, peace, and respect)
- Religious/spiritual/cultural needs are met (3)
- Patient's and/or family's wishes are honored (3)
- Patient was not successfully resuscitated, but staff tried their best (2)
- Music is allowed (1)
- Environment is quiet (1)
- Staff does not panic (1)
- Family does not panic (1) or scream or cry out loud in distress (1)

IMPLICATIONS FOR NURSING PRACTICE: The results of this study offer information applicable to EOL care in the critical care setting. The author suggested that there is a need to recognize that palliative care in the ICU can coexist with curative care. The author concluded, "Critical care nurses have an opportunity to provide excellent EOL care for their patients, but they must first understand what constitutes a good death; obtaining this information will help facilitate compassionate EOL care, which will ultimately improve the nursing care of dying patients and their families in the ICU" (p. 97).

Maladaptive Responses to Loss

When, then, is the grieving response considered to be maladaptive? Three types of pathological grief reactions have been described. These include delayed or inhibited grief, an exaggerated or distorted grief response, and chronic or prolonged grief.

Delayed or Inhibited Grief

Delayed or inhibited grief refers to the absence of evidence of grief when it ordinarily would be expected. Many times, cultural influences, such as the expectation to keep a "stiff upper lip," cause the delayed response.

Delayed or inhibited grief is potentially pathological because the person is simply not dealing with the reality of the loss. He or she remains fixed in the denial stage of the grief process, sometimes for many years. When this occurs, the grief response may be triggered,

sometimes many years later, when the individual experiences a subsequent loss. Sometimes the grief process is triggered spontaneously or in response to a seemingly insignificant event. Overreaction to another person's loss may be one manifestation of **delayed grief**.

The recognition of delayed grief is critical because, depending on the profoundness of the loss, the failure of the mourning process may prevent assimilation of the loss and thereby delay a return to satisfying living. Delayed grieving most commonly occurs because of ambivalent feelings toward the lost entity, outside pressure to resume normal function, or perceived lack of internal and external resources to cope with a profound loss.

Distorted (Exaggerated) Grief Response

In the distorted grief reaction, all of the symptoms associated with normal grieving are exaggerated. Feelings of sadness, helplessness, hopelessness, powerlessness, anger, and guilt, as well as numerous somatic complaints, render the individual dysfunctional in terms of management of daily living. Murray, Zentner, and Yakimo (2009) described an exaggerated grief reaction in the following way:

> An intensification of grief to the point that the person is overwhelmed, demonstrates prolonged maladaptive behavior, manifests excessive symptoms and extensive interruptions in healing, and does not progress to integration of the loss, finding meaning in the loss, and resolution of the mourning process. (p. 706)

When the exaggerated grief reaction occurs, the individual remains fixed in the anger stage of the grief response. This anger may be directed toward others in the environment to whom the individual may be attributing the loss. However, many times the anger is turned inward on the self. When this occurs, depression is the result. Depressive mood disorder is a type of exaggerated grief reaction.

Chronic or Prolonged Grieving

Some authors have discussed a chronic or prolonged grief response as a type of maladaptive grief response. Care must be taken in making this determination because, as was stated previously, length of the grief response depends on the individual. An adaptive response may take years for some people. A prolonged process may be considered maladaptive when certain behaviors are exhibited. Prolonged grief may be a problem when behaviors such as maintaining personal possessions aimed at keeping a lost loved one alive (as though he or she will eventually reenter the life of the bereaved) or disabling behaviors that prevent the bereaved from adaptively performing activities of daily living are in evidence. Another example is of a widow who refused to participate in family gatherings following the death of her husband. For many years until her own death, she took a sandwich to the cemetery on holidays, sat on the tombstone, and ate her "holiday meal" with her husband. Other bereaved individuals have been known to set a place at the table for the deceased loved one long after the completed mourning process would have been expected.

Normal versus Maladaptive Grieving

Several authors have identified one crucial difference between normal and maladaptive grieving: the loss of self-esteem. Marked feelings of worthlessness are indicative of depression rather than uncomplicated bereavement. Corr and Corr (2013) state, "Normal grief reactions do not include the loss of self-esteem commonly found in most clinical depression" (p. 241). Pies (2013) affirmed:

> Unlike the person with MDD [Major depressive disorder], most recently bereaved individuals are usually not preoccupied with feelings of worthlessness, hopelessness, or unremitting gloom; rather, self-esteem is usually preserved; the bereaved person can envision a "better day;" and positive thoughts and feelings are often interspersed with negative ones.

It is thought that this major difference between normal grieving and a maladaptive grieving response (the feeling of worthlessness or low self-esteem) ultimately precipitates depression, which can be a progressive situation for some individuals. A summary of differences between normal grieving and clinical depression is presented in Table 37-2.

TABLE 37–2 Normal Grief Reactions versus Symptoms of Clinical Depression

NORMAL GRIEF	CLINICAL DEPRESSION
Self-esteem is intact	Self-esteem is disturbed
May openly express anger	Usually does not directly express anger
Experiences a mixture of "good and bad days"	Is in a persistent state of dysphoria
Able to experience moments of pleasure	Anhedonia is prevalent
Accepts comfort and support from others	Does not respond to social interaction and support from others
Maintains feeling of hope	Feelings of hopelessness prevail
May express guilt feelings over some aspect of the loss	Has generalized feelings of guilt
Relates feelings of depression to specific loss experiences	Does not relate feelings to a particular experience
May experience transient physical symptoms	Expresses chronic physical complaints

SOURCES: Corr & Corr (2013); Pies (2013); and Sadock & Sadock (2007).

Application of the Nursing Process

Background Assessment Data: Concepts of Death—Developmental Issues

All individuals have their own unique concept of death, which is influenced by past experiences with death as well as age and level of emotional development. This section addresses the various perceptions of death according to developmental age.

Children

Birth to Age 2

Infants are unable to recognize and understand death, but they can experience the feelings of loss and separation. Infants who are separated from their mother may become quiet, lose weight, and sleep less. Children at this age will likely sense changes in the atmosphere of the home where a death has occurred. They often react to the emotions of adults by becoming more irritable and crying more.

Ages 3 to 5

Preschoolers and kindergartners have some understanding about death but often have difficulty distinguishing between fantasy and reality. They believe death is reversible, and their thoughts about death may include magical thinking. For example, they may believe that their thoughts or behaviors caused a person to become sick or to die.

Children of this age are capable of understanding at least some of what they see and hear from adult conversations or media reports. They become frightened if they feel a threat to themselves or their loved ones. They are concerned with safety issues and require a great deal of personal reassurance that they will be protected. Regressive behaviors, such as loss of bladder or bowel control, thumb sucking, and temper tantrums are common. Changes in eating and sleeping patterns may also occur.

Ages 6 to 9

Children at this age are beginning to understand the finality of death. They are able to understand a more detailed explanation of why or how a person died, although the concept of death is often associated with old age or with accidents. They may believe that death is contagious and avoid association with individuals who have experienced a loss by death. Death is often personified, in the form of a "bogey man" or a monster—someone who takes people away or someone whom they can avoid if they try hard enough. It is difficult for them to perceive their own death. Normal grief reactions at this age include regressive and aggressive behaviors, withdrawal, school phobias, somatic symptoms, and clinging behaviors.

Ages 10 to 12

Preadolescent children are able to understand that death is final and eventually affects everyone, including themselves. They are interested in the physical aspects of dying and the final disposition of the body. They may ask questions about how the death will affect them personally. Feelings of anger, guilt, and depression are common. Peer relationships and school performance may be disrupted. There may be a preoccupation with the loss and a withdrawal into the self. They will require reassurance of their own safety and self-worth.

Adolescents

Adolescents are usually able to view death on an adult level. They understand death to be universal and inevitable; however, they have difficulty tolerating the intense feelings associated with the death of a loved one. They may or may not cry. They may withdraw into themselves or attempt to go about usual activities in an effort to avoid dealing with the pain of the loss. Some teens exhibit acting-out behaviors, such as aggression and defiance. It is often easier for adolescents to discuss their feelings with peers than with their parents or other adults. Some adolescents may show regressive behaviors, whereas others react by trying to take care of their loved ones who are also grieving. In general, individuals of this age group have an attitude of immortality. Although they understand that their own death is inevitable, the concept is so far-reaching as to be imperceptible.

Adults

The adult's concept of death is influenced by experiential, cultural, and religious backgrounds (Murray et al., 2009). Behaviors associated with grieving in the adult were discussed in the section on "Theoretical Perspectives on Loss and Bereavement."

Older Adults

Philosophers and poets have described late adulthood as the "season of loss." Jeffreys (2010) states:

> The grief of older people is unique because of the many non-death losses that are a part of aging. These include physical changes, changes in family, occupational and social roles, relocation and shifts in mental functioning. (p. 18)

By the time individuals reach their 60s and 70s, they have experienced numerous losses, and mourning has become a lifelong process. Those who are most successful at adapting earlier in life will similarly cope better with the losses and grief inherent in aging. Unfortunately, with the aging process comes a convergence of losses, the timing of which makes it impossible for the aging individual to complete the grief process in response to one loss before another occurs. Because grief is cumulative, this can result in **bereavement overload**; the person is less able to adapt and reintegrate, and mental and physical health is jeopardized (Halstead, 2005). Bereavement overload has been implicated as a predisposing factor in the development of depressive disorder in older adults.

Background Assessment Data: Concepts of Death—Cultural Issues

As previously stated, bereavement practices are greatly influenced by cultural and religious backgrounds. It is important for health-care professionals to have an understanding of these individual differences in order to provide culturally sensitive care to their clients. Clinicians must be able to identify and appreciate what is culturally expected or required, because failure to carry out expected rituals may hinder the grief process and result in unresolved grief for some bereaved individuals. Box 37-1 provides a set of guidelines for assessing culturally specific death rituals. Following is a discussion of selected culturally specific death rituals.

African Americans

Customs of bereaved African Americans are similar to those of the dominant American culture of the same religion and social class, with a blending of cultural practices from the African heritage. Most African American Christians are affiliated with the Baptist and Methodist denominations (Campinha-Bacote, 2013). Campinha-Bacote (2013) states:

> One response to hearing about a death of a family member or close member in the African American culture is "falling-out," which is manifested by sudden collapse and paralysis and the inability to see or speak. However, the individual's hearing and understanding remain intact. Health care practitioners must understand the African American culture to recognize this condition as a cultural response to the

death of a family member or other severe emotional shock and not as a medical condition requiring emergency intervention. (p. 106)

Funeral services may differ from the traditional European American service with ceremonies and rituals modified by the musical rhythms and patterns of speech and worship that are unique to African Americans. Feelings are expressed openly and publicly at the funeral, and eulogies are extremely important. Services usually conclude with a viewing of the body and burial at a cemetery. Burial rather than cremation is usually chosen (Asante, 2009).

Many African Americans attempt to maintain a strong connection with their loved ones who have died. This connection may take the form of communication with the deceased's spirit through mediums who are believed to possess this special capability.

Asian Americans

Chinese Americans

Death and bereavement in the Chinese tradition are centered on ancestor worship. Chinese people have an intuitive fear of death and avoid references to it. Tsai (2013) states:

> Many Chinese are hesitant to purchase life insurance because of their fear that it is inviting death. The color white is associated with death and is considered bad luck. Black is also a bad luck color. (p. 189)

In the traditional Chinese culture, people often do not express their emotions openly. Mourners are recognized by black armbands and white strips of cloth tied around their heads (Tsai, 2013). The dead are honored by placing food, money for the person's spirit, or articles made of paper around the coffin.

Japanese Americans

The dominant religion among the Japanese is Buddhism. On death of a loved one, the body is prepared by close family members. This is followed by a 2-day period of visitation by family and friends, during which there is prayer, burning of incense, and presentation of gifts. Funeral ceremonies are held at the Buddhist temple, and cremation is common. The mourning period is 49 days, the end of which is marked by a family prayer service and the serving of special rice dishes. It is believed that at this time, the departed has joined those already in the hereafter. Perpetual prayers may be donated through a gift to the temple (Ito & Hattori, 2013).

Vietnamese Americans

Buddhism is the predominant religion among the Vietnamese. Attitudes toward death are influenced by the Buddhist emphasis on cyclic continuity and reincarnation. Many Vietnamese people believe that birth and death are predestined.

BOX 37-1 Guidelines for Assessing Culturally Specific Death Rituals

DEATH RITUALS AND EXPECTATIONS
1. Identify culturally specific death rituals and expectations.
2. Explain death rituals and mourning practices.
3. What are specific burial practices, such as cremation?

RESPONSES TO DEATH AND GRIEF
4. Identify cultural responses to death and grief.
5. Explore the meaning of death, dying, and the afterlife.

Adapted from Purnell, L.D. (2013). The Purnell model for cultural competence. In L.D. Purnell (Ed.), Transcultural health care: A culturally competent approach (4th ed.). Philadelphia, PA: F.A. Davis.

Most Vietnamese people prefer to die at home, and most do not approve of autopsy. Cremation is common. The final moments before the funeral procession are a time of prayer for the immediate family. Individuals in mourning wear white clothing for 14 days. During the following year, men wear black armbands and women wear white headbands (Mattson, 2013). The 1-year anniversary of an individual's death is commemorated. Clergy should only be called to visit the sick at the request of the client or family, and is usually associated with last rites, especially by Vietnamese people who practice Catholicism. For this reason, hospital visitation by clergy may be very upsetting to clients. Receiving flowers also may be distressing, as flowers usually are reserved for the rites of the dead (Appel, 2013).

Filipino Americans

Following a death in the Filipino community, a wake is held with family and friends. This wake usually takes place in the home of the deceased and lasts up to a week before the funeral. A large proportion of Filipinos are Catholic. Munoz (2013) states:

> Among Catholics, 9 days of novenas are held in the home or in the church. These special prayers ask God's blessing for the deceased. Depending upon the economic resources of the family, food and refreshments are served after each prayer day. Sometimes the last day of the novena takes on the atmosphere of a *fiesta* or a celebration. Filipino families in the United States follow variations of this ritual according to their social and economic circumstances. (p. 242)

Most follow the traditional custom of wearing dark clothing—black armbands for men and black dresses for women—for 1 year after the death, at which time ritualistic mourning officially ends. Emotional outbursts of uncontrolled crying are common expressions of grief. Fainting as a bereavement practice is not uncommon (Munoz, 2013). Burial of the body is most common, but cremation is acceptable.

Jewish Americans

Traditional Judaism believes in an afterlife, where the soul continues to flourish, although today, many dispute this interpretation (Selekman, 2013). However, most Jewish people show little concern about life after death and focus is concentrated more on how one conducts one's present life. Taking one's own life is forbidden, and ultraconservative Jewish people may deny the person who commits suicide full burial honors; however, the more liberal view is to emphasize the needs of the survivors.

A dying person is never left alone. At death, the face is covered with a cloth, and the body is treated with respect. Autopsy is only allowed if it is required by law, the deceased person has requested it, or it may save the life of another (Selekman, 2013).

For the funeral, the body is wrapped in a shroud and placed in a wooden, unadorned casket. No wake and no viewing are part of a Jewish funeral. Cremation is prohibited. Selekman (2013) states:

> After the funeral, mourners are welcomed to the home of the closest relative. Water to wash one's hands before entering is outside the front door, symbolic of cleansing the impurities associated with contact with the dead. The water is not passed from person to person, just as it is hoped that the tragedy is not passed. At the home, a meal is served to all the guests. This "meal of condolence" or "meal of consolation" is traditionally provided by the neighbors and friends. (p. 350)

The 7-day period beginning with the burial is called *shiva*. During this time, mourners do not work, and no activity is permitted that diverts attention from thinking about the deceased. Mourning lasts 30 days for a relative and 1 year for a parent, at which time a tombstone is erected and a graveside service is held (Selekman, 2013).

Mexican Americans

Most Mexican Americans view death as a natural part of life. The predominant religion is Catholic, and many of the death rituals are a reflection of these religious beliefs. A vigil by family members is kept over the sick or dying person. Following the death, large numbers of family and friends gather for a *velorio*, a festive watch over the body of the deceased person (Zoucha & Zamarripa, 2013). Evening group prayers (*novenario*) follow for 9 days following the burial (Salazar, 2009).

Mourning is called *luto* and is symbolized by wearing black, black and white, or dark clothing and by subdued behavior. Often the bereaved refrain from attending movies or social events and from listening to radio or watching television. For middle-aged or elderly Mexican Americans, the period of bereavement may last for 2 years or more. These mourning behaviors do not indicate a sign of respect for the dead; instead, they demonstrate evidence that the individual is grieving for a loved one. Burial is more common than cremation, and often the body is buried within 24 hours of death, which is required by law in Mexico (Zoucha & Zamarripa, 2013).

Native Americans

More than 500 Native American tribes are now recognized by the U.S. government. Although many of the tribal traditions have been modified throughout the years, some of the traditional Native American values have been preserved.

The Navajo of the Southwest, the largest Native American tribe in the United States, do not bury the body of a deceased person for 4 days after death. Beliefs require that a cleansing ceremony take place before burial to prevent the spirit of the dead person from trying to assume control of someone else's spirit (Purnell, 2009). The dead are buried with their shoes on the wrong feet and rings on their index fingers. The Navajo generally do not express their grief openly and are reluctant to touch the body of a dead person. Purnell (2009) states:

> One death taboo involves talking with clients concerning a fatal disease or illness. Effective discussions require that the issue be presented in the third person, as if the illness or disorder occurred with someone else. [The health-care provider must] never suggest that the client is dying. To do so would imply that the provider wishes the client dead. If the client does die, it would imply that the provider may have evil powers. (p. 314)

Nursing Diagnosis/Outcome Identification

From analysis of the assessment data, appropriate nursing diagnoses are formulated for the client and family experiencing grief and loss. From these identified diagnoses, accurate planning of nursing care is executed. Possible nursing diagnoses for grieving persons include:

■ Risk for complicated grieving related to loss of a valued entity/concept; loss of a loved one
■ Risk for spiritual distress related to complicated grief process

The following criteria may be used for measurement of outcomes in the care of the grieving client:

The client:

■ Acknowledges awareness of the loss.
■ Is able to express feelings about the loss.
■ Verbalizes stages of the grief process and behaviors associated with each.
■ Expresses personal satisfaction and support from spiritual practices.

Planning/Implementation

Table 37-3 provides a plan of care for the grieving person. Selected nursing diagnoses are presented, along with outcome criteria, appropriate nursing interventions, and rationales for each.

Table 37-3 | CARE PLAN FOR THE GRIEVING PERSON

NURSING DIAGNOSIS: RISK FOR COMPLICATED GRIEVING

RELATED TO: Loss of a valued entity/concept; loss of a loved one

OUTCOME CRITERIA	NURSING INTERVENTIONS	RATIONALE

Short-Term Goals
• Client will acknowledge awareness of the loss
• Client will express feelings about the loss
• Client will verbalize own position in the grief process
 	
Long-Term Goal
• Client will progress through the grief process in a healthful manner toward resolution.
	1. Assess client's stage in the grief process.
	2. Develop trust. Show empathy, concern, and unconditional positive regard.
	3. 💬 Help the client actualize the loss by talking about it. "When did it happen? How did it happen?" and so forth.
	4. Help the client identify and express feelings. Some of the more problematic feelings include:
	  a. **Anger.** The anger may be directed at the deceased, at God, displaced onto others, or retroflected inward on the self. Encourage the client to examine this anger and validate the appropriateness of this feeling.
		1. Accurate baseline data are required to provide appropriate assistance.
		2. Developing trust provides the basis for a therapeutic relationship.
		3. Reviewing the events of the loss can help the client come to full awareness of the loss.
		4. Until client can recognize and accept personal feelings regarding the loss, grief work cannot progress.
		  a. Many people will not admit to angry feelings, believing it is inappropriate and unjustified. Expression of this emotion is necessary to prevent fixation in this stage of grief.

Continued

Table 37-3 | CARE PLAN FOR THE GRIEVING PERSON—cont'd

OUTCOME CRITERIA	NURSING INTERVENTIONS	RATIONALE
	b. **Guilt.** The client may feel that he or she did not do enough to prevent the loss. Help the client by reviewing the circumstances of the loss and the reality that it could not be prevented.	b. Feelings of guilt prolong resolution of the grief process.
	c. **Anxiety and helplessness.** Help the client to recognize the way that life was managed before the loss. Help the client to put the feelings of helplessness into perspective by pointing out ways that he or she managed situations effectively without help from others. Role-play life events and assist with decision-making situations.	c. The client may have fears that he or she may not be able to carry on alone.
	5. Interpret normal behaviors associated with grieving and provide client with adequate time to grieve.	5. Understanding of the grief process will help prevent feelings of guilt generated by these responses. Individuals need adequate time to adjust to the loss and all its ramifications. This involves getting past birthdays and anniversaries of which the deceased was a part.
	6. Provide continuing support. If this is not possible by the nurse, then offer referrals to support groups. Support groups of individuals going through the same experiences can be very helpful for the grieving individual.	6. The availability of emotional support systems facilitates the grief process.
	7. Identify pathological defenses that the client may be using (e.g., drug/alcohol use, somatic complaints, social isolation). Assist the client in understanding why these are not healthy defenses and how they delay the process of grieving.	7. The bereavement process is impaired by behaviors that mask the pain of the loss.
	8. Encourage the client to make an honest review of the relationship with the lost entity. Journal keeping is a facilitative tool with this intervention.	8. Only when the client is able to see both positive and negative aspects related to the loss will the grieving process be complete.

Table 37-3 | CARE PLAN FOR THE GRIEVING PERSON—cont'd

NURSING DIAGNOSIS: RISK FOR SPIRITUAL DISTRESS

RELATED TO: Complicated grief process

OUTCOME CRITERIA	NURSING INTERVENTIONS	RATIONALE
Short-Term Goal • Client will identify meaning and purpose in life, moving forward with hope for the future. **Long-Term Goal** • Client will express achievement of support and personal satisfaction from spiritual practices.	1. Be accepting and nonjudgmental when client expresses anger and bitterness toward God. Stay with the client. 2. Encourage the client to ventilate feelings related to meaning of own existence in the face of current loss. 3. Encourage the client as part of grief work to reach out to previously used religious practices for support. Encourage client to discuss these practices and how they provided support in the past. 4. Assure the client that he or she is not alone when feeling inadequate in the search for life's answers. 5. Contact spiritual leader of client's choice, if he or she requests.	1. The nurse's presence and nonjudgmental attitude increase the client's feelings of self-worth and promote trust in the relationship. 2. Client may believe he or she cannot go on living without the lost entity. Catharsis can provide relief and put life back into realistic perspective. 3. Client may find comfort in religious rituals with which he or she is familiar. 4. Validation of client's feelings and assurance that they are shared by others offer encouragement and an affirmation of acceptability. 5. These individuals serve to provide relief from spiritual distress and often can do so when other support persons cannot.

Evaluation

In the final step of the nursing process, a reassessment is conducted to determine if the nursing actions have been successful in achieving the objectives of care. Evaluation of the nursing actions for the grieving client may be facilitated by gathering information using the following types of questions:

■ Has the client discussed the recent loss with staff and family members?

■ Is the client able to verbalize feelings and behaviors associated with each stage of the grieving process and recognize his or her own position in the process?

■ Has obsession with and idealization of the lost entity subsided?

■ Is anger toward the loss expressed appropriately?

■ Is the client able to participate in usual religious practices and feel satisfaction and support from them?

■ Is the client seeking out interaction with others in an appropriate manner?

■ Is the client able to verbalize positive aspects about his or her life, past relationships, and prospects for the future?

Additional Assistance

Hospice

Hospice is a program that provides palliative and supportive care to meet the special needs of people who are dying and their families. Hospice care provides physical, psychological, spiritual, and social care for the person for whom aggressive treatment is no longer appropriate. Various models of hospice exist, including freestanding institutions that provide both inpatient and home care, those affiliated with hospitals and nursing homes in which hospice services are provided within the institutional setting, and hospice organizations that provide home care only. Historically, the hospice movement in the United States has evolved mainly as a system of home-based care.

Hospice helps clients achieve physical and emotional comfort so that they can concentrate on living life as fully as possible. Clients are urged to stay active for as long as they are able—to take part in activities they enjoy, and to focus on the quality of life.

The National Hospice and Palliative Care Organization (NHPCO) (2000) has published standards of care based on principles that are directed at the hospice program concept. These principles of care are presented in Box 37-2.

Hospice follows an interdisciplinary team approach to provide care for the terminally ill individual in the familiar surroundings of the home environment. The interdisciplinary team consists of nurses, attendants (homemakers, home health aides), physicians, social workers, volunteers, and health-care workers from other disciplines as required for individual clients.

The hospice approach is based on seven components: the interdisciplinary team, pain and symptom management, emotional support to client and family, pastoral and spiritual care, bereavement counseling, 24-hour on-call nurse/counselor, and staff support. These are the ideal, and not all hospice programs may include all of these services.

Interdisciplinary Team

Nurses

A registered nurse usually acts as case manager for care of hospice clients. The nurse assesses the client's and family's needs, establishes the goals of care, supervises and assists caregivers, evaluates care, serves as client advocate, and provides educational information as needed to client, family, and caregivers. He or she also provides physical care when needed, including IV therapy.

BOX 37-2 Principles of Care—National Hospice and Palliative Care Organization

ACCESS, RIGHTS AND ETHICS
Access: The hospice offers palliative care to terminally ill patients and their families regardless of age, gender, nationality, race, creed, sexual orientation, disability, diagnoses, availability of primary caregiver or ability to pay.
Rights: The hospice respects and honors the rights of each patient and family it serves.
Ethics: The hospice assumes responsibility for ethical decision-making and behavior related to the provision of hospice care.

BEREAVEMENT CARE AND SERVICES
Addressing issues related to loss, grief and bereavement begins at the time of admission to the hospice with the initial assessment and continues throughout the course of care. Bereavement services are provided to help patients, families and caregivers cope with the multitude of losses that occur during the illness and eventual death of the patient. Bereavement services are offered based on a number of factors including the individual assessment, intensity of grief, coping ability of the survivors and their needs, as perceived by each patient, family and caregiver.

CLINICAL CARE AND SERVICES
The desired outcomes of hospice intervention are safe and comfortable dying, self-determined life closure and effective grieving, all as determined by the patient and family/caregivers. The interdisciplinary team identifies, assists and respects the desires of the patient and family/caregivers in the facilitation of these outcomes through treatment, prevention and promotion of strategies based on continuous assessment.

COORDINATION AND CONTINUITY OF CARE
The hospice provides coordinated and uninterrupted service and assures continuity of care across settings from admission through discharge and subsequent bereavement care.

HUMAN RESOURCES
Hospice organizational leaders ensure that the number and qualifications of staff and volunteers are appropriate to the scope of care and services provided by the hospice program.

INTERDISCIPLINARY TEAM
The hospice interdisciplinary team, in collaboration with the patient, family and caregiver, develops and maintains a patient, family and caregiver-directed, individualized, safe and coordinated plan of palliative care.

LEADERSHIP AND GOVERNANCE
Hospice has an organizational leadership structure that permits and facilitates action and decision making by those individuals closest to any issue or process.

MANAGEMENT OF INFORMATION
The hospice identifies and collects information needed to operate in an efficient manner. Such information is handled in a manner that respects the patient's, family's and hospice's confidentiality.

PERFORMANCE IMPROVEMENT AND OUTCOMES MEASUREMENT
The hospice defines a systematic, planned approach to improving performance. This approach is authorized and supported by the governing body and leaders.

SAFETY AND INFECTION CONTROL
The hospice provides for the safety of all staff and promotes the development and maintenance of a safe environment for patients and families served.

Adapted from *National Hospice and Palliative Care Organization (2000).* Standards of Practice for Hospice Programs. *Alexandria, VA: Author. Item No. 711077,* available from NHPCO 1-800-646-6460.

Attendants

These individuals are usually the members of the team who spend the most time with the client. They assist with personal care and all activities of daily living. Without these daily attendants, many individuals would be unable to spend their remaining days in their home. Attendants may be noncertified and provide basic housekeeping services; they may be certified nursing assistants who assist with personal care; or they may be licensed vocational or practical nurses who provide more specialized care, such as dressing changes or tube feedings.

Physicians

The client's primary physician and the hospice medical consultant have input into the care of the hospice client. Orders may continue to come from the primary physician, whereas pain and symptom management may come from the hospice consultant. Ideally, these physicians attend weekly client care conferences and provide in-service education for hospice staff as well as others in the medical community.

Social Workers

The social worker assists the client and family members with psychosocial issues, including those associated with the client's condition, financial issues, legal needs, and bereavement concerns. The social worker provides information on community resources from which client and family may receive support and assistance. Some of the functions of the nurse and social worker may overlap at times.

Trained Volunteers

Volunteers are vital to the hospice concept. They provide services that may otherwise be financially impossible. They are specially selected and extensively trained, and they provide services such as transportation, companionship, respite care, recreational activities, light housekeeping, and in general are sensitive to the needs of families in stressful situations.

Rehabilitation Therapists

Physical therapists may assist hospice clients in an effort to minimize physical disability. They may assist with strengthening exercises and provide assistance with special equipment needs. Occupational therapists may help the debilitated client learn to accomplish activities of daily living as independently as possible. Other consultants, such as speech therapists, may be called upon for the client with special needs.

Dietitian

A nutritional consultant may be helpful to the hospice client who is experiencing nausea and vomiting, diarrhea, anorexia, and weight loss. A nutritionist can ensure that the client is receiving the proper balance of calories and nutrients.

Counseling Services

The hospice client may require the services of a psychiatrist or psychologist if there is a history of mental illness, or if neurocognitive disorder or depression has become a problem. Other types of counseling services are available to provide assistance in dealing with the special needs of each client.

Pain and Symptom Management

Improved quality of life at all times is a primary goal of hospice care. Thus, a major intervention for all caregivers is to ensure that the client is as comfortable as possible, whether experiencing pain or other types of symptoms common in the terminal stages of an illness.

Emotional Support

Members of the hospice team encourage clients and families to discuss the eventual outcome of the disease process. Some individuals find discussing issues associated with death and dying uncomfortable, and if so, their decision is respected. However, honest discussion of these issues provides a sense of relief for some people, and they are more realistically prepared for the future. It may even draw some clients and families closer together during this stressful time.

Pastoral and Spiritual Care

Hospice philosophy supports the individual's right to seek guidance or comfort in the spiritual practices most suited to that person. The hospice team members help the client obtain the spiritual support and guidance for which he or she expresses a preference.

Bereavement Counseling

Hospice provides a service to surviving family members or significant others after the death of their loved one. This is usually provided by a bereavement counselor, but when one is not available, volunteers with special training in bereavement care may be of service. A grief support group may be helpful for the bereaved and provide a safe place for them to discuss their own fears and concerns about the death of a loved one.

Twenty-Four-Hour On-Call

The standards of care set forth by NHPCO state that care shall be available 24 hours a day, 7 days a week. A nurse or counselor is usually available by phone or for home visits around the clock. The knowledge that emotional or physical support is available at any time, should it be required, provides considerable support and comfort to significant others or family caregivers.

Staff Support

Team members (all who work closely and frequently with the client) often experience emotions similar to those of the client or their family and/or significant others. They may experience anger, frustration, or fears of death and dying—all of which must be addressed through staff support groups, team conferences, time off, and adequate and effective supervision. Burnout is a common problem among hospice staff. Stress can be reduced, trust enhanced, and team functioning more effective if lines of communication are kept open among all members (medical director through volunteer), if information is readily accessible through staff conferences and in-service education, and if staff know they are appreciated and feel good about what they are doing.

Advance Directives

The term **advance directive** refers to either a living will or a durable power of attorney for health care (also called a health-care proxy). Either document allows an individual to provide directions about his or her future medical care.

A living will is a written document made by a competent individual that provides instructions that should be used when that individual is no longer able to express his or her wishes for health-care treatment. The durable power of attorney for health care is a written form that gives another person legal power to make decisions regarding health care when an individual is no longer capable of making such decisions. Some states have adopted forms that combine the intent of the durable power of attorney for health care (i.e., to have a proxy) and the intent of the living will (i.e., to state choices for end-of-life medical treatment).

Doctors usually follow clearly stated directives. It is important that the physician be informed that an advance directive exists and what the specific wishes of the client are. In most states, health-care professionals are legally bound to honor the client's wishes (Norlander, 2008). In 1991, the U.S. Congress passed the *Patient Self-Determination Act*. This legislation requires that all health-care facilities that receive Medicare or Medicaid funds must advise clients of their rights to refuse treatment, to make advance directives available to clients on admission, and to keep records of whether a client has an advance directive or a designated health-care proxy (Sadock & Sadock, 2007).

Catalano (2012) notes that unless a natural death act has been enacted into law by a state, the living will has no mechanism of legal enforcement. These laws have been called "pull the plug" statues and have various names in different states, such as "Removal of Life Support Systems Act" (Connecticut), "Natural Death Act" (Washington), "Declaration of Death Act" (New Jersey), and "Medical Treatment Decision Act" (Arizona) (Mantel, 2013). Catalano (2012) states:

> In some states, a living will is considered only advisory and the physician has the right to comply with the living will or treat the client as the physician deems most appropriate. There is no protection for nurses or other health care practitioners against criminal or civil liability in the execution of living wills in states without a natural death act. (p. 155)

Norlander (2008, p. 20) suggests the following reasons why advance directives sometimes are not honored:

■ The advance directive is not available at the time treatment decisions need to be made. This is especially true in emergency situations.

■ The advance directive is not clear. Statements such as "no heroic measures" can be interpreted in many different ways.

■ The health-care proxy is unsure of the client's wishes.

Advance directives allow the client to be in control of decisions at the end of life. It is also a way to spare family and loved ones the burden of making choices without knowing what is most important to the person who is dying.

IMPLICATIONS OF RESEARCH FOR EVIDENCE-BASED PRACTICE

Douglas, R., & Brown, H.N. (2002). Patients' attitudes toward advance directives. *Journal of Nursing Scholarship, 34*(1), 61-65.

DESCRIPTION OF THE STUDY: This study was conducted to investigate hospitalized patients' attitudes toward advance directives. It explored patients' reasons for completing or not completing advance directive forms, and examined demographic differences between patients who did and did not complete advance directive forms. Subjects consisted of a convenience sample of 30 hospitalized patients. Criteria required that the patients (1) speak English, (2) be at least 18 years of age, (3) be oriented to time and place, and (4) have been approached by an RN regarding advance directives, as documented in the patient chart. Data were collected over a 3-week period in the oncology and medical-telemetry units of a teaching hospital in central North Carolina. Interviews were conducted using an adapted advance directive attitude survey (ADAS) in which subjects were asked five general questions regarding perceptions of personal health, whether they had ever received information on advance directives, whether they had ever completed an advance directive, and whether they had ever had a discussion with either their primary physician or family members

IMPLICATIONS OF RESEARCH FOR EVIDENCE-BASED PRACTICE—cont'd

about end-of-life care. Demographic data were also obtained. The tool was based on a 4-point Likert scale from 1 (strongly disagree) to 4 (strongly agree). Higher scores indicate more favorable attitudes toward advance directives.

RESULTS OF THE STUDY: Subjects ranged in age from 24 to 85 years, with a mean age of 57 years. Nineteen were Caucasian, 10 were African American, and 1 was Hispanic. Ten had completed grade school or junior high, 13 completed high school, 4 completed college, and 3 had master's degrees or beyond. Twelve subjects had been diagnosed with cancer; 5 with respiratory disorders; 4 with sickle cell disease; 3 with cardiac disorders; 2 with vascular disorders; and 1 each with gastrointestinal, musculoskeletal, neurological, and dermatological disorders. Twenty-three subjects had received information on advance directives and 7 said they had received no information. Thirteen of the subjects had completed advance directives and 17 had not.

Participants with the highest mean scores were African American, female, aged 35 to 49 years, with a high school education. No subject in the 20 to 30 age group had completed an advance directive, whereas 62 percent of subjects over age 65 had done so. The two people with the lowest scores both disagreed with the statement that an advance directive would make sure that their family knew what treatment they desired and they would receive the treatment they desired. The 13 participants who had

completed advance directives cited the following reasons for doing so: (a) desire not to be placed on life support, (b) desire to name someone to make decisions in event of incapacitation, (c) desire to make decisions easier for spouse or family, (d) failing health, and (e) advancing age. The 17 who had not completed advance directives cited the following reasons: (a) keep putting it off, (b) not necessary at this point in my life, (c) uncomfortable making decisions about life support, (d) never heard of advance directives before, (e) form was too long, (f) trust husband to make those decisions, and (g) advance directives are unnecessary.

IMPLICATIONS FOR NURSING PRACTICE: The authors suggested that nurses need to explain what advance directives are when asking patients if they have an advance directive. They stated: "[Nurses] can explore alternative ways to educate patients about advance directives (e.g., videotape), and follow up with patients who have requested information to see if they have additional questions or need assistance completing an advance directive." They also suggested that nurses need to inform physicians when patients have advance directives. As patient advocates, nurses have the responsibility for making sure that patients understand the purpose of advance directives and what is involved in completing an advance directive, and for ensuring that patients' end-of-life care is executed according to their wishes.

Summary and Key Points

■ Loss is the experience of separation from something of personal importance.

■ Loss is anything that is perceived as such by the individual.

■ Loss of any concept of value to an individual can trigger the grief response.

■ Elisabeth Kübler-Ross identified five stages that individuals pass through on their way to resolution of a loss. These include denial, anger, bargaining, depression, and acceptance.

■ John Bowlby described similar stages that he identified in the following manner: stage I, numbness or protest; stage II, disequilibrium; stage III, disorganization and despair; and stage IV, reorganization.

■ George Engel's stages include shock and disbelief, developing awareness, restitution, resolution of the loss, and recovery.

■ J. William Worden, a more contemporary clinician, has proposed that bereaved individuals must accomplish a set of tasks in order to complete the grief process. These four tasks include accepting the reality of the loss, processing the pain of grief, adjusting to a world without the lost entity, and finding an enduring connection with the lost entity in the midst of embarking on a new life.

■ The length of the grief process is highly individual, and it can last for a number of years without being maladaptive.

■ The acute stage of the grief process typically lasts a couple of months, but resolution usually takes much longer.

■ Kübler-Ross suggested that a calendar year of experiencing significant events and anniversaries without the lost entity may be required.

■ Anticipatory grieving is the experiencing of the feelings and emotions associated with the normal grief process in response to anticipation of the loss.

■ Anticipatory grieving is thought to facilitate the grief process when the actual loss occurs.

■ Three types of pathological grief reactions have been described. These include the following:

　■ Delayed or inhibited grief in which there is absence of evidence of grief when it ordinarily would be expected.

　■ Distorted or exaggerated grief response in which the individual remains fixed in the anger stage of the grief process and all of the symptoms associated with normal grieving are exaggerated.

　■ Chronic or prolonged grieving in which the individual is unable to let go of grieving behaviors after an extended period of time and in which behaviors are evident that indicate the bereaved individual is not accepting that the loss has occurred.

■ Several authors have identified one crucial difference between normal and maladaptive grieving: the loss of self-esteem.

■ Feelings of worthlessness are indicative of depression rather than uncomplicated bereavement.

■ Very young children do not understand death, but often react to the emotions of adults by becoming more irritable and crying more. They often believe death is reversible.

■ School-age children understand the finality of death. Grief behaviors may reflect regression or aggression, school phobias, or sometimes a withdrawal into the self.

■ Adolescents are usually able to view death on an adult level. Grieving behaviors may include withdrawal or acting out. Although they understand that their own death is inevitable, the concept is so far-reaching as to be imperceptible.

■ By the time a person reaches the 60s or 70s, he or she has experienced numerous losses. Because grief is cumulative, this can result in bereavement overload. Depression is a common response.

■ Nurses must be aware of the death rituals and grief behaviors common to various cultures. Some of these rituals associated with African Americans, Asian Americans, Filipino Americans, Jewish Americans, Mexican Americans, and Native Americans were presented in this chapter.

■ Hospice is a program that provides palliative and supportive care to meet the special needs of people who are dying and their families.

■ The term *advance directive* refers to either a living will or a durable power of attorney for health care. Advance directives allow clients to be in control of decisions at the end of life and spare family and loved ones the burden of making choices without knowing what is most important to the person who is dying.

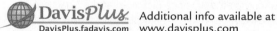 **DavisPlus** DavisPlus.fadavis.com   Additional info available at www.davisplus.com

Review Questions
Self-Examination/Learning Exercise

*Select the answer that is **most** appropriate for each of the following questions.*

1. Which of the following is most likely to initiate a grief response in an individual?
   a. Death of the pet dog
   b. Being told by her doctor that she has begun menopause
   c. Failing an exam
   d. A only
   e. All of the above.

2. Nancy, who is dying of cancer, says to the nurse, "I just want to see my new grandbaby. If only God will let me live until she is born. Then I'll be ready to go." This is an example of which of Kübler-Ross's stages of grief?
   a. Denial
   b. Anger
   c. Bargaining
   d. Acceptance

3. Gloria, a recent widow, states, "I'm going to have to learn to pay all the bills. Hank always did that. I don't know if I can handle all of that." This is an example of which of the tasks described by Worden?
   a. Task I: Accepting the reality of the loss
   b. Task II: Processing the pain of grief
   c. Task III: Adjusting to a world without the lost entity
   d. Task IV: Finding an enduring connection with the lost entity in the midst of embarking on a new life

4. Engel identifies which of the following as successful resolution of the grief process?
   a. When the bereaved person can talk about the loss without crying
   b. When the bereaved person no longer talks about the lost entity
   c. When the bereaved person puts all remembrances of the loss out of sight
   d. When the bereaved person can discuss both positive and negative aspects about the lost entity

Review Questions—cont'd
Self-Examination/Learning Exercise

5. Which of the following is thought to facilitate the grief process?
   a. The ability to grieve in anticipation of the loss
   b. The ability to grieve alone without interference from others
   c. Having recently grieved for another loss
   d. Taking personal responsibility for the loss

6. When Frank's wife of 34 years dies, he is very stoic, handles all the funeral arrangements, doesn't cry or appear sad, and comforts all of the other family members in their grief. Two years later, when Frank's best friend dies, Frank has sleep disturbances, difficulty concentrating, loss of weight, and difficulty performing on his job. This is an example of which of the following maladaptive responses to loss?
   a. Delayed grieving
   b. Distorted grieving
   c. Prolonged grieving
   d. Exaggerated grieving

7. A major difference between normal and maladaptive grieving has been identified by which of the following?
   a. There are no feelings of depression in normal grieving.
   b. There is no loss of self-esteem in normal grieving.
   c. Normal grieving lasts no longer than 1 year.
   d. In normal grief the person does not show anger toward the loss.

8. Which grief reaction can the nurse anticipate in a 10-year-old child?
   a. Statements that the deceased person will soon return
   b. Regressive behaviors, such as loss of bladder control
   c. A preoccupation with the loss
   d. Thinking that they may have done something to cause the death

9. Which of the following is a correct statement when attempting to distinguish normal grief from clinical depression?
   a. In clinical depression, anhedonia is prevalent.
   b. In normal grieving, the person has generalized feelings of guilt.
   c. The person who is clinically depressed relates feelings of depression to a specific loss.
   d. In normal grieving, there is a persistent state of dysphoria.

10. Which of the following is *not* true regarding grieving by an adolescent?
    a. Adolescents may not show their true feelings about the death.
    b. Adolescents tend to have an immortal attitude.
    c. Adolescents do not perceive death as inevitable.
    d. Adolescents may exhibit acting out behaviors as part of their grief.

References

Appel, S.J. (2013). Vietnamese Americans. In J.N. Giger (Ed.), *Transcultural nursing: Assessment and intervention* (6th ed., pp. 426-461). St. Louis, MO: Mosby.

Asante, M.K. (2009). *Contours of the African American culture.* Retrieved from www.asante.net/articles/12/contours-of-the-african-american-culture

Campinha-Bacote, J. (2013). People of African American heritage. In L.D. Purnell (Ed.), *Transcultural health care* (4th ed., pp. 91-114). Philadelphia, PA: F.A. Davis.

Catalano, J.T. (2012). *Nursing now! Today's issues, tomorrow's trends* (6th ed.). Philadelphia, PA: F.A. Davis.

Corr, C.A., & Corr, D.M. (2013). *Death and dying: Life and living* (7th ed.). Belmont, CA: Wadsworth.

Halstead, H.L. (2005). Spirituality in older adults. In M. Stanley, K.A. Blair, & P.G. Beare (Eds.), *Gerontological nursing: A health promotion/protection approach* (3rd ed.). Philadelphia, PA: F.A. Davis.

Ito, M., & Hattori, K. (2013). People of Japanese heritage. In L.D. Purnell (Ed.), *Transcultural health care: A culturally competent approach* (4th ed., pp. 319-338). Philadelphia, PA: F.A. Davis.

Jeffreys, J.S. (2010). Understanding grief in older adults. *Living With Loss Magazine,* Winter 2010. Eckert, CO: Bereavement Publications.

Mantel, D.L. (2013). Laws on death and dying. *Advance for long-term care management*. Retrieved from http://long-term-care.advanceweb.com/Article/Laws-On-Death-Dying-2.aspx

Mattson, S. (2013). People of Vietnamese heritage. In L.D. Purnell (Ed.), *Transcultural health care: A culturally competent approach* (4th ed., pp. 479-480). Philadelphia, PA: F.A. Davis.

Munoz, C.C. (2013). People of Filipino Heritage. In L. D. Purnell (Ed.), *Transcultural health care: A culturally competent approach* (4th ed., pp. 228-249). Philadelphia, PA: F.A. Davis.

Murray, R.B., Zentner, J.P., & Yakimo, R. (2009). *Health promotion strategies through the life span* (8th ed.). Upper Saddle River, NJ: Prentice Hall.

National Hospice and Palliative Care Organization (NHPCO). (2000). *Standards of practice for hospice programs*. Alexandria, VA: NHPCO.

Norlander, L. (2008). *To comfort always: A nurse's guide to end-of-life care*. Indianapolis, IN: Sigma Theta Tau International.

Pies, R.W. (2013). Grief and depression: The sages knew the difference. *Psychiatric Times*, April 29, 2013. Retrieved from www.psychiatrictimes.com/display/article/10168/2140230

Purnell, L.D. (2009). People of Navajo Indian heritage. *Guide to culturally competent health care* (2nd ed. pp. 303-320). Philadelphia, PA: F.A. Davis.

Purnell, L.D. (2013). The Purnell model for cultural competence. In L.D. Purnell (Ed.), *Transcultural health care: A culturally competent approach* (4th ed. pp. 15-44). Philadelphia, PA: F.A. Davis.

Sadock, B.J., & Sadock, V.A. (2007). *Synopsis of psychiatry: Behavioral sciences/clinical psychiatry* (10th ed.). Philadelphia, PA: Lippincott Williams & Wilkins.

Salazar, M.L. (2009). *Life in death: Mexican American grave decorating and funerary rituals*. Unpublished thesis. Department of Anthropology. San Marcos, TX: Texas State University.

Selekman, J. (2013). People of Jewish heritage. In L.D. Purnell (Ed.), *Transcultural health care: A culturally competent approach* (4th ed., pp. 339-356). Philadelphia, PA: F.A. Davis.

Tsai, Hsiu-Min. (2013). People of Chinese heritage. In L.D. Purnell (Ed.), *Transcultural health care: A culturally competent approach* (4th ed., pp. 178-196). Philadelphia, PA: F.A. Davis.

Worden, J. W. (2009). *Grief counseling and grief therapy: A handbook for the mental health practitioner* (4th ed.). New York, NY: Springer.

Zoucha, R., & Zamarripa, C.A. (2013). People of Mexican heritage. In L.D. Purnell (Ed.), *Transcultural health care: A culturally competent approach* (4th ed., pp. 374-390). Philadelphia, PA: F.A. Davis.

Classical References

Bowlby, J. (1961). Processes of mourning. *International Journal of Psychoanalysis, 42,* 22.

Engel, G. (1964). Grief and grieving. *American Journal of Nursing, 64,* 93.

Kübler-Ross, E. (1969). *On death and dying*. New York, NY: Macmillan.

@ INTERNET REFERENCES

- Additional references related to bereavement may be located at the following websites:
  - www.journeyofhearts.org
  - www.nhpco.org
  - www.hospicefoundation.org
  - www.livingwithloss.com
  - www.caringinfo.org
  - www.aahpm.org
  - www.hpna.org

Military Families

38

CHAPTER OUTLINE

Objectives

Homework Assignment

Historical Aspects

Epidemiological Statistics

Application of the Nursing Process

Treatment Modalities

Summary and Key Points

Review Questions

KEY TERMS

deployment

posttraumatic stress disorder

Ready Reserve

veterans

traumatic brain injury

OBJECTIVES

After reading this chapter, the student will be able to:

1. Discuss historical aspects and epidemiological statistics related to members and veterans of the U.S. military.
2. Describe the lifestyle of career military families.
3. Discuss the impact of deployment on families of service members.
4. Discuss concerns of women in the military.
5. Describe combat-related illnesses common in members and veterans of the U.S. military.
6. Apply steps of the nursing process in care of veterans with traumatic brain injury and posttraumatic stress disorder.
7. Discuss various modalities relevant to treatment of traumatic brain injury and posttraumatic stress disorder.

HOMEWORK ASSIGNMENT

Please read the chapter and answer the following questions:

1. Name some positives and negatives associated with the military lifestyle.
2. Describe some behaviors exhibited by school-age children in response to the deployment of a parent.
3. How do the feelings about leaving their children during a deployment differ between men and women service members?
4. Name some symptoms of posttraumatic stress disorder.

Because of U.S. involvement in Iraq and Afghanistan, perhaps at no time in modern history has so much attention been given to what individuals and families experience as a result of their lives in the military. There is an ongoing effort by organizations that provide services for active-duty military personnel and **veterans** of military combat to keep up with the growing demand, and resources for these services will be required for many years to come. The need for mental health-care practitioners will rise as the increasing number of veterans and their family members struggle to cope with their combat-related experiences.

This chapter addresses issues associated with the lives of military families and veterans of military combat. A discussion of nursing care for these individuals is presented, and selected medical treatment modalities are described.

Historical Aspects

"To care for him who shall have borne the battle and for his widow and his orphan."

Abraham Lincoln, 1865

There is little doubt that individuals who survive military combat return from battle with scars—either physical, psychological, or both. Reports of war-related, psychological symptoms have existed in writing throughout the centuries; terms such as "shell shock" and "battle fatigue" have been used to describe these symptoms. Many veterans of World War I and World War II were expected to be stoic, to lock up their feelings, and to never speak of the scenes of carnage and combat that they had witnessed. The abuse of alcohol became a common way to deal with the emotions that they did not feel comfortable discussing. **Posttraumatic stress disorder** (PTSD) has been related to the high rates of alcoholism among veterans, particularly those who have experienced active-duty combat. It has only been in recent history that the invisible wounds of combat veterans have received the treatment they desperately require.

Very little was written about PTSD during the years between 1950 and 1970. This absence was followed in the 1970s and 1980s with an explosion in the amount of research and writing on the subject. Many of the papers written during this time were about Vietnam veterans. Clearly, the renewed interest in PTSD was linked to the psychological casualties of the Vietnam War. The diagnostic category of PTSD did not appear until the third edition of the *Diagnostic and Statistical Manual of Mental Disorders* (*DSM-III*) in 1980, after a need was indicated by increasing numbers of problems with Vietnam veterans and victims of multiple disasters.

Epidemiological Statistics

There are currently about 1.5 million individuals serving in the U.S. Armed Forces in more than 150 countries around the world (USA.gov, 2013). Approximately 15 percent of these are women. Veterans currently number 21.8 million, with about 7 percent being women. In addition, more than 1 million men and women compose the total of the U.S. Military "Ready Reserve" who are members of various components of the National Guard and U.S. Military Reserves (Kapp, 2012). The purpose of the **Ready Reserve** is to "provide trained units and qualified persons available for active duty in the armed forces, in time of war or national emergency, and at such other times as the national security may require, to fill the needs of the armed forces whenever more units and persons are needed than are in the regular components" (Title 10 U.S. Code 10102, 2006).

Since the beginning of the wars in Afghanistan and Iraq in 2001, more than 1.9 million U.S. military personnel have been deployed in 3 million tours of duty lasting more than 30 days as part of Operation Enduring Freedom (OEF) and Operation Iraqi Freedom (OIF) (Institute of Medicine [IOM], 2012). The cost in deaths and physical and psychological injuries cannot be measured.

Application of the Nursing Process

Assessment

The Military Family

The military lifestyle offers both positive and negative aspects to those who choose this way of life. Hall (2011) summarizes a number of pros and cons about what has come to be known as "The Warrior Society." Some advantages include the following:

■ Early retirement compared to civilian counterparts
■ The security of a vast system to meet family needs
■ Job security with a guaranteed paycheck
■ Health-care benefits
■ Opportunities to see areas of the world
■ Educational opportunities

Some disadvantages include the following:

■ Frequent separations and reunions
■ Regular household relocations
■ Living life under the maxim of "the mission must always come first"
■ A pattern of rigidity, regimentation, and conformity in family life
■ Feelings of detachment from nonmilitary community
■ The social effects of "rank"
■ The lack of control over pay, promotion, and other benefits

Mary Wertsch (1996), who conducted a vast amount of research on the culture of the military family, stated, "The great paradox of the military is that its members, the self-appointed front-line guardians of our cherished American democratic values, do not live in democracy themselves" (p. 15). The military is maintained by a rigid authoritarian structure, and these characteristics often extend into the structure of the home.

A class system is strikingly evident in the military, with two distinct subcultures: that of the officer and that of the enlisted ranks. Hall (2011) states:

> The United States has made great strides in the past five decades to affirm and equalize the differences in society, but the assumption of all military systems in the world is that it is essential for the functioning of the organization to maintain a rigid hierarchical system based on dominance and subordination. (p. 38)

Isolation and alienation are common facets of military life. To compensate for the extreme mobility, the focus of this lifestyle turns inward to the military world, rather than outward to the local community. Children of military families almost always report that no matter what school they attend, they feel "different" from the other students (Wertsch, 1996).

These descriptions apply principally to "career" military families. There is another type of military family that has become a familiar part of the American culture in recent years. The military campaigns of OEF and OIF together make up the longest sustained U.S. military operation since the Vietnam War, and they are the first extended conflicts to depend on an all-volunteer military (IOM, 2012). There has been heavy dependence on the National Guard and Reserves, and an escalation in the pace, duration, and number of deployments and redeployments experienced by these individuals. Many had joined the National Guard or Reserves as a second job for financial reasons or for the educational opportunities available to them. Little thought had been given to the possibility of actually fighting in a war. As one anonymous reservist posted on his blog,

> The active forces have the harder role. They're required to be fully ready 24/7/365, and to deploy and fight on much shorter notice than the Reserve [forces]. It's their livelihood and (for many) their career. They're serving full-time; reservists aren't. That was once clearly true. But not really quite true anymore. Many reservists in critically-needed specialties have already served multiple years on active duty since 9/11, and this situation doesn't look to change anytime soon. ("'Kelly Temps' in Uniform," 2012)

In recent years, enlistees in the National Guard and Reserves are being told that they should expect to serve an interval of active duty. Most individuals in the National Guard and Reserves are willing to serve when and where they are needed. However, they consider themselves "part-timers." The extended campaigns of OEF and OIF have changed this part-time concept for many who have served multiple tours of duty, creating a hardship on their families and their civilian careers. Many of these "temporary citizen soldiers," as well as their full-time military counterparts, now carry the physical and psychological scars of battle.

Military Spouses and Children

A military spouse inherently knows and lives with the concept of "mission first." Devries, Hughes, Watson, and Moore (2012) state, "While the military works hard to value the family lives of service members and their welfare, the nature of the job is that the mission trumps all other concerns" (p. 11). However, times have changed from the days when life in the military was viewed as a two-person career, in which a woman was expected to "create the right family setting so that her husband's work reflected his life at home, by staying positive, being interested in his duty, and being flexible and adaptable" (Hall, 2012, p. 148). Many of today's military spouses have their own careers or are pursuing higher levels of education. They do not view the military as a joint career with their service member spouse.

The lives of military spouses and children are clearly affected when the service-member's active duty assignments require frequent family moves. Wakefield (2007) has stated, "The many short-term relationships, complications of spousal employment, university transfer issues, escalated misbehavior of the children, day-care arrangements, spousal loneliness, and increased financial obligations are just some of the issues military personnel face that can lead to frustration." In most instances, when the service member receives orders for a new geographical assignment, the spouse's education, career, or both is put on hold, and the entire family is relocated. Other occasions may arise when the family is unable to immediately follow the service member to the new location. In certain instances, such as when a student may be about to complete a semester or is about to graduate, the service member may proceed to the new assignment without the family. This is difficult for the military spouse who is left alone to care for the children, as well as to deal with all aspects of the move.

Military children face unique challenges. There are 1.9 million children and youth in military families (Department of Defense [DoD], 2012a). They primarily attend civilian public schools where they form a unique subculture among staff and peers who often do not understand their life experiences. Children who grow up in a career military family learn to adapt to changing situations very quickly and to hide a certain level of fear associated with the nomadic lifestyle. Hall (2008) states:

> It is not just a fear of what might happen to their family or their military parents but a fear of the unknown, of not being accepted, of being behind, of not finding friends, or of not being cool. One of the most common concerns expressed by students when they arrive in a new school is who they will eat lunch with. Another reality for student athletes is that a student could be the star of the basketball team in one school and be sitting on the bench at the next. (p. 103)

The Impact of Deployment

Not since the Vietnam War have so many U.S. military families been affected by deployment-related family separation, combat injury, and death. Many service members have been deployed multiple times. Those who are deployed most frequently describe their greatest fear as that of having to leave their spouse and children. Lengthy separations pose many challenges to all members of the family. Spouses undertake all the challenges of managing the household, in addition to assuming the role of the singular parent. The pressure and stress are intense as the spouse attempts to maintain an atmosphere of strength for the children, while experiencing the fears and anxiety associated with the life-threatening conditions facing his or her service member partner.

Approximately 2 million American children have experienced the **deployment** of a parent to Iraq or Afghanistan. More than 48,000 children have either lost a parent or have a parent who was wounded in these conflicts. Smith (2012) states:

> The stress that comes when a family member is deployed is significant, and that stress is multiplied when a loved one is wounded or killed. When parents return from deployment, they are not always the same as they were before. Major injuries, such as loss of a limb, traumatic brain injury, or posttraumatic stress disorder are life-altering, and children often have a hard time understanding the reason for a significant change in the appearance, personality, or behavior of a parent.

The following behaviors have been reported in children in response to the deployment of a parent (American Academy of Child & Adolescent Psychiatry, 2014):

- Infants (birth to 12 months): May respond to disruptions in their schedule with decreased appetite, weight loss, irritability, and/or apathy.
- Toddlers (1 to 3 years): May become sullen, tearful, throw temper tantrums or develop sleep problems.
- Preschoolers (3 to 6 years): May regress in areas such as toilet training, sleep, separation fears, physical complaints, or thumb sucking. May assume blame for parent's departure.
- School-age children (6 to 12 years): Are more aware of potential dangers to parent. May exhibit irritable behavior, aggression, or whininess. May become more regressed and fearful about parent's safety.
- Adolescents (13 to 18 years): May be rebellious, irritable, or more challenging of authority. Parents need to be alert to high-risk behaviors, such as problems with the law, sexual acting out, and drug or alcohol abuse.

Pincus, House, Christenson, and Alder (2013) describe the cycle of deployment in five distinct stages: predeployment, deployment, sustainment, redeployment, and postdeployment.

Predeployment The time frame for this stage is variable, beginning with the receipt of the orders and ending when the service member departs. Family members alternate with feelings of denial and anticipation of loss. The soldier and family get their affairs in order, extended training periods result in long hours apart,

and the anxiety of the anticipated departure promotes stress and irritability among family members.

Deployment This stage includes the time from actual deployment through the first month of separation. Military spouses report feeling disoriented and overwhelmed, and experience a range of emotions including numbness, sadness, loneliness, and abandonment. It is a time of disorganization as the spouse struggles to take charge of the details of living without his or her partner.

Sustainment Sustainment begins about 1 month into the deployment until about a month before the service member's expected return. During this stage, the spouse and children establish new support systems and institute new family routines. Technology makes it possible for the family and service member to keep in touch with each other by phone, video, and e-mail. Despite the difficulties and obstacles encountered, most military families successfully negotiate this stage and anxiously anticipate their loved one's return.

Redeployment This stage is defined as the month before the service member is scheduled to return home. There is excitement and apprehension associated with the homecoming. Pincus and associates (2013) identify concerns such as, "Will he (she) agree with the changes I have made?" "Will I have to give up my independence?" "Will we get along?"

Postdeployment This stage typically lasts 3 to 6 months and begins with the return of the service member to the home station. There is a period of adjustment beginning with the "honeymoon" period, when the spouses reconnect physically, but not necessarily emotionally. The returning service member may desire to "pick up where he or she left off," only to encounter resistance from the spouse who expresses a reluctance to relinquish the degree of independence and autonomy to which he or she has become accustomed during the separation. Pincus and associates (2013) state:

> Postdeployment is probably the most important stage for both soldier and spouse. Patient communication, going slow, lowering expectations, and taking time to get to know each other again is critical to the task of successful reintegration of the soldier back into the family.

Counseling may be required in the event that the service member has been injured or experiences a traumatic stress reaction.

Women in the Military

Women make up approximately 15 percent of the U.S. military and 17 percent of National Guard and Reserve members (Mathewson, 2011). Women have been serving in the military since the time of the Civil War, mostly in the roles of nurses, spies, and support persons. In recent years, the Pentagon relaxed its ban on women serving in combat roles, and "women began to fly combat aircraft, staff missile placements, drive convoys in the desert, and participate in other roles that involved potential combat exposure" (Mathewson, 2011, p. 217). Early in 2013, the Secretary of Defense lifted the ban on combat jobs to women, gradually opening direct combat units to female troops. At the present time, certain specialty positions continue to remain off-limits, although the plan is to integrate women into these positions. Flexibility in the new law exists for exemptions to occur if further assessment reveals that some jobs are inappropriate for women.

Special Concerns of Women in the Military

There are a number of issues of special concern to women in the military, including sexual harassment, sexual assault, differential treatment and conditions, and being a parent.

Sexual Harassment Sexual harassment is defined as "unwanted, unwelcome comments or physical contact of a sexual nature occurring in the workplace" (Mathewson, 2011, p. 221). From statements such as "you look nice this morning" or "hey you smell good" to blatant suggestions or requests for sexual interactions, Wolfe and associates (1998), in a study of women on active duty during the Persian Gulf War, found that both physical and sexual harassment were higher than those typically found in peacetime military samples. Reports by military therapists convey that these women who were sexually harassed while in the military suffer high rates of a range of problems following discharge, including poor self-image, relationship problems, drug use, depression, and PTSD.

Sexual Assault The Department of Defense (DoD, 2012b) reported 2,723 cases of active service member sexual assaults in 2011. Sexual assault is defined as "attempted or completed sexual attack through threat or use of physical force that took place on or off duty during the course of military service" (Mathewson, 2011, p. 221). It is estimated that only about 13 percent of sexual assaults in the military are reported. Reasons for not reporting include fears of causing trouble in their unit, that their commanders and fellow soldiers would turn against them, that they would be passed over for well-deserved promotions, or that they would be transferred and removed from duty altogether (Vlahos, 2012). Some women who have reported the incident to their commanding officers have been told to "forget about it," "buckle up," or "pretend it didn't happen," and are made to feel as though they are the perpetrator instead of the victim. Wolf (2012) describes how the military deals with rape as "a culture of cover-up."

Some women who report their sexual assaults are discharged from the service with psychiatric diagnoses of personality disorder or adjustment disorder. Vlahos (2012) reports:

> For the veteran, getting a personality disorder or adjustment disorder discharge can be catastrophic. Not only does it carry a stigma for future employers, it cuts the veteran off from a series of benefits, including health care and service-related disability compensation.

Although they compose only 15 percent of military personnel, women constitute almost one-fourth of all personality disorder discharges. Survivors of sexual assault in the military report long-lasting effects, including PTSD, depression, suicidal ideation and attempts, eating disorders, anxiety disorders, relationship difficulties, and substance abuse. Wolf (2012) notes that, among military veterans, the leading cause of PTSD for men is combat trauma, whereas for women it is sexual trauma. She states, "Our women veterans are more likely to be traumatized by a sexual assault by a fellow soldier, or a commander, than by their own battlefield or war experiences."

Differential Treatment and Conditions Although their numbers have increased, women still constitute a minority in the military. One female officer accounted that because of the small number of women in any given unit, officers and enlisted personnel are often housed together. She indicated that she missed being with other officers to discuss work and to be able to spend time with her peers. She also reported that the enlisted women were uncomfortable with an officer in their presence.

Women's military careers are often limited by their exclusions from occupational specialties. These sanctions often preclude female officers and enlisted personnel from the most prestigious units and occupations in the military, their participation in which is essential to ascending in the ranks should they choose to make the military a career. However, as stated previously, some changes are currently proposed that, when implemented, will decrease occupational discrimination against women in the military.

Parenting Issues Women's feelings associated with leaving their children often differ from those of men. Women seem to struggle more with guilt feelings for "abandoning" their children, whereas men have stronger emotions tied to a sense of doing their duty. Although men also experience regret at leaving their children, they often rely on the assurance that the children have their mothers to care for them.

Veterans

There are 21.8 million veterans in the United States, 20.2 million male veterans and 1.6 million female

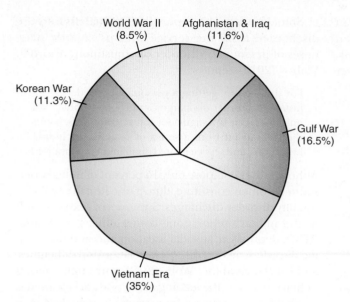

World War II
(8.5%)

Afghanistan & Iraq
(11.6%)

Korean War
(11.3%)

Gulf War
(16.5%)

Vietnam Era
(35%)

FIGURE 38-1 Percentage of veterans according to period of service. (Source: U.S. Census Bureau, 2013).

veterans. Figure 38-1 provides a breakdown by percentage, according to period of service.

Most veterans returning from a combat zone undergo a period of adjustment. Although the majority do not develop a behavioral health condition, most will experience feelings and reactions that may contribute to difficulties with their reintegration into civilian life. Many veterans suffer from migraine headaches and experience cognitive difficulties, such as memory loss. Hypervigilance, insomnia, and jitteriness are common. The Substance Abuse and Mental Health Services Administration (SAMHSA, 2012) states, "Veterans may struggle to concentrate; engage in aggressive behavior, such as aggressive driving; and use alcohol, tobacco, and drugs excessively. However, the intensity and duration of these and other worrisome behaviors can indicate a more serious problem and the need for professional treatment" (p. 1).

Traumatic Brain Injury

The Departments of Veterans Affairs and Defense (DVA/DoD, 2009, p. 16) offer the following definition of **traumatic brain injury** (TBI):

A traumatically induced structural injury and/or physiological disruption of brain function as a result of an external force that is indicated by new onset or worsening of at least one of the following clinical signs, immediately following the event:

■ Any period of loss of or a decreased level of consciousness

■ Any loss of memory for events immediately before or after the injury (posttraumatic amnesia)

■ Any alteration in mental state at the time of the injury (confusion, disorientation, slowed thinking, etc.) (Alteration of consciousness/mental state)

■ Neurological deficits (weakness, loss of balance, change in vision, praxis, paresis/plegia, sensory loss, aphasia, etc.) that may or may not be transient

■ Intracranial lesion

Symptoms may be classified as mild, moderate, or severe, according to severity of symptoms.

In the civilian population, the most common causes of TBI include child abuse in infants and toddlers, motor vehicle accidents in adolescents and young adults, and falls and associated subdural hematomas in older adults (Strong & Donders, 2012). Blasts from explosive devices are the leading cause of TBI for active-duty military personnel in combat (Birk, 2010). TBI also results from penetrating wounds, severe blows to the head with shrapnel or debris, and falls or bodily collisions with objects following a blast. Symptoms of TBI according to level of severity are presented in Table 38-1.

Most soldiers who have sustained a mild TBI improve with no lasting clinical sequelae (DVA/DoD, 2009). Many recover within hours to days, or at most, weeks. In a small minority, symptoms persist from 6 months to a year. The location and severity of the injury are factors that determine the long-term outcome for individuals with TBI. Severity is determined by the nature, speed and location of the impact, and by complications such as hypoxemia, hypotension, intracranial hemorrhage, or increased intracranial pressure (Ribbers, 2013).

The most common long-term sequelae related to TBI include problems with cognition (e.g., thinking, memory, and reasoning) and behavior or mental health (e.g., depression, anxiety, personality changes, aggression, acting out, and social inappropriateness)

TABLE 38-1 Criteria and Symptomatology of Traumatic Brain Injury According to Level of Severity

MILD	MODERATE	SEVERE
Criteria	**Criteria**	**Criteria**
Structural imaging = normal	Structural imaging = normal or abnormal	Structural imaging = normal or abnormal
Loss of consciousness 0–30 min	Loss of consciousness > 30 min and < 24 hrs	Loss of consciousness >24 hrs
Alteration of consciousness/ mental state = a moment up to 24 hrs	Alteration of consciousness/mental state = > 24 hours. Severity based on other criteria.	Alteration of consciousness/mental state = > 24 hours. Severity based on other criteria.
Posttraumatic amnesia = 0–1 day	Posttraumatic amnesia = > 1 and < 7 Days	Posttraumatic amnesia = > 7 days
Glasgow Coma Scale = 13–15	Glasgow Coma Scale = 9–12	Glasgow Coma Scale = < 9
Symptoms	**Symptoms**	**Symptoms**
Headache	Any of the symptoms of mild TBI	Any of the symptoms of mild TBI
Dizziness, ringing in the ears	Headache that gets worse or does not go away	Headache that gets worse or does not go away
Nausea	Repeated nausea and vomiting	Repeated nausea and vomiting
Trouble concentrating, confusion	Seizures	Seizures
Blurred vision	Difficulty awakening from sleep	Inability to awaken from sleep
Changes in sleep patterns	Dilation of one or both pupils of the eyes	Dilation of one or both pupils of the eyes
Mood changes	Slurred speech	Slurred speech
Sensitivity to light or sound	Weakness or numbness in the extremities	Weakness or numbness in the extremities
	Loss of coordination Increased confusion Restlessness Agitation	Loss of coordination Profound confusion Restlessness Agitation

SOURCES: DVA/DoD, 2009; Mayo Clinic, 2012; National Institute of Neurological Disorders and Stroke (NINDS), 2013.

(Ribbers, 2013). Seizures occur in about 15 to 20 percent of individuals with TBI and commonly develop within the first 24 hours following the injury. With mild TBI, seizures usually subside within a week after the initial trauma. The potential for chronic epilepsy increases with severity of the injury.

Language and communication problems, such as aphasia, dysarthria, and dysphasia, can result from TBI (Safaz, Yasar, Tok, & Yilmaz, 2008). Difficulties may also exist in the more subtle aspects of communication, such as body language and nonverbal expression.

Studies show that TBI has long-term adverse effects on social functioning and productivity. Temkin, Corrigan, Dikmen, and Machamer (2009) stated:

Penetrating head injury sustained in wartime is clearly associated with increased unemployment. TBI also adversely affects leisure and recreation, social relationships, functional status, quality of life, and independent living. Although there is a dose-response relationship between severity of injury and social outcomes, there is insufficient evidence to determine at what level of severity the adverse effects are demonstrated. (p. 460)

Neurocognitive disorders, such as Alzheimer's disease (AD) and Parkinson's disease, are related to TBI (Ribbers, 2013). The risk for AD in individuals with moderate TBI is 2.3 times greater than it is in the general population. An association between Parkinson's disease and TBI has also been established. The disorder may develop years after TBI as a result of damage to the basal ganglia (Ribbers, 2013).

Posttraumatic Stress Disorder

Posttraumatic stress disorder (PTSD) is the most common mental disorder among veterans returning from military combat. The DVA (2012) provides the following prevalence estimates:

- Veterans of OEF and OIF, 11 to 20 percent
- Gulf War veterans, 10 percent
- Vietnam veterans, 30 percent

The diagnostic criteria for PTSD from the *Diagnostic and Statistical Manual of Mental Disorders, Fifth Edition (DSM-5)* (2013) are presented in Chapter 28 of this text. The disorder can occur when an individual is exposed to an accident or violence in which there is actual or threatened death or serious injury to the self or others. Symptoms of PTSD include the following:

- Reexperiencing the trauma through flashbacks, nightmares, and intrusive thoughts
- Intensive efforts to avoid activities, people, places, situations, or objects that arouse recollections of the trauma
- Chronic negative emotional state and diminished interest or participation in significant activities
- Aggressive, reckless, or self-destructive behavior
- Hypervigilance and exaggerated startle response
- Angry outbursts, problems with concentration, and sleep disturbances

Symptoms of PTSD may be delayed, in some instances for years. When emotions regarding the trauma are constricted, they may suddenly appear at sometime in the future following a major life event, stressor, or an accumulation of stressors with time that challenge the person's defenses. Symptoms also may be masked by other physical or mental health problems that the veteran may be experiencing. In some instances, the symptoms do not appear to be problematic until the individual begins a readjustment to routine occupational or social functioning.

Reports indicate that some World War II veterans are only now, decades after returning from combat, being diagnosed with PTSD. At the time of their return, rarely did these veterans speak of their war experiences. But in many, the visions of horror have seeped to the surface in nightmares, flashbacks, anxiety, and emotional numbness. In a study at the University of Michigan, Dr. Helen Kales found that, in a group of World War II veterans being treated for depression, 38 percent of them met the criteria for PTSD (Albrecht, 2009). Langer (2011) reported that the PTSD symptoms for these veterans seemed to become more prominent in midlife, and that the most significant precipitant was retirement. For many, their work gave meaning to their lives, and without it the symptoms of depression, anxiety, substance abuse, and PTSD began to emerge. Langer (2011) stated:

> Besides retirement, other precipitants [to PTSD in midlife] include the deaths of friends, one's own deteriorating health, children becoming autonomous, divorce, and other losses associated with aging. Other precipitants include current events that trigger memories of one's own combat experience, e.g., 9/11, and other wars.

Veterans with PTSD experience marital and relationship difficulties, including higher rates of physical and verbal aggression against their partners and children and higher rates of divorce (Monson, Fredman, & Adair, 2008). The burden of caregiving to a partner with PTSD has been noted as an etiological factor in relationship difficulties. The caregiver's perception of how caring for the impaired partner affects their social life, health, or financial status is directly associated with the degree of difficulty experienced in the relationship (Lavender & Lyons, 2012). Some caregivers may experience what has been termed as *secondary trauma* or *vicarious traumatization*, a condition in which somatic symptoms and emotional distress occur as a response to caring for an individual who exhibits the symptoms of PTSD. Secondary symptoms are also common in children with a parent suffering from PTSD. Figley (1998) suggested that family members "experience emotions that are strikingly similar to the victim's. This includes visual images (e.g., flashbacks), sleeping problems, depression, and other symptoms that are a direct result of visualizing the victim's traumatic experiences, exposure to the symptoms of the victim, or both" (pp. 20-21).

Co-occurring disorders are common in individuals with PTSD, including major depressive disorder, substance use disorders, and anxiety disorders. Individuals with TBI also may develop PTSD, depending on the degree of amnesia experienced immediately following the cerebral trauma.

Depression and Suicide

The most recent statistics by SAMHSA indicated that 9.3 percent of U.S. veterans between ages 21 and 39 experienced at least one major depressive episode in the year prior to the survey (SAMHSA, 2012). The survey indicated that female veterans are twice as likely as their male counterparts to suffer from depression. The disorder affects 14.8 million U.S. adults annually, and veterans account for slightly more than 14 percent of the total (National Alliance on Mental Illness [NAMI], 2009). Impairments are observed in the domains of home management, interpersonal relationships, and occupational and social functioning.

Reports by the DoD and VA indicate that the number of suicides among veterans and active-duty military has risen dramatically since 2001, the year that detailed record-keeping began. Suicide among military personnel is closely associated with the diagnoses of substance use disorder, major depressive disorder, PTSD, and TBI. A common theme among investigations of suicide attempts and completed suicides by military service members is marital/relationship distress. Devries and associates (2012) stated:

> From 2005 to 2009, relationship problems were a factor in over 50 percent of the suicides in the Army. The health of our military fighting force is directly related to the health of our military marriages. What we see in the military is a common drama of relationship problems played out in an environment of uncommon stressors. (p. 7)

A study by Jakupcak and associates (2010) concluded that veterans who are unmarried or those who report lower satisfaction with their social support networks are at increased risk for suicide.

Substance Use Disorder

Substance use disorder is a common co-occurring condition with PTSD. One study reports that almost 22 percent of veterans with PTSD also receive a diagnosis of substance use disorder (Brancu, Straits-Troster, & Kudler, 2011). SAMHSA (2012) states that alcohol misuse and abuse, hazardous drinking, and binge drinking are common among OEF and OIF veterans, who often report drinking to numb the agonizing feelings and erase the painful memories related to their combat experiences. One research study of OIF veterans indicated that individuals who were exposed to extreme violence and human trauma were more likely to engage in frequent and heavy drinking than their counterparts who had less exposure to such combat experiences (Killgore et al., 2008).

Substance abuse continues to be a major concern for the military. Although there have been reductions over time in tobacco use and illicit drug use, increases in other areas, such as prescription drug abuse and heavy alcohol use, are an ongoing problem. Alcohol abuse is the most prevalent problem, and referrals for treatment are inadequate (National Institute on Drug Abuse [NIDA], 2011). NIDA (2011) reports, "Research findings highlight the need to improve screening and access to care for alcohol-related problems among service members returning from combat deployments"(p. 1).

Diagnosis/Outcome Identification

Nursing diagnoses are formulated from the data gathered during the assessment phase and with background knowledge regarding predisposing factors to the disorder. Table 38-2 presents a list of selected client behaviors and the NANDA nursing diagnoses that correspond to those behaviors, which may be used in planning assistance for families as they

TABLE 38-2 Nursing Diagnoses: Planning Care for Military Families

RISK FACTORS/ DEFINING CHARACTERISTICS	NURSING DIAGNOSES	OUTCOME CRITERIA
PTSD Rage reactions, aggression, irritability, substance use, flashbacks, startle reaction	Risk for other-directed violence	Client will demonstrate appropriate coping behaviors. Client will not harm others.
Depression, perception of lack of social support, physical disabilities from combat injuries, feelings of hopelessness	Risk for suicide	Client will not harm self.
Anger, aggression, depression, difficulty concentrating, flashbacks, guilt, headaches, hypervigilance, intrusive thoughts and dreams, nightmares, emotional numbness, panic attacks, substance abuse	Post-trauma syndrome related to having experienced the trauma of military combat	Client will begin a healthy grief resolution, initiating the process of psychological healing. Client will demonstrate ability to deal with emotional reactions in an individually appropriate manner.
Substance abuse	Ineffective coping; ineffective denial	Client will verbalize understanding of the destructiveness of substance abuse and demonstrate a more adaptive method of coping.

Continued

TABLE 38–2 **Nursing Diagnoses: Planning Care for Military Families—cont'd**		
RISK FACTORS/ DEFINING CHARACTERISTICS	NURSING DIAGNOSES	OUTCOME CRITERIA
Confusion, fear, and anxiety among family members and their inability to deal with the affected member's unpredictable behavior; ineffective family decision-making process	Interrupted family processes related to crisis associated with veteran member's illness	Family will verbalize understanding of trauma-related illness, demonstrate ability to maintain anxiety at manageable level, and make appropriate decisions to stabilize family functioning.
TRAUMATIC BRAIN INJURY		
Impaired physical mobility, limited range of motion, decreased muscle strength and control, perceptual or cognitive impairment, seizures	Risk for injury	Client will remain free of physical injury.
Memory deficits; distractibility; altered attention span or concentration; impaired ability to make decisions, problem-solve, reason or conceptualize; personality changes	Disturbed thought processes*	Client will regain cognitive ability to execute mental functions realistic with the extent of the injury.
Inability to perform desired or appropriate activities of daily living	Self-care deficit (specify)	Client performs self-care activities within level of own ability.
Confusion, fear, and anxiety among family members and the inability to adapt to changes associated with veteran member's injury; difficulty accepting/receiving help; inability to express or to accept each others' feelings	Interrupted family processes related to situational transition and crisis; uncertainty about expectations and ultimate outcome	Family will verbalize understanding of trauma-related illness, demonstrate ability to maintain anxiety at manageable level, and make appropriate decisions to stabilize family functioning.
FAMILY MEMBERS' ISSUES		
Regressive behaviors, loss of appetite, temper tantrums, clinging behaviors, guilt and self-blame, sleep problems, irritability, aggression (children)	Risk for delayed development related to feelings of abandonment associated with parent's deployment	Parent/caregiver will identify behaviors at risk and initiate interventions to promote appropriate development. Child will develop healthy coping strategies and resume normal developmental progression.
Rebelliousness, irritability, acting out behaviors, promiscuity, substance use (adolescents)	Ineffective coping related to feelings of abandonment associated with parent's deployment	Client will work through stages of grief associated with the perceived loss and demonstrate healthy, age-appropriate coping strategies.
Depression, anxiety, loneliness, fear, feeling overwhelmed and powerless, anger (spouse/partner)	Risk for complicated grieving related to military deployment of spouse/partner	Client will work through stages of grief, achieve a healthy acceptance, and express a sense of control over the present situation and future outcome.
Anger, anxiety, frustration, ineffective coping, sleep deprivation, somatic symptoms, fatigue (spouse/ partner/caregiver)	Caregiver role strain related to complexity of care-giving responsibilities; lack of respite	Caregiver will demonstrate effective problem-solving skills and develop adaptive coping mechanisms to regain equilibrium

*This diagnosis has been retired from the NANDA-I list of approved diagnoses. It is used in this instance because it is most compatible with the identified behaviors.

confront the unique challenges associated with military life. Outcome criteria are presented for each.

Planning/Implementation/Evaluation

Nurses provide care for service members, veterans, and their families in a variety of settings, including general hospitals, VA hospitals, community health centers, doctors' offices, long-term care centers, and community-based clinics. The care required by the veterans returning from combat in the war on terrorism is complex and multifaceted. War-related physical injuries are often striking and conspicuous in their visibility. However, it is the veteran's *invisible* injuries with which psychiatric/mental health nurses are most often called

upon for treatment. The need for nurses to provide care for the increasing number of veterans with these invisible injuries is intensifying, and the DVA continues to search for more effective ways to ensure that military veterans and families receive the care that they desperately need and deserve. In some instances, this means additional medical skills training for psychiatric nurses in an effort to prepare them for the "polytrauma needs of veterans" (Wynn & Sherrod, 2010).

Interventions for a selected number of nursing diagnoses relevant to veterans and military families are presented in Table 38-3. Evaluation is conducted by reassessing to determine if the nursing actions have been successful in meeting the outcome criteria.

TABLE 38–3 **Nursing Interventions for Veteran Clients and Military Families**	
Post-trauma syndrome (PTSD)	Stay with the client during periods of flashbacks and nightmares and offer reassurance of personal safety. Encourage the client to talk about the traumatic experience at his or her own pace. Discuss maladaptive coping mechanisms being employed. Assist the client in his or her effort to use more adaptive strategies. Include available support systems, and make referrals for additional assistance where required. Help client understand that use of substances merely numbs feelings and delays healing. Refer for treatment of substance use disorder. Discuss use of stress-management techniques, such as deep breathing, meditation, relaxation, and exercise. Administer medications as prescribed, and provide medication education.
Risk for suicide (PTSD, TBI)	Assess degree of risk according to seriousness of threat, existence of a plan, and availability and lethality of the means. Ask directly if person is thinking of acting on thoughts or feelings. Ascertain presence of significant others for support. Determine whether substance use is a factor. Encourage expression of feelings, including appropriate expression of anger. Ensure that environment is safe. Help client identify more appropriate solutions and offer hope for the future. Negotiate a short-term no-suicide contract. (Some clinicians question the effectiveness of this intervention; however, it has proved successful with some individuals.) Involve family/significant others in the planning.
Disturbed thought processes (TBI)	Evaluate mental status, including extent of impairment in thinking ability; remote and recent memory; orientation to person, place, and time; insight and judgment; changes in personality; attention span, distractibility, and ability to make decisions or problem-solve; ability to communicate appropriately; anxiety level; evidence of psychotic behavior . Report to physician any cognitive changes that become obvious. Note behavior indicative of potential for violence and take appropriate action to prevent harm to client and others. Provide safety measures as required. Institute seizure precautions if indicated. Assist with limited mobility issues. Monitor medication regimen. Refer to appropriate rehabilitation providers.
Interrupted family processes (PTSD; TBI)	Encourage the importance of continuous, open communication between family members to facilitate ongoing problem-solving. Assist the family to identify and use previously successful coping strategies. Encourage family participation in multidisciplinary team conference or group therapy.

Continued

TABLE 38–3	**Nursing Interventions for Veteran Clients and Military Families–cont'd**
	Involve family in social support and community activities of their interest and choice.
	Encourage use of stress-management techniques.
	Make necessary referrals (e.g., Parent Effectiveness, specific disease or disability support groups, self-help groups, clergy, psychological counseling, or family therapy).
	Assist family to identify situations that may lead to fear or anxiety.
	Involve family in mutual goal-setting to plan for the future.
	Identify community agencies from which family may seek assistance (e.g., Meals on Wheels, visiting nurse, trauma support group, American Cancer Society, Veterans Administration).
Risk for complicated grieving (family of deployed service member)	Help family members to realize that all of the feelings they are having are a normal part of the grieving process.
	Validate their feelings of anger, loneliness, fear, powerlessness, dysphoria, and distress at separation from their loved one.
	Help parent to understand that children's and adolescents' problematic behaviors are symptoms of grieving, and that they should not be deemed unacceptable and result in punishment, but rather be recognized as having their basis in grief.
	Children should be allowed an appropriate amount of time to grieve. Some experts believe children need at least four weeks to adjust to a parent's deployment (Gabany & Shellenbarger, 2010). Refer for professional help if improvement is not observed in a reasonable period of time.
	Assess if maladaptive coping strategies, such as substance abuse, are being used.
	Identify and encourage clients to employ previously used successful coping strategies.
	Encourage resuming involvement in usual activities.
	Caution against spending too much time alone.
	Suggest keeping a journal of experiences and feelings.
	Refer to other resources, as needed, such as psychotherapy, family counseling, religious references or pastor, or grief support group.
Caregiver role strain (spouse/caregiver of injured service member)	Assess the spouse/caregiver's ability to anticipate and fulfill the injured service member's unmet needs. Provide information to assist the caregiver with this responsibility.
	Ensure that the caregiver encourages the injured service member to be as independent as possible.
	Encourage the caregiver to express feelings and to participate in a support group.
	Provide information or demonstrate techniques for dealing with acting out, violent, or disoriented behavior by the injured service member.
	Identify additional needs and ensure that resources are provided (e.g., physical therapy, occupational therapy, nutritionist, financial and legal help, and respite care).
	Assess for abuse of substances as a coping strategy.
	Refer to counseling or psychotherapy as needed.

Treatment Modalities

Posttraumatic Stress Disorder

Psychosocial Therapies

Cognitive therapy, prolonged exposure therapy, group and family therapy, and eye movement desensitization and reprocessing have all been used successfully in the treatment of PTSD. These therapies are discussed at length in Chapter 28 of this text.

Psychopharmacology

The selective serotonin reuptake inhibitors (SSRIs) are now considered first-line treatment of choice for PTSD because of their efficacy, tolerability, and safety ratings. Other antidepressants that have also been effective include trazadone, the tricyclics amitriptyline and imipramine, and the MAO inhibitor phenelzine. Benzodiazepines are sometimes prescribed for their anti-panic effects, although their addictive properties make them less desirable. Antihypertensives, such as propranolol and clonidine, have been successful in alleviating symptoms such as nightmares, intrusive recollections, hypervigilance, insomnia, startle responses, and angry outbursts.

Complementary Therapies

Acupuncture has been used successfully as an adjunctive therapy for individuals with PTSD. Relaxation techniques have been shown to alleviate symptoms associated with physiological hyperreactivity, and hypnosis may be helpful for symptoms such as pain, anxiety, dissociation, and nightmares (Brancu et al., 2011).

Traumatic Brain Injury

Type of care for the client with TBI depends on severity of the injury and area of the brain involved. Brancu and associates (2011) state, "Since 90 percent of patients have mild cases and experience full recovery, early intervention involving education and a focus on recovery is strongly recommended" (p. 59).

Psychosocial Therapies

Cognitive behavioral therapy (CBT) has been shown to be helpful to individuals with TBI. Scorer (2013) states, "An advantage of [CBT] interventions is that, given their highly structured content, they are amenable to specialized adaptation for memory, attention, and problem solving impairments, reflecting the difficulties people with TBI often experience." Other therapies, such as prolonged exposure therapy, may also work well for veterans with mild TBI and emotional trauma (Brancu et al., 2011).

Rehabilitation Therapies

Rehabilitation therapy is multifaceted and determined by severity and location of the brain damage. Specialists in the care of the individual with TBI may include any or all of the following (Mayo Clinic, 2012):

- **Physiatrist.** A physician trained in the medical specialty of physical medicine and rehabilitation. This physician oversees other professionals involved in the rehabilitation process.
- **Occupational Therapist.** Helps the individual learn, relearn, or improve skills for everyday living.
- **Physical Therapist.** Assists the veteran with mobility and relearning movement patterns, balance, and walking.
- **Recreational Therapist.** Assists with leisure activities.
- **Speech and Language Pathologist.** Helps the person improve communication skills and use assistive communication devices, if necessary.
- **Neuropsychologist or psychiatrist.** Helps the veteran manage behaviors or learn coping strategies, provides talk therapy as needed for emotional and psychological well-being, and prescribes medication as needed.
- **Social Worker or Case Manager.** Coordinates access to services, assists with care decisions and planning, and facilitates communication among various professionals, care providers, and family members.

Psychopharmacology

Medications for the individual with TBI are given to ameliorate specific symptoms. Antidepressants are prescribed for depression, which is very prevalent in individuals with TBI. SSRIs are commonly the antidepressants of choice, although tricyclics and others, such as venlafaxine, trazodone, bupropion, and duloxetine, are also used. Benzodiazepines or SSRIs may be administered for treatment of anxiety symptoms, and antipsychotics are prescribed if aggression, agitation, or psychotic behaviors occur. Anticonvulsants are given if seizures are a problem, and the physician may prescribe skeletal muscle relaxants for muscle spasms or spasticity. Methylphenidate or modafinil has been used to treat attention deficits and hyperactivity, and donepezil has been shown to be effective in enhancing cognitive performance of individuals with TBI (Foster & Spiegel, 2008).

Summary and Key Points

- There are about 1.5 million individuals serving in the U.S. Armed Forces in more than 150 countries around the world.
- Veterans currently number 21.8 million.
- Since the beginning of the wars in Afghanistan and Iraq in 2001, more than 1.9 million U.S. military personnel have been deployed in 3 million tours of duty.
- The military lifestyle offers both positive and negative aspects to those who choose this way of life.
- To compensate for the extreme mobility, the focus of the military lifestyle turns inward to the military world, rather than outward to the local community.
- In the OEF and OIF campaigns, there has been heavy dependence on the National Guard and Reserves, and an escalation in the pace, duration, and number of deployments and redeployments experienced by these individuals.
- Military families face unique challenges, including frequent moves and many separations.
- Children and adolescents exhibit a number of problematic behaviors in response to the separation from a deployed parent.
- The cycle of deployment is described in five distinct stages: predeployment, deployment, sustainment, redeployment, and postdeployment.
- Special concerns of women in the military include sexual harassment, sexual assault, differential treatment and conditions, and issues related to being a parent.
- Although the majority do not develop a behavioral health condition, most veterans returning from a combat zone experience feelings and reactions that may contribute to difficulties with their reintegration into civilian life.
- Traumatic brain injury (TBI) is a traumatically induced structural injury and/or physiological

■ disruption of brain function as a result of an external force to the head.

■ Symptoms of TBI are related to the severity of the injury and the area of the brain that has been injured.

■ The most common long-term sequelae related to TBI include problems with cognition and behavior or mental health.

■ PTSD is the most common mental disorder among veterans returning from military combat.

■ Symptoms of PTSD may occur shortly after the trauma, or they may be delayed, in some instances for years.

■ Depression among military veterans is quite common, and suicide rates among veterans and service members have continued to rise.

■ Substance use disorder is a common co-occurring condition with PTSD.

■ Nursing care of military families and veterans is presented in the context of the six steps of the nursing process.

■ Treatment modalities for PTSD and TBI include psychosocial therapies, psychopharmacology, complementary therapies, and rehabilitation therapies.

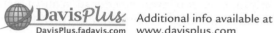 Additional info available at
DavisPlus.fadavis.com   www.davisplus.com

Review Questions
Self-Examination/Learning Exercise

Select the answer that is most appropriate for each of the following questions.

1. Joan's husband, who was deployed to Afghanistan a year ago, is returning home this week. Which of the following postdeployment situations may be likely to occur during the first few months of his return? (Select all that apply.)
   a. A honeymoon period of physical reconnection
   b. Resistance from the spouse regarding possible loss of autonomy
   c. Rejection by the children for perceived abandonment
   d. A period of adjustment to reconnect emotionally

2. Which of the following is the leading cause of TBI in active-duty military personnel in combat?
   a. Military vehicle accidents
   b. Blasts from explosive devices
   c. Falls
   d. Blows to the head from falling debris

3. Leon, a veteran of the war in Iraq, has been diagnosed with PTSD. He is a client of the VA outpatient clinic. He tells the nurse that he experiences panic attacks. Which of the following medications may be prescribed for Leon to treat his panic attacks?
   a. Alprazolam
   b. Lithium
   c. Carbamazepine
   d. Haldol

4. Leon, a veteran of the war in Iraq, has been diagnosed with PTSD. He has been hospitalized after swallowing a handful of his anti-panic medication. His physical condition has been stabilized in the emergency department, and he has been admitted to the psychiatric unit. In developing his initial plan of care, which is the priority nursing diagnosis that the nurse selects for Leon?
   a. Post-trauma syndrome
   b. Risk for suicide
   c. Complicated grieving
   d. Disturbed thought processes

5. Mike was injured during combat in Afghanistan. He has a diagnosis of TBI. Which of the following medications might the physician prescribe to improve Mike's memory and thinking capability?
   a. Carbamazepine
   b. Duloxetine
   c. Donepezil
   d. Bupropion

Review Questions—cont'd
Self-Examination/Learning Exercise

6. Leon, a veteran of the war in Iraq, has been diagnosed with PTSD. He has been hospitalized on the psychiatric unit following an attempted suicide. In the middle of the night, he wakes up yelling and tells the nurse he was having a flashback to when his unit transport drove over an improvised explosive device (IED) and most of his fellow soldiers were killed. He is breathing heavily, perspiring, and his heart is pounding. The nurse's most appropriate *initial* intervention is which of the following?
   a. Contact the doctor on call to report the incident.
   b. Administer the p.r.n. order for chlorpromazine.
   c. Stay with Leon and reassure him of his safety.
   d. Have Leon sit outside the nurses' station until he is calm.

7. Mike, a veteran of combat in Afghanistan, has a diagnosis of mild TBI. The psychiatric home health nurse from the VA medical center is assigned to make home visits to Mike and his wife, Nancy, who is his caregiver. Which of the following would be an appropriate nursing intervention by the home health nurse? (Select all that apply.)
   a. Assess for use of substances by Mike or Nancy.
   b. Encourage Nancy to do everything for Mike to prevent further deterioration in his condition.
   c. Assess Nancy's level of stress and potential for burnout.
   d. Encourage Nancy to allow Mike to be as independent as possible.
   e. Suggest that Nancy ask the physician for a nursing home placement for Mike.

8. Which of the following psychosocial therapies has been shown to be helpful for clients with TBI?
   a. Eye movement desensitization
   b. Psychoanalysis
   c. Reality therapy
   d. Cognitive-behavioral therapy

9. Pam's husband of 1 year left two weeks ago for a year-long deployment in Afghanistan. Pam makes an appointment with the psychiatric nurse practitioner at the Community Mental Health Clinic. She tells the nurse that she can't sleep, has no appetite, is chronically fatigued, thinks about her husband constantly, and fears for his life. Which of the following might the nurse suggest/prescribe for Pam? (Select all that apply.)
   a. A prescription for sertraline, 50 mg/day
   b. Participation in a support group
   c. Resume involvement in usual activities
   d. Perform regular relaxation exercises

References

Albrecht, B. (2009, July 16). Post-traumatic stress disorder hitting World War II veterans. *Cleveland Plain Dealer*, p. A1. Retrieved from http://www.cleveland.com/news/plaindealer/index.ssf?/base/cuyahoga/1247733140222090.xml&coll=2

American Academy of Child & Adolescent Psychiatry. (2014). *Military families resource center*. Retrieved from http://www.aacap.org/AACAP/Families_and_Youth/Resource_Centers/Military_Families_Resource_Center/FAQ.aspx

Birk, M. (2010). Traumatic brain injury. *Army Medicine*. Retrieved from http://www.armymedicine.army.mil/hc/healthtips/08/201003mtbi.cfm

Brancu, M., Straits-Troster, K., & Kudler, H. (2011). Behavioral health conditions among military personnel and veterans: Prevalence and best practices for treatment. *North Carolina Medical Journal, 72*(1), 54-60.

Department of Defense (DoD). (2012b). *Department of Defense annual report on sexual assault in the military, Fiscal year 2011*. Washington, DC: Author.

Department of Defense (DoD). (2012a). *Month of the military child: Saluting our military children*. Retrieved from http://www.dodlive.mil/index.php/2012/04/month-of-the-military-child-saluting-our-military-childre/

Department of Veterans Affairs (DVA). (2012). National Center for PTSD. Retrieved from http://www.ptsd.va.gov/public/pages/how-common-is-ptsd.asp

Department of Veterans Affairs & Department of Defense (DVA/DoD). (2009). *Clinical practice guideline for management of concussion/mild traumatic brain injury*. Retrieved from http://www.healthquality.va.gov/mtbi/concussion_mtbi_full_1_0.pdf

Devries, M.R., Hughes, H.K., Watson, H. & Moore, B.A. (2012). Understanding the military culture. In B.A. Moore (Ed.), *Handbook of counseling military couples* (pp. 7-18). New York, NY: Routledge.

Figley, C. (1998). Burnout as systemic traumatic stress: A model for helping traumatized family members. In C. Figley (Ed.), *Burnout in families: The system costs of caring* (pp. 15-28). Boca Raton, FL: CRC Press.

Foster, M., & Spiegel, D.R. (2008). Use of donepezil in the treatment of cognitive impairments of moderate traumatic brain injury. *Journal of Neuropsychiatry and Clinical Neurosciences, 20*(1), 106.

Gabany, E., & Shellenbarger, T. (2010). Caring for families with deployment stress: How nurses can make a difference in the lives of military families. *American Journal of Nursing, 110*(11), 36-41.

Hall, L.K. (2008). *Counseling military families.* New York, NY: Taylor & Francis.

Hall, L.K. (2011). The military culture, language, and lifestyle. In R.B. Everson & C.R. Figley (Eds.), *Families under fire* (pp. 31-52). New York, NY: Routledge.

Hall, L.K. (2012). The military lifestyle and the relationship. In B.A. Moore (Ed.), *Handbook of counseling military couples* (pp. 137-156). New York, NY: Routledge.

Institute of Medicine (IOM). (2012). Returning home from Iraq and Afghanistan: Preliminary assessment of readjustment needs of veterans, service members, and their families. Washington, DC: The National Academies Press.

Jakupcak, M., Vannoy, S., Imel., Z., Cook, J.W., Fontana, A., Rosenheck, R., & McFall, M. (2010). Does PTSD moderate the relationship between social support and suicide risk in Iraq and Afghanistan war veterans seeking mental health treatment? *Depression and Anxiety, 27*(11), 1001-1005.

Kapp, L. (2012). Reserve component personnel issues: Questions and answers. *Congressional Research Service.* Retrieved from http://www.fas.org/sgp/crs/natsec/RL30802.pdf

"'Kelly Temps' in Uniform." (2012). *This ain't hell, but you can see it from here* [Web log post]. Retrieved from http://thisainthell.us/blog/?p=30410

Killgore, W.D., Cotting, D.I., Thomas, J.L. Cox, A.L., McGurk, D., Vo, A.H., Castro, C.A., Hoge, C.W. (2008) Post-combat invincibility: Violent combat experiences are associated with increased risk-taking propensity following deployment. *Journal of Psychiatric Research, 42*(13), 1112-1121.

Langer, R. (2011). Combat trauma, memory, and the World War II veteran. *War, Literature & the Arts, 23*(1). Retrieved from http://wlajournal.com/23_1/images/langer.pdf

Lavender, J.M., & Lyons, J.A. (2012). Posttraumatic stress disorder. In B.A. Moore (Ed.), *Handbook of counseling military couples* (pp. 183-200). New York, NY: Routledge.

Mathewson, J. (2011). In support of military women and families. In R.B. Everson & C.R. Figley (Eds.), *Families under fire* (pp. 215-235). New York, NY: Routledge.

Mayo Clinic. (2012). Traumatic brain injury. Retrieved from http://www.mayoclinic.com/health/traumatic-brain-injury/DS00552

Monson, C.M., Fredman, S.J. & Adair, K.C. (2008). Cognitive-behavioral conjoint therapy for posttraumatic stress disorder: Application to Operation Enduring and Iraqi Freedom veterans. *Journal of Clinical Psychology, 64*, 958-971.

National Alliance on Mental Illness (NAMI). (2009). Depression and veterans. Retrieved from http://www.nami.org

National Institute of Neurological Disorders and Stroke (NINDS). (2013). *Traumatic brain injury: Hope through research.* Retrieved from http://www.ninds.nih.gov/disorders/tbi/tbi.htm

National Institute on Drug Abuse (NIDA). (2011). *Substance abuse among the military, veterans, and their families.* Washington, DC:

National Institutes of Health. Retrieved from http://www.drugabuse.gov/sites/default/files/veterans.pdf

Pincus, S.H., House, R., Christenson, J., & Alder, L.E. (2013). The emotional cycle of deployment: A military family perspective. *Operation: Military kids.* Retrieved from http://4h.missouri.edu/programs/military/resources/manual/deployment-cycles.pdf

Ribbers, G.M. (2013). Brain injury: Long-term outcome after traumatic brain injury. In J.H. Stone & M. Blouin (Eds.), *International encyclopedia of rehabilitation.* Retrieved from http://cirrie.buffalo.edu/encyclopedia/en/article/338

Safaz, I., Yasar, A.R., Tok, F., & Yilmaz, B. (2008). Medical complications, physical function, and communication skills in patients with traumatic brain injury. *Brain Injury, 22*, 733-739.

Scorer, R. (2013). Psychological therapies for victims of traumatic brain injury. Retrieved from http://www.pannone.com/media/articles/clinical-negligence/medical-negligence/psychological-therapies-for-victims-of-traumatic-brain-injury-and-how-medical-evidence-plays-a-crucial-role

Smith, R. (2012). Military children and families. *Helping Hands for Freedom.* Retrieved from http://helpinghandsforfreedom.org/remaining-programs-2012-arizona-military-children-families/#more-567

Strong, C.H., & Donders, J. (2012). Traumatic brain injury. In B.A. Moore (Ed.), *Handbook of counseling military couples* (pp. 279-294). New York, NY: Routledge.

Substance Abuse and Mental Health Services Administration (SAMHSA). (2012). Behavioral health issues among Afghanistan and Iraq U.S. war veterans. *SAMHSA in Brief, 7*(1).

Temkin, N.R., Corrigan, J.D., Dikmen, S.S., & Machamer, J. (2009). Social functioning after traumatic brain injury. *Journal of Head Trauma Rehabilitation, 24*(6), 460-467.

Title 10 U.S.C. § 10102 (2006 & Supp. 2009). Purpose of Reserve Components. Public Law 103-337, effective February 1, 2010.

U.S. Census Bureau. (2013). Veteran status. *2011 American Community Survey.* Washington, DC: Author.

USA.gov. (2013). Military personnel records and statistics. Retrieved from http://www.usa.gov/Federal-Employees/Active-Military-Records.shtml

Vlahos, K.B. (2012). The rape of our military women. *Anti-War.Com.* Retrieved from http://original.antiwar.com/vlahos/2012/05/14/the-rape-of-our-military-women

Wakefield, M. (2007). Guarding the military home front. *Counseling Today.* Retrieved from http://ct.counseling.org/2007/01/from-the-president-guarding-the-military-home-front

Wertsch, M.E. (1996). *Military brats: Legacies of childhood inside the fortress.* St. Louis, MO: Brightwell.

Wolf, N. (2012). A culture of cover-up: Rape in the ranks of the U.S. military. *The Guardian.* Retrieved from http://www.guardian.co.uk/commentisfree/2012/jun/14/culture-coverup-rape-ranks-us-military

Wolfe, J., Sharkansky, E.J., Read, J.P., Dawson, R., Martin, J.A., & Oimette, P.C. (1998). Sexual harassment and assault as predictors of PTSD symptomatology among U.S. female Persian Gulf military personnel. *Journal of Interpersonal Violence, 13*(1), 40-57.

Wynn, S.T., & Sherrod, R.A. (2010). Providing optimal care for veterans: Preparing psychiatric nurses for complex care. *Journal of Psychosocial Nursing and Mental Health Services, 48*(1), 4-6.

@ INTERNET REFERENCES

- The following websites provide information for and about military service members, their families, and veterans:
  - http://www.va.gov
  - http://www.bpwfoundation.org/index.php/issues/women_veterans
  - http://www.dvnf.org
  - http://www.nvf.org
  - http://www.ptsd.va.gov
  - http://www.ncbi.nlm.nih.gov/pubmedhealth/PMH0001923
  - http://www.mayoclinic.com/health/post-traumatic-stress-disorder/DS00246
  - http://www.cdc.gov/traumaticbraininjury
  - http://www.publichealth.va.gov/vethealthinitiative/traumatic_brain_injury.asp
  - http://www.ninds.nih.gov/disorders/tbi/tbi.htm
  - http://www.militaryfamily.org
  - http://www.woundedwarriorproject.org

MOVIE CONNECTIONS

The Best Years of Our Lives (1946) • *The Deer Hunter* (1978) • *Jarhead* (2005) • *In the Valley of Elah* (2007) • *The Lucky Ones* (2008) • *A Walk in My Shoes* (2010)

Appendix A

Answers to Chapter Review Questions

CHAPTER 1. The Concept of Stress Adaptation
1. b 2. d 3. a 4. b 5. c 6. c, d, b, a

CHAPTER 2. Mental Health/Mental Illness: Historical and Theoretical Concepts
1. c 2. d 3. b 4. a 5. b 6. d 7. c
8. a, b, c, d 9. c 10. b

CHAPTER 3. Theoretical Models of Personality Development
1. b 2. c 3. d 4. b 5. b 6. b 7. a 8. c
9. a 10. b

CHAPTER 4. Concepts of Psychobiology
1. d 2. d 3. a 4. b 5. c 6. a 7. d 8. c
9. b 10. a 11. d 12. a 13. c

CHAPTER 5. Ethical and Legal Issues in Psychiatric/Mental Health Nursing
1. b 2. a 3. c 4. b 5. c 6. d 7. a, b, d
8. b, d 9. a, b 10. c

CHAPTER 6. Cultural and Spiritual Concepts Relevant to Psychiatric/Mental Health Nursing
1. c 2. d 3. a 4. d 5. b 6. c 7. c 8. b
9. b 10. a 11. a 12. d

CHAPTER 7. Relationship Development
1. c 2. a 3. a, b, c 4. b, e 5. b 6. d 7. c
8. b 9. d 10. a, c, d

CHAPTER 8. Therapeutic Communication
1. b 2. a 3. d 4. c 5. a 6. b 7. d 8. a
9. a, b, d 10. b

CHAPTER 9. The Nursing Process in Psychiatric/Mental Health Nursing
1. b 2. a 3. d 4. a 5. c 6. b 7. a, b, c, d
8. d 9. c 10. a, c, d

CHAPTER 10. Therapeutic Groups
1. b 2. d 3. a 4. c 5. c 6. d 7. c 8. b
9. d 10. a

CHAPTER 11. Intervention With Families
1. b 2. c 3. a 4. b 5. d 6. c 7. b 8. c
9. d 10. a

CHAPTER 12. Milieu Therapy—The Therapeutic Community
1. a, b, c 2. b 3. c 4. b 5. a 6. d 7. c
8. b 9. a, b, d, e 10. a, b, c

CHAPTER 13. Crisis Intervention
1. c 2. d 3. a 4. b 5. c 6. a 7. d 8. b
9. b 10. d 11. c 12. c 13. e

CHAPTER 14. Assertiveness Training
1. c 2. a 3. b 4. a 5. a 6. c 7. d 8. a
9. c 10. b

CHAPTER 15. Promoting Self-Esteem
1. b 2. a 3. d 4. c 5. a 6. c 7. b 8. d
9. b 10. a

CHAPTER 16. Anger/Aggression Management
1. b, c 2. c 3. a 4. a, b, d 5. c 6. a, b, c
7. c 8. b 9. b, c, d, e 10. a, b, c

CHAPTER 17. The Suicidal Client
1. b 2. a 3. c 4. a 5. d 6. c 7. c 8. b
9. a, b, c 10. b

CHAPTER 18. Behavior Therapy
1. a 2. a 3. b 4. c 5. a 6. b 7. d
8. f, b, d, a, e, c

CHAPTER 19. Cognitive Therapy
1. c 2. a 3. d 4. b 5. c 6. a 7. d 8. a
9. b 10. c

CHAPTER 20. Electroconvulsive Therapy
1. c 2. b 3. a 4. c 5. d 6. a 7. c 8. d
9. b 10. c

CHAPTER 21. The Recovery Model
1. b, d 2. c 3. d 4. a 5. c

CHAPTER 22. Neurocognitive Disorders
1. c, e 2. d 3. b 4. a, b, e 5. b 6. a, c, e
7. d 8. c 9. a 10. b 11. c, e

CHAPTER 23. Substance-Related and Addictive Disorders
1. a 2. c 3. b 4. b 5. a 6. c 7. a 8. b
9. d 10. a

CHAPTER 24. Schizophrenia Spectrum and Other Psychotic Disorders
1. b **2.** b **3.** c **4.** d **5.** d **6.** a **7.** c **8.** b
9. c **10.** d

CHAPTER 25. Depressive Disorders
1. c **2.** b **3.** a **4.** d **5.** b, c **6.** a, b, c, e
7. a **8.** c **9.** b **10.** d

CHAPTER 26. Bipolar and Related Disorders
1. b **2.** c **3.** a **4.** a, c, d **5.** b **6.** d **7.** b
8. c **9.** a = 3, b = 1, c = 4, d = 2 **10.** c

CHAPTER 27. Anxiety, Obsessive-Compulsive, and Related Disorders
1. d **2.** c **3.** d **4.** a **5.** b **6.** c **7.** a, b, c
8. c **9.** a **10.** b

CHAPTER 28. Trauma- and Stressor-Related Disorders
1. b **2.** c **3.** a **4.** d **5.** b **6.** b **7.** c **8.** a
9. a **10.** d

CHAPTER 29. Somatic Symptom and Dissociative Disorders
1. a **2.** b **3.** d **4.** b **5.** c **6.** d **7.** b **8.** a
9. b **10.** d

CHAPTER 30. Issues Related to Human Sexuality and Gender Dysphoria
1. b **2.** c **3.** a, b, c, d **4.** a **5.** b **6.** d **7.** b
8. d **9.** c **10.** a, b, d, e

CHAPTER 31. Eating Disorders
1. c **2.** a **3.** b **4.** b **5.** c **6.** b **7.** c **8.** b
9. c **10.** a

CHAPTER 32. Personality Disorders
1. d **2.** a **3.** b **4.** d **5.** a **6.** b **7.** c **8.** a
9. d **10.** b

CHAPTER 33. Children and Adolescents
1. b **2.** c **3.** a **4.** b **5.** b **6.** b, c, d **7.** c
8. d **9.** a **10.** b

CHAPTER 34. The Aging Individual
1. c **2.** d **3.** b **4.** a **5.** c **6.** d **7.** a **8.** a
9. c **10.** a

CHAPTER 35. Survivors of Abuse or Neglect
1. b **2.** c **3.** a **4.** d **5.** b **6.** d **7.** a **8.** b
9. b **10.** d

CHAPTER 36. Community Mental Health Nursing
1. a **2.** b **3.** a **4.** c **5.** d **6.** b **7.** c **8.** d
9. a **10.** b

CHAPTER 37. The Bereaved Individual
1. e **2.** c **3.** c **4.** d **5.** a **6.** a **7.** b **8.** c
9. a **10.** c

CHAPTER 38. Military Families
1. a, b, d **2.** b **3.** a **4.** b **5.** c **6.** c
7. a, c, d **8.** d **9.** a, b, c, d

Bonus Chapters on DavisPlus:

Psychopharmacology
1. a **2.** c **3.** d **4.** b **5.** c **6.** b **7.** a **8.** b
9. d **10.** b

Relaxation Therapy
1. a, b, e **2.** a, b, d **3.** a **4.** c **5.** d

Complementary Therapies
1. a, c, e, f **2.** a, b, d **3.** c, d **4.** a, d, e
5. c **6.** d **7.** a **8.** b **9.** a, b, c **10.** c

Forensic Nursing
1. c **2.** b **3.** a, b, e **4.** a, d, e **5.** c **6.** d
7. d **8.** b **9.** a, c, d, e **10.** c

Appendix B

Examples of Answers to Communication Exercises

Chapter 22. Neurocognitive Disorders

1. "Mrs. B. you are not in a restaurant. This is the General Hospital. I am your nurse, Mary. How may I help you?" (Reality orientation.)
2. "Mrs. B. you have already eaten your breakfast. Would you like a snack?"
"Please tell me what it was like when you lived on the farm." (Reminiscing.)

Chapter 23. Substance-Related and Addictive Disorders

1. "Tom, you are here because it has been determined that drinking alcohol is causing problems for you at home and at your work." (Confronting reality.)
2. "Tom, you are experiencing symptoms related to your body's withdrawal from alcohol. When did you have your last drink? I will bring you a cup of coffee." (Confrontation with caring.)
3. "You are feeling angry toward your boss and your wife, but your drinking is apparently interfering with your job and your marriage. Unless you abstain from alcohol, you are at risk of losing both." (Confronting reality.)

Chapter 24. Schizophrenia Spectrum and Other Psychotic Disorders

1. "I know that you believe what you are saying is true, but I find it very hard to accept." (Voicing doubt.)
"Please understand that you are safe here." (Reassurance of safety.)
2. The nurse should slowly and carefully approach Hal so that he is not startled by his or her presence. "Hal, are you hearing the voices again? What do you hear the voices saying to you?" (Encouraging description of perceptions. This type of information may help to protect the client and others from potential violence associated with command hallucinations.)
"I know the voices seem real to you, but I do not hear any voices speaking." (Presenting reality.)
3. "I don't understand what you are saying, Hal. What message do you want to give me? Might you be telling me that you are lonely?" (Seeking clarification; attempting to translate words into feelings.)

Chapter 25. Depressive Disorders

1. "You have had a lot of losses. You are feeling very much alone right now." (Verbalizing the implied.)
2. "You feel sad because you can no longer do the things that you used to do . . . the things that made you feel good about yourself." (Statement that focuses on feelings.)
3. Direct questions assessing suicide potential: "Are you or have you been thinking about harming yourself? Do you have a plan for doing so? Have you ever acted on that plan?"
Demonstrations of genuine concern and caring: "I care about you. I will stay here with you."
Expressions of empathy: "It must be frightening to feel so all alone. But you are not alone. There are many people who care about you, and I am one of those people."

Chapter 32. Personality Disorders

1. "My name is Nancy. I am your nurse on this shift, and you will be in my care until 11 p.m. You may ask for me by my name if you have any requests." (Giving information.)
2. "You were arrested because you broke the law." (Confronting reality.)
3. "I do not give out personal information to patients, and I do not go out with patients. I hope that you will be able to get your life straightened out in a positive way." (Confrontation with caring.)

Chapter 35. Survivors of Abuse or Neglect

1. "You are not to blame. You do not deserve to be abused in this way. He is responsible for his behavior."
2. "There are places you can go where you and your children will be safe. I will give you that information."
"You will need to consider if you want to press charges against him."
3. "You must consider the safety of yourself and your children. You have the phone number of the Safe House. It is your decision what to do now."

Appendix C

Mental Status Assessment

Gathering the correct information about the client's mental status is essential to the development of an appropriate plan of care. The mental status examination is a description of all the areas of the client's mental functioning. The following are the components that are considered critical in the assessment of a client's mental status. Examples of interview questions and criteria for assessment are included.

Identifying Data

1. Name
2. Gender
3. Age
   a. How old are you?
   b. When were you born?
4. Race/culture
   a. What country did you (your ancestors) come from?
5. Occupational/financial status
   a. How do you make your living?
   b. How do you obtain money for your needs?
6. Educational level
   a. What was the highest grade level you completed in school?
7. Significant other
   a. Are you married?
   b. Do you have a significant relationship with another person?
8. Living arrangements
   a. Do you live alone?
   b. With whom do you share your home?
9. Religious preference
   a. Do you have a religious preference?
10. Allergies
    a. Are you allergic to anything?
    b. Foods? Medications?
11. Special diet considerations
    a. Do you have any special diet requirements?
    b. Diabetic? Low sodium?
12. Chief complaint
    a. For what reason did you come for help today?
    b. What seems to be the problem?
13. Medical diagnosis

General Description

Appearance

1. Grooming and dress
   a. Note unusual modes of dress.
   b. Evidence of soiled clothing?
   c. Use of makeup?
   d. Neat; unkempt?
2. Hygiene
   a. Note evidence of body or breath odor.
   b. Condition of skin, fingernails
3. Posture
   a. Note if standing upright, rigid, slumped over.
4. Height and weight
   a. Perform accurate measurements.
5. Level of eye contact
   a. Intermittent?
   b. Occasional and fleeting?
   c. Sustained and intense?
   d. No eye contact?
6. Hair color and texture
   a. Is hair clean and healthy-looking?
   b. Greasy, matted, tangled?
7. Evidence of scars, tattoos, or other distinguishing skin marks
   a. Note any evidence of swelling or bruises.
   b. Birth marks?
   c. Rashes?
8. Evaluation of client's appearance compared with chronological age

Motor Activity

1. Tremors
   a. Do hands or legs tremble?
      • Continuously?
      • At specific times?
2. Tics or other stereotypical movements
   a. Any evidence of facial tics?
   b. Jerking or spastic movements?
3. Mannerisms and gestures
   a. Specific facial or body movements during conversation?
   b. Nail biting?
   c. Covering face with hands?
   d. Grimacing?

4. Hyperactivity
   a. Gets up and down out of chair.
   b. Paces.
   c. Unable to sit still.
5. Restlessness or agitation
   a. Lots of fidgeting.
   b. Clenching hands.
6. Aggressiveness
   a. Overtly angry and hostile.
   b. Threatening.
   c. Uses sarcasm.
7. Rigidity
   a. Sits or stands in a rigid position.
   b. Arms and legs appear stiff and unyielding.
8. Gait patterns
   a. Any evidence of limping?
   b. Limitation of range of motion?
   c. Ataxia?
   d. Shuffling?
9. Echopraxia
   a. Evidence of mimicking the actions of others?
10. Psychomotor retardation
    a. Movements are very slow.
    b. Thinking and speech are very slow.
    c. Posture is slumped.
11. Freedom of movement (range of motion)
    a. Note any limitation in ability to move.

Speech Patterns

1. Slowness or rapidity of speech
   a. Note whether speech seems very rapid or slower than normal.
2. Pressure of speech
   a. Note whether speech seems frenzied.
   b. Unable to be interrupted?
3. Intonation
   a. Are words spoken with appropriate emphasis?
   b. Are words spoken in monotone, without emphasis?
4. Volume
   a. Is speech very loud? Soft?
   b. Is speech low-pitched? High-pitched?
5. Stuttering or other speech impairments
   a. Hoarseness?
   b. Slurred speech?
6. Aphasia
   a. Difficulty forming words
   b. Use of incorrect words
   c. Difficulty thinking of specific words
   d. Making up words (neologisms)

General Attitude

1. Cooperative/uncooperative
   a. Answers questions willingly.
   b. Refuses to answer questions.

2. Friendly/hostile/defensive
   a. Is sociable and responsive.
   b. Is sarcastic and irritable.
3. Uninterested/apathetic
   a. Refuses to participate in interview process.
4. Attentive/interested
   a. Actively participates in interview process.
5. Guarded/suspicious
   a. Continuously scans the environment.
   b. Questions motives of interviewer.
   c. Refuses to answer questions.

Emotions

Mood

1. Depressed; despairing
   a. An overwhelming feeling of sadness
   b. Loss of interest in regular activities
2. Irritable
   a. Easily annoyed and provoked to anger.
3. Anxious
   a. Demonstrates or verbalizes feeling of apprehension.
4. Elated
   a. Expresses feelings of joy and intense pleasure.
   b. Is intensely optimistic.
5. Euphoric
   a. Demonstrates a heightened sense of elation.
   b. Expresses feelings of grandeur ("Everything is wonderful!").
6. Fearful
   a. Demonstrates or verbalizes feeling of apprehension associated with real or perceived danger.
7. Guilty
   a. Expresses a feeling of discomfort associated with real or perceived wrongdoing.
   b. May be associated with feelings of sadness and despair.
8. Labile
   a. Exhibits mood swings that range from euphoria to depression or anxiety.

Affect

1. Congruence with mood
   a. Outward emotional expression is consistent with mood (e.g., if depressed, emotional expression is sadness, eyes downcast, may be crying).
2. Constricted or blunted
   a. Minimal outward emotional expression is observed.
3. Flat
   a. There is an absence of outward emotional expression.

4. Appropriate
   a. The outward emotional expression is what would be expected in a certain situation (e.g., crying upon hearing of a death).
5. Inappropriate
   a. The outward emotional expression is incompatible with the situation (e.g., laughing upon hearing of a death).

Thought Processes

Form of Thought

1. Flight of ideas
   a. Verbalizations are continuous and rapid, and flow from one to another.
2. Associative looseness
   a. Verbalizations shift from one unrelated topic to another.
3. Circumstantiality
   a. Verbalizations are lengthy and tedious, and because of numerous details, are delayed reaching the intended point.
4. Tangentiality
   a. Verbalizations that are lengthy and tedious, and never reach an intended point
5. Neologisms
   a. The individual is making up nonsensical-sounding words, which only have meaning to him or her.
6. Concrete thinking
   a. Thinking is literal; elemental.
   b. Absence of ability to think abstractly.
   c. Unable to translate simple proverbs.
7. Clang associations
   a. Speaking in puns or rhymes; using words that sound alike but have different meanings.
8. Word salad
   a. Using a mixture of words that have no meaning together; sounding incoherent.
9. Perseveration
   a. Persistently repeating the last word of a sentence spoken to the client. (e.g., Ns: "George, it's time to go to lunch." George: "lunch, lunch, lunch, lunch") .
10. Echolalia
    a. Persistently repeating what another person says.
11. Mutism
    a. Does not speak (either cannot or will not).
12. Poverty of speech
    a. Speaks very little; may respond in monosyllables.
13. Ability to concentrate and disturbance of attention
    a. Does the person hold attention to the topic at hand?
    b. Is the person easily distractible?
    c. Is there selective attention (e.g., blocks out topics that create anxiety)?

Content of Thought

1. Delusions (Does the person have unrealistic ideas or beliefs?)
   a. Persecutory: A belief that someone is out to get him or her is some way (e.g., "The FBI will be here at any time to take me away.").
   b. Grandiose: An idea that he or she is all-powerful or of great importance (e.g., "I am the king...and this is my kingdom! I can do anything!").
   c. Reference: An idea that whatever is happening in the environment is about him or her (e.g., "Just watch the movie on TV tonight. It is about my life.").
   d. Control or influence: A belief that his or her behavior and thoughts are being controlled by external forces (e.g., "I get my orders from Channel 27. I do only what the forces dictate.").
   e. Somatic: A belief that he or she has a dysfunctional body part (e.g., "My heart is at a standstill. It is no longer beating.").
   f. Nihilistic: A belief that he or she, or a part of the body, or even the world does not exist or has been destroyed (e.g., "I am no longer alive.").
2. Suicidal or homicidal ideas
   a. Is the individual expressing ideas of harming self or others?
3. Obsessions
   a. Is the person verbalizing about a persistent thought or feeling that he or she is unable to eliminate from their consciousness?
4. Paranoia/suspiciousness
   a. Continuously scans the environment.
   b. Questions motives of interviewer.
   c. Refuses to answer questions.
5. Magical thinking
   a. Is the person speaking in a way that indicates his or her words or actions have power? (e.g., "If you step on a crack, you break your mother's back!")
6. Religiosity
   a. Is the individual demonstrating obsession with religious ideas and behavior?
7. Phobias
   a. Is there evidence of irrational fears (of a specific object, or a social situation)?
8. Poverty of content
   a. Is little information conveyed by the client because of vagueness or stereotypical statements or clichés?

Perceptual Disturbances

1. Hallucinations (Is the person experiencing unrealistic sensory perceptions?)
   a. Auditory (Is the individual hearing voices or other sounds that do not exist?)
   b. Visual (Is the individual seeing images that do not exist?)
   c. Tactile (Does the individual feel unrealistic sensations on the skin?)
   d. Olfactory (Does the individual smell odors that do not exist?)
   e. Gustatory (Does the individual have a false perception of an unpleasant taste?)
2. Illusions
   a. Does the individual misperceive or misinterpret real stimuli within the environment? (Sees something and thinks it is something else?)
3. Depersonalization (altered perception of the self)
   a. The individual verbalizes feeling "outside the body;" visualizing him- or herself from afar.
4. Derealization (altered perception of the environment)
   a. The individual verbalizes that the environment feels "strange or unreal." A feeling that the surroundings have changed.

Sensorium and Cognitive Ability

1. Level of alertness/consciousness
   a. Is the individual clear-minded and attentive to the environment?
   b. Or is there disturbance in perception and awareness of the surroundings?
2. Orientation. Is the person oriented to the following?
   a. Time
   b. Place
   c. Person
   d. Circumstances

3. Memory
   a. Recent (Is the individual able to remember occurrences of the past few days?)
   b. Remote (Is the individual able to remember occurrences of the distant past?)
   c. Confabulation (Does the individual fill in memory gaps with experiences that have no basis in fact?)
4. Capacity for abstract thought
   a. Can the individual interpret proverbs correctly?
      • "What does 'no use crying over spilled milk' mean?"

Impulse Control

1. Ability to control impulses. (Does psychosocial history reveal problems with any of the following?)
   a. Aggression
   b. Hostility
   c. Fear
   d. Guilt
   e. Affection
   f. Sexual feelings

Judgment and Insight

1. Ability to solve problems and make decisions
   a. What are your plans for the future?
   b. What do you plan to do to reach your goals?
2. Knowledge about self
   a. Awareness of limitations
   b. Awareness of consequences of actions
   c. Awareness of illness
      • "Do you think you have a problem?"
      • "Do you think you need treatment?"
3. Adaptive/maladaptive use of coping strategies and ego defense mechanisms (e.g., rationalizing maladaptive behaviors, projection of blame, displacement of anger)

Appendix D

DSM-5 Classification*

ICD-9-CM codes are provided, followed by ICD-10-CM codes in parentheses.

Neurodevelopmental Disorders

Intellectual Disabilities

319 (___.__)	Intellectual Disability (Intellectual Developmental Disorder)
	Specify current severity:
317 (70)	Mild
318.0 (71)	Moderate
318.1 (72)	Severe
318.2 (73)	Profound
315.8 (F88)	Global Developmental Delay
319 (F79)	Unspecified Intellectual Disability (Intellectual Developmental Disorder)

Communication Disorders

315.39 (F80.9)	Language Disorder
315.39 (F80.0)	Speech Sound Disorder
315.35 (F80.81)	Childhood-Onset Fluency Disorder (Stuttering) Note: Later-onset cases are diagnosed as 307.0 (F98.5) adult-onset fluency disorder.
315.39 (F80.89)	Social (Pragmatic) Communication Disorder
307.9 (F80.9)	Unspecified Communication Disorder

Autism Spectrum Disorder

299.00 (F84.0)	Autism Spectrum Disorder *Specify* if: Associated with a known medical or genetic condition or environmental factor; Associated with another neurodevelopmental, mental, or behavioral disorder *Specify* current severity for Criterion A and Criterion B: Requiring very substantial

support, Requiring substantial support, Requiring support
Specify if: With or without accompanying intellectual impairment, With or without accompanying language impairment, With catatonia (use additional code 293.89 [F06.1])

Attention-Deficit/Hyperactivity Disorder

___.__ (___.__)	Attention-Deficit/Hyperactivity Disorder
	Specify whether:
314.01 (F90.2)	Combined presentation
314.00 (F90.0)	Predominantly inattentive presentation
314.01 (F90.1)	Predominantly hyperactive/impulsive presentation
	Specify if: In partial remission *Specify* current severity: Mild, Moderate, Severe
314.01 (F90.8)	Other Specified Attention-Deficit/Hyperactivity Disorder
314.01 (F90.9)	Unspecified Attention-Deficit/Hyperactivity Disorder

Specific Learning Disorder

___.__ (___.__)	Specific Learning Disorder *Specify* if:
315.00 (F81.0)	With impairment in reading (*specify* if with word reading accuracy, reading rate or fluency, reading comprehension)
315.2 (F81.81)	With impairment in written expression (*specify* if with spelling accuracy, grammar and punctuation accuracy, clarity or organization of written expression)
315.1 (F81.2)	With impairment in mathematics (*specify* if with number sense, memorization of arithmetic facts, accurate or fluent calculation, accurate math reasoning)
	Specify current severity: Mild, Moderate, Severe

*Reprinted with permission from the *Diagnostic and Statistical Manual of Mental Disorders, Fifth Edition* (Copyright 2013). American Psychiatric Association.

Motor Disorders

315.4 (F82)	Developmental Coordination Disorder
307.3 (F98.4)	Stereotypic Movement Disorder *Specify* if: With self-injurious behavior, Without self-injurious behavior *Specify* if: Associated with a known medical or genetic condition, neurodevelopmental disorder, or environmental factor *Specify* current severity: Mild, Moderate, Severe

Tic Disorders

307.23 (F95.2)	Tourette's Disorder
307.22 (F95.1)	Persistent (Chronic) Motor or Vocal Tic Disorder *Specify* if: With motor tics only, With vocal tics only
307.21 (F95.0)	Provisional Tic Disorder
307.20 (F95.8)	Other Specified Tic Disorder
307.20 (F95.9)	Unspecified Tic Disorder

Other Neurodevelopmental Disorders

315.8 (F88)	Other Specified Neurodevelopmental Disorder
315.9 (F89)	Unspecified Neurodevelopmental Disorder

Schizophrenia Spectrum and Other Psychotic Disorders

The following specifiers apply to Schizophrenia Spectrum and Other Psychotic Disorders where indicated:

[a] *Specify* if: The following course specifiers are only to be used after a 1-year duration of the disorder: First episode, currently in acute episode; First episode, currently in partial remission; First episode, currently in full remission; Multiple episodes, currently in acute episode; Multiple episodes, currently in partial remission; Multiple episodes, currently in full remission; Continuous; Unspecified

[b] *Specify* if: With catatonia (use additional code 293.89 [F06.1])

[c] *Specify* current severity of delusions, hallucinations, disorganized speech, abnormal psychomotor behavior, negative symptoms, impaired cognition, depression, and mania symptoms

301.22 (F21)	Schizotypal (Personality) Disorder
297.1 (F22)	Delusional Disorder [a, c] *Specify* whether: Erotomanic type, Grandiose type, Jealous type, Persecutory type, Somatic type, Mixed type, Unspecified type *Specify* if: With bizarre content
298.8 (F23)	Brief Psychotic Disorder [b, c] *Specify* if: With marked stressor(s), Without marked stressor(s), With postpartum onset
295.40 (F20.81)	Schizophreniform Disorder [b, c] *Specify* if: With good prognostic features, Without good prognostic features
295.90 (F20.9)	Schizophrenia [a, b, c]
___.__ (___.__)	Schizoaffective Disorder [a, b, c] *Specify* whether:
295.70 (F25.0)	Bipolar type
295.70 (F25.1)	Depressive type
___.__ (___.__)	Substance/Medication-Induced Psychotic Disorder [c] Note: See the criteria set and corresponding recording procedures for substance-specific codes and ICD-9-CM and ICD-10-CM coding. *Specify* if: With onset during intoxication, With onset during withdrawal
___.__ (___.__)	Psychotic Disorder Due to Another Medical Condition [c] *Specify* whether:
293.81 (F06.2)	With delusions
293.82 (F06.0)	With hallucinations
293.89 (F06.1)	Catatonia Associated With Another Mental Disorder (Catatonia Specifier)
293.89 (F06.1)	Catatonic Disorder Due to Another Medical Condition
293.89 (F06.1)	Unspecified Catatonia Note: Code first 781.99 (R29.818) other symptoms involving nervous and musculoskeletal systems.
298.8 (F28)	Other Specified Schizophrenia Spectrum and Other Psychotic Disorder
298.9 (F29)	Unspecified Schizophrenia Spectrum and Other Psychotic Disorder

Bipolar and Related Disorders

The following specifiers apply to Bipolar and Related Disorders where indicated:

[a] *Specify*: With anxious distress (*specify* current severity: mild, moderate, moderate-severe, severe); With mixed

features; With rapid cycling; With melancholic features; With atypical features; With mood-congruent psychotic features; With mood-incongruent psychotic features; With catatonia (use additional code 293.89 [F06.1]); With peripartum onset; With seasonal pattern

___.__ (___.__) Bipolar I Disorder [a]
___.__ (___.__) Current or most recent episode manic
296.41 (F31.11) Mild
296.42 (F31.12) Moderate
296.43 (F31.13) Severe
296.44 (F31.2) With psychotic features
296.45 (F31.73) In partial remission
296.46 (F31.74) In full remission
296.40 (F31.9) Unspecified
296.40 (F31.0) Current or most recent episode hypomanic
296.45 (F31.73) In partial remission
296.46 (F31.74) In full remission
296.40 (F31.9) Unspecified
___.__ (___.__) Current or most recent episode depressed
296.51 (F31.31) Mild
296.52 (F31.32) Moderate
296.53 (F31.4) Severe
296.54 (F31.5) With psychotic features
296.55 (F31.75) In partial remission
296.56 (F31.76) In full remission
296.50 (F31.9) Unspecified
296.7 (F31.9) Current or most recent episode unspecified
296.89 (F31.81) Bipolar II Disorder [a]
Specify current or most recent episode: Hypomanic, Depressed
Specify course if full criteria for a mood episode are not currently met: In partial remission, In full remission
Specify severity if full criteria for a mood episode are not currently met: Mild, Moderate, Severe
301.13 (F34.0) Cyclothymic Disorder
Specify if: With anxious distress
___.__ (___.__) Substance/Medication-Induced Bipolar and Related Disorder
Note: See the criteria set and corresponding recording procedures for substance-specific codes and ICD-9-CM and ICD-10-CM coding.
Specify if: With onset during intoxication, With onset during withdrawal

293.83 (___.__) Bipolar and Related Disorder Due to Another Medical Condition
Specify if:
(F06.33) With manic features
(F06.33) With manic- or hypomanic-like episode
(F06.34) With mixed features
296.89 (F31.89) Other Specified Bipolar and Related Disorder
296.80 (F31.9) Unspecified Bipolar and Related Disorder

Depressive Disorders

The following specifiers apply to Depressive Disorders where indicated:
[a] Specify: With anxious distress (specify current severity: mild, moderate, moderate-severe, severe); With mixed features; With melancholic features; With atypical features; With mood-congruent psychotic features; With mood-incongruent psychotic features; With catatonia (use additional code 293.89 [F06.1]); With peripartum onset; With seasonal pattern

296.99 (F34.8) Disruptive Mood Dysregulation Disorder
___.__ (___.__) Major Depressive Disorder [a]
___.__ (___.__) Single episode
296.21 (F32.0) Mild
296.22 (F32.1) Moderate
296.23 (F32.2) Severe
296.24 (F32.3) With psychotic features
296.25 (F32.4) In partial remission
296.26 (F32.5) In full remission
296.20 (F32.9) Unspecified
___.__ (___.__) Recurrent episode
296.31 (F33.0) Mild
296.32 (F33.1) Moderate
296.33 (F33.2) Severe
296.34 (F33.3) With psychotic features
296.35 (F33.41) In partial remission
296.36 (F33.42) In full remission
296.30 (F33.9) Unspecified
300.4 (F34.1) Persistent Depressive Disorder (Dysthymia) [a]
Specify if: In partial remission, In full remission
Specify if: Early onset, Late onset
Specify if: With pure dysthymic syndrome; With persistent major depressive episode; With intermittent major depressive episodes, with current episode; With intermittent major

depressive episodes, without current episode
Specify current severity: Mild, Moderate, Severe

625.4 (N94.3)   Premenstrual Dysphoric Disorder

___.__ (___.__)   Substance/Medication-Induced Depressive Disorder
Note: See the criteria set and corresponding recording procedures for substance-specific codes and ICD-9-CM and ICD-10-CM coding.
Specify if: With onset during intoxication, With onset during withdrawal

293.83 (___.__)   Depressive Disorder Due to Another Medical Condition
Specify if:

(F06.31)   With depressive features

(F06.32)   With major depressive-like episode

(F06.34)   With mixed features

311   (F32.8)   Other Specified Depressive Disorder

311   (F32.9)   Unspecified Depressive Disorder

Anxiety Disorders

309.21 (F93.0)   Separation Anxiety Disorder

312.23 (F94.0)   Selective Mutism

300.29 (___.__)   Specific Phobia
Specify if:

(F40.218)   Animal

(F40.228)   Natural environment

(___.__)   Blood-injection-injury

(F40.230)   Fear of blood

(F40.231)   Fear of injections and transfusions

(F40.232)   Fear of other medical care

(F40.233)   Fear of injury

(F40.248)   Situational

(F40.298)   Other

300.23 (F40.10)   Social Anxiety Disorder (Social Phobia)
Specify if: Performance only

300.01 (F41.0)   Panic Disorder

___.__ (___.__)   Panic Attack Specifier

300.22 (F40.00)   Agoraphobia

300.02 (F41.1)   Generalized Anxiety Disorder

___.__ (___.__)   Substance/Medication-Induced Anxiety Disorder
Note: See the criteria set and corresponding recording procedures for substance-specific codes and ICD-9-CM and ICD-10-CM coding.
Specify if: With onset during intoxication, With onset during withdrawal, With onset after medication use

293.84 (F06.4)   Anxiety Disorder Due to Another Medical Condition

300.00 (F41.9)   Unspecified Anxiety Disorder

Obsessive-Compulsive and Related Disorders

The following specifier applies to Obsessive-Compulsive and Related Disorders where indicated:

[a] *Specify* if: With good or fair insight, With poor insight, With absent insight/delusional beliefs

300.3 (F42)   Obsessive-Compulsive Disorder [a]
Specify if: Tic-related

300.7 (F45.22)   Body Dysmorphic Disorder [a]
Specify if: With muscle dysmorphia

300.3 (F42)   Hoarding Disorder [a]
Specify if: With excessive acquisition

312.39 (F63.3)   Trichotillomania (Hair-Pulling Disorder)

698.4 (L98.1)   Excoriation (Skin-Picking) Disorder

___.__ (___.__)   Substance/Medication-Induced Obsessive-Compulsive and Related Disorder
Note: See the criteria set and corresponding recording procedures for substance-specific codes and ICD-9-CM and ICD-10-CM coding.
Specify if: With onset during intoxication, With onset during withdrawal, With onset after medication use

294.8 (F06.8)   Obsessive-Compulsive and Related Disorder Due to Another Medical Condition
Specify if: With obsessive-compulsive disorder-like symptoms, With appearance preoccupations, With hoarding symptoms, With hair-pulling symptoms, With skin-picking symptoms

300.3 (F42)   Other Specified Obsessive-Compulsive and Related Disorder

300.3 (F42)   Unspecified Obsessive-Compulsive and Related Disorder

Trauma- and Stressor-Related Disorders

313.89 (F94.1) Reactive Attachment Disorder
Specify if: Persistent
Specify current severity: Severe

313.89 (F94.2) Disinhibited Social Engagement Disorder
Specify if: Persistent
Specify current severity: Severe

309.81 (F43.10) Posttraumatic Stress Disorder (includes Posttraumatic Stress Disorder for Children 6 Years and Younger)
Specify whether: With dissociative symptoms
Specify if: With delayed expression

308.3 (F43.0) Acute Stress Disorder

___.__ (___.__) Adjustment Disorders
Specify whether:

309.0 (F43.21) With depressed mood
309.24 (F43.22) With anxiety
309.28 (F43.23) With mixed anxiety and depressed mood
309.3 (F43.24) With disturbance of conduct
309.4 (F43.25) With mixed disturbance of emotions and conduct
309.9 (F43.20) Unspecified

309.89 (F43.8) Other Specified Trauma- and Stressor-Related Disorder
309.9 (F43.9) Unspecified Trauma- and Stressor-Related Disorder

Dissociative Disorders

300.14 (F44.81) Dissociative Identity Disorder
300.12 (F44.0) Dissociative Amnesia
Specify if:
300.13 (F44.1) With dissociative fugue
300.6 (F48.1) Depersonalization/Derealization Disorder
300.15 (F44.89) Other Specified Dissociative Disorder
300.15 (F44.9) Unspecified Dissociative Disorder

Somatic Symptom and Related Disorders

300.82 (F45.1) Somatic Symptom Disorder
Specify if: With predominant pain
Specify if: Persistent
Specify current severity: Mild, Moderate, Severe

300.7 (F45.21) Illness Anxiety Disorder
Specify whether: Care seeking type, Care avoidant type

300.11 (___.__) Conversion Disorder (Functional Neurological Symptom Disorder)
Specify symptom type:

(F44.4) With weakness or paralysis
(F44.4) With abnormal movement
(F44.4) With swallowing symptoms
(F44.4) With speech symptom
(F44.5) With attacks or seizures
(F44.6) With anesthesia or sensory loss
(F44.6) With special sensory symptom
(F44.7) With mixed symptoms
Specify if: Acute episode, Persistent
Specify if: With psychological stressor (specify stressor), Without psychological stressor

316 (F54) Psychological Factors Affecting Other Medical Conditions
Specify current severity: Mild, Moderate, Severe, Extreme

300.19 (F68.10) Factitious Disorder (includes Factitious Disorder Imposed on Self, Factitious Disorder Imposed on Another)
Specify Single episode, Recurrent episodes

300.89 (F45.8) Other Specified Somatic Symptom and Related Disorder
300.82 (F45.9) Unspecified Somatic Symptom and Related Disorder

Feeding and Eating Disorders

The following specifiers apply to Feeding and Eating Disorders where indicated:
[a] *Specify* if: In remission
[b] *Specify* if: In partial remission, In full remission
[c] *Specify* current severity: Mild, Moderate, Severe, Extreme

307.52 (___.__) Pica [a]
(F98.3) In children
(F50.8) In adults
307.53 (F98.21) Rumination Disorder [a]
307.59 (F50.8) Avoidant/Restrictive Food Intake Disorder [a]
307.1 (___.__) Anorexia Nervosa [b, c]
Specify whether:
(F50.01) Restricting type
(F50.02) Binge-eating/purging type
307.51 (F50.2) Bulimia Nervosa [b, c]
307.51 (F50.8) Binge-Eating Disorder [b, c]
307.59 (F50.8) Other Specified Feeding or Eating Disorder
307.50 (F50.9) Unspecified Feeding or Eating Disorder

Elimination Disorders

307.6 (F98.0)	Enuresis *Specify* whether: Nocturnal only, Diurnal only, Nocturnal and diurnal
307.7 (F98.1)	Encopresis *Specify* whether: With constipation and overflow incontinence, Without constipation and overflow incontinence
___.__ (___.__)	Other Specified Elimination Disorder
788.39 (N39.498)	With urinary symptoms
787.60 (R15.9)	With fecal symptoms
___.__ (___.__)	Unspecified Elimination Disorder
788.30 (R32)	With urinary symptoms
787.60 (R15.9)	With fecal symptoms

Sleep-Wake Disorders

The following specifiers apply to Sleep-Wake Disorders where indicated:

a *Specify* if: Episodic, Persistent, Recurrent
b *Specify* if: Acute, Subacute, Persistent
c *Specify* current severity: Mild, Moderate, Severe

780.52 (G47.00)	Insomnia Disorder a *Specify* if: With non-sleep disorder mental comorbidity, With other medical comorbidity, With other sleep disorder
780.54 (G47.10)	Hypersomnolence Disorder b, c *Specify* if: With mental disorder, With medical condition, With another sleep disorder
___.__ (___.__)	Narcolepsy c *Specify* whether:
347.00 (G47.419)	Narcolepsy without cataplexy but with hypocretin deficiency
347.01 (G47.411)	Narcolepsy with cataplexy but without hypocretin deficiency
347.00 (G47.419)	Autosomal dominant cerebellar ataxia, deafness, and narcolepsy
347.00 (G47.419)	Autosomal dominant narcolepsy, obesity, and type 2 diabetes
347.10 (G47.429)	Narcolepsy secondary to another medical condition

Breathing-Related Sleep Disorders

327.23 (G47.33)	Obstructive Sleep Apnea Hypopnea c
___.__ (___.__)	Central Sleep Apnea *Specify* whether:
327.21 (G47.31)	Idiopathic central sleep apnea
786.04 (R06.3)	Cheyne-Stokes breathing
780.57 (G47.37)	Central sleep apnea comorbid with opioid use Note: First code opioid use disorder, if present. *Specify* current severity
___.__ (___.__)	Sleep-Related Hypoventilation *Specify* whether:
327.24 (G47.34)	Idiopathic hypoventilation
327.25 (G47.35)	Congenital central alveolar hypoventilation
327.26 (G47.36)	Comorbid sleep-related hypoventilation *Specify* current severity
___.__ (___.__)	Circadian Rhythm Sleep-Wake Disorders a *Specify* whether:
307.45 (G47.21)	Delayed sleep phase type *Specify* if: Familial, Overlapping with non-24-hour sleep-wake type
307.45 (G47.22)	Advanced sleep phase type *Specify* if: Familial
307.45 (G47.23)	Irregular sleep-wake type
307.45 (G47.24)	Non-24-hour sleep-wake type
307.45 (G47.26)	Shift work type
307.45 (G47.20)	Unspecified type

Parasomnias

___.__ (___.__)	Non-Rapid Eye Movement Sleep Arousal Disorders *Specify* whether:
307.46 (F51.3)	Sleepwalking type *Specify* if: With sleep-related eating, With sleep-related sexual behavior (sexsomnia)
307.46 (F51.4)	Sleep terror type
307.47 (F51.5)	Nightmare Disorder b, c *Specify* if: During sleep onset *Specify* if: With associated non-sleep disorder, With associated other medical condition, With associated other sleep disorder
327.42 (G47.52)	Rapid Eye Movement Sleep Behavior Disorder
333.94 (G25.81)	Restless Legs Syndrome
___.__ (___.__)	Substance/Medication-Induced Sleep Disorder Note: See the criteria set and corresponding recording procedures for substance-specific codes and ICD-9-CM and ICD-10-CM coding.

Specify whether: Insomnia type, Daytime sleepiness type, Parasomnia type, Mixed type
Specify if: With onset during intoxication, With onset during discontinuation/withdrawal

780.52 (G47.09)	Other Specified Insomnia Disorder
780.52 (G47.00)	Unspecified Insomnia Disorder
780.54 (G47.19)	Other Specified Hypersomno-lence Disorder
780.54 (G47.10)	Unspecified Hypersomnolence Disorder
780.59 (G47.8)	Other Specified Sleep-Wake Disorder
780.59 (G47.9)	Unspecified Sleep-Wake Disorder

Sexual Dysfunctions

The following specifiers apply to Sexual Dysfunctions where indicated:

 a *Specify* whether: Lifelong, Acquired
 b *Specify* whether: Generalized, Situational
 c *Specify* current severity: Mild, Moderate, Severe

302.74 (F52.32)	Delayed Ejaculation a, b, c
302.72 (F52.21)	Erectile Disorder a, b, c
302.73 (F52.31)	Female Orgasmic Disorder a, b, c
	Specify if: Never experienced an orgasm under any situation
302.72 (F52.22)	Female Sexual Interest/Arousal Disorder a, b, c
302.76 (F52.6)	Genito-Pelvic Pain/Penetration Disorder a, c
302.71 (F52.0)	Male Hypoactive Sexual Desire Disorder a, b, c
302.75 (F52.4)	Premature (Early) Ejaculation a, b, c
___.__ (___.__)	Substance/Medication-Induced Sexual Dysfunction c
	Note: See the criteria set and corresponding recording procedures for substance-specific codes and ICD-9-CM and ICD-10-CM coding.
	Specify if: With onset during intoxication, With onset during withdrawal, With onset after medication use
302.79 (F52.8)	Other Specified Sexual Dysfunction
302.70 (F52.9)	Unspecified Sexual Dysfunction

Gender Dysphoria

___.__ (___.__)	Gender Dysphoria
302.6 (F64.2)	Gender Dysphoria in Children

Specify if: With a disorder of sex development

302.85 (F64.1)	Gender Dysphoria in Adolescents and Adults
	Specify if: With a disorder of sex development
	Specify if: Posttransition
	Note: Code the disorder of sex development if present, in addition to gender dysphoria.
302.6 (F64.8)	Other Specified Gender Dysphoria
302.6 (F64.9)	Unspecified Gender Dysphoria

Disruptive, Impulse-Control, and Conduct Disorders

313.81 (F91.3)	Oppositional Defiant Disorder
	Specify current severity: Mild, Moderate, Severe
312.34 (F63.81)	Intermittent Explosive Disorder
___.__ (___.__)	Conduct Disorder
	Specify whether:
312.81 (F91.1)	Childhood-onset type
312.82 (F91.2)	Adolescent-onset type
312.89 (F91.9)	Unspecified onset
	Specify if: With limited prosocial emotions
	Specify current severity: Mild, Moderate, Severe
301.7 (F60.2)	Antisocial Personality Disorder
312.33 (F63.1)	Pyromania
312.32 (F63.2)	Kleptomania
312.89 (F91.8)	Other Specified Disruptive, Impulse-Control, and Conduct Disorder
312.9 (F91.9)	Unspecified Disruptive, Impulse-Control, and Conduct Disorder

Substance-Related and Addictive Disorders

The following specifiers and note apply to Substance-Related and Addictive Disorders where indicated:

 a *Specify* if: In early remission, In sustained remission
 b *Specify* if: In a controlled environment
 c *Specify* if: With perceptual disturbances
 d The ICD-10-CM code indicates the comorbid presence of a moderate or severe substance use disorder, which must be present in order to apply the code for substance withdrawal.

Substance-Related Disorders

Alcohol-Related Disorders

___.__ (___.__)	Alcohol Use Disorder a, b
	Specify current severity:
305.00 (F10.10)	Mild
303.90 (F10.20)	Moderate
303.90 (F10.20)	Severe

303.00 (___.__)   Alcohol Intoxication
   (F10.129)   With use disorder, mild
   (F10.229)   With use disorder, moderate
      or severe
   (F10.929)   Without use disorder
291.81 (___.__)   Alcohol Withdrawal [c, d]
   (F10.239)   Without perceptual
      disturbances
   (F10.232)   With perceptual disturbances
___.__ (___.__)   Other Alcohol-Induced
   Disorders
291.9 (F10.99)   Unspecified Alcohol-Related
   Disorder

Caffeine-Related Disorders

305.90 (F15.929)   Caffeine Intoxication
292.0 (F15.93)   Caffeine Withdrawal
___.__ (___.__)   Other Caffeine-Induced
   Disorders
292.9 (F15.99)   Unspecified Caffeine-Related
   Disorder

Cannabis-Related Disorders

___.__ (___.__)   Cannabis Use Disorder [a, b]
   Specify current severity
305.20 (F12.10)   Mild
304.30 (F12.20)   Moderate
304.30 (F12.20)   Severe
292.89 (___.__)   Cannabis Intoxication [c]
   Without perceptual
   disturbances
   (F12.129)   With use disorder, mild
   (F12.229)   With use disorder,
      moderate or severe
   (F12.929)   Without use disorder
   With perceptual disturbances
   (F12.122)   With use disorder, mild
   (F12.222)   With use disorder,
      moderate or severe
   (F12.922)   Without use disorder
292.0 (F12.288)   Cannabis Withdrawal [d]
___.__ (___.__)   Other Cannabis-Induced
   Disorders
292.9 (F12.99)   Unspecified Cannabis-Related
   Disorder

Hallucinogen-Related Disorders

___.__ (___.__)   Phencyclidine Use Disorder [a, b]
   Specify current severity:
305.90 (F16.10)   Mild
304.60 (F16.20)   Moderate
304.60 (F16.20)   Severe
___.__ (___.__)   Other Hallucinogen Use
   Disorder [a, b]
   Specify the particular
   hallucinogen

   Specify current severity:
305.30 (F16.10)   Mild
304.50 (F16.20)   Moderate
304.50 (F16.20)   Severe
292.89 (___.__)   Phencyclidine Intoxication
   (F16.129)   With use disorder, mild
   (F16.229)   With use disorder, moderate
      or severe
   (F16.929)   Without use disorder
292.89 (___.__)   Other Hallucinogen
   Intoxication
   (F16.129)   With use disorder, mild
   (F16.229)   With use disorder, moderate
      or severe
   (F16.929)   Without use disorder
292.89 (F16.983)   Hallucinogen Persisting
   Perception Disorder
___.__ (___.__)   Other Phencyclidine-Induced
   Disorders
___.__ (___.__)   Other Hallucinogen-Induced
   Disorders
292.9 (F16.99)   Unspecified Phencyclidine-
   Related Disorder
292.9 (F16.99)   Unspecified Hallucinogen-
   Related Disorder

Inhalant-Related Disorders

___.__ (___.__)   Inhalant Use Disorder [a, b]
   Specify the particular inhalant
   Specify current severity:
305.90 (F18.10)   Mild
304.60 (F18.20)   Moderate
304.60 (F18.20)   Severe
292.89 (___.__)   Inhalant Intoxication
   (F18.129)   With use disorder, mild
   (F18.229)   With use disorder, moderate
      or severe
   (F18.929)   Without use disorder
___.__ (___.__)   Other Inhalant-Induced
   Disorders
292.9 (F18.99)   Unspecified Inhalant-Related
   Disorder

Opioid-Related Disorders

___.__ (___.__)   Opioid Use Disorder [a]
   Specify if: On maintenance
   therapy, In a controlled
   environment
   Specify current severity:
305.50 (F11.10)   Mild
304.00 (F11.20)   Moderate
304.00 (F11.20)   Severe
292.89 (___.__)   Opioid Intoxication [c]
   Without perceptual
   disturbances
   (F11.129)   With use disorder, mild

(F11.229)   With use disorder,
moderate or severe
(F11.922)   Without use disorder
292.0 (F11.23)   Opioid Withdrawal [d]
___.__ (___.__)   Other Opioid-Induced Disorders
292.9 (F11.99)   Unspecified Opioid-Related
Disorder

Sedative-, Hypnotic-, or Anxiolytic-Related Disorders

___.__ (___.__)   Sedative, Hypnotic, or Anxiolytic
Use Disorder [a, b]
Specify current severity:
305.40 (F13.10)   Mild
304.10 (F13.20)   Moderate
304.10 (F13.20)   Severe
292.89 (___.__)   Sedative, Hypnotic, or Anxiolytic
Intoxication
(F13.129)   With use disorder, mild
(F13.229)   With use disorder, moderate
or severe
(F13.929)   Without use disorder
292.0 (___.__)   Sedative, Hypnotic, or Anxiolytic
Withdrawal [c, d]
(F13.239)   Without perceptual
disturbances
(F13.232)   With perceptual
disturbances
___.__ (___.__)   Other Sedative-, Hypnotic-, or
Anxiolytic-Induced Disorders
292.9 (F13.99)   Unspecified Sedative-,
Hypnotic-, or Anxiolytic-
Related Disorder

Stimulant-Related Disorders

___.__ (___.__)   Stimulant Use Disorder [a, b]
Specify current severity:
___.__ (___.__)   Mild
305.70 (F15.10)   Amphetamine-type
substance
305.60 (F14.10)   Cocaine
305.70 (F15.10)   Other or unspecified
stimulant
___.__ (___.__)   Moderate
304.40 (F15.20)   Amphetamine-type
substance
304.20 (F14.20)   Cocaine
304.40 (F15.20)   Other or unspecified
stimulant
___.__ (___.__)   Severe
304.40 (F15.20)   Amphetamine-type
substance
304.20 (F14.20)   Cocaine
304.40 (F15.20)   Other or unspecified
stimulant
292.89 (___.__)   Stimulant Intoxication [c]

Specify the specific intoxicant
292.89 (___.__)   Amphetamine or other
stimulant, Without perceptual
disturbances
(F15.129)   With use disorder, mild
(F15.229)   With use disorder,
moderate or severe
(F15.929)   Without use disorder
292.89 (___.__)   Cocaine, Without perceptual
disturbances
(F14.129)   With use disorder, mild
(F14.229)   With use disorder,
moderate or severe
(F14.929)   Without use disorder
292.89 (___.__)   Amphetamine or other
stimulant, With perceptual
disturbances
(F15.122)   With use disorder, mild
(F15.222)   With use disorder,
moderate or severe
(F15.922)   Without use disorder
292.89 (___.__)   Cocaine, With perceptual
disturbances
(F14.122)   With use disorder, mild
(F14.222)   With use disorder, moderate
or severe
(F14.922)   Without use disorder
292.0 (___.__)   Stimulant Withdrawal [d]
Specify the specific substance
causing the withdrawal
syndrome
(F15.23)   Amphetamine or other
stimulant
(F14.23)   Cocaine
___.__ (___.__)   Other Stimulant-Induced
Disorders
292.9 (___.__)   Unspecified Stimulant-Related
Disorder
(F15.99)   Amphetamine or other
stimulant
(F14.99)   Cocaine

Tobacco-Related Disorders

___.__ (___.__)   Tobacco Use Disorder [a]
Specify if: On maintenance therapy,
In a controlled environment
Specify current severity:
305.1 (Z72.0)   Mild
305.1 (F17.200)   Moderate
305.1 (F17.200)   Severe
292.0 (F17.203)   Tobacco Withdrawal [d]
___.__ (___.__)   Other Tobacco-Induced
Disorders
292.9 (F17.209)   Unspecified Tobacco-Related
Disorder

Other (or Unknown) Substance-Related Disorders

___.__ (___.__)	Other (or Unknown) Substance Use Disorder [a, b]
	Specify current severity:
305.90 (F19.10)	Mild
304.90 (F19.20)	Moderate
304.90 (F19.20)	Severe
292.89 (___.__)	Other (or Unknown) Substance Intoxication
(F19.129)	With use disorder, mild
(F19.229)	With use disorder, moderate or severe
(F19.929)	Without use disorder
292.0 (F19.239)	Other (or Unknown) Substance Withdrawal [d]
___.__ (___.__) ·	Other (or Unknown) Substance-Induced Disorders
292.9 (F19.99)	Unspecified Other (or Unknown) Substance-Related Disorder

Non-Substance-Related Disorders

312.31 (F63.0)	Gambling Disorder [a]
	Specify if: Episodic, Persistent
	Specify current severity: Mild, Moderate, Severe

Neurocognitive Disorders

___.__ (___.__)	Delirium
	[a] Note: See the criteria set and corresponding recording procedures for substance-specific codes and ICD-9-CM and ICD-10-CM coding.
	Specify whether:
___.__ (___.__)	Substance intoxication delirium [a]
___.__ (___.__)	Substance withdrawal delirium [a]
292.81 (___.__)	Medication-induced delirium [a]
293.0 (F05)	Delirium due to another medical condition
293.0 (F05)	Delirium due to multiple etiologies
	Specify if: Acute, Persistent
	Specify if: Hyperactive, Hypoactive, Mixed level of activity
780.09 (R41.0)	Other Specified Delirium
780.09 (R41.0)	Unspecified Delirium

Major and Mild Neurocognitive Disorders

Specify whether due to: Alzheimer's disease, Frontotemporal lobar degeneration, Lewy body disease, Vascular disease, Traumatic brain injury, Substance/medication use, HIV infection, Prion disease, Parkinson's disease, Huntington's disease, Another medical condition, Multiple etiologies, Unspecified

[a] *Specify* Without behavioral disturbance, With behavioral disturbance. *For possible major neurocognitive disorder and for mild neurocognitive disorder, behavioral disturbance cannot be coded but should still be indicated in writing.*

[b] *Specify* current severity: Mild, Moderate, Severe. *This specifier applies only to major neurocognitive disorders (including probable and possible).*

Note: As indicated for each subtype, an additional medical code is needed for probable major neurocognitive disorder or major neurocognitive disorder. An additional medical code should *not* be used for possible major neurocognitive disorder or mild neurocognitive disorder.

Major or Mild Neurocognitive Disorder Due to Alzheimer's Disease

___.__ (___.__)	Probable Major Neurocognitive Disorder Due to Alzheimer's Disease [b]
	Note: Code first 331.0 (G30.9) Alzheimer's disease.
294.11 (F02.81)	With behavioral disturbance
294.10 (F02.80)	Without behavioral disturbance
331.9 (G31.9)	Possible Major Neurocognitive Disorder Due to Alzheimer's Disease [a, b]
331.83 (G31.84)	Mild Neurocognitive Disorder Due to Alzheimer's Disease [a]

Major or Mild Frontotemporal Neurocognitive Disorder

___.__ (___.__)	Probable Major Neurocognitive Disorder Due to Frontotemporal Lobar Degeneration [b]
	Note: Code first 331.19 (G31.09) frontotemporal disease.
294.11 (F02.81)	With behavioral disturbance
294.10 (F02.80)	Without behavioral disturbance
331.9 (G31.9)	Possible Major Neurocognitive Disorder Due to Frontotemporal Lobar Degeneration [a, b]
331.83 (G31.84)	Mild Neurocognitive Disorder Due to Frontotemporal Lobar Degeneration [a]

Major or Mild Neurocognitive Disorder With Lewy Bodies

___.__ (___.__)	Probable Major Neurocognitive Disorder With Lewy Bodies [b]
	Note: Code first 331.82 (G31.83) Lewy body disease.
294.11 (F02.81)	With behavioral disturbance
294.10 (F02.80)	Without behavioral disturbance

331.9 (G31.9)   Possible Major Neurocognitive Disorder With Lewy Bodies [a, b]

331.83 (G31.84)   Mild Neurocognitive Disorder With Lewy Bodies [a]

Major or Mild Vascular Neurocognitive Disorder

___.__ (___.__)   Probable Major Vascular Neurocognitive Disorder [b]
Note: No additional medical code for vascular disease.

290.40 (F01.51)   With behavioral disturbance

290.40 (F01.50)   Without behavioral disturbance

331.9 (G31.9)   Possible Major Vascular Neurocognitive Disorder [a, b]

331.83 (G31.84)   Mild Vascular Neurocognitive Disorder [a]

Major or Mild Neurocognitive Disorder Due to Traumatic Brain Injury

___.__ (___.__)   Major Neurocognitive Disorder Due to Traumatic Brain Injury [b]
Note: For ICD-9-CM, code first 907.0 late effect of intracranial injury without skull fracture. For ICD-10-CM, code first S06.2X9S diffuse traumatic brain injury with loss of consciousness of unspecified duration, sequela.

294.11 (F02.81)   With behavioral disturbance

294.10 (F02.80)   Without behavioral disturbance

331.83 (G31.84)   Mild Neurocognitive Disorder Due to Traumatic Brain Injury [a]

Substance/Medication-Induced Major or Mild Neurocognitive Disorder [a]

Note: No additional medical code. See the criteria set and corresponding recording procedures for substance-specific codes and ICD-9-CM and ICD-10-CM coding.
Specify if: Persistent

Major or Mild Neurocognitive Disorder Due to HIV Infection

___.__ (___.__)   Major Neurocognitive Disorder Due to HIV Infection [b]
Note: Code first 042 (B20) HIV infection.

294.11 (F02.81)   With behavioral disturbance

294.10 (F02.80)   Without behavioral disturbance

331.83 (G31.84)   Mild Neurocognitive Disorder Due to HIV Infection [a]

Major or Mild Neurocognitive Disorder Due to Prion Disease

___.__ (___.__)   Major Neurocognitive Disorder Due to Prion Disease [b]
Note: Code first 046.79 (A81.9) prion disease.

294.11 (F02.81)   With behavioral disturbance

294.10 (F02.80)   Without behavioral disturbance

331.83 (G31.84)   Mild Neurocognitive Disorder Due to Prion Disease [a]

Major or Mild Neurocognitive Disorder Due to Parkinson's Disease

___.__ (___.__)   Major Neurocognitive Disorder Probably Due to Parkinson's Disease [b]
Note: Code first 332.0 (G20) Parkinson's disease.

294.11 (F02.81)   With behavioral disturbance

294.10 (F02.80)   Without behavioral disturbance

331.9 (G31.9)   Major Neurocognitive Disorder Possibly Due to Parkinson's Disease [a, b]

331.83 (G31.84)   Mild Neurocognitive Disorder Due to Parkinson's Disease [a]

Major or Mild Neurocognitive Disorder Due to Huntington's Disease

___.__ (___.__)   Major Neurocognitive Disorder Due to Huntington's Disease [b]
Note: Code first 333.4 (G10) Huntington's disease.

294.11 (F02.81)   With behavioral disturbance

294.10 (F02.80)   Without behavioral disturbance

331.83 (G31.84)   Mild Neurocognitive Disorder Due to Huntington's Disease [a]

Major or Mild Neurocognitive Disorder Due to Another Medical Condition

___.__ (___.__)   Major Neurocognitive Disorder Due to Another Medical Condition [b]
Note: Code first the other medical condition.

294.11 (F02.81)   With behavioral disturbance

294.10 (F02.80)   Without behavioral disturbance

331.83 (G31.84)   Mild Neurocognitive Disorder Due to Another Medical Condition [a]

Major or Mild Neurocognitive Disorder Due to Multiple Etiologies

__._ (__._)	Major Neurocognitive Disorder Due to Multiple Etiologies [b] Note: Code first all the etiological medical conditions (with the exception of vascular disease).
294.11 (F02.81)	With behavioral disturbance
294.10 (F02.80)	Without behavioral disturbance
331.83 (G31.84)	Mild Neurocognitive Disorder Due to Multiple Etiologies [a]

Unspecified Neurocognitive Disorder

799.59 (R41.9)	Unspecified Neurocognitive Disorder [a]

Personality Disorders

Cluster A Personality Disorders

301.0 (F60.0)	Paranoid Personality Disorder
301.20 (F60.1)	Schizoid Personality Disorder
301.22 (F21)	Schizotypal Personality Disorder

Cluster B Personality Disorders

301.7 (F60.2)	Antisocial Personality Disorder
301.83 (F60.3)	Borderline Personality Disorder
301.50 (F60.4)	Histrionic Personality Disorder
301.81 (F60.81)	Narcissistic Personality Disorder

Cluster C Personality Disorders

301.82 (F60.6)	Avoidant Personality Disorder
301.6 (F60.7)	Dependent Personality Disorder
301.4 (F60.5)	Obsessive-Compulsive Personality Disorder

Other Personality Disorders

310.1 (F07.0)	Personality Change Due to Another Medical Condition *Specify* whether: Labile type, Disinhibited type, Aggressive type, Apathetic type, Paranoid type, Other type, Combined type, Unspecified type
301.89 (F60.89)	Other Specified Personality Disorder
301.9 (F60.9)	Unspecified Personality Disorder

Paraphilic Disorders

The following specifier applies to Paraphilic Disorders where indicated:

[a] *Specify* if: In a controlled environment, In full remission

302.82 (F65.3)	Voyeuristic Disorder [a]
302.4 (F65.2)	Exhibitionistic Disorder [a]

Specify whether: Sexually aroused by exposing genitals to prepubertal children, Sexually aroused by exposing genitals to physically mature individuals, Sexually aroused by exposing genitals to prepubertal children and to physically mature individuals.

302.89 (F65.81)	Frotteuristic Disorder [a]
302.83 (F65.51)	Sexual Masochism Disorder [a] *Specify* if: With asphyxiophilia
302.84 (F65.52)	Sexual Sadism Disorder [a]
302.2 (F65.4)	Pedophilic Disorder *Specify* whether: Exclusive type, Nonexclusive type *Specify* if: Sexually attracted to males, Sexually attracted to females, Sexually attracted to both *Specify* if: Limited to incest
302.81 (F65.0)	Fetishistic Disorder [a] *Specify*: Body part(s), Nonliving object(s), Other
302.3 (F65.1)	Transvestic Disorder [a] *Specify* if: With fetishism, With autogynephilia
302.89 (F65.89)	Other Specified Paraphilic Disorder
302.9 (F65.9)	Unspecified Paraphilic Disorder

Other Mental Disorders

294.8 (F06.8)	Other Specified Mental Disorder Due to Another Medical Condition
294.9 (F09)	Unspecified Mental Disorder Due to Another Medical Condition
300.9 (F99)	Other Specified Mental Disorder
300.9 (F99)	Unspecified Mental Disorder

Medication-Induced Movement Disorders and Other Adverse Effects of Medication

332.1 (G21.11)	Neuroleptic-Induced Parkinsonism
332.1 (G21.19)	Other Medication-Induced Parkinsonism
333.92 (G21.0)	Neuroleptic Malignant Syndrome
333.72 (G24.02)	Medication-Induced Acute Dystonia
333.99 (G25.71)	Medication-Induced Acute Akathisia
333.85 (G24.01)	Tardive Dyskinesia
333.72 (G24.09)	Tardive Dystonia
333.99 (G25.71)	Tardive Akathisia
333.1 (G25.1)	Medication-Induced Postural Tremor

333.99 (G25.79)   Other Medication-Induced Movement Disorder

___.__ (___.__)   Antidepressant Discontinuation Syndrome

995.29 (T43.205A)   Initial encounter
995.29 (T43.205D)   Subsequent encounter
995.29 (T43.205S)   Sequelae

___.__ (___.__)   Other Adverse Effect of Medication

995.20 (T50.905A)   Initial encounter
995.20 (T50.905D)   Subsequent encounter
995.20 (T50.905S)   Sequelae

Other Conditions That May Be a Focus of Clinical Attention

Relational Problems

Problems Related to Family Upbringing

V61.20 (Z62.820)   Parent-Child Relational Problem
V61.8 (Z62.891)   Sibling Relational Problem
V61.8 (Z62.29)   Upbringing Away From Parents
V61.29 (Z62.898)   Child Affected by Parental Relationship Distress

Other Problems Related to Primary Support Group

V61.10 (Z63.0)   Relationship Distress With Spouse or Intimate Partner
V61.03 (Z63.5)   Disruption of Family by Separation or Divorce
V61.8 (Z63.8)   High Expressed Emotion Level Within Family
V62.82 (Z63.4)   Uncomplicated Bereavement

Abuse and Neglect

Child Maltreatment and Neglect Problems

Child Physical Abuse, Confirmed
995.54 (T74.12XA)   Initial encounter
995.54 (T74.12XD)   Subsequent encounter

Child Physical Abuse, Suspected
995.54 (T76.12XA)   Initial encounter
995.54 (T76.12XD)   Subsequent encounter

Other Circumstances Related to Child Physical Abuse
V61.21 (Z69.010)   Encounter for mental health services for victim of child abuse by parent
V61.21 (Z69.020)   Encounter for mental health services for victim of non-parental child abuse
V15.41 (Z62.810)   Personal history (past history) of physical abuse in childhood
V61.22 (Z69.011)   Encounter for mental health services for perpetrator of parental child abuse

V62.83 (Z69.021)   Encounter for mental health services for perpetrator of non-parental child abuse

Child Sexual Abuse, Confirmed
995.53 (T74.22XA)   Initial encounter
995.53 (T74.22XD)   Subsequent encounter

Child Sexual Abuse, Suspected
995.53 (T76.22XA)   Initial encounter
995.53 (T76.22XD)   Subsequent encounter

Other Circumstances Related to Child Sexual Abuse
V61.21 (Z69.010)   Encounter for mental health services for victim of child sexual abuse by parent
V61.21 (Z69.020)   Encounter for mental health services for victim of non-parental child sexual abuse
V15.41 (Z62.810)   Personal history (past history) of sexual abuse in childhood
V61.22 (Z69.011)   Encounter for mental health services for perpetrator of parental child sexual abuse
V62.83 (Z69.021)   Encounter for mental health services for perpetrator of nonparental child sexual abuse

Child Neglect, Confirmed
995.52 (T74.02XA)   Initial encounter
995.52 (T74.02XD)   Subsequent encounter

Child Neglect, Suspected
995.52 (T76.02XA)   Initial encounter
995.52 (T76.02XD)   Subsequent encounter

Other Circumstances Related to Child Neglect
V61.21 (Z69.010)   Encounter for mental health services for victim of child neglect by parent
V61.21 (Z69.020)   Encounter for mental health services for victim of non-parental child neglect
V15.42 (Z62.812)   Personal history (past history) of neglect in childhood
V61.22 (Z69.011)   Encounter for mental health services for perpetrator of parental child neglect
V62.83 (Z69.021)   Encounter for mental health services for perpetrator of nonparental child neglect

Child Psychological Abuse, Confirmed
995.51 (T74.32XA)   Initial encounter
995.51 (T74.32XD)   Subsequent encounter

Child Psychological Abuse, Suspected
995.51 (T76.32XA)   Initial encounter
995.51 (T76.32XD)   Subsequent encounter

Other Circumstances Related to Child Psychological Abuse
V61.21 (Z69.010)   Encounter for mental health services for victim of child psychological abuse by parent
V61.21 (Z69.020)   Encounter for mental health services for victim of non-parental child psychological abuse
V15.42 (Z62.811)   Personal history (past history) of psychological abuse in childhood
V61.22 (Z69.011)   Encounter for mental health services for perpetrator of parental child psychological abuse
V62.83 (Z69.021)   Encounter for mental health services for perpetrator of nonparental child psychological abuse

Adult Maltreatment and Neglect Problems

Spouse or Partner Violence, Physical, Confirmed
995.81 (T74.11XA)   Initial encounter
995.81 (T74.11XD)   Subsequent encounter

Spouse or Partner Violence, Physical, Suspected
995.81 (T76.11XA)   Initial encounter
995.81 (T76.11XD)   Subsequent encounter

Other Circumstances Related to Spouse or Partner Violence, Physical
V61.11 (Z69.11)   Encounter for mental health services for victim of spouse or partner violence, physical
V15.41 (Z91.410)   Personal history (past history) of spouse or partner violence, physical
V61.12 (Z69.12)   Encounter for mental health services for perpetrator of spouse or partner violence, physical

Spouse or Partner Violence, Sexual, Confirmed
995.83 (T74.21XA)   Initial encounter
995.83 (T74.21XD)   Subsequent encounter

Spouse or Partner Violence, Sexual, Suspected
995.83 (T76.21XA)   Initial encounter
995.83 (T76.21XD)   Subsequent encounter

Other Circumstances Related to Spouse or Partner Violence, Sexual
V61.11 (Z69.81)   Encounter for mental health services for victim of spouse or partner violence, sexual
V15.41 (Z91.410)   Personal history (past history) of spouse or partner violence, sexual
V61.12 (Z69.12)   Encounter for mental health services for perpetrator of spouse or partner violence, sexual

Spouse or Partner Neglect, Confirmed
995.85 (T74.01XA)   Initial encounter
995.85 (T74.01XD)   Subsequent encounter

Spouse or Partner Neglect, Suspected
995.85 (T76.01XA)   Initial encounter
995.85 (T76.01XD)   Subsequent encounter

Other Circumstances Related to Spouse or Partner Neglect
V61.11 (Z69.11)   Encounter for mental health services for victim of spouse or partner neglect
V15.42 (Z91.412)   Personal history (past history) of spouse or partner neglect
V61.12 (Z69.12)   Encounter for mental health services for perpetrator of spouse or partner neglect

Spouse or Partner Abuse, Psychological, Confirmed
995.82 (T74.31XA)   Initial encounter
995.82 (T74.31XD)   Subsequent encounter

Spouse or Partner Abuse, Psychological, Suspected
995.82 (T76.31XA)   Initial encounter
995.85 (T76.31XD)   Subsequent encounter

Other Circumstances Related to Spouse or Partner Abuse, Psychological
V61.11 (Z69.11)   Encounter for mental health services for victim of spouse or partner psychological abuse
V15.42 (Z91.411)   Personal history (past history) of spouse or partner psychological abuse
V61.12 (Z69.12)   Encounter for mental health services for perpetrator of spouse or partner psychological abuse

Adult Physical Abuse by Nonspouse or Nonpartner, Confirmed

995.81 (T74.11XA)	Initial encounter
995.81 (T74.11XD)	Subsequent encounter

Adult Physical Abuse by Nonspouse or Nonpartner, Suspected

995.81 (T76.11XA)	Initial encounter
995.81 (T76.11XD)	Subsequent encounter

Adult Sexual Abuse by Nonspouse or Nonpartner, Confirmed

995.83 (T74.21XA)	Initial encounter
995.83 (T74.21XD)	Subsequent encounter

Adult Sexual Abuse by Nonspouse or Nonpartner, Suspected

995.83 (T76.21XA)	Initial encounter
995.83 (T76.21XD)	Subsequent encounter

Adult Psychological Abuse by Nonspouse or Nonpartner, Confirmed

995.82 (T74.31XA)	Initial encounter
995.82 (T74.31XD)	Subsequent encounter

Adult Psychological Abuse by Nonspouse or Nonpartner, Suspected

995.82 (T76.31XA)	Initial encounter
995.82 (T76.31XD)	Subsequent encounter

Other Circumstances Related to Adult Abuse by Nonspouse or Nonpartner

V65.49 (Z69.81)	Encounter for mental health services for victim of nonspousal adult abuse
V62.83 (Z69.82)	Encounter for mental health services for perpetrator of nonspousal adult abuse

Educational and Occupational Problems

Educational Problems

V62.3 (Z55.9)	Academic or Educational Problem

Occupational Problems

V62.21 (Z56.82)	Problem Related to Current Military Deployment Status
V62.29 (Z56.9)	Other Problem Related to Employment

Housing and Economic Problems

Housing Problems

V60.0 (Z59.0)	Homelessness
V60.1 (Z59.1)	Inadequate Housing
V60.89 (Z59.2)	Discord With Neighbor, Lodger, or Landlord

V60.6 (Z59.3)	Problem Related to Living in a Residential Institution

Economic Problems

V60.2 (Z59.4)	Lack of Adequate Food or Safe Drinking Water
V60.2 (Z59.5)	Extreme Poverty
V60.2 (Z59.6)	Low Income
V60.2 (Z59.7)	Insufficient Social Insurance or Welfare Support
V60.9 (Z59.9)	Unspecified Housing or Economic Problem

Other Problems Related to the Social Environment

V62.89 (Z60.0)	Phase of Life Problem
V60.3 (Z60.2)	Problem Related to Living Alone
V62.4 (Z60.3)	Acculturation Difficulty
V62.4 (Z60.4)	Social Exclusion or Rejection
V62.4 (Z60.5)	Target of (Perceived) Adverse Discrimination or Persecution
V62.9 (Z60.9)	Unspecified Problem Related to Social Environment

Problems Related to Crime or Interaction With the Legal System

V62.89 (Z65.4)	Victim of Crime
V62.5 (Z65.0)	Conviction in Civil or Criminal Proceedings Without Imprisonment
V62.5 (Z65.1)	Imprisonment or Other Incarceration
V62.5 (Z65.2)	Problems Related to Release From Prison
V62.5 (Z65.3)	Problems Related to Other Legal Circumstances

Other Health Service Encounters for Counseling and Medical Advice

V65.49 (Z70.9)	Sex Counseling
V65.40 (Z71.9)	Other Counseling or Consultation

Problems Related to Other Psychosocial, Personal, and Environmental Circumstances

V62.89 (Z65.8)	Religious or Spiritual Problem
V61.7 (Z64.0)	Problems Related to Unwanted Pregnancy
V61.5 (Z64.1)	Problems Related to Multiparity
V62.89 (Z64.4)	Discord With Social Service Provider, Including Probation Officer, Case Manager, or Social Services Worker
V62.89 (Z65.4)	Victim of Terrorism or Torture
V62.22 (Z65.5)	Exposure to Disaster, War, or Other Hostilities

V62.89 (Z65.8)   Other Problem Related to Psychosocial Circumstances

V62.9 (Z65.9)   Unspecified Problem Related to Unspecified Psychosocial Circumstances

Other Circumstances of Personal History

V15.49 (Z91.49)   Other Personal History of Psychological Trauma

V15.59 (Z91.5)   Personal History of Self-Harm

V62.22 (Z91.82)   Personal History of Military Deployment

V15.89 (Z91.89)   Other Personal Risk Factors

V69.9 (Z72.9)   Problem Related to Lifestyle

V71.01 (Z72.811)   Adult Antisocial Behavior

V71.02 (Z72.810)   Child or Adolescent Antisocial Behavior

Problems Related to Access to Medical and Other Health Care

V63.9 (Z75.3)   Unavailability or Inaccessibility of Health Care Facilities

V63.8 (Z75.4)   Unavailability or Inaccessibility of Other Helping Agencies

Nonadherence to Medical Treatment

V15.81 (Z91.19)   Nonadherence to Medical Treatment

278.00 (E66.9)   Overweight or Obesity

V65.2 (Z76.5)   Malingering

V40.31 (Z91.83)   Wandering Associated With a Mental Disorder

V62.89 (R41.83)   Borderline Intellectual Functioning

NANDA Nursing Diagnoses: Taxonomy II

Domains, Classes, and Diagnoses

Domain 1: Health Promotion

Class 1: Health Awareness

Deficient diversional activity
Sedentary lifestyle

Class 2: Health Management

Deficient community health
Risk-prone health behavior
Ineffective health maintenance
Readiness for enhanced immunization status
Ineffective protection
Ineffective self-health management
Readiness for enhanced self-health management
Ineffective family therapeutic regimen management

Domain 2: Nutrition

Class 1: Ingestion

Insufficient breast milk
Ineffective infant feeding pattern
Imbalanced nutrition: Less than body requirements
Imbalanced nutrition: More than body requirements
Readiness for enhanced nutrition
Risk for imbalanced nutrition: More than body requirements
Impaired swallowing

Class 2: Digestion

Class 3: Absorption

Class 4: Metabolism

Risk for unstable blood glucose level
Neonatal jaundice
Risk for neonatal jaundice
Risk for impaired liver function

Class 5: Hydration

Risk for electrolyte imbalance
Readiness for enhanced fluid balance
Deficient fluid volume
Risk for deficient fluid volume
Excess fluid volume
Risk for imbalanced fluid volume

Domain 3: Elimination and Exchange

Class 1: Urinary Function

Functional urinary incontinence
Overflow urinary incontinence
Reflex urinary incontinence
Stress urinary incontinence
Urge urinary incontinence
Risk for urge urinary incontinence
Impaired urinary elimination
Readiness for enhanced urinary elimination
Urinary retention

Class 2: Gastrointestinal Function

Constipation
Perceived constipation
Risk for constipation
Diarrhea
Dysfunctional gastrointestinal motility
Risk for dysfunctional gastrointestinal motility
Bowel incontinence

Class 3: Integumentary Function

Class 4: Respiratory Function

Impaired gas exchange

Domain 4: Activity/Rest

Class 1: Sleep/Rest

Insomnia
Sleep deprivation
Readiness for enhanced sleep
Disturbed sleep pattern

Class 2: Activity/Exercise

Risk for disuse syndrome
Impaired physical mobility
Impaired bed mobility
Impaired wheelchair mobility
Impaired transfer ability
Impaired walking

Class 3: Energy Balance

Disturbed energy field
Fatigue
Wandering

Class 4: Cardiovascular/Pulmonary Responses

Activity intolerance
Risk for activity intolerance
Ineffective breathing pattern
Decreased cardiac output
Risk for ineffective gastrointestinal perfusion
Risk for ineffective renal perfusion
Impaired spontaneous ventilation
Ineffective peripheral tissue perfusion
Risk for decreased cardiac tissue perfusion
Risk for ineffective cerebral tissue perfusion
Risk for ineffective peripheral tissue perfusion
Dysfunctional ventilatory weaning response

Class 5: Self-Care

Impaired home maintenance
Readiness for enhanced self-care
Bathing self-care deficit
Dressing self-care deficit
Feeding self-care deficit
Toileting self-care deficit
Self-neglect

Domain 5: Perception/Cognition

Class 1: Attention

Unilateral neglect

Class 2: Orientation

Impaired environmental interpretation syndrome

Class 3: Sensation/Perception

Class 4: Cognition

Acute confusion
Chronic confusion
Risk for acute confusion
Ineffective impulse control
Deficient knowledge
Readiness for enhanced knowledge
Impaired memory

Class 5: Communication

Readiness for enhanced communication
Impaired verbal communication

Domain 6: Self-Perception

Class 1: Self-Concept

Hopelessness
Risk for compromised human dignity
Risk for loneliness
Disturbed personal identity
Risk for disturbed personal identity
Readiness for enhanced self-concept

Class 2: Self-Esteem

Chronic low self-esteem
Situational low self-esteem

Risk for chronic low self-esteem
Risk for situational low self-esteem

Class 3: Body Image

Disturbed body image

Domain 7: Role Relationships

Class 1: Caregiving Roles:

Ineffective breastfeeding
Interrupted breastfeeding
Readiness for enhanced breastfeeding
Caregiver role strain
Risk for caregiver role strain
Impaired parenting
Risk for impaired parenting
Readiness for enhanced parenting

Class 2: Family Relationships:

Risk for impaired attachment
Interrupted family processes
Readiness for enhanced family processes
Dysfunctional family processes

Class 3: Role Performance:

Ineffective relationship
Readiness for enhanced relationship
Risk for ineffective relationship
Ineffective role performance
Parental role conflict
Impaired social interaction

Domain 8: Sexuality

Class 1: Sexual Identity

Class 2: Sexual Function

Sexual dysfunction
Ineffective sexuality pattern

Class 3: Reproduction

Ineffective childbearing process
Readiness for enhanced childbearing process
Risk for ineffective childbearing process
Risk for disturbed maternal/fetal dyad

Domain 9: Coping/Stress Tolerance

Class 1: Post-Trauma Responses

Post-trauma syndrome
Risk for post-trauma syndrome
Rape-trauma syndrome
Relocation stress syndrome
Risk for relocation stress syndrome

Class 2: Coping Responses

Ineffective activity planning
Risk for ineffective activity planning
Anxiety
Defensive coping

Ineffective coping
Readiness for enhanced coping
Ineffective community coping
Readiness for enhanced community coping
Compromised family coping
Disabled family coping
Readiness for enhanced family coping
Death anxiety
Ineffective denial
Adult failure to thrive
Fear
Grieving
Complicated grieving
Risk for complicated grieving
Readiness for enhanced power
Powerlessness
Risk for powerlessness
Impaired individual resilience
Readiness for enhanced resilience
Risk for compromised resilience
Chronic sorrow
Stress overload

Class 3: Neurobehavioral Stress

Autonomic dysreflexia
Risk for autonomic dysreflexia
Disorganized infant behavior
Risk for disorganized infant behavior
Readiness for enhanced organized infant behavior
Decreased intracranial adaptive capacity

Domain 10: Life Principles

Class 1: Values

Readiness for enhanced hope

Class 2: Beliefs

Readiness for enhanced spiritual well-being

Class 3: Value/Belief/Action Congruence

Readiness for enhanced decision making
Decisional conflict
Moral distress
Noncompliance
Impaired religiosity
Readiness for enhanced religiosity
Risk for impaired religiosity
Spiritual distress
Risk for spiritual distress

Domain 11: Safety/Protection

Class 1: Infection

Risk for infection

Class 2: Physical Injury

Ineffective airway clearance
Risk for aspiration

Risk for bleeding
Impaired dentition
Risk for dry eye
Risk for falls
Risk for injury
Impaired oral mucous membrane
Risk for perioperative positioning injury
Risk for peripheral neurovascular dysfunction
Risk for shock
Impaired skin integrity
Risk for impaired skin integrity
Risk for sudden infant death syndrome
Risk for suffocation
Delayed surgical recovery
Risk for thermal injury
Impaired tissue integrity
Risk for trauma
Risk for vascular trauma

Class 3: Violence

Risk for other-directed violence
Risk for self-directed violence
Self-mutilation
Risk for self-mutilation
Risk for suicide

Class 4: Environmental Hazards

Contamination
Risk for contamination
Risk for poisoning

Class 5: Defensive Processes

Risk for adverse reaction to iodinated contrast media
Latex allergy response
Risk for latex allergy response
Risk for allergy response

Class 6: Thermoregulation

Risk for imbalanced body temperature
Ineffective thermoregulation
Hypothermia
Hyperthermia

Domain 12: Comfort

Class 1: Physical Comfort

Acute pain
Chronic pain
Nausea
Readiness for enhanced comfort
Impaired comfort

Class 2: Environmental Comfort

Readiness for enhanced comfort
Impaired comfort

Class 3: Social Comfort

Social isolation
Impaired comfort
Readiness for enhanced comfort

Domain 13: Growth/Development

Class 1: Growth

Risk for disproportionate growth

Class 2: Development

Delayed growth and development
Risk for delayed development

SOURCE: *NANDA International. (2012). Nursing Diagnoses: Definitions & Classification 2012-2014.* Hoboken, NJ: Wiley-Blackwell. With permission.

Appendix F

Assigning Nursing Diagnoses to Client Behaviors

Following is a list of client behaviors and the NANDA nursing diagnoses that correspond to the behaviors and that may be used in planning care for the client exhibiting the specific behavioral symptoms.

BEHAVIORS	NANDA NURSING DIAGNOSES
Aggression; hostility	Risk for injury; Risk for other-directed violence
Anorexia or refusal to eat	Imbalanced nutrition: Less than body requirements
Anxious behavior	Anxiety (Specify level)
Confusion; memory loss	Confusion, acute/chronic; Impaired memory; Disturbed thought processes*
Delusions	Disturbed thought processes*
Denial of problems	Ineffective denial
Depressed mood or anger turned inward	Complicated grieving
Detoxification; withdrawal from substances	Risk for injury
Difficulty accepting new diagnosis or recent change in health status	Risk-prone health behavior
Difficulty making important life decision	Decisional conflict
Difficulty sleeping	Insomnia; Disturbed sleep pattern
Difficulty with interpersonal relationships	Impaired social interaction; Ineffective relationship
Disruption in capability to perform usual responsibilities	Ineffective role performance
Dissociative behaviors (depersonalization; derealization)	Disturbed sensory perception (kinesthetic)*
Expresses feelings of disgust about body or body part	Disturbed body image
Expresses anger at God	Spiritual distress
Expresses lack of control over personal situation	Powerlessness
Fails to follow prescribed therapy	Ineffective self-health management; Noncompliance
Flashbacks, nightmares, obsession with traumatic experience	Post-trauma syndrome
Hallucinations	Disturbed sensory perception (auditory; visual)*
Highly critical of self or others	Low self-esteem (chronic; situational)
HIV positive; altered immunity	Ineffective protection
Inability to meet basic needs	Self-care deficit (feeding; bathing; dressing; toileting)
Loose associations or flight of ideas	Impaired verbal communication
Loss of a valued entity, recently experienced	Risk for complicated grieving

Continued

BEHAVIORS	NANDA NURSING DIAGNOSES
Manic hyperactivity	Risk for injury
Manipulative behavior	Ineffective coping
Multiple personalities; gender dysphoria	Disturbed personal identity
Orgasm, problems with; lack of sexual desire; erectile dysfunction	Sexual dysfunction
Overeating, compulsive	Risk for imbalanced nutrition: More than body requirements
Phobias	Fear
Physical symptoms as coping behavior	Ineffective coping
Potential or anticipated loss of significant entity	Grieving
Projection of blame; rationalization of failures, denial of personal responsibility	Defensive coping
Ritualistic behaviors	Anxiety (severe); Ineffective coping
Seductive remarks; inappropriate sexual behaviors	Impaired social interaction
Self-inflicted injuries (non-life-threatening)	Self-mutilation; Risk for self-mutilation
Sexual behaviors (difficulty, limitations, or changes in; reported dissatisfaction)	Ineffective sexuality pattern
Stress from caring for chronically ill person	Caregiver role strain
Stress from locating to new environment	Relocation stress syndrome
Substance use as a coping behavior	Ineffective coping
Substance use (denies use is a problem)	Ineffective denial
Suicidal gestures/threats; suicidal ideation	Risk for suicide; Risk for self-directed violence
Suspiciousness	Ineffective coping; Disturbed thought processes*
Vomiting, excessive, self-induced	Risk for deficient fluid volume
Withdrawn behavior	Social isolation

*These diagnoses have been retired from the NANDA-I list of approved nursing diagnoses.

Glossary

A

abandonment. A unilateral severance of the professional relationship between a health-care provider and a client without reasonable notice at a time when there is still a need for continuing health care.

abreaction. "Remembering with feeling;" bringing into conscious awareness painful events that have been repressed, and reexperiencing the emotions that were associated with the events.

abuse. To use wrongfully or in a harmful way. Improper treatment or conduct that may result in injury.

acquired immunodeficiency syndrome (AIDS). A condition in which the immune system becomes deficient in its efforts to prevent opportunistic infections, malignancies, and neurological disease. It is caused by the human immunodeficiency virus (HIV), which is passed from one individual to another through body fluids.

acupoints. In Chinese medicine, acupoints represent areas along the body that link pathways of healing energy.

acupressure. A technique in which the fingers, thumbs, palms, or elbows are used to apply pressure to certain points along the body. This pressure is thought to dissolve any obstructions in the flow of healing energy and to restore the body to a healthier functioning.

acupuncture. A technique in which hair-thin, sterile, disposable, stainless-steel needles are inserted into points along the body to dissolve obstructions in the flow of healing energy and restore the body to a healthier functioning.

adaptation. Restoration of the body to homeostasis following a physiological and/or psychological response to stress.

addiction. A compulsive or chronic requirement. The need is so strong as to generate distress (either physical or psychological) if left unfulfilled.

adjustment. The process of modifying one's behavior in changed circumstances or an altered environment in order to fulfill psychological, physiological, and social needs.

adjustment disorder. A maladaptive reaction to an identifiable psychosocial stressor that occurs within 3 months after onset of the stressor. The individual shows impairment in social and occupational functioning, or exhibits symptoms that are in excess of a normal and expectable reaction to the stressor.

advance directive. A legal document that a competent individual may sign to convey wishes regarding future health-care decisions intended for a time when the individual is no longer capable of informed consent. It may include one or both of the following: (1) a living will, in which the individual identifies the type of care that he or she does or does not wish to have performed, and (2) a durable power of attorney for health care, in which the individual names another person who is given the right to make health-care decisions for the individual who is incapable of doing so.

advocacy. The act of pleading for, supporting, or representing a cause or individual. Advocacy in nursing applies to any act in which the nurse is serving in the best interests of the patient, from simple procedures such as hand washing to protect the patient from infection to complex ethically and morally charged issues in which certain clients are unable to advocate for themselves. Nurses also advocate for their patients indirectly by serving in organizations that support and serve to improve health care for all individuals, and by participating in policy-making legislation that affects health care of the public.

affect. The behavioral expression of emotion; may be appropriate (congruent with the situation); inappropriate (incongruent with the situation); constricted or blunted (diminished range and intensity); or flat (absence of emotional expression).

affective domain. A category of learning that includes attitudes, feelings, and values.

aggression. Harsh physical or verbal actions intended (either consciously or unconsciously) to harm or injure another.

aggressiveness. Behavior that defends an individual's own basic rights by violating the basic rights of others (as contrasted with **assertiveness**).

agoraphobia. The fear of being in places or situations from which escape might be difficult (or embarrassing) or in which help might not be available in the event of a panic attack.

agranulocytosis. Extremely low levels of white blood cells. Symptoms include sore throat, fever, and malaise. This may be a side effect of long-term therapy with some antipsychotic medications.

AIDS. See **acquired immunodeficiency syndrome (AIDS).**

akathisia. Restlessness; an urgent need for movement. A type of extrapyramidal side effect associated with some antipsychotic medications.

akinesia. Muscular weakness; or a loss or partial loss of muscle movement; a type of extrapyramidal side effect associated with some antipsychotic medications.

Alcoholics Anonymous (AA). A major self-help organization for the treatment of alcoholism. It is based on a 12-step program to help members attain and maintain sobriety. Once individuals have achieved sobriety, they in turn are expected to help other alcoholic persons.

allopathic medicine. Traditional medicine. The type traditionally, and currently, practiced in the United States and taught in U.S. medical schools.

alternative medicine. Practices that differ from usual traditional (allopathic) medicine.

altruism. One curative factor of group therapy (identified by Yalom) in which individuals gain self-esteem through mutual sharing and concern. Providing assistance and support to others creates a positive self-image and promotes self-growth.

altruistic suicide. Suicide based on behavior of a group to which an individual is excessively integrated.

amenorrhea. Cessation of the menses; may be a side effect of some antipsychotic medications.

amnesia. An inability to recall important personal information that is too extensive to be explained by ordinary forgetfulness.

amnesia, generalized. The inability to recall anything that has happened during the individual's entire lifetime.

amnesia, localized. The inability to recall all incidents associated with a traumatic event for a specific time period following the event.

amnesia, selective. The inability to recall only certain incidents associated with a traumatic event for a specific time period following the event.

amphetamine. A racemic sympathomimetic amine that acts as a central nervous system stimulant. It (and its derivatives, such as methamphetamine and dextroamphetamine) is a commonly abused substance, but has therapeutic use in the treatment of narcolepsy and attention-deficit/hyperactivity disorder.

andropause. A term used to identify the male climacteric. Also called *male menopause*. A syndrome of symptoms related to the decline of testosterone levels in men. Some symptoms include depression, weight gain, insomnia, hot flashes, decreased libido, mood swings, decreased strength, and erectile dysfunction.

anger. An emotional response to one's perception of a situation. Anger has both positive and negative functions.

anger management. The use of various techniques and strategies to control responses to anger-provoking situations. The goal of anger management is to reduce both the emotional feelings and the physiological arousal that anger engenders.

anhedonia. The inability to experience or even imagine any pleasant emotion.

anomic suicide. Suicide that occurs in response to changes that occur in an individual's life that disrupt cohesiveness from a group and cause that person to feel without support from the formerly cohesive group.

anorexia. Loss of appetite.

anorexiants. Drugs that suppress appetite.

anorgasmia. Inability to achieve orgasm.

anosmia. Inability to smell.

anticipatory grief. A subjective state of emotional, physical, and social responses to an anticipated loss of a valued entity. The grief response is repeated once the loss actually occurs, but it may not be as intense as it might have been if anticipatory grieving has not occurred.

antisocial personality disorder. A pattern of socially irresponsible, exploitative, and guiltless behavior, evident in the tendency to fail to conform to the law, develop stable relationships, or sustain consistent employment; exploitation and manipulation of others for personal gain is common.

anxiety. Vague diffuse apprehension that is associated with feelings of uncertainty and helplessness.

aphasia. Inability to communicate through speech, writing, or signs, caused by dysfunction of brain centers.

aphonia. Inability to speak.

apraxia. Inability to carry out motor activities despite intact motor function.

arbitrary inference. A type of thinking error in which the individual automatically comes to a conclusion about an incident without the facts to support it, or even sometimes despite contradictory evidence to support it.

ascites. Excessive accumulation of serous fluid in the abdominal cavity, occurring in response to portal hypertension caused by cirrhosis of the liver.

assault. An act that results in a person's genuine fear and apprehension that he or she will be touched without consent. Nurses may be guilty of assault for threatening to place an individual in restraints against his or her will.

assertive behavior. Behavior that enables individuals to act in their own best interests, to stand up for themselves without undue anxiety, to express their honest feelings comfortably, or to exercise their own rights without denying those of others.

assessment. A systematic, dynamic process by which the registered nurse, through interaction with the patient, family, groups, communities, populations, and health-care providers, collects and analyzes data. Assessment may include the following dimensions: physical, functional, psychosocial, emotional, cognitive, sexual, cultural, age-related, environmental, spiritual/transpersonal, and economic (ANA Standards of Practice, 2010).

associative looseness. Sometimes called loose associations, a thinking process characterized by speech in which ideas shift from one unrelated subject to another. The individual is unaware that the topics are unconnected.

ataxia. Muscular incoordination.

attachment theory. The hypothesis that individuals who maintain close relationships with others into old age are more likely to remain independent and less likely to be institutionalized than those who do not.

attention-deficit/hyperactivity disorder. A disorder that is characterized by a persistent pattern of inattention and/or hyperactivity and impulsivity, or both. Motor activity is excessive, and the ability to concentrate is impaired.

attitude. A frame of reference around which an individual organizes knowledge about his or her world. It includes an emotional element and can have a positive or negative connotation.

autism. A focus inward on a fantasy world, while distorting or excluding the external environment; common in schizophrenia.

autism spectrum disorder. A disorder that is characterized by impairment in social interaction skills and interpersonal communication, and a restricted repertoire of activities and interests.

autocratic. A leadership style in which the leader makes all decisions for the group. Productivity is very high with this type of leadership, but morale is often low because of the lack of member input and creativity.

autoimmunity. A condition in which the body produces a disordered immunological response against itself. In this situation, the body fails to differentiate between what is normal and what is a foreign substance. When this occurs, the body produces antibodies against normal parts of the body to such an extent as to cause tissue injury.

automatic thoughts. Thoughts that occur rapidly in response to a situation, and without rational analysis. They are often negative and based on erroneous logic.

autonomy. Independence; self-governance. An ethical principle that emphasizes the status of persons as autonomous moral agents whose right to determine their destinies should always be respected.

aversive stimulus. A stimulus that follows a behavioral response and decreases the probability that the behavior will recur; also called punishment.

axon. The cellular process of a neuron that carries impulses away from the cell body.

B

battering. A pattern of repeated physical assault, usually of a woman by her spouse or intimate partner. Men are also battered, although this occurs much less frequently.

battery. The unconsented touching of another person. Nurses may be charged with battery should they participate in the treatment of a client without his or her consent and outside of an emergency situation.

behavior modification. A treatment modality aimed at changing undesirable behaviors, using a system of reinforcement to bring about the modifications desired.

behavior therapy. A form of psychotherapy, the goal of which is to modify maladaptive behavior patterns by reinforcing more adaptive behaviors.

behavioral objectives. Statements that indicate to an individual what is expected of him or her. Behavioral objectives are a way of measuring learning outcomes, and are based on the affective, cognitive, and psychomotor domains of learning.

belief. A belief is an idea that one holds to be true. It can be rational, irrational, taken on faith, or a stereotypical idea.

beneficence. An ethical principle that refers to one's duty to benefit or promote the good of others.

bereavement overload. An accumulation of grief that occurs when an individual experiences many losses over a short period of time and is unable to resolve one before another is experienced. This phenomenon is common among the elderly.

binge and purge. A syndrome associated with eating disorders, especially bulimia nervosa, in which an individual consumes thousands of calories of food at one sitting, and then purges through the use of laxatives or self-induced vomiting.

bioethics. The term used with ethical principles that refer to concepts within the scope of medicine, nursing, and allied health.

biofeedback. The use of instrumentation to become aware of processes in the body that usually go unnoticed and to bring them under voluntary control (e.g., the blood pressure or pulse); used as a method of stress reduction.

bipolar disorder. Characterized by mood swings from profound depression to extreme euphoria (mania), with intervening periods of normalcy. Psychotic symptoms may or may not be present.

body image. One's perception of his or her own body. It may also be how one believes others perceive his or her body. (See also **physical self**.)

borderline personality disorder. A disorder characterized by a pattern of intense and chaotic relationships, with affective instability, fluctuating and extreme attitudes regarding other people, impulsivity, direct and indirect self-destructive behavior, and lack of a clear or certain sense of identity, life plan, or values.

boundaries. The level of participation and interaction between individuals and between subsystems. Boundaries denote physical and psychological space individuals identify as their own. They are sometimes referred to as limits. Boundaries are appropriate when they permit appropriate contact with others while preventing excessive interference. Boundaries may be clearly defined (healthy) or rigid or diffuse (unhealthy).

bulimia. Excessive, insatiable appetite.

C

cachexia. A state of ill health, malnutrition, and wasting; extreme emaciation.

cannabis. The dried flowering tops of the hemp plant. It produces euphoric effects when ingested or smoked and is commonly used in the form of marijuana or hashish.

carcinogen. Any substance or agent that produces or increases the risk of developing cancer in humans or lower animals.

case management. A health-care delivery process, the goals of which are to provide quality health care, decrease fragmentation, enhance the client's quality of life, and contain costs. A case manager coordinates the client's care from admission to discharge and sometimes following discharge. Critical pathways of care are the tools used for the provision of care in a case management system.

case manager. The individual responsible for negotiating with multiple health-care providers to obtain a variety of services for a client.

catastrophic thinking. Always thinking that the worst will occur without considering the possibility of more likely, positive outcomes.

catatonia. A type of psychological disturbance that is typified by stupor or excitement. Stupor is characterized by extreme psychomotor retardation, mutism, negativism, and posturing; excitement by psychomotor agitation, in which the movements are frenzied and purposeless. Catatonic symptoms may be associated with other mental or physical disorders.

catharsis. One curative factor of group therapy (identified by Yalom), in which members in a group can express both positive and negative feelings in a nonthreatening atmosphere.

cell body. The part of the neuron that contains the nucleus and is essential for the continued life of the neuron.

Centers for Medicare and Medicaid Services (CMS). The division of the U.S. Department of Health and Human Services responsible for Medicare funding.

child sexual abuse. Any sexual act, such as indecent exposure or improper touching to penetration (sexual intercourse), that is carried out with a child.

chiropractic medicine. A system of alternative medicine based on the premise that the relationship between structure and function in the human body is a significant health factor and that such relationships between the spinal column and the nervous system are important because the normal transmission and expression of nerve energy are essential to the restoration and maintenance of health.

Christian ethics. The ethical philosophy that states one should treat others as moral equals, and recognize the equality of other persons by permitting them to act as we do when they occupy a position similar to ours; sometimes referred to as "the ethic of the golden rule."

circadian rhythm. A 24-hour biological rhythm controlled by a "pacemaker" in the brain that sends messages to other systems in the body. Circadian rhythm influences various regulatory functions, including the sleep-wake cycle, body temperature regulation, patterns of activity such as eating and drinking, and hormonal and neurotransmitter secretion.

circumstantiality. In speaking, the delay of an individual to reach the point of a communication, owing to unnecessary and tedious details.

civil law. Law that protects the private and property rights of individuals and businesses.

clang association. A pattern of speech in which the choice of words is governed by sounds. Clang associations often take the form of rhyming.

classical conditioning. A type of learning that occurs when an unconditioned stimulus (UCS) that produces an unconditioned response (UCR) is paired with a conditioned stimulus (CS), until the CS alone produces the same response, which is then called a conditioned response (CR). Pavlov's example: food (i.e., UCS) causes salivation (i.e., UCR); ringing bell (i.e., CS) with food (i.e., UCS) causes salivation (i.e., UCR), ringing bell alone (i.e., CS) causes salivation (i.e., CR).

codependency. An exaggerated dependent pattern of learned behaviors, beliefs, and feelings that make life painful. It is a dependence on people and things outside the self, along with neglect of the self to the point of having little self-identity.

cognition. Mental operations that relate to logic, awareness, intellect, memory, language, and reasoning powers.

cognitive. Relating to the mental processes of thinking and reasoning.

cognitive development. A series of stages described by Piaget through which individuals progress, demonstrating at each successive stage a higher level of logical organization than at each previous stage.

cognitive domain. A category of learning that involves knowledge and thought processes within the individual's intellectual ability. The individual must be able to synthesize information at an intellectual level before the actual behaviors are performed.

cognitive maturity. The capability to perform all mental operations needed for adulthood.

cognitive therapy. A type of therapy in which the individual is taught to control thought distortions that are considered to be a factor in the development and maintenance of emotional disorders.

colposcope. An instrument that contains a magnifying lens and to which a 35-mm camera can be attached. A colposcope is used to examine for tears and abrasions inside the vaginal area of a sexual assault victim.

common law. Laws that are derived from decisions made in previous cases.

communication. An interactive process of transmitting information between two or more entities.

community. A group of people living close to and depending to some extent on each other.

compensation. An ego defense mechanism in which an individual covers up a real or perceived weakness by emphasizing a trait one considers more desirable.

complementary medicine. Practices that differ from usual traditional (allopathic) medicine, but may in fact supplement it in a positive way.

compounded rape reaction. Symptoms that are in addition to the typical rape response of physical complaints, rage, humiliation, fear, and sleep disturbances. They include depression and suicide, substance abuse, and even psychotic behaviors.

compulsions. Unwanted repetitive behavior patterns or mental acts (e.g., praying, counting, repeating words silently) that are intended to reduce anxiety, not to provide pleasure or gratification (APA, 2013). They may be performed in response to an obsession or in a stereotyped fashion.

concept mapping. A diagrammatic teaching and learning strategy that allows students and faculty to visualize interrelationships between medical diagnoses, nursing diagnoses, assessment data, and treatments. A diagram of client problems and interventions.

concrete thinking. Thought processes that are focused on specifics rather than on generalities and immediate issues rather than eventual outcomes. Individuals who are experiencing concrete thinking are unable to comprehend abstract terminology.

conditioned response. In classical conditioning, a response that is a *learned* response (not reflexive) following repeated exposure to a target stimulus.

conditioned stimulus. In classical conditioning, an unrelated stimulus that is presented to a subject with a target stimulus, and that, with repeated exposure, comes to elicit the same response as the original target stimulus.

confabulation. Creating imaginary events to fill in memory gaps.

confidentiality. The right of an individual to the assurance that his or her case will not be discussed outside the boundaries of the health-care team.

contextual stimuli. Conditions present in the environment that support a focal stimulus and influence a threat to self-esteem.

contingency contracting. A written contract between individuals used to modify behavior. Benefits and consequences for fulfilling the terms of the contract are delineated.

controlled response pattern. The response to rape in which feelings are masked or hidden, and a calm, composed, or subdued affect is seen.

counselor. One who listens as the client reviews feelings related to difficulties he or she is experiencing in any aspect of life; one of the nursing roles identified by H. Peplau.

countertransference. In psychoanalytic theory, countertransference refers to the counselor's behavioral and emotional response to the client. These responses may be related to unresolved feelings toward significant others from the counselor's past, or they may be generated in response to the client's behavior toward the counselor.

covert sensitization. An aversion technique used to modify behavior that relies on the individual's imagination to produce unpleasant symptoms. When the individual is about to succumb to undesirable behavior, he or she visualizes something that is offensive or even nauseating in an effort to block the behavior.

criminal law. Law that provides protection from conduct deemed injurious to the public welfare. It provides for punishment of those found to have engaged in such conduct.

crisis. Psychological disequilibrium in a person who confronts a hazardous circumstance that constitutes an important problem which for the time he or she can neither escape nor solve with usual problem-solving resources.

crisis intervention. An emergency type of assistance in which the intervener becomes a part of the individual's life situation. The focus is to provide guidance and support to help mobilize the resources needed to resolve the crisis and restore or generate an improvement in previous level of functioning. Usually lasts no longer than 6 to 8 weeks.

critical pathways of care. An abbreviated plan of care that provides outcome-based guidelines for goal achievement within a designated length of time.

culture. A particular society's entire way of living, encompassing shared patterns of belief, feeling, and knowledge that guide people's conduct and are passed down from generation to generation.

curandera. A female folk healer in the Latino culture.

curandero. A male folk healer in the Latino culture.

cycle of battering. Three phases of predictable behaviors that are repeated over time in a relationship between a batterer and a victim: tension-building phase; the acute battering incident; and the calm, loving, respite (honeymoon) phase.

cyclothymic disorder. A chronic mood disturbance involving numerous episodes of hypomania and depressed mood, of insufficient severity or duration to meet the criteria for bipolar disorder.

D

date rape. A situation in which the rapist is known to the victim. This may occur during dating or with acquaintances or schoolmates. (Also called *acquaintance rape.*)

decatastrophizing. In cognitive therapy, with this technique the therapist assists the client to examine the validity of a negative automatic thought. Even if some validity exists, the client is then encouraged to review ways to cope adaptively, moving beyond the current crisis situation.

defamation of character. An individual may be liable for defamation of character by sharing with others information about a person that is detrimental to that person's reputation.

deinstitutionalization. The removal of mentally ill individuals from institutions and the subsequent plan to provide care for these individuals in the community setting.

delayed grief. The absence of evidence of grief when it ordinarily would be expected.

delayed ejaculation. Delayed or absent ejaculation, even though the man has a firm erection and has had more than adequate stimulation.

delirious mania. A grave form of mania characterized by severe clouding of consciousness and representing an intensification of the symptoms associated with mania. The symptoms of delirious mania have become relatively rare since the availability of antipsychotic medications.

delirium. A state of mental confusion and excitement characterized by disorientation for time and place, often with hallucinations, incoherent speech, and a continual state of aimless physical activity.

delusions. False personal beliefs, not consistent with a person's intelligence or cultural background. The individual continues to have the belief in spite of obvious proof that it is false and/or irrational.

dementia. See **neurocognitive disorder.**

dendrites. The cellular processes of a neuron that carry impulses toward the cell body.

denial. Refusal to acknowledge the existence of a real situation and/or the feelings associated with it.

density. The number of people in a given environmental space, influencing interpersonal interaction.

depersonalization. An alteration in the perception or experience of the self so that the feeling of one's own reality is temporarily lost.

depression. An alteration in mood that is expressed by feelings of sadness, despair, and pessimism. There is a loss of interest in usual activities, and somatic symptoms may be evident. Changes in appetite and sleep patterns are common.

derealization. An alteration in the perception or experience of the external world so that it seems strange or unreal.

detoxification. The process of withdrawal from a substance to which one has become addicted.

diagnosis related groups (DRGs). A system used to determine prospective payment rates for reimbursement of hospital care based on the client's diagnosis.

Diagnostic and Statistical Manual of Mental Disorders, Fifth Edition (DSM-5). Standard nomenclature of emotional illness published by the American Psychiatric Association (APA) and used by all health-care practitioners. It classifies mental illness and presents guidelines and diagnostic criteria for various mental disorders.

dichotomous thinking. In this type of thinking, situations are viewed in all-or-nothing, black-or-white, good-or-bad terms.

directed association. A technique used to help clients bring into consciousness events that have been repressed. Specific thoughts are guided and directed by the psychoanalyst.

disaster. A natural or man-made occurrence that overwhelms the resources of an individual or community, and increases the need for emergency evacuation and medical services.

discriminative stimulus. A stimulus that precedes a behavioral response and predicts that a particular reinforcement will occur. Individuals learn to discriminate between various stimuli that will produce the responses they desire.

disengagement. In family theory, disengagement refers to extreme separateness among family members. It is promoted by rigid boundaries or lack of communication among family members.

disengagement theory. The hypothesis that there is a process of mutual withdrawal of aging persons and society from each other that is correlated with successful aging. This theory has been challenged by many investigators.

displacement. Feelings are transferred from one target to another that is considered less threatening or neutral.

dissociation. The splitting off of clusters of mental contents from conscious awareness, a mechanism central to hysterical conversion and dissociative disorder.

distraction. In cognitive therapy, when dysfunctional cognitions have been recognized, activities are identified that can be used to distract the client and divert him or her from the intrusive thoughts or depressive ruminations that are contributing to the client's maladaptive responses.

disulfiram. A drug that is administered to individuals who abuse alcohol as a deterrent to drinking. Ingestion of alcohol while disulfiram is in the body results in a syndrome of symptoms that can produce a great deal of discomfort, and can even result in death if the blood alcohol level is high.

domains of learning. Categories in which individuals learn or gain knowledge and demonstrate behavior. There are three domains of learning: affective, cognitive, and psychomotor.

double-bind communication. An emotionally distressing situation in which an individual receives conflicting messages in the communication process, whereby one message is negated by another. This creates a condition in which a successful response to one message results in a failed response to the other.

dual diagnosis. A client has a dual diagnosis when it is determined that he or she has a coexisting substance disorder and mental illness. Treatment is designed to target both problems.

dysthymia. A depressive neurosis. The symptoms are similar to, if somewhat milder than, those ascribed to major depression. There is no loss of contact with reality.

dystonia. Involuntary muscular movements (spasms) of the face, arms, legs, and neck; may occur as an extrapyramidal side effect of some antipsychotic medications.

E

echolalia. The parrot-like repetition, by an individual with loose ego boundaries, of the words spoken by another.

echopraxia. An individual with loose ego boundaries attempting to identify with another person by imitating movements that the other person makes.

ego. One of the three elements of the personality identified by Freud as the rational self or "reality principle." The ego seeks to maintain harmony between the external world, the id, and the superego.

ego defense mechanisms. Strategies employed by the ego for protection in the face of threat to biological or psychological integrity. (See individual defense mechanisms.)

egoistic suicide. The response of an individual who feels separate and apart from the mainstream of society.

electroconvulsive therapy (ECT). A type of somatic treatment in which electric current is applied to the brain through electrodes placed on the temples. A grand mal seizure produces the desired effect. This is used with severely depressed patients refractory to antidepressant medications.

emaciated. The state of being excessively thin or physically wasted.

emotional abuse. A pattern of behavior on the part of the parent or caretaker that results in serious impairment of the child's social, emotional, or intellectual functioning.

emotional neglect. A chronic failure by the parent or caretaker to provide the child with the hope, love, and support necessary for the development of a sound, healthy personality.

empathy. The ability to see beyond outward behavior, and sense accurately another's inner experiencing. With empathy, one can accurately perceive and understand the meaning and relevance in the thoughts and feelings of another.

enmeshment. Exaggerated connectedness among family members. It occurs in response to diffuse boundaries in which there is overinvestment, overinvolvement, and lack of differentiation between individuals or subsystems.

esophageal varices. Veins in the esophagus become distended because of excessive pressure from defective blood flow through a cirrhotic liver.

essential hypertension. Persistent elevation of blood pressure for which there is no apparent cause or associated underlying disease.

ethical dilemma. A situation that arises when on the basis of moral considerations an appeal can be made for taking each of two opposing courses of action.

ethical egoism. An ethical theory espousing that what is "right" and "good" is what is best for the individual making the decision.

ethics. A branch of philosophy dealing with values related to human conduct, to the rightness and wrongness of certain actions, and to the goodness and badness of the motives and ends of such actions.

ethnicity. The concept of people identifying with each other because of a shared heritage.

evaluation. The process of determining the progress toward attainment of expected outcomes, including the effectiveness of care (ANA, 2010).

exhibitionistic disorder. A paraphilic disorder characterized by a recurrent urge to expose one's genitals to a stranger.

expressed response pattern. Pattern of behavior in which the victim of rape expresses feelings of fear, anger, and anxiety through such behavior as crying, sobbing, restlessness, and tenseness; in contrast to the rape victim who withholds feelings in the **controlled response pattern**.

extinction. In behavior therapy, the gradual decrease in frequency or disappearance of a response when the positive reinforcement is withheld.

extrapyramidal symptoms (EPS). A variety of responses that originate outside the pyramidal tracts and in the basal ganglion of the brain. Symptoms may include tremors, chorea, dystonia, akinesia, akathisia, and others. May occur as a side effect of some antipsychotic medications.

F

factitious disorder. Factitious disorders involve conscious, intentional feigning of physical or psychological symptoms. Individuals with factitious disorder pretend to be ill in order to receive emotional care and support commonly associated with the role of "patient."

false imprisonment. The deliberate and unauthorized confinement of a person within fixed limits by the use of threat or force. A nurse may be charged with false imprisonment by placing a patient in restraints against his or her will in a non-emergency situation.

family. Two or more individuals who depend on one another for emotional, physical, and economical support. The members of the family are self-defined (Kaakinen, Hanson, & Denham, 2010).

family structure. A family system in which the structure is founded on a set of invisible principles that influence the interaction among family members. These principles are established over time and become the "laws" that govern the conduct of various family members.

family system. A system in which the parts of the whole may be the marital dyad, parent-child dyad, or sibling groups. Each of these subsystems is further divided into subsystems of individuals.

family therapy. A type of therapy in which the focus is on relationships within the family. The family is viewed as a system in which the members are interdependent, and a change in one creates change in all.

fetishistic disorder. A paraphilic disorder characterized by recurrent sexual urges and sexually arousing fantasies involving the use of nonliving objects.

"fight-or-flight" syndrome. A syndrome of physical symptoms that results from an individual's real or perceived notion that harm or danger is imminent.

flexible boundary. A personal boundary is flexible when, because of unusual circumstances, individuals can alter limits that they have set for themselves. Flexible boundaries are healthy boundaries.

flooding. Sometimes called *implosion therapy*, this technique is used to desensitize individuals to phobic stimuli. The individual is "flooded" with a continuous presentation (usually through mental imagery) of the phobic stimulus until it no longer elicits anxiety.

focal stimulus. A situation of immediate concern that results in a threat to self-esteem.

Focus Charting®. A type of documentation that follows a data, action, and response (DAR) format. The main perspective is a client "focus," which can be a nursing diagnosis, a client's concern, a change in status, or a significant event in the client's therapy. The focus cannot be a medical diagnosis.

folk medicine. A system of health care within various cultures that is provided by a local practitioner, not professionally trained, but who uses techniques specific to that culture in the art of healing.

forensic. Pertaining to the law; legal.

forensic nursing. The application of forensic science combined with the bio-psychological education of the registered nurse, in the scientific investigation, evidence collection and preservation, analysis, prevention and treatment of trauma and/or death related medical-legal issues.

free association. A technique used to help individuals bring to consciousness material that has been repressed. The individual is encouraged to verbalize whatever comes into his or her mind, drifting naturally from one thought to another.

frotteuristic disorder. A paraphilic disorder characterized by the recurrent preoccupation with intense sexual urges or fantasies involving touching or rubbing against a nonconsenting person.

fugue. A sudden unexpected travel away from home or customary work locale with the assumption of a new identity and an inability to recall one's previous identity; usually occurring in response to severe psychosocial stress.

G

gains. The reinforcements an individual receives for somaticizing.

Gamblers Anonymous (GA). An organization of inspirational group therapy, modeled after Alcoholics

Anonymous (AA), for individuals who desire to, but cannot, stop gambling.

gender. The condition of being either male or female.

gender dysphoria. A sense of discomfort associated with an incongruence between biologically assigned gender and subjectively experienced gender.

general adaptation syndrome. The general biological reaction of the body to a stressful situation, as described by Hans Selye. It occurs in three stages: the alarm reaction stage, the stage of resistance, and the stage of exhaustion.

generalized anxiety disorder. A disorder characterized by chronic (at least 6 months), unrealistic, and excessive anxiety and worry.

genetics. Study of the biological transmission of certain characteristics (physical and/or behavioral) from parent to offspring.

genogram. A graphic representation of a family system. It may cover several generations. Emphasis is on family roles and emotional relatedness among members. Genograms facilitate recognition of areas requiring change.

genotype. The total set of genes present in an individual at the time of conception, and coded in the DNA.

genuineness. The ability to be open, honest, and "real" in interactions with others; the awareness of what one is experiencing internally and the ability to project the quality of this inner experiencing in a relationship.

geriatrics. The branch of clinical medicine specializing in the care of the elderly and concerned with the problems of aging.

gerontology. The study of normal aging.

geropsychiatry. The branch of clinical medicine specializing in psychopathology of the elderly.

gonorrhea. A sexually transmitted disease caused by the bacterium *Neisseria gonorrhoeae* and resulting in inflammation of the genital mucosa. Treatment is through the use of a combination of antibiotics. Serious complications occur if the disease is left untreated.

"granny-bashing." Media-generated term for abuse of the elderly.

"granny-dumping." Media-generated term for abandoning elderly individuals at emergency departments, nursing homes, or other facilities—literally leaving them in the hands of others when the strain of caregiving becomes intolerable.

grief. A subjective state of emotional, physical, and social responses to the real or perceived loss of a valued entity. Change and failure can also be perceived as losses. The grief response consists of a set of relatively predictable behaviors that describe the subjective state that accompanies mourning.

grief, exaggerated. A reaction in which all of the symptoms associated with normal grieving are exaggerated out of proportion. Pathological depression is a type of exaggerated grief.

grief, inhibited. The absence of evidence of grief when it ordinarily would be expected.

group. A collection of individuals whose association is founded on shared commonalities of interest, values, norms, or purpose. Membership in a group is generally by chance (born into the group), by choice (voluntary affiliation), or by circumstance (the result of life-cycle events over which an individual may or may not have control).

group therapy. A therapy group, founded in a specific theoretical framework, led by a person with an advanced degree in psychology, social work, nursing, or medicine. The goal is to encourage improvement in interpersonal functioning.

gynecomastia. Enlargement of the breasts in men; may be a side effect of some antipsychotic medications.

H

hallucinations. False sensory perceptions not associated with real external stimuli. Hallucinations may involve any of the five senses.

hepatic encephalopathy. A brain disorder resulting from the inability of the cirrhotic liver to convert ammonia to urea for excretion. The continued rise in serum ammonia results in progressively impaired mental functioning, apathy, euphoria or depression, sleep disturbances, increasing confusion, and progression to coma and eventual death.

HIV-associated neurocognitive disorder. A neuropathological syndrome, possibly caused by chronic HIV encephalitis and myelitis and manifested by cognitive, behavioral, and motor symptoms that become more severe with progression of the disease.

home care. A wide range of health and social services that are delivered at home to recovering, disabled, chronically or terminally ill persons in need of medical, nursing, social, or therapeutic treatment and/or assistance with essential activities of daily living.

homocysteine. An amino acid produced by the catabolism of methionine. Elevated levels may be linked to increased risk of cardiovascular disease.

homosexuality. A sexual preference for persons of the same gender.

hospice. A program that provides palliative and supportive care to meet the special needs arising out of the physical, psychosocial, spiritual, social, and economic stresses that are experienced during the final stages of illness and during bereavement.

humors. The four body fluids described by Hippocrates: blood, black bile, yellow bile, and phlegm.

Hippocrates associated insanity and mental illness with these four fluids.

hypersomnia. Excessive sleepiness or seeking excessive amounts of sleep.

hyperactivity. Excessive psychomotor activity that may be purposeful or aimless, accompanied by physical movements and verbal utterances that are usually more rapid than normal. Inattention and distractibility are common with hyperactive behavior.

hypertensive crisis. A potentially life-threatening syndrome that results when an individual taking monoamine oxidase (MAO) inhibitors eats a product high in tyramine. Symptoms include severe occipital headache, palpitations, nausea and vomiting, nuchal rigidity, fever, sweating, marked increase in blood pressure, chest pain, and coma. Foods with tyramine include aged cheeses or other aged, overripe, and fermented foods; broad beans; pickled herring; beef or chicken liver; preserved meats; beer and wine; yeast products; chocolate; caffeinated drinks; canned figs; sour cream; yogurt; soy sauce; and some over-the-counter cold medications and diet pills.

hypnosis. A treatment for disorders brought on by repressed anxiety. The individual is directed into a state of subconsciousness and assisted, through suggestions, to recall certain events that he or she cannot recall while conscious.

hypomania. A mild form of mania. Symptoms are excessive hyperactivity, but not severe enough to cause marked impairment in social or occupational functioning or to require hospitalization.

hysteria. A polysymptomatic disorder characterized by recurrent, multiple somatic complaints often described dramatically.

I

id. One of the three components of the personality identified by Freud as the "pleasure principle." The id is the locus of instinctual drives; is present at birth; and compels the infant to satisfy needs and seek immediate gratification.

identification. An attempt to increase self-worth by acquiring certain attributes and characteristics of an individual one admires.

illusion. A misperception of a real external stimulus.

implosion therapy. See **flooding**.

impulsive. The urge or inclination to act without consideration to the possible consequences of one's behavior.

incest. Sexual exploitation of a child under 18 years of age by a relative or non-relative who holds a position of trust in the family.

informed consent. Permission granted to a physician by a client to perform a therapeutic procedure, prior to which information about the procedure has been presented to the client with adequate time given for consideration about the pros and cons.

insomnia. Difficulty initiating or maintaining sleep.

insulin coma therapy. The induction of a hypoglycemic coma aimed at alleviating psychotic symptoms; a dangerous procedure, questionably effective, no longer used in psychiatry.

integration. The process used with individuals with dissociative identity disorder in an effort to bring all the personalities together into one; usually achieved through hypnosis.

intellectualization. An attempt to avoid expressing actual emotions associated with a stressful situation by using the intellectual processes of logic, reasoning, and analysis.

interdisciplinary care. A concept of providing care for a client in which members of various disciplines work together with common goals and shared responsibilities for meeting those goals.

intimate distance. The closest distance that individuals will allow between themselves and others. In the United States, this distance is 0 to 18 inches.

intoxication. A physical and mental state of exhilaration and emotional frenzy or lethargy and stupor.

introjection. The beliefs and values of another individual are internalized and symbolically become a part of the self, to the extent that the feeling of separateness or distinctness is lost.

isolation. The separation of a thought or a memory from the feeling, tone, or emotions associated with it (sometimes called *emotional isolation*).

J

justice. An ethical principle reflecting that all individuals should be treated equally and fairly.

K

Kantianism. The ethical principle espousing that decisions should be made and actions taken out of a sense of duty.

kleptomania. A recurrent failure to resist impulses to steal objects not needed for personal use or monetary value.

Korsakoff's psychosis. A syndrome of confusion, loss of recent memory, and confabulation in alcoholics, caused by a deficiency of thiamine. It often occurs together with Wernicke's encephalopathy and may be termed *Wernicke-Korsakoff syndrome*.

L

laissez-faire. A leadership type in which the leader lets group members do as they please. There is no direction from the leader. Member productivity and morale may be low, owing to frustration from lack of direction.

lesbian. A female homosexual.

libel. An action with which an individual may be charged for sharing with another individual, in writing, information that is detrimental to someone's reputation.

libido. Freud's term for the psychic energy used to fulfill basic physiological needs or instinctual drives such as hunger, thirst, and sexuality.

limbic system. The part of the brain that is sometimes called the "emotional brain." It is associated with feelings of fear and anxiety; anger and aggression; love, joy, and hope; and with sexuality and social behavior.

long-term memory. Memory for remote events, or those that occurred many years ago. The type of memory that is preserved in the elderly individual.

loss. The experience of separation from something of personal importance.

luto. In the Mexican-American culture, the period of mourning following the death of a loved one which is symbolized by wearing black, black and white, or dark clothing and by subdued behavior.

M

magical thinking. A primitive form of thinking in which an individual believes that thinking about a possible occurrence can make it happen.

magnification. A type of thinking in which the negative significance of an event is exaggerated.

maladaptation. A failure of the body to return to homeostasis following a physiological and/or psychological response to stress, disrupting the individual's integrity.

malpractice. The failure of one rendering professional services to exercise that degree of skill and learning commonly applied under all the circumstances in the community by the average prudent reputable member of the profession with the result of injury, loss, or damage to the recipient of those services or to those entitled to rely upon them.

managed care. A concept purposefully designed to control the balance between cost and quality of care. Examples of managed care are health maintenance organizations (HMOs) and preferred provider organizations (PPOs). The amount and type of health care that the individual receives is determined by the organization providing the managed care.

mania. A manifestation of bipolar disorder in which the predominant mood is elevated, expansive, or irritable. Motor activity is frenzied and excessive. Psychotic features may or may not be present.

marital rape. Sexual violence directed at a marital partner against that person's will.

marital schism. A state of severe chronic disequilibrium and discord within the marital dyad, with recurrent threats of separation.

marital skew. A marital relationship in which there is lack of equal partnership. One partner dominates the relationship and the other partner.

Medicaid. A system established by the federal government to provide medical care benefits for indigent Americans. The Medicaid program is jointly funded by state and federal governments, and coverage varies significantly from state to state.

Medicare. A system established by the federal government to provide medical care benefits for elderly Americans.

meditation. A method of relaxation in which an individual sits in a quiet place and focuses total concentration on an object, word, or thought.

melancholia. A severe form of major depressive episode. Symptoms are exaggerated, and interest or pleasure in virtually all activities is lost.

menopause. The period marking the permanent cessation of menstrual activity; usually occurs at approximately 48 to 51 years of age.

mental health. The successful adaptation to stressors from the internal or external environment, evidenced by thoughts, feelings, and behaviors that are age-appropriate and congruent with local and cultural norms.

mental illness. Maladaptive responses to stressors from the internal or external environment, evidenced by thoughts, feelings, and behaviors that are incongruent with the local and cultural norms, and interfere with the individual's social, occupational, and/or physical functioning.

mental imagery. A method of stress reduction that employs the imagination. The individual focuses imagination on a scenario that is particularly relaxing to him or her (e.g., a scene on a quiet seashore, a mountain atmosphere, or floating through the air on a fluffy white cloud).

meridians. In Chinese medicine, pathways along the body in which the healing energy (qi) flows, and which are links between acupoints.

migraine personality. Personality characteristics that have been attributed to the migraine-prone person. The characteristics include perfectionistic, overly conscientious, somewhat inflexible, neat and tidy, compulsive, hard worker, intelligent, exacting, and places a very high premium on success, setting high (sometimes unrealistic) expectations on self and others.

milieu. French for "middle"; the English translation connotes "surroundings, or environment."

milieu therapy. Also called therapeutic community, or therapeutic environment, this type of therapy consists of a scientific structuring of the environment in order to effect behavioral changes and to improve the individual's psychological health and functioning.

minimization. A type of thinking in which the positive significance of an event is minimized or undervalued.

mobile outreach units. Programs in which volunteers and paid professionals drive or walk around and seek out homeless individuals who need assistance with physical or psychological care.

modeling. Learning new behaviors by imitating the behaviors of others.

mood. An individual's sustained emotional tone, which significantly influences behavior, personality, and perception.

moral behavior. Conduct that results from serious critical thinking about how individuals ought to treat others; reflects respect for human life, freedom, justice, or confidentiality.

moral-ethical self. That aspect of the personal identity that functions as observer, standard setter, dreamer, comparer, and most of all evaluator of who the individual says he or she is. This component of the personal identity makes judgments that influence an individual's self-evaluation.

mourning. The psychological process (or stages) through which the individual passes on the way to successful adaptation to the loss of a valued entity.

multidisciplinary care. A concept of providing care for a client in which individual disciplines provide specific services for the client without formal arrangement for interaction between the disciplines.

Munchausen syndrome. See **factitious disorder.**

N

narcissism. Self-love or self-admiration.

narcissistic personality disorder. A disorder characterized by an exaggerated sense of self-worth. These individuals lack empathy and are hypersensitive to the evaluation of others.

narcolepsy. A disorder in which the characteristic manifestation is sleep attacks. The individual cannot prevent falling asleep, even in the middle of a sentence or performing a task.

natural law theory. The ethical theory that has as its moral precept to "do good and avoid evil" at all costs. Natural law ethics are grounded in a concern for the human good, that is based on people's ability to live according to the dictates of reason.

negative reinforcement. Increasing the probability that a behavior will recur by removal of an undesirable reinforcing stimulus.

negativism. Strong resistance to suggestions or directions; exhibiting behaviors contrary to what is expected.

neglect of a child. *Physical neglect* of a child includes refusal of or delay in seeking health care, abandonment, expulsion from the home or refusal to allow a runaway to return home, and inadequate supervision. *Emotional neglect* refers to a chronic failure by the parent or caretaker to provide the child with the hope, love, and support necessary for the development of a sound, healthy personality.

negligence. The failure to do something that a reasonable person, guided by those considerations that ordinarily regulate human affairs, would do, or doing something that a prudent and reasonable person would not do.

neologism. New words that an individual invents that are meaningless to others, but have symbolic meaning to the psychotic person.

neurocognitive disorder. Global impairment of cognitive functioning that is progressive and interferes with social and occupational abilities.

neuroendocrinology. The study of hormones functioning within the neurological system.

neuroleptic. Antipsychotic medication used to prevent or control psychotic symptoms.

neuroleptic malignant syndrome (NMS). A rare but potentially fatal complication of treatment with neuroleptic drugs. Symptoms include severe muscle rigidity, high fever, tachycardia, fluctuations in blood pressure, diaphoresis, and rapid deterioration of mental status to stupor and coma.

neuron. A nerve cell; consists of a cell body, an axon, and dendrites.

neurosis. An unconscious conflict that produces anxiety and other symptoms and leads to maladaptive use of defense mechanisms.

neurotic disorder. A psychiatric disturbance, characterized by excessive anxiety and/or depression, disrupted bodily functions, unsatisfying interpersonal relationships, and behaviors that interfere with routine functioning. There is no loss of contact with reality.

neurotransmitter. A chemical that is stored in the axon terminals of the presynaptic neuron. An electrical impulse through the neuron stimulates the release of the neurotransmitter into the synaptic cleft, which in turn determines whether or not another electrical impulse is generated.

nonassertive. Individuals who are nonassertive (sometimes called passive) seek to please others at the expense of denying their own basic human rights.

nonmaleficence. The ethical principle that espouses abstaining from negative acts toward another, including acting carefully to avoid harm.

nursing diagnosis. A clinical judgment about individual, family, or community responses to actual and potential health problems/life processes. Nursing diagnoses provide the basis for selection of nursing interventions to achieve outcomes for which the nurse is accountable.

Nursing Interventions Classification (NIC). A comprehensive, research-based, standardized classification of interventions that nurses perform.

Nursing Outcomes Classification (NOC). A comprehensive, standardized classification of patient/client outcomes developed to evaluate the effects of nursing interventions (Moorhead et al., 2008).

nursing process. A dynamic, systematic process by which nurses assess, diagnose, identify outcomes, plan, implement, and evaluate nursing care. It has been called "nursing's scientific methodology." Nursing process gives order and consistency to nursing intervention.

O

obesity. The state of having a body mass index of 30 or above.

object constancy. The phase in the separation/individuation process when the child learns to relate to objects in an effective, constant manner. A sense of separateness is established, and the child is able to internalize a sustained image of the loved object or person when out of sight.

obsessions. Unwanted, intrusive, persistent ideas, thoughts, impulses, or images that cause marked anxiety or distress. Common ones include repeated thoughts about contamination, doubts, a need to have things in a particular order, aggressive or sexual impulses, and fears of harm to oneself or others (APA, 2013).

obsessive-compulsive disorder. Recurrent thoughts or ideas (obsessions) that an individual is unable to put out of his or her mind, and actions that an individual is unable to refrain from performing (compulsions). The obsessions and compulsions are severe enough to interfere with social and occupational functioning.

oculogyric crisis. An attack of involuntary deviation and fixation of the eyeballs, usually in the upward position. It may last for several minutes or hours and may occur as an extrapyramidal side effect of some antipsychotic medications.

operant conditioning. The learning of a particular action or type of behavior that is followed by a reinforcement.

opioids. A group of compounds that includes opium, opium derivatives, and synthetic substitutes.

orgasm. A peaking of sexual pleasure, with release of sexual tension and rhythmic contraction of the perineal muscles and pelvic reproductive organs.

osteoporosis. A reduction in the mass of bone per unit of volume that interferes with the mechanical support function of bone. This process occurs because of demineralization of the bones, and is escalated in women about the time of menopause.

outcomes. End results that are measurable, desirable, and observable, and translate into observable behaviors.

overgeneralization. Also called "absolutistic thinking." With overgeneralization, sweeping conclusions are made based on one incident—an "all or nothing" type of thinking.

overt sensitization. A type of aversion therapy that produces unpleasant consequences for undesirable behavior. An example is the use of disulfiram therapy with alcoholics, which induces an undesirable physical response if the individual has consumed any alcohol.

P

palilalia. Repeating one's own sounds or words (a type of vocal tic associated with Tourette's disorder).

panic. A sudden overwhelming feeling of terror or impending doom. This most severe form of emotional anxiety is usually accompanied by behavioral, cognitive, and physiological signs and symptoms considered to be outside the expected range of normalcy.

panic disorder. A disorder characterized by recurrent panic attacks, the onset of which are unpredictable, and manifested by intense apprehension, fear, or terror, often associated with feelings of impending doom, and accompanied by intense physical discomfort.

paradoxical intervention. In family therapy, "prescribing the symptom." The therapist requests that the family continue to engage in the behavior that they are trying to change. Tension is relieved, and the family is able to view more clearly the possible solutions to their problem.

paralanguage. The gestural component of the spoken word. It consists of pitch, tone, and loudness of spoken messages, the rate of speaking, expressively placed pauses, and emphasis assigned to certain words.

paranoia. A term that implies extreme suspiciousness. In schizophrenia, paranoia is characterized by persecutory delusions and hallucinations of a threatening nature.

paraphilic disorder. Repetitive behaviors or fantasies that involve nonhuman objects, real or simulated suffering or humiliation, or nonconsenting partners.

parasomnia. Unusual or undesirable behaviors that occur during sleep (e.g., nightmares, sleep terrors, and sleepwalking).

passive-aggressive behavior. Behavior that defends an individual's own basic rights by expressing resistance to social and occupational demands. Sometimes called *indirect aggression*, this behavior takes the form of sly, devious, and undermining actions that express the opposite of what the person is really feeling.

pathological gambling. A failure to resist impulses to gamble, and gambling behavior that compromises, disrupts, or damages personal, family, or vocational pursuits.

pedophilic disorder. Recurrent urges and sexually arousing fantasies involving sexual activity with a prepubescent child.

peer assistance programs. A program established by the American Nurses Association to assist impaired nurses. The individuals who administer these efforts are nurse members of the state associations, as well as nurses who are in recovery themselves.

perseveration. Persistent repetition of the same word or idea in response to different questions.

personal distance. The distance between individuals who are having interactions of a personal nature, such as a close conversation. In the U.S. culture, personal distance is approximately 18 to 40 inches.

personal identity. An individual's self-perception that defines his or her functions as observer, standard setter, and self-evaluator. It strives to maintain a stable self-image and relates to what the individual strives to become.

personal self. See **personal identity**.

personality. Deeply ingrained patterns of behavior, which include the way one relates to, perceives, and thinks about the environment and oneself.

personalization. Taking complete responsibility for situations without considering that other circumstances may have contributed to the outcome.

pharmacoconvulsive therapy. The chemical induction of a convulsion, used in the past for the reduction of psychotic symptoms; a type of therapy no longer used in psychiatry.

phencyclidine. An anesthetic used in veterinary medicine; used illegally as a hallucinogen, referred to as PCP or angel dust.

phenotype. Characteristics of physical manifestations that identify a particular genotype. Examples of phenotypes include eye color, height, blood type, language, and hairstyle. Phenotypes may be genetic or acquired.

phobia. An irrational fear.

physical neglect of a child. The failure on the part of the parent or caregiver to provide for a child's basic needs, such as food, clothing, shelter, medical-dental care, and supervision.

physical self. A personal appraisal by an individual of his or her physical being; includes physical attributes, functioning, sexuality, wellness-illness state, and appearance.

PIE charting. More specifically called "APIE," this method of documentation has an assessment, problem, intervention, and evaluation (APIE) format and is a problem-oriented system used to document nursing process.

positive reinforcement. A reinforcement stimulus that increases the probability that the behavior will recur.

postpartum depression. Depression that occurs during the postpartum period. It may be related to hormonal changes, tryptophan metabolism, or alterations in membrane transport during the early postpartum period. Other predisposing factors may also be influential.

posttraumatic stress disorder (PTSD). A syndrome of symptoms that develop following a psychologically distressing event that is outside the range of usual human experience (e.g., rape, war). The individual is unable to put the experience out of his or her mind, and has nightmares, flashbacks, and panic attacks.

posturing. The voluntary assumption of inappropriate or bizarre postures.

preassaultive tension state. Behaviors predictive of potential violence. They include excessive motor activity, tense posture, defiant affect, clenched teeth and fists, and other arguing, demanding, and threatening behaviors.

precipitating event. A stimulus arising from the internal or external environment that is perceived by an individual as taxing or exceeding his or her resources and endangering his or her well-being.

predisposing factors. A variety of elements that influence how an individual perceives and responds to a stressful event. Types of predisposing factors include genetic influences, past experiences, and existing conditions.

Premack principle. This principle states that a frequently occurring response (R1) can serve as a positive reinforcement for a response (R2) that occurs less frequently. For example, a girl may talk to friends on the phone (R2) only if she does her homework (R1).

premature ejaculation. Ejaculation that occurs with minimal sexual stimulation or before, upon, or shortly after penetration and before the person wishes it.

premenstrual dysphoric disorder. A disorder that is characterized by depressed mood, anxiety, mood swings, and decreased interest in activities during the week prior to menses and subsiding shortly after the onset of menstruation.

priapism. Prolonged painful penile erection; may occur as an adverse effect of some antidepressant medications, particularly trazodone.

primary neurocognitive disorder (NCD). NCD, such as Alzheimer's disease, in which the NCD itself is the major sign of some organic brain disease not directly related to any other organic illness.

primary gain. The receipt of positive reinforcement for somaticizing by being able to avoid difficult situations because of physical complaint.

primary prevention. Reduction of the incidence of mental disorders within the population by helping individuals to cope more effectively with stress and by trying to diminish stressors within the environment.

privileged communication. A doctrine common to most states that grants certain privileges under which health-care professionals may refuse to reveal information about and communications with clients.

problem-oriented recording (POR). A system of documentation that follows a subjective data, objective data, assessment, plan, implementation, and evaluation (SOAPIE) format. It is based on a list of identified patient problems to which each entry is directed.

prodromal syndrome. A syndrome of symptoms that often precede the onset of aggressive or violent behavior. These symptoms include anxiety and tension, verbal abuse and profanity, and increasing hyperactivity.

progressive relaxation. A method of deep muscle relaxation in which each muscle group is alternately tensed and relaxed in a systematic order with the person concentrating on the contrast of sensations experienced from tensing and relaxing.

projection. Attributing to another person feelings or impulses unacceptable to oneself.

prospective payment. The program of cost containment within the health-care profession directed at setting forth preestablished amounts that would be reimbursed for specific diagnoses.

pseudocyesis. A condition in which an individual has nearly all the signs and symptoms of pregnancy but is not pregnant; a conversion reaction.

pseudodementia. Symptoms of depression that mimic those of neurocognitive disorder (NCD).

pseudohostility. A family interaction pattern characterized by a state of chronic conflict and alienation among family members. This relationship pattern allows family members to deny underlying fears of tenderness and intimacy.

pseudomutuality. A family interaction pattern characterized by a facade of mutual regard with the purpose of denying underlying fears of separation and hostility.

pseudoparkinsonism. A side effect of some antipsychotic medications. Symptoms mimic those of Parkinson's disease, such as tremor, shuffling gait, drooling, and rigidity.

psychiatric home care. Care provided by psychiatric nurses in the client's home. Psychiatric home care nurses must have physical and psychosocial nursing skills to meet the demands of the client population they serve.

psychobiology. The study of the biological foundations of cognitive, emotional, and behavioral processes.

psychodrama. A specialized type of group therapy that employs a dramatic approach in which patients become "actors" in life situation scenarios. The goal is to resolve interpersonal conflicts in a less-threatening atmosphere than the real-life situation would present.

psychodynamic nursing. Being able to understand one's own behavior, to help others identify felt difficulties, and to apply principles of human relations to the problems that arise at all levels of experience.

psychoimmunology. The study of the implications of the immune system in psychiatry.

psychomotor domain. A category of learning in which the behaviors are processed and demonstrated. The information has been intellectually processed, and the individual is displaying motor behaviors.

psychomotor retardation. Extreme slowdown of physical movements. Posture slumps; speech is slowed; digestion becomes sluggish. Common in severe depression.

psychophysiological. Referring to psychological factors contributing to the initiation or exacerbation of a physical condition. Either a demonstrable organic pathology or a known pathophysiological process is involved.

psychosis. A mental state in which there is a severe loss of contact with reality. Symptoms may include delusions, hallucinations, disorganized speech patterns, and bizarre or catatonic behaviors.

psychosomatic. See **psychophysiological.**

psychotic disorder. A serious psychiatric disorder in which there is a gross disorganization of the personality, a marked disturbance in reality testing, and the impairment of interpersonal functioning and relationship to the external world.

psychotropic medication. Medication that affects psychic function, behavior, or experience.

public distance. Appropriate interactional distance for speaking in public or yelling to someone some distance away. U.S. culture defines this distance as 12 feet or more.

purging. The act of attempting to rid the body of calories by self-induced vomiting or excessive use of laxatives or diuretics.

pyromania. An inability to resist the impulse to set fires.

Q

qi. In Chinese medicine, the healing energy that flows through pathways in the body called *meridians.* (Also called "chi").

R

rape. The expression of power and dominance by means of sexual violence, most commonly by men over women, although men may also be rape victims. Rape is considered an act of aggression, not of passion.

rapport. The development between two people in a relationship of special feelings based on mutual acceptance, warmth, friendliness, common interest, a sense of trust, and a nonjudgmental attitude.

rationalization. Attempting to make excuses or formulate logical reasons to justify unacceptable feelings or behaviors.

reaction formation. Preventing unacceptable or undesirable thoughts or behaviors from being expressed by exaggerating opposite thoughts or types of behaviors.

receptor sites. Molecules that are situated on the cell membrane of the postsynaptic neuron that will accept only molecules with a complementary shape. These complementary molecules are specific to certain neurotransmitters that determine whether an electrical impulse will be excited or inhibited.

reciprocal inhibition. Also called counterconditioning, this technique serves to decrease or eliminate a behavior by introducing a more adaptive behavior, but one that is incompatible with the unacceptable behavior (e.g., introducing relaxation techniques to an anxious person; relaxation and anxiety are incompatible behaviors).

reframing. Changing the conceptual or emotional setting or viewpoint in relation to which a situation is experienced and placing it in another frame that fits the "facts" of the same concrete situation equally well or even better, and thereby changing its entire meaning. The behavior may not actually change, but the consequences of the behavior may change because of a change in the meaning attached to the behavior.

regression. A retreat to an earlier level of development and the comfort measures associated with that level of functioning.

relaxation. A decrease in tension or intensity, resulting in refreshment of body and mind. A state of refreshing tranquility.

religion. A set of beliefs, values, rites, and rituals adopted by a group of people. The practices are usually grounded in the teachings of a spiritual leader.

religiosity. Excessive demonstration of or obsession with religious ideas and behavior; common in schizophrenia.

reminiscence therapy. A process of life review by elderly individuals that promotes self-esteem and provides assistance in working through unresolved conflicts from the past.

repression. The involuntary blocking of unpleasant feelings and experiences from one's awareness.

residual stimuli. Certain beliefs, attitudes, experiences, or traits that may contribute to an individual's low self-esteem.

retrograde ejaculation. Ejaculation of the seminal fluid backwards into the bladder; may occur as a side effect of antipsychotic medications.

right. That which an individual is entitled (by ethical, legal, or moral standards) to have, or to do, or to receive from others within the limits of the law.

rigid boundaries. A person with rigid boundaries is "closed" and difficult to bond with. Such a person has a narrow perspective on life, sees things one way, and cannot discuss matters that lie outside his or her perspective.

ritualistic behavior. Purposeless activities that an individual performs repeatedly in an effort to decrease anxiety (e.g., hand washing); common in obsessive-compulsive disorder.

S

safe house or shelter. An establishment set up by many cities to provide protection for battered women and their children.

scapegoating. Occurs when hostility exists in a marriage dyad and an innocent third person (usually a child) becomes the target of blame for the problem.

schemas (also called *core beliefs*). Cognitive structures that consist of the individual's fundamental beliefs and assumptions, which develop early in life from personal experiences and identification with significant others. These concepts are reinforced by further learning experiences and in turn, influence the formation of other beliefs, values, and attitudes.

schizotypal personality disorder. A disorder characterized by odd and eccentric behavior, not decompensating to the level of schizophrenia.

secondary NCD. Neurocognitive disorder (NCD) that is caused by or related to another disease or condition, such as HIV disease or a cerebral trauma.

secondary gain. The receipt of positive reinforcement for somaticizing through added attention, sympathy, and nurturing.

secondary prevention. Health care that is directed at reduction of the prevalence of psychiatric illness by shortening the course (duration) of the illness. This is accomplished through early identification of problems and prompt initiation of treatment.

selective abstraction (sometimes referred to as "mental filter"). A type of thinking in which a conclusion is drawn based on only a selected portion of the evidence.

self-concept. The composite of beliefs and feelings that one holds about oneself at a given time, formed from perceptions of others' reactions. The self-concept consists of the physical self, or body image; the personal self or identity; and the self-esteem.

self-consistency. The component of the personal identity that strives to maintain a stable self-image.

self-esteem. The degree of regard or respect that individuals have for themselves. It is a measure of worth that they place on their abilities and judgments.

self-expectancy. The component of the personal identity that is the individual's perception of what he or she wants to be, to do, or to become.

self-ideal. See **self-expectancy.**

sensate focus. A therapeutic technique used to treat individuals and couples with sexual dysfunction. The technique involves touching and being touched by another and focusing attention on the physical sensations encountered thereby. Clients gradually move through various levels of sensate focus that progress from nongenital touching to touching that includes the breasts and genitals; touching done in a simultaneous, mutual format rather than by one person at a time; and touching that extends to and allows eventually for the possibility of intercourse.

seroconversion. The development of evidence of antibody response to a disease or vaccine. The time at which antibodies may be detected in the blood.

sexual assault nurse examiner (SANE). A clinical forensic registered nurse who has received specialized training to provide care to the sexual assault victim.

sexual exploitation of a child. The inducement or coercion of a child into engaging in sexually explicit conduct for the purpose of promoting any performance (e.g., child pornography).

sexual masochism disorder. Sexual stimulation derived from being humiliated, beaten, bound, or otherwise made to suffer.

sexual sadism disorder. Recurrent urges and sexually arousing fantasies involving acts (real, not simulated) in which the psychological or physical suffering (including humiliation) of the victim is sexually exciting.

sexuality. Sexuality is the constitution and life of an individual relative to characteristics regarding intimacy. It reflects the totality of the person and does not relate exclusively to the sex organs or sexual behavior.

shaman. The Native American "medicine man" or folk healer.

shaping. In learning, one shapes the behavior of another by giving reinforcements for increasingly closer approximations to the desired behavior.

shelters. A variety of places designed to help the homeless, ranging from converted warehouses that provide cots or floor space on which to sleep overnight to significant operations that provide a multitude of social and health-care services.

"ship of fools." The term given during the Middle Ages to sailing boats filled with severely mentally ill people who were sent out to sea with little guidance and in search of their lost rationality.

shiva. In the Jewish-American culture, following the death of a loved one, *shiva* is the 7-day period beginning with the burial. During this time, mourners do not work, and no activity is permitted that diverts attention from thinking about the deceased.

short-term memory. The ability to remember events that occurred very recently. This ability deteriorates with age.

silent rape reaction. The response of a rape victim in which he or she tells no one about the assault.

slander. An action with which an individual may be charged for orally sharing information that is detrimental to a person's reputation.

social distance. The distance considered acceptable in interactions with strangers or acquaintances, such as at a cocktail party or in a public building. U.S. culture defines this distance as 4 to 12 feet.

social phobia. The fear of being humiliated in social situations.

social skills training. Educational opportunities through role play for the person with schizophrenia to learn appropriate social interaction skills and functional skills that are relevant to daily living.

Socratic questioning (also called *guided discovery*). When the therapist questions the client with Socratic questioning, the client is asked to describe feelings associated with specific situations. Questions are stated in a way that may stimulate in the client a recognition of possible dysfunctional thinking and produce a dissonance about the validity of the thoughts.

somatization. A method of coping with psychosocial stress by developing physical symptoms.

specific phobia. A persistent fear of a specific object or situation, other than the fear of being unable to escape from a situation (agoraphobia) or the fear of being humiliated in social situations (social phobia).

spirituality. The human quality that gives meaning and sense of purpose to an individual's existence. Spirituality exists within each individual regardless of belief system and serves as a force for interconnectedness between the self and others, the environment, and a higher power.

splitting. A primitive ego defense mechanism in which the person is unable to integrate and accept both positive and negative feelings. In the view of these individuals, people—including themselves—and life situations are either all good or all bad. This trait is common in borderline personality disorder.

statutory law. A law that has been enacted by legislative bodies, such as a county or city council, state legislature, or the U.S. Congress.

statutory rape. Unlawful intercourse between a person who is over the age of consent and a person who is under the age of consent. Legal age of consent varies from state to state. An individual can be arrested for statutory rape even when the interaction has occurred between consenting individuals.

stereotyping. The process of classifying all individuals from the same culture or ethnic group as identical.

stimulus. In classical conditioning, that which elicits a response.

stimulus generalization. The process by which a conditioned response is elicited from all stimuli *similar* to the one from which the response was learned.

store-front clinics. Establishments that have been converted into clinics that serve the homeless population.

stress. A state of disequilibrium that occurs when there is a disharmony between demands occurring within an individual's internal or external environment and his or her ability to cope with those demands.

stress management. Various methods used by individuals to reduce tension and other maladaptive responses to stress in their lives; includes relaxation exercises, physical exercise, music, mental imagery, or any other technique that is successful for a person.

stressor. A demand from within an individual's internal or external environment that elicits a physiological and/or psychological response.

sublimation. The rechanneling of personally and/or socially unacceptable drives or impulses into activities that are more tolerable and constructive.

subluxation. The term used in chiropractic medicine to describe vertebrae in the spinal column that have become displaced, possibly pressing on nerves and interfering with normal nerve transmission.

substance abuse. Use of psychoactive drugs that poses significant hazards to health and interferes with social, occupational, psychological, or physical functioning.

substance addiction. Physical addiction is identified by the inability to stop using a substance despite attempts to do so; a continual use of the substance despite adverse consequences; a developing tolerance; and the development of withdrawal symptoms upon cessation or decreased intake. Psychological addiction is said to exist when a substance is perceived by the user to be necessary to maintain an optimal state of personal well-being, interpersonal relations, or skill performance.

substitution therapy. The use of various medications to decrease the intensity of symptoms in an individual who is withdrawing from, or experiencing the effects of excessive use of, substances.

subsystems. The smaller units of which a system is composed. In family systems theory, the subsystems are composed of husband-wife, parent-child(ren), or sibling-sibling.

sundowning. A phenomenon in neurocognitive disorder (NCD) in which the symptoms seem to worsen in the late afternoon and evening.

superego. One of the three elements of the personality identified by Freud that represents the conscience and the culturally determined restrictions that are placed on an individual.

suppression. The voluntary blocking from one's awareness of unpleasant feelings and experiences.

surrogate. One who serves as a substitute figure for another.

symbiotic relationship. A type of "psychic fusion" that occurs between two people; it is unhealthy in that severe anxiety is generated in either or both if separation is indicated. A symbiotic relationship is normal between infant and mother.

sympathy. The actual sharing of another's thoughts and behaviors. Differs from **empathy**, in that with empathy one experiences an objective understanding of what another is feeling, rather than actually sharing those feelings.

synapse. The junction between two neurons. The small space between the axon terminals of one neuron and the cell body or dendrites of another is called the synaptic cleft.

syphilis. A sexually transmitted disorder caused by the spirochete *Treponema pallidum* and resulting in a chancre on the skin or mucous membranes of the sexual organs. If left untreated, it may become systemic. End-stage disease can have profound effects, such as blindness or insanity.

systematic desensitization. A treatment for phobias in which the individual is taught to relax and then asked to imagine various components of the phobic stimulus on a graded hierarchy, moving from that which produces the least fear to that which produces the most.

T

tangentiality. The inability to get to the point of a story. The speaker introduces many unrelated topics, until the original topic of discussion is lost.

tardive dyskinesia. Syndrome of symptoms characterized by bizarre facial and tongue movements, a stiff neck, and difficulty swallowing. It may occur as an adverse effect of long-term therapy with some antipsychotic medications.

technical expert. Peplau's term for one who understands various professional devices and possesses the clinical skills necessary to perform the interventions that are in the best interest of the client.

temperament. A set of inborn personality characteristics that influence an individual's manner of reacting to the environment, and ultimately influences his or her developmental progression.

territoriality. The innate tendency of individuals to own space. Individuals lay claim to areas around them as their own. This phenomenon can have an influence on interpersonal communication.

tertiary gain. The receipt of positive reinforcement for somaticizing by causing the focus of the family to switch to the individual and away from conflict that may be occurring within the family.

tertiary prevention. Health care that is directed toward reduction of the residual effects associated with severe or chronic physical or mental illness.

therapeutic communication. Caregiver verbal and nonverbal techniques that focus on the care receiver's needs and advance the promotion of healing and change. Therapeutic communication encourages exploration of feelings and fosters understanding of behavioral motivation. It is nonjudgmental, discourages defensiveness, and promotes trust.

therapeutic community. Also called *milieu therapy*, this approach strives to manipulate the environment so that all aspects of the client's hospital experience are considered therapeutic.

therapeutic group. Differs from group therapy in that there is a lesser degree of theoretical foundation. Focus is on group relations, interactions between group members, and the consideration of a selected issue. Leaders of therapeutic groups do not require the degree of educational preparation required of group therapy leaders.

therapeutic relationship. An interaction between two people (usually a caregiver and a care receiver) in which input from both participants contributes to a climate of healing, growth promotion, and/or illness prevention.

thought-stopping technique. A self-taught technique that an individual uses each time he or she wishes to eliminate intrusive or negative, unwanted thoughts from awareness.

time out. An aversive stimulus or punishment during which the individual is removed from the environment where the unacceptable behavior is being exhibited.

token economy. In behavior modification, a type of contracting in which the reinforcers for desired behaviors are presented in the form of tokens, which may then be exchanged for designated privileges.

tolerance. The need for increasingly larger or more frequent doses of a substance in order to obtain the desired effects originally produced by a lower dose.

tort. The violation of a civil law in which an individual has been wronged. In a tort action, one party asserts that wrongful conduct on the part of the other has caused harm, and compensation for harm suffered is sought.

transference. Transference occurs when a client unconsciously displaces (or "transfers") to the nurse or therapist feelings formed toward a person from his or her past.

transgenderism. A disorder of gender identity or gender dysphoria (unhappiness or dissatisfaction with one's gender) of the most extreme variety. The individual, despite having the anatomical characteristics of a given gender, has the self-perception of being of the opposite gender, and may seek to have gender changed through surgical intervention.

transvestic disorder. Recurrent urges and sexually arousing fantasies involving dressing in the clothes of the opposite gender.

triangles. A three-person emotional configuration that is considered the basic building block of the family system. When anxiety becomes too great between two family members, a third person is brought in to form a triangle. Triangles are dysfunctional in that they offer relief from anxiety through diversion rather than through resolution of the issue.

Trichotillomania (hair-pulling disorder). The recurrent failure to resist impulses to pull out one's own hair.

type A personality. The personality characteristics attributed to individuals prone to coronary heart disease, including excessive competitive drive, chronic sense of time urgency, easy anger, aggressiveness, excessive ambition, and inability to enjoy leisure time.

type B personality. The personality characteristics attributed to individuals who are not prone to coronary heart disease; includes characteristics such as ability to perform even under pressure but without the competitive drive and constant sense of time urgency experienced by the type A personality. Type Bs can enjoy their leisure time without feeling guilty, and they are much less impulsive than type A individuals; that is, they think things through before making decisions.

type C personality. The personality characteristics attributed to the cancer-prone individual. Includes characteristics such as suppression of anger, calm, passive, puts the needs of others before his or her own, but holds resentment toward others for perceived "wrongs."

type D personality. Personality characteristics attributed to individuals who are at increased risk of cardiovascular morbidity and mortality. The characteristics include a combination of negative emotions and social inhibition.

tyramine. An amino acid found in aged cheeses or other aged, overripe, and fermented foods; broad beans; pickled herring; beef or chicken liver; preserved meats; beer and wine; yeast products; chocolate; caffeinated drinks; canned figs; sour cream; yogurt; soy sauce; and some over-the-counter cold medications and diet pills. If foods high in tyramine content are consumed while an individual is taking MAO inhibitors, a potentially life-threatening syndrome called hypertensive crisis can result.

U

unconditional positive regard. Carl Rogers' term for the respect and dignity of an individual regardless of his or her unacceptable behavior.

unconditioned response. In classical conditioning, an unconditioned response refers to a reflexive response to a specific target stimulus.

unconditioned stimulus. In classical conditioning, a specific stimulus that elicits an unconditioned, reflexive response.

undoing. A mechanism used to symbolically negate or cancel out a previous action or experience that one finds intolerable.

universality. One curative factor of groups (identified by Yalom) in which individuals realize that they are not alone in a problem and in the thoughts and feelings they are experiencing. Anxiety is relieved by the support and understanding of others in the group who share similar experiences.

utilitarianism. The ethical theory that espouses "the greatest happiness for the greatest number." Under this theory, action would be taken based on the end results that will produce the most good (happiness) for the most people.

V

values. Personal beliefs about the truth, beauty, or worth of a thought, object, or behavior, that influence an individual's actions.

values clarification. A process of self-discovery by which people identify their personal values and their value rankings. This process increases awareness about why individuals behave in certain ways.

velorio. In the Mexican-American culture, following the death of a loved one, the *velorio* is a festive watch by family and friends over the body of the deceased person before burial.

veracity. An ethical principle that refers to one's duty to always be truthful.

voyeuristic disorder. Recurrent urges and sexually arousing fantasies involving the act of observing unsuspecting people, usually strangers, who are either naked, in the process of disrobing, or engaging in sexual activity.

W

waxy flexibility. A condition by which the individual with schizophrenia passively yields all movable parts of the body to any efforts made at placing them in certain positions.

Wernicke's encephalopathy. A brain disorder caused by thiamine deficiency and characterized by visual disturbances, ataxia, somnolence, stupor, and, without thiamine replacement, death.

withdrawal. The physiological and mental readjustment that accompanies the discontinuation of an addictive substance.

word salad. A group of words that are put together in a random fashion without any logical connection.

Y

yin and yang. The fundamental concept of Asian health practices. Yin and yang are opposite forces of energy such as negative/positive, dark/light, cold/hot, hard/soft, and feminine/masculine. Food, medicines, and herbs are classified according to their yin and yang properties and are used to restore a balance, thereby restoring health.

yoga. A system of beliefs and practices, the ultimate goal of which is to unite the human soul with the universal spirit. In Western countries, yoga uses body postures, along with meditation and breathing exercises, to achieve a balanced, disciplined workout that releases muscle tension, tones the internal organs, and energizes the mind, body, and spirit, so that natural healing can occur.

Index

Page numbers followed by f denote figures; those followed by t denote tables; those followed by b denote boxes.

O